NURSING DIAGNOSIS & INTERVENTION

PLANNING FOR PATIENT CARE

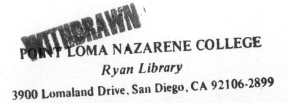

NURSING DIAGNOSIS & INTERVENTION

PLANNING FOR PATIENT CARE

GERTRUDE K. McFARLAND, DNSc, RN, FAAN
Health Scientist Administrator
Nursing Research Study Section
Division of Research Grants
National Institutes of Health
USPHS, US Department of Health and Human Services
Bethesda, Maryland

ELIZABETH A. McFARLANE, DNSc, RN
Associate Professor and Associate Dean for Academic Affairs
School of Nursing
The Catholic University of America
Washington, DC

SECOND EDITION

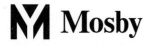 Mosby

St. Louis Baltimore Boston Chicago London Philadelphia Sydney Toronto

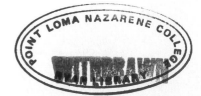

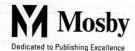

M Mosby

Dedicated to Publishing Excellence

Publisher: Alison Miller
Editor: Terry Van Schaik
Developmental Editor: Janet Livingston
Project Manager: Mark Spann
Designer: Gail Morey Hudson
Manufacturing Supervisor: Mary Stueck

SECOND EDITION

Printed in the United States of America

Mosby–Year Book, Inc.
11830 Westline Industrial Drive
St. Louis, Missouri 63146

ISBN 0-8016-6703-8

———

93 94 95 96 97 CL/DC 9 8 7 6 5 4 3 2 1

Contributors

NOLA M. BECKET, MS, RN

Nursing Quality Assurance Coordinator,
University Hospital,
Oregon Health Sciences University,
Portland, Oregon

SUSAN L. CARLSON, MSN, RN, CS

Education Coordinator,
Fairfax Hospital,
Falls Church, Virginia

SISTER KAREN CHAMPAGNE, MSN, RN, OP

QA/QI Coordinator,
St. Anne's Hospital,
Fall River, Massachussetts

HELENE MILLIKEN CLARK, PhD, MSN, RN, C

Assistant Professor and Coordinator of
Adult Health Nursing, School of Nursing,
The Catholic University of America,
Washington, D.C.

DOROTHY M. CRAIG, MScN, RN

Associate Professor, Faculty of Nursing,
University of Toronto,
Toronto, Ontario, Canada

CAROLYN S. D'AVIS, MSN, RN

Coordinator for Baccalaureate Program,
School of Nursing,
The Catholic University of America,
Washington, D.C.

JACQUELINE DIENEMANN, PhD, RN

Associate Professor, School of Nursing,
Johns Hopkins University,
Baltimore, Maryland

PHYLLIS A. ENFANTO, MS, RN, CCRN

Critical Care Nurse Educator,
St. Elizabeth's Hospital,
Boston, Massachusetts

MARGARET I. FITCH, PhD, RN

Oncology Nurse Researcher,
Toronto-Bayview Regional Cancer Center/Sunnybrook
Health Science Center;
Assistant Professor, Faculty of Nursing,
University of Toronto,
Toronto, Ontario, Canada

MARGIE L. FRENCH, MS, RN, CS*

Clinical Specialist in Gerontological Nursing;
Clinical Manager,
Rehabilitation Unit/Vancouver Division,
Department of Veterans Affairs Medical Center,
Portland, Oregon

---

*The opinions expressed in chapters written by the contributors designated by an asterisk are those of the authors and do not necessarily reflect those of the National Institutes of Health or Food and Drug Administration, USPHS, U.S. Department of Health and Human Services; the Veterans Administration; or the Army or Department of Defense.

CRISTINE M. GALANTE, PhD, RN,*

LTC(P), Army Nurse Corps;
Senior Health Program Analyst,
Office of the Assistant Secretary of Defense
(Health Affairs),
Washington, D.C.

PATRICIA M. GARVER, DNSc, RN, CS

Department of Human Services,
Geriatric Home Care,
Arlington, Virginia

LAUREL S. GARZON, DNSc, RN

Assistant Professor, School of Nursing,
Old Dominion University,
Norfolk, Virginia

ELIZABETH KELCHNER GERETY, MS, RN, CS, FAAN*

Clinical Nurse Specialist, Psychiatry,
Psychiatry Consultation Service,
Portland Veterans Affairs Medical Center,
Portland, Oregon;
Instructor, Department of Mental Health Nursing,
School of Nursing,
Oregon Health Sciences University,
Portland, Oregon

JANE E. GRAYDON, PhD, RN

Associate Professor, Faculty of Nursing;
Chair, Department of Nursing Science,
School of Graduate Studies,
University of Toronto,
Toronto, Ontario, Canada

PAULINE McKINNEY GREEN, PhD, RN

Assistant Professor, College of Nursing,
Howard University,
Washington, D.C.

JANICE C. HALLAL, DNSc, RN

Associate Professor, School of Nursing
The Catholic University of America,
Washington, D.C.

LINDA K. HEITMAN, MSN, RN

Clinical Nurse Specialist,
Regional Heart Center Coordinator,
Southeast Missouri Hospital,
Cape Girardeau, Missouri

SONIA D. HINDS, MSN, RN

Acting Co-Director, Nursing Education Branch,
Office of Chief Clinical Officer,
D.C. Commission on Mental Health Services,
Washington, D.C.

LOIS M. HOSKINS, PhD, RN

Associate Professor, School of Nursing,
The Catholic University of America,
Washington, D.C.

KAREN E. INABA, MS, RN, CS

Psychiatric Consultation-Liaison
Clinical Nurse Specialist, Oregon Health Sciences
University Hospital, Portland, Oregon;
Assistant Professor, Department of
Mental Health Nursing, School of Nursing,
Oregon Health Sciences University,
Portland, Oregon

SHIRLEY A. JACKSON, MS, RN, CCRN

Critical Care Clinical Nurse Specialist,
Department of Education, Elliot Hospital,
Manchester, New Hampshire

JACQUELINE L. KARTMAN, MS, RNC, CCRN

Clinical Nurse Specialist, Intensive Care,
Lutheran Hospital-La Crosse,
La Crosse, Wisconsin

MAUREEN A. KNIPPEN, DNSc, RN*

Consumer Safety Officer,
Food and Drug Administration,
Division of Drug Marketing, Advertising, and
Communications, Office of Drug Standards,
Kensington, Maryland

CANDICE S. KORB, MS, RN

Nursing Instructor,
School of Nursing,
Marymount University,
Arlington, Virginia

CAROL E. KUPPERBERG, MSN, RN

Home Care Case Manager,
Children's Home Health Care Services,
Children's National Medical Center,
Washington, DC

LORNA LARSON, DNSc, RN

Formerly Program Analyst,
Quality Assurance Division,
D.C. Commission of Mental Health Services,
Washington, D.C.

CAROL LAWSON, MSc, RN

Nursing Consultant,
Montreal, Quebec, Canada

PRISCILLA LeMONE, RN, DSN

Assistant Professor, School of Nursing,
University of Missouri-Columbia,
Columbia, Missouri

MARGARET LUNNEY, PhD, RN, CS

Associate Professor,
Hunter-Bellevue School of Nursing,
Hunter College of the City University of New York,
New York, New York

MARY MARIANI, MSN, RN

Clinical Manager,
Psychiatric Intensive Case,
Management Services/IBM Division,
American PsychManagement, Inc.
Arlington, Virginia

MARY E. MARKERT, MN, RN

Psychiatric Clinical Administer,
Saint Elizabeth's Campus,
D.C. Commission on Mental Health Services,
Washington, D.C.

SISTER JUDITH MARONI, CSJ, DNSc, RN, CS

Assistant Professor, School of Nursing,
University of Pittsburgh,
Pittsburgh, Pennsylvania

GERTRUDE K. McFARLAND, DNSc, RN, FAAN*

Health Scientist Administrator,
Nursing Research Study Section,
Division of Research Grants,
National Institutes of Health, USPHS,
U.S. Department of Health and Human Services,
Bethesda, Maryland

ELIZABETH A. McFARLANE, DNSc, RN

Associate Professor and Associate Dean for
Academic Affairs, School of Nursing,
The Catholic University of America,
Washington, D.C.

MARGARET J. McGOVERN, MScN, RN

Executive Director, Bereaved Families of
Ontario-Metro Toronto,
Toronto, Ontario, Canada;
Assistant Professor, Faculty of Nursing,
University of Toronto,
Toronto, Ontario, Canada

KAREN A. McWHORTER, MN, RN*

Clinical Specialist in Gerontological Nursing,
Consultant Geriatric Mental Health,
Department of Veterans Affairs Medical Center,
Nursing Home Care Unit/Vancouver Division,
Portland, Oregon

JOAN MESCH, MS, RN, CNA*

Clinical Manager, Surgical Intensive Care Unit,
Portland Veterans Affairs Medical Center,
Portland, Oregon

VICTORIA L. MOCK, DNSc, RN, OCN

Assistant Professor, School of Nursing,
Boston College,
Boston, Massachusetts

MARTHA M. MORRIS, EdD, RN

Director, Department of Nursing,
Maryville College,
St. Louis, Missouri

M. ELETTA MORSE, MSN, RN, ANP-C

Geriatric Clinical Nurse Specialist,
Alexandria Hospital,
Alexandria, Virginia

CHARLOTTE E. NASCHINSKI, MS, RN*

Deputy Director,
Continuing Health Professional Education,
Uniformed Services University of the Health Sciences,
U.S. Department of Defense,
Bethesda, Maryland

JOYCE NEUMANN, MS, RN, OCN

Clinical Nurse Specialist,
Bone Marrow Transplant Unit,
The University of Texas,
M.D. Anderson Cancer Center,
Houston, Texas

COLLEEN K. NORTON, MSN, RN, CCRN

Clinical Assistant Professor, School of Nursing,
The Catholic University of America,
Washington, D.C.

LINDA O'BRIEN-PALLAS, PhD, RN

Assistant Professor and Career Scientist,
Co-Director, Quality of Worklife Research Unit,
Faculty of Nursing, University of Toronto,
Toronto, Ontario, Canada

ANNETTE M. O'CONNOR, PhD, RN

Associate Professor, School of Nursing,
University of Ottawa,
Ottawa, Ontario, Canada

BARBARA E. POKORNY, MSN, RN, CS

Family Nurse Practitioner,
Community Health Center of New London,
New London, Connecticut

M. GAIE RUBENFELD, MS, RN

Assistant Professor, Department of Nursing Education,
Eastern Michigan University,
Ypsilanti, Michigan

ANDREA BOURQUIN RYAN, MSN, RN

Clinical Specialist,
Washington Hospital Center,
Washington, D.C.

SISTER MARIA SALERNO, OSF, DNSc, RNC

Associate Professor, School of Nursing,
The Catholic University of America,
Washington, D.C.

ROSEMARIE F. DiMAURO SATYSHUR, DNSc, RN

Assistant Professor,
School of Nursing,
The Catholic University of America,
Washington, D.C.

MARY ANN KADOW SCHROEDER, DNSc, RN

Associate Professor, School of Nursing,
The Catholic University of America,
Washington, D.C.

CAROLE A. SHEA, PhD, RN, CS

Associate Dean of Academic Affairs,
College of Nursing, Northeastern University,
Boston, Massachusetts

SISTER MAURITA SOUKUP, DNSc, CCRN, RN

Director-Eastern Iowa Heart Institute,
St. Luke's Hospital;
Adjunct Faculty of Nursing, Mt. Mercy College,
Cedar Rapids, Iowa;
Adjunct Faculty of Nursing, University of Iowa,
Iowa City, Iowa

KAREN A. STEVENS, PhD, RN

Associate Professor, Department of Nursing,
Bowie State University,
Bowie, Maryland

SYLVIA RAE STEVENS, MS, RN, CS

Adjunct Assistant Professor, School of Nursing,
The Catholic University of America,
Washington, D.C.

BARBARA L. STRUNK, AB, BSN, CETN

Enterostomal Therapy Nurse, University Hospital,
Oregon Health Sciences University,
Portland, Oregon

KRISTY SWIECH, MS, RN

Clinical Instructor,
Boston University Medical Center,
Boston, Massachusetts

JEAN O. TROTTER, MS, RN, C

Health Care Consultant, Specialist in Home Care,
Trotter Health Care Consultants,
Columbia, Maryland

JOAN C. VELOS, MSN, RN, CRNP

Cardiothoracic and Vascular Nurse Practitioner,
Louis F. Plzak, Jr. MD, PA,
Bryn Mawr, Pennsylvania

KARIN von SCHILLING, MScN, RN

Professor Emeritus, School of Nursing,
Faculty of Health Sciences, McMaster University,
Hamilton, Ontario, Canada

ELEANOR A. WALKER, PhD, RNC

Associate Professor and
Coordinator, Graduate Program,
Department of Nursing,
Bowie State University,
Bowie, Maryland

EVELYN L. WASLI, DNSc, RN

Chief Nurse,
Emergency Psychiatric Response Division,
D.C. Community Mental Health Services,
Washington, D.C.

JUDITH H. WATT-WATSON, MScN, RN

Clinical Associate Professor, Faculty of Nursing,
University of Toronto,
Toronto, Ontario, Canada

JANET R. WEBER, EdD, MSN, RN

Assistant Professor, Department of Nursing,
Southeast Missouri State University,
Cape Girardeau, Missouri

LINDA K. WEINBERG, MSN, CRN, CNA

Nurse Manager,
Anne Arundel Medical Center,
Annapolis, Maryland

TO

**ALL PROFESSIONAL NURSES AND
NURSING STUDENTS**

who use and test
nursing diagnoses in practice

Preface

Nurses engaged in contemporary practice use the nursing process in their delivery of care. The nursing process is a problem-solving process and includes the commonly accepted components of (1) assessment, (2) nursing diagnosis, (3) planning, (4) implementing, and (5) evaluating. Nursing diagnosis is a critical link in this nursing process. Developments in nursing diagnosis continue to be stimulated by the work of the North American Nursing Diagnosis Association (NANDA).

This book provides comprehensive information that will enhance the understanding of all currently accepted NANDA nursing diagnoses. Chapter 1 presents the historical evolution of nursing diagnosis as a critical nursing activity and the development of a diagnostic taxonomy. Nursing diagnosis as an essential element of the nursing process and the 11 Functional Health Patterns are described in Chapter 2. These 11 Functional Health Patterns—Health Perception–Health Management Pattern, Nutritional and Metabolic Pattern, Elimination Pattern, Activity-Exercise Pattern, Sleep-Rest Pattern, Cognitive-Perceptual Pattern, Self-Perception–Self-Concept Pattern, Role–Relationship Pattern, Sexuality-Reproductive Pattern, Coping–Stress Tolerance Pattern, and Value–Belief Pattern—serve as an organizing framework for categorizing all the approved NANDA diagnoses that are presented in this book. The relative ease with which nurses can understand this framework and apply it in a variety of settings has prompted its use in classifying the nursing diagnoses.

Comprehensive content is presented on each nursing diagnosis, including:

1. Definition and overview that integrates theory and research findings of the nursing diagnosis; including developmental, family, community, and cultural considerations
2. Assessment, including assessment strategies and guides defining characteristics, related factors, and related medical and psychiatric diagnoses
3. Examples of specific nursing diagnoses
4. Description of planning and implementation with an emphasis on rationale, including boxed nursing care guidelines
5. Evaluation
6. Case studies with plan of care, which are boxed so they are easy to locate, provide an example for individualizing care for patients with a particular nursing diagnosis

This book will assist nurses and nursing students in conducting a comprehensive assessment; formulating a nursing diagnosis; and planning, implementing, and evaluating nursing care. The book is intended to encourage nurses in contributing to the ongoing development and classification of nursing diagnoses.

ACKNOWLEDGMENT

We are grateful to our many nurse colleagues who continue to stimulate our thinking about the development of nursing science and in particular nursing diagnoses. Sincere appreciation is extended to our many contributors who are experts in nursing diagnosis and practice. To our families—husband Al McFarland and husband and sons Tom, Mike, Denis, and Matt McFarlane—for their tolerance and patience during this project. Finally, our gratitude is extended to the Mosby staff—Terry Van Schaik, Editor, and Janet Livingston, Developmental Editor, Nursing Division, for their encouragement, support, and skills.

Gertrude K. McFarland
Elizabeth A. McFarlane

Contents

Nursing Diagnosis: Past and Present Perspectives

The North American Nursing Diagnosis Association (NANDA) defines *nursing diagnosis* as a "clinical judgment about individual, family, or community responses to actual or potential health problems/life processes. Nursing diagnoses provide the basis for selection of nursing interventions to achieve outcomes for which the nurse is accountable".[7] The term *nursing diagnosis* provides nurses with an accurate description of a critical nursing activity. The American Nurses' Association (ANA) has reinforced this view through the publication of *Nursing: A Social Policy Statement* and *Standards of Clinical Nursing Practice*.

Nursing: A Social Policy Statement presents a definition of nursing in terms of provision of care. Nursing is defined as "the diagnosis and treatment of human responses to actual or potential health problems."[4] The definition reflects four defining characteristics of nursing: the *phenomena* of which nurses should be aware, that is, human responses to actual or potential health problems; *theory,* which is used to sharpen observations and therefore enhance an understanding of the phenomena of concern to nurses; *actions,* which are taken to ameliorate, improve, or correct conditions, to prevent illness, and to promote health; and beneficial *effects* that occur because of nursing actions and relate to the identifiable human responses. The relationship among the defining characteristics of nursing, the nursing process, and the standards of care is shown in Fig. 1. Diagnosis—the culmination of assessing and the

impetus for outcome identification and planning—should reflect an understanding of the phenomena of concern as the focus for nursing action.

The acceptance of nursing diagnosis as a critical nursing activity and a vital link in the nursing process has received further support from the ANA through the development and publication of standards that provide direction for professional nursing practice. The ANA began work on the development of standards of practice in the late 1960s. The results of those initial efforts were published in 1973 as the *Standards of Nursing Practice.* [5] More recently, the Standing Committee on Nursing Practice Standards and Guidelines, under the ANA Congress of Nursing Practice, recommended that the standards be revised. The committee, a subsequent Task Force on Nursing Practice Standards, and numerous specialty nursing organizations and groups collaborated in "the development of standards that are applicable to all nurses engaged in clinical practice."[3]

The outcomes of the ANA's most recent efforts were published in December, 1991 as *Standards of Clinical Nursing Practice*. The publication presents both "Standards of Care" that describe "a competent level of nursing care as demonstrated by the nursing process, involving assessment, diagnosis, outcome identification, planning, implementation, and evaluation"[3] and "Standards of Professional Performance" that describe "a competent level of behavior in the professional role—

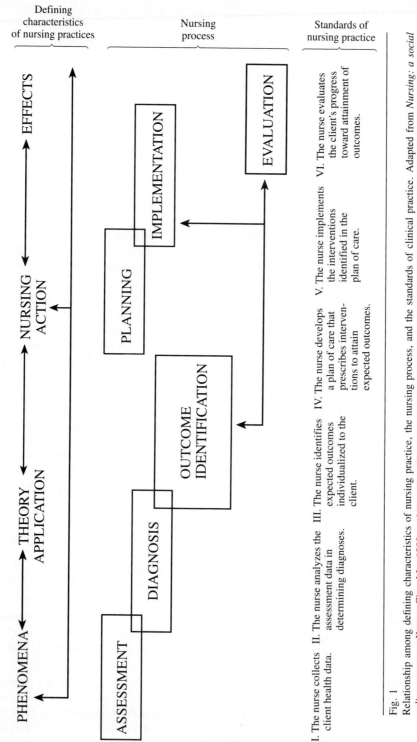

Fig. 1
Relationship among defining characteristics of nursing practice, the nursing process, and the standards of clinical practice. Adapted from *Nursing: a social policy statement*, Kansas City, Mo, 1980, and *American Nurses' Association and Standards of Clinical Practice*, Kansas City, Mo, 1991, American Nurses' Association.

including activities related to quality of care, performance appraisal, education, collegiality, ethics, collaboration, research, and resource utilization".[3] Both sets of standards include criteria by which each identified standard is measured. Nursing diagnosis is explicitly defined in the Standards as "a clinical judgment about the client's response to actual or potential health conditions or needs" and is the focus of Standard II, which is titled "Diagnosis" and states that "the nurse analyzes the assessment data in determining diagnoses." The importance of the nursing diagnoses is further emphasized in Standard III, which focuses on Outcome Identification and includes a measurement criterion stating that "outcomes are derived from the diagnoses."

The American Association of Critical-Care Nurses (AACN) also has recognized nursing diagnosis as a vital link in the nursing process. In the association's publication, *Outcome Standards for Nursing Care of the Critically Ill,*[2] nursing diagnosis was used as a framework for conceptualizing nursing practice. Selected nursing diagnoses are presented with related outcome standards and outcome criteria as well as nursing interventions and monitoring guidelines. AACN considered the use of nursing diagnosis as an organizing framework to be a bold step that could provoke controversy, yet nursing diagnosis was recognized as a component of nursing practice that provided a link between process and outcome as essential indicators of quality of care.

More recently, the Joint Commission on Accreditation of Healthcare Organizations (JCAHO) recognized nursing diagnosis in the publication of its Nursing Care Standards in the Accreditation Manual for Hospitals (AMH), 1991 edition.[17] Specific reference to nursing diagnosis is made through the requirement that six elements of documentation be included in the patient's medical record: (1) the initial assessments and reassessments; (2) the **nursing diagnoses** and/or patient care needs; (3) the interventions identified to meet the patient's nursing care needs; (4) the nursing care provided; (5) the patient's response to, and the outcomes of, the care provided; and (6) the

abilities of the patient and/or, as appropriate, his/her significant other(s) to manage continuing care needs after discharge. A revision made to one of the nursing care standards (NC 1.3.5) published in the AMH, 1991 edition, places further emphasis on the role of nursing diagnosis in nursing care planning. The standard as published in the 1992 edition reads: N.C. 1.3.5 Nursing care data related to patient assessments, *the nursing diagnoses and/or patient needs,* nursing interventions, and patient outcomes are permanently integrated into the clinical information system (for example, the medical record). (Italics indicate the inserted revision.)[16]

Although it is apparent that nursing diagnosis recently has come to be accepted as a pivotal force in the nursing process, the use of the term *diagnosis* by nurses has gradually become accepted over the past four decades.

DIAGNOSIS REVISITED

During the 1950s, Virginia Fry[11] introduced the term *nursing diagnosis* in the literature. She described the first major task in developing a creative approach to nursing as the formulation of a nursing diagnosis and the development of an individualized care plan. This suggestion was not supported by ANA's Model Practice Act of 1955, which included the following statement: "The foregoing shall not be deemed to include acts of diagnosis or prescription of therapeutic or corrective measures."[18] Thus, nurses hesitated to use the term nursing diagnosis; instead of diagnosing responses to health problems, they described their activity as determining the nursing problems of the patient or family. Abdellah's definition of *nursing problem* as "a condition faced by the patient or family which the nurse can assist him or them to meet through the performance of her professional functions"[1] suggests that the nurse must determine the problem and derive a focus for the planning of nursing interventions. Nurses made conclusions from the phenomena they observed. In essence, they were diagnosing the patient's or family's problems based on the assessment data they had gathered.

Although there were few references to nursing diagnosis in the nursing literature of the 1960s, the efforts supporting inclusion of it in nursing terminology were apparent. Two articles published in the *American Journal of Nursing* in the early 1960s countered the arguments that only physicians should diagnose. Chambers[9] even provided a working definition of nursing diagnosis: "a careful investigation of the facts to determine the nature of a nursing problem." The term *problem* refers to a patient's specific need that requires nursing intervention in order to be met. Komorita[23] reviewed the proposed descriptions of nursing diagnosis and offered her own definition: "Nursing diagnosis should be a conclusion based on scientific determination of an individual's nursing needs, resulting from critical analysis of his behavior, the nature of his illness, and numerous other factors which affect his condition. This conclusion should then serve as a guide for nursing care." This definition foreshadowed the use of diagnosis as recommended in the *Standards of Nursing Practice* in 1973. Yet nurses and other health care professionals in the 1960s appear to have been uncomfortable with the term and continued to differ in opinion concerning its use.

Myra Levine[25] confronted the difficulties that nurses had in accepting and using the term nursing diagnosis by proposing a new nursing term that described the scientific approach to planning and providing nursing care. The word proposed was *trophicognosis*. Its derivation is from the Greek words *trophikos techne,* which mean the "art of nursing," and the suffix *-gnosis,* which signifies "the knowledge of." Levine offered the definition of trophicognosis as "a nursing care judgment arrived at by the scientific method."

As the profession of nursing continued to struggle with terminology, Lester King, M.D., published his article "What is Diagnosis?" in the *Journal of the American Medical Association.* King's article refutes the argument that only physicians can diagnose. He wrote that "although diagnosis ordinarily has medical connotations, this is not essential, for the term involves activities by no means unique to medicine." He described three criteria or components that must be present to make a diagnosis: (1) there must be a preexisting series of categories or classes that provide a reference for the diagnosis, (2) there must be a particular entity that is to be diagnosed, and (3) there must be a deliberate judgment that the assessed phenomenon or response belongs in a particular category or class. These criteria or components address the need for a classification system or taxonomy.

A CLASSIFICATION SYSTEM FOR NURSING DIAGNOSES

Nurses recognized the need for a taxonomic system that would provide a frame of reference for nursing diagnoses, and efforts to create such a system of classification for nursing diagnoses were initiated. In October 1973, 100 interested nurses participated in the First National Conference on Classification of Nursing Diagnoses. The purpose of the conference was "to initiate the process of preparing an organized, logical, comprehensive system for classifying those health problems or health states diagnosed by nurses and treated by means of nursing intervention."[13] Although several classification systems had been discussed at the conference, none was selected for use. At the conclusion of the conference, the participants realized that the development of a system for classifying nursing diagnoses and the process for identifying diagnostic labels were just beginning. One hundred nursing diagnoses were proposed and described at the conference, but no attempt was made to categorize these. However, participants agreed that such efforts would continue at subsequent conferences.

Significant progress occurred in the 17 months between the first and second conferences. The Clearinghouse-National Group for Classification of Nursing Diagnoses was established at St. Louis University School of Nursing, and plans to publish a newsletter were made. The Clearinghouse assumed responsibility for coordinating data collection for a project that would "accumulate data on nursing diagnoses identified on a wide range of patients in many nursing care organizations across the country."[12] These data were analyzed and used to evaluate the diagnoses identified at the First National Conference and to identify more diagnoses.

In March 1975, 119 nurses who represented nursing practice, education, and research convened for the Second National Conference on Classification of Nursing Diagnoses in St. Louis, Missouri. Three conference objectives were established[12]:

1. To consider further issues relevant to the development of nomenclature and taxonomy of those health conditions diagnosed by nurses
2. To revise or evaluate those diagnoses identified at the First National Conference on Classification of Nursing Diagnoses
3. To identify and describe additional diagnoses

Although information was shared about the process of taxonomic development, many issues related to the introduction of a taxonomic system remained unsolved. Those attending the conference did make progress in the areas of evaluation of the diagnoses identified at the first conference and identification of new diagnoses. Thirty-seven diagnostic labels or categories were accepted at the Second Conference. It should be noted that acceptance was relative to particular diagnostic concepts. Nurses were cautioned that the "approved" labels with their defining characteristics were neither exhaustive nor mutually exclusive. In essence, specific diagnostic labels with defining characteristics were accepted with the recognition that further data were needed to substantiate and support the validity of the diagnostic labels or categories. The participants at the conference identified an additional 19 labels that were recommended for consideration at future conferences.

Considerable progress toward the development of a system of classification of nursing diagnoses occurred at the Third and Fourth National Conferences,[21] which were held in 1978 and 1980. At the Third Conference, 14 nurse theorists met for the purpose of reaching consensus on a framework to place diagnostic terms into a taxonomy. After the theorists' initial efforts, three clinical specialists worked with the theorists at the Fourth Conference, and conscientious efforts were made to integrate the views of practitioners with the nurse theorists' framework. Participants at the Third and Fourth Conferences witnessed the maturing of the nursing diagnosis movement. The conference agenda included the presentation of papers that reflected theoretical and practical perspectives in the classification and use of nursing diagnoses. Five research papers on the development and use of nursing diagnosis were presented at each of the two conferences.

Concurrent with the contributions that resulted from the conferences, the nursing literature of the 1970s reflected not only the growing acceptance of the term nursing diagnosis, but also the increased application of nursing diagnosis in clinical practice and education. Journal articles increased in frequency, books addressing a theoretical and practical knowledge base were published, and in 1979 an issue of *Advances in Nursing Science,* a scholarly journal, featured theoretical and research-based articles on nursing diagnosis.[10] This growing acceptance and interest indicated that support existed for a professional organization committed to the development of a diagnostic taxonomy.

ONGOING EFFORTS IN TAXONOMY DEVELOPMENT

The formal organization of the North American Nursing Diagnosis Association (NANDA) was presented to the participants at the Fifth National Conference on Classification of Nursing Diagnoses in April 1982, and the bylaws were accepted by the members later that year. The purpose of the association, as described in the bylaws, is "to develop, refine, and promote a taxonomy of nursing diagnostic terminology of general use to professional nurses."[20] The Fifth Conference also provided a forum for the presentation of the outcome of the nurse theorists' work since the preceding conference. A diagnostic framework that identified the health of unitary man/human as the phenomenon of concern to nursing was presented to the participants. Nine interactional patterns were proposed as concepts inherent to the diagnostic framework. These patterns, described as patterns of unitary persons at the Sixth Conference and renamed the nine central human response patterns at the Seventh Conference, are presented in the box at right.

The Sixth and Seventh Conferences convened in 1984 and 1986, respectively. The proceedings from the two conferences[15,29] documented the ongoing development of a taxonomy and presented research studies on the identification and validation of nursing diagnoses. The foundational work for the emerging taxonomy was presented at the Sixth Conference, and Taxonomy I was presented at the Seventh Conference with subsequent approval by NANDA members. The effect of nursing diagnosis on clinical practice and education can be seen through the breadth of issues related to nursing diagnosis that were addressed at the conferences: diagnosis related groups (DRGs), cost reimbursement, quality assurance, clinical competence, and computerization. Although no new diagnoses were presented at the Sixth Conference, 22 diagnoses were presented at the Seventh Conference. Twenty-one of these were accepted by the members of NANDA and added to the list of diagnostic categories that had been developed and refined through the previous conferences.

The list of diagnoses was expanded further in 1988. Fifteen new diagnoses and two recommendations for revisions of diagnoses accepted at earlier conferences were presented at the Eighth Conference on Classification of Nursing Diagnoses in March of that year.[8] All but one of the proposed new diagnoses were accepted by the members of NANDA. The need to continue work on Taxonomy I was evident at the Eighth Conference, and minor revisions were made, resulting in Taxonomy I Revised (Appendix A).

The Ninth Conference on Classification of Nursing Diagnoses convened in 1990.[7] Two new nursing diagnoses were presented at the confer-

---

❖ HUMAN RESPONSE PATTERNS

1. Exchanging—mutual giving and receiving
2. Communications—sending
   Communicating—sending messages
3. Relating—establishing bonds
4. Valuing—assigning relative worth
5. Choosing—selection of alternatives
6. Moving—activity
7. Perceiving—reception of information
8. Knowing—meaning associated with information
9. Feeling—subjective awareness of information

---

ence; both were accepted by NANDA members after the conference, bringing the total of diagnostic labels that have been approved for clinical use and testing to 100. Of special interest to those in attendance were two major topics: (1) the work of the Diagnosis Review Committee and the NANDA board of directors on developing a working definition of nursing diagnosis, clarification of terms used in relation to nursing diagnoses, and refinement of the nursing diagnosis submission guidelines and diagnostic review process; and (2) the work of the Taxonomy Committee on the development of Taxonomy II and the submission of the International Classification of Diseases-Tenth Edition (ICD-10) of "Conditions that Necessitate Nursing Care."

NANDA's Taxonomy Committee has identified and continues its work on several issues that must be resolved to further develop and refine the taxonomic system for nursing diagnoses. While work on Taxonomy II continues,[19,33] five specific issues are being addressed: levels of abstraction of diagnoses, the placement of wellness-related diagnoses, methods for testing the taxonomic structure and classification scheme, use of the structure in practice, and revision or deletion of diagnoses that do not meet the criteria specified in NANDA's definition of nursing diagnoses. Also, the probability of occurrence of possible nursing diagnosis not yet approved should be established in order to support the diagnostic review process and further development of the taxonomy.

CLASSIFICATION SYSTEMS USED IN PRACTICE

Attempts at developing a diagnostic classification system have not been limited to the work done through the Conferences on Classification of Nursing Diagnoses. Several proponents of nursing diagnosis have identified the need to develop categories of nursing diagnoses that would be meaningful to the practicing nurse. One of the most notable of these systems for categorization is the Functional Health Patterns proposed by Marjory Gordon.[14] These 11 patterns provide a structure for assessment, that is, the initial and continued health status evaluation of a person, family, or community. In addition to supporting a deliberative and systematic assessment, the functional health patterns have been described as having the following advantages[14]:

1. Not having to be continually relearned (application is expanded as clinical knowledge accumulates)
2. Leading directly to nursing diagnosis
3. Encompassing a holistic approach to human functional assessment in any setting and with any age-group at any point in the health-illness continuum

The relative ease with which the nurse can understand this framework and apply it in a variety of settings has prompted its acceptance as a valuable guide for assessment. Appendix B presents the categorization of NANDA-accepted nursing diagnoses according to Gordon's Functional Health Patterns.

A second organizing framework, particularly useful to nurses practicing in community health settings, is the classification scheme developed and used by the Visiting Nurse Association of Omaha.[27] This classification scheme focuses on nursing problems (or nursing diagnoses) and has three basic components: problem classification scheme, problem rating scale for outcomes, and intervention scheme. The problems are divided into the four domains representative of community health nursing practice: environmental, psychosocial, physiological, and health behaviors. Use of the classification scheme has positively influenced the agency's orientation plan, clinical record, computerized management information system, and quality assurance program.

In an effort to develop a classification of home health Medicare patients that would assist in predicting the need for nursing and other home health services, Saba[31] surveyed 646 home health agencies. The agencies collected data on the entire episode of home health care from admission to discharge of 8,961 study patients. Twenty Home Health Care Components were developed and served as a framework for the classification and coding of nursing diagnoses/patient problems and nursing interventions. The resulting nursing diagnosis classification scheme consists of 145 nursing diagnoses (50 two-digit major categories divided into 95 three-digit subcategories), and "was used to code the 40,361 nursing diagnoses and/or patient problems collected from the study patients."[31] Saba's Nursing Diagnoses for Home Health Care: Classification and Coding Scheme is presented in Appendix C.

The need to identify the phenomena or human responses of concern for psychiatric and mental health nursing practice prompted the formation of a task force in 1984 to guide the development of a classification system useful to psychiatric and mental health nurses.[26] This endeavor was supported by the Executive Committee of the Division of Psychiatric and Mental Health Nursing Practice of the American Nurses' Association. The task force studied both the NANDA taxonomy and the classification system presented in the third edition of the *Diagnostic and Statistical Manual of Mental Disorders* (DSM-III) and noted that "the defining characteristics of the NANDA nursing diagnoses and the diagnostic criteria of the DSM-III psychiatric diagnoses are actually human responses."[26] The work of the task force has resulted in the delineation of three generic response classes by which the system is organized: individual, interpersonal-family, and community-environment. Within each generic response class, response patterns are being developed. Although many of the NANDA diagnostic labels can be found in this classification system, additional, more specific, diagnoses have been included.

The relationship between the NANDA and ANA psychiatric-mental health taxonomic systems is vividly described by Vincent and Coler[32] "as an actual tree, the NANDA taxonomic labels are the roots; the ANA psychiatric-mental health taxa, the supporting branches; the fruit, the NANDA diagnostic labels." The need for a practice-relevant classification system useful to pediatric nurse practitioners has also been identified, with initial work on development of such a system completed.[6] Other specialty nursing organizations and groups can be expected to call for development of taxonomic structures that address unique needs and requirements.

Efforts are also ongoing in the development of classification systems of patient outcomes and nursing interventions. Lang and Marek[24] emphasize the importance of patient outcomes as descriptors and referents for measuring nursing practice. They present an initial classification of outcome indicators made up of 15 categories: physiological, psychosocial, functional, behavioral, knowledge, symptom control, home maintenance, well-being, goal attainment, patient satisfaction, safety, nursing diagnosis resolution, frequency of service, cost, and rehospitalization. McCloskey and colleagues[28] are focusing their work on the development of a standardized language for nursing interventions. They identify eight reasons for developing a classification system of nursing interventions. These reasons relate to the need to standardize nomenclature about nursing treatment; address the links among diagnoses, treatments, and outcomes; facilitate the development of information systems; facilitate teaching of decision making; assist in determining costs of nursing services; assist in planning for resources; provide a language to communicate the unique functions of nursing; and articulate with classification systems of other health care providers.

Although some may view the energy invested in developing different classification systems as detracting from the development of a unified diagnostic taxonomy, such efforts have opened the lines of communication. Nurses' expectations and needs of such a system have become apparent. The major contribution has been the development of "competing" diagnostic classification systems that resulted from the collaborative efforts of NANDA, ANA, and other groups of nurses. As an example, the ANA[30] has identified an activity critical to the future of nursing: "the implementation of standards of practice through the development of criteria related to specific nursing diagnoses." This activity must draw from the collective wealth of nursing knowledge and understanding that resides in the membership of ANA, NANDA, and other professional organizations. It will be through such collaboration that the seeds of nursing diagnosis, which were planted in the 1950s, will continue to germinate and take root. The use and ongoing evaluation of nursing diagnosis will enrich the fields of nursing education, practice, and research.

REFERENCES

1. Abdellah FG: Methods of identifying covert aspects of nursing problems, *Nurs Res* 6(1):4-23, 1957.
2. American Association of Critical-Care Nurses: *Outcome standards for nursing care of the critically ill,* Laguna Niguel, Calif, 1990, The Association.
3. American Nurses' Association: Standards of clinical nursing practice, Kansas City, Mo, 1991, The Association.
4. American Nurses' Association: *Nursing: a social policy statement,* Kansas City, Mo, 1980, The Association.
5. American Nurses' Association: *Standards of nursing practice,* Kansas City, Mo, 1973, The Association.
6. Burns C: Development and content validity testing of a comprehensive classification of diagnoses for pediatric nurse practitioners, *Nurs Diag* 2:95-103, 1991.
7. Carroll-Johnson RM: *Classification of nursing diagnoses: proceedings of the Ninth Conference,* Philadelphia, 1991, JB Lippincott.
8. Carroll-Johnson RM: *Classification of nursing diagnoses: proceedings of the Eighth Conference,* Philadelphia, 1989, JB Lippincott.
9. Chambers W: Nursing diagnosis, *Am J Nurs* 62(11):102-104, 1962.
10. Chinn PL, editor: Nursing diagnosis, *Adv Nurs Sci* 2(1):1, 1979.
11. Fry VS: The creative approach to nursing, *Am J Nurs* 53(3):301-302, 1953.
12. Gebbie KM: *Summary of the Second National Conference: classification of nursing diagnoses,* St Louis, 1976, Clearinghouse-National Group for Classification of Nursing Diagnoses.

13. Gebbie KM and Lavin MA: *Classification of nursing diagnoses: proceedings of the First National Conference,* St Louis, 1975, Mosby–Year Book.
14. Gordon M: *Nursing diagnosis: process and application,* New York, 1987, McGraw-Hill.
15. Hurley ME: *Classification of nursing diagnoses: proceedings of the Sixth Conference,* St Louis, 1986, Mosby–Year Book.
16. Joint Commission on Accreditation of Healthcare Organizations: *Accreditation manual for hospitals,* Oakbrook Terrace, Ill, 1992, The Commission.
17. Joint Commission on Accreditation of Healthcare Organizations: *Accreditation manual for hospitals,* Oakbrook Terrace, Ill, 1991, The Commission.
18. Kelly LY: Nursing practice acts, *Am J Nurs* 74:1310-1319, 1974.
19. Kerr M and others: Committee report: from Taxonomy I to Taxonomy II, *Nurs Diag* 2:131-136, 1991.
20. Kim MJ, McFarland GK, and McLane AM: Classification of nursing diagnoses: proceedings of the Fifth National Conference, St Louis, 1984, Mosby–Year Book.
21. Kim MJ and Moritz DA: *Classification of nursing diagnoses: proceedings of the Third and Fourth National Conferences,* New York, 1982, McGraw-Hill.
22. King LS: What is a diagnosis? *JAMA* 202:154-157, 1967.
23. Komorita NI: Nursing diagnosis, *Am J Nurs* 63(12): 83-85, 1963.
24. Lang NM and Marek KD: The classification of patient outcomes, *J Prof Nurs* 6:158-163, 1990.
25. Levine ME: Trophicognosis: an alternative to nursing diagnosis. In *American Nurses' Association Regional Clinical Conference (2): Exploring progress in medical-surgical nursing,* New York, 1966, The Association.
26. Loomis ME and others: Development of a classification system for psychiatric/mental health nursing: individual response class, *Arch Psychiatr Nurs* 1(1):16-24, 1987.
27. Martin KS and Scheet NJ: *The Omaha system: applications for community health nursing,* Philadelphia, 1992, WB Saunders.
28. McCloskey JC and others: Classification of nursing interventions, *J Prof Nurs* 6:151-157, 1990.
29. McLane AM: *Classification of nursing diagnoses: proceedings of the Seventh Conference,* St Louis, 1987, Mosby–Year Book.
30. Phaneuf MC: *Issues in professional nursing practice: 7. Standards of nursing practice,* Kansas City, Mo, 1985, American Nurses' Association.
31. Saba VK: The classification of home health care nursing diagnoses and interventions, *Caring Magazine* 50-57, March 1992.
32. Vincent KG and Coler MS: A unified nursing diagnostic model, *Image: J Nurs Schol* 22:93-95, 1990.
33. Warren JJ and Hoskins LM: The development of NANDA's nursing diagnosis taxonomy, *Nurs Diag* 1:162-168, 1990.

2

Nursing Diagnosis: The Critical Link in the Nursing Process

PROFESSIONAL TRENDS

A number of professional trends have led to the acceptance of the nursing diagnosis as a component of the nursing process. As described in Chapter 1, the National Conferences on the Classification of Nursing Diagnoses focused on the need to specify more clearly what nurses contribute to resolve specific patient problems and the need to store such information by means of automated record keeping. Each national conference* has built on previous work in the identification and development of nursing diagnoses and has served to further institutionalize the acceptance of nursing diagnosis as a critical link in the nursing process. Ongoing research on the identification and development of nursing diagnoses also is now published in *Nursing Diagnosis,* the new official Journal of the North American Nursing Diagnosis Association; e.g., Chang, et al.,[7] Hardy,[13] and Gift et al.[10]

The American Nurses' Association, through its published standards for generic and specialty nursing, lent considerable support to the acceptance of the nursing diagnosis as a part of the nursing process,[2] as did the ANA publication *Nursing: A Social Policy Statement.*[1] Nursing is defined in that document as "the diagnosis and treatment of human responses to actual or potential health problems" (p. 9). "Diagnosis is a beginning effort to objectify a perceived difficulty or need by naming it, as a basis for understanding and taking action to resolve the concern. A nurse's conceptualization or diagnosis of a presenting condition is a way of ascribing meaning to it" (p. 11).

Other professional trends have increased the use of nursing diagnoses as part of the nursing process in clinical practice. Among them are state nurse practice acts that hold the nurse accountable for nursing diagnosis in clinical practice, as well as professional standards. The Joint Commission on Accreditation of Healthcare Organizations 1992 Standard NC.1.3.5 states, for example: "Nursing care data related to patient assessments, the nursing diagnoses and/or patient needs, nursing interventions and patient outcomes are permanently integrated into the clinical information system (for example, the medical record)."[21, p. 6]

Pressure for the use and adoption of nursing diagnoses also comes from current endeavors such as computerized nursing care records, reimbursement models based on nursing diagnoses, patient classification based on nursing diagnoses, and standardized methods of reporting nursing information, as in the Minimum Nursing Data Set.

NURSING PROCESS—A PROBLEM-SOLVING PROCESS

The nursing process is a problem-solving process that nurses apply in rendering nursing care to patients. The commonly accepted components of the nursing process are (1) assessment (data collection), (2) nursing diagnosis (problem identification), (3) planning (goal setting), (4) implementing (nursing intervention and treatment), and (5) evaluating. The diagram in Chapter 1 clearly shows the relationship between components of the nursing process and the standards of nursing prac-

---

*References 5,6,8,9,14,16-18

tice previously discussed. The diagram shows that nursing diagnosis provides a clear focus for care planning, that is, for goal setting and the selection of nursing interventions. In other words, the symptoms of conditions diagnosed can be alleviated or modified by nursing actions. Therefore nursing diagnosis is a critical link in the nursing process.

DEFINITION OF NURSING DIAGNOSIS

An officially accepted definition of the concept of nursing diagnosis was approved by the Ninth Conference of NANDA.[19] This definition states that "Nursing Diagnosis is a clinical judgment about individual, family, or community responses to actual or potential health problems/life processes. Nursing diagnoses provide the basis for selection of nursing interventions to achieve outcomes for which the nurse is accountable."[p. 5]

This definition serves as the definition for understanding the use of nursing diagnosis in this text. An example of a nursing diagnosis is Dysfunctional Grieving, or, if the related factor has been identified, Dysfunctional Grieving related to inadequate social supports. Of course, more than one related factor could be involved, in which case the nursing diagnosis could be Dysfunctional Grieving related to inadequate social supports and inability to attend to grieving because of other tasks. An alternate way of addressing multiple related factors is to state each as a separate nursing diagnosis, such as (1) Dysfunctional Grieving related to inadequate social supports and (2) Dysfunctional Grieving related to inability to attend to grieving because of other tasks.

The Nursing Diagnosis Category

To further understand the concept of nursing diagnosis the three essential components known as PES[11] are explored.

Health Problems

P refers to the health problems or health state of an individual, family, or community expressed in a short, clear, and precise word, words, or phrase. Examples of such health states or problems as exemplified by nursing diagnoses categories are High Risk for Injury, Anxiety, and Knowledge Deficit (Specify). Note that High Risk for Injury refers to a "high risk for" rather than actual problem. The majority of nursing diagnosis labels could, in fact, be considered both high risk for or actual, for instance, High Risk for Sleep Pattern Disturbance or Sleep Pattern Disturbance.

Related Factors

E, the second component, stands for related factors. Related factors are any internal or external elements that have an effect on the person, family, or community and contribute to the existence of, or maintenance of, the person's health problem. They are "factors which appear to show some type of patterned relationship with the nursing diagnosis. Such factors may be described as antecedent to, associated with, related to, contributing to, or abetting."[19, p. 5] Related factors, where applicable and when they can be identified, should be as concise as possible and included in the nursing diagnostic statement.

Because additional research is needed on the related factors for any one of the NANDA nursing diagnoses, the identification of the related factors is somewhat tentative. Linking the health problem or nursing diagnosis category with only one related factor may imply a single cause, which can inhibit the implementation of holistic nursing care. Thus at times the use of the nursing diagnosis category itself (such as Diversional Activity Deficit) may be sufficient as a working nursing diagnosis for a patient and can provide direction for planning care without narrowing the focus to only one aspect of a larger, more complex health problem. Multiple specific nursing diagnostic statements that include very specific related factors can also be formulated to capture the complex needs of a specific patient.

In the care plans for the case studies in this text, usually one specific nursing diagnosis is the focus of planning. This is to help the reader understand the particular nursing diagnosis category under discussion and does not imply that additional nursing diagnoses should not also be identified and used to develop the care plan.

This logic can be taken a step further. It may at times be important to use a diagnostic category at a higher level of abstraction in the NANDA taxonomy to capture the essence of complexities and interrelatedness of a patient's health state, thereby providing direction for holistic nursing intervention. An example of such a nursing diagnosis is Altered Self-Concept. Body Image Disturbance, Personal Identity Disturbance, Self-Esteem Disturbance: Chronic Low, and Self-Esteem Disturbance: Situational have all been identified as components of the self-concept and have been incorporated into nursing diagnoses in previous NANDA work, thereby clarifying the abstract diagnosis Altered Self-Concept. Currently, Body Image Disturbance, Personal Identity Disturbance, Self-Esteem Disturbance: Chronic Low, and Self-Esteem Disturbance: Situational are listed under Altered Self-Concept in the NANDA taxonomy.

An even higher level of abstraction may be very useful in some clinical situations. Much is being written in the literature about Functional Health Patterns, one of which is the Self-Perception-Self-Concept pattern. In one text,[11] 12 nursing diagnostic labels are identified as a part of this pattern, among them being Self-Esteem Disturbance, Body Image Disturbance, and Personal Identity Disturbance. If in time, clinical observation and testing lend credence to this classification scheme, then the functional pattern, that is, the Self-Perception-Self-Concept Pattern, may itself be a useful nursing diagnosis in the clinical arena, especially in those clinical conditions where a very abstract nursing diagnosis would be useful to holistically capture very complex and interrelated elements. In this text, the Functional Health Patterns serve as an organizing framework for the NANDA nursing diagnoses that are addressed later in the chapter.

In the Nursing Care Guidelines in this text the level of abstraction addressed is at the nursing diagnosis category level; that is, nursing interventions are identified for nursing diagnoses such as Personal Identity Disturbance or Impaired Verbal Communication. Thus a nurse or student nurse can select nursing interventions from these guidelines to develop a plan of care for a patient, for example, with a nursing diagnosis of Personal Identity Disturbance.

Whether a "related to" phrase is added to the nursing diagnosis category along with a related factor for a given patient must be determined by a practicing nurse who has clinical judgment and experience. The related factor determined from the assessment data by the nurse further directs the selection of the nursing interventions made from the Nursing Care Guidelines; i.e., the practicing nurse tailors the nursing interventions to the specific nursing diagnosis and needs of an individual patient. Examples of this are provided in the Case Study with Plan of Care in each chapter.

Defining Characteristics

S, the third component, stands for defining characteristics. These are the cluster of subjective and objective signs and symptoms indicating the presence of a condition that corresponds to a given nursing diagnosis. Considerable research[12,15] is currently underway in validating nursing diagnoses so that eventually the cluster of defining characteristics identified for a given nursing diagnosis category will be supported. For the moment, however, some of the defining characteristics are based on clinical observation and group consensus. The clinician must use clinical reasoning to formulate the most appropriate nursing diagnosis or diagnoses for a given patient. To review, the usual way of stating a nursing diagnosis is not to include the signs and symptoms in the diagnoses but rather to state the nursing diagnosis category plus the related factor or factors if known.

Critical Versus Supporting Defining Characteristics. Some authors differentiate defining characteristics that are critical for formulating a given nursing diagnosis from those defining characteristics that are supporting but not critical. For example, Gordon[11, p. 17] states that "critical defining characteristics are the major criteria for diagnostic judgment. They are found nearly always when the diagnosis is present and are absent when the diagnosis is absent . . . When a patient manifests signs and symptoms that correspond to the critical defining characteristics then the use of the diagnostic category is appropriate." Caution is warranted in such an approach, however. Differentiating critical defining characteristics from supporting characteristics at this stage of the art and science of nursing diagnosis should be considered developmental because there is little research on which to base such differentiation.

NURSING PROCESS AND PLANNING FOR PATIENT CARE
Assessment

The first phase of the nursing process is assessment. The purpose of this phase is to collect data about a patient, family, or community to (1) assess the wellness state and desire for additional health lifestyle improvements, (2) assess for risk factors to identify potential nursing diagnoses, (3) assess for any alterations in the wellness state, as well as the response to these alterations and any nurse or medical therapy already implemented to determine the patient's, family's, or community's actual nursing diagnoses, (4) assess strengths and potential strengths, along with a history of coping strategies used, and (5) assess the patient's family, health care, and other relevant resources available, and other relevant environmental factors.

There are a number of variables to keep in mind while assessing a patient, family, or community. (1) The patient, family, or community must always be viewed holistically, while considering the uniqueness during the assessment process. It is thus important to collect data on the physiological, sociocultural, spiritual, psychological, developmental, and environmental aspects of functioning as relevant, assessing wellness and

strengths, patterns, alterations, and risk factors. (2) The nurse must be aware of self so he/she can be as objective as possible and understand the patient, family, or community from the patient's, family's, or community's own perspective. Yura and Walsh[25, p. 111] describe this well: "The nurse maintains a clear distinction between meaning that originates in him or herself and that which originates in the patient. The nurse attempts to understand these meanings at a particular moment with the idea that this understanding is subject to correction and change as new data become available." This will enable the nurse to collect objective data and differentiate between the cues actually manifested by the patient, family, or community, and nursing judgments or inferences made about these cues. (3) The interview and data collection process, including any guides or tools developed, must be adapted to the patient's or family's setting, that is, home versus hospital. (4) The setting in which the interview is conducted must be conducive to the collection of the nursing data—there should be minimal interruptions and noise, pleasant decor, comfortable seats, and a comfortable temperature. (5) A number of data collection strategies should be used, such as the nursing interview and history; observation; physical examination; medical records, including previous nursing notes and care plans; interview of family members and significant others; observation of the environment and collaboration with nurse colleagues and other health team members on a one-to-one basis or in patient care planning conferences. Communicating effectively and observing systematically are, of course, very important throughout the entire assessment process.

The Initial Interview

The assessment phase includes both a general initial interview and a focused assessment. The initial data-based interview focuses on the patient, family, or community, and allows the nurse to collect data for the second phase of the nursing process—nursing diagnosis. A sample interview guide for an adult patient appears in Appendix D. Because of their apparent relevance to clinical practice, the Functional Health Patterns are useful in categorizing the NANDA nursing diagnoses[11] (Appendix B) and providing some conceptual direction for the initial assessment of a patient. There are 11 functional health patterns[11], each of which is defined below with the purpose of assessing the pattern. An assessment guide based on the Functional Health Patterns is presented in Appendix C.[23]

The Functional Health Patterns. The *Health Perception–Health Management Pattern* refers to the patient's perceptions of his/her own health state and how his/her health goals and beliefs shape personal health care practices. The purpose of the assessment is to determine past and current health-seeking behaviors, compliance with both nursing and medical treatment recommendations, resources available for health maintenance, injury prevention practices, and whether and how the patient is seeking a higher level of well-being.

The *Nutritional and Metabolic Pattern* refers to the biopsychosocial states linked to food and water supply and the patient's nutrient and fluid intake. The purpose of assessment is to determine the patient's functional or dysfunctional fluid and food patterns along with possible reasons, condition of the skin as a reflection of nutrition, and metabolic problems in temperature regulation. Weight, temperature, diet, fluid intake, and skin integrity are all assessed.

The *Elimination Pattern* describes a patient's urinary and bowel elimination patterns. The purpose of the assessment is to determine the adequacy of these patterns by assessing urinary and bowel routines, habits, and practices.

The *Activity-Exercise Pattern* refers to a patient's motivation and capability to engage in energy-consuming activities and conditions that affect these activities. The purpose of the assessment is to determine the patient's desire, choice, and actual involvement in leisure, work, self-care, and exercise. Also assessed are nursing diagnoses that can influence the activity pattern, such as tissue perfusion, cardiac output, breathing pattern, and gas exchange.

The *Sleep-Rest Pattern* refers to the patient's rest and sleep perceptions and practices. The purpose of the assessment is to determine the quality of the sleep and rest, as well as the patient's methods for promoting rest and sleep.

The *Cognitive-Perceptual Pattern* refers to the ability of the patient to perceive, understand, remember, and make decisions about information from the internal and external environment. The purpose of the assessment is to determine the status of the five senses and the use of any aids (for example, a hearing aid), degree of discomfort or pain, any perceptual alterations, and the patient's ability to understand, make decisions, and use good judgment. Also assessed is the patient's understanding of health care self-management practices and knowledge.

The *Self-Perception—Self-Concept Pattern* includes the patient's patterns of perception, attitudes, and self-competency. The purpose of the assessment is to determine the patient's attitudes and beliefs about personal abilities, identity, self-worth, and body image. Emotions and feelings such as grieving, anxiety, hopelessness, and powerlessness are also assessed.

The *Role-Relationship Pattern* involves the patient's needs and actual interactions with others at work, in the family, or in the community. The purpose of the assessment is to determine the patient's role and responsibility at work, in the family, or in social life, including his/her communication skills and patterns. Areas in which the patient is adequate or experiences difficulty are both assessed. Also assessed are risk factors for self-harm and potential for inflicting physical harm on others.

The *Sexuality-Reproductive Pattern* refers to the patient's actual and perceived satisfaction or dysfunction in sexuality or reproduction. The purpose of assessment is to determine the patient's degree of satisfaction or dissatisfaction in fulfilling sexual and reproductive needs. Assessed are the patient's reproductive pattern and associated problems and concerns.

The *Coping—Stress Tolerance Pattern* refers to the patient's or family's adaptive or maladaptive response to stress and challenging life events.

The purpose of the assessment is to determine the nature and degree of stressors, stress response, and coping patterns. Assessed are perceptions of the stress and coping strategies and the resources available to the patient and family.

The *Value-Belief Pattern* includes the beliefs and values that guide a person's choices and lifestyle. The purpose of the assessment is to determine these life beliefs and values, including spiritual, religious, and philosophical beliefs.

The Focused Assessment. The general initial interview can often determine the need for a focused assessment involving the collection of very specific data about alterations in a particular functional pattern, and more specifically, in a given diagnostic category. This focused assessment either rules out or validates the alterations or potential alterations in health or the desire for additional health seeking opportunities as suggested by the data gathered during the initial interview. Each of the following nursing diagnosis sections in the text contains an assessment with specific questions and tools for a focused assessment, along with clearly identified defining characteristics and related factors for each diagnostic category. A focused assessment can be completed as part of the initial interview if the data already collected suggest the need. Another focused assessment should be conducted after the initial one as additional data indicate a change in the patient's condition. The patient's verbalizations or information from other sources, such as the family or other health care team members, can all indicate a need for this second focused assessment.

Formulating Nursing Diagnoses

To formulate accurate nursing diagnoses with a given patient, family, or community, the nurse must consider a number of important factors. Knowledge of nursing science and other related biopsychosocial sciences is important for the practicing nurse to move from the assessment phase of the nursing process to formulating accurate nursing diagnoses. Clinical practice guided by experienced faculty, clinical nurse specialists, and experienced clinicians facilitates growth and assurance of the nurse's diagnostic reasoning skills. The opportunity to practice in a protected setting such as the classroom or the continuing education workshop likewise facilitates growth in the nurse's ability to formulate accurate nursing diagnoses. Equally essential is the need for the practicing nurse to consult quality nursing practice reference texts and manuals, which should be found in every health care setting library, and to consult with nurse peers, nurse consultants and specialists, and other health team members, either individually or in nursing staff or team conferences. It is likewise important to understand that the nursing diagnosis or diagnoses that the nurse formulates when beginning to care for a patient are working diagnoses subject to change and ongoing revision: The nurse may identify alternative explanations and confirm or rule these out based on the data initially available, the nurse may obtain more data about the patient over time, or the patient's condition may change. Indeed, unless openness to alternative explanations is maintained, one alternative may be overvalued, and the resulting narrow focus may not allow for all data to be considered, thus causing an inaccurate nursing diagnosis. Finally, the nurse's ability to understand the clinical reasoning process is an asset when the nurse actually assumes responsibility for formulating accurate nursing diagnoses in the clinical setting.

Diagnosis as a Process. One of the most commonly accepted models of diagnosis as a process contains four activities—collecting information, interpreting the information, clustering the information, and naming the cluster—occurring as an ongoing cyclical process that involves both cognitive and perceptual activities.[11] Data collected by means of the strategies discussed above and in subsequent sections need to be interpreted to have meaning. Gordon elucidates: "To interpret means to assign meaning to a cue or determine what is significant."[11, p. 212] Interpretation involves the ability to (1) pay attention to and recognize diagnostic cues, (2) clarify or search for a clearer understanding of the cues, (3) verify or double-check the cues, (4) recognize the direct or concealed meaning of the cues, and (5) evaluate the cues so that the initial cues are put together to have meaning.

In evaluating cues, the observed baseline data are compared with population norms or standards. The baseline data are also very useful in ongoing monitoring of the patient's progress. Through inferential reasoning, the nurse determines whether the cues fall within the expected norms or indicate some type of health problem. Interpretation must also take into account the whole patient situation and environment. Diagnostic hypotheses (the possible meanings of a cue or cue cluster) are then formed, providing further structure to the diagnostic tasks. Checkpoints for hypothesis generation and testing include the following[11]:

1. Has the collected data been clarified and verified?
2. Has attention been given to diagnostic cues in the data that have been collected?
3. Have the cues been interpreted for meaning and compared against norms?
4. Have the cues been adequately analyzed for the possibility of alternative explanations?
5. Have the defining characteristics for the hypotheses being tested been addressed?
6. Objectively, are sufficient cues or defining characteristics present to formulate tentative nursing diagnoses?

The diagnostic process involves ongoing information clustering, that is, relating and clustering the collected cues. The generated diagnostic hypothesis facilitates this activity. The collected cues may not always lead directly and easily to the formulation of a nursing diagnosis. Inconsistencies among cues may be the result of (1) conflicting reports from health care team members, the patient, or the family, (2) measurement errors resulting from miscommunication or faulty instruments, (3) faulty expectations resulting from a nurse's lack of experience or knowledge, or (4) unreliable information.[11] Besides resolving such inconsistencies the clinician must weigh cues so he/she can arrive at the best working hypothesis and eventually name and formulate the actual nursing diagnostic statement that is the very best

statement possible until an even more precise one can be formulated.

As previously described, the nursing diagnostic statement includes the health problem along with the related factor or factors when known. The health problem can be selected from the list of NANDA nursing diagnosis categories (Each is discussed in depth in the following sections) if the cluster of signs and symptoms collected during assessment corresponds, at least in part, to the defining characteristics for a given nursing diagnosis category. Not all of the defining characteristics for a specific nursing diagnosis need be observed in, or reported by, a patient in order to use the diagnosis, but this determination requires clinical expertise and knowledge. Based on the collected data, the related factor or factors can also be identified. Common related factors for each of the nursing diagnoses in the following chapters are listed and can be used in formulating a specific nursing diagnosis if supported by the collected data.

In addition to naming the actual specific nursing diagnosis (for instance, Dysfunctional Grieving related to multiple unresolved previous losses), other assessment conclusions can be reached at the naming stage of the diagnostic process. First, the assessment conclusion often results in more than one nursing diagnosis, and they must be prioritized to identify those requiring immediate intervention. The assessment may also determine that the patient does not have an actual or evident health problem. The patient's history, current lifestyle, and other data sources may present evidence of risk factors, and the assessment conclusion may indicate a high risk nursing diagnosis such as High Risk for Violence: Self-Directed related to lengthy history of violent behavior. Depending on the patient's identified risk factors, any of the nursing diagnoses can be high risk such as High Risk for Social Isolation. Such diagnoses address the preventive aspect of nursing care. A health promotion diagnosis may also result from the assessment, e.g., Health Seeking Behaviors (Specify).

Planning

The third phase of the nursing process is planning. "Planning is the determination of a plan of action to assist the client toward the goal of optimal wellness based on the highest level of fulfillment [in relation to the Functional Health Patterns] and to resolve the nursing diagnosis [or diagnoses]."[25, p. 138] The formulated nursing diagnosis or diagnoses provide direction to the planning process and in selecting nursing interventions to achieve the desired outcomes. In other words, patient goals—referred to as *expected patient outcomes* in many contemporary practice settings and in this text—are developed for each of the nursing diagnoses formulated for a given patient. For each nursing diagnosis, one or more expected patient outcomes may be identified. The expected patient outcomes are desirable and measurable patient health states, including biological or physiological, psychological, sociocultural, and spiritual aspects, and the knowledge or skills related to these health states. The expected patient outcomes denote progress toward the resolution or modification of the condition that corresponds to an actual nursing diagnosis, the prevention of a condition that corresponds to a high risk for a nursing diagnosis, or progress toward a higher level of optimal wellness in a patient who is healthy but desires to engage in further health seeking behaviors. In a deteriorating health state or terminal illness, the expected patient outcome may be directed toward achieving satisfactory adaptation or coping.

The development of expected patient outcomes is guided by a number of factors. (1) They should be stated in patient behavioral terms, with measurable verbs, and be specific in content. For example, "The patient will [expected patient outcome]." or "The patient will be able to [expected patient outcome]." Examples of expected patient outcomes for a patient with the nursing diagnosis of Post-Trauma Response could be to resolve the physiological changes suffered in the trauma, to express feelings about the effect of the trauma on personal lifestyle, to experience increasingly longer periods free of impaired concentration, to maintain old and develop new interpersonal relationships, to abstain from drugs and alcohol, and to integrate the traumatic experience into the patient's lifestyle and perception of self. For a patient with a nursing diagnosis of Impaired Verbal Communication, the expected patient outcomes could include to attend to, perceive, and process relevant stimuli; to send precise, understandable messages using congruent verbal and nonverbal communications; and to send and receive feedback. (2) The development of any expected patient outcome is guided by the formulated nursing diagnosis, including the related factor if identified and stated. This is evident because the desired overall outcome is to modify or resolve the condition that corresponds to an actual nursing diagnosis or, in the case of a potential nursing diagnosis, to prevent the occurrence of the actual condition in a patient with known risk factors. (3) The overall database collected during both the initial interview and focused assessment is also critically important, because the expected patient outcomes must be realistic and attainable for a given patient and take into account his/her strengths and potential, lifestyle, family, living arrangements, and the community in which the patient resides. (4) Expected patient outcomes can be developed as both short-term and long-term outcomes and must be reviewed or modified as the patient progresses. This is especially important when the nursing diagnosis itself is modified or resolved. (5) A time frame can be specified wherein the expected patient outcome or outcomes should be achieved for a particular patient. (6) If the focus is the family or community, expected outcomes refer to achievable behaviors for the family or community. That is, the phrase for the family would be "The family will [expected family outcome]" or "The family will be able to [expected family outcome]." For example, for the nursing diagnosis Ineffective Family Coping: Compromised, an expected family outcome could be to promote health to maintain family integrity or to use additional resources to preserve family supportive capacity.

In each of the sections of this text, sample expected patient outcomes are identified. Based on the data collected on a given patient and the actual nursing diagnosis formulated, these expected patient outcomes can be selected and used in developing a patient care plan.

Major Expected Patient Outcomes are identified for each nursing diagnosis in the Nursing Care Guidelines and are further discussed in each Planning and Implementation with Rationale section of each subsequent chapter in this text.

The planning process also involves selecting nursing interventions (the action the nurse must take or assist the patient in taking) to achieve the specified expected patient outcome or outcomes. Nursing interventions are categorized by the level of assistance that the nurse offers the patient; these categories range from interventions that the nurse totally performs for a patient who is unable to assist to those that offer support and encouragement for a patient who actively participates in his/her own care. Nursing interventions involve ongoing assessment and monitoring, coordination of resources and health care services, emotional support or therapy, guidance or counseling, teaching, acting for or doing for the patient, collaborating with the patient, referring the patient to other health team members, monitoring the environment, and supporting and teaching the family. Similar to the expected patient outcomes, nursing diagnoses and the related factors guide the selection of nursing interventions. The intended result of the implementation of the nursing interventions is to meet the expected patient outcomes.

In each of the nursing diagnosis sections of this book, sample nursing interventions are clearly identified in the Nursing Care Guidelines and discussed in detail, including the rationale for their use in the Planning and Implementation with Rationale section. These nursing interventions are useful in developing a patient's plan of care and must be selected based on a particular patient's specific nursing diagnostic statement and expected outcomes, along with such collected data as the patient's particular strengths, coping skills, and resources available.

Approaches to writing actual nursing orders differ. Nursing orders can be stated more gener-

ally, as in the multiple sample interventions described in the following sections. Or these nursing interventions can be specified further into behaviors tailored to a particular patient. For example, one expected patient outcome for the nursing diagnosis Altered Nutrition: Less than Body Requirements listed in this text is that the patient will improve and maintain food intake to meet metabolic demands. Among the nursing interventions identified for this expected patient outcome is to encourage verbalization by the patient and his/her family of preferred mealtimes, meal locations, and food likes and dislikes. Developed into a more specific nursing order, this nursing intervention could be "Meet with Mrs. Karen J. and her husband on Wednesday afternoon during visiting hours to discuss preferred mealtimes, meal locations, and food likes and dislikes." Or "Schedule procedures so they do not conflict with mealtimes" can be developed into a more specific nursing order, such as "Schedule Mrs. Karen J. for a chest x-ray examination at 10 AM on Friday." Carnevali[4] advocates that nursing orders include the date, an action or directive verb, the action and when it should occur, how frequently and how long the action should occur, where the action is to take place, and the nurse's signature. The nursing interventions in the following sections can serve as useful guidelines if such specific nursing orders are desired.

Based on the collected data, a number of nursing diagnoses may be formulated for a particular patient. In the planning phase, attention must be given to assigning priority to these concomitant nursing diagnoses because it may be unreasonable to develop and implement expected patient outcomes and a corresponding plan of action for each of them. Therefore the nurse, in collaboration with the patient, may need to determine which nursing diagnoses should be addressed first in the care plan.

Implementing

Implementing is the fourth phase of the nursing process and "is the initiation and completion of actions necessary to accomplish the defined goal of optimal wellness for the client."[25, p. 154] Depending on the nature of the patient's problem and on his/her condition, ability, and resources, as well as the nature of the action planned, the nursing care plan may be implemented primarily by the nurse or by the nurse in collaboration with the patient, the patient's family, community resources, or other health care team members to whom selected aspects of care are delegated. Yura and Walsh[25, p. 154] further note that "the implementation phase for the nursing process draws heavily on the intellectual, interpersonal, and technical skills of the nurse. Decision making, observation, and communication are significant skills enhancing the success of actions." The nursing care plan serves as a blueprint for action, and the nurse must monitor the patient's progress and achievement of the specified expected outcomes.

For each nursing diagnosis in the following sections, a sample Case Study with Plan of Care follows the description of the case study. The sample care plan is designed to help the reader understand the nursing diagnosis on which the section focuses and is not intended to address other nursing diagnoses that could also be formulated for the specific patient in the case study.

JCAHO recognizes nursing diagnoses and requires that the "primary place to document the nursing process is a patient's medical record, either directly or by reference to some document or standard of care", i.e., it must be shown that a plan of care is in place.[3, p. 35]

The following quote provides an excellent conclusion to the implementation section of the nursing process:

The success or failure of the nursing care plan depends on the nurse's intellectual, interpersonal, and technical abilities. This includes the ability to judge the value of new data that become available to the nurse during implementation, and the nurse's innovative and creative ability in making adaptations to compensate for unique characteristics—physical, emotional, cultural, and spiritual—that become known during interaction with the client. The nurse must have the ability to react

to verbal and nonverbal cues, validating inferences based on observation. Paramount during the interaction is the nurse's acceptance of himself or herself as a person and the confidence in his or her ability to perform the independent nursing functions inherent in the planned action, recognizing those that are interdependent. . . The nurse must have a realistic understanding of self, recognizing and accepting strengths and limitations; be convinced of his or her own personal worth and find meaning in his or her life; meet his or her own human needs reasonably well. . . . The more wholesome the nurse's view of himself or herself as a person and the stronger the philosophy of life, the less likely the client will experience depersonalizing encounters with the nurse.[25, p. 154]

Evaluating

The fifth phase of the nursing process is evaluating, which follows the implementation phase. In the implementation phase, the patient is monitored and data are collected to determine whether progress toward the achievement of the expected patient outcomes is being made, and in turn, whether the patient's condition has improved. This improvement can relate to actual nursing diagnoses being modified or resolved, actual nursing diagnoses being prevented in the case of potential nursing diagnoses, or health seeking behaviors being enhanced in the case of the patient with the nursing diagnosis of Health Seeking Behaviors. Specific outcome criteria can be delineated to indicate whether the stated expected patient outcomes are being achieved.

Each of the following sections contains a description of relevant criteria that must be monitored to evaluate a patient's progress. Evaluation is very important in the nursing process because it is on the results of evaluation that nursing diagnoses are reexamined and perhaps restated, expected patient outcomes are altered, and different nursing interventions are implemented.

The work of NANDA in identifying and developing nursing diagnoses and a taxonomy is an evolving, ever-changing process. Although the past 20 years of effort have resulted in a clinically useful list of nursing diagnoses and a beginning taxonomy, ongoing clinical observation and research will result in deletions, modifications, and additions to this system.

Nurse researchers are encouraged to continue the progress in research on nursing diagnosis, as reflected in the review of nursing diagnosis research by Gordon[12] and Kim[15] in the *Annual Review of Nursing Research*.

The practicing nurse is encouraged to use the nursing diagnoses recently developed and to test them in clinical practice, providing feedback to the professional organization when changes are needed in the system.

Specialty organizations—e.g., the ANA Council of Psychiatric Mental Health Nursing, which has been working since 1984 to develop a "comprehensive working list on the phenomena of concern for psychiatric mental health (PMH) nurses"[20]—are encouraged to submit their work to NANDA for inclusion in the NANDA Taxonomy.

Finally, the nurse should keep in mind that the processes of clinical decision making and diagnostic reasoning are very complex and that more nursing research is needed to understand these complex processes. As the NANDA Taxonomy of nursing knowledge evolves in practice, nursing will continue to evolve as a true profession.[22,24]

REFERENCES

1. American Nurses' Association: *Nursing: a social policy statement,* Kansas City, Mo, 1980, The Association.
2. American Nurses' Association: *Standards of nursing practice,* Kansas City, Mo, 1973, The Association.
3. Brider P: Who killed the nursing care plan? *Am J Nurs, 91* (5):35-39, 1991.
4. Carnevali D: *Nursing care planning: diagnosis and management,* Philadelphia, 1983, JB Lippincott.
5. Carroll-Johnson RM (editor): *Classification of nursing diagnoses: proceedings of the Ninth Conference,* Philadelphia, 1991, JB Lippincott.
6. Carroll-Johnson RM: *Classification of nursing diagnoses: proceedings of the Eight Conference,* Philadelphia, JB Lippincott, 1989.
7. Chang BL and others: Self-care deficit with etiologies: reliability of measurement, *Nurs Diag,* vol 1, no 1, pp. 31-36, 1990.
8. Gebbie KM: *Summary of the Second National Conference,* St Louis, The Clearinghouse—National Group for Classification of Nursing Diagnoses, 1976.
9. Gebbie K and Lavin M: *Classification of nursing diagnoses: proceedings of the First National Conference,* St Louis, 1975, Mosby–Year Book.
10. Gift AF, Nield M: Dyspnea: a case for nursing diagnosis status, *Nurs Diag,* vol 2, no 2, pp. 66-71, 1991.
11. Gordon M: *Nursing diagnoses: process and application,* New York, 1987, McGraw-Hill.
12. Gordon M: Nursing diagnosis, *Annu Rev Nurs Res 3:* 127-146, 1985.
13. Hardy MA: A pilot study of the diagnosis and treatment of impaired skin integrity: dry skin in older persons, *Nurs Diagn,* vol. 1(2):57-63, 1990.
14. Hurley ME (editor): *Classification of nursing diagnosis: proceedings of the Sixth Conference,* St Louis, 1986, Mosby–Year Book.
15. Kim MJ: Nursing diagnosis, *Annu Rev Nurs Res 7:*117-142, 1989.
16. Kim MJ, McFarland GK, McLane AM (editors): *Classification of nursing diagnosis: proceedings of the Fifth National Conference,* St Louis, 1984, Mosby–Year Book.
17. Kim MJ, Moritz DA (editors): *Classification of nursing diagnosis: proceedings of the Third and Fourth Conferences,* New York, 1982, McGraw Hill.
18. McLane AM (editor): *Classification of nursing diagnosis: proceedings of the Seventh Conference,* St Louis, 1988, Mosby–Year Book.
19. North American Nursing Diagnosis Association: *Taxonomy I revised—1990—with official nursing diagnoses,* St. Louis, 1990, NANDA.
20. O'Toole AW, Loomis ME: Revision of the phenomena of concern for psychiatric mental health nursing, *Arch Psychiatr Nurs III* (5):288-299, 1989.
21. Parsek JD: Did JCAHO abolish care plans? *Am Nurs 23*(8):6, 1991.
22. Sheppard KC: Endorsement of the NANDA taxonomy, *Dimens Oncol Nurs, III* (4):29-34, 1989.
23. Weber J: *Nurses' handbook of health assessment,* Philadelphia, 1988, JB Lippincott.
24. Westfall U and others: Activating clinical inferences: a component of diagnostic reasoning in nursing, *Res Nurs Health 9*(4):269-277, 1986.
25. Yura H and Walsh M: *The nursing process: assessing, planning, implementing, evaluating,* Norwalk, Conn, 1988, Appleton & Lange.

I

HEALTH PERCEPTION— HEALTH MANAGEMENT PATTERN

Altered Health Maintenance

Altered Health Maintenance is the inability to identify, manage, or seek help to maintain health.[3]

OVERVIEW

Few diagnostic categories fall so clearly within the scope of nursing practice as does Altered Health Maintenance. Nurses have traditionally been concerned with assisting individuals, their families, or groups in achieving optimum health. Given today's health care environment of diminishing resources, Altered Health Maintenance assumes even greater relevance. Recommendations published in *Nursing's Agenda For Health Care Reform* [1] call for a plan to convert "a system that focuses on the costly treatment of illness to a system that emphasizes primary health care services and the promotion, restoration, and maintenance of health." Nurses must understand the meaning of Altered Health Maintenance and explore the probable causes that contribute to its existence.

Economic, political, and social factors may prevent individuals from maintaining an acceptable level of wellness or even a state of "health" that is understood to mean disease-free. Our life span has increased, leading to greater health care needs[9] and fewer resources to meet these needs.

By 2000, people over age 65 will represent an estimated 13% of the population of the United States, in contrast to 8% in 1950.[12] As the "graying of America" continues, so does the demand for nurses who are educated in and informed of this older population's needs.[2]

The nursing diagnosis of Altered Health Maintenance is not limited to the aged population. Today, fewer people have adequate financial resources to pay for even essential health care services and "More than 60 million Americans are either uninsured or underinsured."[1] Additionally, the costs of health care are increasing. "Health care expenditures in the United States are approaching 12% of the gross national product,"[1] an increase of more than 100% since 1965.[8]

As the cost of health care continues to escalate, the number of persons in the United States without resources to pay for medical care will grow. These individuals will likely turn to the self-care mode of health care treatment. The nurse's role in self-care is to teach the person to strengthen skills that he/she already possesses, thereby increasing maximum independence.[9] Education and support accomplish the goals of this aspect of health maintenance.

Responsibility for health maintenance falls primarily on adults because they are legally bound to care for dependent children. However, Altered Health Maintenance is an appropriate diagnosis for minors who exhibit some defining characteristics, such as lack of adequate immunizations, frequent infections, or inadequate accident prevention practices. After diagnosing Altered Health Maintenance, the nurse intervenes by counseling and educating the responsible adult or minor and

I

the adult with impaired cognitive abilities such as those seen with mental retardation or addictive behaviors.

NANDA accepted Altered Health Maintenance as a diagnosis in 1982.[6] Little research has been done on assessment, interventions, or evaluation of interventions. One possible reason for the lack of research may be the broad scope of the diagnosis.

A study conducted to determine the incidence of nursing diagnoses in a psychiatric ward in Taiwan found that of 56 patients assessed in a 1-year period, 24 were diagnosed with Altered Health Maintenance. The two nursing diagnoses identified most frequently were Altered Thought Processes (51 patients) and Sleep Pattern Disturbance (47 patients).[11]

ASSESSMENT

Learning the individual's perception of his/her health status is the first step when assessing Health Perception-Health Management Pattern. This functional health pattern is assessed, according to Gordon,[4] "to obtain data about general perceptions, general health management, and preventive practices." The nurse must consider cultural factors. Presumptions made about a patient's culture may lead to a misdiagnosis of an actual problem or the identification of a "problem" that is simply an ethnic variant. The nurse should interpret the meaning of behaviors, beliefs, and practices from a holistic viewpoint and avoid grouping individuals according to their culture.[7]

Another pitfall to avoid while assessing patients is misinterpreting subjective and objective data as defining characteristics of this nursing diagnosis. For instance, if a patient arrives in the hospital for a cardiac catheterization and states, "They say I've got a little heart trouble, but, ya' know, a guy has to die from something," several questions need to be answered to make an accurate nursing diagnosis. Without further clarification, it may appear that the patient is denying his illness, lacks knowledge regarding his illness, or believes that he has little control of his health. Additional assessment of his behavior may validate his casual

attitude as a coping mechanism that compensates for the overwhelming fear of being hospitalized for a potentially life-threatening condition. Isolated cues or responses may initially be misleading, and a premature conclusion or incorrect nursing diagnosis may result.

Altered Health Maintenance has an extremely broad conceptual base and seems to lack the specificity found in more concrete, physiological diagnoses, such as Chronic Pain or Ineffective Airway Clearance. "Altered Health Maintenance transcends disease-related categories,"[10] age groups, and cultures. The unit for analysis may be an individual, family, or community, and suggested assessment questions for each category are available.[4] Although the related factors contributing to Altered Health Maintenance are extremely varied, the nurse must identify the factor(s) contributing to the occurrence of the diagnosis in a particular patient so that he/she can implement appropriate interventions. The defining characteristics that can lead the nurse to make this diagnosis are also varied.

❖ Defining Characteristics

The presence of the following defining characteristics indicates that the patient may be experiencing Altered Health Maintenance:

- Frequent infections, anorexia, obesity, head aches, or malaise
- Poor diet
- Lack of adequate immunizations
- Need for alcohol, drugs, or tobacco
- Emotional fragility or behavior disorders
- Verbalization of inaccurate information
- Inability to take responsibility for basic health practices
- Inadequate accident prevention practices
- Lack of knowledge regarding basic health practices
- Lack of adaptive behavior
- Failure to manage stress
- Lack of equipment, finances, and/or other resources
- Lack of adequate housing
- Illiteracy

❖ **Related Factors**

The following related factors are associated with Altered Health Maintenance:

- Lack of gross and/or fine motor skills
- Unachieved developmental skills
- Inability to make judgments
- Inadequate information
- Failure to practice age-related preventive measures
- Lack of perceived threat to health
- Perceptual or cognitive impairment
- Poor learning skills
- Ineffective coping (individual or family)
- Emotional difficulties
- Failure to assume responsibility for primary prevention
- Alteration in communication skills
- Loss of independence
- Inadequate resources
- Changing support systems
- Lack of access to health care services
- Disabling spiritual distress
- Dysfunctional grieving

❖ **Related Medical/Psychiatric Diagnoses**

The following are examples of related medical/psychiatric diagnoses for Altered Health Maintenance:

- Accidental poisoning
- Acute trauma
- Alcohol dependence
- Alzheimer's disease
- Anorexia nervosa
- Chronic renal failure
- Coronary artery disease
- Dementia
- Diabetes mellitus
- Drug overdose
- Failure to thrive
- Hypothermia
- Malignant hypertension
- Malnutrition
- Mental retardation
- Mood disorders
- Mumps
- Obesity
- Personality disorders
- Rubella
- Rubeola
- Schizophrenia
- Spinal cord injury
- Traumatic head injury

NURSING DIAGNOSES

Examples of *specific* nursing diagnoses for Altered Health Maintenance are:

1. Altered Health Maintenance related to inability to secure adequate permanent housing for self and family.
2. Altered Health Maintenance related to lack of knowledge regarding required childhood immunizations.
3. Altered Health Maintenance related to failure to manage demands of work, family, and home.
4. Altered Health Maintenance related to inability to transport self to clinic for weekly appointments.

PLANNING AND IMPLEMENTATION WITH RATIONALE

After identifying the nursing diagnosis Altered Health Maintenance, the nurse establishes a plan of care to resolve the problem or change the patient's unhealthful behavior. Realistic and measurable expected patient outcomes are determined. The nursing actions or interventions are aimed at alleviating or reducing the factors responsible for or contributing to the Altered Health Maintenance.

The boxed Nursing Care Guidelines illustrate realistic expected outcomes and appropriate nursing interventions for Altered Health Maintenance when it results from lack of adequate resources or materials necessary for discharge to home from a hospital. The overall nursing implementation is to coordinate appropriate referrals. The patient must first recognize that he/she will need help after returning home. The nursing strategy to accomplish this outcome includes further assessment of the patient's home situation. This allows both the nurse and the patient to explore the appropriate referrals and clarify the patient's perceptions of his/her abilities. *These interventions will help the patient anticipate the realities of his/her home environment. Specifically, the physical layout of the home as it relates to the patient's present needs and functional abilities must be anticipated.* Discussing inconsistencies between needs and abilities gives the nurse an understanding of the patient's perception of his/her capabilities. This knowledge is helpful when evaluating the patient's strengths and limitations. *"The strengths of the client must be systematically identified and utilized to promote client independence."* [5]

The second expected patient outcome in the Nursing Care Guidelines is that the patient will participate in the decision-making process regarding discharge plans. *Driving the trend toward health promotion, disease prevention, and optimal functioning are early hospital discharge and greater reliance on home care by family, friends, and community-based services.*[5] *Interventions that focus on self-care also promote personal responsibility for health and wellness. With these interventions, the nurse demonstrates the value placed on the patient's autonomy and independence.*

EVALUATION

Evaluation determines the effectiveness of the nursing interventions. The predicted changes specified in the expected patient outcomes are reviewed. Ideally the expected patient outcomes are accomplished and the problem is resolved, but in actual practice some changes in the plan of care will most likely be needed.

Evaluation of the expected patient outcome that the patient will identify the need for assistance in obtaining appropriate referrals for discharge is usually accomplished by listening to the patient and/or family to determine if they agree with the referrals for discharge. Sometimes negotiation among the patient, nurse, physician, and other health professionals is needed when the plan is not mutually accepted. The ultimate goal of discharge is to return the patient to a safe environment. However, there may be a fine line between the patient's independence and his/her safety. The

❖ NURSING CARE GUIDELINES

Nursing Diagnosis: Altered Health Maintenance Related to Lack of Adequate Resources/Materials Necessary for Discharge to Home

Expected Patient Outcomes	Nursing Interventions
The patient will identify the need for assistance in obtaining appropriate referrals for discharge.	• Discuss the physical layout of the home, noting the presence and the number of steps as well as the location of rooms in relation to present needs and functional ability. • Address issues concerning discharge: ability to care for personal needs, ambulatory status, medication therapy, follow-up treatment, and availability of friends or family to assist the patient. • Discuss any inconsistencies between needs and ability to care for self. • Encourage the patient and family to verbalize concerns regarding discharge.
The patient will actively participate in the decision-making process regarding discharge plans.	• Communicate the expectation that the patient and/or family will be involved in decision-making • Discuss the referrals necessary for discharge, such as social services, meal preparation, home health supplies, and professional health services. • Coordinate all referrals. • Document and report discharge plans. • Keep the patient and his/her family informed of discharge plans and status.

❖ CASE STUDY WITH PLAN OF CARE

Mr. Marty M. is brought into the emergency department of a large city hospital. His friend tells the triage nurse that Mr. M.'s cough has become much worse in the last few days, and therefore he has been unable to work. His friend reports, "Marty just ain't himself, he's laying around a lot and won't eat much either." Mr. M. was reluctant to seek medical attention, but his friend insisted. He is admitted to the hospital to rule out a medical diagnosis of upper respiratory infection, anemia, or malnutrition. The patient's chief complaint is: "I get so tired these days, I can't catch my breath after walking a little bit. I can't work when I feel this bad, and lately my cough is worse. Maybe I just need some vitamins or something." The medical history indicates that Mr. M. drinks approximately 4 to 6 beers per day, and he has smoked one pack of cigarettes per day for 41 years. He was hospitalized 5 years before with acute GI bleeding and was told that he had the "start" of emphysema. He was advised to stop smoking and drinking. Mr. M. has been divorced for 15 years.

He has four adult children, none of whom he has seen or heard from in over 5 years. He lives in a boarding house and works as a temporary unskilled laborer for various local construction companies. If the work is available, Mr. M. usually works 30 hours per week. He explains, "I make enough to live on," but admits that he worries about the time when he will be unable to work. He and his friends from the boarding house frequently get together to play cards or drink beer at a nearby tavern. When he is not working, Mr. M. usually stays around the lounge of the boarding house to watch television or visit with the other residents. A physical examination determines that Mr. M. is an alert 59-year-old white male with a blood pressure of 128/88 mm Hg; temperature of 100.2° F; pulse of 96/min and regular; respirations of 32/min and shallow; productive cough of brownish colored sputum; coarse, moist breath sounds on auscultation; height of 5'8"; weight of 132 pounds; and stool negative for blood.

PLAN OF CARE FOR MR. MARTY M.

Nursing Diagnosis: *Altered Health Maintenance Related to Lack of Perceived Threat to Health*

Expected Patient Outcomes	Nursing Interventions
Mr. M. will identify behaviors that contribute to alteration in health maintenance.	• Discuss with Mr. M. his perception of his current health status, such as his diminished functional ability. • Clarify misunderstandings or misinformation regarding probable reasons for his deteriorating health. • Help Mr. M. to examine the factors in his life that may contribute to acute and/or chronic illness. • Use active listening and encourage Mr. M. to verbalize his feelings about making a decision to change his lifestyle.
Mr. M. will verbalize desire to participate in health maintenance process to reduce or eliminate risk factors (alcohol and tobacco use and inadequate calorie intake).	• Assist Mr. M. in setting realistic and attainable short- and long-term goals, such as smoking one less cigarette per day. • Help Mr. M. to assess personal strengths and weaknesses. • Discuss possible ways of using strengths to enhance health maintenance efforts. • Explore with Mr. M. methods to correct the behaviors that impede health maintenance. • Provide Mr. M. with emotional support and encouragement in making his own decisions.
Mr. M. will demonstrate the ability to manage health maintenance as evidenced by his participation in initiating appropriate referrals.	• Support Mr. M. in his efforts to change his lifestyle. • Provide Mr. M. with appropriate referrals and community resources, such as public health services, veterans assistance, and local self-help groups.
Mr. M. will identify probable future health maintenance needs.	• Help Mr. M. establish a self-monitoring follow-up plan to include a social support network. • Reinforce the benefits of maintaining or improving health status (for example, the ability to remain employed and living independently).

nurse best evaluates the patient's active participation in the decision-making process regarding his or her discharge plans by observing the patient's and/or family's behavior and level of involvement.

REFERENCES

1. American Nurses Association: Nursing's agenda for health care reform, pp. 2, 5, *Am Nurs,* June, 1991.
2. Eliopoulos C: *Gerontological nursing,* ed 2, Philadelphia, 1987, JB Lippincott.
3. Gordon M: *Manual of nursing diagnosis: 1991-1992,* St Louis, 1991, Mosby–Year Book.
4. Gordon M: *Nursing diagnosis: process and application,* ed 2, p. 102, New York, 1987, McGraw-Hill.
5. Houldin A, Saltstein S, and Ganley K: *Nursing diagnoses for wellness: supporting strengths,* Philadelphia, 1987, JB Lippincott.
6. Kim M, McFarland G, and McLane A: *Classification of nursing diagnosis: proceedings of the Fifth National Conference,* St Louis, 1984, Mosby–Year Book.
7. Mardiros M: Cultural differences in decision making. In Hannah K, Reimer M, Mills W, and Letourneau S (editors), *Clinical judgment and decision making: the future with nursing diagnosis* (pp. 318-322), New York, 1987, John Wiley & Sons.
8. National Center for Health Statistics: *Health, United States,* 1990 (DHHS Publication No. PHS 91-1232), Washington, DC: U.S. Government Printing Office.
9. Pearlmutter D: Megatrends and health care in the late 1980s, *JEN 13*(1):38, 1987.
10. Ryan P: Altered health maintenance. In Thompson J, and others (editors): *Mosby's manual of clinical nursing* (pp. 1609-1611), St Louis, 1989, Mosby–Year Book.
11. Tsai SL: Incidence of nursing diagnosis in a psychiatric ward in Taiwan. In Hannah K, Reimer M, Mills W, and Letourneau S, (editors): *Clinical judgment and decision making: the future with nursing diagnosis* (pp. 187-190), New York, John Wiley & Sons.
12. U.S. Department of Health & Human Services: *Healthy people 2000: national health promotion and disease prevention objectives* (DHHS Publication No. PHS 91-50213), Washington, DC: U.S. Government Printing Office.

Noncompliance (Specify)

Noncompliance (Specify) is the state in which an individual who has expressed the desire and intent to adhere to a therapeutic recommendation does not adhere to the recommendation.

OVERVIEW

Use of the terms *compliance* and *noncompliance* was frequently debated in the 1970s and early 1980s. Some health care providers thought that these terms were judgmental and that they automatically placed blame on a patient who failed to comply with or adhere to a therapeutic recommendation. Haynes, Taylor, and Sackett[10] attempted to dispute the "unhealthy connotations" of the terms and presented a definition of compliance that they felt was nonjudgmental. Compliance was defined "as the extent to which a person's behavior (in terms of taking medications, following diets, or executing lifestyle changes) coincides with medical or health advice."[9] It was further noted that the term *adherence* could be used interchangeably with the term *compliance*.

Haynes, Taylor, and Sackett's definition implies that compliance can vary in degree. The extent to which a person's behavior coincides with the therapeutic recommendation may range from not following any of the aspects of the recommendation to following the total therapeutic plan. The challenge to health care providers is to identify the variables or factors that will contribute to or interfere with a person's ability or readiness to comply with therapeutic recommendations. To meet this challenge, several models that focus on health behavior and compliance have been proposed. Specific models that have been used in nursing practice and research are presented; these models attempt to identify specific variables and their relationship to compliant behavior.[4,6,10]

Interaction Model of Client Health Behavior. Cox[4] specifies three elements in the interaction model of client health behavior: (1) client singularity, (2) client-professional interaction, and (3) health outcomes, one of which is adherence to the recommended care regimen. Client singularity includes four background variables (demographic characteristics, social influence, previous health care experience, and environmental resources) and three internal personal variables (intrinsic motivation, cognitive appraisal, and affective response). These background and personal variables not only interact and influence one another, but they also interact with and have an effect on client-professional interaction.

Client-professional interaction involves affective support, health information, decisional control, and professional and technical competencies. These elements also interact with one another and, with the personal variables, influence all aspects of health outcome. Health outcome comprises the use of health care resources and clinical health status indicators, the severity of the health care problem, adherence to the recommended care regimen, and satisfaction with care. This model offers direction either for the initial assessment, which may indicate that attainment of a desired health outcome is jeopardized, or for a reassessment, which is performed to determine why the intended health outcome was not achieved. Cox has applied the interaction model of client health behavior to a study of community-based elders.[5]

Interactionist Model for Compliance/Noncompliance. Dracup and Meleis[6] have proposed an interactionist model for compliance/noncom-

I

pliance that is based on role theory and is founded on three assumptions: (1) "the act of compliance or noncompliance is an outcome of a health transaction;" (2) three conditions should be present before behavior can be analyzed in terms of compliance or noncompliance: (a) the patient is a partner in any attempt to increase compliance, (b) the diagnosis must be correct, and (c) the proposed therapy must benefit the patient; and (3) compliance is a result of the patient's interaction with significant others and the environment.

Within the model, four components are identified and their relationship to compliance and noncompliance delineated:

1. *Compliance role enactment.* Compliance involves behaviors and activities that are demanded by the performance of a new role (for instance, participating in regular exercise or omitting the consumption of certain foods).
2. *Self-concept.* The sick role or the at-risk role must be incorporated into the patient's self-concept for compliance to occur.
3. *Counter-roles.* To enhance compliance, health professionals, spouses, and significant others should reinforce the compliant role of the patient and assume roles that are congruent to or complementary with all of the patient's roles.
4. *Evaluation.* The patient's roles (behaviors related to the therapeutic recommendations) and the counter-roles that others have assumed should be periodically evaluated to promote behaviors of compliance.

In essence, "the individual who complies with health regimens must identify himself with a compliance role, have access to cues and behaviors of the proposed role, receive cues from others to enact such a role, and evaluate himself and others vis-a-vis that role."[6] This interactionist model of compliance/noncompliance can guide the nurse in assessing the degree of success a patient may have in assuming and maintaining behaviors of compliance.

Health Belief Model. The health belief model (HBM), like the models previously discussed, is an interactive model in which each variable affects the others. The original HBM was developed to predict preventive health behavior and was later revised to explain and predict compliant behavior.[1,13] The revised HBM (see the figure on p. 29) has provided a conceptual framework for examining the multiple variables, their interaction, and their effect on compliant behavior. It can be used as a guide for assessing and evaluating a patient's readiness to undertake the recommended compliant behavior and for determining the presence of factors that can hinder or assist the patient's adherence to the therapeutic recommendation.

To determine a patient's readiness to undertake the recommended compliant behavior, three areas should be examined: the patient's health-oriented motivations, the value the person places on reducing the illness threat (perceived susceptibility and severity), and the person's belief that compliant behavior can reduce the illness threat (perceived benefits and costs). Rosenstock[12] proposes that self-efficacy should be added to the beliefs necessary for compliant behavior. "The belief in one's personal self-efficacy is the conviction that one is capable of carrying out the health recommendation. Patients may believe in the effectiveness or benefits of a regimen but still not comply with it if they do not believe they have the ability to follow it."

Although the nurse may determine that a person is ready to undertake compliant behaviors, factors may be present that will prevent the internalization of such behaviors. Demographic and personal factors can have such an effect. For example, the very young and the very old may have difficulty in understanding and performing specific behaviors, or a specific cultural heritage may make it difficult to accept certain compliant behaviors.[11] Additional factors that can enhance or hinder the person's readiness to follow the therapeutic recommendation have been categorized as structural factors (such as the complexity, side effects, and duration of the proposed therapeutic regimen), attitudinal factors (such as satisfaction with health care providers and facilities), personal

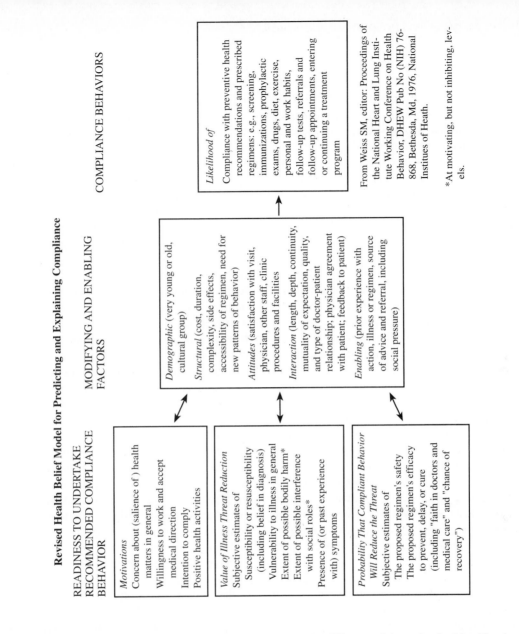

Revised Health Belief Model for Predicting and Explaining Compliance

READINESS TO UNDERTAKE RECOMMENDED COMPLIANCE BEHAVIOR

Motivations
Concern about (salience of) health matters in general
Willingness to work and accept medical direction
Intention to comply
Positive health activities

Value of Illness Threat Reduction
Subjective estimates of
Susceptibility or resusceptibility (including belief in diagnosis)
Vulnerability to illness in general
Extent of possible bodily harm*
Extent of possible interference with social roles*
Presence of (or past experience with) symptoms

Probability That Compliant Behavior Will Reduce the Threat
Subjective estimates of
The proposed regimen's safety
The proposed regimen's efficacy to prevent, delay, or cure (including "faith in doctors and medical care" and "chance of recovery")

MODIFYING AND ENABLING FACTORS

Demographic (very young or old, cultural group)
Structural (cost, duration, complexity, side effects, accessibility of regimen, need for new patterns of behavior)
Attitudes (satisfaction with visit, physician, other staff, clinic procedures and facilities)
Interaction (length, depth, continuity, mutuality of expectation, quality, and type of doctor-patient relationship; physician agreement with patient; feedback to patient)
Enabling (prior experience with action, illness or regimen, source of advice and referral, including social pressure)

COMPLIANCE BEHAVIORS

Likelihood of
Compliance with preventive health recommendations and prescribed regimens: e.g., screening, immunizations, prophylactic exams, drugs, diet, exercise, personal and work habits, follow-up tests, referrals and follow-up appointments, entering or continuing a treatment program

From Weiss SM, editor: Proceedings of the National Heart and Lung Institute Working Conference on Health Behavior, DHEW Pub No (NIH) 76-868, Bethesda, Md, 1976, National Institues of Heath.

*At motivating, but not inhibiting, levels.

interaction factors (such as the quality and type of relationship with the health care providers), and enabling factors (such as prior experience with the illness or illness threat and actual compliance behaviors).

Models such as the three presented reflect the complexity inherent in attempting to identify the variables that may influence whether a person is successful in adopting compliance behaviors. The nurse can use a single model or a combination of models to guide the collection of data that will help determine why a person who has been an informed, willing participant in the identification of therapeutic goals and has indicated a desire to comply does not comply with the therapeutic recommendation.

ASSESSMENT

To make the nursing diagnosis of Noncompliance, the nurse must collect subjective and objective data that indicate the patient's nonadherence to the recommended therapeutic regimen. Suggested in the definition of the diagnosis is that the patient must be aware of the recommendations

I

and express an intention to follow them. This means that the patient's abilities, inabilities, desires, and intentions must be assessed before the therapeutic recommendation is made. Although it may seem that such an assessment would initially identify the patients expected to be compliant, it is important to acknowledge that a patient's motivation, the estimate of susceptibility to an illness, or the estimate of the efficacy of the therapy may change. Factors that initially promoted compliance, such as a positive nurse-patient relationship, can also change.

Thus when caring for a patient who has willingly assumed the responsibility of following a particular therapeutic recommendation, the nurse must provide ongoing assessment to determine whether characteristics indicating noncompliance become apparent. Two defining characteristics directly indicate that the patient is not adhering to the therapeutic recommendation: (1) the nurse observes noncompliant behavior, and (2) the patient or significant others make statements that describe the patient's noncompliant behavior. Other defining characteristics include results of objective tests that reveal noncompliant behavior (for example, physiological measures or detection markers), evidence of the development of complications or exacerbation of symptoms that the recommended therapy should prevent or control, failure to progress or achieve therapeutic goals, and failure to keep appointments or follow through on referrals.

Once the nurse has determined that the patient is not complying, the nurse must seek to identify the factor or factors contributing to the noncompliant behavior. The contributing or related factors for noncompliance can be categorized into three groups: personal factors, interpersonal factors, and environmental factors.

Personal factors are the related factors intimate to the patient. These include one's values; one's beliefs about health, the illness threat, and the therapy; one's ability to implement the recommended therapy; and one's ability to integrate the compliance role into one's existing repertoire of roles. The nurse assesses whether the therapeutic recommendation is compatible with the patient's

general health motivations, cultural influences, and spiritual beliefs. The patient's developmental level in terms of age, physical ability, and emotional maturity must also be considered. The patient's appraisal of the illness threat and the costs and benefits of the therapeutic recommendation will also affect his/her willingness to initiate or continue to incorporate positive behaviors into his/her daily routine.

Burke and Walsh[2] have identified four personal factors that may influence the frail elderly patient's willingness to adhere to a prescribed medication regimen: (1) the prescribed medication may be too expensive; (2) the medication, in terms of administration requirements or therapeutic or side effects, may interfere with usual daily activities; (3) the medication may make the patient feel ill; and (4) the patient may view the medication as ineffective. These same factors can also be applied to other age groups and expanded to incorporate therapeutic recommendations other than medication. For example, prescribed activity/exercise and dietary recommendations may be viewed as expensive (e.g., cost involved in special diets), ineffective (e.g., the effects of diet or exercise not being felt immediately), interfering with usual daily activity (e.g., the need to change usual routine to incorporate new activities or exercise program), and causing one to feel worse than before (e.g., soreness experienced when embarking on a new exercise regimen).

Interpersonal factors refer to those factors involving relationships with others. The helpfulness of the support offered by others, including health care providers, and the satisfaction gained from it are critical to enhance compliant behavior. If relationships are nonsupportive or unsatisfactory and messages that are meant to support the patient in assuming compliant behaviors are unclear, the patient may feel inadequate and not even attempt to comply with the therapeutic recommendation.

Environmental factors can create barriers to the patient's desire and intent to comply. Such barriers can be in the home (such as inadequate food storage and preparation facilities to provide a special diet), the community (such as unsafe streets that interfere with participating in prescribed exercise), and the health care facility (such as noisy, crowded waiting rooms that cause an already anxious patient to become more anxious). The distance the patient must travel to keep appointments or to have prescriptions for medications refilled and the availability and cost of transportation can have a negative effect on the patient's initial intention to participate in follow-up care.

The detection of defining characteristics and related factors of noncompliance depends on a thorough health assessment.[3,8,10,14] The nurse must employ well-developed intellectual, interpersonal, and technical skills to elicit the data needed to make the diagnosis Noncompliance and to plan, implement, and evaluate care that will enhance the patient's ability to adopt compliance behaviors for optimal wellness.

❖ Defining Characteristics

The presence of the following defining characteristics indicates that the patient may be experiencing Noncompliance:
- Objective tests indicating noncompliant behavior (physiological measures or detection of markers)
- Evidence of development of complications
- Evidence of exacerbation of symptoms
- Display of noncompliant behavior
- Statements by the patient or significant others describing noncompliant behavior
- Failure to keep appointments or follow through on referrals
- Failure to progress or achieve therapeutic goals

❖ Related Factors

The following related factors are associated with Noncompliance:
Personal factors
- Incongruence between the therapeutic recommendation and the patient's personal value system
- Conflicts with general health motivations, cultural influences, or spiritual beliefs
- Developmental level (very young or very old)
- Perception that self is nonsusceptible or invulnerable to the illness threat
- Perception that the costs outweigh the bene-

fits of the therapeutic recommendations
- Perception that the therapeutic recommendations are ineffective
- Previous unsuccessful experience with a therapeutic recommendation
- Experiencing side effects from therapy
- Knowledge or skill deficit
- Not identifying self with a compliance role

Interpersonal factors
- Nonsupportive family or significant others
- Unsatisfactory relationship with health care providers
- Confusion resulting from unsuccessful communication of health information
- Lack of confidence in professional and technical capabilities of health care providers

Environmental factors
- Nontherapeutic environment of the home, community, or health care facility
- Distance or lack of transportation prevent the patient from keeping appointments or following through on referrals

❖ Related Medical/Psychiatric Diagnoses

The following are examples of related medical/psychiatric diagnoses (Patients with medical and psychiatric diagnoses of actual or potential health problems that require an incorporation of therapeutic recommendations into their present life patterns may experience Noncompliance. The health problems may be chronic or acute and may incorporate therapeutic recommendations that are intended to prevent the development of or progression of the medical or psychiatric problem.):
- Coronary heart disease
- Diabetes mellitus
- Eating disorders (e.g., obesity, anorexia nervosa)
- Hypertension
- Substance abuse disorders (e.g., alcoholism)

NURSING DIAGNOSES

Examples of *specific* nursing diagnoses for Noncompliance are:
- Noncompliance with prescribed medications related to knowledge deficit secondary to complexity of medication regimen.

I

❖ *NURSING CARE GUIDELINES*

Nursing Diagnosis: Noncompliance related to personal factors that impede adherence to therapeutic recommendation

Expected Patient Outcomes	Nursing Interventions
	Related to conflicts with value system
The patient will resolve conflicts between his or her personal values and the therapeutic recommendation.	• Explore with the patient the incongruence between values (e.g., general health beliefs and spiritual and cultural influences) and recommended therapy. • Evaluate with the patient specific existing conflicts. • Explore with the patient the possibility of altering or revising the therapeutic recommendation so that it is compatible with his/her values.
	Related to perceived nonsusceptibility to illness threat
The patient will accept that he/she is susceptible to the illness threat.	• Explore with the patient the factors that put him/her at risk for illness or that indicate the presence of illness or disease. • Explain to the patient the signs, symptoms, and risk factors for the illness threat.
	Related to perception that the costs of the therapeutic recommendation outweigh the benefits
The patient will identify benefits of the therapy that outweigh the costs and inconveniences.	• Explore what the patient identifies as benefits and costs of the therapy. • Explore with the patient ways to reduce the identified costs of therapy (e.g., side effects, inconveniences, changing a comfortable lifestyle, or actual financial costs). • Explain the benefits of the therapy to the patient, emphasizing the therapy's contributions to the patient's maintaining or regaining health and a sense of well-being.
	Related to knowledge or skill deficit about therapeutic recommendation
The patient will feel capable of following the therapeutic recommendation.	• Explain to the patient the principles and any required procedures related to the therapy. • Provide the patient with an opportunity to describe and demonstrate the "what, why, and how" of the therapeutic recommendation. • Explain ways in which the recommendation can be incorporated into the patient's daily routine. • Include the patient's significant others during explanations about the recommendation.

- Noncompliance with recommended activity/exercise regimen related to muscular discomfort experienced after initial implementation of recommended regimen.
- Noncompliance with prescribed diet related to confusion resulting from communication of information about expected results of prescribed diet.
- Noncompliance with recommendation to quit smoking related to perception that a high weight gain is a necessary consequence for one who quits smoking.

PLANNING AND IMPLEMENTATION WITH RATIONALE

In planning care for the patient diagnosed as noncompliant, *the nurse and the patient should focus their attention on the long-term goal of patient compliance with the therapeutic recommendation.* If this goal is mutually acceptable, nursing interventions will be directed toward eliminating or reducing the factors that contribute to the noncompliant behavior. The nurse and the patient must work together in identifying patient outcomes and nursing interventions that will support achievement of this long-term goal. Specifically, the nurse can guide the patient in (1) appraising readiness to incorporate the therapeutic recommendations into the present life pattern, (2) enacting strategies for change, and (3) integrating the change into the existing life pattern.[7]

To address the personal factors that contribute to noncompliance, expected outcomes may focus on one or more of the following: the patient's motivation to protect or restore health, the patient's acceptance that he or she is susceptible to the illness threat or actually has a disease, the patient's belief that the benefit of following the therapeutic recommendation outweighs its associated costs and inconveniences, and the patient's belief that he/she is capable of following the therapeutic recommendation, that is, able to assume the compliance role.[12] To achieve such outcomes, *the patient's unique needs, beliefs, and preferences about the therapeutic recommendation must be addressed.* It is also essential that the patient understand the principles of the recommended therapy and be able to perform procedures required by the recommendations. If the recommended therapy is complex, the patient should be gradually taught elements or components of the therapy and allotted adequate time to incorporate each component into the newly acquired role of compliance.

For the patient whose noncompliance stems from interpersonal factors, the expected outcomes must focus on eliminating or controlling nonsupportive and unsatisfactory relationships with significant others and health care providers. The nurse should work with the patient in determining how these relationships can be improved so that they will support the patient's compliance. Providers and significant others can enhance compliance by being responsive to the patient's needs, by acknowledging the patient's successful efforts, and by reinforcing the "what, why, and how" of the therapeutic recommendation. If a patient expresses a lack of confidence in health care providers, the nurse should explore the situation and give the patient information that will correct misconceptions or offer the needed support to correct the situation.

Environmental factors that impede a patient's intention and desire to comply should be addressed by altering the environment to enhance compliance and controlling or eliminating the environmental conditions that create barriers to compliant behavior. For example, the nurse can explore the options available to the patient who lacks the facilities to prepare an appropriate diet. Guidance might be provided about simplifying the purchase, storage, and preparation of required foods. Other options, such as eating out and having meals delivered to the home, should also be explored.

For the patient who lacks the transportation necessary for keeping appointments, the nurse should explore public and private transportation services. If cost is a factor, the nurse may refer the patient to social services so that adequate transportation arrangements can be made. When the environmental factors threatening compliance

I

❖ *CASE STUDY WITH PLAN OF CARE*

Mrs. Nancy L. is a 38-year-old African-American woman who considers herself to be in good health. Last month she visited a women's health clinic for her annual physical examination and Papanicolaou smear. Initial evaluation at the clinic revealed the following data: blood pressure of 154/92 supine and 148/98 standing, height of 5'3", and weight of 172 pounds. History, physical examination findings, and laboratory results were negative except for obesity and mild hypertension. The clinic notes indicated that "Mrs. L. was counseled about a dietary restriction of sodium and the need for weight loss." Mrs. L. reports that her mother had high blood pressure, and her mother had to take medication that made her feel worse. Mrs. L.'s mother died at the age of 64 after a stroke. The prospect of controlling her blood pressure through dietary restrictions appears to appeal to Mrs. L. She states that she really wants to lose weight because she is uncom-

fortable and unhappy with herself. Mrs. L. lives with her husband and three daughters, aged 18, 17, and 15. The entire family is overweight, and their meals consist mainly of convenience foods. Mrs. L. returned to the clinic 1 month after her initial visit to have her blood pressure and weight monitored. Her blood pressure remained the same as the previous visit, and she had lost a half-pound. Mrs. L. stated that she had hoped she would be able to lose weight and that she felt very discouraged by her lack of progress. She admitted that her diet continued to consist mainly of convenience foods. Although she had attempted to prepare low-calorie meals for herself, she found that she was "tempted" to eat the food she prepared for her family. When asked why she prepared separate meals for the family, she responded, "They told me that they don't want to eat diet food and that I shouldn't diet because they love me the way I am."

PLAN OF CARE FOR MRS. NANCY L.

Nursing Diagnosis: *Noncompliance with Dietary Recommendation Related to Lack of Support of Family Members*

Expected Patient Outcomes

Mrs. L. will prepare and eat meals that meet requirements for reduced sodium and calorie intake.

Nursing Interventions

- Review with Mrs. L. a 1200 calorie, low-sodium diet.
- Discuss with Mrs. L. foods that she should avoid because of sodium content (e.g., processed luncheon meats, pickles, and canned and frozen foods).
- Work with Mrs. L. and her family to prepare a weekly meal plan that is appealing and provides essential nutrients while reducing sodium and calorie content.
- Meet with Mrs. L. and her family to discuss the relationship between hypertension and obesity and between hypertension and high sodium intake.
- Emphasize to the family the importance of their role in supporting Mrs. L.
- Discuss with Mrs. L. a progressive plan that will include increasing her usual amount of exercise.
- Stress the importance of frequent monitoring of weight and encourage Mrs. L. to visit the clinic weekly to be weighed.
- Assess Mrs. L.'s need for support through a "self-help" group that focuses on good nutrition and weight loss.
- Assist Mrs. L. in contacting the local "self-help" group that she might find supportive.

exist in the health care facility, the staff should be realistic in their assessment of the situation and creative in determining an appropriate solution. For example, an alternative waiting area could be found for the patient who is bothered by the noisy, crowded waiting room.

Because the variables that influence whether a person will comply with a therapeutic recommendation are numerous and their interaction complex, the nurse must consider the specific needs of the patient in planning and implementing care. The Nursing Care Guidelines focus on personal factors that can interfere with a patient's desire to comply and are intended to provide general examples of patient outcomes and nursing interventions.

EVALUATION

The patient's achievement of the expected patient outcomes should be a reliable indicator that the identified contributing or related factors have been controlled or eliminated. However, it is necessary for the nurse to continue an ongoing assessment. The patient's actual and potential compliance behavior must be continually evaluated.

The presence of characteristics that reflect continuing noncompliance should be investigated. If the patient continues to have difficulty adhering to the therapeutic recommendations, the nurse must seek to validate the related factors that were initially identified as contributing to the noncompliance. If the related factors are assessed as accurate, the chosen nursing interventions should be reviewed and evaluated.

Such an evaluation may indicate that the interventions were inadequate for a particular patient. For example, a patient seen in an outpatient clinic and diagnosed with noncompliance related to a skill deficit could have a learning disability of which the nurse is unaware. The patient may have been attentive to the explanation of principles and the demonstration of procedures and even able to initially return the demonstration. The patient may have expressed confidence, stating that he is capable of implementing the procedure. However, when the patient tries to perform the procedure on the following day, he is unable to recall the steps of the procedure. Although the nurse and the patient may have been confident that the expected outcome had been achieved before the patient left the clinic the previous day, it becomes obvious that evaluating the patient's attainment of new information must continue over time. This situation emphasizes the importance of collecting assessment data that reflects the uniqueness of each patient and planning care that is tailored to each patient.

REFERENCES

1. Becker MH and others: Patient perceptions and compliance: recent studies of the health belief model. In Haynes RB, Taylor DW, and Sackett DL (editors): *Compliance in health care,* Baltimore, 1979, The Johns Hopkins University Press.
2. Burke MM, Walsh MB: *Gerontologic nursing: care of the frail elderly,* St Louis, 1992, Mosby–Year Book.
3. Carroll-Johnson RM: *Classification of nursing diagnoses: proceedings of the Eighth Conference,* Philadelphia, 1989, JB Lippincott.
4. Cox CL: An interaction model of client behavior: theoretical prescription for nursing, *Adv Nurs Sci* 5:41-56, 1982.
5. Cox CL: The interaction model of client behaviors: application to the study of community based elders, *Adv Nurs Sci* 9:40-57, 1986.
6. Dracup KA and Meleis AI: Compliance: an interactionist approach, *Nurs Res* 31:31-36, 1982.
7. Fleury JD: Empowering potential: a theory of wellness motivation, *Nurs Res* 40:286-291, 1991.
8. Gordon M: *Manual of nursing diagnosis,* 1991-1992, St Louis, 1991, Mosby–Year Book.
9. Haynes RB: Introduction. In Haynes RB, Taylor DW, and Sackett DL (editors): *Compliance in health care,* Baltimore, 1979, The Johns Hopkins University Press.
10. Haynes RB, Taylor DW, and Sackett DL (editors): *Compliance in health care,* Baltimore, 1979, The Johns Hopkins University Press.
11. Hymovick DP, Hagopian GA: *Chronic illness in children and adults: a psychosocial approach,* Philadelphia, 1992, WB Saunders.
12. Rosenstock IM: Enhancing compliance with health recommendations, *J Pediatr Health Care* 2(2):67-72, 1988.
13. Weiss SM (editor): Proceedings of the National Heart and Lung Institute Working Conference on Health Behavior, DHEW Pub No (NIH) 76-868, Bethesda, Md, May 12-16, 1975, National Institutes of Health.
14. Whitley GG: Noncompliance: an update, *Iss Ment Health Nurs* 12:229-238, 1991.

Altered Protection

Altered Protection is the state in which an individual experiences a decrease in the ability to guard the self from internal or external threats, such as illness or injury.[3]

OVERVIEW

Altered Protection is a nursing diagnosis that can be applied to diverse patient populations in both acute and chronic settings. Protection refers to the ability to guard oneself from danger or injury and to the ability to provide a safe environment. Patients who are at risk for Altered Protection include those with cancer, especially lymphoma, leukemia, and multiple myeloma; immune diseases, such as acquired immunodeficiency syndrome (AIDS); and coagulation disorders, such as disseminated intravascular coagulopathy (DIC). Altered protection is also a concern when administering certain medications, such as antineoplastics, corticosteroids, immunotherapeutic agents, thrombolytic enzymes, antibiotics, and anticoagulants. Also at risk are patients who are undergoing general surgery, radiation[7] or organ transplantation, are under 2 or over 60 years of age, are malnourished, are experiencing stressful situations, have an excessive intake of alcohol, have a hypersensitive[5] reaction to harmless agents, are drug abusers, or have burns, especially over more than 20% of total body surface.

The immune response is a normal protective mechanism. Protective mechanisms in human beings function in several ways, including destroying the threatening agent and preparing an area to make it less likely to be attacked. The components of the immune system include the lymph nodes, the thymus, the spleen, and the tonsils.

Immunity protects the body against foreign materials, invasion by microbial agents, and proliferation of mutant cells. When it is deficient, inappropriate, or misdirected, this response can cause disease.[8]

The three types of immune cells are the macrophage, the B lymphocyte, and the T lymphocyte. The macrophages, the mature monocytes, surround, engulf, and dispose of microorganisms and cellular debris. They remove foreign waste products from the body. The antigen is processed in the macrophage, and the macrophage transfers the antigen to the lymphocyte. Lymphocytes originate in the bone marrow and make up about 25% to 30% of the total white blood cell count. The two types of lymphocytes are B cells and T cells. The T lymphocytes, produced by the bone marrow, mature under the influence of the thymus gland. They account for 70% to 80% of the blood lymphocytes. When the T cells are exposed to an antigen, they divide rapidly and produce new T cells sensitized to that antigen. Types of T cells include killer cells, helper cells, and suppressor cells.[2] The killer cells adhere to the surface of the invading cell and disrupt its membrane, thereby altering its intracellular environment and killing it. The helper cells stimulate the B lymphocytes to differentiate into antibody producers. The suppressor cells function to reduce the humoral response, a hypersensitivity response.

The B lymphocytes are also produced in the bone marrow and mature either in the bone marrow or somewhere else in the body. B cells have a life span of about 7 days, have on their surface antigen and immunoglobulins (causing antibody formation), and when examined appear larger than the T cells. The B cell population is high in certain tissues, such as the tonsil and the spleen, and low in the circulating blood volume.[8] B lymphocytes include the plasma cells and memory cells. Plasma cells synthesize and secrete copious amounts of antibodies. The memory cells develop into antibody-secreting cells when reexposed to a specific antigen.

Through examination of the immune response, one can identify those patients at high risk for Altered Protection. Patients with cancer, especially lymphoma, leukemia, and multiple myeloma, and patients receiving cancer chemotherapy and radiotherapy are at high risk for the development of immunosuppression. Patients with lymphoma experience malignancies in the lymphocytes, thereby affecting the immunological defense. Leukemia involves the replacement of bone marrow with malignant, immature white cells. A multiple myeloma is a malignant neoplasm of the bone marrow. Patients on chemotherapy and radiotherapy experience damage to normal cells as well as malignant cells. Bone marrow cells are specifically vulnerable because they reproduce rapidly.

The acquired immunodeficiency syndrome (AIDS) destroys the cell-mediated immune system. AIDS is caused by the human immunodeficiency virus (HIV). HIV affects the helper T lymphocytes and the macrophages. These cells are responsible for cell-mediated immunity, which, when weakened, will cause a variety of opportunistic infections. HIV also attacks the bone marrow. Patients with blood dyscrasias such as disseminated intravascular coagulopathy (DIC) are also at risk for altered protection. DIC causes an excessive stimulation of the body's clotting response, thereby predisposing the patient to disseminated thrombosis and bleeding.

The effects of corticosteroids, immunotherapeutic agents, antibiotics, anticoagulants, and thrombolytic medications must also be examined in relation to this nursing diagnosis. Corticosteroids cause an increase in susceptibility to infection as well as the side effects of immunosuppression. Anticoagulant therapy and thrombolytic enzymes increase the risk of injury and bleeding by

delaying coagulation of the blood. Antibiotic therapy with medications such as penicillin and the cephalosporins can cause superinfections. Tetracycline and chloramphenicol therapy can cause an inhibition of cellular immunity.[4]

The patient with a history of alcoholism should be examined for signs and symptoms of Altered Protection. Abnormalities found in patients with alcoholism include anemias, difficulties in counteracting infection, and interference in the clotting mechanism. Alcohol also interferes with the delivery of folate to the bone marrow precursors.[6] Stress may also be considered a risk factor for altered protection because of its effects on the immune system. Stress will cause an increase in the production of corticosteroids, which in turn will lower the body's defense mechanisms. Stress also causes a decrease in the production of T cells and macrophages, thereby decreasing the body's ability to recognize antigens, permitting the spread of infection. Malnutrition may also cause a secondary immunosuppression because of the loss of or inadequate synthesis of the immunoglobulins.[2] The immune system is poorly developed in the very young and somewhat deteriorated in the elderly, predisposing them to an increased incidence of autoimmune disease. The patient with burns, most specifically full thickness burns greater than 10% or partial thickness burns greater than 20% of total body surface area burned, is also at high risk for Altered Protection because normal skin function is either diminished or lost, causing loss of protective barriers, resulting in such responses as loss of temperature control, fluid volume imbalance, and susceptibility to infection.

ASSESSMENT

Assessment of the patient with altered protection begins by obtaining a thorough patient history. After obtaining demographic data, the nurse should obtain the chief complaint of the patient. The nurse should record the complaint using the patient's own words and and should describe the patient's perception of the problem. Patients with Altered Protection may present with a varying number of complaints, depending on the etiology of the problem. The patient with AIDS, for example, may present with complaints of fever, malaise, tender and swollen lymph nodes, and diarrhea. The patient with DIC may complain of bleeding that is diverse and unrelated. It is important to explore the presenting problem in terms of the "PQRST" phenomena: (1) provocative and palliative—what initiates the complaint and what makes it feel better, (2) the quality and quantity of discomfort, (3) the region and radiation of the complaint, (4) the severity based on a scale of 1 to 10, and (5) the timing—when does it start, how long does it last, and how often does it occur.[1]

The nurse then obtains the patient's history. Important data related to Altered Protection includes information on childhood illnesses, surgery or injuries, allergies, medications the patient has been taking, diet, and use of alcohol. In addition, the nurse must assess the patient's response to the health problem and the ability to cope with any limitations. The history should also incorporate a description of a typical day in his/her life, with a focus on activities, dietary habits, exercise, stressors, and sleep patterns. Family history should include the incidence of cancer and anemia, and the age, health status, and cause of death of the immediate family members.

The next step in assessment is an objective review of all the systems. The nurse should note the patient's weight and any history of weakness and fatigue. Vital signs are taken and recorded. The assessment of the ears, eyes, nose, and throat is useful in revealing the occurrence of headaches, frequent colds, nosebleeds, frequent sore throats, and bleeding from the gums. Lymph nodes in the neck may be swollen and painful in the patient with altered protection. A respiratory and cardiovascular assessment will determine the presence of a cough; the color, odor, and consistency of the sputum; the presence of dyspnea and orthopnea; and complaints of palpitations, wheezing, and edema of the extremities. The patient may be anorexic, dehydrated, nauseous, and vomiting. Blood may be present in the stools. Genitourinary

assessment might demonstrate frequent urination, with complaints of burning and the presence of blood in the urine. The nurse assesses the integumentary system, most specifically the skin and mucous membranes. Surgical or traumatic wounds, burn injuries, or pressure sores breach the body's physical defenses.[4] The patient with Altered Protection should be examined for muscle or joint pains and signs of easy bruising or bleeding. The postoperative patient may show signs of impaired healing.

Laboratory data to be evaluated include the CBC with differential, with emphasis on the red blood cell count; hemoglobin, hematocrit, and the white blood cell count. The red blood cell count may be decreased because of bone marrow suppression. The hemoglobin and hematocrit may be abnormally low because of a bleeding disorder. The white blood cell count is generally increased in infection and decreased with bone marrow suppression and certain medications. Prothrombin time (PT), coagulation, and partial thromboplastin time (PTT) may be increased or decreased depending on the disorder. Chest x-ray changes may be subtle in the patient with Altered Protection. No one diagnostic measure is totally adequate for making the diagnosis of Altered Protection. The nurse must be aware of the trends in laboratory data and combine them with clinical findings.

❖ Defining Characteristics

The presence of the following defining characteristics indicates that the patient might be experiencing Altered Protection:

- Impaired healing
- Altered clotting
- Maladaptive stress response
- Neuro-sensory alterations
- Impaired or lost skin barrier
- Chilling
- Perspiring
- Dyspnea
- Cough
- Itching
- Restlessness
- Insomnia
- Fatigue
- Anorexia
- Weight loss
- Weakness
- Immobility
- Disorientation
- Pressure sores
- Frequent infections
- Altered CBC and coagulation profile

❖ **Related Factors**

The following related factors are associated with Altered Protection:
- Age under 2 or over 60
- Inadequate nutrition
- Alcohol abuse
- Drug abuse
- Abnormal blood profiles
- Drug therapies
- Surgery
- Radiation
- Cancer
- Immune disorders
- Burns

❖ **Related Medical/Psychiatric Diagnoses**

The following are examples of related medical/psychiatric diagnoses for Altered Protection:
- Acquired Immunodeficiency Syndrome (AIDS)
- Acute or chronic conditions resulting in altered immune response
- Allergic disorders with integumentary or respiratory responses
- Anemias
- Burns
- Cancer requiring treatment with chemotherapy or radiotherapy
- Diabetes
- Disseminated intravascular coagulation (DIC)
- Eating disorders
- Leukemia
- Lupus erythematosus
- Major depression
- Malnutrition
- Psychoactive substance use disorder
- Rheumatoid arthritis

NURSING DIAGNOSES

Examples of *specific* nursing diagnoses for Altered Protection are:
- Altered Protection related to loss of skin barrier in 20% full-thickness burn injury.
- Altered Protection related to general surgical procedure and multiple invasive lines.
- Altered Protection related to increased intake of alcohol and decreased intake of nutrients.

- Altered Protection related to lowered defense mechanisms associated with increased stress.

PLANNING AND INTERVENTIONS WITH RATIONALE

Nursing interventions for the patient with Altered Protection will differ based on the related factor involved but should include the following: (1) monitoring and treating the defining characteristics of altered protection, (2) maintenance of adequate nutrition, (3) promotion of adequate rest, safety, and stress control; (4) promotion of wound healing, (5) control of bleeding and eventual freedom from bleeding, and (6) education regarding the risk factors involved in altered protection.

The nurse should assess and monitor defining characteristics. Vital signs are taken at least every 4 hours with emphasis on the trends in respiratory rate and body temperature. Laboratory data on the hemoglobin, hematocrit, white and red blood cell count, and coagulation profile are obtained and observed for abnormalities. The guaiac test is done on stool and gastric secretions. The nurse monitors the patient for the presence of any symptoms of an acute infection, such as sore throat, tender and swollen lymph nodes, weakness and fatigue, and diarrhea. The patient's skin should remain intact; when this is not possible, wounds, burned areas, and pressure sores are monitored for signs of healing. *Accurate and continuous assessment and monitoring promotes early diagnosis of Altered Protection.*

Adequate nutrition is promoted and maintained. Intake, output, and the patient's weight are monitored on a daily basis. In the presence of anorexia, nausea, and vomiting, the patient may be able to tolerate only liquids, but a regular diet should be resumed as soon as possible, as *it promotes vitamin, mineral, and nitrogen balance.* In the presence of inadequate nutrition, total parenteral nutrition may be necessary.

Adequate rest, safety, and stress control are important aspects of nursing care. Narcotics, if ordered, are given to *control pain* and *promote rest.* They are administered with care so as not to overmedicate the patient, thereby interfering with mobility, coughing, and deep breathing. Measures such as back rubs and position changes *help to promote comfort*. Stress control begins with the patient recognizing the stress and the factors that precipitate it. Stress management can be fostered in the hospital setting through meditation, diversional activities such as reading and watching television, and relaxation tapes. The patient's environment should be examined for unsafe conditions *to prevent accidents or trauma*.

Promotion of wound healing is essential in the postoperative patient, the patient with burns, and the patient with pressure sores. The patient's position is changed at least every 2 hours. Aseptic technique during all dressing changes and wound care *prevents contamination*. Continuous observation and care of wounds and monitoring of the color, odor, and consistency of the drainage *assures early detection of wound infections*. Use of egg crates and pressure mattresses *prevents pressure sores*.

Measures to prevent abnormal clotting and bleeding are essential to the nursing care of certain patients with Altered Protection. All stools and gastric secretions are monitored for the presence of blood. The coagulation profile is observed for abnormalities. Irritated oral mucous membranes are treated with warm saline rinses. Sites

❖ NURSING CARE GUIDELINES
Nursing Diagnosis: Altered Protection

Expected Patient Outcomes	Nursing Interventions
The patient will maintain adequate protection as measured by: temperature less than 99.8° F; hemoglobin, hematocrit, white cell count, red cell count, and coagulation profile within normal limits; absence of swollen lymph nodes, weakness, and fatigue; and intact skin.	• Record vital signs every 4 hours, or as indicated. • Monitor blood work as ordered, observing trends. • Assess the lymphatic system, documenting the presence of swollen and painful lymph nodes. • Observe the patient's activity level and document the presence of any weakness and fatigue. • Assess the patient's wounds and/or skin for signs of redness, purulent discharge, odor, and integrity. • Change the patient's position, if bedridden, every 2 hours. • Apply egg crate or air mattress to the patient's bed when indicated.
The patient will demonstrate adequate nutrition and hydration as measured by: weight maintained at desired level for height and body build; absence of anorexia, nausea, and vomiting, an intake equal to output; and verbalization of behaviors necessary to maintain body weight.	• Identify patients at risk for inadequate nutrition. • Record patient's weight every 24 hours. • Record caloric count daily for 3 days. • Record intake and output every 8 hours. • Determine patient's cultural and personal food preferences, and provide if diet permits. • Offer small frequent meals composed of foods that are not likely to cause intolerances, and avoid foods such as hot, spicy foods and high-fiber foods. • Educate the patient and significant others on well-balanced meals associated with diet prescribed. • Examine medications the patient is taking for evidence of side effects that interfere with diet. • Offer fluids.

❖ *NURSING CARE GUIDELINES—cont'd*

Expected Patient Outcomes	Nursing Interventions
The patient will maintain adequate rest, freedom from injury, and control of stressors as measured by: reports of adequate sleep, absence of injury, and control of stress response.	• Observe rest and sleep patterns. • Space nursing care activities to allow patient several 2-hour rest periods each day and longer hours of sleep at night. • Observe patient for signs of fatigue. • Provide a quiet environment along with relaxation strategies such as back rubs. • Assess patient's environment for signs of unsafe practices. • Assess level of stress in the patient. • Assist the patient in recognition of stressors. • Assist the patient in identifying coping strategies to deal with stressors. • Implement stress-reduction techniques, such as relaxation therapy and meditation, while the patient is in the hospital.
Skin integrity will remain intact as measured by: absence of redness, swelling, pain and purulent discharge from wounds; absence of redness and breakdown in pressure areas; and intact skin.	• Assess wound every shift for signs of infection. • Maintain aseptic technique during treatments and dressing changes. • Change position every 2 hours, massaging all bony prominences. • Institute active and passive range-of-motion exercises. • Assess skin for signs of reddened or blanched areas. • Avoid overuse of soap and rinse and dry skin thoroughly. • Massage skin with lubricant or lotion if indicated.
The patient will demonstrate absence of abnormalities in bleeding and clotting as measured by: normal bleeding and clotting times, absence of bleeding from invasive sites and mucous membranes, and absence of blood in fluids and waste products.	• Monitor prothrombin time, partial thromboplastin time, and coagulation studies. • Assess urine, stool, and gastric secretions for signs of bleeding. • Apply pressure to invasive sites, injection sites, and wounds. • Avoid the use of intramuscular injections and promote use of the oral and intravenous routes. • Offer meticulous and careful mouth care. • Educate the patient regarding bleeding precautions. • Avoid the use of rectal and vaginal suppositories. • Monitor menstrual flow when indicated. • Avoid trauma by maintaining a safe environment. • Institute blood and body fluid precautions.
The patient will have adequate knowledge to foster protection as measured by his or her description of the actions that will foster adaptive protection.	• Assess the patient's level of knowledge and readiness to learn. • Identify family members and significant others who should participate in learning. • Assess the environment for distractions that might hinder learning. • Assess the patient's and significant others' motivation and anxiety level. • Provide the necessary information to foster protection. • Provide written information for the patient. • Promote wellness through instruction and example.

I

of invasive procedures, such as central lines and arterial lines are examined routinely; intramuscular injections are kept to a minimum. When injections are necessary, pressure is applied for several minutes after medication administration. Blood products, if ordered, are administered according to hospital procedure. Substances containing aspirin are avoided, and the use of vaginal or rectal suppositories and tampons is limited or prohibited. The patient is encouraged to shave with an electric razor. *These measures promote safety in the patient at high risk for Altered Protection.*

Education is offered to the patient and family or significant other. The patient is taught to recognize signs and symptoms of bleeding and is encouraged to maintain a safe environment and to avoid trauma. Blood and body fluid precautions may be necessary in the hospital as well as the home. The patient is encouraged to avoid contact with people with viral or bacterial infections. The patient is taught guidelines that address the trans-

mission and prevention of communicable diseases. The patient's knowledge of the disease and treatment should be assessed and the necessary information provided. *Patient/family education provides the necessary information to foster adaptation to an illness, and promotes participation and some sense of control in the patient.*

EVALUATION

Patients with altered protection should demonstrate optimal nutrition, fluid and electrolyte balance, and the absence of nosocomial infections. The patient should have adequate sleep periods and be free from injury. Skin integrity will be maintained, and bleeding will be minimal or absent. The patient and significant others will know information that is essential to maintaining optimal protection. If the expected outcomes are not achieved, the care plan should be reassessed and revised as necessary, taking into consideration specifics of each patient situation.

❖ *CASE STUDY WITH PLAN OF CARE*

Mr. Charles Y. is a 38-year-old psychologist who was diagnosed as HIV positive 2 years ago. Mr. Y. has a successful independent practice composed mostly of people who are recovering from alcoholism. In his free time, he enjoys the opera and old movies, plays racquetball occasionally, and likes to cook. Mr. Y. owns a condominium where he lives with Bob, his significant other. Mr. Y. is of English ancestry and active in the Episcopalian church. He is one of three children, and both of his parents are alive and well.

Mr. Y. has been experiencing periods of low-grade temperature and chills for about 3 months. He developed an elevated temperature (102° to 103°), night sweats, intermittent chest pain, a persistent nonproductive cough, and profound anorexia 2 weeks ago. Bob encouraged Mr. Y. to seek help at a nearby clinic, where the tentative diagnosis of pneumocystis carinii pneumonia was made. He was admitted to a medical floor of a nearby medical center.

Mr. Y. is anxious and upset on admission. His physical assessment reveals a mildly undernourished, diaphoretic male. Mr. Y. complains of tightness in his chest. The nurse auscultates rales one third up the base of the right lung. Initial laboratory data reveals an Hgb of 10.2, Hct of 35, po_2 of 76, and T cell count of 250 T cells/uL. Admission orders include complete bed rest, an IV infusion of 5% D/W to be infused at 125 cc/hour, and blood and body fluid precautions. Nasal oxygen is initiated at 3 liters, and Mr. Y. is scheduled for a chest x-ray and bronchoscopy. His medications include Bactrim IV, Pentamidine IV, and Tylenol by mouth for a temperature greater than 101°. The primary nursing diagnosis for Mr. Y. is Altered Protection related to immunosuppressed status and inadequate nutrition. Patients like him could have many needs and many nursing diagnoses, such as impaired gas exchange, social isolation, and possible ineffective individual coping.

I

PLAN OF CARE FOR MR. CHARLES Y.

Nursing Diagnosis: *Altered Protection Related to Immunosuppressed Status and Inadequate Nutrition.*

Expected Patient Outcomes	Nursing Interventions
Mr. Y. will regain adaptive protection as measured by: temperature less than 99.8°; Hgb, Hct, and T cell count increasing toward normal range; and absence of weakness and fatigue.	• Monitor vital signs, especially temperature, every 4 hours. • Monitor Hgb, Hct, and white blood cell count daily. • Institute blood and body fluid precautions. • Instruct patient and significant others about infection control. • Administer antipyretics when appropriate. • Encourage intake of fluids. • Space nursing care activities to allow for periods of rest alternating with activity for the patient. • Assist patient in identifying and coping with stressors.
Mr. Y. will demonstrate adequate nutrition and hydration as measured by: achievement of optimal nutrition, no evidence of further weight loss, intake that equals output, and electrolytes within normal limits.	• Assess weight daily. • Monitor intake and output. • Assess electrolytes, particularly potassium, sodium, and chlorides. • Place Mr. Y. on a 3-day calorie count to help identify his nutritional needs. • Encourage family and significant others to bring in Mr. Y.'s favorite foods. • Encourage snacks and nutritional foods. • Consult with dietician for specific diet prescription.
Mr. Y. will acquire sufficient knowledge to foster protection as evidenced by verbalization about the transmission of the virus, signs and symptoms of opportunistic infections, and infection control precautions.	• Evaluate Mr. Y.'s knowledge of the HIV virus and its affect on protective mechanisms. • Determine Mr. Y.'s level of anxiety and the affect that it has on his readiness to learn. • Instruct Mr. Y. and his significant other on signs and symptoms of opportunistic infections, when to seek help, and infection control precautions. • Evaluate the effect of the instruction on Mr. Y.'s knowledge base and reinstruct as necessary. • Provide Mr. Y. with methods for acquiring additional information after discharge.

REFERENCES

1. Bates B: *A guide to physical examination and history taking,* Philadelphia, 1991, JB Lippincott.
2. Bullock B and Rosenthal P: *Pathophysiology: adaptation and alterations in function,* Boston, 1984, Little, Brown.
3. Carroll-Johnson RM: *Classification of nursing diagnoses: proceedings of the Ninth Conference,* Philadelphia, 1991, JB Lippincott.
4. Hudak C, Gallo B, and Bent J: *Critical care nursing: a holistic approach,* ed 3, Philadelphia, 1990, JB Lippincott.
5. Ignatavicius DD and Bayne MV: *Medical-surgical nursing: a nursing process approach,* Philadelphia, 1991, WB Saunders.
6. Luckman J and Sorenson K: *Medical-surgical nursing: a psychophysiologic approach,* Philadelphia, 1987, WB Saunders.
7. Lunney M: Nursing diagnosis: refining the system, *Am J Nurs,* March, p. 456, 1982.
8. Porth C: *Pathophysiology: concepts of altered health status,* Philadelphia, 1990, JB Lippincott.

High Risk for Infection

High Risk for Infection is the state in which an individual has an increased susceptibility for invasion by pathogenic and/or opportunistic organisms.

OVERVIEW

High Risk for Infection is a nursing diagnosis that is pertinent for a broad spectrum of patients in varied settings. Depending on the degree of interaction between the host, the infectious organism, and the environment, any patient can have the potential to develop an infection. Infectious organisms are present at all times in the atmosphere and in our bodies. For an infectious disease to develop, the delicate balance among host, organism, and environment must be upset. This imbalance can result from three factors: a change in the host that decreases existing defense mechanisms; an increase in the virulence of the infectious agent; or an environmental factor that influences the host, the disease-producing organism, or both. Therefore, to identify patients who are at High Risk for Infection, one must examine all three components of the triad.

Bacteria, viruses, chlamydia, rickettsiae, fungi, protozoa, arthropods, and helminths are all organisms that can infect humans. Within these categories exist pathogenic and nonpathogenic organisms. Pathogenicity refers to the ability of an organism to cause disease. Nonpathogenic organisms include those that normally exist in or on the body; these organisms are called normal flora. Normal flora do not usually cause disease unless host susceptibility increases. An infectious disease that develops in this manner is called an opportunistic infection. One example is the destruction of normal flora in the vaginal tract through the use of antimicrobial agents. These lactobacilli normally produce an environmental pH that is nonconducive to the growth of yeast cells. When the normal flora is destroyed, Candida albicans can proliferate and cause a secondary or opportunistic vaginal infection. One must remember that almost all normally nonpathogenic organisms can become pathogenic.

Pathogens also can normally reside in the environment and the body without causing disease. One such organism is the varicella-zoster virus, which remains dormant in the nerve cells after recovery from chickenpox. These pathogens result in shingles when virulence or host susceptibility changes. Virulence is the degree to which an organism can cause disease. It is determined not only by the number of organisms present but also by the organism's ability to adhere to host cells, produce toxins, avoid phagocytosis, produce immunologic injury, and mutate.[12,14]

An infectious disease occurs when a pathogen gains entry into a host and produces local, systemic, or focal effects. This process occurs through a sequence of events. First, the organism lives in a reservoir, living or nonliving, where it may multiply. It leaves the reservoir through a portal of exit and is transmitted to the host through a portal of entry. Transmission can occur by direct contact, either through touching or by droplet; by indirect contact, such as through food or airborne organisms; or by vectors, such as mosquitos. After gaining access to the host, the pathogen multiplies, evades host defense mechanisms, penetrates and spreads through tissue by secreting enzymes, and may produce endotoxins or exotoxins.[8] These enzymes and toxins, in combination with the host's response, cause the symptoms associated with the infectious disease.

Infection is resisted through the body's defense mechanisms. These include physical or mechanical barriers, chemical barriers, and cellular defenses. The skin and mucous membranes provide physical barriers as long as they remain intact. Mucous and ciliary action in the respiratory tract sweep organisms along to be eliminated by coughing or sneezing or through the gastrointestinal tract. Saliva, urine, and tears serve as barriers by washing organisms away. The acid PH of the skin and gastrointestinal and genitourinary tracts creates an environment that is unfavorable for the growth of certain microorganisms, as does the presence of enzymes, fatty acids, and some protein substances in bodily secretions.

If an infectious organism succeeds in breaking through these barriers, nonspecific and specific cellular defense mechanisms respond. As host cells are damaged, blood flow to the area increases through vasodilation in response to substances released by the destroyed cells. Vascular permeability also increases, allowing the release of fluid and phagocytic cells into the tissue. These actions result in the erythema, warmth, and edema that occurs with infection. Phagocytic cells, which include both neutrophils and macrophages, engulf and digest or kill the invading organisms. In addition, the macrophages degrade destroyed host cells and function in the specific immune response described below. Debris of this phagocytic activity results in the formation of pus in localized infections.

Cell-mediated immunity and humoral immunity make up the body's specific immune response. Cell-mediated immunity involves T-lymphocytes. Macrophages present the foreign substance or antigen to the T-lymphocytes. In response, helper T-cells release lymphokines that stimulate B-cells, stimulate cytotoxic and suppressor T-cells, further activate the macrophage system, and help produce the above described nonspecific actions.[6]

Humoral immunity involves B-lymphocytes, the white blood cells that produce antibodies. Antibodies are protein substances that assist in fight-

ing infection. They can act directly by causing agglutination, precipitation, or neutralization of the antigenic material present on invading organisms or by lysis of the organisms. Most of the activity against these infectious agents, however, is through activation of the complement system by antibody-antigen complexes. On activation, the complement system, which consists of enzyme precursors, produces lysis, agglutination, phagocytosis, and neutralization of invading organisms as well as chemotaxis, activation of mast cells and basophils, and other inflammatory effects.[6]

The white blood cells involved in the different immune responses are produced, stored, and matured in various body structures such as the bone marrow, thymus, spleen, and lymph nodes. During infection these structures are stimulated to produce and release white blood cells. This action results in an overall increase in the white blood cell count above the normal 5,000 to 10,000 cells/mm^3 and/or a shift in the differential cell count. A shift to the left in the differential is typically seen with bacterial infections where the increase in the number of white blood cells is due to an increase in the number of neutrophils, specifically immature cells or bands. Parasitic infections will cause an increase in the number of eosinophils. After production, the white blood cells depend on adequate blood and lymph circulation for transportation to the body sites where they are needed.

The possibility for infection to occur increases whenever any of the body's defense mechanisms are compromised. Compromised defense mechanisms occur not only with a break in the physical barriers of the skin and mucous membranes, but also with alterations in pH, production of enzymes and protein substances, blood, blood-forming organs, and circulation.

The last component of the triad of infection is the environment. Weather can affect the ability of microorganisms to exist, proliferate, and be transmitted through the air. Reservoirs for pathogens include water and decaying materials. Hospitals, specifically, are breeding grounds for pathogenic organisms. Nosocomial, or hospital-acquired in-

I

fections, pose a threat to all hospitalized patients.

Sanitation and hygiene practices are important safeguards against the proliferation and transmission of infectious organisms. This component involves many socioeconomic aspects. Education, economic status, culture, and religion can affect nutrition, hygiene, sanitation practices, willingness to seek information, access to agencies concerned with protection against and treatment for infections, and the ability to participate in programs that decrease risk for infection.

ASSESSMENT

Assessment and interventions must include all three components of the triad: pathogen, host, and environment. When assessing for a High Risk for Infection, one must first obtain a nursing history. Although all the functional health patterns can provide pertinent data, those that are most important to assess include the following: health perception-health management pattern, nutritional and metabolic pattern, sexuality-reproductive pattern, and value-belief pattern.[5] In addition, general information such as age, allergies, and even local address can contribute information for determining a risk for infection.

Assessment of the health perception-health management pattern includes any existing health problems that could decrease resistance to infection, such as diabetes mellitus, congestive heart failure, peripheral vascular disease, or cancer. The nurse should note any treatments or medications that increase risk. These risks include radiation therapy, chemotherapy, antimicrobial therapy, or any recent invasive procedures. The nurse should investigate recent contacts with infectious persons or environments, including travel to areas known to have certain diseases (such as malaria, cholera, or typhoid fever) endemic in the population. Past infectious diseases, as well as participation in immunization programs, should be documented.

Assessment of the nutritional and metabolic pattern could identify nutritional deficits that decrease resources the body needs to produce the components that help to resist infection. In addi-

tion, drug and alcohol use are associated with increased risk for infection.

Sexuality patterns and history of sexual abuse can help to determine the risk for sexually transmitted diseases or past trauma. Multiple sexual partners or homosexual and/or bisexual lifestyles, as well as illicit drug use, are most important to assess in determining the risk for HIV transmission.

Assessment of the value-belief pattern may indicate the potential for compliance or noncompliance with prescribed interventions that may be contrary to one's beliefs. For example, a person who fasts extensively and is prescribed a high-calorie diet may be reluctant to follow the prescribed diet. Of particular importance is the assessment of a person's value system and religious affiliation.

After obtaining a history, one should assess subjective and objective data within the nutritional and metabolic pattern, elimination pattern, activity-exercise pattern, sleep-rest pattern, and cognitive-perceptual pattern. Vital signs, condition of the skin, enlarged lymph nodes, breath sounds, any discharge, and complaints of pain, weakness, lethargy, or malaise are important to note. The CBC, electrolyte values, and urinalysis results are laboratory data to be evaluated as indicators of nutrition, immune function, and presence of infection. The nurse should observe personal hygiene, including cleanliness and condition of the mouth and teeth.

By gathering these data, the nurse may identify risk factors for the development of infection. Age itself is a risk factor. Normal skin changes that occur with aging, such as thinning, affect the skin's ability to act as a barrier against microorganisms. In addition, production of secretions and blood flow decreases, as does the rate of tissue regeneration.[10] At the opposite end of the age continuum are infants, who are also at risk because of their immature immune systems and thin, easily damaged epithelial tissues.

Nutritional status can greatly increase a person's susceptibility to infection. For example, vitamins A, B, and C all help in the maintenance of skin and mucous membranes, the healing of wounds, and the response to inflammation. Protein also contributes to these activities, in addition to being involved with the immune response. Production of bone marrow and liver, spleen, and lymphoid tissues depends on adequate protein and iron stores. These are the tissues from which phagocytes and lymphocytes arise. In addition, an infectious state or other medical condition increases metabolic demands and so further depletes nutritional stores.[7]

Medical conditions and treatments can also compromise the body's defense mechanisms in other ways. Chemotherapy, radiation therapy, and any condition affecting the spleen, bone marrow, or liver can decrease the production of white blood cells. Diabetes mellitus, rheumatoid arthritis, and certain medications decrease the ability of white blood cells to reach the infection site. Phagocytosis may be ineffective in a person who has Hodgkin's disease, cirrhosis, or lupus erythematosus.[4] Renal insufficiency causes the accumulation of toxins, which may destroy the various defense mechanisms.

Cancer presents many problems that lead to an increased risk for infection. Persons with cancer have increased nutritional needs and therefore are at risk for malnutrition and cachexia. Obstruction of both lymph and blood circulation may decrease the ability to bring the necessary white blood cells and antibodies to the site of infection and also decrease drainage from these sites. All treatments for cancer, including surgery, radiation, and chemotherapy, further compromise a person's ability to resist and combat infection. Some types of cancer can directly affect the body's ability to produce the cells involved in the immune response. These include leukemia, lymphoma, and myeloma.

Acquired immunodeficiency syndrome, AIDS, is caused by the human immunodeficiency virus (HIV). This virus affects the T-4 helper cells, which are lymphocytes involved in the immune response. The HIV causes these cells to replicate the virus, after which the T-4 helper cells die prematurely or are inactivated. Eventually, the person develops an immunodeficiency state and is unable to resist infections and the growth of neoplasms. Some of the infections and neoplasms associated with AIDS are pneumocystis carinii, candidiases, cytomegalovirus, Kaposi's sarcoma, and non-Hodgkin's lymphoma.

Any type of invasive procedure, such as surgery, urinary catheterization, or central access lines, breach the first line of defense, which is the skin and mucous membranes. This breach allows microorganisms access to the body. In addition, specific problems accompany each type of procedure.

Faulty surgical and aseptic technique, as well as the presence of an infection preoperatively, greatly increase the risk for infection in surgical patients. A decrease in the function of T-lymphocytes has been documented after the use of general anesthesia.[9]

Urinary catheterization may cause trauma to the urethra, thereby allowing microorganisms access. In addition, the catheter provides direct access to the bladder, a normally sterile environment. Microorganisms may travel along the catheter into the bladder and eventually to the kidneys. Urinary catheterization also bypasses the mechanical action of voiding, which usually sweeps bacteria through the urethra and provides an acid pH that is detrimental to the existence of microorganism.

Endotracheal procedures tend to dry out the mucous membranes. They also provide direct access to the respiratory tract. By bypassing and damaging the cilia, the procedure does not allow foreign material and debris to be swept up and out of the lower airway.

Central access lines, both venous and arterial, may contribute to infection in the body by allowing organisms to travel through the insertion site and along the catheter. These catheters further increase the risk for infection by promoting the formation of clots. Blood clots in and around the catheter, as well as the presence of moisture under the dressing, allow for bacterial growth.[1,11,13]

Also at risk are those persons who are not able to protect themselves. This inability may result from physiological factors leading to hospitalization, where they must rely on others for care. It may also stem from a Knowledge Deficit. This deficit may be related to lack of knowledge regarding prevention of infection or inability to understand or carry out instructions.

The presence of an infection increases the risk for further infection in a person who has decreased defense mechanisms. The clinician can identify an infection by an assessment of physiological signs and symptoms and laboratory data.

Hematological studies indicate the presence of an infection by an elevated white blood cell count and sedimentation rate. Other specimens and tests are specific to areas of infection. X-ray examinations can indicate cysts, infiltrates, and bone abnormalities. A urinalysis, culture, and sensitivity test identifies urinary tract infections. Sputum, stool, and blood cultures indicate infections in their respective sites. Studies of cerebral spinal fluid can indicate both bacterial and viral infections in the central nervous system.

Physiological signs and symptoms that indicate infection include subjective data such as complaints of pain or muscle aches, malaise, and lethargy. Objective data might reveal an elevated temperature, pulse, respiratory rate, and blood pressure; decreased urinary output indicative of dehydration; warm flushed skin; drainage; neck rigidity; rashes; and enlarged lymph nodes. These characteristics can result from either the toxins produced by the organisms or the activities of the person's defense mechanisms. By obtaining an in-depth history and assessment of risk factors, one can determine those persons at High Risk for Infection.

❖ Risk Factors

The presence of the following behaviors, conditions, or circumstances render the patient more vulnerable to a High Risk for Infection:

- Age (e.g., the very young, the very old)
- Inadequate physical barriers
- Inadequate chemical barriers
- Inadequate cellular response
- Radiation therapy
- Medications (e.g., antibiotics, steroids)
- Malnutrition
- Hospitalization
- Unsanitary living conditions
- Inadequate acquired immunity
- Acute and chronic illnesses
- Invasive procedures
- Chemotherapy
- Lack of immunizations
- Knowledge deficit

❖ Related Medical/Psychiatric Diagnoses

The following are examples of related medical/psychiatric diagnoses for High Risk for Infection:

- AIDS
- Aplastic anemia
- Burns
- Cancer
- Cirrhosis
- Congestive heart failure
- Connective tissue disorders (e.g., rheumatoid arthritis, lupus erythematosus)
- Diabetes mellitus
- Fractures
- Hodgkin's disease
- Immunodeficiency states
- Leukemia
- Lymphoma
- Myeloma
- Peripheral vascular disease
- Renal insufficiency
- Skin disorders (e.g., psoriasis, herpes zoster, impetigo, rashes)
- Splenectomy or anomalies of the spleen
- Trauma

Psychiatric disorders interfering with adequate nutrition (e.g., bipolar disorder, depressive disorder, delusional disorder (paranoid disorder) may relate to High-Risk for Infection.

NURSING DIAGNOSES

Examples of *specific* nursing diagnoses for High Risk for Infection are:

- High risk for infection related to decreased nutrition.
- High risk for infection related to decreased immune function.
- High risk for infection related to altered skin integrity.
- High risk for infection related to poor hygiene.

PLANNING AND IMPLEMENTATION WITH RATIONALE

Interventions for persons with High Risk for Infection address three areas: (1) assessing risk factors, (2) reducing risk factors, and (3) promoting wellness.[3]

The nurse continues and expands the baseline assessment for the duration of patient care. Continuous monitoring for signs and symptoms of infection in all patients is essential. As procedures and medications are introduced, the nurse must identify potential sites for infections. Furthermore, nutritional and immune status can weaken with increased demands on metabolism and immune responses. *The nurse must document this information at least every shift or out-patient visit to identify changes from the baseline assessment.*

Reduction of risk factors involves promoting those activities that support normal defense mechanisms. Pathologic organisms are spread by direct contact through touching; therefore, handwashing remains one of the single most important interventions performed by health care workers and taught to individuals. In addition to handwashing, the current Centers for Disease Control (CDC) guidelines call for wearing gloves whenever contact with blood and body fluids, including saliva, is possible. Masks and protective eyewear should be used when droplets of body fluids may be generated, and gowns worn when it is likely that uniforms may become contaminated. Gloves should be changed and hands washed after each patient contact.[2] In addition, proper isolation procedures should be known and followed for those persons at risk for infection and for those with an existing infection.

All clinicians should carefully follow hospital policy for changing intravenous and central access tubings, solutions, and dressings. *This usually involves changing solution bottles every 24 hours and tubing and dressings every 24 to 48 hours to decrease the opportunity for the growth of organisms. Aseptic technique is extremely important in the prevention of nosocomial infections when dealing with any invasive procedure, including changing intravenous lines and bottles and doing dressing changes.*

All patients at risk for development of respiratory infections, including postoperative patients, people with preexisting respiratory and cardiovascular problems, and persons with decreased mobility, must be encouraged to cough, practice deep breathing exercises, and use respiratory aids, such as incentive spirometers. *These activities decrease the pooling of secretions and promote oxygen exchange and should be done at least every hour.*

When not contraindicated, ambulation also helps to prevent respiratory problems, in addition to preventing venous stasis, which could lead to clot formation. If ambulation is contraindicated, position changes and extremity exercises should be performed at least hourly. Elevating the head of the bed and sitting in a chair can also be used to prevent these problems, but they should not be used in place of ambulation.

Promoting personal and oral hygiene in all patients, particularly those anticipating invasive procedures, helps maintain the skin and mucous membranes. It also reduces the number of microorganisms present on these surfaces. Skin care and oral hygiene should be done at least once every day. Daily baths should be carefully evaluated in elderly patients because of the drying effect that occurs with bathing. Skin creams and lubricants should be used on dry skin to prevent cracking. Skin surfaces are to be kept dry, and contact between skin surfaces minimized. Hygiene also includes daily perineal care for all patients. Cleansing with warm water and careful drying is suggested for patients with retention catheters[4]. *Urinary systems should be kept closed and below the level of the bladder to prevent backflow of urine.*

Knowledge of side effects of all medications is important to identify those that might depress patients' immune systems or promote growth of opportunistic organisms. One must also adhere to administration guidelines for antimicrobials in order to maintain a therapeutic level at all times. That is, nurses should administer antibiotics around the clock at equal time intervals.

Because nutrition plays such an important role in maintaining the body's defense mechanisms, the nurse must continually promote adequate diet and fluid intake for all patients. The diet must be nutritionally complete with sufficient calories to

I

prevent use of existing body reserves for energy. It should be high in vitamin C, protein, and iron to promote healing and maintain the structures of the immune system. Fluid intake should be at least 2400 ml per day, unless contraindicated, to prevent dehydration.

Promotion of wellness is accomplished mainly through teaching. *Hygiene, sanitation, and proper food handling are areas to be addressed to promote public health.* Promotion of wellness includes maintenance of safe water supplies and hand-washing after using restrooms and before handling food. *Proper storage and cooking of food avoids spoilage that can lead to the transmission of disease.*

Health teaching should include information on behaviors that may lead to the inhibition or destruction of normal defense mechanisms. Smoking, substance abuse, fad diets, and unprotected sexual intercourse or multiple sexual partners are examples.

Nurses can be instrumental in the promotion of immunization programs for both children and adults. *Immunizations protect individuals against certain diseases and decrease the potential for transmission of communicable diseases.* Persons anticipating international travel should contact local health departments to determine which vaccines are necessary. High-risk groups, such as children, the elderly, and the debilitated, should be assessed and educated regarding necessary immunizations. Nurses should provide instruction about potential side effects of vaccines and what to do if they develop, as well as the need to follow through on immunization series in order to receive full protection.

EVALUATION

The nurse can evaluate the success of infection control programs by monitoring infection rates on individual, institutional, and community levels. Participation in community immunization and health promotion programs are also indicators the nurse can evaluate. The health care provider and

---

❖ NURSING CARE GUIDELINES
Nursing Diagnosis: High Risk for Infection

Expected Patient Outcomes

The patient will be free of infection as indicated by normal vital signs; normal white blood count; normal sedimentation rate; negative cultures; warm, dry skin; no flushing of skin; no drainage; no rash; no neck rigidity; clear breath sounds; clear, yellow urine; and no chills, pain, malaise, or lethargy.

Nursing Interventions

- Monitor vital signs every 4 hours.
- Monitor laboratory values for indications of infection.
- Monitor and document signs and symptoms of infection every 4 hours.
- Collect specimens as needed to monitor for presence of infection.
- Wash hands between all patient contacts.
- Use appropriate isolation techniques, including masks, gowns, and gloves.
- Encourage coughing and deep breathing and/or use of respiratory aids every hour.
- Encourage ambulation and/or position changes and extremity exercises at least every shift.
- Maintain closed urinary catheter system and provide daily catheter care.
- Monitor medication regimen for side effects and effective schedule.

❖ *NURSING CARE GUIDELINES—cont'd*

Expected Patient Outcomes	Nursing Interventions
The patient's skin and mucous membranes will be intact.	• Use aseptic technique for all invasive procedures and dressing changes. • Observe hospital guidelines for maintenance of intravenous and central lines. • Provide daily skin care and oral hygiene. • Use appropriate antimicrobial solutions and ointments for wound care. • Change soiled dressings as needed. • Schedule and perform position changes every 1-2 hours.
The patient will verbalize risk factors for infection.	• Teach risk factors for infection, including age, nutrition, defense mechanisms, chronic and acute illnesses, invasive procedures, medications, and sexual practices.
The patient will identify preventive measures to reduce the risk of infection.	• Teach coughing and deep breathing exercises, the use of respiratory aids, the need for ambulation, and wound and skin care.
The patient will demonstrate a lifestyle that will promote wellness, including no substance abuse, no smoking, adequate diet and fluid intake, proper skin care and oral hygiene, monogamous sexual relationships and/or the use of condoms, and the maintenance of a clean and safe environment.	• Develop and implement teaching plans regarding proper nutrition, the detrimental effects of smoking and substance abuse, safe sexual practices, personal hygiene, and sanitation. • Participate in community programs for public sanitation, communicable diseases, and health promotion
The patient will participate in immunization programs.	• Encourage participation in immunization programs through individual and community teaching.

the patient can measure individual progress regarding health practices against goals that they have agreed upon. Areas to be addressed include lifestyle, personal hygiene, nutrition, and wound and skin care. Regardless of which method the nurse uses for evaluation, accurate documentation of results remains vital to ensure continuity of successful programs and accurate long-term planning and evaluation.

❖ CASE STUDY WITH PLAN OF CARE

Mrs. Lois S. is a 75-year-old woman who was admitted to the medical-surgical unit after a bowel resection for an obstruction resulting from a malignant lesion. She has a central line through which she receives hyperalimentation at 75 ml/hr. Mrs. S. also has a Foley catheter and a nasogastric tube connected to low intermittent suction. Her medical history reveals no other illnesses or previous surgeries. She does not smoke. Although she is widowed and living by herself, Mrs. S. does have a daughter living in the area. Presently Mrs. S. complains of incisional pain and weakness. Objective data includes a temperature of 98.6° F (37° C), pulse of 80 beats/min, respirations of 20/min, weight of 120 pounds, height of 5'4", white blood cell count of 6,000, hemoglobin of 14 g/dl, and hematocrit of 39%. Her lungs are clear, and her skin is warm, dry, and intact, although she has an abdominal incision that has a dry dressing. Her urine is clear and amber colored.

PLAN OF CARE FOR MRS. LOIS S.

Nursing Diagnosis: High Risk for Infection Related to Surgery, Foley Catheter, Central Line, Age, and Cancer

Expected Patient Outcomes

Mrs. S. will be free of infection as indicated by T 98.6° F (37° C), P 60 to 68, R 16 to 25, BP 120/80, white blood cell count of 4,500 to 10,000/mm³, skin warm and dry; no flushing of skin, urine clear, no redness or edema at central line site, no tenderness, redness, or positive Homan's sign in lower extremities, and no complaint of chills.

Nursing Interventions

- Wash hands and put on gloves before any direct contact with Mrs. S.
- Monitor and document vital signs every 4 hours.
- Monitor CBC when ordered for increase in white blood cell count, sedimentation rate, or decreased Hgb or Hct.
- Monitor and document skin condition, urine color, central line site, breath sounds, condition of lower extremities, and presence of chills every shift.
- Encourage Mrs. S. to cough and deep breathe or use her incentive spirometer very hour.
- Assist Mrs. S. in ambulation at least every shift.
- Administer pain medication before ambulation or respiratory exercise.
- Change hyperalimentation bottle every 24 hours, using aseptic technique.
- Change hyperalimentation tubing and central line dressing every 48 hours, using aseptic technique.
- Maintain closed urinary system below the level of the bladder.
- Assist Mrs. S. in washing with mild soap and water every morning. Ensure adequate towel drying. Apply lotion to areas of dryness.
- Cleanse perineal area with warm water during bath and pat dry.
- Assist Mrs. S. in brushing her teeth once each shift.
- Cleanse and lubricate nares around nasogastric tube at least every day.
- Change nasogastric drainage container every 48 hours.
- Administer 500 mg of ampicillin every 6 hours around the clock. Assess for signs of superinfection or reaction.

Mrs. S. will have a healed incision with no purulent drainage.

- Monitor and document condition of dressing and incision every shift.
- Culture any suspicious drainage, using aseptic technique.
- Using aseptic technique, change soiled or loose dressing.

Mrs. S. will have adequate nutrition as indicated by weight remaining 120 lb, intake equaling output, good skin turgor, Hgb 12 to 16 g/dl, Hct 37% to 47%, and blood sugar 70 to 115 mg/dl.

- Maintain hyperalimentation at 75 ml/hr.
- Assess and document blood sugar by finger-stick every 6 hours.
- Measure and record accurate intake and output every shift.
- Weigh Mrs. S. and record weight every morning at the same time and using the same scale.
- Monitor ordered Hgb and Hct for anemia and dehydration.
- Instruct Mrs. S. on the need for a diet high in protein, vitamin C, and iron.
- Provide fluid intake of at least 2,400 ml/day and instruct on importance of fluid intake.
- Notify Mrs. S.'s physician of any significant changes in her condition.

REFERENCES

1. Bostrom-Ezrati J, Dibble S, Ruzzuto C: Intravenous therapy management: who will develop insertion site symptoms? *Applied Nurs Res* 3(4):146-151, 1990.
2. Centers for Disease Control: Recommendations for prevention of HIV transmission in health-care settings, *Morbidity and Mortality Weekly Report,* Atlanta, 1987, US Department of Health and Human Services.
3. Doenges M, Moorhouse M: *Nurses' pocket guide: nursing diagnoses with interventions,* ed 3, Philadelphia, 1991, FA Davis.
4. Gurevich I, Tafuro P: The compromised host: deficit-specific infection and the spectrum of prevention, *Cancer Nurse* 9(5):263-275, 1986.
5. Gordon M: *Manual of nursing diagnosis: 1991-1992,* St Louis, 1991, Mosby-Year Book.
6. Guyton AC: *Textbook of medical physiology,* ed 8, Philadelphia, 1991, WB Saunders.
7. Keithley JK: Infection and the malnourished patient, *Heart Lung* 12(1):23-27, 1983.
8. Luckmann J, Sorensen KC: *Medical-surgical nursing: a psychophysiological approach,* ed 3, Philadelphia, 1987, WB Saunders.
9. Miller TA: *Physiologic basis of modern surgical care,* St Louis, 1988, Mosby–Year Book.
10. Nagani P: Management of common infections in the elderly outpatient, *Geriatrics* 41(11):67-80, 1986.
11. Parsa MH and others: Intravenous catheter-related infection, *Infect Surg,* 789-798, 1985.
12. Patrick ML and others: *Medical-surgical nursing: pathophysiological concepts,* ed 2, Philadelphia, 1991, JB Lippincott.
13. Petrosino B and others: Infection rates in central venous catheter dressings, *Oncol Nurs Forum* 15(6):709-711, 1988.
14. Porth CM: *Pathophysiology: concepts of altered health states,* ed 3, Philadelphia, 1990, JB Lippincott.

High Risk for Injury

High Risk for Trauma

High Risk for Poisoning

High Risk for Suffocation

High Risk for Injury *is a state in which the individual is at risk for injury as a result of agent and environmental variables interacting with the adaptive and defensive resources of the individual (host).*[16]

High Risk for Trauma *is the accentuated risk of accidental tissue injury, including wounds, burns, and fractures.*[16]

High Risk for Poisoning *is the accentuated risk of accidental exposure to or ingestion of drugs or dangerous products in doses sufficient to cause poisoning.*[16]

High Risk for Suffocation *is the accentuated risk of accidental suffocation caused by an inadequate air supply for inhalation.*[16]

OVERVIEW

The diagnosis of High Risk for Injury is classified by the North American Nursing Diagnosis Association as a higher level diagnosis that may be more specifically described in terms of trauma, poisoning, or suffocation. This chapter presents an overview of injury in general and addresses the diagnoses of High Risk for Trauma, Poisoning, and Suffocation in particular.

Injury in the United States continues to be a se-rious health problem. It is the fourth leading cause of death, accounting for 39.5 deaths per 100,000 people.[21] It is the leading cause of death in children and young adults. The number of persons injured per year is higher for males than females in most age-groups until 54 years of age, when injured females outnumber injured males. Injuries for both males and females rise rapidly after 70 years of age.

Injury and injury prevention are now recognized areas of research and practice, involving the multidisciplinary efforts of physicians, nurses, social workers, and other specialists. Epidemiologists, who study the factors that determine and influence the occurrence of disease and its course, have discussed the theory of injury and published the results of their descriptive research on injuries and the agents that caused them.[3,13,26,28]

Over the years, the concept of accidental injury developed. The word *accident* connoted either a random event or one that resulted from careless, thoughtless, or even sinful behavior.[33] Significant progress has been made in the area of injury control by promoting use of the term *injury* in place of the term *accident. Injury* refers to tissue damage caused by exchanges of environmental energy that are beyond the body's resilient capacity.[14]

The term *injury* is preferred because *accident* implies the idea of chance and passivity in encounters with external forces. Injury is amenable to investigation if it is viewed as having a distinct etiology—the inability to resist energy transfer.

An unfavorable relationship in any injury exists among the variables of host, agent, and environment. The agent-host-environment model, traditionally used to describe communicable diseases, can also be used to understand injuries. The host is the injured person who has certain characteristics such as age, sex, developmental level, neuromuscular status, and coping ability. The agent is the form of energy (kinetic, gravitational, chemical, thermal, electrical, or lack of oxidation) that causes damage to the tissue. The environment is the physical surroundings and psychosocial situation. Physical factors may refer to climate, geography, noxious gases, sharp corners, or broken glass. An example of a psychosocial factor would be a lack of community safety programs or parental supervision.

Until now nursing has approached injury as a behavioral problem and has emphasized the examination of host and environmental factors. Research from other disciplines, such as physical therapy, engineering, ergonomics, and epidemiology, must be examined to fully describe agents of injury. Haddon[14] developed a framework for analyzing factors and the sequence of events in highway crashes. This framework can be applied to any type of injury by examining the host, agent, and environmental factors involved in the three phases of the injury process—preinjury, injury, and postinjury. Approaches to injury control may be directed at any stage of the injury-producing process.[2] Haddon's strategies or countermeasures have served as the basis for many injury prevention programs. The box on p. 56 presents these countermeasures and examples of how they can be implemented.

Injuries resulting from trauma, poisoning, or suffocation seriously affect persons of all ages but especially those belonging to certain developmental groups. Injury from a variety of agent and environmental variables is the leading cause of death in children and young adults. Although trauma is the sixth leading cause of death in those 75 years of age and older, it is the leading cause of death in children.[21] From 1983 to 1987, 6.7 million emergency room visits were for injuries among children age 1 to 4 years old.[9] All children are at risk for injury but certain characteristics place some children at high risk. Recent research by Bijur and colleagues[6] supports earlier research[7,18,26] that the best predictors for injuries for 5 to 10 year old children are: number of injuries before 5 years of age, male sex, aggressive child behavior, young maternal age, and many older and few younger siblings. Children of mothers who are depressed or ill[5,7] have also been found to have higher rates of injury than other children.

Injury that results from poisoning especially affects both the very young and the elderly, who are at risk, respectively, because of motor skill development and sensory and memory changes characteristic of their age-groups. Young children are at risk for poisoning because of heightened curiosity and an inclination to experience new things by tasting and smelling. Accidental poisoning is the major cause of death in children under 5 years of age. The highest incidence occurs in the 2-year-old age-group, followed by the 1-year-old age-group. Elderly persons are at risk for poisoning because they have failing vision and memory and are frequently required to take several medications.

A special case for poison prevention can be made concerning lead poisoning especially in light of the recent announcement of an epidemic of low-level lead poisoning in this country that is causing serious neurological damage in millions of children.[11] Lead is a heavy metal that has no known physiological use. Lead is present in industrialized environments, particularly central cities, because of environmental pollution. Leaded gasolines and lead-based paints are the largest source of pollution.[31] Lead accumulates slowly in the body and is excreted slowly. Repeated exposure to small amounts of lead over many months produces elevated lead levels. Lead is highly

I

❖ COUNTERMEASURES TO REDUCE INJURY

Countermeasure[14]	Example[29]
1. Prevent the marshaling of the hazardous energy form in the first place.	• Do not manufacture handguns. • Do not use flammable materials in houses, furniture, or clothing.
2. Reduce the chances for a potential hazard.	• Reduce the speed that motor vehicles can reach. • Reduce the hardness of playground surfaces. • Reduce the temperature of hot water tanks.
3. Prevent the occurrence of existing hazards.	• Increase road skid resistance. • Lock personal guns at a target range.
4. Modify the potential severity (rate of spatial distribution) of the hazard by altering the source.	• Improve the use of auto seat restraints and child seat restraints. • Produce containers for hot liquids (e.g., coffee and tea) with wide bottoms and large centers of gravity.
5. Separate in time and space the hazard and that which is to be protected.	• Build pedestrian overpasses and underpasses on the heavily used roads. • Designate separate roads for cars and heavy trucks.
6. Separate the hazard and that which is to be protected by interposition of a material barrier.	• Install air bags in vehicles that inflate automatically when a crash occurs. • Install child-proof gates around swimming pools. • Use child-proof tops for medicine and other containers that have poisonous substances.
7. Modify basic qualities of the hazard.	• Use roadside utility poles that break away when struck by a vehicle. • Prohibit hard surfaces, sharp points, and edges on interiors of transportation vehicles and on bicycles, stairs, furniture, and toys.
8. Make that which is to be protected more resistant to damage from the hazard.	• Provide blood-clotting factors to persons with hemophilia. • Install containers that do not rupture for transportation of hazardous materials. • Provide warm-up exercises before athletic competition and prohibit players from playing if they are injured or out of condition.
9. Counter damage already done by environmental hazard.	• Provide strategically placed quick rescue and emergency medical response. • Make burn centers available to those who need them.
10. Stabilize, repair, and rehabilitate the damaged object.	• Provide for rehabilitation and cosmetic surgery. • Increase job training for the disabled.

toxic to the fetal brain and rapidly developing brain cells of young children.[10] Lead poisoning causes toxic effects on the blood, central nervous system, and kidneys, resulting in anemia, kidney damage, learning disabilities, mental retardation, seizures, coma, and possible death. Moderately elevated lead levels have been correlated with the long-term consequences of a seven-fold increase in school dropout rates and reading disabilities.[23]

Despite the landmark OSHA Act[25] that set the lead standard to reduce lead exposure, workers and their families are still exposed to harmful effects from lead. Minorities represent a large percentage of workers in lead smelting industries and small shops where air-borne lead remains a problem.[1,32] Although the problem is now recognized as cutting across all economic levels, poor and minority children are disproportionately affected.[8,11]

The definition of lead toxicity has recently been set at 10 micrograms per deciliter (μg/dL). Anemia is one of the initial signs of the disease. Lead screening includes obtaining an erythrocyte protoporphyrin (EP) level, which measures hemoglobin synthesis. If the EP level is greater than 35 μg/dL, the clinician should obtain the venous blood lead (PbB) level. Therapy for highly elevated lead levels uses chelating agents such as intravenous calcium disodium edetic acid (Ca EDTA) and British anti-lewisite to remove lead from the blood.[4]

Childhood asphyxiation deaths are caused chiefly by the child's choking on an item, by exclusion of air by covering the mouth and nose or exerting pressure on the throat or chest, by entrapment in abandoned refrigerators, and by cave-ins (inhumations). Suffocation by obstruction of the airway is a major cause of death in children 5 years of age and under.[27] Aspiration and lodging of a foreign body into the respiratory tract will cause a degree of airway obstruction, inflammation, edema, and secretions. Causes of suffocation and strangulation fatalities include (1) plastic bags used as mattress protectors, (2) improperly fitting crib mattresses that can cause the infant to become wedged between the mattress and crib frame, (3) plastic storage bags, (4) cribs with widely spaced slats, (5) abandoned refrigerators, dishwashers, and freezers, (6) clothing (such as a cord or hood) catching in play equipment or machinery, (7) bibs, pull toy strings, pacifiers kept on a string around the neck, (8) drape cords, (9) the cave-in of earth or sand or the collapse of a structure, and (10) food items.

Countermeasures were introduced in the 1950s to reduce injuries and deaths from refrigerator and freezer entrapment, plastic bags, intubation, and mechanical strangulation from wedging in infant cribs. There has been a significant decline in incidence in all areas except mechanical strangulation in cribs. This decline appears to result from passive countermeasures such as design changes in refrigerators and freezers built since 1958.

Drowning was the fourth leading cause of unintentional death for all ages in 1991 and the second leading cause for 1- and 2-year-olds[22]. Freshwater aspiration into lung alveoli reduces the normal surface tension of surfactant, causing alveolar collapse, hypoventilation, and pulmonary edema.[20] Aspiration of hypertonic seawater draws fluid from the plasma into alveoli causing pulmonary edema and intrapulmonary shunt. An analysis of regional data by O'Carroll, Alkon, and Weiss[24] found drowning rates highest among 1- to 4-year-olds with backyard swimming pools. Swimming pool fence regulations have not been an effective passive countermeasure to decrease injury; the reasons for this is a subject that needs further exploration.

Overall, the drowning rates for males were three to four times greater than for females. The drowning rate was much greater for both males and females over 70 years of age than for other age and gender groups. In the elderly, the sites of drowning were either private pools or bathtubs. More information is needed about the context in which the elderly drown in bathtubs to specify the exact risk factors for drowning in the elderly.

ASSESSMENT
High Risk for Injury

The role of the nurse in diagnosing High Risk for Injury is to identify the host, agent, and environmental factors as they become evident from

I

the health history and physical assessment of the patient. Cues from the patient, history, and record are grouped together in logical clusters. For example, the identification of any of the risk factors of High Risk for Injury should alert the nurse to investigate other risk factors that could result in trauma (such as wounds, cuts, or falls), poisoning, or suffocation for the purpose of modifying preinjury risk factors that threaten the patient's physical integrity. The following data will assist in evaluating a patient who may be at risk for injury: age and developmental level; incidence of previous injuries; drug therapy; mobility status, including use of ambulatory and restraining devices; presence of paresis, seizure disorder, sensory impairment, or fatigue; and mental status (confusion, impaired memory and judgment, disorientation, inability to understand and follow directions).[12]

In the final phase of assessment, the nurse analyzes the collected and sorted data. The nurse identifies the host, agent, and environmental variables and their interrelationships. The nurse can diagnose High Risk for Injury when the complex interrelationship of the three variables indicates that the individual is at risk for physical injury. If the assessment data indicate High Risk for Injury, the nurse should further assess to determine whether there is high risk for trauma, poisoning, or suffocation.

❖ Risk Factors

The presence of the following behaviors, conditions, or circumstances render the patient more vulnerable to High Risk for Injury:[16]

Host factors
- Developmental age: physiological and psychosocial
- Cognitive or emotional impairment
- Sensory or motor deficits
- Integrative dysfunction
- Tissue hypoxia
- Malnutrition
- Immune response impairment
- Abnormal blood profile
- Osteoporosis

- Central nervous system depressant drugs
- Decreased proprioceptive reflexes
- Impaired cerebral blood flow
- Children: number of injuries sustained before age 5, aggressive behavior, male sex
- Elderly: frail, restricted mobility

Agent factors
- Energy: chemical, electrical, gravitational, mechanical, radiant, or thermal

Environmental factors
- Physical: unsafe design, structure, or arrangement of home and community or unsafe mode of transportation
- Chemical: presence of pollutants, improperly stored poisons, large supplies of drugs, improperly marked and stored drugs, and use of preservatives, cosmetics, and dyes.

❖ Related Medical/Psychiatric Diagnoses

The following are examples of related medical/psychiatric diagnoses for High Risk for Injury:
- Bipolar disorder, manic episode
- Blindness or any disease of the eyes that limits visual acuity
- Blood dyscrasia causing weakness
- Cerebral vascular accident
- Deafness
- Delusional (paranoid) disorder
- Depression
- Neurological and orthopedic disorders causing alterations in sensation or mobility
- Peripheral vascular disease

High Risk for Trauma

The very young and the very old are at accentuated risk for injury. The clinician should carefully assess young children who seem to be "accident prone" for High Risk for Trauma. Children who tend to run rather than walk, who like to climb, and who like to explore unfamiliar places may be especially prone to accidental injury or trauma.[35] Parental awareness of safety factors, such as use of car seats appropriate for the child's age, gates to block steep stairways, and safety measures in kitchens and bathrooms, is especially important.

The frail elderly are also prone to accidents, and the nurse must assess elderly patients' awareness of their own physiological and psychological status as well as their awareness of the environmental factors that make them more "accident prone." The elderly patient with weakness, poor vision, or balancing difficulties has an accentuated risk of injury from falls (gravitational energy), burns (thermal energy), and cuts (mechanical energy). Slippery floors, unanchored rugs, and unsafe window protection are environmental risk factors that increase the likelihood of trauma. Both normal aging processes and pathological processes increase the likelihood of trauma, espe-

cially falls, in the elderly (see the box below).

The incidence of trauma in the elderly from falls is high and the consequences costly. Therefore, the nurse must be knowledgeable in assessing risk factors indicating a high risk for trauma from falls. Farsightedness and a reduction in the amount of light reaching the retina are expected changes in the elderly that contribute to the risk for falls; certain diseases and pathological changes in the elderly, such as glaucoma, cataracts, and vertigo, also increase the risk.

Drop attacks that cause an elderly person to fall are characterized by sudden falls without loss of consciousness, resulting from cerebral ischemia.[17]

❖ CAUSES OF FALLS IN THE ELDERLY BY PROCESS[15,17,30]

Normal Aging Process	Pathological Process
Neurological/sensory changes	
Vision changes: presbyopia (farsightedness) or reduction in light that reaches retina	Vision changes: glaucoma or cataracts
Auditory impairment: decreased acuity	Auditory impairment: vertigo
Central processing: decreased proprioceptive reflexes	Central processing: senile epilepsy, cerebrovascular accident, or neurosyphilis
Musculoskeletal changes	
Fibrotic changes in joints, muscles, tendons, and ligaments	Gait abnormalities: shuffling; waddling; slow, short, deliberate steps; or muscle rigidity
Loss of muscle size, strength, and speed of contraction	Arthritis
	Osteoporosis
Cardiovascular changes	
Impaired regulation of cerebral blood flow	Orthostatic hypotension
	Postprandial hypotension
Decreased baroreceptor sensitivity	
	Carotid sinus hypersensitivity—excessive cardiac slowing or hypotension
Progressive decrease of cerebral blood flow	Supraventricular and ventricular dysrhythmias—sudden reduction in cardiac output or systemic blood pressure
	Drop attacks
Genitourinary/endocrine changes	
Low estrogen in postmenopausal women	Stress incontinence in postmenopausal women

I

Table 1   Effects of Selected Drugs on the Elderly[19]

Drug	Effect

Benzodiazepines
    Diazepam
    Chlordiazepoxide
	Drowsiness

Hypnotics	Drowsiness
Tricyclic antidepressants	Postural hypotension
Antihypertensives	Postural hypotension
Diuretics	Dizziness and hypotension
Antiparkinsonian agents Levodopa	Hypotension or postural hypotension (corrected by decarboxylase inhibitor)

Antineoplastics
    Vincristine
    Vinblastine
    Cisplatin
    Procarbazine
	Peripheral neuropathies

Alcohol	Possible loss of balance

The fibrotic changes in joint and muscle tissue accentuate the normal fibrosis and loss of muscle size, strength, and contraction that accompany advancing age. The gait and posture changes in the elderly in conjunction with degenerative joint disease, osteoporosis, or gait abnormalities contribute to falls. Osteoporosis in postmenopausal women with insufficient estrogen leads to weakened, demineralized bones that can cause both a fall itself or a bone fracture that causes a fall. Endocrine changes in postmenopausal women may cause stress incontinence and may cause these women to rush to the bathroom, thereby resulting in a fall. Normal estrogen levels maintain the tone of urethral tissue necessary for contraction. Low estrogen levels result in flaccid urethral tissue and relaxation of the pelvic floor muscles, which produce leakage of urine.[15] Elderly patients who take certain medications are at risk for falls from the side effects of the drugs. Table 1 lists selected drugs and the side effects they often have on the elderly. These effects put the elderly at greater risk for sustaining trauma, especially as a result of falling.

❖ **Risk Factors**

The presence of the following behaviors, conditions, or circumstances render the patient more vulnerable to High Risk for Trauma[16]:

Host factors

- Weakness
- Poor vision
- Balancing difficulties
- Reduced hand-eye coordination
- Reduced tactile or temperature sensation
- Reduced large-muscle or small-muscle coordination
- Sensory or motor deficits
- Cognitive or emotional difficulties
- Lack of safety education or safety precautions
- Insufficient finances to purchase safety equipment or make necessary repairs
- History of previous trauma

Agent factors

- Energy: gravitational, mechanical, thermal, electrical, or radiant

Environmental factors

- Slippery floors (e.g., those that are wet or highly waxed)
- Snow or ice on stairs or walkway
- Unanchored rugs
- Bathtub without handgrip or antislip equipment
- Use of unsteady ladder or chairs
- Entering unlighted rooms
- Unsturdy or absent handrails along a staircase
- Unanchored electrical wires
- Litter or liquid spills on floors or staircases
- High beds
- Children playing without gates at top of stairs
- Obstructed passageways
- Unsafe window protection in homes with young children
- Inappropriate or faulty call-for-aid mechanisms for bed-resting patient
- Pot handles facing the front of stove
- Bathing in very hot water
- Unsupervised bathing of young children
- Potential igniting of gas leaks
- Delayed lighting of gas burner or oven
- Experimenting with chemicals or gasoline
- Unscreened fireplaces or heaters

- Wearing plastic aprons or flowing clothing around open flame
- Children playing with matches, candles, or cigarettes
- Inadequately stored combustibles or corrosives (e.g., matches, oily rags, or lye)
- Highly flammable children's clothing or toys
- Overloaded fuse box
- Contact with rapidly moving machinery, industrial belts, or pulleys
- Sliding on coarse bed linen or struggling with in-bed restraints
- Faulty electrical plugs, frayed wires, or defective appliances
- Contact with acids or alkalis
- Playing with fireworks or gunpowder
- Contact with intense cold
- Overexposure to sun, sunlamps, or radiotherapy
- Use of cracked dishware or glasses
- Knives stored uncovered
- Guns or ammunition stored unlocked
- Large icicles hanging from roof
- Exposure to dangerous machinery
- Children playing with sharp-edged toys
- High-crime neighborhood
- Driving a mechanically unsafe vehicle
- Driving after drinking alcohol or using drugs
- Driving at excessive speeds
- Driving without necessary visual aids
- Children riding in front seat in car
- Smoking in bed or near oxygen
- Overloaded electrical outlets
- Grease waste collected on stoves
- Use of thin or worn pot holders
- Unrestrained babies riding in car
- Not using seat restraints
- Not using or misusing necessary headgear by cyclists
- Young children carried on adult bicycles
- Unsafe road conditions
- Play or work near vehicle pathways (e.g., driveways, lanes, or railroad tracks)

❖ Related Medical/Psychiatric Diagnoses

The following are examples of related medical/psychiatric diagnoses for High Risk for Trauma:

- Alzheimer's Disease
- Anemia
- Bipolar disorder, manic episode
- Cataracts, glaucoma
- Cerebral vascular accident
- Delusional (paranoid) disorder
- Diabetes
- Epilepsy
- Orthostatic hypotension
- Osteoporosis
- Parkinsonism
- Substance abuse

High Risk for Poisoning

The nurse assesses the patient and environment for risk factors that increase the likelihood of poisoning, such as injury from chemical energy. Patients with cognitive limitations or emotional problems may not take proper precautions because they are not aware of the hazards of certain products or because of impetuous behavior. Characteristics of a child's developmental age, such as exploration associated with toddlers or peer pressure associated with teenagers, increase the likelihood of exposure to poisonous products or illicit drugs. Both the normal impulse of infants to put things in their mouths and children's tendency toward pica (ingestion of nonfood items) place them in danger of poisoning. The nurse should observe the oral habits of the 1- to 6-year-old child and the conditions of the child's housing for evidence of exposure to chemicals, peeling or chipped paint. In the elderly population, reduced vision, glaucoma, or cataracts can cause accidental poisonings if these patients cannot properly see the labeling on their medications.

❖ Risk Factors

The presence of the following behaviors, conditions, or circumstances render the patient more vulnerable to High Risk for Poisoning[16]:

Host factors
- Reduced vision
- Cognitive or emotional difficulties
- Developmental age of child (e.g., crawling infant; exploring toddler; magical, egocentric

thinking of preschool child; or peer pressure of teenage child)
- Occupational setting that does not have adequate safeguards
- Lack of safety or drug education
- Lack of proper precautions
- Insufficient finances

Agent factors
- Chemical energy

Environmental factors
- Large supplies of drugs in the home
- Medicines stored in unlocked cabinets accessible to children or confused persons
- Availability of illicit drugs potentially contaminated by poisonous additives
- Flaking, peeling paint or plaster in environment of young children
- Lack of parental supervision
- Chemical contamination of food and water
- Unprotected contact with heavy metals, chemicals, or inseticides
- Paint or lacquer in poorly ventilated areas or without proper storage
- Presence of poisonous vegetation
- Presence of atmospheric pollutants

❖ Related Medical/Psychiatric Diagnoses

The following are examples of related medical/psychiatric diagnoses for High Risk for Poisoning:
- Depression
- Lead Poisoning
- Mercury Poisoning
- Organophosphate Poisoning
- Psychoactive substance use disorder

High Risk for Suffocation

A number of risk factors for the diagnosis of High Risk for Suffocation are inherent in the developmental characteristics of infants, toddlers, and preschoolers. Children should be assessed for these host characteristics. Children under the age of two commonly pick up items and place them in their mouths; this can be hazardous even if the child is in a "child-safe" environment. Young children who have no fear of harm and do not un-

derstand safety precautions or older children who lack safety education possess important host characteristics that place them at risk for suffocation, choking, aspiration, and submersion accidents. Lack of adult supervision at a pool can result in drowning, especially by children who are unable to swim or who experience difficulty while swimming. Numerous environmental factors place children, adults, and the elderly at risk for accidents that result in asphyxia.

❖ Risk Factors

The presence of the following behaviors, conditions, or circumstances render the patient more vulnerable to High Risk for Suffocation[16]:

Host factors
- Reduced olfactory sensation
- Reduced motor abilities
- Disease or injury processes
- Cognitive or emotional difficulties
- Lack of safety education or precautions
- Lack of awareness of hazards in environment

Agent factors
- Lack of oxygenation

Environmental factors
- Pillow placed in an infant's crib
- Vehicle warming in closed garage
- Children playing with plastic bags or inserting small objects into their mouths or noses
- Discarded or unused refrigerators or freezers without removed doors
- Children left unattended in bathtubs or pools
- Household gas leaks
- Smoking in bed
- Use of fuel-burning heaters not vented to outside
- Low-strung clotheslines
- Pacifier hung on cord around infant's neck
- Eating large mouthfuls of food
- Propped bottle placed in an infant's mouth while the infant is in a crib
- Improperly stored poisonous substances
- Lack of parental supervision
- Lack of safety precautions

❖ **Related Medical/Psychiatric Diagnoses**

The following are examples of related medical/psychiatric diagnoses for High Risk for Suffocation:

- Inhalation Injuries
- Neurological and Pulmonary Impairments affecting ability to swallow or breath (e.g., bronchial asthma, status asthmaticus, myasthenia gravis, cerebral vascular accident)
- Tetanus

NURSING DIAGNOSES

Examples of *specific* diagnoses for High Risk for Injury, High Risk for Trauma, High Risk for Poisoning, and High Risk for Suffocation are:

- High Risk for Injury related to decreased vision
- High Risk for Trauma related to peer pressure and impetuous behavior
- High Risk for Poisoning related to housing with peeling paint and extensive renovations
- High Risk for Suffocation related to lack of awareness of hazards in environment

PLANNING AND IMPLEMENTATION WITH RATIONALE

Planning for all four diagnoses includes making decisions about the desired patient outcomes and appropriate interventions for each diagnosis. There is a direct relationship between patient outcomes and interventions. Interventions may be thought of as the means to the end, that is, the behavioral outcome that is desired in the patient. In planning interventions for High Risk for Injury in general or in terms of trauma, poisoning, or suffocation, the nurse chooses actions most likely to prevent patient injury. It is important to tailor planned interventions to individual patients. If possible, planning should include the patient and his or her family, who may then assist in planning and implementation.

The clinician must plan and implement strategies or countermeasures aimed at the agent causing the injury so that the host is protected from the agent, the environment is altered, or both. For example, to achieve the patient outcome of "No falls experienced while in the hospital," interventions aimed at the agent (gravitational energy) to prevent trauma from falling in the hospitalized toddler may be very different from those for the elderly. The reason for choosing a particular intervention will vary in different situations. For example, the rationale for reducing an environmental factor that contributes to falls in young children by the intervention "Remove clutter from the floor" is that *young children are unable to comprehend the consequences of walking directly on objects*. In the elderly, the rationale for the same intervention is that *the normal aging process causes elderly persons to be farsighted and to have a decreased amount of light reaching the retina, reducing their ability to see items in their path*. The presence of glaucoma or cataracts in the elderly further decreases vision. Removing objects in the environment is an example of one of Haddon's countermeasures.[14] This countermeasure is aimed at preventing harm from the agent of injury (gravitational energy) by separating in time and space the hazard and the person to be protected.

The planning and implementation phases of the nursing process for High Risk for Injury, High Risk for Trauma, High Risk for Poisoning, and High Risk for Suffocation end with the development of the plan of nursing care and documentation of the nurse's completed actions and the patient's responses to those actions.[34] Nursing Care Guidelines are presented for planning care for patients at risk for trauma, poisoning (lead), and suffocation. The focus of the expected patient outcome identified in each of the Nursing Care Guidelines is to prevent a specific injury, that is, to prevent trauma, poisoning, and suffocation.

EVALUATION

The nurse evaluates the plan of care both during and following implementation. The nurse focuses her evaluation on the patient's response to nursing interventions in relation to predetermined desired patient outcomes. The key determination to make when evaluating High Risk for Injury, Trauma, Poisoning, and Suffocation is whether the patient suffered an injury. For less discrete de-

Text continued on p. 67.

I

❖ *NURSING CARE GUIDELINES: HIGH RISK FOR TRAUMA*
Nursing Diagnosis: High Risk for Trauma

Expected Patient Outcomes	Nursing Interventions
	Host
Accidental injury will be prevented in the patient at risk.	• Screen the patient for presence of risk factors for trauma from falling: assess patient characteristics such as age, developmental level, mental ability, emotional state, socioeconomic status, mobility, strength, and capacity to carry out tasks.
	• Determine if history or presence of disease increases risk for trauma from falls.
	• Identify contributing factors.
	• Document findings on patient record.
	• Educate the patient and family by explaining the risk factors that contribute to increased risk of injury, and the necessary safety precautions to alleviate these.
	Agent
	• Identify agent of injury.
	• Implement countermeasures to prevent injury caused by agent of injury. For example, thermal agent—modify the rate or spatial distribution of energy from its source by installing safety faucets to prevent burns from hot water; gravitational agent—increase resistance to damage from energy source by requesting consult for physical or occupational therapy.
	Environment
	• Identify and remove hazards in the environment that precipitate falls.
	• Explain safety reasons for altering the environment and prevent possible injury by providing general safety information.
	• Provide specific anticipatory guidance about safety.
	• Identify community resources for elderly, e.g., Meals on Wheels, Emergency Life Alarm.

❖ *NURSING CARE GUIDELINES: HIGH RISK FOR POISONING*

Nursing Diagnosis: *High Risk for Poisoning related to ingestion of lead resulting from lack of awareness of home hazards*

Expected Patient Outcomes	Nursing Interventions
The patient will not ingest or be exposed to substances containing lead.	*Host* • Screen for listlessness, anorexia, pallor, pica (eating of nonfood items), or mouthing nonfood items. • Ask parents if the child eats well-balanced meals; complains of stomachaches; has hard, infrequent bowel movements; is irritable, distracted, or hyperactive; has changed in sleep pattern; or has forgotten any motor activities previously mastered. • Refer children with positive screening to a physician for evaluation. • Monitor laboratory results for levels of hematocrit, hemoglobin, lead, FEP, and calcium in the urine. *Agent* • Determine agent factor responsible for injury—chemical (lead metal). • Implement countermeasures to prevent injury from lead through lead abatement programs and parent-child education programs. *Environment* • Assess and monitor family structure. • Identify passive parent, patterns of parent-child interaction, and family stressors. • Identify adults in home who work in industries where exposure is likely and who may bring lead dust home via skin and clothing. • Identify lead environment—old, flaking, chipped paint; plaster chips; colored newsprint; cigarette butts and ashes; water from lead pipes or lead soldered pipes; soil; food grown in soil with heavy lead content; leaded gasoline; and foreign-made ceramic dishes or toys. • Identify sources of lead in air—exposure to a smelting factory, burning of leaded objects, or living near a busy street or public garage, living in older housing undergoing renovation. • Assess parents' present level of understanding of lead poisoning and educate as needed. • Provide anticipatory guidance on patterns of normal growth and development and the hazards for lead poisoning and their relationship to nutrition and development. • Suggest activities for parents that promote parent-child interaction and decrease pica behavior in child. • Refer to public health nurse for follow-up.

I

❖ *NURSING CARE GUIDELINES FOR SUFFOCATION*

Nursing Diagnosis: High Risk for Suffocation related to lack of awareness of environmental hazards

Expected Patient Outcomes	Nursing Interventions
Suffocation will be prevented in the child and adult at risk.	**Host** • Assess and monitor personal characteristics: age, developmental level, mental status, muscle strength, coordination, temperament, knowledge, capacity to protect self from suffocation **Agent** • Determine possible causes of lack of oxygenation that result in airway obstruction or aspiration and hypoxemia. • Use countermeasures to prevent or reduce injury from lack of oxygenation, such as placing a fence around swimming pools, child-proofing the surroundings, and providing swimming instruction. • Teach emergency rescue to parents, caregivers, siblings, and the community. • Perform Heimlich maneuver or cardiopulmonary resuscitation if needed. **Environment** • Identify environmental hazards that cause suffocation. • Alter environment by removing hazards. • Determine parents' knowledge of safety precautions appropriate for child's developmental level. • Inform parents of common items that pose safety problems. Inform about safety precautions and teach them to routinely check and childproof the environment. • Work toward community support for environmental measures known to be effective in reducing injury.

❖ *CASE STUDY WITH PLAN OF CARE*

Ms. Estelle J. is an 84-year-old woman with failing vision who resides in a local nursing home. Ms. J. was walking down the corridor when she suddenly fell, striking her head on the floor. There were no seizures and no loss of consciousness. She was brought to the emergency room via ambulance. Physical assessment revealed the following findings: Frail, elderly female with blood pressure 140/90, pulse 96, unlabored respirations of 24 per minute, temperature 99 degrees. Skin—pale, swelling, and bruise on right side of forehead. Chest—clear. Extremities—peripheral pulses 1+, slight ankle edema. Mental status—awake but dis-oriented. Follows commands poorly. Pupils 4–5 cm, equal, round, reactive to light and accommodation. Spontaneous movement of all extremities. Lower extremities—slight quadricep weakness. Reflexes—+2, intact, and symmetrical. Lab results: electrolytes WNL, Tests: CT scan—negative. Physician orders include: Transfer to nursing unit for observations. Soft diet. Activity—OOB in chair BID. Commode with assistance. On the nursing unit Ms. J. repeatedly tried to get out of bed on her own. The following care plan was developed for Ms. J.

PLAN OF CARE FOR MS. ESTELLE J.

Nursing Diagnosis: High Risk for Trauma related to history of falls and disorientation

Expected Patient Outcomes	Nursing Interventions
Trauma will be prevented as evidenced by absence of falls.	**Host** • Identify Ms. J. as a high risk for falls and document. • Assess and monitor neurological status. • Orient Ms. J. to time, place, and person each time you approach her. • Explain procedures to Ms. J. before starting them. • Instruct Ms. J. to use call bell for requesting assistance. • Instruct Ms. J. to remain in bed. **Agent** • Implement countermeasures to prevent injury from fall caused by gravity, such as altering floor surface characteristics by not waxing floors and increasing Ms. J.'s flexibility and mobility through exercise. **Environment** • Keep light on at night and bed rails up when Ms. J. is unattended. • Keep bed in low position with wheel locked. • Encourage Ms. J. to void before retiring. • Offer assistance to Ms. J. in getting out of bed every 2-3 hours to use the commode to prevent her from getting up on her own. • Use nonskid slippers. • Request order for family member, staff member, or companion to stay with Ms. J. at all times.

sired outcomes, one must determine whether the desired outcomes have been achieved completely, partially, or not at all. The following important questions should be answered when evaluating the care for patients with these diagnoses: Were the desired outcomes (prevention of) trauma, poisoning, or suffocation) achieved and to what extent? What data support this? Were the interventions effective in preventing injury? If not, why? Is a different plan needed? What data support this? Was the plan of care communicated and carried out? Was the patient and his or her family included in the initial planning? What barriers exist to the implementation of planned care? Was the correct person or health-team member chosen to carry out a particular action? Is the diagnosis High Risk for Injury legitimate for this patient or is a reassessment needed to obtain more subjective and objective data to confirm the diagnosis?

Documentation of the usefulness of interventions in the achievement of outcomes and answers to the pertinent questions previously listed will prompt the nurse to decide to (1) continue the current plan with periodic reassessment, (2) modify the plan, or (3) terminate the plan if it is no longer needed.

REFERENCES

1. Alexander D: Chronic lead exposure. A problem for minority workers, *Amer Assoc of Occupat Health Nurs* 37(3):105-108, 1989.
2. Baker SM: Injury control. In Sartwell P, ed: *Maxcy-Rosenau Preventive medicine and public health,* New York, 1973, Appleton-Century-Crofts.
3. Baker SM, O'Neill B, Ginsburg M, Li G: *The injury fact book,* ed 2, New York, 1991, Oxford University Press.
4. Barker PO, Lewis DA: The management of lead exposure in pediatric populations, *Nurs Pract* 15(12):8-16, 1990.
5. Beautrais AL, Ferguson DM, Shannon FT: Accidental child poisoning in the first three years of life, *Aust Pediatr J* 17:104-109, 1981.

6. Bijur P, Golding J, Goldacre M: Persistence of occurrence of injury: can injuries of preschool children predict injuries of school-age children?, *Pediatrics* 82(5):707-712, 1988.

7. Brown GW, Davidson S: Social class, psychiatric disorder of mother and accidents to children, *Lancet* 1:378-380, 1978.

8. Centers for Disease Control: *Strategic plan for the elimination of childhood lead poisoning,* Atlanta, 1991, Department of Health and Human Services.

9. Centers for Disease Control: Playground-related injuries in preschool-aged children–United States, 1983-1987, *Morbidity and Mortality Weekly Report* 37:629-632, 1988.

10. Dietrich K, Kraft K, Bornschein R: Low level fetal exposure effect on neurobehavioral development in early infancy, *Pediatrics* 5:721-730, 1988.

11. Environmental Defense Fund: *Legacy of lead: America's continuing epidemic of childhood lead poisoning,* Washington, DC, 1990, Environmental Defense Fund.

12. Fife D, Solomon P, Stanton M: A falls/risk program: code orange for success, *Nurs Manage* 15(11):50-53, 1984.

13. Gallagher S, Finneson K, Guyer B: The incidence of injuries among 87,000 Massachusetts children and adolescents: results of the 1980-81 statewide childhood injury prevention program surveillance system, *Am J Public Health* 74(12):1340-1347, 1984.

14. Haddon W: On the escape of tigers: an ecologic note, *Am J Public Health* 60(12):2229-2234, 1970.

15. Irrgang S: Classifications of urinary incontinence, *J Enterstomal Ther* 13(2):62-65, 1986.

16. Kim M, McFarland G, McLane A: *Pocket guide to nursing diagnoses,* ed 4, St. Louis, 1991, Mosby–Year Book.

17. Lipsitz L: Abnormalities in blood pressure homeostasis that contribute to falls in the elderly, *Clin Geriatr Med* 1(3):637-643, 1985.

18. Manhiemer DI, Dewey J, Mellinger GD: *50,000 child-years of accidental injury,* Public Health Rep 81, 519-533, 1966.

19. McDonald JB: The role of drugs in the elderly, *Clin Geriatr Med* 1(3):621-633, 1985.

20. Modell JH, Boyen PG: Drowning and near-drowning. In Shoemaker WC and others, editors: *Textbook of critical care,* Philadelphia, 1989, WB Saunders Co.

21. National Center for Health Statistics: Advance Report of Final Mortality Statistics, 1989, *Monthly Vital Statistics Report* 40(8) Supp. 2, 1992.

22. National Safety Council: *Accident facts,* Itasca, Il, 1992 National Safety Council.

23. Needleman et al.: The long-term effects of exposure to low doses of lead in childhood, *NEJM* 32:83-88, 1990.

24. O'Carroll PW, Alkon E, Weiss B: Drowning mortality in Los Angeles County, 1976 to 1984, *JAMA* 260(2):380-383, 1984.

25. Occupational Safety and Health Administration, US Dept. of Labor: *Occupational exposure to lead,* Federal Register 1978, 43:54353-54616.

26. Rivara FP: Epidemiology of childhood injuries I: Review of current research and presentation of conceptual framework, *Am J Dis Child* 136(5):399-405, 1982.

27. Rivara FP, Bergman AB, LoGerfo JP: Epidemiology of childhood injuries II: Sex differences in injury rates, *Am J of Dis Child* 136(6):502-506, 1982.

28. Robertson L: Injury epidemiology and the reduction of harm. In Mechanic D, editor: *Handbook of health, health care, and the health professions.* New York, 1984, The Free Press.

29. Robertson L: *Injuries: Causes, control strategies and public policy,* Lexington, Mass, 1983, Lexington Books.

30. Rodstein M: Accidents among the aged. In Reichel W, ed: *Clinical aspects of aging,* Baltimore, 1983, Williams & Wilkins.

31. US Department of Health and Human Services, Public Health Service, Centers for Disease Control: *Preventing lead poisoning in young children,* Atlanta, 1985.

32. US Department of Equal Employment Opportunity Commission: Job patterns for minorities and women in private industry, Washington, DC, 1980.

33. Waller JA: Prevention of premature death and disability due to injury. In Last J, editor: *Maxcy-Rosenau Public health and preventive medicine,* New York, 1986, Appleton-Century-Crofts.

34. Yura H, Walsh MB: *The nursing process,* ed 5, Norwalk, Conn, 1985, Appleton-Century-Crofts.

35. Zuckerman BS, Duby JC: Developmental approach to injury prevention, *Pediatr Clin North Am* 32(1):17-29, 1985.

Health Seeking Behaviors (Specify)

Health Seeking Behaviors (Specify) is the state in which a client with stable health actively seeks ways to alter personal health habits and/or the environment to achieve optimal health.

OVERVIEW

Ellis[11] notes that although promoting human health has always been a goal of nursing, the concept of "health" is only gradually developing importance as more emphasis is placed on the health of individuals, families, groups, and communities. To work with clients who wish to work toward optimal health, an understanding of health, health promotion, and factors related to the adoption of positive personal health habits is essential.

To date, the nursing literature offers no consensus definition of *health*. The nurse theorists' definitions of health differ and include stability,[23] adaptation,[18,31] wholeness or integrity,[25] and functional independence.[15] Other common descriptions of health are absence of disease, being successful and happy, and self-actualization. Smith[34] identified four models of health: (1) the eudaemonistic model, in which health is self-actualization, (2) the adaptive model, in which health is flexible adaptation to the environment, (3) role performance, or the ability to carry out social roles, and (4) the clinical model, in which health is the absence of signs or symptoms of disease or disability. Epp[12] has defined health also as a resource for living and managing one's surroundings. Meleis[21] notes that because nursing is practiced in many different clinical areas and in many different countries, each with its own cultural patterns, many definitions of health are required.

In current literature, optimal health or wellness is defined as being unique to each client and dependent on his/her definition of health.[19] The uniqueness occurs because each person constantly interacts with the environment, and the relationship between the client and the environment (including family, peers, and the community) will affect both the choice of a definition of health and the choice of health behaviors.[20]

When Smith's four models of health[34] are used to examine a client's progression toward health, the eudaemonistic model seems to most strongly espouse the client's potential to achieve total well-being. In this model, Pender[28] perceives the person as motivated by a desire to grow, express his or her potential, and attain a better quality of life. In the adaptive model, a need to gain or maintain stability motivates the person. In the role performance model, a need to gain mastery over a specific set of skills motivates the person. In the clinical model, prevention of disease motivates the person. Moch[22] believes that illness can initiate a growth experience for patients, therefore nurses should offer opportunities for patients to increase their health even while they are receiving treatment for their disease. Both health promotion and disease prevention can lead to increased health status based on the client's definition of health.

Laffrey[19] emphasizes that although health is now viewed as a human right, individuals should assume the responsibility for their own health. Nurses can work as partners with clients while assisting them to achieve health. The nurse's role in this partnership should include not only understanding the client's current definition of health but also, when necessary providing information about other dimensions of health, which may help the client to reach his/her potential.

Although health promotion and primary prevention are closely linked, Stachtchenko and Jenicek[35] differentiate between the two terms. They note that reducing the risk of disease is the basis of disease prevention whereas increasing well being is the basis for health promotion. The essential aspects of health promotion include enabling change in lifestyle behaviors and political action directed at "healthy" policy.[35] Other authors concur that health promotion focuses on well-being and use the terms "well-being," "actualization,"[27,28] and "high-level wellness"[37] to define *health promotion*. Perhaps for nursing, the concept of health promotion as the process of enabling people to increase control over and improve their health[26] provides the clearest direction.

Some health behaviors that affect health have been the focus of research studies. To date, research has mainly focused on health behaviors that significantly affect mortality. Breslow and Enstrom[7] studied seven health practices: never having smoked cigarettes, regular physical activity, moderate or no use of alcohol, 7 to 8 hours of sleep per day, maintaining proper weight, eating breakfast, and not eating between meals. The number of these health practices is inversely related to age-adjusted mortality rates. Belloc[2] found that five practices—smoking, weight control, drinking, hours of sleep, regularity of meals, and physical activity—also are inversely related to age-adjusted mortality rates.

More recent studies of women have found that never having smoked cigarettes is related to lower mortality.[6] A decrease in physical activity for elderly women and a history of cigarette smoking for elderly men were associated with subsequent physical limitations.[5] The link of smoking with lung cancer has been well substantiated, and many authorities have described smoking as North America's greatest health risk. In developing a health habits scale, Williams and others[36] found smoking to be independent of other health behaviors. They concluded that health habits may not form a unitary construct.

A few studies have looked at persons who practice health behaviors. Among the elderly, married men practiced more health behaviors, such as eating properly and obtaining adequate rest and exercise, than did women or single men.[8] Norman,[24] in a review of current studies, notes that socioeconomic status is a particularly reliable indicator of how an individual will behave in health matters—the higher one's income, the more likely one is to engage in positive health practices. This behavior may be related to the educational level associated with the socioeconomic status. Individuals who believe in health promotion activities are also more likely to practice them than those who do not.[38]

Although most of the population could benefit from health promotion, the nurse may have to target his/her interventions toward those who are known to have fewer positive health practices or those whose health practices may compromise their health. These persons would include, for example, people from lower socioeconomic groups, teens who smoke and drink or develop poor nutritional practices, adults with sedentary lifestyles, people under severe stress (such as single parents or elderly caregivers), and women whose children have left home and for whom, therefore, self-actualization has become important. However, programs that simply aim at changing personal behavior without recognizing the complex relationship of behavior to cultural, psychosocial, and environmental factors and public policy are unlikely to succeed.[1,13] The nurse's role may need to extend to advocacy and social action.[9]

A few studies have examined factors that influence health behaviors. Social support positively affects the practice of healthy lifestyle behaviors.[3,16] Social interaction itself is a positive health behavior; increased mortality rates occur among those with few social ties.[32] Zimmerman and Connor[39] suggest that timing of support may be critical. Hannah[14] found that the selection of health-promoting behaviors is related to a person's immediate concerns about health and assessment of his/her present health status, not to a concern about long-term outcomes. One study found motivation to be the most important factor in positive responses to cues for health promotion.[17]

In summary, the literature has identified a number of factors that affect how the individual progresses toward optimal health, health behaviors that affect health, and significant factors that affect health behavior. The client who wishes to attain health may be an individual, a family, or a group. The term "client" reflects a health orientation, as opposed to the term "patient," which has an illness orientation.

ASSESSMENT

Assessment should begin with an investigation into the current health and social status. This should include a review of body systems; health perception, practices, and risks: supporting systems; social, cultural, and financial status; and the environment. An assessment of family functioning and developmental status will be important, as well as the individual assessment of family members.

To assist the client in moving toward higher levels of health, the nurse must understand the meaning of health for the client. The nurse needs to assess the client's values so that any changes in health practices will not conflict with these values. For example, the man who values time with his wife and family is unlikely to forfeit time with them to attend an exercise program even though he is highly motivated to increase his physical activity.

The nurse should assess any factors that the client feels will interfere with his ability to engage in specific health-promoting behaviors. The nurse and client can then discuss strategies to reduce or eliminate these barriers.

The nurse should assess the client's environment for both support and stress. First, the nurse should determine the client's support systems, including the degree of support available to the client to initiate and maintain health-promoting behaviors. Second, the nurse should assess the environment for noxious stressors that could be reduced or eliminated.

To assist the client in achieving higher levels of health, the nurse may provide the client with information about specific health behaviors and environmental factors and their influence on health status. This information may assist the client in determining the behaviors he or she wishes to adopt or reduce. When the client is exposed to multiple risk factors, the nurse can assist the client in assigning priority to the choices so that he or she does not become overwhelmed.

The major characteristic of the client seeking ways to move toward optimal health is an expressed desire to seek a higher level of wellness. Observed behaviors that alert the nurse to the client's desire to seek a higher level of wellness include, for example, the client's switching to nutritious snacks rather than eating donuts and drinking coffee. Joining a weight-control group or rising early to jog are also behavioral indicators of a desire to move toward optimal health—indicators that the nurse should explore with the client. Other behaviors that identify health seeking clients include a request for information about community resources that could aid in their pursuit of health and a struggle with a difficult behavior change, such as stopping smoking without professional assistance.

Although some clients will be interested in reducing threats to their health and may request that the nurse guide them to change old behavior patterns and maintain new ones, many clients will not be aware of how their behaviors affect their health. Persons with sedentary lifestyles, in high-stress occupations, and whose high alcohol intake is associated with "business transactions" may see no reason to change their lifestyles until they are exposed to consciousness-raising information or they suffer an assault to their health.

An expressed desire to participate in decisions about their health and to gain control of their health practices, as well as behavior that implies such a desire (for example, questioning health care practices or requesting and clarifying information and alternatives), also identifies clients

I

who are likely seeking to move toward optimal health. The expression of concern about environmental conditions, such as noxious fumes from a local chemical plant or about inadequate recreational areas for children, also characterizes clients who may wish to lobby for changes in their environments that will affect health and move clients closer to their optimal level of wellness.

In summary, nurses need to be aware of the variety of ways in which clients communicate their desire to move toward higher levels of wellness. The nurse who notes only verbalized desires will overlook many clients. Behavioral clues, including behavior change and information-seeking behavior, can be excellent defining characteristics of health seeking clients for the alert nurse.

A number of factors will affect the desire to move to a higher level of wellness. Confidence in one's ability to grow and change is a major one. The longer the client has carried out a health-compromising behavior, the harder it will be for him/her to change. Also, the client who has suffered no noticeable ill effects may see no reason to change.

Support for the behavioral change will also be important. Family and friends can sabotage good intentions by encouraging old behaviors that they enjoyed with the client, such as drinking alcohol or smoking. Friends and family can also be positive forces, providing social interaction to reinforce positive health behaviors. Economic support is important because the low wage earner may be unable to increase nutritious foods in the diet or take vacations from a stressful work place.

Cultural factors may relate to behaviors that impact on health. For example, dietary patterns associated with cultural identity may be difficult to change. Attendance at group programs that provide support for behavior change may be denied to women whose cultural norms do not encourage women to leave home alone.

Time may also affect behavior change. For the single parent or the harassed executive, finding or taking the time for oneself is often difficult. Therefore behavioral changes that can be easily worked into busy schedules are the most likely to be maintained.

Age and educational level have been highly correlated with positive health behaviors, as has socioeconomic status.[24] However, research suggests that the educational level underlying the socioeconomic status is the most likely reason for the positive health behavior. Recent research also suggests that health behavior is related to a person's perceptions and concerns about his or her own health.[14]

Legislation has a major effect on health behaviors. Seat belt and children's car seat legislation has enforced behavior change. Anti-smoking bylaws have also enforced reduction or elimination of smoking in the work place. The nurse should work with clients motivated to move toward higher levels of health by this type of legislation. The nurse can assist these clients to achieve their desired goal. When the behavioral change is accomplished, it likely becomes its own motivator.

Many of the clients who wish to progress toward optimal health will not have any medical diagnosis or condition. Often clients recognize that their health is their own responsibility, and they initiate steps to control it. In reviewing their lifestyle, they decide to change their behaviors to reduce health risks or move toward self-actualization.

A client with a chronic health problem should be stabilized before undertaking difficult lifestyle changes. These clients will likely be unable to manage significant behavior changes because they are coping with major stressors from their illness. One research study identified a relationship between good health status, perceived control over future health, and health practices.[29]

Many assessment tools are available. Some address only specific health behaviors, whereas others are more comprehensive. The comprehensive tools have been developed for use in large-scale surveys. The nurse should select tools for assessment carefully because many tools address only components of current health status, and most tools do not consider the client's definition of health, health values, and the environmental factors. The tools, however, can serve as a useful review and as an educational tool about practices that affect health. Pender's lifestyle and health habit assessment[28] has ten sections that address general competence in self-care, nutritional practices, physical and recreational activity, sleep patterns, stress management, self-actualization, sense of purpose, relationships with others, and use of the health care system. The nurse can use the client's score on this assessment tool to determine areas in which to encourage health-protecting or health-promoting behaviors. Two programs for computerized assessments are the Lifestyle Assessment[33] and the Rhode Island Wellness program.[30] Both of these programs allow the client to review and document his/her health behaviors and receive an assessment of the health risk that results.

❖ Defining Characteristics

The presence of the following defining characteristics indicates that the patient may be experiencing Health Seeking Behaviors.
- Verbalized or otherwise expressed desire to initiate change or modify a health behavior.
- Desire to attain/maintain optimum physical capacity.
- Desire to attain/maintain optimum psychological well being.

❖ Related Factors

The following related factors are associated with Health Seeking Behaviors:
- Lethargy
- Reduced lung capacity
- Shortness of breath
- Excess body fat
- Degree of self efficacy
- Anxiety related to risks to health
- Perceived control of health
- Degree of self confidence
- Feeling stressed
- Age
- Educational level
- Socioeconomic status
- Definition of health
- Relating cultural practices to current environment
- Perceived lack of inner strength
- Perceived loss of contact with desired religion

❖ Related Medical/Psychiatric Diagnosis

The following are examples of related medical/psychiatric diagnoses for Health Seeking Behaviors (Specify):
- Anemia
- Angina pectoris
- Anxiety
- Coronary bypass
- Hypertension
- Irritable bowel syndrome
- Myocardial infarct
- Obesity
- Ulcer, peptic
- Varicose veins

NURSING DIAGNOSES

Examples of *specific* nursing diagnoses for Health Seeking Behaviors (Specify) are:
- Health Seeking Behavior (engage in strenuous physical activity 3 × week for at least 20 minutes) related to feeling stressed and desire to increase feelings of well-being.
- Health Seeking Behavior (reduce fat consumption) related to reducing excess body fat and risk for cardiovascular disease.
- Health Seeking Behavior (effectively manage daily stressors) related to feeling stressed from full-time job and family responsibilities.
- Health Seeking Behavior (lobby for workplace smoking policy) related to perceived control of health and reducing risks from second-hand smoke.

PLANNING AND IMPLEMENTATION WITH RATIONALE

The expected client outcomes may directly relate to specific goals established for a specific behavior (for example, quitting smoking by an agreed date). In general terms, this outcome can be the reduction or elimination of a specific behavior by a specific date or the adoption and regular use of a specific behavior by a specific date. Other outcomes that indicate the behavior change has had an effect include maintenance of the chosen health behavior for 1 year, expressed satisfaction with behavior change, verbalized feelings of increased energy, verbalized feelings of increased self-confidence, and satisfaction, with a move toward optimizing potential.

I

I

Once the nurse and client have established the expected outcomes, they will plan the strategies to reach these goals. The strategies must be acceptable to the client and fit with the client's lifestyle.

The nurse's roles of teacher and counselor are important in implementation.[10] *The nurse may also assist the client in developing new skills to initiate and maintain chosen behaviors.* For example, the person who smokes cigarettes to reduce stress will need to learn other ways to manage stress. The client who wishes to eat nutritiously but is not aware of which foods to include in a balanced diet will require knowledge from a food guide and encouragement to develop skill in using food exchanges.

Information about community resources may be required. For example, clients who wish to stop smoking or lose weight may desire to become involved in a group program to learn with and re-

ceive support from other members.

For the client with a limited support system, the nurse may enlist the support of significant persons in the client's life or refer the client to a self-help or support group. These groups are very helpful in the management of stress and emotional concerns. One successful program described in the literature offers a combination of information, assessment, referral, and support on an individual and group basis.[4]

An important expected client outcome is: The client will initiate, reduce, or eliminate a specific behavior by a specific date. Once that outcome has been established the nurse will assist the client to establish a behavior pattern that the client finds acceptable and does not conflict with his/her values or cultural beliefs. The nurse should teach or reinforce skills that are required to carry out the behavior. The nurse should discuss potentially helpful support systems and community resources

---

❖ NURSING CARE GUIDELINES

Nursing Diagnosis: *Health Seeking Behaviors (Specify)*

Expected Client Outcomes	**Nursing Interventions**
The client will initiate, reduce, or eliminate a specific behavior by a specific date.	• Establish pattern of behavior to be undertaken. • Determine that pattern fits client's values and cultural patterns. • Assist client with skill development required to carry out chosen behavior. • Establish a supportive environment. • Address knowledge deficits related to resources to assist with behavior change. • Provide information about anticipated consequences of behavior change.
The client will regularly engage in a specific behavior by a specific date and will maintain the chosen behavior for 1 year.	• Monitor progress and motivation to continue with behavior. • Provide support and encouragement to maintain progress. • Identify client's perceived benefits. • Identify client's perceived barriers to continuing behavior. • Develop strategies with client to reduce or eliminate barriers.
The client will express satisfaction with behavior change and will verbalize feelings of increased energy.	• Evaluate with client feelings and perceived benefits of behavior change.

❖ CASE STUDY WITH PLAN OF CARE

Mrs. Frances B. is a 30-year-old mother of two sons, 8 and 6 years of age. Mrs. B. has been separated from her husband for 1 year and works full-time to support herself and her family. Mrs. B.'s health is stable; she smokes one package of cigarettes per day and has recently felt she "needed a drink" when she arrived home every night from work. Mrs. B. works as a computer technician and has few social or recreational pursuits. She is concerned about her lack of patience with her children and has called the local health department because she felt unable to tolerate her children's behavior. She appears pale, with dark circles around the eyes; she stands 5'5" and weighs approximately 120 pounds. Mrs. B. has never had any major health problems. A review of her body systems does not reveal any physical problem. However, Mrs. B. reports feeling overwhelmed by her responsibilities and not sleeping well. She also reports that she has recently started drinking two to four drinks almost every night and, in the past 2 to 3 months, has increased her smoking to one and a half packages per day. Since her separation, she feels that her old friends have ignored her, and she has little interaction with peers except at work. Mrs. B. says that she used to enjoy golf but now finds she cannot afford this activity. Her family lives in a distant city, so Mrs. B. has no family support available. She recognizes that her children's behavior is normal, but she finds it difficult to tolerate. Health to Mrs. B. means the ability to fulfill her various role expectations: employee, breadwinner, mother, and homemaker. She values her family and feeling confident in her roles. Together, the nurse and Mrs. B. identified a number of stressors that could impact on her health: smoking one and a half packages of cigarettes per day, lack of social interaction, lack of time for self, her job as a computer operator, increased alcohol intake, lack of physical exercise, and lack of social support. The nurse and Mrs. B. discussed the relationship between stress and health. Mrs. B. expressed a desire to change her lifestyle. The nurse and Mrs. B. agreed that the stressors should be assigned priority as follows: lack of social support, lack of social interaction, lack of time for self, increased alcohol intake, smoking, and the computer job.

PLAN OF CARE FOR MRS. FRANCES B.

Nursing Diagnosis: *Health Seeking Behaviors (Related to Marital Breakup and Heavy Family Demands)*

Expected Client Outcomes	**Nursing Interventions**
Mrs. B. will attend meetings of support groups routinely.	• Perform ongoing assessment of Mrs. B.'s knowledge of stress and stress management.
Mrs. B. will express satisfaction with her ability to accept support and help from others.	• Assess Mrs. B.'s knowledge of community support groups for single parents, and inform Mrs. B about Parents Without Partners (social activities, support programs, family activities, and emergency support network).
Mrs. B. will express feelings of well-being.	• Determine Mrs. B.'s level of comfort in attending meetings.
Mrs. B. will express satisfaction with role function.	• Role play situations that Mrs. B. might encounter in the first meeting.
Mrs. B. will report confidence in her ability to manage children's behavior.	• Assist Mrs. B. with time management skills to help her to find free time to attend meetings and plan time for herself. • Refer Mrs. B. to the volunteer babysitting services for support programs.

and make referrals if needed. The nurse should review anticipated consequences of the behavior change with the client. *It is unlikely that an individual will maintain a behavior change if it greatly interferes with a daily schedule, strongly held values, or cultural beliefs. As well, clients may feel that they do not have the specific skills required to carry out the behavior or the support from significant others that will assist them, at difficult times, in maintaining the behavior. Community support services can often fill this gap.*

A second important expected client outcome is: The client will regularly engage in a specific behavior by a specific date and will maintain the chosen behavior for 1 year. The nurse will maintain contact with the individual over the first year of a behavior change. The nurse will monitor progress and encourage the client to continue the behavior. Problems that are encountered can be discussed and strategies implemented to reduce or eliminate their effect. The nurse will also assist the client to articulate the benefits of the behavior pattern. *Many clients find it difficult to maintain a behavior change over a long period. Continued interest and support from the nurse will be an important factor in behavior maintenance. Without assistance to problem solve or examine the benefits of the behavior pattern, the client may return to old patterns of unhealthful lifestyles.*

Finally, an important expected outcome is that the client will express satisfaction with behavior change and will verbalize feelings of increased energy. The nurse will evaluate with the client his/her feelings about the behavior and the benefits of the change. *For the behavior to become integrated into the lifestyle of the client, the client will need to feel satisfied with the behavior and be able to articulate positive effects of the behavior change.*

EVALUATION

The nurse will evaluate with the client the extent to which the established outcomes have been met. If the outcomes have been fulfilled, the nurse will ask the client to evaluate his/her satisfaction with the planned strategies and whether other interventions could have helped. If outcomes have not been met, the nurse will ask the client to determine why they were not met. The client should (1) feel satisfied with his/her move toward health, (2) feel competent to maintain chosen health behaviors, and (3) feel motivated to continue to grow toward or through self-actualization.

REFERENCES

1. Anderson ET, McFarlane JM: *Community as client*, Philadelphia, 1988, JB Lippincott.
2. Belloc NB: Relationship of health practices and mortality, *Prev Med* 2:67-81, 1973.
3. Berkman LF, Syme SL: Social networks, host resistance, and mortality: a nine year follow-up study of Alameda County residents, *Am J Epidemio* 109(2):186-204, 1979.
4. Black A: Health Styles: moving beyond disease prevention, *Can Nurse* 80(4):18-20, 1984.
5. Branch L: Health practices and incident disability among the elderly, *Am J Public Health* 75(12):1436-1439, 1985.
6. Branch LG, Jette AM: Personal health practices and mortality among the elderly, *Am J Public Health* 74(10):1126-1129, 1984.
7. Breslow L, Enstrom JE: Persistence of health habits and their relationship to mortality, *Pre Med* 9:469-483, 1980.
8. Brubacher BH: Health promotion: a linguistic analysis, *ANS* 5(3):209-221, 1983.
9. Butterfield PG: Thinking upstream: nurturing a conceptual understanding of the societal context of health behavior, *ANS* 12(2):1-8, 1990.
10. Cox CL: An interaction model of client health behavior: theoretical prescription for nursing, *ANS* 5(1):41-56, 1982.
11. Ellis R: Conceptual issues in nursing, *Nurs Outlook* 30(7):406-410, 1982.
12. Epp J: *Achieving health for all: a framework for health promotion, health & welfare Canada*, Ottawa, Canada, 1986, Supply and Services Canada.
13. Hancock T: Healthy women and the future, *Health Care Women Int* 8:249-260, 1987.
14. Hannah TE: Health behavior: the role of health as a personal life concern, *Can J Public Health* 78:165-167, 1987.
15. Henderson V: *Nature of nursing*, New York, 1966, MacMillan Publishing.
16. Hubbard P, Muhlenkamp A, Brown N: The relationship between social support and self-care practices, *Nurs Res* 33(5):266-270, 1984.
17. Kelly RB, Zyzanski SJ, Alemagno SA: Prediction of motivation and behavior change following health promotion: role of health beliefs, social support, and self-efficacy, *Soc Sci Med* 32(3):311-320, 1991.

18. King IMA: *A theory for nursing: systems, concepts, processes,* New York, 1981, John Wiley & Sons.

19. Laffrey SC: Health promotion: relevance for nursing, *Top Clin Nurs* 7(2):29-38, 1985.

20. Laffrey SC, Loveland-Cherry CJ, Winkler SJ: Health behavior: evolution of two paradigms, *Public Health Nurs* 3(2):92-100, 1986.

21. Meleis AI: Being and becoming healthy: the core of nursing knowledge, *Nurs Sci Quart* 3(3):107-114, 1990.

22. Moch SM: Health within illness: conceptual evolution and practice possibilities, *ANS* 11(4):23-31, 1989.

23. Neuman B: *The Neuman systems model: application to nursing education and practice,* Norwalk, Conn, 1989, Appleton & Lange.

24. Norman R: Health behavior: the implications of research, *Health Prom* 25(1,2):2-9, 1986.

25. Orem D: *Nursing: concepts of practice,* St Louis, 1991, Mosby–Year Book.

26. Ottawa Charter for Health Promotion: *Health promotion,* 1(4):iii-v, 1986, Health and Welfare Canada.

27. Pender NJ: Health promotion and illness prevention. In Werley HH, Fitzpatrick JJ (editors): *Annual review of nursing research* vol 2, New York, 1987, Springer Publishing.

28. Pender NJ: *Health promotion in nursing practice,* ed 2, Norwalk, Conn, 1987, Appleton & Lange.

29. Rakowski W: Personal health practices, health status and expected control over future health, *J Comm Health* 11(3):189-203, 1986.

30. Rhode Island Department of Health: *Wellness check program,* Rhode Island, 1983.

31. Roy C: *Introduction to nursing: an adaptive model,* ed 2, Englewood Cliffs, NJ, 1983, Prentice Hall.

32. Schoenbach V, Berton BH, Fredman L, Kleinbaum DG: Social ties and mortality in Evans County, Georgia, *Am J Epidemiol* 123(4):577-591, 1986.

33. Skinner HA, Allen BA, McIntosh MC, Palmer WH: Lifestyle assessment: applying computers in family practice, *Br Med J* 290:212-216, 1985.

34. Smith JA: The idea of health: a philosophical inquiry, *ANS* 3(3):43-50, 1981.

35. Stachtchenko S, Jenicek M: Conceptual differences between prevention and health promotion: research implications for community health programs, *C J Public Health* 81(Jan/Feb):53-59, 1990.

36. Williams RL and others: Development of a health habits scale, *Res Nurs Health* 14:145-153, 1991.

37. World Health Organization: *Health promotion: a discussion document on the concept and principle,* Copenhagen, 1984, The Organization.

38. Yoder LE, Jones SL, Jones PK: The association between health care behavior and attitudes, *Health Values* 9(4):24-31, 1985.

39. Zimmerman RS, Connor C: Health promotion in context: the effects of significant others on health behavior change, *Health Edu Q* 16(1):57-75, 1989.

I

Ineffective Management of Therapeutic Regimen

Ineffective Management of Therapeutic Regimen is a pattern of regulating and integrating into daily living a program for treatment of illness and the sequelae of illness that is unsatisfactory for meeting specific health goals.[13]

OVERVIEW

Therapeutic regimens are sets of rules, or habits, of diet, exercise, and manner of living that are intended to improve health and treat or cure disease.[20] The nursing focus of helping persons to manage therapeutic regimens has been explicit and implicit in the nursing literature, particularly in books and articles on chronic illness and descriptions of nursing care for persons with specific health problems such as diabetes.* That nurses help people to manage therapeutic regimens is also evident in other types of sources, e.g., books on culture.[2]

A diagnosis that was reported by Lunney in 1982, Alteration in Management of Illness, provided the basis for this diagnosis.[12] Methods of concept development, i.e., analysis and synthesis of the literature, were used to identify the definition and defining characteristics of the diagnosis.[21]

Making a diagnosis pertaining to client management of therapeutic regimen requires collaboration between nurse and the client.[6,8] Clients participate by making decisions about the fit of therapeutic regimens with their lifestyle and by acting on their decisions. Because the agent for management of therapeutic regimen is the client,

the concept of management of therapeutic regimen includes ability and actions to regulate or integrate therapeutic regimens into daily activities and willingness to pursue improvements in management behaviors.

Nurses' use of this diagnosis assumes that the client is able to manage a therapeutic regimen. If developmental status, cognitive deficits, physical handicaps, or other stable factors prevent clients from managing therapeutic regimens, the diagnosis does not apply except, perhaps, to justify ongoing nursing care for management of therapeutic regimens.

In comparison with the diagnosis of Noncompliance, a related concept, the diagnosis of management of therapeutic regimen is more comprehensive because its' focus is overall self-regulation and integration based on client values and goals rather than merely the compliance to others' instructions.[9] The concept of management of therapeutic regimen implies client decision making and participation in which adherence/nonadherence may be a partial consideration.

The diagnosis of Ineffective management of therapeutic regimen is appropriate for use with individuals, families, and communities. Individuals need to perform health-related regimens in ways that will produce positive outcomes and incorporate them within activities of daily living. These can be relatively simple regimens, such as taking digoxin after assessing pulse rate, to complex regimens, such as management of peritoneal dialysis. Families need to develop, support, and integrate regimens into family life.[1,3] Communities need to develop health care programs and policies for communities groups and populations.[16]

---

*References 5, 7, 10, 11, 15, 17, 18, 19.

I

A national sample of 58 expert nurses from **26** states, the District of Columbia, and Canada who were working in community settings validated this diagnosis.[13] These experts had an impressive amount of experience in helping clients to manage therapeutic regimens (M = 18.8 years), were educated at the baccalaureate degree or higher (77% had Masters or Doctoral degrees), and had a broad base of experiences in working with all developmental stages and in many types of nursing. The Fehring Validation Model was used for analysis of data.[4] Subjects rated each defining characteristic on a scale of one (almost never present) to five (almost always present). The weighted means of these responses were computed to differentiate defining characteristics as major, minor, and low relevance. One defining characteristic was identified as major with a validity index of over .80 (see below). The remaining five defining characteristics were validated as minor, i.e., the weighted means were between .50 and .79.

ASSESSMENT

Assessment of the defining characteristics may be accomplished early in data collection or may require a broad base of data from the eleven functional health patterns. Since the first of the Functional health patterns deals with Health Management, including management of therapeutic regimens, data collection in this pattern may yield sufficient cues to infer that management of therapeutic regimen is ineffective (or effective). However, data generated during assessment of other patterns should either support or refute initial impressions. The diagnosis should be considered as a hypothesis until integration of the therapeutic regimen with daily living is verified through other patterns. For example, a client may first report that taking blood pressure medication is not a problem and later report that sleep pattern is disturbed by having to get up to the bathroom, or recreational trips cannot be made because of poor bladder control. Subsequent data that indicates difficulty with integrating the therapeutic regimen into daily living should raise a suspicion that management of therapeutic regimen needs to be addressed. This suspicion is then validated with the client.

Making this diagnosis requires skill in taking health histories and establishing trusting relationships with clients. A nonjudgmental, caring approach will provide an environment for clients to reveal their everyday patterns of self-management. The diagnosis is based on everyday patterns rather than on observable behavior, therefore the meaning of nonverbal behavior that is incongruent with verbal data should be validated with the client, e.g., a client who says she is on a low salt diet has a packaged coffee cake on the table.

The major defining characteristic—**choices of daily activities for meeting the goals of a treatment or prevention program are ineffective**—reflects that desire and behavior are incongruent. The client may agree to manage, or take charge of, the illness regimen and set goals accordingly, but such agreement does not mean that goals are being met. When clients agree that behaviors can improve, it increases the need to focus on this diagnosis.

The defining characteristic, **acceleration of illness symptoms,** is a cue that the client may need assistance from nurses to manage the regimen, e.g., a diabetic who has a respiratory problem.[14] Because the effectiveness of management of therapeutic regimen is judged relative to specific health goals, defining characteristics include evidence that treatment goals are not being met. Treatment goals usually include controlling the negative effects of illness on daily living and the progression of illness, reducing risk factors for illness and its sequelae, and optimizing activities of daily living with consideration of illness-related needs.

Because health goals should include the integration of illness regimens with daily routines, the defining characteristic—**verbalized that did not take action to include treatment regimens in daily routines**—indicates that client behaviors may be ineffective. Sources on management of chronic illnesses describe a multitude of factors that interfere with integration of treatment regimens in daily routines, including stigma, cultural traditions, and deficits in community resources.[11,15]

An **expressed desire to manage the treatment of illness and prevention of sequelae** may be a request for help in accomplishing these goals. At the very least, this cue should be assessed in making the diagnosis, since client management of therapeutic regimens is probably not possible without the desire to do so.

The defining characteristics—**verbalized difficulty with regulation/integration of treatment or prevention regimen**—is a cue that the person may need help to achieve treatment goals. If clients do not offer this information, nurses, in assessing for the diagnosis, can seek the data by asking appropriate questions, e.g., "how difficult has it been to change your diet?," or validating the meaning of observations.

The defining characteristic—**verbalized that did not take action to reduce risk factors for progression of illness and sequelae**—indicates that health protection is not sufficient. Strategies in the categories of primary, secondary, and tertiary prevention may be indicated depending on the health problem. For example, managing stress, developing an exercise routine, and stopping smoking may prevent progression of heart disease.

Further research is needed to determine if other defining characteristics are appropriate for this diagnosis. Three additional defining characteristics were recommended by individual nurse experts.[13] These are anxiety, reluctance to discuss therapeutic regimen, and incongruence of verbal and nonverbal behaviors. These behaviors may reflect personal conflict between health behavior and values and/or unwillingness to share information about self-management. One explanation for unwillingness to share information is the overall emphasis in the health care system on compliance.[9] If clients expect nurses to focus on compliance, and, perhaps, use power differences to coerce compliance, they may avoid discussing management issues.

❖ **Defining Characteristics**

The presence of the following defining characteristics indicates that the patient may be experiencing Ineffective Management of Therapeutic Regimen.

Major

- Choices of daily living are ineffective for meeting the goals of a treatment or prevention program

Minor

- Acceleration (expected or unexpected) of illness symptoms
- Verbalized desire to manage the treatment of illness or prevention

- Verbalized difficulty with regulation/integration of one or more prescribed regimens for treatment of illness and its effects or prevention of complications
- Verbalized that did not take action to include treatment regimens in ADL
- Verbalized that did not take action to reduce risk factors for progression of illness and sequelae

❖ **Related Factors**

The following related factors are associated with Ineffective Management of Therapeutic Regimen.

- Perceived seriousness
- Perceived susceptibility
- Perceived barriers
- Perceived benefits
- Powerlessness
- Knowledge deficits
- Mistrust of regimen and/or health care personnel
- Decisional conflicts
- Ineffective communication

- Social support deficits
- Family patterns of health care
- Family conflict
- Economic difficulties
- Complexity of therapeutic regimen
- Inadequate number and types of cues to action
- Excessive demands made on individual or family
- Complexity of health care system

❖ Related Medical/Psychiatric Diagnoses

The following are examples of related medical/psychiatric diagnoses for Ineffective Management of Therapeutic Regimen.

- Alzheimer's disease
- Arthritis
- Cancer
- Coronary artery heart disease
- Depression
- Diabetes mellitus
- Inflammatory bowel disease
- Manic-depression
- Nephritis
- Otitis media
- Peripheral vascular disease
- Rheumatic fever

NURSING DIAGNOSES

Examples of *specific* nursing diagnoses for Ineffective Management of Therapeutic Regimen are:

- Ineffective Management of Therapeutic Regimen related to powerlessness regarding illness symptoms
- Ineffective Management of Therapeutic Regimen related to knowledge deficit regarding medications
- Ineffective Management of Therapeutic Regimen related to inaccurate symptom beliefs
- Ineffective Management of Therapeutic Regimen related to social support deficits

PLANNING AND IMPLEMENTATION WITH RATIONALE

Client expected outcomes that are associated with this diagnosis represent improvements in health behaviors that are consistent with health-related goals. Illness is considered as a dimension of health, therefore illness-related goals are subsumed within health-related goals. The expected outcomes stated here are generic to any health problem. In actual client situations, the expected outcomes should be stated according to specific changes in health behavior as well as specific health goals. The generic client outcomes are (1) describes nutrition, activity/exercise, and/or sleep/rest patterns that are consistent with health-related goals, (2) describes medication-taking that is consistent with health-related goals, and (3) verbalizes a feeling of power/control for management of therapeutic regimens.

Nursing interventions for these expected outcomes require a high degree of interpersonal skills. The trusting relationship that was begun during the diagnostic process needs to continue as the client and nurse work together in designing improved health behaviors. *In a mutually trusting relationship, a person can share perceived difficulties, successes, and failures*. The nurse needs to demonstrate respect and trust in the client's decisions through verbal and nonverbal behaviors. For example, if the client refuses to follow particular advice, the nurse should avoid showing anger or hurt feelings. Words, voice control, and body language should continue to show awareness that the power of self-management is within the client, not the nurse, and that the nurse is there as a helper. Knowledge of cultural variations in health management and tolerance for decisions based on individual, family, or cultural factors will help nurses to work with clients on self-management. Types of interventions that are frequently used with this diagnosis are active listening, contracting, values clarification, and culture brokerage.

Nursing interventions to accomplish the first expected outcome are those that help persons to change patterns. A need to integrate therapeutic regimens, e.g., diet, exercise, rest, into daily living is a challenge for all persons because previous habits have already been established based on values and lifestyle. The nurse's acknowledgement of the challenge may be perceived as supportive by the client. *Perceptions of being supported by others are associated with meeting health-related goals*. Other types of social support should be identified and mobilized. Values clarification can be used to identify values that are inconsistent with current behaviors, e.g., the value of controlling blood pressure may be inconsistent with the client's response to stress. Other methods that increase self-awareness, such as body scanning for symptoms may be warranted. *Symptom awareness and beliefs may be inaccurate*.

Nursing interventions for the second expected outcome include helping the client to develop sufficient knowledge bases and daily habits so the goals of taking medications are met and the dangers are minimized. *Medications are foreign sub-*

stances, many of which are harmful or have un-wanted side effects and adverse effects. Although the intention of taking medications is to achieve positive outcomes, self-management practices, such as changing dosages or times and mixing with over-the-counter drugs, may defeat the purpose of taking medications. Other times, self-management practices that differ from medical prescriptions may be better for the client than what was prescribed. In these instances, the nurse can act as advocate for the client or, preferably, help the client with self-advocacy, in reporting this information to the physician or nurse who prescribed the drug. *Self-advocacy promotes on-*

❖ NURSING CARE GUIDELINES

Nursing Diagnosis: *Ineffective Management of Therapeutic Regimen*

Expected Outcomes	Nursing Interventions
Describe nutrition, activity/ exercise, and/or sleep/rest patterns that are consistent with health-related goals.	• Review client's health (and illness) values. • Identify client perceptions of illness progression, match client perceptions with illness trajectory. • Review association between the symptoms that are experienced by the client, client beliefs about the symptoms, and client actions in response to symptoms; provide information or methods to improve accuracy of symptom beliefs and selection of actions. • Assist client to describe daily routines that would be more consistent with health-related goals (specific patterns to be improved depend on the clinical situation, e.g., with diabetis or heart disease, all three patterns may be considered, with myasthenia gravis, the focus may only be on the balance of activity and rest). • Work with client to select changes that are possible, considering factors such as lifestyle (homeless, drug addiction, 12-hour work shifts, single parent, etc.), culture, family dynamics. • Acknowledge the difficulty of changing daily habits and provide support for client efforts. • Provide information to make changes easier, e.g., using lemon or vinegar instead of salt. • Use formal or informal contracting to facilitate desired changes, consider the use of rewards as positive reinforcement. • Identify community resources that will help client repattern, e.g., self help groups, home care.
Describe medication-taking that is consistent with health related goals.	• Analyze current medication-taking practices, including prescribed and over-the-counter drugs. Review client knowledge and beliefs of drugs and drug interactions. With client, determine changes needed in current practices, e.g., dosage, time, methods of taking. • Assist with repatterning through schedules, reminders, associating medications with other activities such as meals. • In the home, ask to see all drugs even drugs not currently taking; discuss advisability of discarding old drugs.

Continued.

I

❖ *NURSING CARE GUIDELINES— cont'd*

Nursing Diagnosis: *Ineffective Management of Therapeutic Regimen*

Expected Outcomes	Nursing Interventions
Verbalize a feeling of power for management of the therapeutic regimen.	• Assist client to evaluate physical strength and design ways to improve strength, e.g., balance activity with rest. • Review social networks and supports, e.g., do a genogram, help client to mobilize supports, support psychological stamina. • Treat the client with utmost respect and dignity at all times to support self esteem; show recognition of other aspects of personhood besides the illness, assist with changes in body image and role performance. • Teach positive self-talk • Discuss and plan energy conservation • Provide information, verbally & in writing, on all aspects of illness regimen, including the rationale for all changes in behavior • Reinforce feelings of competence, mastery, self-efficacy • Identify and support client coping strategies, within usual coping style, that are working to maintain control

going ability to negotiate with health providers for services and resources that are needed. If medication-taking has been working to accomplish the goals and differs from the medical prescription, e.g., client takes a lower dosage of hypertensive drugs, it is probably best to report this to the health provider rather than suggesting that the client take the prescribed dosage. Overall, nursing advice on medication-taking should be based on thorough understanding of the drugs that the client is taking now and others that are in the home, knowledge of each drug, drug interactions, and diagnosis of possible side effects and adverse effects. Drug dosages that the client has been taking for a few days or more should not be increased or decreased, even to follow a prescription, without consulting the health provider who prescribed the drug.

Nursing interventions for the third executed outcome include actions to empower the client for self-management. A useful model for helping clients to attain and maintain a sense of power is Miller's model for coping with chronic illness.[15] Using this model, the nurse fosters the person's resources for power which are physical strength, psychological stamina-social support, positive self concept, energy, knowledge and insight, motivation, and belief system-hope. *Maximizing a person's power resources facilitates the person's ability to cope with illness. Coping with illness includes many specific tasks, including modifying daily routines to accommodate therapeutic regimens.*[15] The nurse should note that knowledge is only one of the power resources. *Knowledge is necessary but not sufficient for management of therapeutic regimens.* Supporting the client's individual coping style (approach, avoidance, or nonspecific) and effective coping strategies also enhances the nurse's ability to foster a sense of power.

EVALUATION

The expected outcomes related to this diagnosis are evaluated by maintaining a continued relationship with the client and speaking to the client, either in person or by phone, regarding improvements in management strategies. With shortened hospital stays, hospital nurses may have to refer

I

❖ *CASE STUDY WITH PLAN OF CARE*

Mrs. Sarah E. is a 74-year-old female who has been hypertensive for 15 years and was admitted three days ago for hypertensive crisis. A review of health patterns prior to hospitalization reveals that most of the time she took medications as prescribed, but, at times, she did not get new prescriptions filled in time and omitted some dosages. She has a low salt diet and understands it, but often does not follow it. Since her husband's death two years ago, she has been living with her son and daughter-in-law, Jane. She has not spoken with Jane about her health related needs because she thinks that Jane does not want her to live with them, and she does not have experience in relationships with younger women. Jane does all the shopping and cooking in the family. Jane has not approached Mrs. E. about the illness regimen.

PLAN OF CARE FOR MRS. SARAH E.

Nursing Diagnosis: Ineffective management of therapeutic regimen related to communication gap between Mrs. E. and daughter-in-law.

Expected Outcomes	Nursing Interventions
Mrs. E. will set up a meeting among herself, daughter-in-law, and nurse for discharge planning.	• After validating the diagnosis with Mrs. E., discuss the rationale for ongoing effective management including taking meds, low salt diet, weight control, and stress management.[17] • Assess and support power resources, such as physical strength, self esteem, belief system, etc. • Provide information as needed for stress management, e.g., dealing with family conflict. • Review the various ways that Mrs. E. can communicate her needs to Jane. • Assist Mrs. E. to select a specific means of asking Jane to meet with her and nurse for planning future strategies, e.g., ask Mrs. E. to rehearse what she would say, offer ideas as needed.
Mrs. E. will plan strategies for future management with daughter-in-law (and, perhaps, son).	• During the meeting, support Mrs. E. as she tells her daughter-in-law about her illness regimen and problem solves with her regarding the best ways to manage. • Consider ways of increasing independence of Mrs. E. • Discuss the role of son in helping mother with therapeutic regimen. • Refer to home care if nursing diagnosis is not resolved.

patients to home care for follow-up and evaluation. For persons with chronic illnesses, ongoing connections with self help groups and support groups are excellent ways to facilitate continued management, especially when there are changes in health status. If the client is unable to report improvements in health behaviors as planned, the nurse and client should consider whether the goals/objectives are still plausible considering health potentials and is additional assistance needed from the nurse or others.

REFERENCES

1. Bomar PJ: *Nurses and family health promotion: Concepts, assessment, and interventions,* Baltimore, 1989, Williams & Wilkins.
2. Boyle JS, Andrews MM: *Transcultural concepts in nursing care.* Boston, 1989, Scott, Foresman/Little, Brown.
3. Evans BS: The family as a unit in the management of diabetes, *Home Healthcare Nurse* 6(5):10-13, 1988.
4. Fehring R: Methods to validate nursing diagnoses, *Heart & Lung* 16:625-629, 1987.
5. Frenn MD, Borgeson DS, Lee HA, Simandl G: Lifestyle changes in a cardiac rehabilitation program, *Journal of Cardiovascular Nursing* 3(2):43-55, 1989.

6. Fromer MJ: Paternalism in health care, *Nursing Outlook* 29:284-290, 1981.
7. Germain CP, Nemchik RM: Diabetes self-management and hospitalization, *Image: The Journal of Nursing Scholarship* 20(2):74-78, 1988.
8. Kim HS: Collaborative decision making in nursing practice: A theoretical framework, In PL Chinn, *Advances in nursing theory development* (271-283), Rockville, MD, 1983, Aspen.
9. Kontz MM: Compliance redefined and implications for home care, *Holistic Nursing Practice* 3(2):54-64, 1989.
10. Laffrey SC, Crabtree MK: Health and health behavior of persons with chronic cardiovascular disease, *International Journal of Nursing Studies* 25(1):41-52, 1988.
11. Lubkin IM: *Chronic illness: Impact and interventions,* ed 2, Boston, 1990, Jones & Bartlett.
12. Lunney M: Nursing diagnosis: Refining the system, *American Journal of Nursing* 82:456-459, 1982.
13. Lunney M: *The concept of management of therapeutic regimen: Validation of four nursing diagnoses,* Unpublished paper submitted to NANDA, 1991.
14. Mackowiak L, McCarthy R: Managing diabetes on "sick days," *American Journal of Nursing* 88(7):950-951, 1989.
15. Miller JF: *Coping with chronic illness: Overcoming powerlessness,* ed 2, Philadelphia, 1992, FA Davis.
16. Pender NJ: *Health promotion in nursing practice,* ed 2, Norwalk, CT, 1987, Appleton-Lange.
17. Powers MJ, Jalowiec A: Profile of the well-controlled, well-adjusted hypertensive patient, *Nursing Research* 36:106-110, 1987.
18. Snyder TE: An exercise program for dialysis patients, *American Journal of Nursing* 89:362-364, 1989.
19. Strauss AL, Glaser BG: *Chronic illness and the quality of life,* St Louis, 1975, Mosby–Year Book.
20. Thorndike EL, Barnhart CL: *Scott, Foresman Advanced Dictionary,* Glenview, Il, 1979, Scott, Foresman.
21. Walker L, Avant K: *Strategies for theory construction in nursing,* ed 2, Norwalk, CT, 1988, Appleton-Lange.

II

NUTRITIONAL AND METABOLIC PATTERN

Altered Nutrition: High Risk for More Than Body Requirements

Altered Nutrition: More Than Body Requirements

Altered Nutrition: Less Than Body Requirements

Altered Nutrition: High Risk for More Than Body Requirements *is the state in which an individual is at risk of experiencing an intake of nutrients that exceeds metabolic needs.*

Altered Nutrition: More than Body Requirements *is the state in which an individual is experiencing an intake of nutrients that exceeds metabolic needs.*

Altered Nutrition: Less Than Body Requirements *is the state in which an individual experiences an intake of nutrients insufficient to meet metabolic needs.*

OVERVIEW

Nutrition is the "sum of the processes by which a living organism ingests, digests, absorbs, transports, uses, and excretes nutrients and their metabolites".[25] Alterations in nutrition, either more than or less than body requirements, may be the result of a wide variety of physiologic, psychologic, sociocultural, and environmental factors.

Altered Nutrition: High Risk for More than Body Requirements or Altered Nutrition: More than Body Requirements is a human response prevalent in the United States today. Approximately 25% of the adults and 5% to 15% of the children in the United States have excess body weight, and another 33% face a constant battle to keep their weight within the limits considered normal.[14] This health problem continues to rise in spite of the numerous commercial diets and exercise facilities available.

All activities require energy in the form of calories derived from carbohydrates, protein, and fat. A state of energy balance can be calculated by comparing energy intake with energy output. Body fat is formed and weight increases when one consumes more calories than are expended. For example, if a person consumes 500 extra cal-

II

ories a day for 7 days with no increase in exercise, he or she will gain 1 pound of body fat, which is equal to 3,500 calories.[12] *Overweight* is defined as weight in excess of one's desired weight in comparison with recommended weight for age; *obesity* is an excess of body fat.[4] Obesity is categorized as follows:

- Mild obesity: 120% to 140% of ideal body weight.
- Moderate obesity: 141% to 200% of ideal body weight.
- Severe or morbid obesity: >200% of ideal body weight.

Overeating was long believed to be the main cause of weight gain and obesity, but now several theories have been formulated to attempt to explain the etiology of this problem. The theories can be grouped into four categories: (1) hereditary, (2) environmental, (3) physiologic, and (4) psychologic.

Heredity is a major factor in determining whether an adult will be obese. Successions of family generations tend to show the same amount of weight gain and body configuration, supporting heredity as a strong influence in obesity. Obese children do tend to have parents who are also overweight or obese.[31] When one parent is obese, children have a 40% chance of also being obese; when both parents are obese the chance increases to 80%.[4] Research has indicated that adopted children have different patterns of weight gain than their adoptive parents and siblings.[17] The "fat cell" theory supports the belief that obese individuals of all ages tend to have more fat cells than do children and adults of normal weight. Although cell size can decrease with dieting, the number of fat cells remains constant, making weight loss difficult because of the energy needed by these cells.[5]

Home, work, and sociocultural environment also influence the type and amount of food one consumes and the activity in which one participates. Fatness tends to be passed from generation to generation, making the eating habits and customs of a family important environmental factors when considering a risk for obesity. For example,

unattended bottle feeding of infants, using food as a comfort measure, overfeeding, and valuing chubbiness in babies are contributors to early development of obesity.[31] Using food as a reward for good behavior and allowing children to eat nutritionally inadequate foods can result in excess weight in later years.[3,24] An association also exists between hours of television viewing and obesity in adolescents.[10] Another environmental factor that influences weight gain is level of income and educational level. For women, the lower the income and education, the greater the incidence of obesity. For men, obesity is more common in higher income brackets and with higher educational levels et al.[16]

Physiologic bases for obesity include the set point theory, thermogenesis, and endocrine imbalances. The set point theory states that each person has an ideal biological weight, established by biological or genetic factors and controlled by the hypothalamus. When fat stores fall below a certain level, the body adjusts its metabolic rate to maintain its adipose tissue, making it impossible for some people to lose weight.[5] Thermogenesis is heat production that rids the body of excess energy. People of normal weight have an increase in thermogenesis after eating, whereas obese people tend to have a lower thermogenic response to eating. This may be due to a lower availability of adenosine diphosphate–burning sites, which are responsible for utilizing energy not associated with physical activity.[30] An insufficiency of thyroid hormone may lower basal metabolic rate, leading to weight gain. Obesity is also related to adipose and muscle cell insulin resistance, contributing to non–insulin dependent diabetes mellitus.

Psychologic causes for obesity are more difficult to identify. Research has found that persons with strong support systems, positive self-esteem, and healthy relationships participate in lifestyles and eating habits that promote health.[18,23] Positive correlations have also been found between depression and weight gain,[26] and between negative body-image and overweight in females.[27]

Altered Nutrition: Less Than Body Requirements is found in all age groups, at any point on the health-illness continuum, and in all sociocultural and economic classes. Persons most at risk for nutritional deficits are those with low income, the elderly, and hospitalized patients. The last group is especially prone to have a deficit in nutrition, with some degree of malnutrition reported in 12% to 48% of newly admitted patients. Additionally, nutritional parameters have been found to deteriorate in more than 50% of all inpatients receiving care.[6,20]

When the intake of nutrients is at a level of less than body requirements, certain adaptive changes take place. Glycogen stores are depleted during starvation, and the fasting body begins to break down proteins and fats to maintain blood glucose levels. As the body loses its protein and fat stores, a negative nitrogen balance results. Healthy individuals of normal weight can lose only 35% to 40% of their normal weight. This figure represents about one third of total body protein, with loss exceeding this amount being fatal. If the person is deficient in nutrients and weight, a smaller loss is critical.[12]

Nutritional deficits may be classified as either primary or secondary. Primary deficiencies are the result of failure to meet normal nutritional needs because of an inadequate food intake. The deficit may result from poor food habits, lack of knowledge about selecting and preparing foods, inadequate economic resources, and/or lack of facilities to prepare and store food.[19] Secondary nutritional deficits occur when other factors interfere with the utilization of nutrients, even though the diet is sufficient.[25] Interference with nutrient utilization places an individual at risk for pathophysiologic changes and can occur in such varied states as growth spurts, pregnancy, chemical dependency, anorexia nervosa, disease, and pharmacotherapeutic treatments.

ASSESSMENT

Relevant assessment tools and guides for this cluster of nursing diagnoses are: (1) a nursing history with dietary intake data, (2) anthropometric measurements, and (3) biochemical findings.

Each of these assessments will be discussed in this section.

The Nursing History

The nursing history with dietary intake information provides supporting data for the diagnoses. The nurse should include age, gender, past and present medical history, drug use, family history and structure, religious and cultural background, and income. Specific questions to be asked related to the patient's ability to chew and swallow; appetite; food preferences and intolerances; and bowel habits.[9] The dietary assessment guides used as part of the history are:

- The 24-hour food recall to record all types and amounts of food eaten in the past 24 hours,
- The food frequency record, with a checklist to indicate how often specific foods or general food groups are eaten, and
- A food record, which is a diary of all food and beverages consumed over a specific period of time (usually 3 to 7 days).

A dietary log may be useful in assessing nutritional habits and status. The patient should keep this log for at least 2 weeks, and it should include: time of day food is eaten, minutes spent eating, activity while eating, location of meals, type and quantity of food, other people present, feelings about the experience while eating, and daily weight. The patient should hang the log in an easily seen place so that it is convenient to use. At first the patient may dislike the work involved in keeping the dietary log, but this activity serves as a basis for the plan of care and is essential for mutual exploration by the patient and nurse of alternatives to modify past eating behaviors.

Subjective data also includes eating patterns (time of day, type of preparation, setting, reason for eating). Any cultural or religious influences on dietary habits should be explored. Information obtained from these guides is highly subjective and depends on normal cognitive function.

During the nursing history assessing the patient's level of motivation is pertinent. What value does the patient see in weight gain or loss? Does the patient feel capable of gaining or losing weight? What reasons does the patient verbalize for wanting to gain or lose weight?[21] If reasons are based on social or family pressure, the patient will probably not succeed.

The nurse can assess the patient's body image and self-esteem by listening to the patient talk about self and interactions with others. What is the patient's level of socialization? Does this patient have meaningful goals for self and feel accepted by others? Social and family support is essential for adjusting one's weight.

Anthropometric Measurements

Objective data can be obtained through anthropometric measurements, including height, weight, skin (fat) folds, and arm circumference, using the following guidelines:

Height: Height should be measured with the patient barefoot and standing as straight as possible with feet, buttocks, and head touching the wall.

Weight: Weight should be taken at the same time each day, wearing minimal clothing. The Metropolitan Life Insurance (1983) table (Table 1) can be used as a reference for ideal weight. However, tables such as this do not consider age factors or body fat content. Another method of calculating ideal adult body weight follows:
- Men: allow 106 pounds for 5 feet of height, add 6 pounds for each additional inch over 5 feet, and subtract 10% for small frame or add 10% for large frame;
- Women: allow 100 pounds for 5 feet of height, add 5 pounds for each additional inch over 5 feet, and subtract 10% for small frame or add 10% for large frame.

Triceps skinfold: Triceps skinfold (TSF) is measured by using plastic or metal calipers to measure a skin fold on the nondominant arm. With the arm in a dependent position, grasp a fold of skin at the midpoint on the posterior aspect of the upper arm. Apply the caliper and take a reading after waiting 3 seconds. Fat stores (and triceps skinfold measurements) increase with obe-

Table 2   Height and Weight Tables for Adults

	MEN				WOMEN		
Height	Small Frame	Medium Frame	Large Frame	Height	Small Frame	Medium Frame	Large Frame
5'2"	128-134	131-141	138-150	4'10"	102-111	109-121	118-131
5'3"	130-136	133-143	140-153	4'11"	103-113	111-123	120-134
5'4"	132-138	135-145	142-156	5'10"	104-115	113-126	122-137
5'5"	134-140	137-148	144-160	5'1"	106-118	115-129	125-140
5'6"	136-142	139-151	146-164	5'2"	108-121	118-132	128-143
5'7"	138-145	142-154	149-168	5'3"	111-124	121-135	131-147
5'8"	140-148	145-157	152-172	5'4"	114-127	124-138	134-151
5'9"	142-151	148-160	155-176	5'5"	117-130	127-141	137-155
5'10"	144-154	151-163	158-180	5'6"	120-133	130-144	140-159
5'11"	146-157	154-166	161-184	5'7"	123-136	133-147	143-163
6'0"	149-160	157-170	164-188	5'8"	126-139	136-150	146-167
6'1"	152-164	160-174	168-192	5'9"	129-142	139-153	149-170
6'2"	155-168	164-178	172-197	5'10"	132-145	142-156	152-173
6'3"	158-172	167-182	176-202	5'11"	135-148	145-159	155-176
6'4"	162-176	171-187	181-207	6'0"	138-151	148-162	158-179

Source of basic data: 1979 Build Study, Society of Actuaries and Association of Life Insurance Medical Directors of America, 1980.
Reproduced with permission of the Metropolitan Life Insurance Company (copyright 1983).

sity and decrease with successful weight loss or long-standing malnutrition. The following may be used for reference in evaluation of TSF anthropometric readings:[15]

	Adult TSF (mm)		
	Standard reference	>90%	<60%
Men	12.5	> 11.3	< 7.5
Women	16.5	> 14.9	< 9.9

Midarm muscle circumference: A measurement of midarm muscle circumference (MAMC) reflects muscle mass status. The nurse uses a tape measure to measure the circumference of the nondominant arm at the midpoint (which is half-way between the acrominal process and the olecranon process). MAMC decreases with severe muscle-wasting in protein-calorie malnutrition and increases with obesity and muscle hypertrophy. The following may be used for reference in evaluation of MAMC anthropometric readings:[15]

	Adult MAMC (cm)		
	Standard reference	>90%	<60%
Men	25.3	>22.8	<15.2
Women	23.2	>20.9	<13.9

Other calculations and assessments: It is also important to calculate caloric requirements to determine an adequate weight-loss or weight-gain plan. Several factors can alter caloric requirements, including age, gender, and state of health. The United States Department of Agriculture's (USDA) guideline to calculate calorie requirements is to multiply ideal body weight (Table 2) by the number of pounds designated for the patient's gender and level of activity (Table 3). These measurements provide an objective baseline for the nurse and patient as the plan of care is developed.

Physical assessments provide important find-

Table 3 USDA Guidelines for Calculating Caloric Requirements

	Activity Level		
Sex	Sedentary	Moderate	Heavy
Males	16	21	28
Females	14	18	22

Data from Dudek G: *Nutrition handbook for nursing practice,* Philadelphia, 1987, JB Lippincott.

ings, especially for the patient who is malnourished. Physical assessments that indicate nutritional status that is less than body requirements are summarized in Table 4.

Biochemical Data

Biochemical data, especially useful for nutritional deficits, are serum albumin (normal = 4 to 5 g/dl) and transferring (normal = 205 to 410 mg/dl). A low total lymphocyte count is also commonly found when nutrition is less than body requirements. Nitrogen balance can be measured and used as an indicator of anabolism or catabolism of protein. A negative nitrogen balance indicates a catabolic state in which protein is lost from muscles and other tissues and metabolic demands are not being met.[9]

Altered Nutrition: High Risk for More than Body Requirements
❖ Risk Factors

The presence of the following behaviors, conditions, or circumstances render the patient more vulnerable to Altered Nutrition: High Risk for More than Body Requirements:

- Obesity in one or both parents
- Rapid growth in infants/children
- Solid foods as major food source before 5 months of age
- Dysfunctional eating patterns
- Eating in response to cues other than hunger
- Using food for rewards
- Low self-esteem

II

Table 4 Physical Assessments Indicative of Altered Nutrition: Less Than Body Requirements

Body Area Assessed	Abnormal Data
Hair	Dull, dry, brittle, sparse
Eyes	Xerophthalmia; Bitot's spots; increased vascularity; keratomalacia
Lips, buccal cavity	Cheilosis; angular fissures; red, swollen lesions
Tongue	Smooth, swollen, beefy red, atrophic papillae
Gums	Spongy, recessed, bleed easily
Skin	Rough, dry, pale, petechiae; lacking subcutaneous fat; loss of turgor
Muscles	Wasted, flaccid; tenderness; weakness; loss of tone
Nervous system	Decreased or absent knee and ankle reflexes; lethargy; irritability
Cardiovascular	Cardiomegaly; bradycardia at rest and tachycardia with exercise; hypotension
Skeletal	Prominent ribs, scapula; bowed legs or knock-knees
Abdomen	Enlarged, hepatomegaly

❖ **Related Medical/Psychiatric Diagnoses**

The following are examples of related psychiatric/medical diagnoses for Altered Nutrition: High Risk for More Than Body Requirements:

- Cushing's syndrome
- Hypothalamic disorders
- Hypothyroidism
- Major depression
- Non–insulin dependent diabetes mellitus

❖ **Defining Characteristics**

The presence of the following defining characteristics indicates that the patient may be experiencing Altered Nutrition: More Than Body Requirements:

- Weight 10% to 20% over ideal for height and body frame
- Triceps >15 mm in males; >25 mm in females
- Dysfunctional eating patterns
- Sedentary lifestyle

❖ **Related Factors**

The following related factors are associated with Altered Nutrition: More Than Body Requirements:

- Intake greater than metabolic need
- Heredity; obesity in parents
- Lower metabolic rate
- Income
- Educational level
- Eating patterns
- Family customs
- Family values

- Thermogenetic response
- Stress
- Depression
- Lack of support systems
- Low self-esteem

❖ **Related Medical/Psychiatric Diagnoses**

The following are examples of related medical/psychiatric diagnoses for Altered Nutrition: More Than Body Requirements:

- Hypercholesteremia
- Hypertension
- Hypothyroidism
- Non–insulin dependent diabetes mellitus
- Polycythemia vera

Altered Nutrition: Less than Body Requirements
❖ **Defining Characteristics**

The presence of the following defining characteristics indicates that the patient may be experiencing Altered Nutrition: Less Than Body Requirements:

- 10% to 20% below ideal body weight
- Low serum albumin
- Low serum transferring
- Triceps skinfold or arm circumference <60% standard
- Sore, inflamed buccal cavity
- Weak chewing or swallowing muscles
- Abdominal cramping/pain
- Poor muscle tone
- Altered taste sensation
- Lack of interest in food
- Lack of information
- Perceived inability to ingest food
- Aversion to food

❖ Related Factors

The following related factors are associated with Altered Nutrition: Less Than Body Requirements:

- Stress
- Peer pressure
- Poor living conditions
- Inadequate income
- Pregnancy
- Homelessness
- Social influences
- Lack of transportation
- Lack of knowledge

❖ Related Medical/Psychiatric Diagnoses

The following are examples of related medical/psychiatric diagnoses for Altered Nutrition: Less Than Body Requirements:

- Achlorhydria
- Acquired immunodeficiency syndrome
- Allergies
- Burns
- Cancer
- Chemotherapy
- Cirrhosis
- Congenital anomalies
- Diarrhea
- Eating disorders (anorexia nervosa, bulimic disorder)
- Edentulous condition
- Endocrine disorders
- Gastrointestinal surgery
- Major depression
- Parasite infestation
- Radiation therapy
- Substance use disorders

NURSING DIAGNOSES

Examples of *specific* nursing diagnoses for Altered Nutrition: High Risk for More Than Body Requirements are:

- Altered Nutrition: High Risk for More Than Body Requirements related to lifestyle that includes frequent fast-food meals
- Altered Nutrition: High Risk for More Than Body Requirements related to habit of eating high-calorie foods while watching television and aversion to exercise

Examples of *specific* nursing diagnoses for Altered Nutrition: More Than Body Requirements are:

- Altered Nutrition: More Than Body Requirements related to sedentary lifestyle and lack of knowledge about diet and exercise
- Altered Nutrition: More Than Body Requirements related to dysfunctional patterns of eating

Examples of *specific* nursing diagnoses for Altered Nutrition: Less Than Body Requirements are:

- Altered Nutrition: Less Than Body Requirements related to loss of appetite secondary to chemotherapy
- Altered Nutrition: Less Than Body Requirements related to difficulty swallowing secondary to radiation therapy
- Altered Nutrition: Less Than Body Requirements related to low income and lack of transportation to buy food

PLANNING AND IMPLEMENTATION WITH RATIONALE
Altered Nutrition: High Risk For More Than Body Requirements

The implications of obesity for health are an important component in teaching the client with Altered Nutrition: High Risk for More Than Body Requirements. *Patient/health education is the teaching-learning process of influencing patient and family behavior through changes in knowledge, attitudes, and beliefs.*[7] Education should include an explanation of what obesity is and what specific factors increase the potential for its development. The implications for health include a discussion of the effects of excess body weight on the cardiovascular system, on longevity, and on mental health.

Behavioral modification begins with self-monitoring. The patient should keep a dietary log for 1 week. *Patient and nurse analysis of the log will demonstrate eating patterns, including which stimuli lead to eating, types of foods eaten, what precipitates eating, most likely times and places for eating, and amount of exercise.* Patterns of food intake that result in obesity can be identified and a plan made for modifications.

The patient must know how to make proper food choices when developing menus. *By knowing basic body requirements, the patient can make informed choices for meals and snacks.* The nurse should teach about the four food groups; the distribution of proteins, carbohydrates, and fats in foods that are a part of the patient's normal diet; and the requirements for this specific patient.

The nurse should help the patient identify and plan modifications of behaviors that are associated with excess food intake. This may include such modifications as eating only when sitting at the table with a complete place setting, eliminating reading or watching television while eating, taking small bites and chewing thoroughly, placing the fork on the plate between bites, drinking water before and during meals, and learning the difference between appetite and hunger. *All of these behaviors are helpful in controlling the amount of food intake.*

Physical activity is an essential component in any weight-control program. The exercise program should be based on activities identified in the health history or dietary log, and should include gradual increments in increased exercise. *Exercise, when a part of a diet program, increases weight loss through loss of fat rather than muscle and also improves muscle tone, cardiopulmonary status, and mental attitude.*[28]

Individuals who become overweight or obese often have lower self-esteem than those of normal weight. *A higher level of self-esteem may enhance motivation to lose weight.*[2] The nurse should include in a teaching plan mutual goal setting that is realistic in terms of actual food intake, change in eating behaviors, and exercise program. *Unrealistic expectations about weight loss or exercise capability may lead to feelings of defeat and failure, which in turn can cause the patient to give up and return to previous weight increasing behaviors.*

Altered Nutrition: More Than Body Requirements

Counseling and referrals for social support are essential in promoting successful, long-lasting, healthy eating habits. An individual's eating behaviors are influenced by people with whom he/she interacts daily.[13] People who influence food choices include the spouse, family members, coworkers, colleagues, and peers. Other influences on eating behaviors include ethnic and cultural

backgrounds, family traditions, age group, and environmental factors such as type of employment and hours worked. The spouse and family must understand and be involved in the patient's weight-loss program for success in meeting goals. Patients should be encouraged to participate in weight-loss competitions at their place of employment, and to join community programs such as Weight Watchers or Take Off Pounds Sensibly (TOPS).

Monitoring patient activities will identify behaviors that can be changed or that increase caloric expenditure. For example, the patient may decide to park the car a longer distance from work and walk the remaining distance or take stairs rather than ride elevators. The patient may also become involved in a regular exercise program at a community recreation center. Before participating in any exercise program, the patient should have a thorough health assessment, following the recommendations of the American College of Sports Medicine. The behavior changes that are mutually agreed on should be written in contract form; allowing some type of reward for each successful behavior change may facilitate patient compliance. *Eating and exercise habits are learned behaviors and can be modified by specific behavioral strategies.*

The nurse has an important role in teaching the patient how to restrict calories and maintain a nutritionally sound diet.[21] Calories should come from all four food groups and not fall below 1,000 to 1,200 calories per day for women and 1,200 to 1,500 calories per day for men. To calculate calorie restriction, determine the recommended caloric requirement for ideal body weight and subtract the necessary number of calories per day for desired weight loss (for example, 500 calories per day results in a weight loss of one pound per week; 1,000 calories per day results in a weight loss of two pounds per week).[12] Encourage patients to read food labels and to be aware of calorie and fat content of foods. *The patient should consume only enough calories to promote a one- to two-pound weight loss each week. Limiting fat intake can greatly decrease calorie intake.*

❖ *NURSING CARE GUIDELINES*

Nursing Diagnosis: Altered Nutrition: High Risk for More Than Body Requirements

Expected Patient Outcomes	Nursing Interventions
The patient will identify own risk factors and defining characteristics that promote potential for weight gain.	• Teach the patient hereditary, environmental, physiological, and psychological factors that predispose to weight gain. • Discuss the patient's current health status in relation to defining characteristics and risk factors of this diagnosis.
The patient will monitor own eating habits and activities for 1 week, then identify behaviors that need modification to prevent weight gain.	• Explain the process of keeping a daily diary. • Contact the patient midweek to determine compliance and offer assistance. • Analyze the diary with the patient, and assist with identification of needed behavioral changes.
The patient will develop 1-week menus based on own caloric and nutritional needs.	• Teach the patient his or her normal weight range, four basic food groups, recommended caloric intake, and use of food substitution/exchanges.
The patient will change two eating-related behaviors per week that might cause weight gain.	• Discuss the effects on intake of concurrent activities, rigid eating schedule, rapid eating, and varied eating locations. • Assist the patient in choosing behaviors to be changed. • Positively reinforce each successful behavior change. • Support the patient through each failure.
The patient will establish a physical activity routine, reaching 20 to 30 minutes duration four or five times per week.	• Teach the patient initial steps: using stairs instead of elevator, walking to destinations. • Start the patient on a regular walking program, with gradually increasing distances. • Investigate more vigorous activities with the patient, with the advice of a physician.
The patient will show evidence of improved self-image by making positive statements about self and taking initiative in setting goals.	• Use a nonjudgmental approach toward the patient's behavior. • Avoid critical comments when the patient fails to meet specific goals. • Encourage realistic short-term goals. • Establish a reward system with the patient. • Encourage the patient to make choices and take responsibility for actions.

II

❖ *NURSING CARE GUIDELINES*

Nursing Diagnosis: *Altered Nutrition: More Than Body Requirements*

Expected Patient Outcomes	Nursing Interventions
The patient will identify some form of social support for dieting and exercise.	• Inform the patient of the significance of social support in influencing eating and exercise habits. • Provide information on community programs. • Inform the family of their role in the patient's success. • Explore programs at the patient's work setting.
The patient will monitor weight, diet, and exercise activities for 2 weeks to identify those activities and eating habits that can be changed to reduce calorie intake and increase energy expenditure.	• Teach the patient the methods and significance of self-assessment and rewards in promoting weight loss.
The patient will reduce calorie intake by 500 calories a day for each pound of weight loss per week.	• Teach the patient how to calculate ideal body weight and calorie restriction. • Teach the patient methods of decreasing calorie intake.
The patient will participate in a plan of exercise for 20 to 30 minutes three to four times a week.	• Assist the patient with developing an individualized exercise plan.
The patient will verbalize an improvement in feelings about self.	• Allow the patient to make decisions in planning care. • Encourage rewards for success.

Obese people often resist exercise because of embarrassment caused by poor body image and/or discomfort caused by excess weight. The patient should start any exercise program slowly and build up to 20 to 30 minutes of exercise three to four times a week. Elevating the resting heart rate to between 40% and 60% of its maximum rate will burn up stored fat as energy. *Exercise increases metabolic rate, suppresses appetite, reduces fat percentage, lowers blood pressure, lowers serum glucose and lipid levels, relieves tension, and improves self-concept.*[29]

Altered Nutrition: Less Than Body Requirements

The plan of care to improve nutrition for patients with Altered Nutrition: Less Than Body Requirements must include activities to meet a variety of physical and psychosocial needs. In most instances, expected patient outcomes are long-term, with improvement taking 6 to 18 months' time. Despite this long time period, nursing interventions are beneficial in meeting nutritional needs and in coordinating nutritional care activities at any level of deficiency.

❖ *NURSING CARE GUIDELINES*

Nursing diagnosis: *Altered Nutrition: Less Than Body Requirements*

Expected Patient Outcomes	Nursing Interventions
The patient will identify the factors that cause nutritional deficits.	• Discuss with the patient significant risk factors. • Document nutritional status with physical assessments, anthropometric measurements, nursing history, and food history and patterns.
The patient will improve and maintain food intake to meet metabolic demands.	• Encourage verbalization by the patient and the family of preferred mealtimes, meal locations, and food likes and dislikes. • Monitor and document daily weight, laboratory data, and food consumed. • Provide personal care and environment conducive to enhanced appetite: oral hygiene, clean surroundings, and encouragement of family members to bring food from home and visit during mealtimes. • Schedule procedures so they do not conflict with meals. • Administer ordered medications for pain or nausea.
The patient will participate in activities necessary to reduce or eliminate risk factors.	• Teach the patient and the family nutritional guidelines, risk factors, and self-care activities. • Refer as needed to physician, dietitian, social worker, minister, support groups, and/or community agencies.

The reasons for nutritional deficits as well as significant risk factors should be discussed with the patient. *The patient will identify factors causing nutritional deficits; understanding the cause of problems often helps reduce anxiety and facilitates compliance with the plan of care).*[8]

Interventions to facilitate improved nutrition are both independent and collaborative. Independent interventions include oral hygiene, positioning, food service, and schedule coordination. *Good oral hygiene improves the taste of food, making it more palatable, and also helps prevent oral infections. Proper positioning is necessary for chewing and swallowing. Foods that are palatable and of correct texture and temperature can improve appetite. Procedures should be scheduled so they do not interfere with mealtimes.*[19] Environmental interventions to improve appetite and food intake include the elimination or reduction of un-

pleasant sights, sounds, and odors to make eating more pleasurable.

Psychosocial support can be provided by therapeutic communications, by encouraging participation in meals by family members or other significant others, and by referrals to community agencies, therapists, or other health care providers (such as social workers, dietitians, or ministers). The patient should always be involved to increase self-esteem and to promote psychological security. *Psychosocial support reduces stress, increases socialization, and facilitates meeting love and belonging needs.*

Diet teaching involves the nurse, the patient, and other members of the health-care team. *The patient and family must be actively involved in the plan to improve compliance and to promote independent self-care.*[32] Included in the plan should be nutritional guidelines, risk factors, and self-care activities to improve nutrition. If nutritional status does not improve, referrals should be made for supplemental or parenteral feedings, psychological counseling, and/or community support systems.

EVALUATION
Altered Nutrition: High Risk For More Than Body Requirements

The plan of care for the patient with Altered Nutrition: High Risk for More Than Body Requirements requires ongoing evaluation throughout the implementation period. The nurse and patient should meet at least once each week to evaluate the previous week and plan the following week's activities. Evaluation should include food choices, eating-related behavior changes, and amount of physical activity. The nurse facilitates change by encouraging the patient to evaluate self in a positive manner, focusing on successes and finding alternative approaches to failure.

Altered Nutrition: More Than Body Requirements

The nurse and the patient mutually evaluate the plan of care for the Altered Nutrition: More Than Body Requirements. Progress is measured by the goals that have been established for weight loss. The nurse and patient together must decide which goals are being met, which are not, and which require modification. They should consider the following: Is the patient's desired weight being attained? Is the patient modifying eating behaviors? Is the patient participating in a regular exercise program? Is the patient's nutritional status adequate? Does the patient feel better about self?

Altered Nutrition: Less Than Body Requirements

The nursing care plan for Altered Nutrition: Less Than Body Requirements is successful if the patient can verbally identify the factors causing the nutritional deficit, is actively involved in activities that decrease or eliminate risk factors, and demonstrates improved or normal physical nutritional status.

❖ *CASE STUDY WITH PLAN OF CARE*

Juanita L., a 56-year-old widow, was born and raised in Puerto Rico until age 20, when she came to New York to live. She is the mother of 7 children, all of whom live within 10 miles of her apartment. Mrs. L. is the manager of the housekeeping department of a major hotel. Because she had been having frequent headaches, Mrs. L. came to the neighborhood clinic to have her blood pressure taken. Physical findings on her initial visit included a blood pressure of 156/90, respirations of 24/minute, and radial pulse of 84/minute. Her height was 5 feet 2 inches, weight 160 pounds, TSF 30 mm, and MAMC 25 cm. Mrs. L. drives a car to and from work, where she often spends 10 to 12 hours on the job. Her job responsibilities require her to sit for long periods of time doing paper work and mak-ing telephone calls. After work, Mrs. L. spends most evenings relaxing at home watching television. Most meals are from fast-food restaurants or the hotel employee canteen. Mrs. L. spends her weekends cooking for her children and their families. She states "We always have a big family get-together on Sundays at my place. I cook traditional family foods for us, and we just sit, visit, and eat all day." Caloric intake is estimated to be 2,800 calories per day; caloric requirement is 1,680 calories per day. Mrs. L. tells the nurse, "I keep gaining weight! I try not to order french fries at lunch—I just eat hamburgers, but I still keep gaining weight! I do try to buy all 'no-cholesterol' foods though."

II

PLAN OF CARE FOR MRS. JUANITA L.

Nursing diagnosis: *Altered Nutrition: More Than Body Requirements Related To Excessive Caloric Intake and Sedentary Lifestyle*

Expected Patient Outcomes	Nursing Interventions
Mrs. L. will verbalize desire to lose weight and identify relationship of obesity to hypertension and diabetes.	• Explore with Mrs. L. reasons she wants to lose weight. • Teach Mrs. L. the effects of obesity on current health status.
Mrs. L. will become involved with a support system in which to develop healthy eating patterns.	• Refer Mrs. L. to Weight Watchers or TOPS. Ask the patient to bring her husband to the clinic to discuss the importance of weight loss for the patient.
Mrs. L. will identify ways to change current dietary and activity patterns by monitoring dietary and activity patterns for 2 weeks.	• Explain the purpose of self-monitoring, and offer alternate suggestions for current patterns contributing to obesity.

Continued.

II

Expected Patient Outcomes	Nursing Interventions
Mrs. L. will reduce calorie intake to 1,180 calories a day by eating foods from all four food groups, eating low-fat and low-calorie foods, waiting 10 minutes when hunger pains occur before eating, avoiding skipping meals, and eating sitting down in one place.	• Teach Mrs. L. the importance of eating from all four food groups and which are low-calorie foods.
Mrs. L. will modify current activities as evidenced by walking for activities previously done by car, exercising for 20 to 30 minutes four times a week, starting an alternate hobby (instead of baking), and shopping for low-calorie foods.	• Teach Mrs. L. benefits of exercise on weight, health, and sense of well-being: explore alternate forms of exercise the patient enjoys and feels comfortable doing, and teach the patient not to shop while hungry, to use a list, and to buy low-calorie foods for snacks.

REFERENCES

1. Abraham S: Obese and overweight adults in the United States, *Vital Health Statistics* (DHHS Pub. No. 83 -1983), Hyattsville, Md, 1983, U.S. Public Health Service, National Center for Health Statistics.
2. Allan JD: Women who successfully manage their weight, *West J Nurs Res* 11(6):657-675, 1989.
3. Anderson JJ: The status of adolescent nutrition, *Nutr Today* 26(2):7-10, 1991.
4. Beare PE, Myers JL: *Principles and practice of adult health nursing,* St Louis, 1990, CV Mosby.
5. Bronwell KD: The psychology and physiology of obesity: implications for screening and treatment, *J Am Dietet Assoc* 84:406, 1984.
6. Butterworth C: The skeleton in the hospital closet, *Nutr Today* 9(2):4-8, 1974.
7. Carpentio LJ: *Nursing diagnosis: application to clinical practice,* ed 3, Philadelphia, 1989, JB Lippincott.
8. Carpenito LJ: *Nursing care plans and documentation: nursing diagnoses and collaborative problems,* Philadelphia, 1991, JB Lippincott.
9. Curtas S, Chapman G, and Meguid MM: Evaluation of nutritional status, *Nurs Clin North Am* 24:301-313, 1989.
10. Dietz WH: You are what you eat—what you eat is what you are, *J Adolesc Health Care* 11:76-81, 1990.
11. Dudek G: *Nutrition handbook for nursing practice,* Philadelphia, 1987, JB Lippincott.
12. Escheleman MM: *Introductory nutrition and diet therapy,* ed 2, Philadelphia, 1991, JB Lippincott.
13. Farthing MC: Current eating patterns of adolescents in the United States, *Nutr Today* 26(2):35-39, 1991.
14. Foreyt JP: Nine questions most often asked by physicians, *Consultant* 30(6):53-59, 1990.
15. Fuller J, Schaller-Ayers J: *Health assessment: a nursing approach,* Philadelphia, 1990, JB Lippincott.
16. Garn SM, Bailey SM, Cole PE, & Higgins ITT: Level of education, level of income, and level of fatness in adults, *Am J Clin Nutr* 30(5):721-725, 1977.
17. Greenwood MR: *Genetic and metabolic aspects in obesity,* New York, 1983, Churchill-Livingston.
18. Hubbard P, Muhlenkamp AF, and Brown N: The relationship between social support and self-care practice, *Nurs Res* 33:266, 1984.
19. Iverson-Carpenter MS, and others: Fulfilling nutritional requirements, *J Gerontol Nurs* 14(4): 16-24, 1988.
20. Kamath SK, and others: Hospital malnutrition: a 33-hospital screening study, *J Am Dietet Assoc* 86(2):203-206, 1986.
21. McBride AB: Fat: a woman's issue in search of a holistic approach to treatment, *Holistic Nurs Pract* 3(1):9-15, 1988.
22. Metropolitan Life Insurance Company: *Height and weight tables,* 1983.
23. Muhlenkamp AF, Sayles JA: Self-esteem, social support, and positive health practices, *Nurs Res* 35:334, 1986.
24. National Dairy Council: Children's health issues, *Dairy Council Digest* 61(6):31-36, 1990.
25. Phipps WJ, Long BC, Woods NF, and Cassmeyer VL: *Medical-surgical nursing: concepts and clinical practice,* St Louis, 1991, CV Mosby.
26. Polivy J, Herman CP: Clinical depression and weight change: a complex relation, *J Abnorm Psychol* 85:338, 1976.
27. Popkess-Vawter S: Assessment of positive and negative body image in normal weight and overweight females. In Carroll-Johnson RM (ed): *Classification of nursing diagnoses: proceedings of the Eighth Conference,* Philadelphia, 1989, JB Lippincott.
28. Pratt C: Weight reduction: its role in health promotion, *Fam Comm Health* 12(1):67-71, 1989.
29. Segal KR, Xavier Pi-Sunyer F: Exercise and obesity, *Med Clin North Am,* 73:217-235, 1989.
30. Schultz LO: Brown adipose tissue: regulation of thermogenesis and implications for obesity, *J Am Dietet Assoc* 87:761, 1987.
31. Sherman JB, Alexander MA: Obesity in children: a research update, *J Pediatr Nurs* 5(3):161-167, 1990.
32. Wilson PR, Herman J, and Chubon SJ: Eating strategies used by persons with head and neck cancer during and after radiotherapy, *Cancer Nurs* 14(2):98-104, 1991.

II

Ineffective Breastfeeding

Ineffective Breastfeeding is the state in which the mother, infant, or family experience dissatisfaction or difficulty with the breastfeeding process.

OVERVIEW

Lactation is a normal physiological process, and "it is reasonable to suppose that the milk of each species is well adapted to the particular needs of that species."[21] However, the art of breastfeeding is a maternal behavior that is easily influenced by external factors. "Breastfeeding is important for maternal and child health in every culture, and it is essential that women who choose to breastfeed are given the assistance necessary for doing so successfully and exclusively . . . "[18]

In North America in the 1970s, the incidence of breastfeeding was quite low (28% in the United States[21] and 25% in Canada[11]). However, more recently the Canadian incidence of breast-feeding was 70%.[9] Similar observations have been made in the United States.[1] Because there has been no cultural expectation to breastfeed, new mothers and their families have received little or no information, support, or encouragement from health professionals to engage in this activity. In the 1990s more mothers are initiating breastfeeding; many, however, are discontinuing the practice before the 4- to 6-month period recommended by both the American Academy of Pediatrics and the Canadian Paediatric Society;[21] both state that human breast milk is the ideal and only food necessary for the human infant in the first 4 to 6 months of life. Why then are mothers discontinuing breastfeeding in the first few days, weeks, or months after they give birth? An authoritative study reveals that one of the most common reasons for discontinuing breastfeeding is a perceived or actual insufficient supply of breast milk.[17] Other reasons cited include returning to work outside the home, little or no support from partner or significant members of the extended family, nipple soreness, and a lack of knowledge about breastfeeding.[1,18,22,23]

ASSESSMENT

The major defining characteristic of ineffective breastfeeding is expressed dissatisfaction with the breastfeeding process. In the mother, this may manifest as a desire to stop breastfeeding or anxiety about the infant's well-being. In the partner or family, it may manifest as an actual lack of support for the mother's efforts or lack of confidence that the mother can adequately feed the child. The infant may not be gaining weight adequately and may be apathetic or extremely fussy.

Several minor defining characteristics may reveal ineffective breastfeeding. An inadequate milk supply can influence breastfeeding behavior. Evidence is increasing that certain anatomical and hormonal factors affect lactation.[19] A subsequent pregnancy has been know to markedly decrease the maternal breast milk supply.[19]

Recognition of the infant's contribution to breastfeeding success is increasing. The nurse must assess the infant's breastfeeding behavior along with the mother's.[25]

The infant's inability to suck properly may cause an inability to correctly attach to the mother's nipple, which is another defining characteristic.[25] Also, the infant may be unable to correctly attach to the mother's nipple because of genetic, iatrogenic, or positioning problems; an anatomical problem in the mother, such as an inverted nipple or one that tends to retract; or an anatomical problem in the infant, such as a cleft lip or palate. Breast shape seems to have some effect on lactation.[18]

Oxytocin release, stimulated in the mother by thoughts of her infant or by the infant suckling at her breast, is responsible for the ejection of breast milk.[13] When oxytocin stimulates the release of milk, the milk may leak from the breast that is not being used. Studies have shown that it may take 2 or more minutes of sucking for a continuous flow from the milk-producing cells.[13] If oxytocin release is inadequate, then mothers will have Ineffective Breastfeeding.

The infant may demonstrate nonsustained suckling at the breast, that is, sucking for short periods of time and then stopping. The infant prefers continuous feeding without a break for the mother, and he or she may cry when put down. There is slow or no weight gain. However, one must remember that breastfeeding infants do not regain their weight as rapidly as bottle-fed infants. Related factors may include a premature infant or an infant with a heart defect; both of these conditions will cause the infant to be fatigued.[13]

Occasionally infants will only suck from one breast though both may be offered. Observation of both breasts may reveal that one nipple is retracted or inverted. The infant will find that sucking from the normal nipple produces more milk with less work, so he or she will then show a definite preference for it. Also, the mother may offer only one breast to suckle because of a sore nipple on one side.[26]

The nurse may consider a diagnosis of Ineffective Breastfeeding when observing a newborn infant who is breastfeeding less than seven times in 24 hours. The successfully breastfed infant will sleep for periods of 2 to 3 hours[13] between feedings and breastfeed with eyes closed. The emptying time of the stomach for breast milk is about 1½ hours. The nurse should encourage feedings at least every 2 to 3 hours until a breastfeeding routine is established, especially in the newborn.

Nipple soreness is quite common in the first 2 weeks of breastfeeding.[13,17,26] Bleeding, cracks,

or fissures in the nipple, and pain for the duration of breastfeeding may accompany prolonged, persistent soreness. The nurse can assess the actual condition of the nipple by observation and the presence of pain by careful questioning of the mother. Assessing the positioning of the infant at the breast will reveal whether incorrect positioning is the primary cause.[18,22]

In the absence of physiological causes such as sore nipples, the mother may show reluctance to breastfeed her baby because she has internalized some of the North American culture's ambivalent feelings about breastfeeding.[3,4,9] Although breastfeeding is now believed to be the method of choice for infant feeding, the female breast is still seen as a sexual object that is often the partner's exclusive domain. A mother's handling of her breasts will provide a clue to her feelings. Discussing how she made her decision to breastfeed, her partner's feelings, and those of her extended family will be part of the assessment process.

The nurse may consider a diagnosis of Ineffective Breastfeeding when the infant exhibits fussiness and crying within the first hour after breastfeeding and does not respond to other comfort measures or when the infant arches and cries at the breast and resists latching on. Infants who wake within the first hour may not have had sufficient milk. Usually breast milk is not totally digested for at least 1½ hours.[13] The infant needs to suckle at each breast for a sufficient length of time to receive the hind milk, which is rich in fat and comes at the end of the feeding. The fat content of breast milk not only provides the calories infants need, but also satiates them. Sucking time should not be limited.[7] The nurse needs to consider variables specific to each infant. Some infants may stretch, extending their heads and arching their backs as they resist latching on to the breast. These infants may actually seem to be pulling away from the mother and her breast. In these circumstances, assessment includes a check for a neurological defect.

Perceived inadequate milk supply may influence breastfeeding behavior. For a variety of reasons that may be psychological, a mother may believe that her milk cannot be as nutritious for her child as a scientifically prepared formula.[13,17] Because the present cultural norm in some communities is to breastfeed, a mother may discover that an insufficient milk supply is a socially acceptable reason for ceasing breastfeeding when she has no true personal commitment to breastfeed. Issues to consider when determining whether the mother perceives inadequate milk supply and related factors that actually affect the volume of milk supply to consider include: (1) inadequate knowledge of breast milk production,[25] (2) socioeconomic status of mother (which may correlate to her nutrition intake), (3) drug use by the mother (prescribed by the physician or self-prescribed),[13] and (4) inadequate knowledge of the growth spurts that all babies have at different times in the first 6 months of life.[17]

Studies by Atkinson and associates[13] have shown that the milk of mothers who have premature infants is higher in protein nitrogen than milk of mothers with full-term infants. The protein requirement of premature infants is higher than full-term infants.[24] The other advantages of breast milk, such as the immunological factors, will be of value to the premature infant too. However, the premature infant may not be sufficiently strong to suck to initiate milk production. This situation will require that the mother learn hand expression, storage, and how to maintain an adequate milk supply at the time she is adjusting to the fact that she has an infant at risk.

An infant anomaly, such as a cleft lip or palate, may interfere with the sucking reflex. Observation of the infant will include making sure that the infant's tongue is around the mother's nipple and areola, using the mother's breast to secure adequate suction. A cardiac defect may decrease the infant's energy level so that sucking for a period long enough to obtain sufficient milk may be difficult. Assessment includes the amount of time the infant sucks at each breast and how frequently the infant feeds. An infant with Down syndrome or a neurological impairment may have poor muscle tone, which may interfere with the sucking reflex.

Maternal breast anomaly, infections, or previous breast surgery may influence ability to breastfeed. Breast anomalies include nipples that are flat, inverted, or in rare situations completely absent. Sucking for the infant is quite difficult because the infant has nothing on which to latch. Occasionally the very large, pendulous breast is too heavy for the baby to hold in his/her mouth. The nipple is lost, and the infant becomes frustrated. A physical assessment of the nipple and areola, especially prenatally, is imperative. Interference with breastfeeding may occur after cosmetic surgery, including breast augmentation and reduction, but this depends on the type of surgery performed.[19] What has to be assessed is interference with milk production and its delivery to the nipple for the infant to suck.

Interruption of breastfeeding related to maternal or infant needs will influence successful breastfeeding. Temporary interruptions in breastfeeding may result if the infant develops breast milk jaundice; if the mother develops sore, cracked nipples;[17] if the mother or infant becomes ill; or if a mother with mastitis develops an abscess and needs medical intervention.[13] If medical intervention includes a prescription for medication, the effect of the medication on breastfeeding should be determined.[5] If the infant develops a preference for the breastfeeding substitute, the resumption of breastfeeding becomes difficult. Assessing the length of the interruption and keeping it to a minimum is most important.[26] Mothers returning to work outside of the home may temporarily interrupt the rhythm established by the breastfeeding dyad.

The influence of previous breastfeeding failure will depend on the reason for the failure, how the mother accepted the situation, and the support she received from her support system in dealing with resultant feelings of guilt. Her level of self-esteem in the mothering role will contribute to her success or lack thereof. A detailed history of previous births will elicit this information.

The use of supplemental feedings with an artificial nipple may impair breastfeeding. Two barriers to successful breastfeeding are introduced with this one action—the infant will not continue to suck for a sufficient length of time on the breast to increase the milk supply,[13] and nipple confusion occurs. An infant has to work harder to receive breast milk than to receive a breast milk substitute. The infant will learn to prefer the latter and refuse to nurse at the breast.[13] It is well documented that early and frequent supplementation of breastfeeding and introduction of bottles and pacifiers leads to early discontinuation of breastfeeding.[20]

A poor reflex, which may be caused by genetic or developmental problems in the infant, will influence breastfeeding. Genetic or developmental problems will be recognizable by observation. Some infants are ineffective sucklers because of illness, prematurity, or sedation.[17] The nurse needs knowledge of the sucking reflex and the fact that not all infants are born with an instinctive and correct sucking pattern to assist in making this diagnosis.

North American families do not have role models against which to measure breastfeeding success. Most extended family members, especially the infant's grandmothers, did not breastfeed their babies. Studies have demonstrated that partner and family support and encouragement directly affect breastfeeding success. Conversely, lack of support, jealousy of the partner for the mother-infant dyad, and doubt about the mother's ability to adequately nourish the infant will all contribute to breastfeeding failure.[4,13,17] The availability of support from the family and partner will influence breastfeeding success.

Closely related to support is the realization that breastfeeding is a learned process for the mother.[15] In the second half of the century, new mothers have moved away from their traditional sources of assistance. Women in the middle part of the century lost the knowledge and skills to assist breastfeeding mothers. The American Academy of Pediatrics and the Canadian Paediatric Society stated that schools should provide education for the public and health professionals to increase breastfeeding success.[21] Knowledge deficits about milk composition, the milk ejection reflex, proper

sucking, and frequency of breastfeeding adversely affect the duration of breastfeeding.[13]

Few medical diagnoses should interfere with the breastfeeding process. In one study, 94% of the mothers sampled were able to breastfeed successfully when circumstances were favorable.[21] Mothers with breast cancer should not breastfeed their infants; they should receive treatment immediately.[13] With the advent of AIDS, questions have arisen about infected mothers breastfeeding their infants. In countries such as Canada and the United States HIV-infected (human immunodeficiency virus) mothers have been advised against breastfeeding their infants when safe alternatives are available. HIV has been isolated in breast milk. The nurse should determine the source of breastfeeding substitutes, as part of an assessment strategy. Discussion continues regarding the best advice for breastfeeding women.[8]

Several excellent assessment tools that assist in establishing breastfeeding success or impairment are recorded in the literature:

Lawrence[13]: Parameters for evaluation of breastfed infants.

Matthew[16]: Instrument to measure maternal satisfaction and neonates' feeding behaviors (IBFAT, Infant Breastfeeding Assessment Tool).

Riordan[24]: Assessment forms for indicating nipple function and breastfeeding evaluation, and a hospital breastfeeding teaching checklist.

Shrago and Bocar[25]: Systematic Assessment of the Infant at Breast (SAIB).

❖ Defining Characteristics

The presence of the following defining characteristics indicates that the mother may be experiencing Ineffective Breastfeeding.

- Unsatisfactory breastfeeding process
- Actual or perceived inadequate milk supply
- Inability of the infant to attach to maternal nipple correctly
- No observable signs of oxytocin release
- Nonsustained suckling at the breast
- Suckling at only one breast per feeding

II

- Breastfeeding less than seven times in 24 hours
- Persistence of sore nipples beyond the infant's first week of life
- Infant exhibiting fussiness and crying within the first hour after breastfeeding
- Unresponsiveness of the infant to other comfort measures
- Infant arching and crying at the breast
- Resistance of the infant to latch on to breast
- Maternal reluctance to put infant to breast[11]

❖ Related Factors

The following related factors are associated with Ineffective Breastfeeding:

- Prematurity or infant anomaly
- Maternal breast anomaly
- Previous breast surgery
- Infant receiving supplemental feedings with artificial nipple
- Poor infant sucking reflex
- History of breastfeeding failure
- Knowledge deficit
- Nonsupportive partner or family
- Interruption in breastfeeding
- Medical conditions (e.g., AIDS or breast cancer)
- Incongruent cultural norms and expectations

❖ Related Medical/Psychiatric Diagnoses

The following are examples of medical/psychiatric diagnoses for Ineffective Breastfeeding:

For Mother
- Anxiety disorder
- Breast cancer
- Catatonic schizophrenia
- Fibrocystic breast disease
- Infection of nipples
- Paranoid schizophrenia
- Postpartum depression
- Substance abuse
- Low birth weight
- Neurological impairments
- Poor infant sucking reflex
- Major depression
- Mastitis

For Infant
- Cardiovascular impairments
- Congenital oral anomalies (e.g., cleft palate)

NURSING DIAGNOSES

Examples of *specific* nursing diagnoses for Ineffective Breastfeeding are:
- Ineffective Breastfeeding related to poor infant sucking reflex
- Ineffective Breastfeeding related to knowledge deficit
- Ineffective Breastfeeding related to poor positioning
- Ineffective Breastfeeding related to sore nipples
- Ineffective Breastfeeding related to inadequate milk production

PLANNING AND IMPLEMENTATION WITH RATIONALE

The ultimate expected outcome is successful breastfeeding in which the adult members of the family are satisfied with the process and are having minimal difficulty. The infant is content and gaining weight according to accepted standards.[13] The defining characteristics and related factors in the individual family situation will influence the nursing response to assist families to reach this outcome. A discussion of interventions associated with various related factors follows.

Families, the public at large, and health professionals need information about the advantages of breastfeeding, the physiology of lactation, and the emotional and social factors that influence lactation.[1,10,12] The majority of issues and related factors surrounding the diagnosis of Ineffective Breastfeeding could be prevented by education and skills development at appropriate intervals during the perinatal period. Some nursing interventions are appropriate in the prenatal period, whereas others are appropriate in the immediate postpartum period, both in the hospital and immediately after discharge.

Studies have shown that the maternity nurse has not significantly increased his/her breastfeeding knowledge over the past 10 years. Studies consistently demonstrate low mean scores (approximating 50%) on questionnaires designed to test breastfeeding knowledge.[1]

Duration of breastfeeding does not cause sore nipples.[14] Many mothers have soreness in the first week of breastfeeding when the ductules are not yet filled with milk.[13] Mothers need reassurance and information at this time. *Continuing soreness of the nipple is thought to result from incorrect positioning of the infant at the breast.* The following technique is recommended:[14,18]

Sitting upright in bed with her back and arms supported, the mother positions the infant across her abdomen on the side so that the infant's face, chest, genitals, and knees are all facing her. The infant should not have to turn the neck to feed. If the mother brings her knees up, she will support the infant in this position (and relieve the strain on her back). A pillow under the infant and across the mother's abdomen will assist a mother who has had a cesarean delivery. Once the baby is positioned, the mother gives attention to her nipple and areola. The mother should spread her fingers around the breast, with her thumb above the breast and the four fingers below supporting it. *She should be careful not to exert pressure on the breast with any of her fingers because this may lead to a plugged duct.* [22]

The mother may then be instructed to gently tickle the infant's upper lip *to elicit the rooting reflex.* The infant will present a wide open mouth. The mother will then draw the infant's whole body toward her own until the infant's nose is just touching her breast. The mother may need to support her breast during feedings until the infant's suckling is stronger. The mother needs to be sure that the infant is not pulling down on her breast and that the infant has all of the nipple and at least some of the areola in the mouth. Positioning of the infant on the breast can vary so that pressure is distributed more evenly all around the nipple and areola. Observation of the baby's sucking pattern will confirm if the baby's position is correct.[7] Prenatal preparation does not seem to prevent sore nipples.[27] Air-drying of nipples for up to 15 minutes after each feeding can be encouraged. Nipple shields should not be used unless other interventions are not working.[13] Pumping

without a shield has been demonstrated to yield statistically larger milk volumes.[2]

Situations that may be linked to faulty sucking reflex include prematurity or infants with congenital oral anomalies, cardiac defects, or neurological impairments. If the infant has difficulty with the sucking reflex, the nurse should observe the position of the infant's tongue. The wide open mouth should latch on to the breast with the tongue below the nipple and extended over the lower gum and the lower lip extended out rather than in over the lower gums. The nipple and areola are drawn well into the infant's mouth so that the gums compress the areola behind the nipple, forcing the milk gathered in the breast's sinuses into the back of the infant's mouth.[18,22] *Milk is being ingested if the infant is swallowing. If the infant's suction is inadequate, the breast will easily pull away from the infant's mouth.* "In the absence of audible swallowing, a digital suck assessment can be performed . . . To perform a digital suck assessment, the nurse uses a finger covered with a well-fitting glove or finger cot and gently tickles the infant's lips to elicit mouth opening. The finger is then inserted in the infant's mouth. Normally, the infant's tongue curls around the examining finger, forming a trough beneath the finger. The tongue and lips form a complete seal around the finger, with noticeable negative pressure exerted on the finger in a rhythmic pattern . . . "[25]

If the infant has an oral defect, suction may be achieved by bringing the infant closer and having the soft breast tissue fill in for the absence, such as occurs with a cleft lip. *Assisting the mother to position her nipple away from the cleft palate or using a plastic dental plate appliance that covers the cleft palate may assist in achieving and maintaining suction.* [26] Because the infant may tire more quickly from this very hard work, "switch" breastfeeding may be recommended.[26] The infant may be switched back and forth from breast to breast so that the volume of milk received per feeding is maximized. Milk collects in both breasts at several times during a feeding and can

II

pool in the sinuses in the "off" interval.

The milk ejection reflex is "a nerve reflex from the breast to the hypothalamus causing the release of oxytocin by the posterior pituitary gland. Elicited by the infant's suckling, or sometimes even by the mother's thoughts of her baby, this reflex initiates the flow of milk."[26]*Interference with the milk ejection reflex may produce a crying infant in a short time after feeding, an actual reduction in milk production, or weight loss or slow weight gain in the infant.* Limiting the breastfeeding time on each breast to less than 5 minutes does not allow sufficient time to stimulate milk production. *Oxytocin, which activates the milk ejection reflex, may require 2 or more minutes of sucking for full response, peaking at 6 to 10 minutes.* [25]

The foremilk, which collects in the lactiferous sinuses immediately behind the areola between feeds, is more dilute and less fatty than the hind milk. The hind milk is stored in the milk ducts of the breast until oxytocin secreted by the pituitary gland stimulates the myoepithelial cells to contract and eject the milk from the ducts.[13] The infant will not be satisfied until he or she receives the milk with the higher protein and fat content. This milk also supplies most of the calories to ensure weight gain. Milk production is directly related to the complete emptying of both breasts at each feeding. The mother should be encouraged to be as comfortable and relaxed as possible before she breastfeeds. At least initially, she should be encouraged to feed every 2 to 3 hours or on demand if the infant does not sleep for long periods. The infant's crying may stimulate oxytocin release, causing milk ejection.

Several of the problems previously discussed will influence the milk supply. Inhibited milk ejection reflex, incomplete emptying of the breasts, the mother's ingestion of certain drugs, and the mother's diet and smoking behaviors all directly affect the volume of breast milk produced. Initially, a distinction must be made between an infant who normally gains weight slowly and one who is not thriving because of an insufficient milk supply. If the infant appears satisfied even though he or she is thin and gains weight slowly, the infant probably is a slow weight gainer. An assessment of the family's history may reveal that one of the parents was also thin.

Breast milk substitutes, whether infant formula or glucose water, have a significant effect on breast milk supply. They should be avoided, at least in the first month of life. *Besides causing nipple confusion for the infant, these substitutes increase the time between feedings, which in turn negatively influences the stimulation of the breast to produce milk. The early introduction of bottles themselves and pacifiers should be avoided as their use interferes with the prolactin reflex, which influences milk production.*[20]

The mother's diet and general well-being affect the volume of milk produced.[28] Malnutrition does seem to reduce the quantity of milk. Further research is necessary to assess the value of maternal diet supplementation, because studies to date have produced some conflicting results.[13] Health professionals and families who encourage and support the new mother will help her by increasing her confidence in her body's ability to feed the infant. The nurse should encourage the extended family to offer practical assistance to the mother to allow the mother to rest, establish her breast milk, and look after her infant. A nursing supplementation device may be used to supply breast milk pumped from the mother's breast to an infant who needs the extra nourishment and did not empty the breasts at a previous feeding.[6]

EVALUATION

Expected outcomes have been achieved when the mother and family are satisfied with the breastfeeding experience. Families will have sufficient, relevant, correct, and appropriate information to sustain breastfeeding.

Mothers will have confidence in their ability to nurture their infants. Nipple or breast soreness will be eliminated, and infants will suckle effectively. Milk production and ejection will be sufficient so that the family is happy and the baby is thriving (demonstrating an adequate weight gain appropriate to the age and initial birth weight).

II

❖ NURSING CARE GUIDELINE

Nursing Diagnosis: Ineffective Breastfeeding

Expected Patient Outcomes	Nursing Interventions
The family will have the knowledge and skills to ensure breastfeeding success.	• Provide education and hands-on practical demonstrations.
The mother's soreness will be contained or eliminated.	• Demonstrate proper positioning of the infant at breast and educate the mother about nipple care (e.g., air-drying, no special preparation before feeding, and as a last resort, nipple shields).
The infant will suck correctly with the tongue in proper position and suction being achieved.	• Observe the infant sucking and demonstrate technique for effective latching on and methods to ensure suction taught. • Encourage "switch" breastfeeding. • Perform digital suck assessment if audible swallowing not heard.
The mother will understand the relationship of the milk ejection reflex to milk production, and she will be sufficiently relaxed to allow the milk ejection reflex to occur.	• Explain physiology of milk ejection reflex, including importance of frequency and adequacy of feeding time. • Support and encourage the mother in building confidence.
The mother will have sufficient milk to satisfy the infant's needs, and the infant will gain weight at a pace congruent with established growth charts.	• Assess techniques used by the mother. • Chart the infant's weight gain. • Do a family history. Help the mother to eliminate breastfeeding substitutes. • Review the maternal diet, well-being, lifestyle habits, and adjust these if necessary. • Demonstrate the use of a supplemental feeding device.

❖ CASE STUDY WITH PLAN OF CARE

"But everyone said it's so natural to breastfeed, and I want to do what is best for my baby," stated Mrs. Patricia M., who is a 28-year-old primiparous mother who attended prenatal classes. She learned about the advantages of breastfeeding for herself and her baby and the importance of rooming in and demand feeding. She was ready for this experience, except her episiotomy hurt. She had attempted to feed her new son after delivery, but he really only licked at the nipples, preferring to examine his new surroundings. Mrs. M. was excited about breastfeeding initially. However, this is her third day after giving birth, and the baby is still not latching on properly. The nurses are saying that the baby has lost weight and is dehydrated. Mrs. M. is be

Continued.

II

❖ *CASE STUDY WITH PLAN OF CARE— cont'd*

ginning to doubt her decision not to let the baby have glucose water in the nursery. Her breasts are getting hard and sore. The nurse observed Mrs. M.'s current status and did an initial assessment using the previously defined criteria. She determined that: (1) Mrs. M. is excited; she is probably tired and may even be dehydrated unless she has been encouraged to take fluids during and after her labor, (2) because of the soreness of her episiotomy, she is lying lopsided in bed, and (3) the baby is having difficulty latching on to the breast. The nursery staff state the baby has continued to lose weight. Based on these data, the nurse established that Mrs. M.'s ability to breastfeed was impaired by poor latching on of the infant, poor positioning, and lack of confidence in herself. Engorgement of the breasts was evident.

PLAN OF CARE FOR MRS. PATRICIA M.

Nursing Diagnosis: *Ineffective Breastfeeding related to positioning of mother, engorgement of breasts, inadequate sucking reflex of baby, and insecure mother*

Expected Patient Outcomes	Nursing Interventions
Mrs. M. will maintain a position that is comfortable and supportive.	• Change the height of the bed, and support Mrs. M. with pillows. • Educate Mrs. M. about the various positions for holding the baby at the breast.
Mrs. M.'s breasts will no longer be engorged and sore as evidenced by infant's ability to breastfeed. Mother's pain will be relieved.	• Demonstrate hand expression of some milk to soften breasts sufficiently to allow the infant to grasp the nipple and areola and establish suction.
Mrs. M.'s baby will establish effective sucking as evidenced by audible swallowing, content baby.	• Properly position the baby's body in relation to Mrs. M.'s body. • Demonstrate the proper technique; e.g., the baby's tongue should be under the nipple; the nipple and some of the areola should be in the baby's mouth. • Observe the infant to assess for proper suction and swallowing.
Mrs. M. will adjust her lifestyle in order to promote a satisfying breastfeeding experience.	• Encourage Mrs. M. to drink an adequate amount of fluids and eat a balanced diet. • Encourage Mrs. M. to get adequate rest and sleep.
Mrs. M. will be confident in her ability to breastfeed her baby as evidenced by her expression of same on hospital discharge.	• Encourage, support, and praise Mrs. M. for her efforts. • Reassure Mrs. M. that the difficulties that she is experiencing are not unusual. • Chart the infant's weight gain and inform Mrs. M. as progress is made. • Refer Mrs. M. to community nursing agency. • Provide Mrs. M. with educational materials as desired.

REFERENCES

1. Anderson E, Geden E: Nurses' knowledge of breastfeeding, *J Obstet Gynecol Neonatal Nurs* 20(1):58-63, 1991.
2. Auerbach KG: The effect of nipple shields on maternal milk volume, *J Obstet Gynecol Neonatal Nurs* 19(5):419-427, 1990.
3. Bottorff JL, Morse JM: Mothers' perceptions of breast milk, *J Obstet Gynecol Neonatal Nurs* 19(6):518-527, 1990.
4. Brack DC: Social forces, feminism and breastfeeding, *Nurs Outlook* 23(8):556-561, 1975.
5. Briggs GC, Freeman RK, and Yaffee SJ: *Drugs in pregnancy and lactation,* ed 3, Baltimore, 1990, Williams & Wilkins.
6. Edgehouse L, Radzyminski SG: A device for supplementing breast-feeding, *MCN* 15:34-35, 1990.
7. Enkin M, Keirse MJ, and Chalmers I: *A guide to effective care in pregnancy and childbirth,* New York, 1989, Oxford Press.

8. Heymann SF: Modeling the impact of breast-feeding by HIV-infected women on child survival, *Am J Public Health* 80(11):1305-1309, 1990.

9. Hewat R: More effective education for breastfeeding women, *Can Nurse* 81(1):38-40, 1985.

10. Huggins K: *The nursing mother's companion,* Boston, 1990, Harvard Common Press.

11. Komuvesh M: *Infant nutrition: a guide for health professionals,* Toronto, 1984, Ontario Ministry of Health.

12. La Leche League International: *The womanly art of breastfeeding,* ed 5, Franklin Park, Ill, 1991, The League.

13. Lawrence RA: *Breastfeeding: a guide for the medical profession,* ed 3, St Louis, 1989, CV Mosby.

14. L'Esperance C, Frantz K: Time limitation for early breastfeeding, *J Obstet Gynecol Neonatal Nurs* 14(2):114-118, 1985.

15. Marmet C, Shell E: Training neonates to suck correctly, *MCN* 9:401-407, 1984.

16. Matthew MK: Mothers' satisfaction with their neonates' breastfeeding behaviours, *J Obstet Gynecol Neonatal Nurs* 20(1):49-55, 1991.

17. Minchin M: *Breastfeeding matters,* North Sydney, Australia, 1985, George Allen & Unwin.

18. Minchin MK: Positioning for breastfeeding, *Birth* 16(2):67-80, 1989.

19. Neifert MR, Seacat JM: Lactation insufficiency: a rational approach, *Birth* 14(4):182-188, 1987.

20. Newman J: Breastfeeding problems associated with the early introduction of bottles and pacifiers, *J Hum Lact* 6(2):59-63, 1990.

21. Nutrition Committee of the Canadian Paediatric Society and the Committee on Nutrition of the American Academy of Pediatrics: Breast-feeding, *Pediatrics* 62(4):591-601, 1978.

22. Renfrew MJ: Positioning the baby at the breast: more than a visual skill, *J Hum Lact* 5(1):13-15, 1989.

23. Renfrew M, Fisher C, and Arms S: *Bestfeeding: getting breastfeeding right for you,* Berkeley, Calif, 1990, Celestial Arts.

24. Riordan J: *A practical guide to breastfeeding,* St Louis, 1983, CV Mosby.

25. Shrago L, Bocar D: The infant's contribution to breastfeeding, *J Obstet Gynecol Neonatal Nurs* 19(3):209-215, 1990.

26. US Department of Health and Human Services: *Report of the Surgeon General's Workshop on Breastfeeding and Human Lactation,* Rockville, Md, 1985.

27. Walker M, Driscoll JW: Sore nipples: the new mother's nemesis, *MCN* 14:260-265, 1989.

28. Worthington-Roberts BS, Vermeersch J, and Williams SR: *Nutrition in pregnancy and lactation,* ed 4, St Louis, 1989, Mosby–Year Book.

II

Effective Breastfeeding

Effective Breastfeeding is the state in which a mother-infant dyad/family exhibits adequate proficiency and satisfaction with breastfeeding behaviors.[4]

OVERVIEW

Breastfeeding is an interactive process with both psychological and physiological dimensions. The benefits to both the mother and infant have been documented.[1] The most effective measure of successful breastfeeding is its intended outcome, that is, the development of a healthy infant. With successful breastfeeding, assessment of the infant would demonstrate an infant with adequate weight gain as well as daily stools and urine output. The mother's milk production and effective nursing techniques must meet the newborn's needs for adequate caloric and fluid intake.

Each female breast is divided into 15 to 20 glandular lobes. Each lobe contains many alveoli, which are the milk producing structures. Muscle tissue surrounding the alveoli squeezes the alveoli and causes milk to enter ducts and to be carried to the sinuses behind the nipple. During pregnancy estrogen and progesterone have effects on the breast tissue. Estrogen causes the duct system to expand while progesterone stimulates increases in alveolar size. After birth, separation of the placenta causes the anterior pituitary to release prolactin, which stimulates milk production by the alveoli. When sucking occurs the posterior pituitary releases oxytocin, which acts on the muscle tissue around the alveoli, causing the muscle tissue to contract and milk to be released into the ducts and sinuses behind the nipple for the infant. The let-down reflex is an involuntary reflex that causes the pituitary to release oxytocin; sucking and the smell, cry, and touch of the infant initiate the reflex. Inhibitors of the reflex are pain, stress, fear, and anxiety. Interventions, such as making the mother more comfortable and the room quieter and less bright, gentle stroking of the breast, and warm compresses or showers may stimulate the let-down reflex.

The infant's ability to "latch-on" and suck is crucial to effective breastfeeding. Immediately after the birth the infant has a period during which it is quietly alert. During this period breastfeeding may be begun as the infant searches the environment for sounds and voices. Rooting may be stimulated to encourage the infant to latch-on and nurse. The presence in the infant of maternal sedatives within several hours of birth may affect an infant's readiness to nurse in the early postpartal period.[8,9] If this is the case the mother should be encouraged to try to initiate nursing after a short time. The infant's sucking controls the amount of milk produced. Putting the baby to breast on demand supports continued production of an adequate milk supply.[3]

Three types of milk are produced in the initial process of establishing lactation. Colostrum, a thick yellowish fluid, contains more protein, fat-soluble vitamins, and minerals than the milk produced later. This early form of milk contains high levels of immunoglobulin, which impart immunity to factors to which the mother has been exposed. The colostrum is expressed during pregnancy and is replaced by transitional milk several days after birth. Transitional milk contains lactose, high levels of fat, and water-soluble vitamins and is high in calories to enhance growth, which is rapid in early infancy. Mature milk, which appears after 2 weeks, is thin and watery.

Mothers often question its nutritive ability based on its appearance.[6] Mature breast milk, however, contains adequate calories for the baby.

Infant formulas have been developed to deliver the same calorie-to-fluid intake ratio as the breast milk standard. Infant formulas may contain a higher percentage of calories from protein and stress immature kidneys with the metabolism of the waste products of protein breakdown. Infant nutitional needs include 50 to 55 calories per pound of weight each day and 64 to 73 milliliters per pound of weight each day to produce a weight gain of one ounce per day for the first 6 months, and half of that amount the last 6 months of the first year.[1]

The American Academy of Pediatrics[1] recommends the use of breast milk exclusively for the first 6 months of life. The advantages to the infant are nutritional, immunologic and psychological. Breast milk contains easily digestible fatty acids, amino acids, lipids, and lactose. The whey-protein-to-casein-protein ratio helps the infant to use all the formula by complete digestion. The more easily absorbed breast milk leaves the stomach sooner, and the infant may require more frequent feeding than a formula-fed infant.[5] The iron content of breast milk is related to the mother's nutritional state. If the mother's iron stores are sufficient, the breast milk will contain adequate amounts of iron for the developing infant. Although the levels of iron in breast milk are lower than in iron-fortified formulas, the iron in breast milk is more readily absorbed. The mother's nutritional state affects her ability to produce milk that is nutritionally adequate for the baby.[8,9]

The mother's immunologic factors are transferred to the infant in breast milk. The early milk contains high levels of antiviral, antibacterial, and antigenic-inhibiting factors. The infant uses the benefit of this inheritance during the first year of life.[19]

Breastfeeding has psychological advantages in the promotion of the attachment of mother to infant and infant to mother. The direct skin-to-skin contact of breastfeeding and the frequency of this contact facilitate the development of the relationship.[6] Breastfeeding experience helps the mother reconcile the differences between the fantasized infant of pregnancy and the reality of the newborn.[7]

The decision to breastfeed is usually made by the end of the second trimester based on the family needs, advice of relatives, and cultural norms, and less on a basis of knowledge about breastfeeding.[7,9] The role of family and friends and the experiences communicated to the new mother on selection of feeding methods have been described. Difficulty in establishing effective breastfeeding may occur when a mother chooses to nurse solely on the advice of a support person and never examines her own feelings concerning this method of feeding.[10] The development of problems, such as nipple tenderness and engorgement, may affect the desire to nurse.[8,9,12,15] The mother's knowledge level about the common problems of breastfeeding and the self-care measures that may remedy them may indicate the need for additional support through education about nursing.[2,7,11,21]

Cultural norms and expectations play a role in the development of effective breastfeeding.[8-10] A culture that encourages breastfeeding may assist the mother in continuing to nurse if difficulties arise in achieving the success valued by the culture. Western societies encourage the mother to nurse soon after birth and to continue as long as desired. The hospital environment may not facilitate the early initiation of nursing, and nursing past the first year often draws frowns.[2] In Western societies babies may be nursed as long as 4 years, but most have been weaned by several months after birth.[16] The social pressure to wean a child may be felt through stares and polite suggestions concerning the welfare of both mother and baby. Mothers in Asian cultures are also subject to the influences of culture. Often these mothers do not nurse their infants until the mature milk has begun because they believe that colostrum cannot nourish the baby. Many women supplement breastfeeding with formula and do not pump their breasts for relief of engorgement or for the storage of milk for their infant.[14-17] Early introduction of solid foods is encouraged in some rural Western cultures based on the desire for healthy infants. The myth that a fat infant is a healthy infant supports this practice. The American Academy of Pediatrics[1] recommends that no solids be introduced until the fifth to sixth month. Understanding the culturally prescribed beliefs about breastfeeding may assist the nurse in addressing needs and concerns in a culturally appropriate manner.

ASSESSMENT

By historical data gathering and by physical examination of the breasts, the nurse may assess the physical capability to breastfeed effectively. Historical information related to previous breastfeeding experiences and any history of breast disorders can be collected during a prenatal visit if the mother seeks prenatal care. This information is placed on the prenatal record, and the nurse assisting at the time of birth may refer to it. If prenatal access to the mother is limited because of delayed prenatal care or other reasons, this information should be collected on admission to the birthing area. Information related to prenatal education, knowledge of breastfeeding, and support from significant others for nursing may be assessed.

Information about previous pregnancies and postpartal experiences may provide insight into the postpartal course. Mothers may have elected to change the method of feeding with subsequent pregnancies and may be novices at nursing although multiparous. Previous history of breast disease can be obtained, including recent or current episodes of acute mastitis and chronic fibrocystic breast disease. Although neither of these precludes breastfeeding entirely, the extent and severity of symptoms may affect the mother's ability to nurse effectively. Review of the breast changes associated with pregnancy in preparation for nursing includes the increased size of the breast usually noted at 20 weeks, nodular texture of the breast, darkness of the areola and nipple, and tingling of the breast. Physical examination of the breast includes inspection of the surface of the breast for irregularities of shape and size,

nonsymmetrical dimpling of the skin, venous pattern prominence associated with pregnancy, and hyperpigmentation of the areola and nipple. Palpation of the breast is done for irregularities of texture (normally feels nodular as tubercles of Montgomery enlarge), unilateral masses, pain in the breast, colostrum that may be present after the twelfth week of the pregnancy, and striae on the breasts. In addition, the size, shape, and ability of the nipple to become erect for latching-on can be determined. After feedings, nipples may be assessed for the presence of redness or cracking.

Psychosocial factors may affect a mother's readiness for nursing as well as potential for success. Personal factors such as maturity level, dependency needs, anxiety, and low self-esteem have been associated with breastfeeding difficulty.[5,19,21] Personal attitudes related to the advantages and disadvantages of breastfeeding may lead to the establishment of effective breastfeeding. Beliefs that the breastfeeding is demanding, inconvenient, embarrassing, and uncomfortable and that bottle feeding is more convenient have been associated with difficulty in breastfeeding. The attitudes and beliefs of family, friends, and spouse can affect the ability to breastfeed successfully.[11,16] Cultural differences influence who the most important source of support will be for the mother: a close friend for blacks, the mother's mother for Mexican-Americans, and the male partner for whites.[11] Stress and conflict within the changing marital relationship can affect the mother's ability to nurse successfully.

The infant's behavior may affect the success of breastfeeding. Weak or ineffective sucking affects the establishment of lactation. The infant's excessive crying, irritability, and passivity have been associated with breastfeeding difficulties.[18] After breastfeeding has been initiated, assessment of infant growth, urinary output, quantity and characteristics of stools, and contentment with feeding provides indicators of the effectiveness of breastfeeding.

❖ Defining Characteristics

The presence of the following defining characteristics indicates that the patient may be experiencing Effective Breastfeeding:

For Mother
- Signs and/or symptoms of oxytocin release (let-down or milk ejection reflex)
- Infant correctly positioned at breast and stimulation of rooting reflex
- Nursing infant on demand
- Continued nursing of infant after early postpartal period
- Comments about satisfaction with breastfeeding

For Infant
- Adequate weight gain
- Soft stools
- More than six wet diapers per day of unconcentrated urine
- Latches onto nipple
- Sucks vigorously
- Regular and sustained suckling at the breast (8 to 10 times in 24 hours)
- Eagerness to nurse
- Content after feeding

❖ Related Factors

The following related factors are associated with Effective Breastfeeding:

For Mother
- Normal breast structure
- Basic breastfeeding knowledge
- Maternal confidence
- Support sources

For Infant
- Normal infant oral structure
- Infant gestational age greater than 34 weeks

❖ Related Medical/Psychiatric Diagnoses

The following are examples of related medical/psychiatric diagnoses that are unlikely to be present for Effective Breastfeeding:

For Mother
- Advanced fibrocystic disease of breast
- Bipolar disorder, manic

- Carcinoma of breast
- Cleft palate
- Infant prematurity

NURSING DIAGNOSES

Examples of *specific* nursing diagnoses for Effective Breastfeeding are:
- Effective Breastfeeding related to maternal confidence
- Effective Breastfeeding related to normal infant oral structure

PLANNING AND IMPLEMENTATION WITH RATIONALE

Nursing planning and care affect a mother's ability to achieve Effective Breastfeeding.[3,11] Planning nursing care to assist the mother to maintain effective breastfeeding involves the collaboration of the mother, spouse or support person, and other nurses caring for the mother. *The primary outcome of nursing care is the demonstration of breastfeeding that is physically effective and satisfying to both the mother and the infant. To achieve this outcome,* the nurse performs initial assessment of knowledge and experiences of breastfeeding. Based on these data, the nurse begins to teach the mother and support person, if desired, the techniques of breastfeeding, including: nipple stimulation, latching-on of infant to nipple, stimulation of let-down reflex, infant positioning for feeding, alternation of breasts for initiation of each feeding, removal of infant from the breast by breaking suction, breast care, and cleaning of hands and breasts before nursing. After the teaching of these techniques through demonstrations and/or media, the nurse observes the mother-infant couple breastfeeding to determine the use of information in the performance of breastfeeding and proficiency. Mothers have reported concerns related to privacy when nursing during hospitalization. Placing signs on the door or curtains within the room may ensure privacy.

Successful nursing requires that the mother's nutritional intake be adequate. The nurse teaches the mother about the need to consume an extra 500 calories a day, increase fluid intake (an extra two glasses a day), and limit caffeine and foods that are highly seasoned or make the mother uncomfortable. Discussion with the mother about concerns related to energy level, need for rest, relief from discomfort, physical strength, and lifestyle changes *helps identify factors that may affect the mother's ability to nurse successfully.*[2,5,6,20] *To assist the mother in the continuation of breastfeeding after the early postpartal period,* the nurse should initiate teaching that includes scheduling of mother's rest when infant sleeps, planned assistance with infant care, plans for self-care, strategies to maintain family relationships, tech-

II

II

niques for expression and storage of breast milk, signs of engorgement and infections, and techniques for returning to work and continuing to nurse.[3,6,7,13,17]

To determine if the infant is growing as expected with breastfeeding, the infant is assessed for normal growth and development. The mother learns how to determine if the infant is thriving on breastfeeding. Expectations for the infant include 8 to 12 soft to liquid nonodorous stools per day, 6 to 8 wet diapers a day, tendency to quiet after nursing, vigorous suck, need for nonnutritive sucking, and generally healthy appearance. The nurse provides sources of support within the community for the breastfeeding mother *as resources to help answer questions or address concerns and to assist the mother in continuing to breastfeed after early postpartal period.*

The mother who is unable to breastfeed the baby because of infection, infant prematurity, or maternal illness uses the breast pump to stimulate lactation.[10,21] The milk may be stored (if not con-

---

❖ NURSING CARE GUIDELINES
Nursing Diagnosis: *Effective Breastfeeding*

Expected Patient Outcomes	Nursing Interventions
The mother will communicate knowledge of breastfeeding techniques, breastfeed infant successfully, and be satisfied with the experience.	• Determine mother's knowledge and experience with breastfeeding. • Teach the mother and significant others about techniques of breastfeeding: positions for feeding, positions to enable infant to grasp most of areola, need to change positions to avoid or reduce nipple tenderness, use of both breasts at each feeding, stimulation of let-down response, removal from breast by breaking suction, fact that time limits no longer are recommended in early breastfeeding, cleaning of hands and breasts before nursing, and breast care. • Teach techniques for let-down response: warm shower, warm compresses, relaxation, imagery, closeness with infant, cry of the infant, and infant suckling. • Teach mother about her nutritional needs: an extra 500 calories a day, increased fluid intake (extra two glasses of fluids a day), limited caffeine, well-balanced diet, and avoidance of foods that make mother uncomfortable (such as highly seasoned foods). • Encourage mother to describe her feelings about breastfeedings. • Encourage discussion of accommodation of infant feeding and other demands on mother's time. • Encourage discussion of cultural and familial influences on success of breastfeeding. • Encourage discussion of concerns related to energy level, need for rest, and physical strength.
The infant will grow and develop within developmental expectations.	• Teach mother and significant others expectations for breastfed infants: 8 to 12 stools a day or as few as one a day, soft to liquid nonodorous stools, habit of nursing every 2 to 3 hours, 6 to 8 wet diapers a day, restful after nursing, need for nonnutritive sucking, generally healthy appearance.

❖ *NURSING CARE GUIDELINES— cont'd*
Nursing Diagnosis: Effective Breastfeeding

Expected Patient Outcomes	Nursing Interventions
Mother-infant dyad will continue breastfeeding after early postpartal period.	• Assist mother and family in planning for home care: need to rest when infant sleeps, assistance with infant care by significant others, need for self-care to regain energy, maintenance of family relationships, techniques for expression and storage of breast milk, signs of engorgement and infections, and planning for nursing and working. • Provide a quiet, private environment for nursing. • Encourage mother to verbalize her concerns and feelings about breastfeeding and her abilities to breastfeed. • Provide written information about sources of support within the community for the breastfeeding mother.

❖ *CASE STUDY WITH PLAN OF CARE*

Mrs. Roberta R. just delivered the R.'s first child, a 7-pound, 2-ounce boy who is judged to be well in all respects after a 12-hour labor. This is Mrs. R.'s first pregnancy, and she has had no risk factors except a maternal age of 38 years. The couple had indicated in the prenatal record and on admission that they had selected breastfeeding as their method of infant feeding. With this knowledge, as well as her assessment of the couple's readiness to breastfeed, the nurse encouraged Mrs. R. to try breastfeeding the baby in the birthing room. The mother held their son close to her side and stroked him as both parents spoke with him. The infant gazed up at the parents in an alert state as the mother stroked his cheek with her erect nipple. The infant rooted toward the nipple and latched-on with subsequent sucking. The parents touched each other and smiled. The couple planned a hospital stay of 24 hours before returning home. After delivery, mother and baby were transferred to the mother-baby unit. In this unit, mother and baby, as well as father, are able to be together to gain familiarity with parenting in a supportive environment. The nurse from the birthing area reported to the nurse in the mother-baby unit that breastfeeding was begun in the birthing room and the infant nursed briefly.

CARE PLAN FOR THE R. FAMILY

Nursing Diagnosis: Effective Breastfeeding related to initiation of breastfeeding with demonstrated beginning level proficiency and satisfaction with breastfeeding behaviors.

Expected Patient Outcomes	Nursing Interventions
Mrs. R. will describe techniques of breastfeeding such as positions for nursing, rotation of nursing positions, on-demand feeding	• Educate Mrs. R. and her husband regarding techniques of breastfeeding after assessment of their knowledge level including the following: positions for nursing (cradle-hold, football hold, side-lying); assisting infant to grasp entire areola; rotation of nursing positions to prevent nipple soreness; offering alternate breasts initially at each feeding; on-demand feeding to establish milk supply; stimulation of the let-down reflex with nipple stimulation, sucking, warm compresses, and relaxation; information that limiting nursing time is not recommended.

Expected Patient Outcomes	Nursing Interventions
Mrs. R. will breastfeed infant successfully as evidenced by let-down, latching on, alternating nipples, on-demand nursing, positions of infant, and normal weight gain of infant.	• Teach Mrs. R. about factors that indicate her infant has been breastfed successfully: newborn weight gain as expected by norms; demonstration of successful latching-on, removal from the breast, and let-down of milk. • Observe infant to determine whether he nurses at each breast at each feeding and that the infant is restful after each feeding. • Observe mother and infant for successful breastfeeding: let-down, latching-on, alternating nipples, on-demand nursing, positions of infant. • Assess Mrs. R.'s cultural and familial supports for successful breastfeeding.
Breastfeeding will be a satisfying experience for Mrs. R. as evidenced by expressions of satisfaction with choice to nurse her baby and continued breastfeeding when difficulties arise, such as sore nipples.	• Provide a quiet, private environment for nursing. • Provide positive feedback. • Assist Mrs. R. in addressing problems as they arise and planning actions to address them. For example, for problems with let-down when nipples are sore, use warm shower, warm compresses, relaxation, imagery, closeness with the infant, continued sucking, and Vitamin E.
Infant's growth will be within normal developmental expectations: loses no more than 10% of body weight within 3 days of delivery, weight is within the 10th and 90th percentiles.	• Educate Mrs. R. about nutritional needs of the nursing mother: extra 500 calories/day, increased fluid intake, limited caffeine, and well-balanced diet; avoidance of foods that affect mother, such as beans that produce gas. • Encourage Mrs. R. to feed baby on demand to produce the balance of milk production and the infant's needs.
Mrs. R. and her baby will continue to nurse after the early postpartal period.	• Teach Mrs. R. about expectations for the breastfed baby after returning home: as many as 8 to 12 stools/day, as few as one stool/day, soft to liquid nonodorous stools, nursing at least every 2 to 3 hours unless sleeping, 6 to 8 wet diapers/day, tendency to quiet after nursing, and need for nonnutritive sucking. • Assist mother to plan help at home. • Assist mother to plan for rest at home. • Provide resources in the community for help with breastfeeding problems.

traindicated because of infection or medications) and used to feed the baby later.

EVALUATION

The nurse will evaluate with the mother the extent to which the expected outcomes have been met. If the outcomes have been met, data to support this evaluation will include subjective statements of the mother, observations of the mother and infant, and observations and statements of the family members. The mother should continue to (1) demonstrate successful latching-on, let-down of milk, positioning of infant, and removal from the breast, (2) verbalize satisfaction with breastfeeding, (3) nurse infant after postpartal hospital discharge, (4) plan for assistance at home, and (5) have infant whose growth is consistent and within norms. If outcomes have not been met, the nurse will ask the mother to discuss her perceived reasons for not being able to meet goals.

REFERENCES

1. American Academy of Pediatrics, Committee on Fetus and Newborn: *Guidelines for perinatal care,* ed 2, Elk Grove Village, Illinois, 1988, APP.
2. Anderson E: Nurses' knowledge of breastfeeding, *J Obstet Gynecol Neonat Nurs* 20(1):58-64.
3. Boonin A: Hospital practices and breastfeeding duration: a meta-analysis of controlled trials, *Birth* 16(2):64, 1989.
4. Carroll-Johnson RM (editor) *Classification of nursing diagnoses: proceedings of the Ninth Conference* Philadelphia, 1991, JB Lippincott.
5. Chapman J, Macey M, and Keegan M: Concerns of breastfeeding mothers from birth to four months, *Nurs Res* 24(6):374, 1985.
6. Graef P and others: Postpartum concerns of breastfeeding mothers, *J Nurse-Midwifery* 33(20):62, 1988.
7. Grossman LK: The effect of postpartal lactation counseling on the duration of breastfeeding in low-income women, *Am J Dis Child* 144(4):471, 1990.
8. Hill PD: Potential indicators of insufficient milk supply syndrome, *Res Nurs Health* 14(1):11-19.
9. Hill PD: Predictors of breastfeeding deviation among WIC and non-WIC mothers, *Pub Health Nurs* 8(1):46-52.
10. Kaufman KJ: Influence of the social network on choice and duration of breastfeeding in mothers of pre-term infants, *Res Nurs Health* 12(3):149, 1989.
11. Kearney M: Identifying psychosocial obstacles to breastfeeding success, *J Obstet Gynecol Neonat Nurs* March/April, 98, 1988.
12. L'Esperance C, Frantz K: Time limitation for early breastfeeding, *J Obstet Gynecol Neonat Nurs* 14:114, 1985.
13. Mansfead A, Proffitt C, and Smith J: Predicting and understanding mothers infant-feeding intentions and behavior: testing the theory of reasoned action, *J Pers Soc Psych* 44:657, 1983.
14. Matulonis K, Mose J: Weaning patterns of first time mothers, *Matern Child Nurs* 14(3):188, 1989.
15. Moon JL: Breast engorgement: contributing variables and variables amenable to nursing intervention, *J Obstet Gynecol Neonat Nurs* 18(4):309, 1989.
16. Morse J, Harrison M: Social coercion for weaning, *J Nurse-Midwifery* 32:204, 1987.
17. Morse JM: Intending to breastfeed and work, *Obstet Gynecol Neonat Nursing* 18(6):493, 1989.
18. Neifert M, Seacat J: Practical aspects of breastfeeding the premature infant, *Perinatol-Neonatal* 12:24, 1988.
19. Riordan J, Countryman B: Basics of breastfeeding. Part V: self care for continued breastfeeding problems and solutions, *J Obstet Gynecol Neonat Nurs* 9:357, 1980.
20. Williams KM: Weaning patterns of first-time mothers, *Matern Child Nurs* 14(3):188, 1989.
21. Woldt EH: Breastfeeding support groups in the NICU, *Neonat Net* 9(5):53-56, 1991.

II

High Risk for Aspiration

High Risk for Aspiration is the state in which an individual is at risk for entry of gastrointestinal secretions, oropharyngeal secretions, solid, or fluids into tracheobronchial passages.[21]

OVERVIEW
Aspiration of Gastrointestinal Secretions

Aspiration of gastrointestinal contents results in a severe chemical burn of the lung. The severity of injury to the lung increases as the pH of the aspirate falls below 2.5; however, little additional damage to the lung occurs as the pH falls below 1.5.[18] The initial response to aspiration of acid is an intense bronchospasm. Loss of alveolar-capillary integrity and exudation of fluid and protein into the alveoli and bronchi lead to increased lung weight, decreased pulmonary compliance, and pulmonary edema. Loss of intravascular volume into the alveoli and bronchi results in hemoconcentration, hypotension, and shock.[1] The pulmonary artery pressure initially elevates as a result of hypoxia, parenchymal changes resulting from edema and inflammation, local atelectasis, congestion and thromboses in the pulmonary microvessels, and the local release of vasoactive substances by damaged tissue. However, as the exudation of fluid into the lung depletes the intravascular volume, a decrease in cardiac output and a decrease in pulmonary artery and systemic pressures occurs.[7] Hypoxemia is caused by pulmonary edema, decreased surfactant activity, reflex airway closure, alveolar hemorrhage, and hyaline membrane formation.[2] Diffuse alveolar-capillary damage, pulmonary edema, and arterial hypoxemia refractory to treatment may lead to the development of adult respiratory distress syndrome.[7]

Clinical manifestations of aspiration of acid include acute dyspnea; bronchospasm; frothy pink, sputum; tachypnea; cyanosis; fever; tachycardia; hypoxemia (Po_2 ranging from 35 to 50 mm Hg); and hypotension. The chest radiograph shows infiltrates in one or both of lower lobes.[2] Acute respiratory decompensation is short-lived and easier to reverse when neutral clear liquids are aspirated rather than gastric acid.[18]

Aspiration of Oropharyngeal Secretions

Aspiration of oropharyngeal secretions occurs in 45% of normal adults during sleep and in 70% of patients with depressed consciousness.[9] Bacterial aspiration initially results in pneumonitis characterized by the presence of edema and phagocytes within the alveoli. Untreated pneumonitis may progress to necrotizing pneumonia or lung abscess. Necrotizing pneumonia is a suppurative, lobar process. Tissue necrosis results in consolidation and the development of multiple cavities less than 1 cm in diameter. In the formation of a lung abscess the cavities are greater than 1 cm in diameter and communicate with a bronchus. The extent of the lung abscess is usually limited by a surrounding area of fibrosis, which does not occur in necrotizing pneumonia. Gradual extension of the bacterial infection to the pleura results in pleural thickening and fibrosis, whereas rapid involvement of the pleura leads to empyema. Clinical manifestations include fever, cough, sputum, pleuritic chest pain, weight loss, and leukocytosis.[2]

Aspiration of Solids

Solid material obstructing the airway above the larynx and inhibiting closure of the glottis is an extreme emergency characterized by acute asphyxia, aphonia, cyanosis, and air hunger. At first, hypercapnia and hypoxemia stimulate respiration. Lack of treatment results in respiratory depression, asphyxia, and death. The only effective therapy is to dislodge the solid material; this is frequently accomplished by performing the Heimlich maneuver.[7]

Aspiration of small, solid particles results in airway obstruction, inflammation, hemorrhage, and granuloma formation.[7,16] If the particle is not removed soon after aspiration, infection can ensue.[7] Clinical manifestations include severe dyspnea, cyanosis, wheezing, chest pain, and vomiting. The chest radiograph shows atelectasis or obstructive emphysema.[2] High Risk for Aspiration exists in a variety of settings and disease states. Nursing care should be directed toward the identification of patients at risk and the implementation of measures to prevent aspiration.

ASSESSMENT

Many risk factors predispose a patient to a High Risk for Aspiration. Identification and observation of the patient at risk may prevent its occurrence. Conditions that predispose a patient to aspirate include those causing (1) reduced levels of consciousness resulting in compromise of glottic closure and the cough reflex, (2) dysphagia from neurologic deficits or esophageal disorders, (3) mechanical disruption of the glottic closure or the lower esophageal sphincter because of the presence of a tracheostomy tube, an endotracheal tube, or a nasoenteral feeding tube, and (4) pharyngeal anesthesia.[2]

Patients with altered levels of consciousness are predisposed to aspirate because their cough and gag reflexes are depressed. Metheny, Eisenberg, and Spies[12] reported that all of the patients in their study with nasogastric tubes who aspirated were less than alert with altered protective pharyngeal reflexes. This study substantiated the need to feed such patients into the intestine rather than the stomach. Nurses should use nasogastric feedings only in patients who are alert and have intact gag and cough reflexes.

Endotracheal intubation helps prevent aspiration of saliva or regurgitated material when the balloon cuff is adequately inflated.[19] The following factors place the patient with a tracheostomy at greater risk for aspiration: (1) sensory and motor function necessary for swallowing may be disrupted, (2) pharyngeal desensitization may occur because normal airflow through the upper airways is absent, and (3) the tracheostomy tube may anchor the airway in such a way as to interfere with normal airway closure during swallowing.[6,19] Hyperinflation of the balloon cuff may cause mucosal damage or esophageal obstruction with subsequent aspiration. The risk of mucosal damage or esophageal obstruction has been minimized by the use of high-volume, low-pressure cuffs. In addition, high-volume, low-pressure balloon cuffs tend to conform to the shape of the trachea and act as a mechanical barrier to aspiration.[6]

Decreased gastric pH, increased gastric volume, increased intragastric pressure, decreased tone of the lower esophageal sphincter, and depressed function of the laryngeal closure reflex predispose a patient to aspiration. Patients with duodenal ulcer, gastric ulcer, gastritis, esophagitis, or obesity have decreased gastric pH. An increase in acid production has been reported in patients with feelings of resentment and hostility, feelings of anxiety, sustained family difficulties, and psychological treatment. An increase in gastric volume may occur as a result of gastric hypersecretion or delayed gastric emptying. Gastric emptying is frequently delayed at the onset of labor. A decrease in lower esophageal tone increases the risk for esophageal reflux, which may result in regurgitation of gastric contents and subsequent aspiration. Patients at risk for depressed function of the laryngeal closure reflex include those receiving general anesthesia, narcotic sedation, or 50% nitrous oxide–oxygen sedation (dental patients), the intoxicated trauma patient, and the elderly.[7,10]

Aspiration is often difficult to detect and treat. Therefore the nurse must direct his/her interventions toward accurate identification of the patient at risk and implementation of nursing measures to prevent its occurrence.

II

❖ **Risk Factors[4,21]**

The presence of the following behaviors, conditions, or circumstances render, the patient more vulnerable to High Risk for Aspiration:

- Reduced level of consciousness
- Depressed cough and gag reflex
- Presence of tracheostomy or endotracheal tube
- Incomplete lower esophageal sphincter
- Presence of gastrointestinal tubes
- Tube feedings
- Medication administration
- Situations hindering elevation of upper body
- Increased intragastric pressure

- Increased gastric residual volume
- Decreased gastrointestinal motility
- Delayed gastric emptying
- Impaired swallowing
- Facial/oral/neck surgery or trauma
- Wired jaws
- Cardiopulmonary arrest
- Pregnancy, labor, emergency caesarean section
- Preexisting pulmonary disease

❖ **Related Medical/Psychiatric Diagnoses**

The following are examples of related medical/psychiatric diagnoses for High Risk for Aspiration:[2,16]

Altered level of consciousness:
- Alcoholic intoxication
- Cerebrovascular accident
- Diabetic coma
- Drug overdose
- General anesthesia
- Seizures

Dysphagia secondary to

Esophageal disorder:
- Achalasia
- Bowel obstruction
- Diverticula
- Foreign body, tumor, adenopathy
- Gastroesophageal reflux
- Neoplasm

Neurologic disorder:
- Multiple sclerosis
- Myasthenia gravis
- Parkinson's disease
- Pseudobulbar palsy

- Scleroderma
- Stricture
- Tracheoesophageal fistula

Protracted vomiting

NURSING DIAGNOSES

Examples of *specific* nursing diagnoses for patients at High Risk for Aspiration are:
- High Risk for Aspiration related to altered level of consciousness
- High Risk for Aspiration related to the presence of a nasoenteral feeding tube
- High Risk for Aspiration related to dysphagia
- High Risk for Aspiration related to decreased gastrointestinal motility

PLANNING AND IMPLEMENTATION WITH RATIONALE

The mortality rate secondary to aspiration ranges from 55% to 70%.[7] *The nurse should direct his/her interventions for a patient with High Risk for Aspiration toward preventing aspiration.* Proper identification and observation of patients at risk are essential.

In caring for a patient with an endotracheal or tracheostomy tube, the nurse should suction secretions using sterile technique at least every 2 hours, or more frequently if necessary, to maintain airway patency and to clear secretions. After suctioning the endotracheal or tracheostomy tube, the nurse should remove secretions from the mouth and pharynx. The nurse should provide good oral hygiene. To facilitate making a diagnosis of aspiration, the nurse can place a small amount of blue food coloring on the posterior portion of the patient's tongue every 4 to 6 hours;[6] *the presence of blue dye in pulmonary secretions is a positive sign for aspiration.*

Enteral feedings have been an effective physiological means of providing nutrition to patients who are unable to eat. Tube feedings may also supplement oral or parenteral nutrition. Nurses can administer the feedings through a nasogastric, nasointestinal, gastrostomy (surgical or percutaneous), jejunostomy, or gastrostomy/jejunostomy feeding tube.[5] Metheny and others[12] report that *aspiration occurs less frequently with small-bore nasointestinal tubes than with large-bore nasogastric tubes.* Adding blue food coloring to enteral formulas can help in making a diagnosis of aspiration; if the patient aspirates the formula, the nurse can easily detect the formula in the patient's pulmonary secretions.[3] Testing pulmonary secretions for the presence of glucose is another method that aids in the diagnosis of aspiration. Isolated episodes of pulmonary secretions containing 90 mg/dl of glucose or less do not usually cause clinical symptoms. If pulmonary secretions have 130 mg/dl of glucose or greater, feeding should be discontinued.[20]

To prevent aspiration, nurses should administer intermittent tube feedings with the patient's head of the bed elevated at least 45 degrees during and at least 1 hour after the feeding.[8] The head of the bed should be elevated at all times during continuous feedings.

It is essential that nurses perform a gastrointestinal assessment before the start of enteral feedings and every 4 hours during continuous feeding.[11] *Feedings should not be administered when hypoactive or absent bowel sounds, abdominal distention, nausea, or active vomiting are present.* The findings indicate decreased gastric motility.

The nurse should assess the gastric residual volume before beginning enteral feedings because of *the increased risk of vomiting and subsequent aspiration when a large gastric volume is present.* Nurses should not give intermittent tube feedings when the gastric residual volume is greater than 100 ml. The nurse should reassess the gastric residual volume at the next scheduled feeding time. *If residuals of greater than 100 ml are found on two successive checks,* the nurse should notify the physician and discontinue the feeding.[5] *In patients receiving continuous feedings, a residual that is 10% to 20% greater than the flow rate per hour is significant; the feeding should be stopped until the residual has cleared.* It is frequently difficult to accurately assess gastric residual volumes in patients with small-bore feeding tubes because these tubes tend to collapse when negative pressure is applied. Therefore, the nurse should perform serial measurements of the abdominal girth in addition to assessments of gastric residual volumes. The nurse should discontinue tube feedings when the abdominal girth measures 8 to 10 cm above the baseline measurement.[3]

Many nurses have used the auscultatory method to confirm placement of gastric feeding tubes. However, Metheny and others[13] demonstrated that *auscultation is not a reliable method to differentiate gastric from intestinal feeding tube placement, nor gastric from respiratory placement of feeding tubes.* Metheny and others[14,15] reported that assessment of the pH of aspirates from feeding tubes provides a safe and cost-effective method to ascertain feeding tube placement, but the most accurate method for determining placement of small-bore nasogastric and nasointestinal feeding tubes is by radiography.

It is essential that the *patient with impaired swallowing receive adequate nutrition but not aspirate the feedings.* The patient should be in a sitting position while he/she eats. Foods should be served at the proper temperature in a form that is easy for the patient to chew and swallow, such as a mechanical soft diet or pureed foods. The nurse should observe the patient for signs of aspiration while he/she eats.

Aspiration may occur in the patient who has undergone cardiopulmonary resuscitation. Should vomiting occur during cardiopulmonary resuscitation, turn the patient to the side and sweep out the mouth before continuing resuscitative efforts. After cardiopulmonary resuscitation, the nurse should assess the patient for signs and symptoms of aspiration. *Gastric distention frequently occurs during cardiopulmonary resuscitation, and a nasogastric tube may be needed to decompress the stomach.* [17]

Expected patient outcomes and associated nursing interventions are presented for patients at High Risk for Aspiration. The nurse directs his/her interventions toward identification and observation of these patients and to the prevention of aspiration.

Text continued on p. 126.

❖ NURSING CARE GUIDELINES

Nursing Diagnosis: High Risk for Aspiration

Expected Patient Outcomes	Nursing Interventions

Nursing Interventions

For the patient with an endotracheal or tracheostomy tube

The patient will not aspirate food, fluids, or secretions.

- Using sterile technique, suction the patient's airway every 2 hours or more frequently if necessary to maintain adequate airway patency and remove secretions.
- Maintain good oral hygiene for the patient and remove secretions from his/her mouth and pharynx as necessary.
- Place a small amount of blue food coloring on the posterior portion of the patient's tongue every 4-6 hours, assess the patient's pulmonary secretions for the presence of blue dye.

For the patient receiving enteral nutrition

- Position the patient so that he or she is sitting with the head of the bed elevated at least 45 degrees during and at least 1 hour after intermittent tube feedings; the head of the bed should be elevated at all times during the administration of continuous tube feedings.
- Assess the patient's abdomen for bowel sounds and abdominal distention.
- Check the patient's gastric residual volume before intermittent tube feedings and every 4 hours with continuous feedings.
- Add blue food coloring to enteral formulas; assess the patient's pulmonary secretions for the presence of blue dye.
- Check the patient's tracheal aspirate every 6 hours for the presence of glucose.
- Tube feedings should be administered at room temperature; intermittent feedings should be administered slowly; continuous feedings should be administered via an infusion pump and the infusion rate checked hourly.

For the patient with impaired swallowing

- Assess the patient's ability to chew and swallow.
- The patient should be in a sitting position while he/she eats.
- Provide foods that are easy to chew and swallow, such as a mechanical soft diet or pureed foods.
- Observe the patient eat, and assess for signs of aspiration; suction equipment should be readily available in the event that aspiration occurs.

For the patient requiring cardiopulmonary resuscitation

- Clear the patient's mouth and pharynx of any vomitus.
- Decompress the patient's stomach during or after cardiopulmonary resuscitation as necessary (Hospital policy will determine whether this is a nursing function.)
- After cardiopulmonary resuscitation, assess the patient for signs and symptoms of aspiration.

❖ CASE STUDY WITH PLAN OF CARE

Mr. Fred B., a 74-year-old male, was admitted to the hospital for evaluation of exertional angina. Cardiac catheterization revealed a critical stenosis in the left main coronary artery as well as severe triple-vessel coronary artery disease. He elected coronary artery bypass grafting. He was extubated on the first postoperative day and transferred to the intermediate surgical care unit on the second postoperative day. The afternoon of the second postoperative day he had an expressive aphasia and dysphagia. The result of a computed tomographic scan of the head was unremarkable. The cerebrovascular accident was attributed to a small embolus. It was necessary to place a Dobbhoff tube to supplement nutrition with tube feedings. Mr. B. is currently recuperating satisfactorily from his surgery and cerebrovascular accident after being transferred to the general floor. Past medical history includes gastritis. Past surgical history includes right-sided inguinal herniorrhaphy, transurethral prostatectomy, and hemorroidectomy. Mr. B. has no known allergies. Medications given were dipyridamole USP (Persantine), 75 mg three times a day; digoxin, 0.25 mg daily; metoprolol tartrate (Lopressor), 50 mg twice a day; and ranitidine hydrochloride (Zantac), 150 mg twice a day. Mr. B. is a retired sheet metal worker. He bowls once a week in a league and plays softball in spring and summer. Mr. B. lives with his wife, who is in good health. His only son died of a cerebrovascular accident. Three daughters and 18 grandchildren are alive and well. His father died at age 45 years of carcinoma of the larynx, and his mother died at age 55 years of a myocardial infarction. Results of physical examination were as follows: temperature, 98.8° F; heart rate, 82 beats/min and regular; blood pressure, 140/86 mm Hg; height, 5′11″; weight, 212 pounds; head, normocephalic; cranial nerves, gag reflex absent (glossopharyngeal [IX] cranial nerve); heart, regular rhythm with no murmurs; lungs, clear to auscultation and percussion; neck, grade II/VI right carotid bruit, but none on the left; abdomen, bowel sounds present, no palpable masses, and no tenderness; liver and spleen, not palpable; musculoskeletal, freely movable joints; pulses, 2 + femoral, popliteal, posterior tibial, and dorsalis pedal pulses bilaterally; no peripheral edema. Identification of patient risk factors is essential to the prevention of aspiration. Mr. B. has the following risk factors that predispose him to aspiration: absent gag reflex, dysphagia, presence of a nasointestinal tube, gastritis, mental and physical stress caused by stroke and surgery, and a debilitated condition after the stroke and surgery.

PLAN OF CARE FOR MR. FRED B.

Nursing Diagnosis: High Risk for Aspiration related to multiple factors

Expected Patient Outcomes	Nursing Interventions
Mr. B. will receive adequate nutrition to maintain bodily functions, and he will not aspirate.	• Ensure that Mr. B is in a sitting position while he is eating. • Assess Mr. B.'s abdomen for bowel sounds and abdominal distention; inquire as to the presence of gastrointestinal discomfort (namely, nausea, vomiting, diarrhea, or constipation). • Assess Mr. B.'s ability to chew and swallow. • Serve foods at the proper temperature that are easy to chew and swallow. • Add blue food coloring to the enteral formula; check Mr. B.'s pulmonary secretions for the presence of blue dye. • Before tube feedings check the gastric residual volume; if it is greater than 100 ml, do not give the tube feeding. • Observe Mr. B. for aspiration while he is eating and during tube feedings. • Maintain calorie count, daily weights, and intake and output measurements.
Mr. B. will have a patent airway and an effective breathing pattern.	• Assess respiratory status: check rate and depth of breathing; auscultate and percuss lung fields; and assess for signs of bronchospasm, dyspnea, tachypnea, tachycardia, wheezing, rales, rhonchi, cyanosis, fever, leukocytosis, and an infiltrate on the chest radiograph. • Maintain Mr. B.'s body position so as to protect his airway. • Assist Mr. B. in expectorating secretions. • Check pulmonary secretions for the presence of glucose.

EVALUATION

Because aspiration is often difficult to detect, the nurse must have a high degree of suspicion of its potential in patients who are at risk. Assess vital signs and breath sounds regularly. Symptoms of bronchospasm, dyspnea, tachypnea, tachycardia, wheezing, rales, rhonchi, cyanosis, and fever may occur several hours after the event. The chest radiograph will show a diffuse alveolar infiltrate in the affected area.[7] Adding a small amount of blue food coloring to the enteral formula or to the posterior portion of the tongue will facilitate early detection of aspiration in patients receiving enteral nutrition. Check pulmonary secretions for blue food coloring and/or the presence of glucose. The presence of blue food coloring or glucose in pulmonary secretions indicates aspiration. It is important to be aware that a small amount of blood in the pulmonary secretions will render a false positive result on the glucose test.[12]

REFERENCES

1. Awe WC, Fletcher WS, and Jacob SW: The pathophysiology of aspiration pneumonitis, *Surgery* 60:232, 1966.
2. Bartlett JG: Aspiration pneumonia. In Baum GL and Wolinsky E (editors): *Textbook of pulmonary diseases,* ed 4, Boston/Toronto, 1989, Little, Brown.
3. Bernard M, Forlaw L: Complications and their prevention. In Rombeau JL, Caldwell MD (editors): *Enteral and tube feeding,* Philadelphia, 1984, WB Saunders.
4. Breslin EH, Lery MJ: Prevention and treatment of aspiration pneumonitis secondary to massive gastric aspiration, *Crit Care Q* 6:73, 1983.
5. Eisenberg P: Enteral nutrition. Indications, formulas, and delivery techniques, *Nurs Clin North Am* 24:315, 1989.
6. Elpern EH, Jacobs ER, and Bone RC: Incidence of aspiration in tracheally intubated adults, *Heart Lung* 16:527, 1987.
7. Epstein PE: Aspiration diseases of the lungs. In Fishman AP (editor): *Pulmonary diseases and disorders,* ed 2, New York, 1988, McGraw-Hill Book Co.
8. Heitkemper MM, Williams S: Prevent problems caused by enteral feedings, *J Gerontol Nurs* 11:25, 1985.
9. Huxley EJ and others: Pharyngeal aspiration in normal adults and patients with depressed consciousness, *Am J Med* 64:564, 1978.
10. Kinni ME, Stout MM: Aspiration pneumonitis: predisposing conditions and prevention, *J Oral Maxillofac Surg* 44:378, 1986.
11. Kohn CL, Keithley JK: Enteral nutrition. Potential complications and patient monitoring, *Nurs Clin North Am* 24:339, 1989.
12. Metheny NA, Eisenberg P, and Spies M: Aspiration pneumonia in patients fed through nasoenteral tubes, *Heart Lung* 15:256, 1986.
13. Metheny N, McSweeney M, Wehrle MA, and Wiersema L: Effectiveness of the auscultatory method in predicting feeding tube location, *Nurs Res* 39:262, 1990.
14. Metheny N, Williams, P, Wiersema L, and others: Effectiveness of pH measurements in predicting feeding tube placement, *Nurs Res* 38:280, 1989.
15. Metheny N and others: Detection of inadvertent respiratory placement of small-bore feeding tubes. A report of 10 cases, *Heart Lung* 19:631, 1990.
16. Pennza PT: Aspiration pneumonia, necrotizing pneumonia, and lung abscess, *Emer Med Clin North Am* 7:279, 1989.
17. Sommers MS: Trauma after cardiopulmonary resuscitation, *Heart Lung* 20:287, 1991.
18. Teabeaut JR: Aspiration of gastric contents: an experimental study, *Am J Pathol* 28:51, 1952.
19. Von Hippel A: *A manual of thoracic surgery,* ed 2, Anchorage, 1986, Stone Age Press.
20. Winterbauer RH and others: Aspirated nasogastric feeding solution detected by glucose strips, *Ann Intern Med* 95:67, 1981.
21. Wooldridge J: Nursing diagnosis: potential for aspiration. In Carroll-Johnson RM (editor): Classification of nursing diagnoses: proceedings of the Eighth Conference, Philadelphia, 1989, LB Lippincott.

Impaired Swallowing

Impaired Swallowing is the state in which an individual has decreased ability to pass fluids or solids from the mouth to the stomach.[7]

OVERVIEW

Impaired Swallowing is a human response that crosses virtually all age-groups and is associated with a broad range of medical illnesses. Impaired Swallowing historically has been associated primarily with medical diagnoses such as stroke and cancer of the head and neck. However, the literature indicates that impaired swallowing exists as an actual or potential nursing diagnosis for a much larger patient population than that historically identified.[8,14,19] Discussion of the normal swallowing process is an essential first step in the discussion of this impairment.

Swallowing results from a series of complex actions that reflect the intricate anatomy of the oral and pharyngeal structures, multiple neural mechanisms, characteristics of the bolus, and factors specific to the patient, e.g., the physical, cognitive, and emotional level of function.[1] A complete swallowing cycle lasts an average of 5 to 10 seconds and occurs in four stages: oral preparatory, oral, pharyngeal, and esophageal.[11]

In the oral preparatory stage, food or liquid is masticated and/or manipulated. Lip closure keeps the bolus within the oral cavity, and lingual lateralization maneuvers the bolus to and from the teeth and mixes it with saliva. The oral stage begins when the tongue propels the bolus in an upward and backward motion and ends when the bolus enters the pharynx. These two stages are under voluntary control. The pharyngeal stage begins with triggering of the pharyngeal swallow, which is mediated by the action of the medulla

and characterized by a series of neuromuscular events.[11] The esophageal phase is marked by peristaltic wave action of the esophagus that moves the bolus through it to the stomach. Table 6 details the nerves that support the activities in each of the swallowing stages.[13]

Impaired Swallowing is seen commonly in patients with an inadequate cough or gag reflex, a speech disorder, abnormal oral secretions (for instance, scant or thick), musculoskeletal deficits, or impaired neurological functioning. A diverse group of medical diagnoses includes impaired swallowing as a symptom or outcome. Rubin and others[17] group these diagnoses as either structural or neuromuscular with the former being further divided into intrinsic or extrinsic in nature. Table 7 provides selected examples of these disorders. Lust and others'[14] list of medical diagnoses focuses on psycho-developmental disorders such as mental retardation, developmental disablement, and dementia.

In children congenital anomalies such as cleft lip or palate, as well as cerebral palsy and Down syndrome, can contribute to impaired swallowing.[18] Many traumatically brain-injured individuals have problems with oral intake associated with impaired swallowing. Lazarus and Logemann[10] examined the frequency of swallowing disorders in a group of 53 traumatic brain-injury individuals ranging in age from 4 to 69 years. Among the nine different types of disorders identified, the most frequently occurring were delayed triggering of the pharyngeal swallow and reduced tongue control. Impaired Swallowing is increasingly being identified as related to medical problems found in the multihandicapped, mentally retarded population, where the leading cause of death is

Table 5 Cranial Nerve Functions in Swallowing

Stage	Structures	Nerves	Functions
Oral Preparatory	Lips	V, VII	Keeps bolus in oral cavity
	Tongue	VII, IX	Manipulates bolus
Oral	Lips	V, VII	Begins swallowing
	Soft palate	VII, IX, X	Assists separation of oral/nasal cavity
	Cheeks	V, VII	Controls bolus movement when chewing
	Tongue	VII, IX	Collects/moves bolus
Pharyngeal	Oropharynx	IX, X,	Moves bolus to hypopharynx
	Hypopharynx	X, XI	Moves bolus into esophagus
Esophageal	Esophagus	X	Moves bolus into stomach

Table 6 Medical Diagnoses Associated with Impaired Swallowing

Structural Disorders	Neuromuscular Disorders
Intrinsic	Oropharyngeal anesthesia
Inflammatory disorders	Cerebrovascular accident
Oropharyngeal tumors	Amyotrophic lateral sclerosis (ALS)
Esophageal webs/ cancer	Cranial neuropathies
Zenker's diverticulum	Parkinson's disease
Extrinsic	Brain stem tumors
Compression by lesions	Myasthenia gravis
Respiratory tract malignancy	Esophageal motility disorders
Mediastinal tumors	Traumatic brain injury

asphyxia, often related to the aspiration of food.[2,14]

Weiden and Harrigan[20] caution that the presence of Impaired Swallowing should not be dismissed as relating to an emotional disturbance. In discussing patients with drug-induced impaired swallowing, they note that both Parkinson's disease and tardive dyskinesia can cause eating and swallowing disturbances. Psychotropic medications and most anticholinergic agents may impair the gag reflex and thus contribute to Impaired Swallowing.

The nurse must have a clear and complete knowledge base regarding normal swallowing to be effective in identifying impairments. The timely and accurate identification of patients with or at increased risk for impaired swallowing is the focus of the nursing assessment.

ASSESSMENT

Meeroff[15] notes that a detailed patient history can greatly assist in formulating the causes of Impaired Swallowing and offers a detailed history and assessment algorithm to guide the physician in this process. Such a systematic approach also can be applied by the nurse to pinpoint related factors. Loustau and Lee[13] suggest that reflexes, speech/voice, secretions, supporting muscles, and orientation are five broad areas around which to organize nursing assessment of patients having or suspected of having impaired swallowing.

Assessment begins with identification of existing health deficits that may increase the patient's risk of having or developing impaired swallowing. Whereas patients who have had cerebrovascular accidents are often the most severely affected group, other high-risk populations may not be so obvious.[6] Loustau and Lee[13] address this problem, proposing a five-dimensional approach to assessment. Similarly, Gordon[4] proposes assessment based on 11 areas applicable to all patients. Because of their relevance to clinical practice and ability to provide conceptual direction for patient assessment, Gordon's Functional Health Patterns[4] will guide the remainder of the discussion on assessment.

Assessment of the health perception/health

management pattern includes determination of the patient's perception of swallowing ability and what measures are used to assist swallowing. The quality of the patient's diet, along with a history of weight changes, body temperature, and skin integrity provide important assessment data for the nutritional/metabolic pattern. Discussing favorite foods and/or having the patient list the types of food and fluids consumed in an average day give important clues as to the presence of a swallowing disorder.

Patients with Impaired Swallowing also may demonstrate changes in their elimination pattern. A careful history of bowel and bladder patterns can assist in determining the duration and intensity of a swallowing impairment. Similarly, identifying changes in the patient's activity/exercise pattern permits discussion of the patient's goals and level of satisfaction with his/her current health status.

Assessment of the patient's cognitive/perceptual pattern is especially important when an Actual or High Risk for Impaired Swallowing exists. The status of the patient's senses and perception of pain aid in defining the level of impairment. Memory, judgment, ability to concentrate, and decision-making skills will determine the appropriateness of self-care–focused education interventions.

Assessment of the sleep/rest pattern provides valuable information for the appropriate timing of care interventions, as well as identifying when the patient is at an optimum ability to participate in care. Similarly, the patient's emotions and feelings, associated with the self-perception/self-concept pattern, provide important information on the effect of a change in swallowing ability on personal identity and body image. Such assessment data are vital, especially if interventions such as the placement of nasogastric or other alimentary system tubes is being considered.

The quality and quantity of the patient's social support system can be identified through assessment of the role relationship pattern. Information about resources for support and assistance in the home is vital to planning for meeting recovery and/or rehabilitation needs of patients recovering from strokes, closed head injuries, or other long-term illnesses that frequently include Impaired Swallowing among their side effects.

Assessment of the sexuality/reproductive pattern in the patient with, or at risk for, Impaired Swallowing most often focuses on the effects of the impairment on physical energy and psychological well-being. Similarly, assessment data related to the patient's coping/stress tolerance pattern can identify the degree to which Actual or High Risk for Impaired Swallowing is of concern to the patient, what other stressors are contributing to this effect, and what patient-directed versus assisted coping mechanisms are appropriate.

Lastly, assessment of the patient's value/belief pattern focuses on identifying the spiritual and philosophical principles that guide the way the patient views life. Assessment data from this pattern can provide invaluable insight into the potential for patient compliance with and/or participation in his/her recovery from or management of a Swallowing Impairment.

Defining characteristics of this diagnosis include both subjective and objective findings. Subjective data collection includes a detailed health history, with a focus on the patient's view of changes in nutritional status (such as weight loss, anorexia), oral health (such as changes in quality/quantity of secretions, pain, bleeding), and speech/voice quality. Objective data focus on the nurse's assessment of the quality of reflexes, head and neck structures, psychoemotional health status, and speech and voice quality.

In gathering subjective data the nurse first must determine the patient's ability to recall, describe, and discuss past and present health status. If the patient displays significant memory impairment, is easily confused, or appears to be expressively or receptively aphasic, subjective data may be limited or may have to be obtained by interviewing a family member or friend. In all cases the nurse should take all necessary steps to maximize the patient's participation in this phase of the assessment process.

Objective data collection begins with a detailed

physical assessment, with attention to clues about overall nutritional health (for instance, oral mucous membranes, height/weight ratio, skin turgor) and neurological and musculoskeletal status. Identification of the status of the gag, cough, and swallowing reflexes and assessment of the quality of mouth and upper airway structures are critical activities in the performance of a comprehensive evaluation of the patient's health. Inspection and palpation are key assessment behaviors.

❖ Defining Characteristics

The presence of the following defining characteristics indicates that the patient may be experiencing Impaired Swallowing:

- Coughing when eating/drinking
- Reduced buccal/facial tone
- Reduced soft palate function
- Delayed/absent swallowing reflex
- History of declining oral intake
- Pain upon swallowing
- Reduced tongue control
- Weight loss
- Choking
- Fear of choking
- Severe depression
- Denies changes in health
- Avoids favorite foods
- Avoids eating with others
- Limits socialization

The following related factors are associated with Impaired Swallowing:

- Neuromuscular dysfunction
- Mechanical obstruction
- Reddened or irritated oropharyngeal cavity
- Developmental disability
- Neurological deficits
- Depression over current change in health
- Absent/loss of social support system
- Loss of cultural incentives related to eating
- Loss of valuing life/survival

❖ Related Medical/Psychiatric Diagnoses

The following are examples of related medical/psychiatric diagnoses:

- Brain stem tumors
- Cerebrovascular accident
- Dementia
- Esophageal cancer
- Mental retardation
- Cleft lip or palate
- Developmental disablement
- Myasthenia gravis
- Parkinson's disease

NURSING DIAGNOSES

Examples of *specific* nursing diagnoses for Impaired Swallowing are:

- Impaired Swallowing related to neuromuscular dysfunction
- Impaired Swallowing related to reddened, irritated oropharyngeal cavity
- Impaired Swallowing related to neurological deficits
- Impaired Swallowing related to developmental disability

PLANNING AND IMPLEMENTATION WITH RATIONALE

Nursing interventions for patients with Impaired Swallowing can be grouped into three major areas: *assessment* of the patient for changes from the initially assessed baseline function or competency regarding swallowing; *implementation and evaluation* of specific treatment measures designed to eliminate or minimize the diagnosis and its effects; and *teaching* the patient and family about the diagnosis and the specific care behaviors to perform in order to eliminate or minimize the diagnosis.

The first expected patient outcome listed in the Nursing Care Guidelines focuses on the quality and quantity of understanding by the patient and family of the specific characteristics of the patient's swallowing impairment. The nursing interventions associated with this outcome ensure that *the patient and family will be provided accurate and timely information about the nature of the impairment.*

The second expected patient outcome focuses on the patient and family's ability to perform care behaviors in support of successful swallowing. The nursing interventions associated with this outcome ensure that *the patient will attain a level of self-care ability that will sustain an acceptable level of health regarding management of swallowing.*

❖ *NURSING CARE GUIDELINES*

Nursing Diagnosis: *Impaired Swallowing*

Expected Patient Outcomes	Nursing Interventions
The patient and family will state correct information regarding the nature of the impairment.	• Perform and document patient assessment using the impaired swallowing protocol. • Validate understanding with the patient and family. • Explain findings to and discuss with the patient and family.
The patient and family will demonstrate correct performance of care behaviors such as selection and preparation of goods, positioning, oral care, and use of assistive devices.	• Teach the patient and family care behaviors. • Observe patient's and family's performance of learned care behaviors.
The patient will be able to swallow selected food and fluids without evidence of choking, coughing, or aspiration.	• Observe performance of swallowing and evaluate problems. • Reteach care behaviors as necessary.

The third expected patient outcome focuses on the degree of resolution of the impairment in swallowing. The nursing interventions associated with this outcome ensure that *the patient will successfully overcome or will be able to manage the impairment alone or will be able to manage it with additional nursing guidance and support.*

EVALUATION

The degree of achievement of expected patient outcomes will vary depending on the nature and intensity of the impairment, the ability of the patient to participate in care, and the presence of other acute and/or chronic health problems that tax resources and capabilities. The nurse can determine if the first listed outcome in the Nursing Care Guidelines is achieved by questioning the patient and family directly and/or by discussing the patient's hospitalization in general and then focusing the discussion on the patient's views regarding his/her Impaired Swallowing. Incorrect or incomplete patient or family statements will require repeat discussion and explanation of findings. If the patient does not achieve this outcome, the nurse must act to ensure that at least one significant other is able to state correct information.[5]

The nurse can determine attainment of the second listed expected outcome by having the patient and/or family respond to "what if" scenarios in discussions of posthospital care, as well as by direct observation of the patient's self-care behaviors.[3,12] If the patient cannot perform his/her own care behaviors or needs assistance to perform them, the nurse must act to ensure that a significant other is knowledgeable and available to assist the patient.

The achievement of the third expected outcome, being able to swallow selected food and fluids without problems, will vary based on the degree of success possible within the limitations of the impairment and the existence of complicating health problems. The nurse can determine the

II

❖ *CASE STUDY WITH PLAN OF CARE*

Mr. Carl M. is being admitted to the ear/nose/throat unit. He is accompanied by his wife, who gives the following medical history: Mr. M. is a 64-year-old retired carpenter who was in reasonably good health until 2 years ago when he suffered a mild stroke. Initially he lost function of his left side and had left facial drooping and moderate expressive aphasia. The wife states that since the stroke he has regained use of his left side but continues to have some facial drooping and intermittently confused speech. He has lost 20 pounds in the last 2 months, and she has noticed that his voice is more hoarse. Mr. M. said that "It hurts sometimes when I swallow" and that he is more tired lately. Today his doctor told him he has a "small cancer" in his throat and has advised radiation therapy as treatment. The couple has two grown sons who live with their families in nearby cities. Mrs. M. is a retired schoolteacher who does church work but is otherwise at home with her husband. She describes her health as very good. Progress notes indicate significant resolution of most stroke-related side effects. The patient smoked 1½ to 2 packs of cigarettes per day for 40 years but quit 2 years ago (after his stroke). He has mild hypertension and uses no alcohol. Blood pressure is 150/90 mm Hg, respirations are 22/min, temperature is 98.2° F., and pulse is 84/min. He is 73 inches tall and weighs 152 pounds (life average, 175 to 180 pounds; down to 170 to 175 pounds since stroke). His voice is hoarse. The physician's note states that Mr. M. has a 3 cm lesion of the left true vocal cord and moderate pharyngeal erythema and tenderness. The tentative medical diagnosis is squamous cell carcinoma of the left true vocal cord.

The medical plan is for a full medical workup with radiation therapy as the treatment of choice. Mr. M's cough and gag reflexes are intact; there is no other evidence of oral disease. Mr. M. teaches basic carpentry part-time at the local high school (now in summer recess) and does "odd jobs" around the house. His hobbies include woodworking and teaching carpentry to his grandsons. Mr. M. enjoys visits from his "students," who often stop by to discuss carpentry projects. He describes wife as "my companion"; their interaction appears very warm and loving. Mr. M. describes frequent contact with his sons' families and reports they help out more since he has been sick. Combined retirement incomes are described as sufficient with "a little extra." Income from teaching usually is spent on grandchildren. Mr. M.'s routine mealtimes are 8 AM, 1 PM, and 6 PM. He has noticed increased difficulty eating fried foods and most meats and now eats more soups, stews, custards, and mashed potatoes ("easier to get down than steak"). His appetite has decreased progressively over the last 2 to 3 months. Mr. M. is generally quiet during the interview and examination but responds verbally in an appropriate manner when talking. He describes present emotional state as "anxious but hopeful" that treatment will be effective, and he indicates a desire to actively participate in his care and health management. He is looking forward to going home on weekends to "see the kids." He expresses concern about the side effects of radiation, such as pain, fatigue, and changes in speech. The nurse made the following diagnosis: Impaired Swallowing related to stroke-related side effects, presence of vocal cord lesion, and common effects of radiation treatment.

PLAN OF CARE FOR MR. CARL M.

Nursing Diagnosis: *Impaired Swallowing related to stroke-related side effects, presence of vocal cord lesion, and common effects of radiation treatment*

Expected Patient Outcomes

Mr. M. and his family will accurately identify and describe current status related to side effects of stroke as evidenced by consistency of patient's description with clinical facts.

Nursing Interventions

- Discuss health history related to current activities of daily living and self-care ability.
- Identify and agree on those areas where help is needed and by whom.
- Discuss and assess effect of the stroke on ability to chew, swallow, control secretions, speak, and maintain weight.

II

Expected Patient Outcomes	Nursing Interventions
Mr. M. will accurately describe current health limitations and abilities related to new health problem as evidenced by consistency of patient's description with clinical facts.	• Discuss and assess effect of new health problem on ability to chew, swallow, speak, control secretions, and maintain weight.
Mr. M. will accurately identify and describe the common side effects of radiation therapy (RXT) and the measures to prevent or minimize these effects.	• Explain RXT (for instance, purpose, uses, and side effects). • Provide copy of patient education literature, and set time to discuss content as evidenced by consistency of patient's description with that explained by the nurse. • Discuss and demonstrate care measures Mr. M. can take to prevent or minimize RXT effects related to swallowing: oral care procedures, use of analgesics, adequate secretions, daily oral examination, dietary supplements, activity and rest needs, and symptoms and emergencies (for instance, performance of Heimlich maneuver). • Set up consult with speech therapy personnel for assessment and treatment as needed.
Mr. M. will maintain adequate nutritional and hydration status (as seen by weight loss of not more than 8 pounds from start to end of treatment), balanced intake and output, and stable physiological parameters (such as electrolytes).	• Weigh Mr. M. daily. • Monitor intake and output, and keep calorie counts. • Assess oral and pharyngeal health daily. • Set up consult with oral hygienist for assessment and fluoride treatments. • Monitor systemic signs of hydration (such as skin turgor, temperature, and blood chemistries).
Mr. M. will demonstrate a stabilized or improved ability to swallow food and fluids as evidenced by demonstrated swallowing ability and the patient's perception of the quality of that ability.	• Encourage Mr. M. to expand and build swallowing skill, and encourage family to reinforce encouragement.
Mr. M. will participate in making plans regarding his care and future as evidenced by the content of conversations with family, friends, healthcare staff, etc.	• Encourage Mr. M. to make plans regarding resuming preillness work and hobbies. • Compliment Mr. M. on his abilities to participate in his care. • Encourage Mr. M. to be active in self-care, and praise his efforts.

quality of achievement of this outcome by direct observation of the patient under a variety of swallowing conditions. A corollary to this outcome is that the patient must consume sufficient quantities of food and fluids to maintain acceptable levels of nutrition and hydration. If this latter condition is not met, the nurse should consider assistive systems, either short term or long term.[9,16]

REFERENCES

1. Bach DB and others: An integrated team approach to the management of patients with oropharyngeal dysphagia, *J Allied Health* 18(5):4459-4468, 1989.
2. Carter G, Jancar J: Mortality in mentally handicapped: fifty year survey of stroke park hospitals, *J Ment Defic Res* 27:143-156, 1983.
3. Donahue PA: When it's hard to swallow: feeding techniques for dysphagia management, *J Gerontol Nurs* 16(4):6-9, 41-42, 1990.
4. Gordon M: *Nursing diagnosis: process and application,* New York, 1987, McGraw-Hill Book Co.
5. Hutchins BF: Establishing a dysphagia family intervention program for head injured patients, *J Head Trauma Rehab* 4(4):64-72, 1989.
6. Kadas N: The dysphagic patient: everyday care really counts, *RN* 46:38, 1983.
7. Kim MJ, McFarland GK, and McLane AM: *Pocket guide to nursing diagnoses,* ed 4, St Louis, 1991, Mosby–Year Book.
8. Krefting L and others: A retrospective analysis of interdisciplinary dysphagia assessment data, *Phys Occup Ther Geriatr* 9(2):79-95, 1991.
9. Lazarus BA, Murphy JB, and Culpepper L: Aspiration associated with long term gastric versus jejunal feedings: a critical analysis of the literature, *Arch Phys Med Rehab* 71:46-52, 1990.
10. Lazarus C, Logemann J: Swallowing disorders in closed head trauma patients, *Arch Phys Med Rehab* 68:79-84, 1987.
11. Lazarus CL: Swallowing disorders after traumatic brain injury, *J Head Trauma Rehab* 4(4):34-41, 1989.
12. Logemann JA and others: The benefits of head rotation on pharyngoesophageal dysphagia, *Arch Phys Med Rehab* 70:767-771, 1989.
13. Loustau A, Lee KA: Dealing with the dangers of dysphagia, *Nurs 85* 15(2):47, 1985.
14. Lust CA, Fleetwood DE, and Molteler EL: Development and implementation of a dysphagia program in a mental retardation residential facility, *Occup Ther Health Care* 6(2/3):153-172, 1989.
15. Meeroff JC: Diagnosis of dysphagia, *Hosp Pract* p 162, April 15, 1985.
16. Mochizuki RM and others: Heparin lock for nighttime intravenous fluid management in a dysphagic patient, *Rehab Nurs* 15(6):322-324, 1990.
17. Rubin M and others: Dysphagia: a clinical guide, *Hosp Med* 20:231, 1984.
18. Schwaab LM, Niman CW, and Gisel E: Tongue movements in normal 2-, 3-, and 4- year-old children: a continuation study, *Am J Occup Ther* 40:180, 1986.
19. Stratton M: Clinical management of dysphagia in the developmentally disabled adult, *Occup Ther Health Care* 6(2/3):143-152, 1989.
20. Weiden P, Harrigan M: A clinical guide for diagnosing and managing patients with drug-induced dysphagia, *Hosp Comm Psychiatry* 37:396, 1986.

Altered Oral Mucous Membrane

Altered Oral Mucous Membrane is a state in which an individual experiences change or damage to the oral mucous membrane.

OVERVIEW

Striated squamous cells make up the epithelium of the oral cavity. Whereas the tissue type is the same as that of the skin, it lacks the keratin (the tough, fibrous protein formed from flattened, dead cells) typically found on the epidermis.[20] These flattened, platelike cells of the oral mucous membrane are easily shed and replaced by division in the deeper germinative epithelial layer.[27] The entire surface of the mucous membrane is replaced approximately every 7 days.[3] When the balance between the cells that are lost and those that are replacing them, is upset, the integrity of the tissue may be compromised.

Like any body tissue, the mucous membranes are subject to changes at the cellular level in response to alterations in the environment. Cellular loss or changes may result from many factors. Mechanical trauma or injury, such as may result from a broken or jagged dentition, habitual cheek biting, a surgical procedure, or an accident, may be the cause.[9,21] Physical injury of the oral mucous membrane also may occur because of the drying effect of certain risk factors; for instance, mouth breathing, continuous flow of oxygen, intermittent suctioning, and decreased intake of nutrients.[7] Physical injuries also may result from significant thermal changes. Extreme heat from hot foods or fluids may cause burns of the oral cavity and destruction of the epithelium. Extreme cold also may cause cellular injury and has a profound drying effect.

Chemical injury of the oral mucous membrane may be the direct result of contact with some irritating substances as in the case of ingestion of alcohol, use of tobacco, intake of acidic food, or the body's production of toxins (for instance, the mucosa becomes inflamed and ulcerated in patients with renal dysfunction when the levels of ammonia and uremic toxins are elevated). Damage to oral tissue also may have an indirect cause; for example, certain drugs (such as chemotherapeutic agents, antibiotics, steroids, and antidepressants) may produce side effects observed in the oral cavity.[4,11,16] Radiation injury also may be a factor in the cellular damage of the oral mucous membranes if the tissues are within the field of treatment, such as in radiation therapy for head and neck cancers, or if the tissues are subject to the long-term effects of ultraviolet radiation, for instance, as occurs in occupations requiring much time outdoors.

Biological agents also are responsible for changes at the cellular level. Micro-organisms, such as *Candida albicans* (fungal), *herpes simplex* (viral), *streptococcus* (gram-positive bacteria), and *Pseudomonas* (gram-negative bacteria), can injure the mucous membranes through a number of mechanisms (such as interference with cellular production of adenosine triphosphate or the release of endotoxins). In addition, these organisms have the ability to replicate, thereby continuing the injurious process.[20,24] In the case of periodontal disease, a chronic inflammatory disease that occurs most frequently in adults, a combination of bacteria and the mucus forming the dental plaque is responsible for the initiation of the disease process.[11,14,28]

Finally, cellular injury of the oral mucous membrane may result from nutritional imbalance. Specifically, deficiencies of several of the B vitamins (riboflavin, niacin, folic acid, vitamin B_{12}

and pyridoxine) or iron may lead to changes in the tissue of the oral cavity.[1]

The effect of these alterations on the tissue of the oral mucous membranes may vary. Atrophy (decrease in size) of the epithelium may result from the aging process, a disease process, or nutritional deficiency.[1,22] Hyperplasia (an increase in the number of cells) may occur. An example is the gingival hyperplasia that occurs in response to inflammation or as fibrous changes, as occurs as a side effect of diphenylhydantoin (Dilantin).[25] Hypertrophy (an increase in the amount of functioning tissue mass of an organ or part) also may occur; for example, mumps causes hypertrophy of the acinar cells of the parotid gland.[17,25] Leukoplakia (a thickened white patch that does not rub off) is an example of the dysplasia (deranged cell growth with a variation of size, shape, and appearance) that may occur in response to chronic irritation or inflammation of the oral mucous membranes. Although dysplasia is an adaptive process, its progression may lead to neoplastic (abnormal new growth) disease.[17,25]

In the presence of one or more of these factors related to cellular injury, the patient may demonstrate the defining characteristics leading to the nursing diagnosis of Altered Oral Mucous Membrane. It is important to note that an interruption in the integrity of the tissue or underlying structures of the oral cavity will increase the patient's risk for infection because of a break in the body's first line of defense. Alteration in the oral mucous membrane can also influence the patient's level of comfort, nutritional status, ability to communicate, fluid balance, sense of taste, and body image.

ASSESSMENT

The nurse may begin the assessment by obtaining subjective information concerning any sensory changes in the oral cavity, such as pain or discomfort, burning, numbness, paresthesia, sensitivity to temperature changes, or impaired taste (dysgeusia). It is important to include the exact location and duration of the identified changes. Ear pain (otalgia) occasionally is experienced as referred pain in patients with lesions in the posterior oral cavity (pharynx, tonsillar region, posterior tongue, or hypopharynx). Other information to obtain includes current medications; a history of trauma (including previous infections or lesions), tobacco use, alcohol ingestion, ingestion of highly seasoned or hot foods, usual dental practices, and any difficulty chewing or swallowing (dysphagia); oral sexual practices; and speech changes or voice impairment (dysphonia).

Physical assessment is conducted by means of inspection and palpation with the use of the following equipment: gloves, a light, a tongue blade, 4 inch × 4 inch gauze, and a dental mirror, if available. A systematic physical assessment of the oral cavity should include data about the following: saliva, lips, buccal mucosa, teeth, gingiva, tongue, hard and soft palates, pharynx, and regional lymph nodes. Some general characteristics of the mucous membranes in the oral cavity are that they are moist, smooth, and pink or coral in color.

One of the first things observed during inspection of the oral cavity is the amount of *saliva* (moisture) on the mucosa. Saliva serves to clean the mouth, regulate the pH, maintain the integrity of the tissue (through glycoprotein that binds to the surface) and teeth, fight bacteria (via immunoglobulins and enzymes), and begin the process of digestion of carbohydrates.[17,27] Approximately 1.5 L of saliva are produced daily, primarily from the parotid, submandibular, and sublingual glands and to a much lesser degree from minor salivary glands, such as the labial, palatal, and buccal glands.[17] The consistency of saliva normally is similar to that of water, and saliva has a pH of 6.0 to 7.0. A decrease in the amount of saliva and the symptom of xerostomia (dry mouth) may be the result of dehydration, anxiety, glandular disease (such as an infection or obstruction of the duct), drug therapy (especially antihistamines, narcotics, antidepressants, and chemotherapeutic agents), radiation therapy, or an endocrine disorder.[17] In response to a decrease in amount, the consistency of the saliva may change from thin and watery to being viscous and ropy. Along with subjective information and visual inspection of the saliva for clarity and consistency, the amount of moisture in the oral cavity can be assessed by running a gloved finger over the surfaces to evaluate for stickiness of the mucous membranes. Because of saliva's functions in the oral cavity, a decrease in saliva has a profound effect on the other structures.

The color of the *mucosa* changes with anemia (pallor), hypoxia (cyanosis), or other pathological conditions. Peutz-Jeghers syndrome, associated with multiple intestinal polyps, may be manifested by pigmented spots on the lips. It is important to note, however, that pigment changes may occur in dark-skinned individuals who have no disease. Purple discoloration of the oral mucosa caused by extravasation of blood in the area is present in purpura. Increased redness and edema of the oral cavity is indicative of stomatitis, an inflammation of the oral mucosa. The term *mucositis* also is used in conjunction with this inflammation, but unless location is specified, it could mean an inflammation of any mucosal surface.[5] (See Table 7 for a suggested scale to use in assessing stomatitis.) Desquamation, a shedding of the epithelial layer, also may occur.

Lesions or ulcers, which may be considered pathological and appear on mucosal surfaces, include herpes simplex, which is characterized by vesicular eruptions that break and crust over; aphthous ulcers (chancre sores), which may be solitary or multiple, small, round or oval, painful, white ulcers surrounded by a halo of reddened mucosa; chancres associated with syphilis, appearing as firm, buttonlike lesions that ulcerate and crust when external; a mucocele, which is a round, regular, translucent, or blue nodule; leukoplakia, a white, thickened plaque over a small area or large patch that has a tendency to progress to malignant growth; or a verrucous (warty) growth. Any plaque, ulcer, or warty growth that does not heal is considered suspicious for cancer and should be evaluated. In addition, the oral mucosa is frequently the site of candidiasis (moniliasis, thrush), a yeast infection characterized by removable, white plaques that resemble milk curds

Table 7 Gradings of Oral Stomatitis

Grade	Description
I	Mild; generalized erythema of oral mucosa
II	Moderate; generalized erythema of oral mucosa and isolated, small ulcerations and/or white patches
III	Severe; confluent ulcerations with white patches covering more than 25% of oral mucosa
IV	Severe; hemorrhagic ulcerations

From Goodman M, Stoner C: Mucous membrane integrity, impairment of, related to stomatitis. In McNally JC, Somerville ET, Miaskowski C, Rostad M (editors): *Guidelines for oncology nursing practice,* ed,[2] Philadelphia, 1991, WB Saunders. Reproduced with permission of the Oncology Nursing Society.

and, less frequently, a shiny erythema. Clinically this may appear on any or all mucosal surfaces in the oral cavity, and *Candida albicans* is frequently the organism identified on culture.[1,24,25,27] Because of the opportunistic nature of fungal infections such as candidiasis, the incidence is increased in patients receiving antibiotics (which destroy the normally inhibitory bacterial flora), immunosuppressive agents (such as corticosteroids or cytotoxic drugs),[25] or in those who are immunocompromised, such as patients with acquired immunodeficiency syndrome. Other microorganisms and the clinical manifestations that may occur include gram-positive bacteria resulting in a dry, brownish yellow, circular, raised eruption; gram-negative bacteria resulting in a creamy white, raised, moist, glistening, nonpurulent, painful ulcer with a reddened base; and *pseudomonas* resulting in a yellow, dry, painless ulcer with defined borders, which may progress to the necrotic center.[15]

The *lips* should be symmetrical in movement. The inner lip is covered by the mucous membrane. Normally the faint vertical lines on the outer lip surface become more prominent with age or with the absence of teeth or dentures.[27] It is important to assess the lip from commissure to commissure and from outer border to inner mucosal surface. Edema of the lip may be in response to injury or may be an allergic reaction. In addition to the previously mentioned lesions and ulcers, abnormalities of the lips may be manifested as fissures, dry crusts, scales, and cracking (angular stomatitis or cheilosis if the angle of the mouth is involved) which may be indicative of dehydration, nutritional deficiency, overclosure of the mouth, or sensitivity reaction to cosmetics or dentifrice[1,24] or may be in response to extreme cold or dryness of the environment.

With the aid of a light and tongue blade for retraction, an inspection of the *buccal mucosa* (internal cheeks) is possible. A bimanual (gloved finger internally and other finger externally) examination is useful for palpation and to detect changes in tissue consistency. The Stensen ducts (opening of the parotid gland) can be seen bilaterally on the surface of buccal mucosa adjacent to the upper second molar. Fordyce spots (yellow-appearing granules on the buccal mucosa and inner lip) are sebaceous glands that are visible in most adults and are considered normal. An occlusion line may also be apparent on the mucosa adjacent to the point where the teeth meet.

The crown of the *tooth* is usually the only part of the tooth visible. Normally the teeth appear shiny and white (although the color may range to yellow or gray), with smooth edges and no debris. Dental caries may appear first as chalky, white deposits on the tooth surface; if caries is allowed to advance, these lesions then become brown or black, soft, and cavitary. Attrition (flattening of the biting surfaces) may be seen in the older adult. If dentures are present, the nurse should assess them for tightness of fit, and the nurse should determine the condition of mucosa on the underlying alveolar ridge, because this is frequently a site of irritation.

The *gingivae* (gums) are normally pink-coral in color and moist, with a stippled surface and a tight margin with the tooth surface. Increased melanin pigment (patchy, brown discoloration) of the gingivae is normal in some adults but also may be associated with Addison's disease. A bluish-black line on the gingivae approximately 1

mm from the margin may indicate lead or bismuth poisoning. Swelling and redness of the gums (gingivitis) occurs in response to irritations. With severe gingivitis the stippling is decreased, the gums may bleed easily, and the interdental papilla (gingiva between the teeth) becomes bulbous. This may occur in periodontal disease, in which the inflammation process (in response to calculus formation) progresses to involve the deeper supporting structures of the teeth. Pockets may form, and the gums are recessed. Halitosis frequently is associated with periodontal disease but also is related to infection and tissue necrosis elsewhere in the cavity. Gingival changes also are common in the patient with leukemia caused by the presence of leukemic infiltrates. These changes may include gingivitis, gingival hyperplasia, hemorrhage, petechiae, and ulcerations.[25]

Movement of the *tongue* should be symmetrical and mobile in all directions. The dorsal and lateral surfaces are slightly rough (papilla) and moist, and occasionally glisten with slight fissures, whereas the ventral surface is smooth with a prominent venous system. With age the papillae become less distinct and the ventral veins may become varicose. Wharton's ducts of the submaxillary gland can be identified under the tongue on the floor of the mouth near the midline on either side of the frenulum (vertical fold under tongue, attaching it to the floor of the mouth). Gauze and a dental mirror may aid in the retraction of the tongue during inspection and palpation of all surfaces. The facial nerve innervates the anterior two thirds of the tongue and should be evaluated for the ability to distinguish sweet, sour, salty, and bitter tastes. It also innervates certain salivary glands. Sour and bitter are the primary tastes associated with the posterior one third and lateral surfaces of the tongue, which is innervated by the glossopharyngeal nerve. Moisture (saliva) in the oral cavity is essential for the person to perceive the taste of a given substance. The sense of taste is generally thought to decrease with age. Taste alteration may be associated with certain medications or radiation therapy and, in the presence of cancer, may result from tumor byproducts. Mouth blindness (ageusia) is associated with the lack of sense of taste, whereas dysgeusia refers to aberrant taste sensation.[1,19] The tongue may become inflamed (glossitis) in response to leukoplakia, ulcers, lesions, or vitamin B deficiency. The tongue also may become smooth in appearance as a result of vitamin deficiencies. Other abnormalities of the tongue include hairy tongue (elongated papillae on the dorsum, usually in response to antibiotic therapy, but also seen in patients with AIDS), geographic tongue (scattered, red, smooth areas on the dorsum), coated tongue (white, excessive appearance caused by keratinization of the papillae in response to an irritant, tobacco, candies, or drugs), and furrowed tongue (deep fissures in the surface that may be the result of dehydration, chronic irritation, or vitamin deficiency).[1,24,25,27]

The mucous membrane covering the *hard palate* is paler and has an irregular texture. The transverse rugae are the ridges on the anterior surface on either side of the linear raphe (the center line of union between the palatine bones). A common abnormality of the hard palate is torus palatinus. This is defined as a bony midline outgrowth that may vary in size. The mucous membranes of the soft palate and uvula are moist, smooth, pink, movable, and symmetrical.

The nurse can examine the *pharynx* during the assessment of the palate, and examination includes the inspection of the uvula, retromolar trigone, anterior and posterior tonsillar pillars, and the posterior pharynx. A tongue blade and light are needed. The tonsils normally may have clefts (crypts) in the surface.

Finally, assessment of the oral cavity should include palpation of the *lymph nodes* of the neck, especially the tonsillar, submaxillary, and submental, because these are the primary routes of internal drainage from the mouth.[1] The presence of palpable nodes (lymphadenectasia) will lend supporting data to clinical findings of inflammation or possible malignancy but may also help to identify areas needing further assessment.

❖ **Defining Characteristics**

The presence of the following defining characteristics indicates that the patient may be experiencing Altered Oral Mucous Membrane:

- Sensory changes: pain, burning taste, paresthesia, numbness, temperature sensitivity
- Decreased moisture: xerostomia, viscous saliva, fissure
- Color changes: erythema, pallor, pigmentation, coated tongue, exudate
- Lesions or ulcers: vesicles, aphthous ulcer, chancre, mucocele, leukoplakia, erythroplakia
- Oral, plaque or dental caries
- Bleeding, hyperemia, or hemorrhage
- Induration of tissue or lymph nodes
- Inflammation or edema: mucositis, stomatitis, gingivitis, glossitis, desquamation
- Halitosis

❖ **Related Factors**

The following related factors are associated with Altered Oral Mucous Membrane:

- Mechanical trauma: surgery, broken teeth, cheek biting, pressure or friction from oral tubes
- Physical injury or drying effect: mouth breathing, oxygen therapy, inadequate intake of nutrients, decreased salivation, temperature extremes
- Chemical trauma: alcohol, tobacco, acidic foods, side effects of medications
- Radiation injury: radiation therapy to the area, prolonged ultraviolet exposure
- Injury from biological agents: microorganisms (bacterial, viral, fungal), ineffective oral hygiene
- Nutritional imbalance: vitamin deficiency, malnutrition

❖ **Related Medical/Psychiatric Diagnoses**

The following are examples of related medical/psychiatric diagnoses for Altered Oral Mucous Membrane:

- Fractured mandible
- Squamous cell carcinoma of the retromolar trigone
- Intracranial tumor
- Herpes simplex viral infection
- Leukoplatia related to chronic tobacco use

NURSING DIAGNOSES

Examples of *specific* nursing diagnoses for Altered Oral Mucous Membrane are:
- Altered Oral Mucous Membrane related to broken teeth
- Altered Oral Mucous Membrane related to mouth breathing
- Altered Oral Mucous Membrane related to acidic foods

PLANNING AND IMPLEMENTATION WITH RATIONALE

The primary outcome of nursing interventions is *to maintain or attain an intact tissue integrity within the oral cavity.* Basic oral hygiene, including brushing with a soft or medium-soft brush and nonabrasive fluoride toothpaste, daily flossing, and oral rinsing, is the most important intervention in the maintenance of a healthy mucous membrane.[3,6,13] Timing of the prescribed mouthcare regimen is important and should take into account patient preferences. Mouthwashes frequently are used before meals *to help freshen the patient's mouth and stimulate the appetite,* and brushing and rinsing after meals and at bedtime *will remove debris and plaque from teeth.* Omission of oral hygiene for longer than 6 hours will nullify past benefits attained.[12] Research indicates that oral hygiene measures administered every 4 hours are the most effective in improving salivation, moisture of the tongue, moisture of the palate, condition of the mucous membrane, and texture and moisture of the lips.[6]

The nursing decision concerning the equipment to be used for cleansing the oral cavity should include assessment data, specifically information about age, present condition of the mouth, and platelet and white blood counts. A soft-bristle brush is especially important in the patient with thrombocytopenia and in the older adult *because of age-related changes of the oral mucosa that*

may be present, such as thinning of the epithelium, a decrease in saliva, and increased susceptibility to injury. [18,27] In the edentulous patient oral hygiene can be accomplished with thorough cleansing of the removed dentures, the use of mouth washes, and cleansing of the mucosal surface with a sponge or soft toothbrush before a denture or bridge is reinserted. Sponge sticks are ineffective in removing debris from tooth surfaces.[5] In patients with severe stomatitis, thrombocytopenia, or neutropenia, a toothbrush may be contraindicated *because of the potential for further damage.* Gauze (4 inches × 4 inches), moistened with normal saline and wrapped around a gloved finger, may be used to remove dental debris.[12] If oral irrigations are ordered or oral rinsing is problematic for reasons related to patient condition, such as altered level of consciousness or wired jaws, additional equipment may be needed. A Water-Pic, power sprayer, Asepto syringe, or elevated enema bag with a catheter tip may be used. Suction with a Tonsil Tip may also be needed if the patient is unable to expectorate. Lemon and glycerin swabs should never be used on inflamed or broken mucous membrane *because of the irritating effects of the lemon and the drying effect of the glycerin.*[5]

When the integrity of the mucous membrane is altered, additional interventions are required for cleansing. *If somatitis is present or if the risk of it occurring is high,* additional use of mouthwashes with normal saline after and between bushings will soothe inflamed mucosa. Warm saline mouthwashes frequently are ordered for the oral patient who has had surgery. Sterile normal saline (0.9% sodium chloride) should be used in the presence of mouth ulcers, severe neutropenia, or recent oral surgery. However, if the sterility of the solution is not a concern, it can be prepared by mixing 1 teaspoon of salt in 1,000 ml (1 quart) of water. Most commercial mouthwashes contain alcohol, which may irritate already inflamed mucosal surfaces. If thick mucous, crust, and/or debris are present, an oxidizing agent is necessary for mechanical debridement. Two commonly used solutions are hydrogen peroxide and normal saline, in a 1:4 ratio, or sodium bicarbonate, 1 teaspoon in 8 ounces of water. Use of these solutions should be followed by rinsing with warm water or normal saline.[15] Use of hydrogen peroxide in the presence of granulation tissue is usually contraindicated, *because it may destroy the new tissue. It also may cause overgrowth of papillae on the tongue and an increased susceptibility to candidiasis if it is not diluted and rinsed properly.* [5] Other agents that may be used in cleansing the oral cavity are dilute acetic acid, dilute chlorhexidine gluconate (Peridex), dilute povidone-iodine (Betadine), sodium perborate (Amosan), carbamide peroxide (Gly-oxide), or the enzyme combination of glucose oxidase and lactoperoxidase (Bioténe). The frequency of the oral hygiene regimen may be increased to every 2 hours and once or twice during the night *if more severe (grade IV) stomatitis is observed.* This would be imperative in the immunocompromised patient; for example, in the patient who is receiving an antimetabolite chemotherapeutic agent. *Because of the ability of Chlorhexidine to bind with the surface of the mucous membrane,* use twice a day is sufficient to provide the desired antibacterial protection.[8] A denture or bridge should not be reinserted if a lesion or severe stomatitis is present.

The maintenance of moisture in the oral cavity is another expected outcome that will contribute to unimpaired tissue integrity. *Fluid balance and the avoidance of dehydration are essential.* Oral rinsing every 2 to 4 hours (as has been described) also *will help prevent xerostomia.* Additional agents available for the prevention or treatment of xerostomia include artificial saliva preparations, which may contain sorbitol, sodium carboxymethylcellulose or mucins,[10] fluoride, and electrolytes (or enzymes) normally found in saliva, or a solution of calcium and phosphate; sugar-free gum or candies to stimulate saliva production; water-soluble emollient for the lips and mucous membrane; and humidification. Oil-based lubricant should be avoided *because of the danger of aspiration pneumonia and its highly flammable nature in the presence of oxygen therapy.* [5] High-moisture foods, those prepared with gravy or sauces, and

extra fluids (if not contraindicated) should be included in the meal planning of patients with xerostomia.

The prevention of infection is an expected outcome of interventions when dealing with any tissue with impaired continuity. Cultures should be obtained at the first sign of a possible infection. If viral infection is suspected culture should be obtained using viral transport medium (calcium alginate swab can inactivate the virus) and kept cold.[28] Antifungal, antiviral, or antibacterial agents then may be ordered depending on the results of culturing. Such agents also may be ordered prophylactically in patients at high risk for infection. Antifungal (Chlotrimazole troches or Nystatin suspension) agents usually are applied topically and also should be applied to any dentures. The patient should avoid eating or drinking for 30 minutes after application.[2]

Interventions targeted for the patient outcome of the absence of discomfort may include the use of topical and/or systemic analgesics, especially before meals, and altering the diet to avoid acidic or spicy foods, extremes in temperature, and foods that are rough in texture. Patients with more severe, generalized oral alterations (for instance, Grade IV: hemorrhagic ulcerations) may require parenteral narcotics (morphine sulfate, meperidine hydrochloride) and nasogastric or parenteral feedings *to relieve oral discomfort and provide nutrition.* In addition, pressure and/or topical thrombin (Thrombostat) may be needed if bleeding persists.

Topical analgesics may vary and frequently are used in combination, which may include drugs from two or more of the following classifications: antihistamine (diphenhydramine hydrochloride); antacid (Milk of Magnesia, Maalox); antiinflammatory (hydrocortisone); topical anesthetic (Dyclonine hydrochloride 0.5%, Xylocaine viscous 2%, Benzocaine 20%); and agents used to form a protective coating (kaolin/pectin, Sucralfate).[2,4] Many of these are not without systemic side effects, which should be taken into consideration. For example, diphenhydramine hydrochloride (Benadryl) can cause drowsiness and cardiovascu-

II

❖ NURSING CARE GUIDELINES

Nursing Diagnosis: *Altered Oral Mucous Membrane related to chemical injury (decreased mucosal cellular replacement) as a result of chemotherapy*

Expected Patient Outcomes	Nursing Interventions
The patient will exhibit unimpaired tissue integrity of oral mucosa as evidenced by moist, pink, smooth mucosal surfaces and the absence of debris on dental surfaces.	• Assess all surfaces or oral cavity at least once a day including color, moisture, presence of lesions or ulcers, discomfort, debris on and odor of all surfaces, and presence of palpable lymph nodes. • Assist the patient to perform oral hygiene every 4 hours (if self-care difficult), while awake, consisting of: brushing with soft-bristle brush and nonabrasive toothpaste; rinsing with normal saline after brushing and every 2 hours between; flossing with unwaxed dental floss every morning; and moisturizing lips with water-soluble jelly or lip balm. • Monitor laboratory values daily, especially white blood cell and platelet counts.
The patient will experience no oral discomfort as evidenced by verbalization of same, ability to verbally communicate needs, and an oral intake of 2 to 3 L of fluid per day and at least 75% of diet.	• Medicate with topical and/or systemic analgesic, as ordered, 30 to 45 minutes before meals. • Assess the patient's ability to communicate and monitor amounts of food and fluid intake; avoid acidic and highly seasoned food, rough textures, and extremes in temperature; consult with dietitian. • Discourage alcohol, smoking, and smokeless tobacco use. • Encourage frequent dental evaluations.
The patient will state signs and symptoms of tissue alterations and purpose of oral hygiene regimen and will demonstrate proper technique.	• Assess the patient's current knowledge regarding oral hygiene. • Discuss changes that may occur (stomatitis, ulcers, infections) related to specific chemotherapeutic agent and the oral hygiene regimen suggested. • Request that the patient demonstrate oral regimen and correct technique when appropriate. • Discuss possible diet changes and medication use.

lar effects. Lidocaine HCl (Xylocaine) can affect the pharyngeal stage of swallowing, causes numbness, and normally should be limited to 120 ml per 24 hours because of its cardiovascular side effects. Antifungal and antibacterial agents frequently are added when hydrocortisone is used *because of the propensity for superinfections to occur.* An example of one of these combinations is "stomatitis cocktail," which is a mixture of equal parts of lidocaine hydrochloride, diphenhydramine

hydrochloride (12.5 mg/ml), and Maalox, with 30 ml to be swished and swallowed every 2 to 4 hours as needed.[15] Anesthetic agents have also been combined with carboxymethylcellulose (Orabase) or hydroxypropylcellulose (Zilactin) to form a film that adheres to mucosal surfaces, *thereby extending the relief obtained in patients with oral ulcers (Grades II-IV).*

Finally, interventions also should be focused on patient knowledge of factors affecting the oral

❖ CASE STUDY WITH PLAN OF CARE

Mr. Joe W., a 76-year-old man, was admitted to the hospital for further evaluation and treatment of a superior right nasal mass. He had sought treatment a week earlier from his private physician for a complaint of a dull, constant headache posterior to his right eye, an increase in lacrimation of the right eye over the past 6 to 7 weeks, and two episodes of epistaxis in the previous week. He was given a prescription of amoxicillin and referred to the University Hospital. His past medical history included coronary artery bypass grafting 3 years past, colectomy for left colon cancer 15 months earlier, and non–insulin-dependent diabetes mellitus diagnosed 9 months earlier. On admission he was alert and oriented, pupils were equal, round, and reactive to light, and extraocular movements of the right eye were decreased on the lateral and medial gaze, with proptosis of the right eye. The oral assessment revealed pink, slightly dry, smooth mucous membranes, teeth in a good state of repair, and tongue with increased rugosity (folds, wrinkles) but supple and with a full range of motion. With exception of an irregular pulse rate of 64/min and an elevated glucose level (366 mg/dl), all other physical findings and laboratory data were within normal limits. Mr. W. had been living with his wife, who was very concerned and supportive, in their own home about 25 miles from the hospital. A magnetic resonance imaging (MRI) scan done the next day revealed an extensive intracranial tumor from the floor of the frontal fossa to the corpus callosum, filling the sphenoid and both ethmoids with erosion of the medial half of the right orbital roof. The tumor was inoperable, and chemotherapy and radiation for palliation were discussed. Mr. W.'s physical condition quickly declined. Within 3 days he became increasingly somno-

lent and developed left-sided weakness. He was started on dexamethasone, 24 mg every 6 hours, and Phenytoin, 200 mg twice a day. Radiation therapy was begun on day 5 of his hospitalization. His blood glucose had to be controlled with sliding-scale insulin coverage after administration of dexamethasone was begun. Nutrition and hydration became a problem because of his decreased level of consciousness. His albumin dropped to 3.4 gm/dl, and his blood urea nitrogen increased to 33 mg/dl by the fifth day. His diet was changed to a pureed-consistency, 2,000-calorie (American Diabetes Association) diet, and an intravenous line was inserted for hydration. An oral assessment on the seventh day revealed generalized stomatitis, the lips were dry and cracked, his tongue had increased fissures, and there was a white, curdlike plaque covering the entire buccal mucosa bilaterally and the lateral surfaces of the tongue. The following care plan was instituted. The alteration in nutrition was dealt with in a separate nursing diagnosis. When the effectiveness of the nursing interventions in meeting the identified patient outcomes was evaluated, the daily oral assessment did indicate gradual improvement. By discharge, 5 days later, Mr. W.'s oral mucosa still had slight erythema, but the candidiasis had subsided. His tongue was moist and without fissures, and his lips were still slightly dry but no longer cracked. The radiation therapist had approved the use of a water-soluble lip balm, because that area was not in the direct field of treatment. Mr. W.'s level of oral comfort remained good, and his wife was able to state the rationale and demonstrate the ability to provide oral hygiene for her husband before discharge. Radiation therapy continued at the local hospital.

CARE PLAN FOR MR. JOE W.

Nursing Diagnosis: *Altered Oral Mucous Membrane**

Expected Patient Outcomes	Nursing Interventions
Mr. W. will exhibit return to moist, pink, smooth, mucosal surfaces without plaque or debris within 7 days.	• Send culture of oral plaque. • Assess oral cavity every shift, and obtain laboratory values daily. • Perform oral hygiene every 4 hours (beginning at 0900) and once during night consisting of brushing with soft-bristle brush, using a sponge on mucosal surfaces; swishing with a solution of 1 teaspoon baking soda and 8 ounces water; rinsing with normal saline; and flossing once a day. • Spray mouth with artificial saliva between oral hygiene procedures.

Continued.

Expected Patient Outcomes	Nursing Interventions
	• Have Mr. W. swish with 5 ml Nystatin (500,000 units) for 2 to 3 minutes and swallow four times a day.
	• Institute aspiration precautions (if level of consciousness decreases) during oral hygiene, including Sims' position, tonsil suction at bedside, and use of toothbrush with built-in vacuum tip, large syringe for rinsing, and cotton or sponge applicator for applying medication.
	• Consult with radiation therapy personnel before applying lip moisturizers; this will be contraindicated if within the field.
Mr. W. will not exhibit signs or symptoms of discomfort, as evidenced by no complaints (dependent on level of consciousness) and no grimacing or restlessness during oral care or swallowing.	• Assess for discomfort. • Monitor intake and output. • Maintain intake (by mouth and intravenous) of 2 to 3 L per day. • Monitor dietary intake to ensure adequate calorie and protein intake.
Mr. W.'s wife will identify contributing factors and be able to state purpose and demonstrate technique of oral hygiene regimen, by discharge.	• Institute a teaching plan with Mr. W.'s wife for home care (include oral hygiene measures).

* Related to physical injury—the drying effect of mouth breathing and dehydration; chemical injury—possible gingival hyperplasia; injury from biological agent—over-growth of *Candida Albicans* secondary to recent antibiotic therapy, immunosuppressive nature of dexamethasone, and increased blood glucose with uncontrolled DM; and radiation injury resulting from radiation therapy to nasal-frontal tumor.

mucosa and on oral self-care techniques as an expected outcome. The teaching plan should include daily oral examination, oral hygiene regimen, suggested diet changes, importance of dental evaluations, the risks associated with tobacco and alcohol use, pain control, medication administration, and side effects.

EVALUATION

Evaluation of the interventions will center on the appearance of the oral mucous membranes, including the absence of defining characteristics; the level of comfort; and the ability of the patient to communicate orally, to consume nutrients, and finally, to incorporate effective oral hygiene techniques into his/her daily routine.

REFERENCES

1. Bates B: *A guide to physical examination and history taking,* ed 4, Philadelphia, 1987, JB Lippincott.
2. Bavier A: Nursing management of acute oral complications of cancer, *NCI Monographs* 9:123, 1990.
3. Beck S: Impact of a systematic oral care protocol on stomatitis after chemotherapy, *Cancer Nurs* 2:185, 1979.
4. Blaney GM: Mouth care—basic and essential, *Geriatr Nurs* 7:242, 1986.
5. Daeffler R: Oral hygiene measures for patients with cancer, *Cancer Nurs* 3:347, 1980 (Part I); 3:427, 1980 (Part II); 4:29, 1981 (Part III).
6. DeWalt E: Effect of timed hygienic measures on oral mucosa in a group of elderly subjects, *Nurs Res* 24:104, 1975.
7. DeWalt E, Haines S: Effects of specified stressors on healthy oral mucosa, *Nurs Res* 18:22, 1969.
8. Ferretti G, Brown A, Raybould T, and Lillich T: Oral antimicrobial agents—Chlorhexidine, *NCI Monographs* 9:51, 1990.

9. Freedman SD, Devine B: A clean break: post op oral care, *Am J Nurs* 87:474, 1987.

10. Greenspan D: Management of salivary dysfunction, *NCI Monographs* 9:159, 1990.

11. Kahn R: Renewing the commitment to oral hygiene, *Geriatr Nurs* 7:244, 1986.

12. Kim MJ, McFarland GK, and McLane AM: *Pocket guide to nursing diagnoses,* ed 2, St Louis, 1987, CV Mosby.

13. Klocke J, Sudduth A: Oral hygiene instruction and plaque formation during hospitalization, *Nurs Res* 18:124, 1969.

14. Longman AJ, DeWalt EM: A guide for oral assessment, *Geriatr Nurs* 7:252, 1986.

15. McNally JC, Somerville ET, Miaskowski C, and Rostad M: Guidelines for oncology nursing practice, ed 2, Philadelphia, 1991, WB Saunders.

16. Niehaus CS, Peterson DE, and Overholser CD: Oral complications in children during cancer therapy, *Cancer Nurs* 10:15, 1987.

17. Ofstehage JC, Magilvy K: Oral health and aging, *Geriatr Nurs* 7(5):238, 1986.

18. Passos J, Brand L: Effects of agents for oral hygiene, *Nurs Res* 15:186, 1966.

19. Phipps WJ, Long BC, and Wood NF: *Medical-surgical nursing,* ed 4, St Louis, 1991, Mosby–Year Book.

20. Porth CM: *Pathophysiology—concepts of altered health states,* Philadelphia, 1986, JB Lippincott.

21. Resio MJ: Nursing diagnosis: alteration in oral/nasal mucous membrane related to trauma of transsphenoidal surgery, *J Neurosci Nurs* 18:112, 1986.

22. Roth PT, Creason NS: Nursing administered oral hygiene: is there a scientific basis? *J Adv Nurs* 11:323, 1986.

23. Saral R: Laboratory techniques for confirmation of herpes simplex virus infection: an overview, *Nurs Acumen* 2(2):4, 1990.

24. Schaaf M, Carl W: Dental oncology. In Holleb AI, Fink DJ, Murphy GP, editors: *Clinical oncology,* Atlanta, 1991, American Cancer Society.

25. Schweiger J and others: Oral assessment: how to do it, *Am J Nurs* 80:654, 1980.

26. Shafer WG, Hine MK, and Levy BM: *Textbook of oral pathology,* ed 4, Philadelphia, 1983, WB Saunders.

27. Squier CA: Mucosal alterations, *NCI Monogr* 9:169, 1990.

28. Thompson J, McFarland G, Hirsch J, Tucker S, Bowers A: *Mosby's manual of clinical nursing,* ed 2, St Louis, 1989, Mosby–Year Book.

29. Williams L, Peterson D, and Overholzer CD: Acute periodontal infection in myelosuppressed oncology patients: evaluation and nursing care, *Cancer Nurs* 5:465, 1982.

II

High Risk for Fluid Volume Deficit

Fluid Volume Deficit (1)

Fluid Volume Deficit (2)

Fluid Volume Excess

High Risk for Fluid Volume Deficit *is a state in which an individual is at risk of experiencing vascular, cellular, or intracellular dehydration.*[12]

Fluid Volume Deficit (1) *is the state in which an individual experiences vascular, cellular, or intracellular dehydration related to failure of regulatory mechanisms.*[12]

Fluid Volume Deficit (2) *is a state in which an individual experiences vascular, cellular, or intracellular dehydration related to active loss of fluids.*[12]

Fluid Volume Excess *is a state in which an individual experiences increased fluid retention and edema.*[12]

OVERVIEW

Body fluids are located within three compartments: extracellular/intravascular space, extracellular/interstitial space, and intracellular space.[4] The volumes of these fluids are maintained by (1) a precise interaction between intake and output via the kidney, (2) insensible losses of the lung and skin, (3) hydrostatic pressure within the vascular compartment, and (4) the osmolarity within each compartment.[4] Two conditions can cause excess in fluid volume: (1) excessive intake of fluids and sodium and (2) retention of fluids by decreased circulation and/or redistribution within the compartments that results in a compromised regulatory mechanism.

Excessive intake of fluids occurs most frequently from over infusion of intravenous solutions (crystalloids) or colloids such as blood and plasma expanders. This excessive intake of fluids expands the intravascular compartment leading to an increased circulating blood volume. Excessive intake of sodium, primarily from a dietary source, increases the osmolarity of the extracellular compartments resulting in fluid movement into this compartment.[18,19]

Retention of fluids by decreased circulation and/or redistribution within the compartments occurs through alteration in the equilibrium between the hydrostatic pressure of the blood and the colloid osmotic pressure within the capillaries. Normally, fluid filters out of the capillary into the tissue spaces via the hydrostatic pressure. Opposing this outward force is the pressure exerted by plasma proteins, colloid oncotic pressure, which pulls water back into the capillary.[4] Any situation that increases hydrostatic pressure or decreases colloid oncotic pressure will result in fluid movement out of the intravascular space and into the interstitial compartment.

Situations that cause an inadequate circulation of blood (for instance, congestive heart failure and venostasis) increase the hydrostatic pressure in the capillaries, resulting in fluid retention and edema.[21] Situations that cause a deficit of plasma proteins in the capillaries (for instance, inadequate protein intake or the inflammatory process) result in a leakage of fluid into the interstitial space, followed by fluid retention and edema. In any of the above conditions one can use the nursing diagnosis of Fluid Volume Excess.

Many factors influence the regulation of water balance. Depletion of the fluid volume (dehydration) stimulates two osmoreceptor sites in the hypothalamus. Stimulation of one site results in a release of antidiuretic hormone (ADH) and in thirst.[4] Stimulation of the other site, referred to as the *thirst center,* results in a thirst sensation.[20] Stimulation of thirst may also result from excess angiotensin II in the body during such clinical conditions as hemorrhage and low blood pressure.[20] The sensation of thirst initiates an individual's desire to take in fluid: in conditions of blunted desire, dehydration may result. The release of ADH increases the resorption of water at the kidney's collecting ducts, thereby decreasing urine output and expanding extracellular volume.[4] Any condition that causes a decrease in ADH secretion or alters the kidney's ability to respond correctly to an increased ADH secretion (such as acute tubular necrosis) leads to an increase in urine output and possible dehydration.

Aldosterone, a hormone secreted by the adrenal gland, increases sodium uptake in the renal tubules.[4] This increase in sodium retention leads to an increase in water retention. In disease states that cause a primary insufficiency of the adrenal gland, aldosterone is not secreted, which leads to decreased sodium and water uptake and then to dehydration.

An elevation in the osmolarity of the extracellular fluid by failure of a regulatory mechanism, which leads to an increase in electrolytes and/or glucose, draws water into the intravascular space. The increase in fluid volume leads to an increased urine output and possible dehydration.

A fluid volume deficit may occur from active loss of fluids from the body or from shifts of fluids within or outside the intravascular space. Active loss of fluids outside the body results in a fluid volume deficit and dehydration. In some situations the intravascular fluid is redistributed within this compartment or into the interstitial space. These situations result in an intravascular fluid volume deficit. In the presence of any of these conditions one can use the nursing diagnosis Fluid Volume Deficit (2). Although both nursing diagnoses Fluid Volume Deficit (1) and Fluid Volume Deficit (2) refer to a loss of fluid with resultant dehydration, only the former occurs in the presence of a failure of regulatory mechanisms. These mechanisms are still functional in patients with a diagnosis of Fluid Volume Deficit (2).

A potential fluid volume deficit may occur in any situation that predisposes an individual to vascular, cellular, or intracellular dehydration. Any situation that leads to the patient's output being potentially greater than the intake may cause these types of dehydration and may lead to the formulation of the nursing diagnosis High Risk for Fluid Volume Deficit

ASSESSMENT

The failure of the mechanisms regulating water balance can lead to a fluid volume deficit. In addition, any pathophysiological state resulting in a decreased mental status (for instance, coma) may blunt the thirst sensation, and dehydration can result. A psychological alteration such as depression also may blunt the thirst sensation.

Diabetes insipidus results from a deficiency in ADH release from the posterior lobe of the pituitary gland. Etiological factors in diabetes insipidus include trauma or surgery to the neurohypophyseal system, inflammatory conditions such as syphilis, tumors of the neurohypophyseal system, and metastatic lesions from the breast or lung.[5] A deficiency in ADH leads to excessive urine output and eventual dehydration.

Primary adrenal insufficiency, also known as Addison's disease, causes a reduction in three principal steroids, one of which is aldosterone.[8] Without sufficient aldosterone, sodium is not retained and is excreted, along with water, in increased amounts. This condition may lead to dehydration.

Diabetic ketoacidosis is a condition in which diabetes mellitus is uncontrolled.[11] A decrease in insulin production or insulin intake leads to hyperglycemia, glycosuria, and acidosis; the result will be increased osmolarity of the intravascular space. The hyperosmolar effect of glucose pulls water from the interstitial space and intracellular areas into the vascular space to be excreted by the kidneys. Eventually this leads to dehydration.

Hyperglycemic hyperosmolar nonketotic coma (HHNK) is characterized by hyperglycemia but without a buildup of ketone acids or without acidosis.[11] As with diabetic ketoacidosis, the hyperosmolar effect of glucose pulls water into the intravascular space to be excreted by the kidneys. This leads to eventual dehydration.

One major related factor that can lead to Fluid Volume Deficit (2) is the active loss of fluid from the body. This can occur in many different situations. Probably the most common situations in which fluid is actively lost from the body are diarrhea, vomiting, and nasogastric suction. Depending on the extent of the diarrhea or vomiting, large amounts of fluid may be lost through these routes, leading to a volume deficit and dehydration. Along with the excessive fluid loss may be a significant loss of electrolytes. The patient with diarrhea loses sodium and potassium and often develops an acidosis. The patient with excessive vomiting loses sodium, chloride, potassium, and magnesium and often develops an alkalosis.[16]

Other causes of active fluid loss are overzealous dialysis, abnormal drainage from wounds, and excessive menstrual flow. Burns over a significant body surface area cause fluid loss from the affected areas.

Shock states, through varying mechanisms, lead to a fluid volume deficit.[17] Hypovolemic shock leads to a volume deficit through active loss from the body as well as internal loss into the interstitial spaces or cavities (as in ascites). Neurogenic shock leads to a pooling of intravascular fluid in the periphery, resulting in an overall deficit in the central circulation. Both septic and anaphylactic shock lead to a redistribution of fluid in the interstitial spaces and a resultant deficit in intravascular volume.

A number of risk factors can lead to the use of the nursing diagnosis High Risk for Fluid Volume Deficit. Extremes of age and extremes of weight predispose an individual to potential fluid loss. Infants and the elderly have a decreased fluid reserve. In addition, the elderly have a decreased sensation of thirst. Excessive losses through normal routes such as diarrhea or vomiting or through abnormal routes such as indwelling tubes (for instance, a nasogastric tube) might lead to dehydration. Deviations affecting access to, intake of, or absorption of fluids also might lead to dehydration. Situations in which an individual might have trouble accessing or taking in fluids include physical immobility, neurological deficits, or psychological deficits (depression). Because the large intestine functions mainly to absorb water (1,800 to 3,000 ml/day), any condition in which part of the large intestine is removed might lead to a fluid volume deficit.

Factors influencing fluid needs (such as infection or hypermetabolic states) and medications (for instance, diuretics or laxatives) might lead to dehydration.[4] Finally, a knowledge deficit related to fluid volume intake places an individual at risk for dehydration.

Other risk factors that may lead to this nursing diagnosis are increased fluid output from any source (normal or abnormal routes) that has the potential to exceed the individual's intake, and an altered intake. Urinary frequency from such situations as diuretic administration and thirst are other risk factors. In addition to assessing the individual for risk factors, the nurse should ask questions regarding a history of vomiting, diarrhea, fevers, large gains or losses in weight, and medication use. Information on current fluid intake should be obtained, and the patient's knowledge related to fluid volume should be ascertained.

Several defining characteristics indicate generalized fluid volume depletion and are common to both nursing diagnoses Fluid Volume Deficit (1) and Fluid Volume Deficit (2). A decrease in intravascular volume may lead to hypotension and decreased venous filling. Decreased venous filling can be assessed through inspection of the jugular veins. With the patient reclining at a 45-degree angle and the head turned slightly away from the side being observed, shine a light tangentially on the jugular veins.[13] A decrease in venous filling will be observed as minimal jugular vein distention.

An increase in pulse rate (tachycardia) results from a reflex stimulation of the sympathetic nervous system in response to hypotension.[4] Dehydration may lead to an increased body temperature, dry skin, dry mucous membranes, and a decreased skin turgor. Laboratory studies may reveal elevated hematocrit and serum sodium levels reflecting the decreased intravascular volume.

Other defining characteristics may be present that reflect a failure of regulatory mechanisms. Dilute urine, increased urine output, and sudden weight loss may be present in patients with diabetes insipidus.[5] Urine with a low specific gravity (1.000 to 1.005) and increased urine outputs as high as 15 to 16 L/day may be present. A reduction in total body water caused by the failure of fluid volume regulatory mechanisms leads to a sudden weight loss.

In contrast, patients with a fluid volume deficit related to active loss of fluids may have a decreased urine output and concentrated urine (specific gravity > 1.015). These individuals may experience a sudden weight loss related to the fluid deficit. The intake and output records may reveal an output far exceeding the intake, especially if the active loss is related to vomiting, hemorrhage, or diarrhea. This weight loss is in contrast to the patient exhibiting a regulatory failure, such as congestive heart failure, that may lead to weight gain and edema.

In addition to objective data from a physical assessment, the nurse must obtain certain subjective data.[7] The nurse should question the patient regarding a history of symptoms such as weight loss, thirst, and polyuria/dysuria. A family or personal history of diabetes mellitus, Addison's disease, head trauma, cancer, and renal disease is important. The nurse also should elicit information on current drug therapy. A history of symptoms such as nausea and vomiting, diarrhea with black or bloody stools, and weight loss may indicate an active fluid loss. The nurse also should ascertain a family or personal history of blood loss, gastrointestinal disorders or surgery, allergies, medications, or alcohol use.

Three related factors, when present in individuals, lead to the nursing diagnosis of Fluid Volume Excess. Excess fluid or sodium intake may occur in isolation or in association with a particular pathophysiological state. Situations occasionally arise whereby individuals take in too much fluid or sodium either by mouth or via intravenous route.[14,18]

Many pathophysiological states result in compromised regulatory mechanisms and thereby in a fluid volume excess. The oliguric and anuric phase of renal failure (acute or chronic) is marked by the inability to excrete sodium and water.[1] In congestive heart failure (CHF) the heart is unable to pump enough blood to meet the metabolic demands of the body.[4] Right ventricular failure leads to a pressure buildup in the ventricle that spreads to the venous system and causes fluid congestion of the liver and peripheral edema. Left ventricular failure results in an increase in left end-diastolic pressure that spreads to the pulmonary circulatory system and causes fluid to exude into the interstitial lung tissue and the alveolar spaces. In venous insufficiency and venostasis the valves in the veins are overstretched and become incompetent, increasing the hydrostatic pressure in the capillaries, resulting in edema from fluid buildup in the interstitial spaces.[2]

Disorders of the liver such as cirrhosis may compromise regulatory mechanisms and lead to a Fluid Volume Excess. Cancer in the liver also may act to narrow or block the capillary branches, causing an increased pressure in them. Resistance to flow in the liver and increased pressure causes protein to leak from the liver into the peritoneal cavity.[19] As this movement of protein continues, intravascular protein diminishes and fluid moves out of the intravascular space and into the interstitial and intracellular spaces. The clinical picture in these individuals is one of peripheral edema and ascites. The inflammatory process leads to regional and generalized edema through vasodilation and increased capillary permeability.[19]

Some hormonal disturbances lead to fluid retention and edema. Altered adrenocortical function in the form of hypersecretion of glucocorticoids from the adrenal cortex results in Cushing's syndrome. Exaggeration of the normal functions of glucocorticoids has many clinical manifestations. One of these is sodium and water retention. Inappropriate release of antidiuretic hormone from the posterior pituitary has many causes. This syndrome of inappropriate antidiuretic hormone leads to overhydration and a decreased serum osmolality.[15] Abnormalities such as cancer and lymphedema prevent the flow of lymph through the lymphatic system, resulting in peripheral edema.[2] During pregnancy, increased venous pressure results from obstruction of the inferior vena cava and iliac veins by the expanding uterus, leading to edema of the lower extremities.[6]

A thorough physical assessment of individuals with any of the related factors just discussed would reveal certain defining characteristics that might lead to the diagnosis of Fluid Volume Excess. Weight gain may indicate fluid retention and edema. Changes in blood pressure, particularly hypertension, may reflect an expansion of the intravascular volume. Restlessness and anxiety may be present as a function of pulmonary congestion with shortness of breath and also may be related to cerebral edema. Fluid overload causes changes in mental status—lethargy and mental confusion with progression to disorientation and coma.

Inspection of the skin may reveal anasarca (a generalized massive edema) or regional areas of edema. There are two types of edema: (1) pitting, resulting from displacement of interstitial fluid after finger pressure on the area, and (2) nonpitting. A subjective measure used to describe pitting edema is based on a scale of 1+ to 4+, with 1+ indicating minimal pitting and 4+ indicating severe pitting.[13]

Several defining characteristics specific to the cardiovascular system may indicate a Fluid Volume Excess. Inspection might reveal jugular venous distention, one indication of increased fluid volume. In the patient with Fluid Volume Excess or right-sided heart failure, a distention of the jugular vein can be induced by manual pressure over the liver. This is termed a *positive hepatojugular reflex*[13] If hemodynamic monitoring is in place, changes in pulmonary capillary wedge pressure (PCWP) and central venous pressure (CVP) can be measured. High CVP and PCWP indicate a Fluid Volume Excess from overhydration or decreased cardiac output.[19]

Auscultation of the heart in an individual with a Fluid Volume Excess might reveal a third heart sound. Although the third heart sound is often a normal occurrence in children and young adults, in older individuals it indicates an increased venous return to the heart.[7]

Assessment of the respiratory system in the individual with a Fluid Volume Excess may reveal a change in respiratory pattern, shortness of breath, orthopnea, and presence of crackles (rales) from fluid buildup in the lung interstitial tissue. A chest radiograph might reveal pulmonary congestion or pleural effusions.[3]

Any impairment in renal function may result in oliguria (urine output < 400 ml/24 hr). Interstitial accumulation of fluid might cause a depletion of the intravascular space, with the result being oliguria. Changes in specific gravity will occur in the patient with renal failure; it will stabilize often at about 1.010 because of the kidney's inability to concentrate urine.[4] In the patient with intravascular depletion and interstitial accumulation, the specific gravity will be elevated.

Laboratory studies may be altered in the individual with Fluid Volume Excess. Sodium, hematocrit, and serum urea nitrogen levels often are low because of a diluted intravascular space. If renal failure is present, then elevated levels of serum creatinine, potasssium, and urea nitrogen can be expected.

In addition to objective data from a physical assessment, certain subjective data must be obtained. The patient should be questioned regarding a history of symptoms such as shortness of breath, weight gain, weakness/fatigue, and edema. A personal history of pregnancy, along with a family or personal history of diabetes, cardiac/renal disease, liver disease, alcoholism, hypertension, malnutrition, or excessive sodium/fluid intake should be ascertained. Information on current drug therapy and dietary intake also should be included.

High Risk for Fluid Volume Deficit
❖ Risk Factors

The following risk factors are associated with High Risk for Fluid Volume Deficit:

- Loss of fluid through abnormal routes
- Factors influencing fluid needs
- Medications
- Deviations affecting access to, intake of, or absorption of fluids
- Altered intake
- Increased fluid output
- Extremes of weight
- Thirst
- Excessive losses through normal routes
- Urinary frequency
- Extremes of age
- Knowledge deficit related to fluid volume

Fluid Volume Deficit (1)
❖ Defining Characteristics

The presence of the following defining characteristics indicates that the patient may be experiencing Fluid Volume Deficit (1):

- Dilute urine
- Possible weight gain
- Decreased venous filling
- Decreased skin turgor
- Increased urine output
- Hypotension
- Increased pulse rate
- Decreased pulse amplitude

- Edema
- Thirst
- Increased temperature
- Weakness
- Narrowed pulse pressure
- Hemoconcentration
- Dry skin
- Dry mucous membranes
- Sudden weight loss

❖ Related Factors

The following related factors are associated with Fluid Volume Deficit (1):

- Failure of regulatory mechanisms related to diabetes insipidus, primary adrenal insufficiency or Addison's disease, diabetic ketoacidosis, or HHNK

Fluid Volume Deficit (2)
❖ Defining Characteristics

The presence of the following defining characteristics indicates that the patient may be experiencing Fluid Volume Deficit (2):

- Decreased urine output
- Output greater that intake
- Decreased venous filling
- Increased serum sodium
- Thirst
- Increased pulse rate
- Decreased pulse amplitude
- Increased body temperature
- Dry mucous membranes
- Dry skin
- Weakness
- Concentrated urine
- Sudden weight loss
- Hemoconcentration
- Hypotension
- Narrowed pulse pressure
- Decreased skin turgor
- Change in mental status

❖ Related Factors

The following related factor is associated with Fluid Volume Deficit (2):

- Active loss of fluid related to diarrhea, vomiting, wound drainage, burns, or hemorrhage.

Fluid Volume Excess
❖ Defining Characteristics

The presence of the following defining characteristics indicates that the patient may be experiencing Fluid Volume Excess:

- Edema
- Anasarca
- Shortness of breath
- Third heart sound
- Abnormal breath sounds (e.g., rales)
- Blood pressure changes
- Hepatojugular reflex
- Urine specific gravity changes
- Altered electrolytes
- Effusion
- Weight gain
- Intake > output
- Pulmonary congestion on x-ray film
- Change in respiratory pattern
- Decreased hemoglobin or hematocrit
- Jugular venous distention
- Oliguria
- Azoturia (nitrogen in urine)
- Mental status change
- Restlessness and anxiety

❖ Related Factors

The following related factors are associated with Fluid Volume Excess:

- Compromised regulatory mechanisms
- Excess fluid intake
- Excess sodium intake

❖ Related Medical/Psychiatric Diagnoses

The following are examples of related medical/psychiatric diagnoses for fluid volume alterations:

- Acute renal failure
- Addison's disease
- Anaphylactic shock
- Bipolar disorder, manic
- Chronic renal failure
- Cirrhosis of the liver
- Congestive heart failure
- Cushing syndrome
- Diabetes insipidus
- Diabetic ketoacidosis
- Hyperglycemic hyperosmolar nonketotic coma (HHNK)
- Hypothyroid
- Hypovolemic shock
- Major depression
- Nephrotic syndrome
- Neurogenic shock
- Paranoid schizophrenia
- Pregnancy
- Psychoactive substance use disorders
- Glomerulonephritis
- Hepatitis
- Septic shock
- Syndrome of inappropriate ADH secretion

NURSING DIAGNOSES

An example of a *specific* nursing diagnosis for High Risk for Fluid Volume Deficit is:

- High Risk for Fluid Volume Deficit related to daily use of diuretics.

An example of a specific nursing diagnosis for Fluid Volume Deficit (1) is:

- Fluid Volume Deficit (1) related to failure of regulatory mechanisms secondary to hyperglycemic, hyperosmolar nonketotic coma (HHNK).

An example of a specific nursing diagnosis for Fluid Volume Deficit (2) is:

- Fluid Volume Deficit (2) related to active loss of body fluids secondary to diarrhea.

An example of a specific nursing diagnosis for Fluid Volume Excess is:

- Fluid Volume Excess related to fluid retention secondary to impaired myocardial contractility.

PLANNING AND IMPLEMENTATION WITH RATIONALE
High Risk for Fluid Volume Deficit

For the patient whose nursing diagnosis is High Risk for Fluid Volume Deficit, certain outcomes indicate that nursing interventions are having an effect. One such expected outcome is that adequate fluid volume will be maintained as evidenced by weight within normal limits and a balanced intake and output record. Nursing interventions toward that end are discussed in the planning and implementation section of the nursing diagnosis Fluid Volume Deficit (1).

The second expected patient outcome is that laboratory study results are within normal limits. The nurse must pay particular attention to the serum electrolyte levels in patients with diarrhea, vomiting, and drainage from gastrointestinal tubes and in those taking diuretics. *Many types of diuretics (loop diuretics, thiazides) may cause the*

❖ *NURSING CARE GUIDELINES*

Nursing Diagnosis: High Risk for Fluid Volume Deficit

Expected Patient Outcomes	Nursing Interventions
The patient will have adequate fluid volume as evidenced by body weight within normal limits for patient.	• Monitor vital signs. • Weigh the patient daily. • Monitor intake and output. • Assess mental status. • Assess for signs of dehydration. • Assess for symptoms of dehydration. • Administer intravenous and oral fluids as ordered.
The patient's laboratory study values will be within normal limits.	• Monitor laboratory results relevant to Fluid Volume Deficit.
The patient and family will demonstrate an adequate knowledge base.	• Assess knowledge base of patient and family. • Provide information concerning cause of this fluid deficit and how to prevent recurrence, rationale for treatment, and discharge plans for fluid intake and medication.

excretion of substances like hydrogen ions, making the patient more alkalotic. Acid–base disturbances may be present in these patients. The nurse should closely monitor arterial blood gases and replace electrolytes as ordered.

A third and final expected patient outcome is the patient's and family's demonstration of an adequate knowledge base related to fluid volume. Discussion of this expected outcome is in the planning and implementation section of the nursing diagnosis Fluid Volume Deficit (1).

Fluid Volume Deficit (1)

For the patient whose nursing diagnosis is Fluid Volume Deficit (1), certain outcomes indicate that nursing interventions are having an effect. One such expected outcome is that the patient will have adequate fluid volume. Toward that end, the nurse should administer ordered medications and treatments aimed at correcting the failure of fluid volume regulatory mechanisms. *In the individual with diabetes insipidus, hormone replacement therapy (usually in the form of synthetic vasopressin) retards abnormal fluid loss by increasing water reabsorption from the renal tubules.*[15] The patient with diabetic ketoacidosis and HHNK can be treated by administration of insulin. *Insulin reverses the hyperglycemia and hyperketonemia by facilitating glucose movement into the cells for use in metabolic functions.*[11] *Finally, primary adrenal insufficiency may be treated with adequate administration of steroids and replacement therapy for the depleted glucocorticoids and mineralocorticoids.*[8] Continuous monitoring of the patient's hemodynamic status, intake and output, weight, and skin turgor will indicate the fluid volume status of the patient. Intravenous or oral administration of fluids will ensure adequate hydration.

The second expected outcome is that laboratory studies will be within normal limits. *Hematocrit, sodium levels, and other electrolytes may increase with underhydration.* As hydration is regained, the laboratory results should reveal a hematocrit and sodium and other electrolyte levels within normal limits.

Third, the patient should have an adequate knowledge base. It is important to assess the

II

❖ NURSING CARE GUIDELINES
Nursing Diagnosis: Fluid Volume Deficit (1)

Expected Patient Outcomes	Nursing Interventions
The patient will have adequate fluid volume as evidenced by body weight within normal limits for patient.	• Monitor vital signs. • Monitor hemodynamic status. • Monitor intake and output. • Weigh the patient daily. • Assess skin turgor. • Administer medications as ordered to prevent further fluid losses. • Administer intravenous and/or oral fluids as ordered.
The patient's laboratory studies will be within normal limits.	• Monitor laboratory results relevant to Fluid Volume Deficit.
The patient will demonstrate an adequate knowledge base.	• Assess knowledge base of the patient and family. • Provide information concerning cause of this fluid deficit and how to prevent recurrence; rationale for treatment; discharge plans for fluid intake and medications (purpose, side effects, and administration); and follow-up care.

knowledge base of both the patient and family before planning and providing education. The nurse should present information on the etiology of the Fluid Volume Deficit, how to prevent recurrence, rationale for treatment, and discharge plans, including fluid intake, medication, and follow-up care. *Providing patients with needed information for self-care is necessary to assure continuity of care from the hospital to home.*[16]

Finally, look for subjective manifestations to be improved or alleviated. The sensation of thirst should disappear as hydration is initiated. The feeling of weakness, caused by dehydration, similarly will disappear as the fluid balance is regained.

Fluid Volume Deficit (2)

For the patient whose nursing diagnosis is Fluid Volume Deficit (2), certain outcomes indicate that nursing interventions are effective. One such expected outcome is that adequate fluid volume will be achieved and maintained as evidenced by

weight within the patient's normal limits and a balanced intake and output record. Nursing interventions toward that end are discussed in this section under Fluid Volume Deficit (1).

The second expected patient outcome is that laboratory study values will be within normal limits. Particular attention must be paid to the serum electrolyte levels in patients with vomiting and diarrhea. *As HCL (an acid) is removed from the stomach through vomiting, the patient may become more alkalotic. As alkalotic substances (bicarbonate, sodium) are removed from the intestinal tract by diarrhea, the patient may become more acidotic.* Acid–base disturbances may be present in these patients, therefore close monitoring of arterial blood gases is essential. Replace electrolytes as indicated and ordered. Follow the hematocrit levels carefully. *They will be elevated in dehydration because of the fluid volume alteration and decreased in hemorrhage.*

Last, a third expected patient outcome is that the patient and family will demonstrate an ade-

❖ *NURSING CARE GUIDELINES*

Nursing Diagnosis: Fluid Volume Deficit (2)

Expected Patient Outcomes	Nursing Interventions
The patient will have adequate fluid volume as evidenced by body weight within normal limits for patient.	• Monitor vital signs, including central venous pressure. • Weigh the patient daily. • Monitor intake and output. • Assess mental status. • Assess for signs of dehydration (skin turgor, dry mucous membranes, moisture of skin). • Assess for symptoms of dehydration (thirst, weakness). • Administer medications as ordered to prevent further fluid losses. • Administer intravenous and/or oral fluids as ordered.
The patient's laboratory study values will be within normal limits.	• Monitor laboratory results relevant to Fluid Volume Deficit.
The patient and family will demonstrate an adequate knowledge base.	• Assess knowledge base of patient and family. • Provide information concerning cause of this fluid deficit and how to prevent recurrence, rationale for treatment, discharge plans for fluid intake, medications (purpose, side effects, administration), and follow-up care.

quate knowledge base. This expected outcome is discussed in the planning and implementation section of the nursing diagnosis Fluid Volume Deficit (1).

Fluid Volume Excess

For the patient whose nursing diagnosis is Fluid Volume Excess, certain outcomes indicate that nursing interventions are having an effect. One such expected outcome is that the body weight will be within the patient's normal limits as determined by weighing him/her daily. Approximately 1 kilogram of weight gain correlates with a 1 liter fluid excess. If weight gain is present, fluid restriction and sodium-restricted diet may be indicated. Diuretics may be ordered to reduce volume. *The nurse must closely monitor intake and output records. These records provide essential information about fluid balance.* [16]

A second expected outcome is that the patient's

hemodynamic status will be restored to a normal (acceptable) range without medication. The nurse must closely monitor the hemodynamic status. *With Fluid Volume Excess caused by overhydration or altered circulation, these values are likely to be elevated.* [9] The physician should be consulted if the values exceed the normal ranges, and inotropic and/or vasodilator agents should be administered.

A third expected outcome is that electrolyte levels will stay within the normal range. The patient's serum electrolytes should be monitored closely, especially the potassium level if the patient is taking diuretics. *Sodium levels will decrease with overhydration secondary to dilution. Potassium levels may decrease in patients on diuretics, as many of these drugs cause excretion of potassium.* [16] Potassium supplements should be administered as ordered. The presence of dilutional hyponatremia indicates a need for fluid restriction.

❖ *NURSING CARE GUIDELINES*

Nursing Diagnosis: *Fluid Volume Excess*

Expected Patient Outcomes	Nursing Interventions
The patient's body weight will be within his or her normal range.	• Weigh the patient daily. • Monitor intake and output. • Restrict fluid intake (intravenous and oral). • Provide sodium-restricted diet. • Administer diuretics as ordered. • Assess for peripheral edema.
The patient's hemodynamic status will be restored to a normal (acceptable) range.	• Monitor hemodynamic status. • Administer inotropic and/or vasodilator agents if ordered.
The patient's electrolyte level will be within normal range.	• Monitor laboratory results relevant to fluid retention.
The arterial blood gases will be within patients' normal limits and chest radiograph and breath sounds will be clear.	• Assess breath sounds. • Monitor arterial blood gases and chest radiographs. • Administer oxygen as ordered.
The patient will describe less dyspnea and will describe increased comfort.	• Provide a position that will help alleviate dyspnea. • Provide support to edematous areas. • Have the patient do passive and active range-of-motion exercises. • Provide good skin care to edematous areas.
The patient will demonstrate an adequate knowledge base.	• Assess knowledge base of the patient and family. • Provide information concerning cause of this fluid excess and how to prevent recurrence; rationale for treatment: and discharge plans for fluid intake, medications (purpose, side effects, administration), and follow-up care.

Fourth, the arterial blood gases will be within normal limits for the patient, and the chest radiograph and breath sounds will be clear. *Fluid overload in the lungs may cause a decreased oxygenation level, pulmonary congestion on the chest radiograph, and crackles (rales) and rhonchi upon pulmonary auscultation.* The patient should indicate reduced dyspnea and describe increased comfort. Toward this end, the nurse should position the patient in an upright position with edematous areas supported. *The most frequently reported position of comfort is leaning forward with arms and upper body supported.*[10] *This position allows maximum lung expansion with reduced energy expediture.* Passive and active range-of-motion exercises should be encouraged if edema is restricting the patient's activity *as muscle movement facilitates venous return and reduces edema.* If skin is edematous, good skin care is essential.

Finally, the patient will demonstrate an adequate knowledge base. An assessment of the patient and family learning needs and readiness to learn is an essential first step. Provide information concerning the cause of this Fluid Volume Excess and how to prevent recurrence; rationale for treatment; and discharge plans for fluid intake, medications, and follow-up care. Providing patients with needed information for self-care is necessary to assure continuity of care from hospital to home.[16]

EVALUATION
High Risk for Fluid Volume Deficit, Fluid Volume Deficit (1), Fluid Volume Deficit (2)

The effectiveness of nursing interventions related to these diagnosis is measured by certain indicators. The patient will have good skin turgor, moist mucous membranes, and normal weight and will deny any sensation of weakness or thirst. The patient will be fully oriented, intake and output will be balanced, and hemodynamics will be stable. Electrolyte levels and the hematocrit will be within normal levels. Last, the patient and family will be able to (a) explain pertinent risk factors for the present High Risk for Fluid Volume Deficit, and (b) explain the reasons for the fluid deficit, rationale for treatment, and discharge plans for fluid and medication regimen.

Fluid Volume Excess

The effectiveness of these nursing interventions is measured by certain indicators. The patient's weight will return to his or her normal range, vital signs and hemodynamic measurements will be within normal limits for the patient. The patient's electrolyte values and arterial blood gases will be within a normal range. The patient will report decreased anxiety, restlessness, and confusion and improved ability to breathe. Breath sounds and chest radiographs will be clear. Peripheral or generalized edema will be resolving. An increase in weight gain and continued abnormal hemodynamic measurements require reevaluation of fluid intake and output. Current medication therapy may need to be reevaluated in conjunction with the physician. If breath sounds and chest radiograph are not clear reevaluate the fluid status as previously discussed. Continued abnormal pulmonary status and electrolyte profile may indicate additional causes and the need to consult the physician.

❖ CASE STUDY WITH PLAN OF CARE

Mr. Joe S., a 55-year-old electrician, was seen in the emergency room with increasing dyspnea on exertion and occasional paroxysmal nocturnal dyspnea. He further reported a new onset of aching abdominal pain and increased peripheral edema. Joe had an anterior myocardial infarction 2 years before this admission, for which furosemide (40 mg twice a day), digoxin (0.125 mg once a day), and a low-sodium diet were prescribed. Physical examination revealed distended neck veins, 3-pitting edema in his lower extremities bilaterally, a positive hepatojugular reflex, and bibasilar crackles (rales). A chest radiograph showed pulmonary congestion. An electrocardiogram revealed sinus rhythm with an occasional premature ventricular contraction. Laboratory studies showed a serum sodium of 130 mEq/L and a potassium level of 3.5 mg/L. A medical diagnosis was made: congestive heart failure with left and right ventricular involvement. Joe was admitted to the telemetry unit for treatment and close observation. Initial vital signs were heart rate, 115 beats/min; respiratory rate, 28 breaths/min; blood pressure, 98/50 mm Hg; and central venous pressure, 16 mm Hg. A nursing diagnosis of Fluid Volume Excess related to congestive heart failure was formulated.

Continued.

CARE PLAN FOR MR. JOE S.

Nursing Diagnosis: Fluid Volume Excess related to congestive heart failure

Expected Patient Outcomes	Nursing Interventions
Mr. S. will maintain a stable hemodynamic status, as evidenced by vital signs and central venous pressure within normal limits.	• Monitor vital signs, including central venous pressure. • Administer diuretics as ordered. • Administer inotropic agents or vasodilators as ordered.
Mr. S.'s body weight will be maintained within his normal range.	• Weigh Mr. S. daily. • Monitor intake and output every shift. • Maintain fluid restriction as ordered. • Provide reduced-sodium diet as ordered. • Assess for peripheral edema bilaterally every shift and as needed.
Mr. S.'s electrolyte levels will remain within a normal range.	• Monitor serum electrolyte levels. • Replace potassium and other electrolytes as ordered. • Monitor blood urea nitrogen and creatinine levels. • Measure urine specific gravity.
Mr. S. will maintain normal (acceptable) pulmonary status as evidenced by arterial blood gases within normal limits, clear breath sounds, and normal chest radiographs.	• Assess breath sounds every 4 hours and as needed. • Monitor chest radiography reports. • Monitor results of arterial blood gases. • Administer oxygen as ordered. • Encourage coughing and deep-breathing exercises every 2 hours and as needed. • Perform incentive spirometry every 2 hours and as needed.
Mr. S. will indicate less dyspnea and will experience more comfort.	• Position Mr. S. to help alleviate dyspnea. • Provide support to edematous areas. • Have Mr. S. do range-of-motion exercises if activity is limited. • Encourage active range of motion. • Provide proper skin care for edematous areas.
Mr. S. and his family will demonstrate adequate knowledge base regarding the diagnosis.	• Explain cause of the fluid volume excess. • Explore the possible causes of the congestive heart failure. • Provide information concerning signs and symptoms of congestive heart failure, diet, medications, activity, and follow-up care. • Ask Mr. S. to demonstrate knowledge before discharge.

REFERENCES

1. Baer C: Acute renal failure, *Nursing 90* 20(6):34, 1990.
2. Blank CA, Irwin GH: Peripheral vascular disorders assessment and intervention, *Nurs Clin North Am* 25 (4):777, 1990.
3. Brenner M, Welliver J: Pulmonary and acid-base assessment, *Nurs Clin North Am* 25 (4):761, 1990.
4. Bullock B, Rosendahl P: *Pathophysiology: adaptations and alterations in function,* Boston, 1988, Little Brown.
5. Cagno J: Diabetes insipidus, *Crit Care Nurs* 9(6):86, 1989.
6. Cohen S, Kenner C, and Hollingsworth A: *Maternal, neonatal and women's health nursing,* Springhouse, PA, 1991, Springhouse Corp.
7. Criscitiello M: Fine-tuning the cardiovascular exam, *Patient Care* 24(1):51, 1990.
8. Epstein C: Fluid volume deficit for the adrenal crisis patient, *Dimen Crit Care Nurs* 10(4):210, 1991.
9. Gawlinski A: Saving the cardiogenic shock patient, *Nurs 89* 19(12): 34, 1989.
10. Gift A: Dyspnea, *Nurs Clin North Am* 25(4):955, 1990.
11. Graves L: Diabetic ketoacidosis and hyperosmolar hyperglycemic nonketotic coma, *Crit Care Nurs Quart* 13(3):50, 1990.
12. Kim MJ, McFarland GK, and McLane AM: *Pocket guide to nursing diagnoses,* ed 4, St. Louis, 1991, CV Mosby.
13. Malasanos L, Barkauskas V, and Stoltenberg-Allen K: *Health assessment,* ed 4, St. Louis, 1990, CV Mosby.
14. Miller L, Holloway N: Water intoxication: psychogenic hyperdipsia, *Crit Care Nurs* 9(7):74, 1989.
15. Patterson L, Noroian E: Diabetes insipidus versus syndrome of inappropriate antidiuretic hormone, *Dimen Crit Care Nurs* 8(4):226, 1989.
16. Potter PA, Perry AG: *Fundamentals of nursing concepts, process and practice,* St. Louis, 1989, CV Mosby.
17. Rice V: Shock, a clinical syndrome: an update part I. An overview of shock, *Crit Care Nurs* 11(4):20, 1991.
18. Rinard G: Water intoxication, *Am J Nurs* 89:1635, 1989.
19. Thompson J, and others: *Mosby's manual of clinical nursing,* ed 2, St Louis, 1989, CV Mosby.
20. Woodtli A: Thirst: a critical care nursing challenge, *Dimen Crit Care Nurs* 9(1):6, 1990.
21. Wright S: Pathophysiology of congestive heart failure, *J Cardiovasc Nurs* 4(3):1, 1990.

II

High Risk for Impaired Skin Integrity

Impaired Skin Integrity

High Risk for Impaired Skin Integrity *is a state in which the individual's skin is at risk of being adversely altered.*

Impaired Skin Integrity *is a state in which the individual's skin is adversely altered.*

OVERVIEW

The functions of the skin are to provide a tough, protective covering for the internal environment of the body, to act as a barrier to the loss of water and electrolytes, to regulate temperature, and to function in excretion, absorption, and sensation.[14] Care of the skin is a basic nursing procedure that requires diligence and advanced assessment skills on the part of the practicing nurse for prevention and adequate treatment.

A number of risk factors have been identified that are thought to predispose an individual to skin breakdown as well as interfere with the healing process of an existing skin impairment. The list can be organized into intrinsic and extrinsic factors. Intrinsic factors relate to the internal physiological functions that have an effect on skin integrity. An example of this is nutritional status. Extrinsic factors generally represent any external force that may adversely affect the skin. Examples of these are prolonged pressure and the presence of moisture.

Overall, the development of impaired skin integrity usually is related to the presence of multiple factors acting on the individual at a given time. The response of the individual to these factors depends on the type of factors present and the individual's position on the health-illness continuum. Nurses must be aware of individuals at risk for impaired skin integrity so that steps can be taken to try to prevent the occurrence of an actual impairment in skin integrity.

The terms *pressure ulcer, decubitus ulcer, and bedsore* often are used interchangeably to describe an area of cellular necrosis. The ulcer represents a break in the integrity of the skin that can progress in severity to affect the epidermis, dermis, subcutaneous tissue, and even the muscle. Incidence rates for decubitus ulcers vary depending on the population studied and the surveying methods used. With respect to the hospitalized patient population, many rates have been reported, but they generally range from 3% to 10% of all hospitalized patients.[13] Actual skin impairments have serious financial, psychological, and social ramifications for the individual and the community at large. Therefore it is imperative that prevention be the primary goal and that individuals with skin impairments be identified and treated promptly.

ASSESSMENT
High Risk for Impaired Skin Integrity

Assessment of individuals at risk for the development of impaired skin integrity is a complex process because of the number of factors involved. For this reason it is not always clear which factors are the most significant contributor to the problem or, in fact, which individuals will go on to develop an impairment.

Intrinsic (internal) factors include altered nutritional states such as malnutrition, emaciation, and obesity. Poor nutrition interferes with the normal tissue integrity and impairs proper wound healing. Specifically, disturbances such as hypoproteinemia; ascorbic acid, iron, and zinc deficiencies; fat and carbohydrate insufficiency; and vitamin A, B, C, D, and K deficiencies may result in impaired tissue regeneration and repair, depending on the type and degree of the deficiency present.[3] Chronic malnutrition results in weight loss (emaciation) and decreased padding from loss of subcutaneous tissue and muscle mass, thereby predisposing the individual to skin impairments or compounding existing ones. The presence of a negative nitrogen balance, which is associated with some nutritional disturbances, predisposes an individual to edema formation, and this makes the skin more vulnerable to injury. Obesity may result in decreased sensation and possibly decreased circulation related to the effects of the additional adipose tissues.[14]

Altered circulation, which accompanies peripheral vascular disease and diabetes, will result in less than optimal blood flow carrying oxygen and nutrients to the skin. This can increase the likelihood of skin breakdown. Altered sensation results in decreased or absent response to various stimuli, such as heat, pressure, and pain, that serve as a warning of potential damage to the skin integrity.

Developmental factors also have an effect on the integrity of the skin. Specific age related changes in the skin, such as loss of dermal thickness, reduction of circulation through the dermis, or decreased or altered pressure perception and light touch response, render the elderly population at risk for impaired skin.[12] Alterations in skin turgor, such as changes in elasticity that may accompany aging, may impair skin integrity. Similarly, infants and small children may be at increased risk for skin breakdown because of excessive skin exposure to urine, which can lead to maceration

of the skin. Conditions that promote itching may impair skin integrity by stimulating scratching of the skin.[14] Medications that give rise to allergic reactions and the release of histamine from cells may cause itching. Immunologic deficits, dry skin, and psychogenic reactions may initiate scratching, which may impair skin integrity.[14]

Extrinsic or external factors also may affect skin integrity. Mechanical factors include shearing forces and friction injuries to the epidermis that are sustained as the individual slides up or down in bed. Scratching represents a potential mechanical cause of impaired skin. Prolonged pressure from physical immobilization, fractures, or restraint may cause impaired skin integrity by impairing circulation to all body parts or dependent areas. When the external pressure exerted on an area of skin is greater than the capillary hydrostatic pressure, capillary obstruction occurs, resulting in a deficiency of nutrition caused by ischemia.[1]

Pressure sustained for more than 1 to 2 hours may result in pathological changes that lead to death in tissues. The presence of moisture on a chronic basis, in the form of urine, perspiration, or humidity, can lead to maceration of the epidermis, which reduces the effectiveness of the skin to resist destruction from other factors.[11] Poor hygiene may contribute to impaired skin by providing an ischemic environment that attracts and fosters the growth and proliferation of bacteria. The heat, exhibited as fever, raises the metabolic needs and the demand for oxygen; this can potentiate tissue ischemia especially if an individual is already in a compromised condition.[11] Fecal incontinence is thought to contribute to skin impairment through exposure of the skin to bacteria and toxins in the stool and through skin maceration.[11]

There are a number of assessment tools described in the literature that have as a goal the prediction or identification of individuals at risk to develop an impairment in skin integrity. Three scales will be discussed here. The best known pressure-ulcer assessment tool is the Norton Scale. Norton and associates pioneered this clinical area with the formation of a scale that determines scores based on five categories: mobility, activity, incontinence, mental status, and physical condition. Some find the categories used by Norton to be confusing, and the tool tends to overpredict in some situations.[6] Gosnell in 1973 introduced a tool that built on Norton's work, and in 1987 Gosnell again released a revised tool. This tool was extended to include a more detailed assessment of the skin, nutrition, and hydration status, and it provided room for documentation of interventions. A third tool, the Braden Scale for Predicting Pressure Sore Risk, was developed in 1987 by Bergstrom and associates. This tool measures six factors: sensory perception, activity, mobility, moisture, friction, and nutrition. Many institutions develop their own risk assessment scale based on components from the tools listed above, and therefore more clinical testing and usage of these tools is needed in the clinical setting.

❖ Risk Factors

The presence of the following behaviors, conditions, or circumstances renders the patient more vulnerable to High Risk For Impaired Skin Integrity:

External (environmental) factors	Internal (somatic) factors
• Hyperthermia/hypothermia	• Medications
• Chemical substance	• Altered nutritional state: (obesity, emaciation, and malnutrition)
• Mechanical factors: shearing forces, pressure, restraints	• Altered circulation
• Radiation	• Decreased sensation
• Physical immobilization	• Skeletal prominence
• Excretions and secretions	• Developmental factors
• Humidity	• Immunologic deficit
	• Alterations in skin turgor (change in elasticity)
	• Excretions and secretions
	• Psychogenic factors
	• Edema

❖ Related Medical/Psychiatric Diagnoses

The following are examples of related medical/psychiatric diagnoses for High Risk for Impaired Skin Integrity:

• Coma state
• Diabetes mellitus
• Obesity

Impaired Skin Integrity

The defining characteristics for Impaired Skin Integrity include disruption of skin integrity, destruction of skin layers, and invasion of body structures.[8] The first defining characteristic is the disruption of the skin surface; this can be caused by the development of primary lesions such as papules, pustules, vesicles, and wheals.

The second defining characteristic involves changes in these lesions that may give rise to secondary lesions that destroy skin layers.[2] The development of a decubitus ulcer or pressure ulcer is the most common example of an actual destruction of skin layers. Other examples include burns and fissures.

The third defining characteristic involves the invasion of body structures. This happens when the primary impairment is so devastating or so resistant to treatment that it penetrates the epidermis, dermis, subcutaneous tissue, and muscle and reaches the internal organs. This commonly occurs through trauma or the progression of a decubitus ulcer.

A number of related factors of intrinsic and extrinsic origin affect the skin and may impair skin integrity. The related factors are similar to the risk factors associated with the diagnosis High Risk for Impaired Skin Integrity and also affect an actual impairment by interfering with healing.

The development of a decubitus ulcer generally occurs in a systematic way that can be expressed through a staging process. Staging ulcers is an important step, because the plan of care should coincide with the stage of the ulcer. Through the years many different staging systems have been described in the literature. Because enterostomal therapy nurses are the leaders in skin care, a staging system devised by the International Association of Enterostomal Therapists (IAET) will be described here.

Stage 1: Erythema not resolving within 30 minutes of pressure relief. Epidermis remains intact. *Reversible with intervention.*

Stage 2: Partial thickness loss of skin layers involving epidermis and possibly penetrating into but not through the dermis. May present as blistering with erythema and/or induration; wound base moist and pink; painful; free of necrotic tissue.

Stage 3: Full-thickness tissue loss extending through dermis to involve subcutaneous tissue. Presents as shallow crater unless covered by eschar. May include necrotic tissue, undermining sinus tract formation, exudate, and/or infection. Wound base is usually not painful.

Stage 4: Deep tissue destruction extending through subcutaneous tissue to fascia and may involve muscle layers, joint, and/or bone. Presents as deep crater, unless covered by eschar. May include necrotic tissue, undermining, sinus tract formation, exudate, and/or infection. Wound base usually is not painful.[7]

❖ Defining Characteristics

The presence of the following defining characteristics indicates that the patient may be experiencing Impaired Skin Integrity:

- Disruption of skin surface
- Destruction of skin layers
- Invasion of body structures

❖ Related Factors

The following related factors are associated with Impaired Skin Integrity:

External (environmental) factors	Internal (somatic) factors
• Hyperthermia/hypothermia	• Medications
• Chemical substance	• Altered nutritional state: obesity, emaciation, malnutrition
• Mechanical factors: shearing forces, pressure, restraints	• Altered circulation
• Radiation	• Decreased sensation
• Physical immobilization	• Skeletal prominence
• Excretions and secretions	• Developmental factors
• Humidity	• Immunologic deficit
	• Alterations in skin turgor (change in elasticity)
	• Excretions and secretions
	• Psychogenic factors
	• Edema

❖ Related Medical/Psychiatric Diagnoses

The following are examples of related medical/psychiatric diagnoses for Impaired Skin Integrity:

- Chicken pox
- Chronic renal failure
- Coma state
- Cirrhosis
- Dermatitis
- Diabetes mellitus
- Diarrhea and dehydration
- Measles
- Obesity
- Paralysis

NURSING DIAGNOSES

Examples of *specific* nursing diagnoses for High Risk for Impaired Skin Integrity are:

- High Risk for Impaired Skin Integrity related to severe malnutrition as evidenced by albumin level of 2.0.
- High Risk for Impaired Skin Integrity related to presence of persistent diarrhea.

Examples of *specific* nursing diagnoses for Impaired Skin Integrity are:

- Impaired Skin Integrity related to prolonged pressure and decreased mobility secondary to fractured hip as evidenced by stage 3 ulcer on sacrum.
- Impaired Skin Integrity related to prolonged urinary incontinence as evidenced by perianal excoriation.

PLANNING AND IMPLEMENTATION WITH RATIONALE
High Risk for Impaired Skin Integrity

Knowledge of the factors that contribute to the development of Impaired Skin Integrity will lead the practitioner to an appropriate plan of care.[10,15] The expected outcome of the plan is the maintenance of intact skin integrity, and the nurse achieves this by performing nursing interventions aimed at reducing or eliminating the risk factors that contribute to impaired skin integrity.[15] The overall plan focuses on (1) conducting a thorough assessment, (2) providing adequate general skin care, (3) preventing unnecessary trauma to the skin, (4) optimizing circulatory status, and (5) optimizing nutritional status.

First, the nurse must thoroughly assess the individual's integument and determine the presence of risk factors, as previously identified, to develop appropriate strategies. The nurse should also inspect the skin for its integrity and absence or presence of redness, blisters, warmth, swelling, and drainage. Capillary refill should also be checked. Monitor laboratory values, as ordered, that have an effect on the integument, and report results to the physician: albumin, uric acid, bilirubin, arterial blood gases, blood urea nitrogen, hemoglobin, and hematocrit.[11] *Assessment of risk factors is essential to planning an appropriate plan of care*. The expected outcome is that individuals at risk for skin breakdown will be identified.

The second step in the plan is to provide good general skin care to all patients at risk for Impaired Skin Integrity. The nurse should keep the skin clean and dry to prevent breakdown of the epidermis from maceration and to limit bacterial growth.[9] Because urinary and fecal incontinence are major causes of skin breakdown, incontinent patients must be identified and kept as dry as possible. The nurse should assess for incontinent episodes with each position change, apply protective creams to the affected area, and in collaboration with the physician, institute measures to control the problem. *Moisture may cause maceration and/or chemical erosion, which contributes to skin breakdown*. The expected outcome is that the skin will remain intact.

Third, the nurse must take measures to avoid unnecessary injury to the patient's skin. Trauma to the tissues has been noted to occur as a result of friction and shearing forces acting on the skin as the patient slides in bed.[11] To lessen the extent of this motion as much as possible, nurses should move patients up in bed by means of a pull sheet so that the patient is not dragged. The use of a footboard or knee gatch is sometimes useful to keep patients from sliding in the bed. The 30-degree Fowler's position should be limited to less than an hour, because this position has been found to destroy tissues.[7] Furthermore, the 90-degree lateral position should be avoided as a preventive technique, because this results in the hastened development of trochanteric and malleolar ulcers because of the vulnerable location. The nurse should use occlusive dressings that act as a second layer of skin and powders applied to the skin to reduce the trauma to the skin in high-risk areas.[7] *Physical trauma from friction and shearing forces contributes to skin breakdown*. The expected outcome is that the skin will remain intact.

Fourth, the nurse must institute measures to increase circulation to all areas of the body to allow for intake of nutrients and removal of waste. Patients should ambulate if possible, and the sitting position should be limited to less than 2 hours. Reposition bedfast patients every 1 to 2 hours and provide range-of-motion exercises with each position change. Use pressure-relieving/reducing mattresses (water mattress, air-fluidized bed, alternating air mattress) as indicated.[4] *Necrosis may occur from high pressure over short periods of time or from low pressure over long periods of time*. The expected outcome is that adequate circulation will be maintained to all areas of the body and the skin will remain intact.

Fifth, in collaboration with the physician identify nutritional deficiencies and implement strategies to improve status. Nutritional deficits are a common problem in hospitalized patients and are a major cause of skin breakdown.[3] Collaborate with the dietitian to provide the patient with a sufficient intake of calories, protein, and fluids. Be aggressive and prompt to report problems with nutrition to the physician so that adequate supplements or alternative feeding methods can be instituted. Monitor problems by assessing daily

❖ NURSING CARE GUIDELINES

Nursing Diagnosis: *High Risk for Impaired Skin Integrity*

Expected Patient Outcomes	Nursing Interventions
The patient's skin will remain intact.	• Assess the patient for the presence of intrinsic/extrinsic risk factors associated with skin breakdown. • Inspect the patient's skin for redness, lesions, blisters, swelling, and drainage and document. • Monitor laboratory values that have an effect on the skin and report to physician: hematocrit/hemoglobin, bilirubin, blood urea nitrogen, albumin, uric acid, and arterial blood gases. • Keep the patient's skin clean and dry. • Cleanse the patient with mild soap promptly after incontinence. • Apply protective creams if reddened areas develop from incontinence. • Consult enterostomal therapy nurse. • Assess patient/family knowledge regarding skin breakdown and preventive care.
Trauma to the patient's skin is minimized.	• Utilize assistive devices and/or techniques to facilitate dependent/independent patient movements, leg trapeze, lifts, turning sheets, transfer boards. • Use powder or cornstarch judiciously on surfaces contacting the skin. • Place footboard on bed. • Use knee gatch when head of bed is elevated. • Limit Fowler's position to less than 1 hour. • Apply clear occlusive dressing to high risk areas of skin.
The patient's circulation will be maximized.	• Ambulate and get patient out of bed if possible. • Limit the sitting position to less than 2 hours. • Reposition the patient every 1 to 2 hours using all four sides. • Provide range-of-motion exercises every 2 hours. • Avoid massaging reddened areas when repositioning patient. • Utilize pressure-relieving device for patients who cannot tolerate turning. • Utilize pressure-reducing device in conjunction with turning schedule.
The patient's nutritional status will be optimized.	• In collaboration with the physician, monitor/assess nutritional parameters: oral/parenteral intake of protein, calories, and fluids; albumin and total protein levels, and daily weights in relation to patient's ideal weight.

weights, dietary intake, and albumin levels. *Optimum tissue hydration and a positive nitrogen balance are critical elements in wound healing.* The expected outcome is that the patient will receive adequate nutritional intake to maintain a positive nitrogen balance.

Impaired Skin Integrity

The nursing goals for the individual with Impaired Skin Integrity are (1) to regain intact skin integrity, (2) to reduce or eliminate factors that contribute to the development or extension of the skin impairment, (3) to increase comfort if pain or itching sensation is present, and (4) to teach the individual or family the plan of care.

First, the nurse should assess the skin impairment for size, depth, presence of redness or drainage, signs of infection, presence of granulation tissue, presence of necrotic tissue, presence of sinus tract, and location. The nurse should identify the cause(s) of the impairment, if possible, to lessen the extent of the impairment. The nurse should document the stage of the ulcer according to a standard staging system, such as the one recommended by the IAET, if the impairment is a decubitus ulcer. *Accurate assessment and regular documentation of skin impairments will result in the provision of better care and improved evaluation of treatments.*

Most impairments in skin integrity will receive some kind of topical treatment that is appropriate for the type of impairment present.[5] The aim of topical therapy is to keep the wound clean and to enhance the normal healing process.[4] Nurses most often are involved in the treatment of decubitus and pressure ulcers and are often responsible for determining an appropriate treatment. Many hospitals employ an enterostomal therapy (ET) nurse who is a specialist in skin care. The ET nurse should collaborate with nursing and medicine departments to recommend an appropriate treatment plan for individual patients. The literature on topical treatments for decubitus ulcers should be reviewed with a critical eye, because much of the literature is not research based. Points to remember when treating decubitus and pressure ulcers

are as follows: (1) the decubitus ulcer heals more slowly, and therefore time must be allowed for a given treatment to take effect before final evaluation or discontinuation of treatment; (2) continuity of treatment between shifts and day to day is important for healing purposes and for proper evaluation of treatment; (3) the choice of treatment should consider the stage, location, and status of the ulcer, secreting or nonsecreting, and the presence or absence of necrotic tissue; and (4) the cause(s) of the ulcer should be considered.

All wounds must be cleansed. Some of the commonly used antimicrobial cleaning agents are providone-iodine, hydrogen peroxide, chlorhexidine gluconate, and acetic acid.[4] There is some debate over the use of these products, because in some cases they are thought to delay wound healing.[4] If these products are used, especially the providone-iodine, they must be diluted before cleaning an open wound. Some practitioners find cleaning superficial ulcers and abrasions with soap and water to be superior to topical antiseptics. Another recommendation is the use of water-based surfactant cleaners such as Cara-Klenz and Shur Clens, which contain wetting agent beads that break down the surface action between water and oil and do not impair healing. Topical therapies for decubitus ulcers have undergone significant changes over time, and research in this area continues to improve as nurses begin to conduct more rigorous studies using control groups.

For almost a decade, the trend in topical therapy has been based on the principles of moist wound healing. Significant developments have occurred in this area. A moist environment is maintained by applying an occlusive, adhesive, moisture vapor film or wafer over the wound and surrounding skin. A moist environment speeds epithelialization, because there is no scab formation, and it allows the individual's own white blood cells (under the dressing) to phagocytize the debris and microorganisms under the wound.[4] Such dressings are available as a thin film or as a thicker wafer and should be applied on the basis of the anatomical location of the ulcer and the contributing factors. These adhesive dressings in-

❖ *NURSING CARE GUIDELINES*
Nursing Diagnosis: Impaired Skin Integrity

Expected Patient Outcomes	Nursing Interventions
The patient will attain intact skin.	• Assess for etiologic factors. • Assess the impairment and document size, depth, presence of redness, drainage, or necrotic tissue, location, presence or absence of granulation tissue, and symptoms of infection. • Control (where possible) factors that contribute to skin impairments (see High Risk for Skin Impairment). • Consult enterostomal therapy nurse. • In collaboration with ET nurse and physician, institute a topical therapy to create a favorable environment for healing. • Use topical therapy to keep the wound surface clean, moist, and free from infection (transparent adhesive, hydrocolloid, gel, or moist gauze dressings).
The patient will achieve comfort through relief of itching.	• Assess causative factors of itching. • Teach patient about itching and the need to refrain from scratching. • Provide mitts for or restrain confused individuals to prevent scratching. • Administer antihistamines and antipruritics as ordered, as needed. • Use distraction techniques to prevent scratching. • Prevent excessive dryness of the skin: bathe only as necessary, use mild soap, lubricate skin after bathing, and maintain adequate hydration status.
The patient or family will demonstrate knowledge of care of the skin.	• Teach the patient and family about general skin care, the mechanism of action and application of treatments, the importance of providing an adequate dietary intake, and measures to prevent skin impairments.

crease patient comfort, reduce friction, can remain in place 1 to 7 days, and have demonstrated success in the treatment of stages 1, 2, and 3 ulcers.[4] For deeper stage 3 and 4 ulcers, absorptive dressings such as gauze, karaya powder, and dressings composed of dextranomer beads or copolymer starches are recommended.

If necrotic tissue is present, the tissue must be removed, or debrided, before healing will begin. Debridement can be achieved by mechanical scrubbing, by use of sharp instruments, and with enzymatic agents such as sutilains (Travase) and fibrinolysin. There are a number of skin-barrier creams and ointments available to protect skin from breakdown from excessive moisture. These can also be applied to stage 1 ulcers (reddened areas) to prevent breakdown.

Second, the plan must incorporate the following principles: providing adequate general skin care, preventing unnecessary trauma to the skin, optimizing circulation status, and optimizing nutritional status (see High Risk for Impaired Skin Integrity). *These components are vital to skin maintenance and restoration.*

II

❖ *CASE STUDY WITH PLAN OF CARE*

Mrs. Vicki W., a 75-year-old woman, was admitted to the medical unit for treatment of severe dehydration. The daughter reported that Mrs. W. had experienced decreased appetite for about 3 weeks and that during the past week she often refused to eat. Furthermore, during the week she began to stay in bed most of the day, getting up only to use the bathroom. Initial assessment revealed a frail, slightly lethargic but oriented elderly woman. Body weight was 90 pounds for a frame of 5'1", skin was flaking off her arms, a 10 cm stage 2 pressure ulcer was located on her left hip, albumin level was 2.7 gm/dl (low), and blood urea nitrogen was 68 mg/dl. One nursing diagnosis was that of Impaired Skin Integrity related to immobility and malnutrition.

PLAN OF CARE FOR MRS. VICKI W.

Nursing Diagnosis: Impaired Skin Integrity related to immobility and malnutrition

Expected Patient Outcomes	Nursing Interventions
Mrs. W. will regain skin integrity.	• Assess, monitor, and document the characteristics of the wound. • Cleanse the wound with soap and water and pat dry. • Apply Op-Site clear occlusive dressing to wound and surrounding tissue. • Consult the enterostomal therapy nurse.
Mrs. W. will demonstrate absence or control of factors that contribute to the formation of the impairment—poor nutrition and immobility.	• Monitor nutritional status. • Follow daily weights, albumin levels, and tolerance to feedings. • Maintain nasogastric tube feedings as ordered. • Maintain hydrating intravenous line as ordered. • Place Mrs. W. on alternating air mattress. • Remove Mrs. W. from her bed and ambulate as tolerated. • Reposition Mrs. W. every 2 hours if necessary. • Add lubricating oil to bath water, apply body lotion after bath, and limit frequency of baths. • Monitor blood chemistries that affect skin and report these: blood urea nitrogen, albumin, hematocrit/hemoglobin, arterial blood gases, uric acid, and bilirubin.

Third, the physician should be involved in devising a plan of care based on the cause, to reduce itching and scratching. Minimize the patient's dry skin if possible by limiting the frequency of baths, using a mild soap sparingly, blotting skin dry after bathing, applying lotion to skin when wet,[14] and maintaining adequate hydration status. Administer antipruritics as ordered to control itching. Remind the patient about the dangers of scratching, for instance, damage to the epidermis and potential for infection. Use mitts and other restraints when needed for young children or confused adults to prevent scratching. Use distraction techniques to remove the individual's focus from the itching sensation. *Reducing damage induced by scratching will preserve the integument.*

The fourth goal is successfully teaching the patient and family about skin care and the impairment. The individual or family should be knowledgeable about general skin care and assessment, use of lubricants, protocol for increasing circulation, importance of nutrition, mechanism of action for topical treatments, the causes of pruritus, interventions that relieve itching, and factors that increase itching. *It is critical to determine the patient/family's knowledge level and availability of resources and to refer them to appropriate sources of assistance.*

EVALUATION

The overall indicator that demonstrates the effectiveness of the nursing interventions for the nursing diagnosis of high risk for impaired skin integrity is the presence of intact skin. By maintaining clean and dry skin, avoiding trauma to the skin, and maximizing circulatory and nutritional status, the nurse increases the patient's resistance to skin breakdown.

The first patient outcome for the patient with impaired skin integrity is to regain skin integrity. Data indicating improvement in this condition are: (1) The impairment in integrity is clean and free of secondary bacterial infection, (2) the impairment in integrity decreases in size, and (3) the skin is warm, dry, and intact. The next expected outcome is that the individual will demonstrate increased comfort through the relief of itching. Data indicating improvement in this status are subjective reports from the individual of relief of itching and the presence of intact skin. The last expected outcome is that the individual or family will demonstrate knowledge of skin care. This is achieved through follow-up observation of a demonstration of skin care by patient or family.

REFERENCES

1. Alterescu V: Etiology and treatment of pressure ulcers, *Decubitus 1* (1):28-35, 1988.
2. Bates B: *A guide to physical examination,* ed 4, Philadelphia, 1987, JB Lippincott.
3. Bobel LM: Nutritional implications in patients with pressure sores, *Nurs Clin North Am* 22(2):379-389, 1987.
4. Fowler E: Equipment and products used in management and treatment of pressure ulcers, *Nurs Clin North Am* 22(2):449-461, 1987.
5. Goodman T, Thomas C, and Rappaport N: Skin ulcers overview, nursing implications, *AORN J* 52(1):24-37, 1990.
6. Gosnell DJ: Assessment and evaluation of pressure sores, *Nurs Clin North Am* 22(2):399-415, 1987.
7. IAET: Standards of care—dermal wounds: pressure sores, *J Enterostom Ther* 15(1):4-17, 1987.
8. Kim MJ, McFarland GK, and McLane AM: *Pocket guide to nursing diagnoses,* ed 4, St Louis, Mosby–Year Book.
9. Kosiak M: Prevention and rehabilitation of pressure ulcers, *Decubitus* 4(2):60-68, 1991.
10. Maklebust J: Impact of AHCPR pressure ulcer guidelines on nursing practice, *Decubitus* 4(2):46-50, 1991.
11. Maklebust J: Pressure ulcer: etiology and prevention, *Nurs Clin North Am* 22(2):356-377, 1987.
12. Matteson MA, McConnell ES: *Gerontological nursing,* Philadelphia, 1988, WB Saunders.
13. Meehan M: Multisite pressure ulcer prevalence survey, *Decubitus* 3(4):14-17, 1990.
14. Phipps NJ, Long BC, Woods NF, and Cassmeyer VL: *Medical surgical nursing concepts and clinical practice,* ed 4, St Louis, 1991, Mosby–Year Book.
15. Van Etten NK, Sexton P, and Smith R: Development and implementation of a skin care program, *Ostomy Wound Management* 27(3):40-54, 1990.
16. Wound Care Update 91, *Nurs 91* 4(4):47-50, 1991.

II

Impaired Tissue Integrity

Impaired Tissue Integrity is the state in which an individual experiences damage (reversible or irreversible) to mucous membrane, corneal, integumentary, or subcutaneous tissue.

OVERVIEW

Tissue impairment is characterized by an inflammatory response to injury regardless of etiology, duration, or extent. Tissue type and extent of damage determine other responses. Damage is reversible if tissue cells remain intact. Epidermal tissues (outer skin layer and cornea) regenerate in a relatively short time when damaged; however, damage to the dermis (inner skin layer) or subcutaneous tissues involving the vasculature requires complex reparative processes.[14]

Upon injury, hemostatic mechanisms, of reflex vasospasm and platelet aggregation prevent excessive blood loss and bacterial invasion. Inflammation stimulated by hypoxia and cellular acidosis follow within 5 to 10 minutes of injury: The release of histamine and bradykinin dilate nearby small blood vessels, which leak serous exudate. This environment enables white blood cells, such as the leukocytes, to enter, debride the wound, and ingest bacteria.[20] The surrounding tissues will be painful, reddened, swollen, and warmer than undamaged tissues.

Irreversible damage results in tissue necrosis appearing as a soft, yellow, fibrous slough or a dry eschar. Eschar, a leathery scab that tenaciously adheres to the bed of a wound, acts like a foreign body. It, and any other necrotic tissue, is a good breeding ground for bacteria. It also prevents the easy migration of epithelial cells across the wound bed.[2] Tissue necrosis may not be visible when only underlying tissues are damaged.

Impaired tissues go through three major phases of healing in response to injury: inflammation, a substrate or exudate phase of about 48 hours duration; proliferation, a phase of collagen synthesis and/or epithelialization lasting about 3 weeks; and remodeling, a maturational phase in which collagen bundles realign, strengthening tissues over months to years.[3]

Tissues require adequate oxygen, nutrients, and a moist environment for optimal healing. Multiple factors may modify these conditions. Age,[6,11] disease and medical treatment,[21] food intake,[22] mood,[7] temperature, activity, and rest influence the rate and quality of tissue repair.[14]

Given optimal conditions, wound contraction begins about the fifth day, thinning and stretching the skin as the wound margins are pulled together. If tissue necrosis has involved the skin's full thickness and deeper structures, scar tissue forms and the wound will take longer to close than with partial-thickness damage. Contractures result when wounded tissues over joints are pulled too tightly. Insufficient closure of wounds results in chronic impairment. With chronic impairments, the skin may be too thin and easily redamaged, or open areas may continue to suppurate. Scar tissue over bony prominences greatly increases the risk of recurrent impairments.

ASSESSMENT

Interpretation of data gathered during assessment determines the plan of care. The nurse (or clinician) must consider the location of tissue impairment, its depth, and the factors related to it in choosing topical care and equipment. The nurse can focus assessment data in two major areas: defining characteristics and related factors. A number of medical and psychiatric diagnoses should alert the clinician to consider the risk or presence of tissue impairment.

In relation to defining characteristics, erythema is indicative of the inflammatory response to tissue injury. Erythema over a bony prominence that does not resolve within 30 minutes of relief of pressure is considered a stage I pressure ulcer.[10] Erythema, induration, edema, exudate, and pain together are associated with infections. The nurse must be aware, however, that exudate and odor, without other signs of infection, do not always indicate an infection. Other possible causes are the desirable autolytic debridement and digestion of necrotic tissue by white blood cells, which accompanies the use of hydrocolloid dressings.[2] The nurse should cleanse the wound before complete assessment.

The nurse must consider the type of tissue disruption. The appearance of the tissue impairment is important in differentiating the etiology. A discrete lesion over a bony prominence could be a pressure ulcer. A red raised rash with eroding skin in the same location may indicate a fungus infection.

The patient's complaints of pain and itching are also helpful cues. Pain in a pressure ulcer indicates that the skin damage may not be full thickness. Absence of pain makes deeper damage probable. Itching of the axilla or the skin under an ostomy appliance could indicate a Candida infection.

Many factors are related to the development of tissue impairment. Because tissues cannot heal without removal of tissue irritants and amelioration of contributing conditions, the success of the treatment plan depends on correct identification of the related factors.

Research is ongoing to establish strong scientific support for many of the above factors. Indications are that no one factor can be identified in an individual case of tissue impairment. For example, the immobile patient may be receiving steroids for COPD and be unable to get out of bed when diarrhea is experienced.

Tissues must receive oxygen via the circulatory system to remain healthy. Extrinsic pressures can close vessels caught between a hard surface and a bony prominence, resulting in a pressure ulcer. The immobile patient is at High Risk for Impaired Tissue Integrity. Intrinsic developments such as peripheral vascular disease or diabetes can cause venous stasis or arterial ulcers.[8,19]

Trauma to tissues, whether accidental or deliberate, can be from three sources: physical, chemical, and biological agents. Sharp or hard objects, such as bedrails, slider boards, or fingernails can damage tissue. Friction against bed sheets will eventually abrade skin. Shearing causes deeper damage when muscle rubs against bony prominences as the head of a bed is raised.[15]

Chemical agents are anything that causes topical irritation to skin, eyes, or mucous membranes, such as soaps or insecticides. Medications are intrinsic chemical agents that may cause tissue reactions. Chemotherapeutic agents, such as 5-FU or Cytoxan, are associated with mucous membrane lesions and skin erythema.

Contact with biologic agents, such as stool or wound drainage, is related to erosion of skin and deeper tissues.[1,15] Tissues become macerated, increasing susceptibility to trauma. Incontinence also increases susceptibility to opportunistic skin infections such as Candida.[16]

Other microorganisms cause tissue impairment. Herpes lesions may look like pressure ulcers. Lack of healing after treatment has been instituted or severe pain may be a clue to culture for herpes. The nurse may be the first to see these infections and must be astute.

Radiation from the sun or radiation therapy damages tissues. Radiation therapy damage can vary from superficial dry skin to deep open draining wounds as tumor cells necrose.[21] In many cases the damage from radiation therapy must run its course. The clinician must assess for other sources of damage to weakened tissues. Radiation therapy can damage tissues permanently. Irradiated tissues are more susceptible to pressure damage. Healing of surgical wounds in areas of previous irradiation is slowed, occasionally resulting in breakdown of incisions.

II

Nutrition is important in keeping tissues healthy and supporting the repair process. Severe protein depletion results in interstitial edema, which prevents efficient tissue oxygenation. Lack of protein, zinc, and vitamins inhibits the repair process.[23] Several studies have found a possible link between malnutrition and tissue break-down.[12,13,17]

Medications have serious effects on tissues. Steroids suppress the inflammatory response necessary for wound healing.[9] Skin also atrophies and becomes very susceptible to extrinsic damage, such as stripping by tape, with long-term use of steroids. Allergic reactions to medication such as antibiotics are sometimes manifest by skin rashes. The effects of chemotherapy were mentioned previously.

Lack of knowledge may be a factor related to tissue impairment. People at risk must know how to prevent tissue problems. A new paraplegic needs to learn how to care for his skin. A person receiving radiation therapy or medications needs information on side effects and tissue-protective strategies.

Emotional states sometimes have a serious effect on self-care ability, even for a person with adequate knowledge of proper skin care. The depressed person may not eat. The hopeless paraplegic may not take the trouble to shift his weight frequently.

Medical and psychiatric diagnoses related to tissue impairment have been discussed previously.[17] In general, four types of conditions should alert the nurse or clinician to consider the risk of Impaired Tissue Integrity: those that impair circulation, compromise mobility, interfere with the body's ability to heal, or affect a person's self-care capacity.

❖ **Defining Characteristics**

The presence of the following defining characteristics indicates that the patient may be experiencing Impaired Tissue Integrity:

- Erythema
- Edema
- Ecchymosis
- Eschar
- Exudate
- Odor
- Induration
- Rashes/blisters/lesions
- Pain
- Itching

❖ **Related Factors**

The following related factors are all associated with Impaired Tissue Integrity:

- Altered circulation
  Immobility
  Disease
- Trauma/irritation
  Incontinence
  Shearing/friction
  Thermal damage
  Radiation (including therapeutic)
  Diarrhea
  Pressure
- Nutritional deficits
- Medication effects; e.g., steroids
- Emotional states
  Depression
  Hopelessness
- Knowledge deficit

❖ **Related Medical/Psychiatric Diagnoses**

The following are related medical/psychiatric diagnoses for Impaired Tissue Integrity:

- Bacterial/viral/fungal infection
- Cancer
- Cardiac disorders
- COPD
- Depression
- Diabetes
- Hematopoietic disorders
- Obsessive-compulsive disorder
- Peripheral vascular disease
- Psychosis
- Spinal cord injuries

NURSING DIAGNOSES

Examples of *specific* nursing diagnoses for Impaired Tissue Integrity are:

- Impaired Tissue Integrity related to radiation therapy.
- Impaired Tissue Integrity related to pressure.
- Impaired Tissue Integrity related to diarrhea.
- Impaired Tissue Integrity related to long-term use of steroids.

PLANNING AND IMPLEMENTATION WITH RATIONALE

Nursing interventions for Impaired Tissue Integrity are focused on optimizing conditions for healing. Treatment centers on removing related causal factors, such as pressure or stool, and creating a moist, protected environment for healing wounds. Additionally, nutritional intervention to support the body's self-healing capacity and self-care instruction may be needed.

Adequate Circulation

Circulation is necessary for the *transport of oxygen and nutrients to tissues*. All external pressures must be reduced below capillary closure. Pressure relief must be provided for the patient while in bed or in the chair, and other sources of pressure on impaired tissues eliminated. Various tools used in patient care, such as temperature probes, cervical collars, tubing, splints, braces, and support stockings, *may restrict circulation, especially over bony prominences,* and should thus be carefully monitored. Moving, which activates a pumping action of skeletal muscles, and pressure relief through passive moving or pressure-relief devices are means to *maintain or improve circulation*. Active movement by the patient who is oriented and physically capable may be enhanced through exercise programs tailored for an individual's age, general health, and freedom of movement. When moving is problematic, assistance or passive movement by the nurse, with or without devices, may be necessary. Options include (1) frequent small body movements (rotating a small soft pillow to shift extremities or pressure gradients on the trunk) accompanied by total body shifts (side-back-side) at least every 2 hours and (2) use of the appropriate pressure-relief device based on patients' individual characteristics.[4]

When mobility is restricted, the use of pressure-relief devices is imperative. Compressible systems such as foam pads and mattresses reduce the peak pressure between the body and supporting surfaces and are appropriate for patients capable of moving. Air mattresses reduce pressures below capillary closure. These systems are appropriate when patients are immobile and unable to shift positions. Airflow and fluidized systems *maintain subcapillary pressure* (except at the heels) at all times by dispersing pressure evenly over the total contact surface, and they are appropriate when the risk of ischemia is very high or when all available support surfaces have impaired tissues.

Patients with poor circulation related to endogenous causes, such as peripheral vascular disease, will also require medical treatment. Elevation of edematous extremities to the level of the heart will *decrease resistance to venous circulation*. Antiembolic devices, such as support hosiery, may be used to apply pressure *to prevent or reduce edema* in extremities.

Tissue Regeneration

Wounds need a moist protected environment to *support granulation and reepithelialization*.[2] The nurse or clinician should carefully select dressings based on specific wound conditions—size (particularly depth), amount of exudate, necrotic tissue, and location on the body.[5] Wounds with extensive necrotic tissues may need active debridement. A wet to dry gauze dressing will unselectively remove tissue from a wound. Absorbent gels, pastes, or granules will *keep a wound moist and help absorb liquified necrotic tissue*. Thick eschar will need surgical debridement.

As necrotic tissue decreases and granulation tissue develops, protection of new tissue and absorption of exudate become the primary goals. Hydrocolloid wafers absorb exudate and form a gel. This gel *keeps the wound moist* and separates easily from the wound, *avoiding trauma to new tissues*. When exudate is minimal, the nurse may use a transparent dressing to *protect the wound and keep it gently moist* during the final phase of contraction and reepithelialization.

Irrigate loose exudate from wounds with each dressing change to *decrease the bacterial population and remove loose foreign bodies* (necrotic tissue, gels, etc.). Antiseptic solutions such as povidone-iodine and hydrogen peroxide traditionally have been used for cleansing wounds; however, their use may be detrimental to healing, at least in clean uninfected wounds, because of damaging effects on new cell growth.[2,18] Normal saline and

II

❖ NURSING CARE GUIDELINES

Nursing Diagnosis: Impaired Tissue Integrity

Expected Patient Outcomes	Nursing Interventions
The patient will have maximized circulation.	• Provide pressure relief in bed, chair, wheelchair. • Assess skin for erythema under braces, tubes, splints, support stockings at least every 8 hours. • Turn patient at least every 2 hours, no matter what type of pressure relief chosen. • Institute passive or active range-of-motion exercises. Choose assistive devices to optimize mobility. • Keep edematous extremities elevated.
The patient will have evidence of tissue regeneration repair.	• Cover wounds with dressings that promote: moist wound healing, mechanical or autolytic debridement, absorption of excess wound drainage. • Adjust type of dressing as wound characteristics change. • Avoid cleaning wounds with substances that damage healing tissues. • Protect tissues from incontinence by using fecal pouch and/or moisture barrier ointments. Avoid diapers if possible. • Collaborate with physician in identifying and treating bacterial, fungal, and viral tissue infections. • Collaborate with dietitian to provide high-protein diet of sufficient calories to support healing.
The patient and/or family will know how to take care of tissues.	• Teach patient/family how to protect tissues from pressure, moisture, incontinence. • Teach patient/family which activities, treatments, medications may have adverse effects on tissue integrity. • Teach patient/family signs and symptoms of Impaired Tissue Integrity.

newly developed nonionic surfactants *cleanse the wound without toxic effects* to granulation tissue.[18]

Adequate nutritional intake and hydration are important for *tissue regeneration* and may require intervention. This may be in the form of patient education or more active assistance, depending on the patient's ability and motivation to eat a proper diet. A high-protein, high-carbohydrate, moderately low-fat diet with adequate calories is needed; supplemental vitamins (especially C and

A) and minerals also may be indicated.[23] Consultation with a dietitian will be helpful if diet is a major factor in individual cases. Nourishments can be planned to supplement meals carefully designed to meet the increased nutrient requirements of healing tissues. Attention to fluid intake for adequate hydration, especially with burns or draining wounds, also is important. Intake of four to six glasses of fluids daily is a minimum requirement that will need to be increased to *replace fluid losses* from tissue damage.

Provide patients with information about factors related to healing and their specific care needs *to enlist cooperation with treatment and prepare for self-care*. Teaching may also include general hygienic instruction. Pace instructions based on patient feedback. Progress from the simple, less-threatening aspects of self-care to the more complex aspects. The nurse may also give care instructions to family members.

EVALUATION

Systematic evaluation focuses on specific outcomes expected as a response to treatments for Impaired Tissue Integrity. Time the frequency of observations to detect both positive and negative changes in impaired tissues, depending on the phase of healing and the extent to which the related factors have been eliminated or controlled.

Adequate Circulation

When oxygen saturation levels and transport are normal, circulation to tissues can be observed in the symmetrical color, brisk capillary refill time (less than 3 seconds), and skin temperature that is slightly cool or warm to touch within expected variations related to the area observed. With adequate circulation, as tissues repair,

swelling (edema) will resolve. The size, shape, and turgor of tissues will change and normalize as swelling decreases. Watch for erythema over bony prominences when repositioning the patient to determine whether pressure relief is adequate.

Tissue Regeneration

Wounds heal in a constant trajectory over time, under optimal conditions. Tissue regeneration in wounds is evidenced by decreasing necrotic tissue as the wound is filled with red or pink, moist, granular tissue. Serial measurements should reveal progressively reduced diameter and depth of wounds over time.

Confirm patient knowledge and skills related to self-care as teaching progresses. Observe the patient's ability to perform care correctly and consistently, and determine perceptions of self-care efficacy. As self-care capacity increases, patients may be involved in caring for their wound in preparation for total self-care when that is indicated.

Impaired Tissue Integrity includes a wide variety of problems, and it needs specification for patient care. The following case study illustrates an individualized plan of nursing care.

❖ *CASE STUDY WITH PLAN OF CARE*

Ms. Helen W. is a 74-year-old woman with a 15-year history of chronic obstructive pulmonary disease. She has taken prednisone for 10 years to control her respiratory symptoms. In the 2 weeks before admission to the hospital she had increasing difficulty breathing. She slept in a recliner chair because she "couldn't get her head high enough to breathe in bed." She reported losing 10 pounds in the last 6 weeks. She was admitted to the hospital 7 days ago for increasing respiratory distress and pitting edema of her lower extremities. On exam, her respirations are 40/minute and labored with rhonchi heard in both lungs. Pitting edema is present

on both lower legs and feet. Her skin is thin, dry, and scaly. She has multiple ecchymotic areas on her arms with a 2 cm skin tear on her right forearm. Her coccyx area has a 2 cm by 3 cm shallow open lesion covered with a thin layer of yellow necrotic tissue. Tube feedings were started 2 days ago. She now has diarrhea, which she cannot control. She is unable to get out of bed without assistance. Her buttocks are erythematous, and an itchy red raised rash with satellite lesions is starting to appear. Her albumin level is 2.5 g/dl (normal is greater than 3.5 g/dl), serum transferrin is 170 mg/dl (normal is greater than 200 mg/dl).

Continued.

PLAN OF CARE FOR MS. HELEN W.

Nursing Diagnosis: *Impaired Tissue Integrity related to pressure, diarrhea, steroid use, malnutrition, edema, and fungus infection*

Expected Patient Outcomes	Nursing Interventions
Ms. W. will exhibit wound healing as evidenced by: disappearance of rash within 7 days; dissolution of necrotic tissue, development of granulation tissue, and epithelialization in 3 to 4 weeks; closure of skin tear within 2 weeks.	• Place fecal pouch around anus as long as diarrhea continues. • Cover coccyx wound with hydrocolloid dressing. Use adhesive remover to gently remove dressing and replace every 2 to 3 days. Place hydrogel dressing over skin tear. Change every day. • Collaborate with physician to treat fungus infection. • Collaborate with dietitian to provide high-protein diet, including tube feeding and oral intake. Assist patient to eat as needed.
Ms. W. will have maximized circulation as evidenced by decreased edema in extremities, absence of erythema over bony prominences.	• Provide pressure relief on bed. • Assist Ms. W. to stay off her back as much as possible. • Place antiembolic equipment or stockings on legs. Remove for 30 minutes very 4 hours. • Keep legs elevated. • Collaborate with physical therapist regarding range of motion.
Ms. W. will demonstrate knowledge of how to prevent damage to her tissues.	• While doing skin/tissue care, show Ms. W. how to prevent damage from pressure and friction. • Teach signs and symptoms of tissue damage. • Teach which equipment and skin care products to use. • Explain the importance of good nutrition and hydration to the maintenance of tissue integrity.

REFERENCES

1. Allman RM and others: Pressure sores among hospitalized patients, *Ann Intern Med* 105:337-342, 1986.
2. Alvarez O, Rozint J, and Meehan M: Principles of moist wound healing: indications for chronic wounds. In Krasner D, editor: *Chronic wound care,* King of Prussia, Penn, 1990, Health Management Publications.
3. Cooper DM: Optimizing wound healing, *Nurs Clin North Am* 25(1):165-180, 1990.
4. Counsell C and others: Interface skin pressures on four pressure-relieving devices, *J Enterostom Ther* 17:150-153, 1990.
5. Fowler EM: Equipment and products used in management and treatment of pressure ulcers, *Nurs Clin North Am* 22(2):449. 1987.
6. Garvin G: Wound healing in pediatrics, *Nurs Clin North Am* 25(1):181-192, 1990.
7. Holden-Lund C: Effects of relaxation with guided imagery on surgical stress and wound healing, *Res Nurs Health* 11:235-244, 1988.
8. Holloway GA: Lower leg ulcers: an overview, *Nurs Clin North Am* 25(1):206-212, 1990.
9. Hotter AN: Wound healing and immunocompromise, *Nurs Clin North Am* 25(1):193-201, 1990.
10. International Association for Enterostomal Therapy: Standards of care. Dermal ulcers: pressure sores, Irvine, Calif, 1987.
11. Jones PL, Millman A: Wound healing and the aged patient, *Nurs Clin North Am* 25(1):263-277, 1990.
12. Kaminski JV, Pinchcofsky-Devin G, and Williams SD: Nutritional management of decubiti ulcers in the elderly, *Decubitus* 2(4):20-30, 1989.
13. Kemp MG and others: Factors that contribute to pressure sores in surgical patients, *Res Nurs Health* 13:293-301, 1990.
14. Krasner D: The physiology of wound healing: an overview. In Krasner D, editor: *Chronic wound care,* King of Prussia, Penn, 1990, Health Management Publications.
15. Maklebust J: Pressure ulcers: etiology and prevention, *Nurs Clin North Am* 22(2):359-378, 1987.
16. McMullen D: Candida albicans and incontinence, *Derm Nurs* 3(1):21-24, 1991.
17. Peiper B and others: Visceral protein nutritional assessment of patients placed on the high or low air-loss bed, *J Enterostom Ther* 17(4):145-149, 1990.

18. Rodeheaver GT: Controversies in topical wound management: wound cleansing and wound disinfection. In Krasner D, editor, *Chronic wound care,* King of Prussia, Penn, 1990, Health Management Publications.

19. Rosenberg CS: Wound healing in the patient with diabetes mellitus, *Nurs Clin North Am* 25(1):247-261, 1990.

20. Sieggreen MY: Healing of physical wounds, *Nurs Clin North Am* 25(1):439-447, 1987.

21. Strohl RA: Radiation skin reactions. *Progressions: Developments in ostomy and wound care,* 1(3):3-12, 1988.

22. Windsor JA, Knight GS, and Hill GL: Wound healing response in surgical patients: recent food intake is more important than nutritional status, *Br J Surg* 75:135-137, 1988.

23. Wroblewski JJ: The nutritional aspects of pressure ulcer care. In Krasner D, editor: *Chronic wound care,* King of Prussia, Penn, 1990, Health Management Publications.

II

High Risk for Altered Body Temperature

Ineffective Thermoregulation

Hyperthermia

Hypothermia

High Risk for Altered Body Temperature is the state in which an individual is more vulnerable to develop failure to maintain temperature within normal range.[5,6]

Ineffective Thermoregulation is the state in which an individual's temperature fluctuates between hypothermia and hyperthermia.[18]

Hyperthermia is the state in which an individual's temperature is elevated above his or her normal range.[18]

Hypothermia is the state in which an individual's temperature is reduced below his or her normal range.[18]

OVERVIEW

The human body is constantly producing and releasing heat. Human beings are homeotherms (warmblooded animals) who are usually able to regulate their body temperature within the relatively narrow range of 97° F to 99.5° F (36° C to 37.5° C) with rectal values 1° F or .6° C higher.[16] Most healthy adults can tolerate extremes of ambient (environmental) temperature for short periods without untoward effects because of the body's beautifully designed control system. This remarkable adaptability may lead healthy persons to feel a false sense of invulnerability and complacency in the face of possible threats to health.

Not all parts of the body have the same temperature. The core body temperature or the internal trunk temperature, generally measured by a rectal thermometer or more recently by the tympanic temperature probe,[14] is usually higher than that of the extremities or body surface temperature, usually measured by an oral or axillary thermometer. Tympanic temperatures are an accurate reflection of core body temperatures and can be measured by an infrared thermometer, which has a short otoscope-type tip. This instrument is easy to use, comfortable for patients, and relatively noninvasive, and takes only 1 to 2 seconds to register.[14] It also utilizes a more accessible site than the rectal area. A drawback of tympanic thermometers is that they are relatively expensive compared with most other thermometers.

Oral temperatures are still the most commonly used readings and are generally satisfactory for most purposes. However, oral temperatures can be lowered by tachypnea (rapid breathing)[12] and after drinking ice water or cold drinks, especially in older patients.[33] These lower surface temperatures do not reflect true body temperatures. Patients with tachypnea may actually have a fever and should have their temperature measured rectally or tympanically. Oral temperature readings should be delayed after cold drinks for at least 15 minutes for persons under 40 years of age; 20 minutes for those 40 to 59 years old, and 30 minutes for persons 60 years and older.[33]

Body temperatures fluctuate in response to activity, environmental temperature changes, and as part of the circadian rhythms of the body, which are the daily 24-hour patterns in some physiological functions.[15,32] Recent studies have focused on the relationship of circadian rhythms to body temperature in the elderly,[10,22,28] the very young,[35] and head-injured patients.[21] This research is adding to knowledge of developmental differences and patient responses to illness and providing a basis for timing of nursing interventions. A general finding regarding the temperature circadian rhythm is that it peaks in the late afternoon or early evening and has a low level in the middle of the night or very early morning. Women tend to have a rise in temperature before ovulation and have wider fluctuations related to the menstrual cycle.[32]

The hypothalamus mediates temperature control through secretion of the TSH-RH (thyroid stimulating hormone-releasing hormone), which initiates a series of actions resulting in heat production and conservation of heat. The hypothalamus also reverses the process and shuts down the TSH-RH pathway, which stimulates heat loss mechanisms.[32] The hypothalamus can be described as a thermostat that sets the body temperature at a certain point and maintains it there. The hypothalamus senses body temperature through its central thermoreceptors and through peripheral receptors in the skin.[34]

Temperature regulation is primarily accomplished through three physiologic mechanisms: *heat production, heat loss, and heat conservation.* [31,32]

Heat production occurs as a result of chemical reactions of metabolism and thermogenesis and skeletal muscle contraction (increased muscle tone and shivering). The chemical reactions are related to maintenance of body metabolism and food metabolism.

Heat loss is accomplished by involuntary physiologic processes of radiation, conduction, convection, evaporation, and adaptation to a warmer climate and by voluntary measures.[31,32,37] *Radiation* loss is through electromagnetic waves coming off a skin surface that is warmer than the surrounding air. *Conduction* is loss by direct molecule transfer to a cooler molecular surface such as water or air. *Convection* is the transfer of heat by currents of liquids or gases. It is the process of exchange by which warmer air of the skin surface is exchanged for the cooler surrounding air. *Evaporation* of heat takes place when body water is lost from the surface of the skin and mucous membrane. The heat is lost in the process of converting body water to gas. Sweating is a major source of heat loss by evaporation.

In addition to these major heat loss mechanisms, a physical adaptation occurs as the body adjusts to a warmer climate over a period of time of about 1 to 6 weeks.[16] At first there is a feeling of weakness and fatigue, which gradually changes as the body gets accustomed to the warmer temperature. Then the person experiences earlier and increased sweating. The heart rate is decreased, slowing the production of heat, and the extracellular and plasma volumes are increased, providing more fluid for evaporation heat loss. The loss of salt in urine and sweat diminishes. The person begins to feel more energy and is able to resume usual activity as the adjustment phase to warm weather is completed.[24] Voluntary measures are those actions that people take in response to increased body temperature, such as slowing down, wearing cooler clothing, and stretching out to increase the body surface area for heat loss.

Heat conservation is achieved through involuntary vasoconstriction at the periphery of the body and voluntary actions of the individual to over-

II

come lower body temperature. Peripheral vasoconstriction helps move blood away from the body surface, where heat can be lost, to the body core. Voluntary behaviors are: adding more clothing, increasing activity to generate more heat, and sometimes curling up in a ball to reduce the surface area for heat loss.

Some developmental differences at both extremes of the life cycle increase the risk for Altered Body Temperature. Infants and the elderly need careful monitoring for body temperature maintenance.[32] Infants are able to produce adequate heat but are predisposed to poor heat conservation and excessive heat loss because of the newborn's relatively large skin surface area compared with body weight and because of the thin subcutaneous fat layer.[3,37] Newborns also have difficulty in getting rid of heat when they are in an overheated environment. Heat loss mechanisms are not as well developed as in the older child or adult.

Heat production in the elderly, on the other hand, is decreased because of slowed metabolic processes and circulation and difficulties in heat conservation caused by diminished responses to environmental temperatures, such as lessened sweating, decreased perception of temperature changes, and desynchronization of circadian rhythms.[1,20,23,28] It takes an elderly person, 70 years or older, nearly twice the time to return to normal core body temperature after exposure to extremes of heat and cold as it does a younger person, and this reaction becomes more pronounced with increasing age.[13] Elderly persons are also at greater risk for adverse effects of heat exposure because of diminished awareness of temperature changes and decreased sensation of thirst, as well as slowed vasomotor responses.[25,29]

Acute and chronic illnesses, surgical procedures,[17] medications, and anesthesia often play a role in increasing the risk for Altered Body Temperature. Some cultural and socioeconomic considerations that may affect a person's capability to maintain a normal body temperature are an adequate diet, exercise, appropriate seasonal clothing, and access to indoor heating and air conditioning. Income, social support, and knowledge of a healthy lifestyle are important components as well, particularly for those segments of the population at greatest risk. A high index of alertness on the part of family and professional caregivers can often make the difference in preventing those at risk from developing thermoregulatory disorders.

Fever or pyrexia is a special case of temperature change in which the set point for body temperature has been elevated, usually in response to a pathological process such as a viral or bacterial infection that produces pyrogens (fever-producing substances). Fever is not necessarily the result of a failure of the body's temperature regulation but more a matter of marshaling the body's defenses by resetting the thermostat at a higher level. Fever can be beneficial to the body by aiding responses to infectious processes.[24] Just raising body temperature may kill many microorganisms and retard the growth and replication of others.[32] Some current therapeutic protocols recommend a watchful monitoring of an elevated temperature in an individual and withholding the administration of antipyretics early on to give the body's defenses a chance to work.[32,37] This approach is reminiscent of the premodern era of treatment when caregivers waited for the fever to "break," signaling the onset of recovery. However, fever can be a serious complication in some patients such as neurosurgical patients, and it is important to determine the cause and initiate prompt appropriate treatment.[9]

Ineffective Thermoregulation

Ineffective Thermoregulation is the state in which there are unstable fluctuations above and below the normal range of body temperature, going between hyperthermia and hypothermia. It tends to occur in premature or newborn infants, in whom the usual temperature control mechanisms are not yet developed, or in very frail elderly individuals, in whom the usual temperature control mechanisms are no longer functioning adequately as a result of degeneration or disease, in response to fluctuations in the environmental temperature. Toxic agents, trauma, tumors, infection, or vascular disease can impair the hypothalamus temperature-control center, which may result in an unstable body temperature condition in which the temperature shifts above and below normal. In addition to noxious agents directly affecting the hypothalamus, abnormal conditions can affect the skin, peripheral nerves, and the autonomic nervous system responses, causing Ineffective Thermoregulation. Although the body has a marvelous adaptability to changes in the environment, including temperature changes, prolonged exposure to temperature extremes can eventually overwhelm the normal control mechanisms.[34]

Hyperthermia

Hyperthermia is the state in which an individual's body temperature is elevated above his or her normal range. Schoessler and others defined *Hyperthermia* as "marked warming of the core temperature."[32] *Hyperpyrexia* is the state when the body temperature reaches a very high elevation. Effects of severe Hyperthermia are coagulation of cell proteins, nerve damage, and death. In the adult, temperatures of 106° F (41° C) produce convulsions, and temperatures of 109° F (43° C) result in death.[32]

Internal causes of Hyperthermia may be located in the hypothalamus itself, such as lesions of the anterior hypothalamus. Alternatively, internal causes may be disorders in the heat-producing mechanisms, such as thyrotoxicosis, or in the heat-loss process, such as circulatory impairment or decrease in sweat production.

A rare inherited disorder that is potentially life threatening is malignant hyperthermia. It is triggered by the use of anesthetic agents and muscle relaxants used with anesthesia. It causes a defect in calcium metabolism that manifests itself by increased muscle contraction, rigidity, increased oxygen consumption, and increased heat production with temperatures that can go as high as 115° F (46° C).[34] If uncontrolled, malignant hyperthermia causes renal failure, neurological damage, heart failure, and disseminated intravascular coagulation (DIC).[26]

Hyperthermia can also be related to exposure to external environmental heat. Three general reactions occur with this type of exposure: heat cramps, heat exhaustion, and heatstroke or sunstroke.[26,32]

Heat cramps and heat exhaustion are conditions usually caused by excessive physical activity or exercise in hot weather. Heat cramps are muscle pains in the extremities or abdomen brought on by sodium chloride depletion as a result of prolonged sweating. Heat exhaustion is more severe than heat cramps. It involves vasomotor collapse with weakness, faintness, headache, and perhaps nausea and vomiting.

Heat cramps and heat exhaustion are treated with fluids containing sodium chloride, rest, and, in the case of emergency heat exhaustion, treatment for shock and transport to to a medical facility for follow-up care. Heat cramps and heat exhaustion can be prevented by using caution regarding vigorous activity in hot weather, attending to adequate fluid intake, and reducing exposure to external heat, especially during peak hours.

Heatstroke is a serious condition that requires emergency treatment. It is associated with retention of excessive body heat. The central temperature control fails to regulate perspiration. Heatstroke is potentially lethal if not reversed quickly. Some associated factors, in addition to exposure to external heat, are cardiovascular disease, alcoholism, obesity, old age, and prior febrile illness.[26] Heatstroke can affect young healthy adults who exercise too vigorously in extremely hot weather. Children are more susceptible than adults to heatstroke because they generate more heat during activity and have less sweating capacity.[32]

Manifestations of heatstroke are hot, dry, flushed skin, dizziness, faintness, confusion, and eventual loss of consciousness. If not treated, the heatstroke victim will die, but with prompt adequate treatment most people recover without ill effects. Treatment consists of cooling by a variety of methods, from an air-cooled room, to wrapping in a cold sheet, to a cooling blanket. Care

II

includes monitoring the cooling process to ensure that a reflex peripheral vasoconstriction does not occur, which will prevent cooling of the body core.[34] The heatstroke victim should not shiver because it raises the temperature. Sometimes the person's temperature control center is permanently damaged, increasing the risk for future episodes of Hyperthermia.

Researchers have linked hemorrhagic shock and encephalopathy to hyperpyrexia in infants and small children.[7,8,11] Infections in children have had a long and well-known association with hyperpyrexia,[2] which in most cases is a completely reversible, non–life-threatening condition.

Hypothermia

Hypothermia is the state in which an individual's body temperature is reduced below his or her normal range. Schoessler and others define Hypothermia as "marked cooling of core temperature."[32] Hypothermia can be accidental or therapeutic. Therapeutic hypothermia is sometimes used during surgery or limb reimplantation to preserve ischemic tissue.[32]

Severe uncontrolled cooling produces vasoconstriction, microcirculatory changes, coagulation, and ischemic tissue damage. *Accidental hypothermia,* a temperature below 95° F (35° C), is usually the result of prolonged exposure to cold environments, such as winter weather or a sudden immersion in a body of cold water. Hypothermia caused by cold water exposure is much more dramatic because water thermal conductivity is 32 times that of air.[34]

Lesions of the posterior hypothalamus can cause a Hypothermia that depends on the environmental temperature. Acute illnesses such as congestive heart failure, uremia, diabetes mellitus, drug overdosage, and acute respiratory failure can result in acute thermoregulatory failure and Hypothermia. Other conditions contributing to a predisposition to Hypothermia are myxedema, cerebrovascular disease, liver disease, Addison's disease, and alcohol ingestion. Unintended Hypothermia can occur with failure to recognize some patient's vulnerability to developing Hypothermia. Studies

of body temperature in surgical patients have identified the elderly as most susceptible to Hypothermia[17] and have demonstrated that not providing extra covering during and after surgery has a significant lowering effect on body temperature in older patients.[38]

Manifestations of Hypothermia are sleepiness, hypotension, cool or cold pale skin, and decreased level of consciousness. Ventricular dysrhythmias and apnea followed by cardiac arrest occur as the Hypothermia deepens. The focus of Treatment is on preventing further progression of the Hypothermia, rewarming, and advanced life-support measures. It is important to proceed gradually with rewarming because complications of acidosis, rewarming shock, dysrhythmia, and deepened Hypothermia may result if the body does not adjust to the rewarming process fairly quickly.[32] Rewarming therapy is controversial and methods vary from passive to active techniques, including invasive procedures.[39] Passive techniques include placing the person in a warm room and wrapping him/her in a blanket. Active techniques include the following: electric blanket, warm objects, warm bath, heated humidified inhalation, intragastric balloon, warm colonic irrigation, peritoneal dialysis or hemodialysis, and extracorporeal blood rewarming (heart/lung bypass). As was true of the other temperature disorders, the elderly and the very young are especially prone to Hypothermia because of altered thermoregulatory mechanisms.

• • •

The four nursing diagnoses related to body temperature are classified as part of the human response pattern labeled *exchanging* by NANDA; these diagnoses involve the process of mutual giving and receiving.[6]

To summarize the preceding discussion, the human temperature response is primarily, if not entirely, in the realm of a physiological reaction of metabolism. It is the giving or receiving of heat by the human body to maintain a stable internal environment that supports vital functions. This continuous process occurs in a variety of ways—

heat is produced as a result of body metabolism, and the amount of heat is regulated by the rate of metabolism. Heat is lost through conduction, convection, radiation, and evaporation. These physiological activities are modified in human beings by functional health patterns, etiologies, related factors, and risk factors. The related factors can be grouped under seven categories: age or developmental stage, weight, exposure to extremes of temperature, activity or exercise, disease and trauma, drugs and/or alcohol, and socioeconomic status. A more detailed discussion of these categories and functional health patterns is provided under Assessment.

ASSESSMENT

Assessing the person for temperature disorders includes identifying the defining characteristics and the related (or risk) factors of the diagnosis through the collection and analysis of subjective and objective data. Subjective data include information gathered from the individual's report of his/her condition through careful interviewing and history taking.

The Functional Health Patterns provide a framework for organizing the subjective data obtained from the patient and/or family during the interview process. Of the 11 functional health patterns, eight have particular relevance for the patient with thermoregulatory problems and would form the basis for a focused interview. They are: Health Perception-Health Management; Nutritional and Metabolic; Activity-Exercise; Cognitive-Perceptual; Self-Perception-Self-Concept; Role-Relationships; Coping-Stress Tolerance; and Value-Belief.

The Health Perception-Health Management pattern is concerned with the person's knowledge and behavior regarding present and past state of health. Assessment of this pattern provides information about acute and chronic conditions that could affect body temperature regulation, previous history of thermoregulatory alterations, use of medications, previous surgery, and other relevant treatments. The nurse assesses health practices, such as avoidance of prolonged exposure to tem-

perature extremes, protective clothing, appropriate heating and cooling systems, and other environmental aspects, to identify specific risk factors for problems with body temperature control. Knowledge of age or developmental aspects related to temperature maintenance would be part of a person's health perception and management.

The Nutritional and Metabolic pattern includes history of weight loss or gain, adequacy of diet, and fluid intake, especially during winter and summer months. The nurse assesses factors that influence nutrition and metabolism, such as skin and oral mucous membrane integrity, ability to obtain and prepare food, and knowledge of a balanced diet. Intake of drugs and alcohol receives special emphasis because these substances can interfere with both nutrition and body temperature. The usual range or average body temperature should be obtained if known.

The Activity-Exercise pattern has an immediate bearing on body temperature regulation. Too much or too little exercise affects the production of body heat. This pattern is especially important when assessing children, who generate more heat during activity, and older people, who tend to produce less heat and are also prone to be less active.[32] The Activity-Exercise pattern is especially important during months of extreme changes in environmental temperature. The nurse must determine physical conditions that inhibit optimum activity, such as chronic respiratory, circulatory, or orthopedic conditions or changes in mental status with a corresponding decrease in alertness.

The Cognitive-Perceptual pattern focuses on the sensory functions of vision, hearing, smell, taste, touch, pain perception, proprioception, and especially temperature sensation. Usually if perception of light touch is present, temperature sensation is intact.[3] The Cognitive-Perceptual pattern also includes the intellectual functions of judgment, memory, attention, and decision-making regarding health behaviors and environmental safety. The nurse should assess knowledge of specific risks, such as hypothermia and hyperthermia, related to environmental temperature changes and knowledge of increased vulnerability

II

resulting from acute and chronic conditions, medications, and alcohol intake.

The Self Perception-Self-Concept pattern offers clues to the competency of the person or family to manage personal life situations. Information about body image, sense of control over conditions, energy levels, moods, and concerns with perceived or real threats to health and well-being can be obtained by assessing this pattern. Young healthy individuals may not see themselves as vulnerable to temperature regulatory problems and take undue risks, such as prolonged exposure to the elements without adequate protection.

The Role-Relationship pattern has an important bearing on resources for prevention as well as early detection, of temperature control disorders. Physiologically the very young and the very old are the most vulnerable members of the population for thermoregulatory alterations. These persons also tend to have more passive roles in society and depend more on others for assistance in meeting their needs for daily living and for socioeconomic support. Hence they are doubly at risk. Adequate food, clothing, and shelter may be at least partially provided by others. Therefore, assessing relationships is an important part of data collection. Mental alertness is diminished in temperature alterations, and the frequent presence of others, who may pick up the early signs of trouble, may be a vital element in survival.

The Coping-Stress Tolerance pattern includes information about current and past stressors and the person's or family's adaptation. Of specific interest are major life events such as loss of significant others, physical or psychological illness or trauma, and moving or relocation. Socioeconomic conditions resulting in lower financial resources and a lower standard of living are quite important in increasing risk in vulnerable people. Elderly persons have been known to lower heat in winter and avoid turning on air conditioning in the summer to save on costs. Some older people may curtail necessary food and clothing because of a lack of funds. Families with small children on reduced incomes are also at risk as they try to keep down expenses. Information about past experiences with similar stress and successful adaptation methods is helpful in assessing current status and resources and in identifying the internal and external factors, risks, and etiology in temperature disorders.

Value-Belief pattern assessment gives an indication of the overall importance, or value, the person or family places on life, health, and well-being and cultural factors that may affect these values. This pattern helps to determine what efforts people are willing to expend to preserve and maintain health and to prevent illness. If a person has a fatalistic attitude about illness or injury or believes that health is not under personal control, it may be difficult to obtain the person's involvement in overcoming risk factors. Information on this pattern can provide knowledge about acceptable resources outside the immediate family unit for physical, as well as spiritual, assistance. Church, religious and civic groups, and community associations are important sources of support for many people. Sometimes the church visitor may be the only contact for a homebound elderly person.

Objective data are facts that the nurse gathers using techniques that do not require cognitive input from the individual, such as physical assessment techniques, laboratory data, and observation of environment. Appropriate, thorough, accurate methods of assessment, as well as adequate background knowledge of physiology, developmental changes, and associated disease or environmental conditions, are essential for correct diagnoses, effective planning, and successful outcomes when caring for people with temperature disorders.

Defining characteristics of three of the body temperature diagnoses can be grouped according to regulatory changes and cognitive changes. High Risk for Altered Body Temperature is not included because it is a potential alteration and the characteristics are not actually present. Regulatory changes identified in Ineffective Thermoregulation are unstable fluctuations above and below the normal range of body temperature, usually occurring in premature or newborn infants or very frail elderly persons in response to fluctua-

II

tions in environmental temperature. Cognitive changes can range from mild drowsiness or listlessness to confusion, disorientation, seizures, and coma, depending on the amount of deviation from normal and the general health of the individual.

Regulatory changes in Hyperthermia are elevated body temperature greater than 99.5° F (37.5° C) orally or 100.5° F (38° C) rectally, warm flushed skin, complaints of generalized or specific aches, and increased heart and respiratory rates. If the temperature remains very high (over 106° F or 41° C) or rises very rapidly, cerebral irritation occurs in some individuals. The nurse may observe cognitive changes in persons with hyperthermia, including restlessness, headache, drowsiness, confusion, and seizures or convulsions.[3,4]

The person with Hypothermia manifests regulatory changes in the same body systems as the person with Hyperthermia. The body temperature is reduced below 97° F (36° C) orally or 98° F (36.6° C) rectally. Other signs are cool skin with pallor; blanching or redness; loss of appetite; decreased sensation of cold; decreased blood pressure, heart, and respiratory rates; and shivering. Cognitive changes are slurred speech, confusion, drowsiness, restlessness, and possible coma.

Assessment of temperature disorders includes a careful investigation of possible related or risk factors. Seven generally accepted areas of risk factors are addressed here.[4,18,31]

Age. Temperature variations are of particular concern for those at either end of the age continuum.[31,32] The very young have immature thermal control mechanisms not yet ready to deal with extremes of temperature. Sweat glands are underdeveloped, and there is less subcutaneous fat, poor vasomotor control, greater heat loss through convection and radiation as a result of a large skin surface compared with body weight and in infants, a lower metabolic rate.[37] Older adults are also at greater risk for thermoregulatory problems.[1,23] Complex, multifactorial changes occur in the elderly that influence temperature maintenance. Many of the same mechanisms influencing temperature instability in the very young are also operative in the very old, but for different reasons. The elderly have lost some of their ability to respond to temperature change. Sweat glands have atrophied, blood vessels are less elastic and do not dilate and constrict as readily, and the metabolic rate is generally lowered among the elderly. The low metabolic rate results partially from a decrease in physical activity and a resultant decrease in heat production.[32]

Weight. Persons who are more than 20% underweight or overweight are more prone to alterations in body temperature. In general those who are overweight may be at risk for hyperthermia because of excess fat, which inhibits release of heat. Those who are underweight are at risk for hypothermia because of decreased body insulation and lower metabolism.

Exposure to Extremes of Temperature. Short-term exposure to moderate changes of external or ambient temperature is generally of little consequence to the healthy person. Prolonged exposure to extremes of environmental temperature can severely tax the body's thermoregulatory mechanisms and leave a person permanently at higher risk for ineffective thermoregulation.[27] Exposure to temperature extremes can also aggravate existing pathological conditions. Wearing of inadequate protective clothing and failure to take measures to limit exposure in extremely hot or cold environments greatly increase the risk of adverse effects of exposure.

Activity or Exercise. Activity tends to increase body temperature. Vigorous exercise such as jogging during hot weather or excessive activity in a person with a fever can increase the body temperature to a dangerous level and cause dehydration. For an elderly person, too little activity or exercise in an environmental temperature that is cold, cool, or even normal can result in below-normal body temperatures.

Disease and Trauma. The presence of acute or chronic disease or injury increases the risk of both hyperthermia and hypothermia. Also, exposure to thermal stress can exacerbate preexisting pathological conditions.[27] Persons with hypertension, cardiovascular disease, respiratory and nervous disorders, thyroid imbalances, autoimmune conditions, and mental conditions are especially vulnerable. Infections are a frequent cause of increased body temperature.

Major trauma can have an effect on temperature regulation. Serious central nervous system injury usually causes a sustained temperature elevation (central hyperthermia), which is difficult to treat. Other types of trauma, such as accidental injury, hemorrhage, thermal burns, and major surgery, can cause hypothermia because of damage to heat conservation systems, which results in excessive heat loss.[30,32]

Drugs and Alcohol. Certain medications, alcohol, and anesthetics can result in temperature regulation problems. Drug groups that contribute to hyperthermia or hypothermia are diuretics, anticholinergics, phenothiazines, antihypertensives, and antidepressants. Many of these drugs cause vasomotor and neurological changes, altered metabolic rates, sedation, and decreased alertness, thereby compromising the body's ability to adapt to environmental temperature variations. Elderly persons often take one or more of these medications.[29,39]

Socioeconomic Status. Low socioeconomic status is a common feature among patients with temperature disorders, especially the elderly.[29] A large number of elderly persons are living at or near the poverty level; they may live in substandard conditions and attempt to conserve limited resources by cutting down on food, heat, and clothing. A number of older people also live alone and may be unaware that they are at greater risk when environmental temperatures are extreme, and therefore they do not take adequate precautions. They are also less likely to be alert to symptoms of impending temperature disorders because of sensory deficits.

Collection of data for assessment of individuals with body temperature disorders is done primarily by interview and physical assessment, plus observation of environmental factors. Measurement of body temperature is obviously of particular importance. Measurement of the core temperature of the body is necessary because the surface or skin temperature is not a good indicator of vital processes. The surface is where heat exchange occurs between the body and environment, but heat production occurs at the core, deep within the body.[3,16,32] Because taking a temperature is such a common practice and is a relatively easy procedure to learn, its importance may not always be recognized.[19] Body temperature is called a vital or cardinal body sign because abnormal temperatures reflect abnormalities within the body. These variations can range from minor temporary disorders, such as a slight respiratory infection, to a serious, life-threatening condition, such as heat stroke or accidental hypothermia.

The two instruments commonly used to measure body temperature are the glass mercury bulb thermometer and the electronic thermometer. Most hospitals and institutions use electronic thermometers because they register more quickly. Glass thermometers are still more commonly used at home, because they are less expensive and do not require special maintenance. Another type of thermometer, sometimes used in ambulatory care departments because it is rapid (45 seconds) and convenient, is the disposable chemical strip thermometer, which is used orally or placed on the forehead or other highly vascular skin surface of the body. Accuracy of this type of thermometer has not yet been well documented.

There are three body sites commonly used for temperature measurement: the oral, rectal, and axillary sites. Although many health professionals consider the rectal route the most accurate, others disagree that this is the preferred method.[19] It is considered to be the most uncomfortable method and can be the most dangerous if not properly done. Complications have occurred as a result of rectal thermometers breaking, being retained or perforating the rectum in infants or neonates.[37] Oral temperatures can also be dangerous for children under 5 years of age and persons who are confused. The oral route is still the preferred method for older children and most adults. The accuracy of the oral route is in question for people who have respiratory problems or are mouth breathers. A recent study found that rapid respirations (tachypnea) affect the accuracy of oral temperature estimation, especially when electronic thermometers are used.[12] Axillary temperatures are recommended for most children under 5 years of age; the readings are accurate enough for most purposes if the temperature is taken properly. The normal temperature varies slightly, depending on the body site used. The normal range for oral temperature is 97.6° to 99.0° F (36.5° to 37.5° C), for rectal is 98.6° to 100.4° F (37.0° to 38.0° C), and for axillary is 96.6° to 98.4° F).(36.0° to 37.0° C). Consult basic nursing texts for detailed procedures on methods of temperature measurement.[36]

The tympanic membrane of the ear is the newest site for body temperature measurement, and this technique seems to be the most accurate noninvasive measurement of core body temperature. It is still relatively expensive, however, because it requires a special instrument and is not yet in general use.[14] For most purposes the three common sites of oral, rectal, and axillary are quite adequate.

In addition to temperature variations that result from the method of measurement and accuracy of the instrument, normal variations relate to age, room temperature, time of day, and activity.[36] Children's temperatures normally run 1° F higher than adults. Sleep and work patterns cause some variation, with the lowest temperature at night and the highest in late afternoon or early evening. Activity increases heat production and body temperature.

HIGH RISK FOR ALTERED BODY TEMPERATURE
❖ Risk Factors

The presence of the following conditions renders the patient more vulnerable to High Risk for Altered Body Temperature:

- Extremes of age
- Exposure to extremes of environmental temperature
- Inactivity or excessive exercise
- Presence of acute/chronic diseases affecting body temperature
- Dehydration
- Intake of medications/alcohol
- Trauma
- Extremes of weight
- Inadequate environmental protection (inappropriate clothing, deficient home heating/cooling)
- Decrease in mental alertness/confusion
- Low socioeconomic status
- Living alone
- Lack of social support

❖ Related Medical/Psychiatric Diagnoses

The following are examples of related medical/psychiatric diagnoses for High Risk for Altered Body Temperature[26,32,34]:

- Accidental hypothermia
- Acute illness (infections)
- Burns
- Central nervous system trauma
- Chronic illness (cardiovascular disorders)
- Dehydration
- Hemorrhagic shock
- Major body trauma
- Malignant hyperthermia
- Malnutrition (underweight, overweight)
- Prematurity

INEFFECTIVE THERMOREGULATION
❖ Defining Characteristics

The presence of the following defining characteristics indicates that the patient may be experiencing ineffective thermoregulation:

- Fluctuations in body temperature above and below the normal range. Also see defining characteristics for Hyperthermia and Hypothermia.

❖ Related Factors

The following related factors are associated with Ineffective Thermoregulation:

- Developmental immaturity: premature or newborn infant
- Previous episode of Hyperthermia/Hypothermia
- Frail elderly
- Fluctuating environmental temperatures
- Disease/illness/trauma affecting temperature regulation (e.g., spinal cord disorder, burns)
- Exposure to toxic agents

• Lack of knowledge or inability to provide adequate protection from changing temperatures

❖ **Related Medical/Psychiatric Diagnoses**

The following are examples of related medical/psychiatric diagnoses for Ineffective Thermoregulation:[26,32,34]

• Exposure to extreme cold or hot environment
• Hypothalamic damage caused by: toxic agent, trauma, tumor, infection, vascular disease

• Peripheral neuropathy
• Skin disorder
• Spinal cord disorder

HYPERTHERMIA

❖ **Defining Characteristics**

The presence of the following defining characteristics indicates that the patient may be experiencing Hyperthermia:

• Increase in body temperature above the normal range
• Increased respiratory rate (tachypnea)
• Increased blood pressure
• Generalized or specific aches
• Drowsiness/restlessness/confusion

• Flushed, warm skin, diaphoresis early stages; hot and dry later
• Increased heart rate (tachycardia)
• Headache
• Muscle rigidity later
• Seizures/convulsions later

❖ **Related Factors**

The following related factors are associated with Hyperthermia:

• Extremes of age
• Inability or decreased ability to sweat
• Dehydration
• Inappropriate clothing

• Increased metabolic rate
• Disease/illness/trauma to CNS
• Medications/anesthetics
• Vigorous activity

• Inadequate intake of fluids

• Exposure to hot environment

❖ **Related Medical/Psychiatric Diagnoses**

The following are examples of related medical/psychiatric diagnoses for Hyperthermia:[26,32,34]

• Anterior hypothalamic lesions
• Decreased cardiac output
• Exposure to hot environment (heat cramps, heat exhaustion, heat stroke)

• Infection
• Malignant hyperthermia
• Thyrotoxicosis

HYPOTHERMIA

❖ **Defining Characteristics**

The presence of the following defining characteristics indicates that the patient may be experiencing Hypothermia:

• Decrease in body temperature below normal range
• Piloerection (goose bumps)
• Decreased heart rate
• Drowsiness/restlessness/confusion

• Cool, pale, blanched, or reddened skin
• Decreased respiratory rate
• Decreased blood pressure
• Coma, later

❖ **Related Factors**

The following related factors are associated with Hypothermia:

• Extremes of age
• Inability or decreased ability to shiver
• Malnutrition
• Alcohol intake
• Exposure to cold environment

• Decreased metabolic rate
• Disease/illness/trauma
• Medications/anesthetics
• Inactivity
• Inadequate clothing

❖ **Related Medical/Psychiatric Diagnoses**

The following are examples of related medical/psychiatric diagnoses for Hypothermia[26,32,34]:

• Acute respiratory failure

• Cerebrovascular disease

- Cirrhosis
- Congestive heart failure
- Diabetes mellitus
- Drug overdose
- Exposure to cold environment
- Myxedema
- Pancreatitis
- Pituitary insufficiency
- Posterior hypothalamic lesions
- Psychoactive substance use disorder (alcohol abuse)
- Spinal cord injury
- Uremia

NURSING DIAGNOSES

Examples of *specific* nursing diagnoses for High Risk for Altered Body Temperature are:

- High Risk for Altered Body Temperature related to prematurity
- High Risk for Altered Body Temperature related to advanced age and presence of neuropathy
- High Risk for Altered Body Temperature related to cerebrovascular disease
- High Risk for Altered Body Temperature related to spinal cord injury

Examples of *specific* nursing diagnoses for Ineffective Thermoregulation are:

- Ineffective Thermoregulation related to premature birth
- Ineffective Thermoregulation related to advanced age (over 90 yr) and presence of burns
- Ineffective Thermoregulation related to spinal cord injury
- Ineffective Thermoregulation related to advanced age and extensive abdominal surgery

Examples of *specific* nursing diagnoses for Hyperthermia are:

- Hyperthermia related to a genetic defect and anesthetic administration (Malignant Hyperthermia)
- Hyperthermia related to vigorous exercise and exposure to hot environment (playing tennis in 98° F weather for 4 hours)
- Hyperthermia in an elderly person related to dehydration from inadequate fluid intake and decreased ability to sweat
- Hyperthermia in an infant related to inappropriate clothing (sweater and heavy blanket wrap) in 90° F temperature

Examples of *specific* nursing diagnoses for Hypothermia are:

- Hypothermia related to alcohol intake and inadequate clothing during winter weather (for a homeless person)
- Hypothermia related to exposure to cold environment (for a child who fell through ice on a pond)
- Hypothermia related to diabetes mellitus and decreased heat in the living quarters during the winter (for an elderly person)
- Hypothermia related to prolonged surgery and a decreased metabolic rate (for a postsurgical patient)

PLANNING AND IMPLEMENTATION WITH RATIONALE

The overall goals for patients with body temperature abnormalities are to achieve and maintain a normal range of temperature before permanent damage occurs to vital organs such as the liver, heart, and central nervous system. The nurse must reduce the harmful effects of thermal variation by monitoring and maintaining the essential functions of regulation, circulation, respiration, nutrition, and fluid balance while providing comfort.[4,18,34]

HIGH RISK FOR ALTERED BODY TEMPERATURE

The nurse should collect data on persons at High risk for Altered Body Temperature to identify the status of the thermoregulatory system.[36] Close monitoring of vital functions is especially important during situations of specific risk such as dehydration, injury, infection, major surgery, or environmental exposure in vulnerable elderly, the very young, and those with compromised neurological or circulatory status.

The nurse should address, whenever possible, risk factors that can be prevented, reduced, or modified. A person may change or eliminate exposure to environmental extremes, dehydration, extremes of activity, and poor nutrition because of education and better use of support systems. The nurse and other care givers should maintain a

❖ NURSING CARE GUIDELINES: HIGH RISK FOR ALTERED BODY TEMPERATURE

Nursing diagnosis: High Risk for Altered Body Temperature related to advanced age and peripheral neuropathy.

Expected Patient Outcomes	Nursing Interventions[18,36]
The patient will maintain normal range of body temperature of 97° F (36° C) to 99.5° F (37.5° C) or normal range for patient.	• Monitor vital signs on a specified schedule. • Assess overall circulatory status: capillary refill, skin and mucous membrane color. • Assess peripheral neurological status and temperature sense. • Monitor fluids and food intake. • Adjust environmental temperature as needed. • Avoid exposure to drafts or overheated areas. • Schedule regular physical activity as permitted. • Provide adequate clothing based on environmental temperature.
The patient and/or significant others will identify risks associated with advanced age, neuropathy, and temperature control.	• Educate patient and significant others regarding risk factors associated with advanced age (changes in circulatory system and nervous system and increased susceptibility to temperature alterations) and methods to compensate for or reduce risks.

high index of alertness for vulnerable persons with one or more risk factors. The goal for the patient at High Risk for Altered Body Temperature is to maintain a normal range of body temperature.

Interventions are directed toward reduction or modification of risk factors wherever possible and close monitoring of vital signs and adequacy of circulation to detect and treat early signs of changes and thus avert adverse complications. Interventions include providing good fluid and nutritional support. The person must maintain an optimum activity level and avoid exposure to temperature extremes. *The nurse must carefully manage chronic and acute health problems to promote a stable physiological condition and reduce the risk of Ineffective Thermoregulation.*

INEFFECTIVE THERMOREGULATION

This diagnosis contains elements of both Hyperthermia and Hypothermia and focuses espe-

cially on the inability of the system to balance itself. The expected patient outcome for these patients is to achieve and maintain a normal, stable range of body temperature. The goal of the interventions is to control the fluctuations between hyperthermia and hypothermia. The nursing measures used as interventions are discussed in the following sections.

HYPERTHERMIA

Extreme variations in temperature are considered medical emergencies. In severe hyperthermia or heat stroke, where the temperature may be 105° F or above, the immediate goal is to reduce the core temperature to 102° F as rapidly as possible *to prevent damage to vital organs, especially the brain and nervous system,* [34] then to reestablish sweating and replace fluids. Nurses monitor the temperature continuously by rectal probe. A patient with severe hyperthermia or heat stroke would be admitted to the intensive care unit and the following temperature-reducing measures may be initiated.

❖ *NURSING CARE GUIDELINES: INEFFECTIVE THERMOREGULATION*

Nursing diagnosis: *Ineffective Thermoregulation in infant related to immature temperature control*[18,37]

Expected Patient Outcomes	**Nursing Interventions**
Achieve and maintain stable optimum range of body temperature for an infant, within 97.7° F (36.5° C) to 99.5° F (37.5° C).	• Initially, monitor vital signs and axillary temperature on a continuous schedule until stabilized, usually about 10 to 12 hours. • During cooling or rewarming procedures monitor axillary temperature and vital signs frequently but at least every 2 hr. • Adjust environmental temperature to infant's needs; may require preheated environment. • Keep infant away from drafts or vents. • Provide appropriate clothing, warmed blanket. • Uncover only one area of body for exam or procedure. • Administer fluids at room temperature. • Monitor skin temperature and relate it to ambient air temperature; decreased skin temperature may indicate radiant heat loss. • Monitor lab values for evidence of instability: BUN (elevated), serum Ph (acidosis), blood glucose (hypoglycemia), serum electrolytes (hyperkalemia). • Refer to nursing interventions specific to hyperthermia and hypothermia as infant's condition warrants.

• Immersing in an ice water bath, covering the patient with a wet sheet and ice chips, using a hypothermia blanket, or sponging continuously with cold water and directing a fan so that it blows on the patient, providing an air current for evaporation of heat.

• *Monitoring vital signs frequently and carefully, taking electrocardiogram (ECG), central venous pressure (CVP), and level of consciousness measures to determine vital organ functioning and watching for dysrhythmias and hypotension.*

• *Maintaining fluid balance initially through IV infusions to replace fluid loss and to maintain adequate circulation and urine output. Fluids must be given slowly to prevent heart and kidney damage resulting from over loading the circulatory system, especially in older patients.*

• *Administering oxygen to supply tissue needs*

because of increased metabolic rate and to prevent heart and respiratory failure. Mechanical ventilation may be necessary for the comatose patient *who is unable to breathe on his own.*

• *Monitoring fluid and electrolyte balance continuously to prevent acidosis, hypocalcemia, hypokalemia, and convulsions from developing by early detection and treatment.* Urinary output is measured frequently *to assess renal and circulatory function.*

Careful monitoring during cooling is very important because a sudden drop in temperature could cause dysrhythmias and circulatory collapse.[34] Antipyretics generally are contraindicated for heat illness.[32] These drugs work by resetting the thermoregulatory setpoint, but that is not the problem in this form of hyperthermia. *The setpoint is normal, but the organism just cannot cope with eliminating enough heat to maintain a normal temperature.*

II

❖ *NURSING CARE GUIDELINES: HYPERTHERMIA*

Nursing Diagnosis: *Hyperthermia related to exposure to a hot environment*[18,34]

Expected Patient Outcomes	Nursing Interventions
The patient will have no signs or symptoms of Hyperthermia: tachypnea, tachycardia, increased blood pressure, hot dry skin, headache, drowsiness, or confusion; temperature will be maintained between 97° F (36° C) and 99.5° F (37.5° C) orally or 98.6° F (37 C) and 100.4° F (38° C) rectally; and vital signs will be within normal limits for patient.	• Apply internal/external cooling measures as ordered: appropriate cold bath, hypothermia blanket, or other means. • Administer IV fluids as necessary. • Measure intake and output, report urine output below .5 ml/kg/hr. • Monitor vital signs continuously or at frequent intervals until stabilized at normal range. • Monitor laboratory studies: ABG, blood and urine tests. • Assess skin color and temperature. • Administer antipyretics if indicated.
The patient and/or significant other will identify factors related to development of Hyperthermia and ways to reduce or modify them.	• Educate patient and/or significant other on personal and environmental factors that can promote Hyperthermia and specific precautions regarding future exposure to extremely hot environment.

In less serious cases of hyperthermia (heat exhaustion or heat shock) the condition develops more slowly over a period of several days and is usually caused by dehydration with corresponding drop in blood volume. For these patients, more moderate treatment and replacement of fluids and electrolytes is indicated. *If treatment and care are initiated early enough, recovery is generally complete.* The elderly and persons exercising vigorously in hot weather are the most common victims.

After the acute phase is over, direct attention to reducing the risk of future episodes.[32,34] *Advise patients to avoid reexposure to high temperatures because they will be hypersensitive to heat for an extended period and in some cases permanently.*[32,34] Stress the importance of reducing ac-

tivity in hot weather, wearing loose comfortable clothing, and maintaining adequate fluid intake. Urge athletes to approach exercise cautiously and allow time for acclimatization.[16,32]

HYPOTHERMIA

Hypothermia can also be severe enough to require emergency care. When the body temperature drops below 91.4° F (31.3° C), vital functions can profoundly deteriorate. The nurse must continuously monitor, carefully rewarm, and give supportive care to the patient.

1. *Monitoring of vital signs is similar to that for hyperthermia, but special attention is given to ECG monitoring because the heart muscle is especially vulnerable to the effects of cold. Fluid balance, urinary output,*

❖ *NURSING CARE GUIDELINES: HYPOTHERMIA*

Nursing Diagnosis: *Hypothermia related to exposure to a cold environment*[18,34]

Expected Patient Outcomes	Nursing Interventions
The patient will have no signs or symptoms of hypothermia: confusion, slurred speech, drowsiness, hypotension, or cardiac dysrhythmias; temperature will be maintained between 97° F (36° C) and 99.5° F (37.5° C) orally or 98.6° F (37° C) and 100.4° F (38° C) rectally; vital signs will be within normal limits for the patient; laboratory values will be within normal limits; and peripheral circulation will be adequate.	• Rewarm body gradually by internal or external methods as appropriate and ordered for slow-onset hypothermia: blankets, warm atmosphere. • Rapid core rewarming done for abrupt-onset hypothermia: hyperthermia blanket, immersion in warm water, or rapid core warming with heated IV fluids, hemodialysis, peritoneal dialysis, gastric and colonic irrigations. • Monitor temperature continuously or every hour, generally with rectal probe until stable at normal range. • Measure vital signs every hour; continuous ECG monitoring; note dysrhythmias. • Maintain patent airway. • Monitor laboratory studies: ABG, serum electrolytes, BUN, glucose; note abnormalities. • Monitor urine every 2 hours for decreased output less than 1 ml/kg/hr. • Provide supportive measures of warm comfortable environment. • Use special care in gentle handling of body because of susceptibility of cold tissues to injury.
The patient and/or significant others will identify factors related to the development of hypothermia and ways to reduce or modify them.	• When physiological condition is stabilized, educate patient and significant others on precautions regarding exposure to extremely cold environments and factors that predispose to development of hypothermia, such as poor nutrition, acute and chronic illness, and inadequate heating systems and clothing. • Emphasize importance of previous episode of hypothermia predisposing to subsequent attacks and need to increase awareness.

blood gases, and blood chemistries are all important indicators of circulatory status, blood pressure, and the presence of hypoxemia and acidosis.

2. Rewarming should be done carefully until normal function returns. *As the body temperature rises, demand for oxygen increases, and cardiac output may not be adequate because of the weakened, cold heart muscle* in cases of chronic or slow develop-

ing Hypothermia. A thermal blanket may be used for external active warming. Internal core rewarming methods such as warm IV fluids, or nasogastric, peritoneal, and rectal warm lavages may also be used. *More rapid measures can be used with abrupt onset hypothermia because pathophysiological changes have not had time to develop.* [34]

3. *Supportive care may include intubation and heated oxygen, electrical defibrillation, and*

careful administration of cardiac drugs because of danger of the bolus effect when circulation returns to normal. Very careful handling is necessary to prevent cardiac dysrhythmias.

Patients who survive Hypothermia usually do not suffer permanent neurological deficits if the body temperature does not fall below 85° F (28.4° C).[16,36] Most thermometers do not register temperatures below 94° F (34.5.° C). When hypothermia is suspected, obtain special thermometers.

In mild cases of hypothermia; passive rewarming measures, such as removing the person's wet clothing and wrapping him or her in a dry blanket, will prevent further drops in temperature and conserve body heat, which will gradually rewarm the person. If the victim is awake and alert, warm fluids may be given, but avoid alcohol consumption. The common belief that alcohol warms is not based on fact. It causes peripheral vasodilation, increasing heat loss from the skin.

EVALUATION

Specific determination of patient outcomes involves ongoing observation and recording of interventions. The primary outcome in each diagnosis is the maintenance of a normal range of body temperature to prevent damage to vital organs, in particular the heart and brain. The normal range of body temperature for most adults is between 97° F and 99.5° F orally and 98.6° F and 100.4° F rectally.

If the body temperature is maintained, the major outcome for High Risk for Altered Body Temperature is achieved. Modifying or eliminating risk factors wherever possible and educating patients and caregivers to have a high degree of alertness for the onset of thermal alterations can enhance vulnerable persons' chances of averting future episodes of thermoregulatory failure and serious complications.

The primary concern in Ineffective Thermoregulation is related to the instability of the regulatory system. If stability within the normal range of temperature can be achieved and maintained, the desired outcome has been reached. In the case of the infant the instability is developmental and will be outgrown, but in the case of the elderly individual it will continue to require close monitoring and continued vigilance.

In severe Hyperthermia and Hypothermia, which are medical emergencies, evaluation of the outcome is done almost simultaneously with the intervention itself. If the outcomes are not being achieved fast enough, or if the patient's condition is deteriorating, more intensive efforts must be made. For instance, if the body temperature is not being lowered in a patient with hyperthermia, the nurse will take more aggressive or additional cooling measures. Continuous monitoring of the patient's physiological and mental status provides the evaluation data for immediate decisions about continuing current management or changing strategies. In critical situations involving life-threatening conditions, nurses and the physician jointly develop this plan. The major responsibility for development in the initial phase rests with the physician. The nurse may assume more responsibility for collecting, interpreting, and reporting clinical data.

After the critical, acute phase has passed and the patient is recovering, he or she should be involved in plans for prevention of recurrence. Expected outcomes to be evaluated at this stage include the patient's and significant other's expressed understanding of the related factors resulting in the temperature alteration and stated plans for maintaining a normal temperature range by avoiding or modifying risk factors.

❖ CASE STUDY WITH PLAN OF CARE

Mrs. Edna G., an 80-year-old widow who lives alone in a small town in upstate New York, arrives at 1 PM by ambulance at the emergency room of the local hospital in a drowsy, confused, disoriented state of consciousness. When her neighbor discovered her shortly after noon, Mrs. G. was lying on her kitchen floor in her nightgown. Her backdoor had been left open; the temperature was cold and wintry. Mrs. G. told her neighbor that she had gone to the door to look for her cat that morning about 9 AM and had become weak and dizzy, so she lay down on the kitchen floor and couldn't get up. The neighbor, noting Mrs. G.'s disorientation, confusion, and slurred speech, called the ambulance, which brought her to the hospital. Mrs. G's medical history includes hypertension treated with diuretics, arteriosclerosis, CHF, and progressive weight loss resulting from poor appetite. The physical findings include a temperature of 93° F rectally; blood pressure 90/60; pulse 45 beats/min, respirations 12/min and shallow; weight 90 pounds; height 5'2"; skin pale and cold with sporadic shivering; reflexes decreased; pupils sluggish and slightly constricted. Information about Mrs. G.'s dietary patterns was contributed by the neighbor because of Mrs. G's confused status. Mrs. G. does not eat much or buy much food. The neighbor takes Mrs. G. to the grocery store once a week, but Mrs. G. expresses concern about food prices and buys very little. Her refrigerator contained a pint of milk, a small can of juice, a bowl of soup, and some leftover vegetables that had spoiled. There was a box of cereal on the shelf and some crackers, but no other food in the house except cat food. Mrs. G. did not go shopping last week because she didn't feel well. Mrs. G. attends church services with a church member who picks her up on Sunday and brings her home. Otherwise she is alone at home, watches TV, and takes care of her cat. The house has become run down and has a cracked window, causing a draft in the kitchen. Mrs. G. doesn't have close family ties. Her husband died 20 years ago and they had no children. She has a niece who lives on the West coast whom she has not seen or heard from since her husband's death. Mrs. G. owns her own house and has a modest but adequate income for routine living expenses from her husband's social security, plus dividends from some utility stocks. Mrs. G. told her neighbor several weeks ago that she is afraid of becoming poor and "going on welfare." She tries to save money by keeping her heating bill down and conserving on food. Some of her clothes are threadbare, but she says she cannot afford new ones.

PLAN OF CARE FOR MRS. EDNA G.

Nursing Diagnosis: *Hypothermia related to cold temperature, cardiovascular disease, hypertension, and malnutrition*

Expected Patient Outcomes	Nursing Interventions
Mrs. G. will have no signs and symptoms of hypothermia in 3-4 hr; no confusion, drowsiness, hypotension, or bradycardia; normal reflexes: pupils react to light and accommodation is present.	• Slowly rewarm Mrs. G. by use of a thermal blanket to increase body temperature 1°-2°/hr. Observe level of consciousness and neurological status.
Mrs. G.'s temperature will be maintained between 98.6° and 100.4° F rectally in 3-4 hr.	• Monitor rectal temperature every hour until stable and within normal limits.
Mrs. G.'s vital signs (blood pressure, pulse, respirations) will be maintained within normal limits in 3-4 hr. No dysrhythmia will be present.	• Monitor vital signs every hour, with continuous ECG monitoring until blood pressure and pulse are within normal limits and stable.

Continued.

II

Expected Patient Outcomes	Nursing Interventions
Mrs. G.'s skin will be warm and pink.	• Support Mrs. G. in a warm, comfortable environment with room temperature at 70°-75° F.
Mrs. G. will return to normal daily activities without complications.	• Gradually increase activities; be gentle in moving and handling body parts.
Mrs. G. will express knowledge of related (risk) factors for development and recurrence of hypothermia: exposure to cold, inadequate clothing, presence of heart disease, inadequate nutrition, and inactivity.	• Discuss related/risk factors for development of hypothermia.
Mrs. G. will discuss a plan of prevention that includes the following: maintaining room temperature between 70° and 75° F; following a diet program with a goal of weight gain with an ideal body weight (IBW) of between 100 and 120 pounds; identifying warm clothing already owned and sources for additional clothing at reasonable cost (such as second-hand shops); describing simple, moderate exercises she can do 3-4 times a week (walking, going up and down stairs, exercise program at senior center); and discussing a schedule of potential daily contacts with neighbors and friends.	• Involve Mrs. G. in discharge and long-term planning regarding prevention of recurrence of hypothermia: contact utility company for senior citizen discount on heating bill; discuss plans for increasing food intake and weight gain; ask Mrs. G. about clothing for keeping warm; suggest exercise to stimulate metabolism; and discuss possible increase in social activities and more frequent contacts with neighbors and friends.

REFERENCES

1. Abrass IB: Disorders of temperature regulation. In Hazzard WR, Andres R, Bierman, EL and Blass JP (editors): *Principles of geriatric medicine and gerontology.* (ed 2) (pp. 1084-1088), New York, 1990, McGraw-Hill.
2. Alpert G, Hibbert E, and Fliesher GR: Case-control study of hyperpyrexia in children, *Pediatr Infect Dis J* 9:161-163, 1990 (From Oski FA, Stockman JA (editors): *The yearbook of pediatrics, 1991,* St Louis, 1991, Mosby–Year Book.)
3. Bates B: *A guide to physical examination and history taking* (ed 5), Philadelphia, 1991, JB Lippincott.
4. Carpenito LJ: *Nursing diagnosis and application to clinical practice* (ed 3), Philadelphia, 1989, JB Lippincott.
5. Carroll-Johnson RM (editor): *Classification of nursing diagnoses: proceedings of the Eighth Conference,* Philadelphia, 1989, JB Lippincott.
6. Carroll-Johnson RM (editor): *Classification of nursing diagnoses: proceedings of the Ninth Conference,* Philadelphia, 1991, JB Lippincott.
7. Chaves-Carballa E, Montes J, Nelson W, and Chrenka B: Hemorrhagic shock and encephalopathy, *Am J Dis Child* 144:1079-1082, 1990.
8. Corrigan J: The 'H' in hemorrhagic shock and encepha-

lopathy syndrome should be hyperpyrexia, *Am J Dis Child* 144:1077, 1990.

9. Cunha B, Tu R: Fever in the neurosurgical patient, *Heart Lung* 17(6):608-611, 1988.

10. Davis C, Lentz M: Circadian rhythms: charting oral temperatures to spot abnormalities, *J Gerontol Nurs* 15(4):34-39, 1989.

11. Dupee C: Hyperpyrexia, hemorrhagic shock and encephalopathy, and creatinine phosphokinase, *Am J Dis Child* 145:719, 1991.

12. Durham M, Swanson B, and Paulford P: Effect of tachypnea on oral temperature estimation, a replication, *Nurs Res* 35(4):211-214, 1986.

13. Ebersole P, Hess P: *Toward healthy aging: Human needs and nursing response* (ed 3), St Louis, 1990, CV Mosby.

14. Erickson R, Yount S: Comparison of tympanic and oral temperatures in surgical patients, *Nurs Res* 40(2):90-93, 1991..

15. Guiffre M and others: The relationship between axillary and core body temperature, *Appl Nurs Res* 3(2):52-55, 1990.

16. Guyton AC: *Textbook of medical physiology* (ed 8), Philadelphia, 1991, WB Saunders.

17. Heidenreich T, Guiffre M: Postoperative temperature measurement, *Nurs Res* 39(3):153-155, 1990.

18. Kim MJ, McFarland G, and McLane A: *Pocket guide to nursing diagnosis* (ed 4), St Louis, 1991, CV Mosby.

19. Kozier B, Erb G, and Oliveri R: *Fundamentals of nursing: concepts, process and practice*, California, 1991, Addison-Wesley.

20. Kramer M, Vandyke J, and Rosen A: Mortality in elderly patients with thermoregulatory failure, *Arch Intern Med* 144:1521-1523, 1989.

21. Lanuza D, Robinson C, Marotta S, and Patel M: Body temperature & heart rate rhythms in acutely head-injured patients, *Appl Nurs Res* 2(3):135-139, 1989.

22. Mason D: Circadian rhythms of body temperature and activation and well-being of older women, *Nurs Res* 37(5):276-281, 1988.

23. Matz R: Hypothermia: mechanisms and countermeasures, *Hosp Pract* 21(1):45-48, 54-58, 63-66, 68-71, 1986.

24. McCance K, Huether S: *Pathophysiology: the biologic basis for disease in adults and children*, St Louis, 1990, CV Mosby.

25. Miescher S, Fortney S: Responses to dehydration and rehydration during heat exposure in young and older men, *Am J Physiol* 257:R1050-R1056, 1989.

26. Phipps W, Long B, Woods N, and Cassmeyer V: *Medical-surgical nursing: concepts and clinical practice* (ed 4), St Louis, 1991, Mosby–Year Book.

27. Ramsey JM: *Basic pathophysiology: modern stress and the disease process*, Menlo Park, Calif, 1982, Addison-Wesley.

28. Richardson GV: Circadian rhythms and aging. In Schneider E, Rowe J (editors): *Handbook of the biology of aging* San Diego, 1990, Academic Press, pp. 275-295.

29. Robbins A: Hypothermia and heat stroke: protecting the elderly patient, Geriatrics 44(1):73-77, 80, 1989.

30. Roberts SL: *Nursing diagnosis and the critically ill patient*, Norwalk, Conn, 1987, Appleton & Lange.

31. Schauf C, Moffett D, and Moffett S: *Human physiology: foundations and frontiers*, St Louis, 1990, CV Mosby.

32. Schoessler M, Ludwig-Beymer P, and Huether S: Pain, temperature regulation, sleep and sensory function. In McCance KL, Huether SE, (editors): *Pathophysiology: the biologic basis for diseases in adults and children*, St Louis, 1990, CV Mosby.

33. Sugarek N: Temperature lowering after iced water: enhanced effects in the elderly, *J Am Geriatr Soc* 34:526-529, 1986.

34. Thelan LA, Davie JK, and Urden LD: *Textbook of critical care nursing; diagnosis and management*, St Louis, 1990, CV Mosby.

35. Thomas K: The emergence of body temperature biorhythm in preterm infants, *Nurs Res* 40(2):98-102, 1991.

36. Thompson J, and others: *Mosby's Manual of Clinical nursing*, St Louis, 1989, CV Mosby.

37. Whaley LF, Wong DF: (ed 2) *Essentials of pediatric nursing*, St Louis, 1989, CV Mosby.

38. White H, and others: Body temperature in elderly surgical patients, *Res Nurs Health* 10:317-321, 1987.

39. Wongsurawat N, Davis B, and Morley J: Thermoregulatory failure in the elderly, *J Am Geriatr Soc* 38(8):899-906, 1990.

II

Interrupted Breastfeeding

Interrupted Breastfeeding is a break in the continuity of the breastfeeding process as a result of the inability or inadvisability to put baby to breast for feeding[27]

OVERVIEW

More and more mothers wish to breast feed and consider it to be central to their relationship with their new baby. Certain conditions can lead to a temporary interruption in breastfeeding, however. Most common is the mother's return to work. Various maternal or neonatal conditions can also lead to an interruption in breastfeeding. To many, the solution is to advise the mother to discontinue nursing. In fact, some argue that efforts to continue breastfeeding may compromise the health of the mother or baby. This perspective ignores the natural aspects of the process and focuses, instead, on negative aspects of the situation. In most cases, the interruption need only be very brief, and breastfeeding can be successfully resumed in a short time. If the mother wishes to continue lactation, the professional nurse can provide information about ways to maintain lactation as well as how to store expressed milk so that it can be fed to the baby until breastfeeding can be resumed.[2,3,11,24]

ASSESSMENT

Given the major defining characteristic that breastfeeding is interrupted, several minor defining characteristics come into play. Basic is the mother's wish to maintain lactation so she can eventually breast feed her baby. As we know, the decision to breast feed, as well as the degree of commitment to maintaining it, is most often influenced by the attitudes and opinions of friends, relatives, and the significant other, as well as by cultural customs. In view of the availability of infant formulas, it is important to assess the commitment and support available to the mother in maintaining breastfeeding when it is interrupted.[16,19,28]

The nurse must be alert to any of the conditions that may lead to a temporary interruption in lactation. In the case of the mother, breastfeeding is often interrupted because of an illness or condition that requires medication and/or hospitalization. Or, the mother returns to work and breastfeeding is interrupted during work hours. For the neonate, not only illnesses and impairments, but also prematurity, often lead to Interrupted Breastfeeding.

Exacerbations of pre-existing medical conditions of the mother may result in Interrupted Breastfeeding. By scrutinizing the history, identification of potential problem areas is possible. In addition to assessing for the development of complications, the nurse needs to determine the effect of ongoing medications on the nursing neonate. It is often the nurse who is aware of the mother's commitment to breastfeeding and who is cognizant of medications which would or would not adversely affect the neonate when nursing.[28]

With the increasing number of diabetic women who can now reproduce, there has been a growing number who desire to breast feed. In addition to the benefits of breast milk for the neonate, breastfeeding is helpful to the mother since it can heighten normalcy in an otherwise high risk pregnancy. Because diabetics are more prone to infections that may lead to interruptions in breastfeeding, assessment of symptoms indicating such infections, and interventions to prevent them, is in-

II

dicated. Assessment of the diabetic state, including dietary intake, can often ward off development of abnormal metabolic states that can influence breast milk and potentially interrupt lactation. Frequent breastfeedings, as well as assessment of neonatal hypoglycemia, can go a long way in avoiding interruptions that occur when the infant needs to be bottle fed for hypoglycemia.[25,26]

Allergic diseases of the mother, especially asthma, often require medications which can affect the nursing neonate. Careful attention to the type of medication as well as assessment of allergic symptoms can lessen the likelihood of interrupting breastfeeding.[25,26]

Whether a mother with kidney disease experiences an interruption in breastfeeding or not depends on the degree of kidney impairment prior to pregnancy. If the impairment was only mild to moderate, breastfeeding can often be maintained without any interruption. But, if there was severe kidney impairment, most clinicians advise new mothers not to breast feed at all. In addition, mothers are usually advised to avoid breastfeeding if hypertension accompanies kidney impairment. Attention to a diagnosis of kidney disease will direct careful postpartum assessment of blood pressure, output, or any accompanying symptoms of complications. Because mothers who have had a renal transplant receive immunosuppressants, questions about the effects of these medications on the infant's immune system arise and many wonder about the advisability of breastfeeding.[25,26]

Mothers who are chronic hypertensives may experience difficulties with control of blood pressure during pregnancy and right after birth. Breastfeeding may be interrupted while the new mother receives medications to maintain or regain blood pressure control. Often, though, medications can be altered and breastfeeding continued.[2]

Whether previous breast surgery leads to cessation, or merely a temporary interruption of breastfeeding, seems to depend on the location and type of surgery. Studies indicate that mastectomies, breast reductions, or even biopsies can lead to

problems with sufficiency of milk supply. In particular, women with periareolar incisions are five times more likely to have lactation insufficiency. Careful scrutiny of the history as well as assessment of the breast itself can provide cues to potential problems. Particularly important is assessment of sufficiency of the milk supply so that the nutritional well being of the infant is assured.[25,26]

Certain conditions associated with pregnancy can also lead to Interrupted Breastfeeding. Primary among these is pregnancy induced hypertension. In particular, administration of magnesium sulfate often interrupts lactation because it is a central nervous system depressant for the baby as well as the mother. Assessment of signs indicating worsening of pregnancy induced hypertension (such as elevated blood pressure, protein in the urine, edema, hyperactive reflexes, reduced output) as well as side effects of the magnesium sulfate (such as depressed respirations and reflexes) is warranted. Some allow breastfeeding to continue while magnesium sulfate is being administered. If so, the infant's behavior should be assessed for effects of the drug.[28]

Infections, or the development of a fever, can also lead to Interrupted Breastfeeding until the source of infection or fever is identified. Common infections are mastitis, endometritis, and cystitis. Careful assessment for infection of the breast (warm, reddened, tender area, fever), uterus (fever, lower abdominal tenderness, foul smelling lochia), or urinary tract (frequency, urgency, dysuria, retention) is advocated.[16,28]

Maternal medications often lead to an interruption in breastfeeding since they can stimulate or inhibit lactation, change the milk composition, or pass into the breast milk thereby affecting the infant. Most drugs do pass into the breast milk, but the actual effect on the baby is dependent on many factors. Some of these factors are the amount/dose, the sucking activity of the infant, functional changes in the gastrointestinal tract of the baby, and the gastrointestinal tract pH of the baby. Most antimicrobials do not pose any risk to the baby, but some, such as chloramphenicol, may result in temporary interruption of breastfeeding. Neurotropic drugs, which are often prescribed for epilepsy, anxiety, depression, and psychoses, are often a concern to health care providers. In reality, though, these drugs are typically of little significance to the nursing infant unless the baby has hepatic insufficiency or immature kidneys. Definitely contraindicated during breastfeeding are anticancer drugs, radioactive drugs, lithium, phenylbutazone, atropine, and ergot alkaloids. In addition, high doses of prednisone necessitate Interrupted Breastfeeding until four hours after each dose.[29] Careful attention to the mother's history as well as medications that may be prescribed can alert the nurse to the necessity for interruptions in lactation as well as provide a basis for assessment of effects on the nursing neonate.

Not only maternal, but neonatal illnesses/conditions can lead to Interrupted Breastfeeding. Primary among these is prematurity of the infant. Many advocate the use of expressed breast milk (in gavage feedings) until actual breastfeeding of the premature can be initiated. It seems that social support of the mother is particularly important during the time breastfeedings are interrupted. During this time, assessment of pumping techniques as well as milk storage is necessary so that the milk supply is adequately stimulated and safe breast milk is provided for the baby. With proper education and assistance, the initiation of breastfeeding of the premature infant can be eased considerably, and the nutritional status of the infant maintained. In the past, many recommended progressing from gavage to bottle feedings before starting breastfeeding, thinking that breastfeeding was more fatiguing to the premature. Several studies have found, however, that breastfeeding is actually less stressful than bottle feeding and advocate progressing right to the breast. Assessment of signs indicating that the premature is ready for breastfeeding allows initiation of the process at a time when the baby is capable and the physiological status is stabilized. Monitoring physiological responses, feeding behaviors, and adequacy of milk supply can then help ensure success of lactation.[17,20,23,32]

Other neonatal conditions, besides prematurity, can also lead to Interrupted Breastfeeding. These include neonatal anomalies (such as cleft lip or palate),[8] neonatal illnesses (such as neonatal sepsis or necrotizing enterocolitis),[1,12] neurological impairments that affect sucking,[22] respiratory problems (such as respiratory distress syndrome or meconium aspiration),[14,34] or common surgical problems (such as gastroschisis, omphalocele, tracheal esophageal fistulas, meconium ileus, imperforate anus, diaphragmatic hernia, meningocele, hydrocephalus).[30] The alarming increase in the number of mothers who abuse alcohol and/or other drugs has contributed to an increase in the number of infants who have fetal alcohol syndrome or experience the effects of withdrawal. Both of these affect sucking and can therefore, interrupt breastfeeding.[9,11,13,18,21] Once these neonatal conditions are resolved or the infant is stabilized, breastfeeding can be resumed. Assessing the progress of breastfeeding is then warranted.

Jaundice is relatively common in neonates, occurring in up to 60% of infants during the first week. Many are of the opinion that evidence of neonatal jaundice warrants interruption of lactation. This is because breastfeeding has been implicated as the causative agent in jaundice. Recent research indicates that breast fed babies typically have fewer stools in the first few days. As a result, some of the conjugated bilirubin in the small bowel is reabsorbed instead of being excreted in the stool, resulting in an increased load for conjugation in the hepatic system. In addition, breastfed babies usually take in fewer calories than bottle-fed babies in the first few days. This results in decreased clearance of bilirubin in the hepatic system. To counteract these two effects, early, frequent breastfeeding is advocated to not only hasten early stools but also to provide calories. It is interesting to note that supplementing breastfeedings with bottle feedings of sterile or glucose water has not been found to reduce the incidence of jaundice. Instead, babies who get supplemental bottles have fewer stools and higher bilirubin levels than those who are breast fed and not supplemented.[4,10,33]

There is a condition called true breast milk jaundice which usually does lead to an interruption in breastfeeding. It occurs in 1% to 3% of breast fed babies. This type of jaundice is characterized by bilirubin levels that begin to rise between 4 and 7 days, that peak around 2 weeks (level at 25-20 mg/dl), and require 4 to 16 weeks to resolve. Etiology of this condition remains elusive. A currently accepted theory suggests that breastfeeding leads to higher levels of free fatty acids than bottle feeding. Interruption of breastfeeding is typically advocated during phototherapy treatment. Formula feedings during treatment are thought to complement the phototherapy by increasing stool excretion as well as by increasing hepatic clearance of bilirubin. Some, however, have proposed more frequent breastfeeding with a supplementation device rather than interrupting breastfeeding to accomplish this purpose.[4,10,33] Because there is a cephalocaudal progression of jaundice as bilirubin rises, observation of the existence of jaundice over the entire body is necessary. Some use an icterometer as an aid to assessment. The presence of bruising and/or cephalhematomas should be noted as well, since both add to the amount of blood that needs to be broken down. Because a bilirubin level that is too high is the culprit in kernicterus, total bilirubin levels need to be assessed by using a transcutaneous bilirubinometer and by doing traditional blood tests.

Relatively common difficulties that contribute to Ineffective Breastfeeding may result in interrupted lactation. These include breast engorgement, sore nipples, inadequate letdown, inadequate suck, or temporary insufficiencies of milk (which often result in supplementation). Assessment includes observation of feeding patterns (frequency, duration) and feeding behaviors. In addition, signs of let-down, indicators of adequacy of milk supply, and signs of infant growth are assessed.

Cesarean birth, breastfeeding, and father's feelings of separation have also been associated with Interrupted Breastfeeding. For some, merely having a cesarean birth may result in pain that interrupts breastfeeding. At times, breastfeeding is interrupted to allow the father an opportunity to lessen feelings of separation by feeding the baby. Breastfeeding more than one infant can lead to interruptions in the process for one baby. One infant may suck less vigorously than the other and need supplementation, or there may be a brief insufficiency of supply for several babies.[31]

❖ **Defining Characteristics**

The presence of the following defining characteristics indicates that the patient may be experiencing Interrupted Breastfeeding*:

Major Defining Characteristic
- Infant not receiving nourishment at the breast for some or all feedings.

Minor Defining Characteristics
- Separation of mother and infant (for some feedings because of maternal illness, neonatal illness, or maternal employment).
- Maternal desire to maintain lactation and provide (or eventually provide) her breastmilk for her infant's nutritional needs.
- Lack of knowledge (or experience) regarding expression, maintenance of supply, or storage of breast milk.

❖ **Related Factors**

The following related factors are associated with Interrupted Breastfeeding*:

Maternal Factors
- Previous breast surgery
- Illness, infection
- Illness associated with pregnancy
- Employment
- Fever, etiology undetermined
- Breastfeeding difficulties (such as sore nipples)
- Admission to hospital or intensive care unit
- Cesarean delivery
- Medication contraindicating breastfeeding
- Father's feelings of separation from infant

Neonatal Factors
- Prematurity
- Anomaly
- Illness
- True breast milk jaundice
- Surgical conditions
- Breastfeeding multiples

---

*Adapted from North American Nursing Diagnosis Association, 1992 Ballot.

❖ Related Medical/Psychiatric Diagnoses

The following are examples of related medical/psychiatric diagnoses for Interrupted Breastfeeding:

Maternal Diagnoses

- Asthma
- Cardiovascular disease
- Diabetes mellitus, inadequate intake, accompanying infections
- Endometritis
- Hypertension requiring medication
- Ingestion of excessive alcohol or illegal drugs
- Kidney disease
- Mastitis
- Medications for psychological conditions
- Pregnancy induced hypertension
- Pulmonary embolism
- Seizure disorders requiring medication
- Simple mastectomy or breast reduction
- Surgical conditions

Neonatal Diagnoses

- Fetal alcohol syndrome
- Hypoglycemia associated with being infant of diabetic mother
- Necrotizing enterocolitis
- Neonatal jaundice
- Neonatal sepsis
- Oral defects, such as cleft palate, lip
- Respiratory problems such as pneumonia, respiratory distress syndrome, or meconium aspiration
- Sucking disorders in a neurologically impaired infant
- True breast milk jaundice
- Withdrawal from drugs as result of maternal abuse

NURSING DIAGNOSES

Examples of *specific* nursing diagnoses for Interrupted Breastfeeding are:

- Interrupted Breastfeeding related to work schedule
- Interrupted Breastfeeding related to pregnancy induced hypertension with administration of magnesium sulfate
- Interrupted Breastfeeding related to neonate requiring surgery for imperforate anus
- Interrupted Breastfeeding related to premature gestation

PLANNING AND IMPLEMENTATION WITH RATIONALE

Overall, the expected outcome after a temporary interruption is successful resumption of breastfeeding. In addition, adequacy of the neonate's intake needs to be assured.

Adequacy of Breasts and Nipples for Breastfeeding

Breast tissue must be sufficient to produce milk. It is rare that it is not, but certain conditions (such as breast surgery) may affect initiation of the process and cause a temporary interruption.[6,25,26] If noninfectious mastitis develops, for example, the nurse needs to ensure frequent pumping with breast massage above the tender area. *This helps reduce stasis and therefore the likelihood of infection.* For engorgement, interventions include frequent pumping, with massage, and application of warm compresses prior to pumping. *These enhance let-down and emptying so that stasis is prevented.* If nipple assessment indicates a flat nipple, trauma, soreness, bruising, or cracking, the nurse intervenes with breast shells (which help nipples evert) and instructions on correct use of the pump. Information about proper care of the nipples is also provided so trauma and the potential for infection is minimized.[35,36]

Providing Quiet, Comfortable Environment

It is a well known fact that emotional factors and anxiety can influence let-down. *Therefore, interventions that assure comfort and relaxation during pumping are essential.* This may not be easy since hospital space is often limited. It is often difficult to find a quiet, private place to pump at work as well. It may require a great deal of ingenuity on the part of the nurse and client to figure out where there is a comfortable, relaxed location for pumping.[17,24,28,35,36]

Stimulating Breasts to Maintain Milk Supply

The impetus for breast milk production is suckling of the infant, which stimulates the prolactin and let-down reflexes. Maintenance of the milk supply, then, requires consistent stimulation of the breast at regular intervals of 2 to 3 hours at first, and then at 3 to 4 hour intervals. Longer intervals between feedings can result in engorgement, stasis, and possible mastitis. In order to initiate the let-down reflex, each breast must be pumped for at least 5 to 10 minutes per session; many recommend at least 10 minutes per breast. For those who are pumping at work, more frequent breastfeeding when at home is advised to help assure sufficient stimulation of the breasts. *Exclusive breastfeeding or pumping for the first 4 to 6 weeks (rather than offering any bottles) assures that the milk supply is well established as well as avoids nipple confusion.*[15] It is now well documented that sucking at the breast is quite different than sucking an artificial nipple. Many believe that these differences confuse the infant, which leads to difficulties in suckling at the breast. Interventions by the nurse include providing information about the frequency/duration of pumping necessary to adequately stimulate the breast. Citing advantages, disadvantages, and costs of various pumps helps the mother to make an informed choice about the type of pump she wants to use. Demonstration of the pump selected, with helpful hints and cautions, aids learning. It is important to caution about potential trauma, which can be inflicted by continuous pumping or by using a pressure that is too high.[3] *By allowing practice, the mother becomes familiar with the pumping procedure at a time when reinforcement for correct performance and answers to questions can be provided.*[3,15,28]

Safety of Milk Supply

If expressed breast milk is to be fed to the infant by bottle or gavage feedings, attention must focus on assuring safety of the milk. Even if milk is discarded, *cleanliness during pumping helps prevent mastitis.* This involves education about the importance of cleanliness, sterilizing or cleaning pump equipment, cleanliness of milk storage containers, as well as proper storage of milk. Discussions about safe storage and cooling help the mother decide on a convenient method for storing her milk. Relaying information about labeling containers promotes use of expressed milk in proper sequence. *To retard growth of microorganisms and avoid contamination of expressed milk,* discussion of the proper temperatures for the refrigerator or freezer as well as the length of time that milk can be stored is necessary. Information about the proper thawing of milk is also included so that safety is maintained.[5,15]

Assuring Successful Resumption of Breastfeeding

Once the need for the temporary interruption of breastfeeding no longer exists, the nurse assists the mother in resuming breastfeeding. Because anxiety and concern over adequacy of milk supply often accompany resumption of breastfeeding, efforts to assist and support the mother are important in assuring success. *Careful assessment of all aspects of breastfeeding (such as position, latch-on, sucking behaviors) provides data for subsequent interventions that can enhance the process.* Hints that aid breastfeeding of babies with particular problems (such as hints for feeding a baby with cleft palate) ease the transition to breastfeeding. Pointing out indicators of let-down as well as the baby's unique sucking behaviors can help the mother attune to, and meet, the nutritive needs of her particular baby. *Positive feedback provides reinforcement for effective breastfeeding.* And, it is always important to determine whether the baby is receiving adequate nutrition.[3,5]

Adequate Maternal Nutritional and Fluid Intake

It is common knowledge that the nutrition and fluid intake of the mother is important in maintaining the quality and quantity of breast milk pumped and subsequently fed to the baby. *Nutrients and fluids are necessary to meet energy,*

Text continued on p. 208.

❖ *NURSING CARE GUIDELINES*
Nursing Diagnosis: Interrupted Breastfeeding

Expected Patient Outcomes	Nursing Interventions
• The mother's breasts will be adequate for breastfeeding as evidenced by: breasts soft immediately after pumping; breasts filling, with ropy texture, after pumping; breasts symmetrical; absence of non-infectious or infectious mastitis; absence of engorgement.	• Assess breasts by observation/palpation for indications of breast milk as well as absence of factors that may hinder breastfeeding (such as non-infectious and infectious mastitis or breast reduction). • For mastitis, teach to pump breasts frequently, massaging above the tender area while pumping. • If breasts are engorged, teach to pump breasts frequently, around the clock. Also instruct to massage breasts and apply warm compresses before pumping, as well as to pump long enough to empty the breasts.
• The mother's nipples will be favorable for breastfeeding as evidenced by nipples everted (not flat or inverted); absence of bruising, cracking, bleeding; minimal soreness occurring only with latch-on or beginning of pumping.	• Assess nipples for ease of latch-on or indications of trauma • Do "pinch" test to determine if nipples are flat or inverted. • If nipples are flat, instruct on use of breast shells between pumpings; pumping will help nipples evert and breast shells apply pressure behind nipple to help it become more prominent. • If nipples are sore, teach how to use pump correctly. • Advise to pump frequently with low pressure and to apply small amount of breast milk to nipples after pumping (lubricates, softens). • Explain that ointments and resting the nipple have not been found to help decrease soreness; continue pumping. • Instruct to avoid soap on nipples since it can dry the epithelium and cause soreness, as well as make it more prone to infection. • Instruct how to air dry nipples after pumping, which helps toughen nipples. • If nipples are bruised, check pumping techniques (high pressure can traumatize). • If nipples are cracked, check pumping techniques, and when baby nurses again, position correctly.
• The mother will secure a comfortable environment for pumping.	Assist the mother to find a comfortable environment for pumping.
• The mother will adequately stimulate and empty her breasts.	• Instruct that a similar quantity of breast milk should be expressed each time; breasts should become soft after pumping, filling and becoming firm again after pumping; breasts should be without symptoms of infectious or noninfectious mastitis.

Continued.

❖ *NURSING CARE GUIDELINES— cont'd*

Nursing Diagnosis: *Interrupted Breastfeeding*

Expected Patient Outcomes	Nursing Interventions
	• Relay information about types of pumps (various hand held and electric); advantages and disadvantages, costs, as well as where to purchase. • Demonstrate, in detail, how to use the pump selected. • For an electric pump, teach to assemble sterile/clean container, tubing, equipment; wash hands and breasts; massage breasts to stimulate let-down; place flange on breasts; turn on and regulate suction so it is gentle, starting with low suction. • For hand, cylinder pump, teach to slide outer cylinder of pump away from breast to create suction. • Instruct to pump every 2-3 or 3-4 hours for at least 10 minutes/ breast.
• The mother will maintain safety of expressed milk.	• Inform about type of container appropriate to store expressed milk (not glass since immunologic factors adhere to glass); most use a small plastic container rather than plastic liners and store milk in single use containers because once thawed, milk cannot be refrozen. • Instruct how to label expressed milk so it can be used in proper sequence to minimize contamination. • Instruct on proper cooling of milk to minimize bacterial growth; keep in cooler in ice or use ice packs during transport. • Teach how to properly freeze milk if necessary; use milk within 2 weeks if in refrigerator freezer or 6 months in deep freeze. • Teach how to sterilize pump equipment and milk containers if necessary; boil for 5 minutes or dishwasher temperature at 180° F. • Teach how to thaw milk appropriately in gradually warming water. • Caution against boiling milk (it destroys immune properties) or heating it in microwave (it can burn the baby).
• The mother will have intake of adequate nutrients and fluids for lactation.	• Obtain typical 24-hour dietary recall. • Analyze recall for adequacy; compare intake with requirements for lactation. • Instruct on changes needed to meet nutritional requirements for lactation. • Individualize teaching to include preferences. • Instruct about adequate fluid intake (10 or more glasses of fluid/ day).

❖ *NURSING CARE GUIDELINES — cont'd*

Nursing Diagnosis: Interrupted Breastfeeding

Expected Patient Outcomes	Nursing Interventions
• The mother will be able to breastfeed again successfully	• Assess for and assist with adequate latch-on (mouth wide open, tongue under nipple, lips everted or flared out, nipple and ¼ to ½ inches of areola in mouth, complete seal). • Assess for, and assist, with correct position at breast (ventral surface of baby to ventral surface of Mom; mouth at level of nipple; without sideways turning of head or extension of trunk/neck so baby does not come off the breast); changes holds from cradle to football (to change area of greatest pressure). • If let-down problem, teach to massage breasts before feeding, use warm compresses before nursing, avoid fatigue, allow sufficient time to stimulate let-down. • Assess for and assist with adequate suck. Instruct to avoid artificial nipples, pacifiers, or breast shields which cause nipple confusion. • Observe for nutritive suck (rhythmic with swallowing after about 3 sucks, or about 1 suck/second; cheeks hollow; no smacking or clicking sounds). • For infant facial nerve problems, use a football hold, then present the nipple by stroking it down over the upper, and then lower, lip's midline. In the cradle hold, place unaffected side down and stroke lower corner of mouth. • Use oral stimulation before the feeding (gently stroke around baby's lips and then gums); next allow baby to suck on mother's finger. • For cleft lip, place nipple to one side of cleft and use mother's thumb to fill the gap and create a seal. For cleft palate, position the nipple to one side of the cleft; keep areola soft so latch-on is easier. Hold in upright position for feeding. Burp baby frequently. Have Mom use a pump, or nipple roll, to elongate nipple. • For a high palate or groove, teach to use supplementer device, and try the sidelying position. • Use a milk incentive of breast milk on lower or upper lip just before latch-on. • Assess for adequate let-down (milk dripping from other breast; areolar fullness; tingling sensation; nutritive suck). • Assess for adequacy of milk supply (appropriate weight gain; 6 wet diapers/day; regular bowel movements; no fussiness after a feeding; awake during feeding; stays on breast; nurses 8 times/day).

growth, and physical activity needs of the baby.[7,15] New mothers are often unaware of nutritional and fluid requirements for lactation. Merely providing this information is often not sufficient to ensure compliance, however. Paying attention to a dietary recall and including food preferences helps individualize teaching so the mother can translate requirements into applicable actions.[28]

EVALUATION

Expected outcomes have been cited in the patient outcome column of the Nursing Guidelines.

Mothers who had their breastfeeding temporarily interrupted by maternal or infant conditions should be guided and supported in the following areas: determining a method of pumping their breasts; being successful in stimulating an adequate milk supply through pumping; maintaining safety of expressed breast milk; maintaining an adequate nutrition and fluid intake for lactation; and successful resumption of breastfeeding. Nursing information, instruction, and support will have helped the mother be successful with breastfeeding even though it was temporarily interrupted.

❖ *CASE STUDY WITH PLAN OF CARE*

Mrs. Monica S. was a 25-year-old, married, primigravida woman who attended childbirth education classes. Long before becoming pregnant, she decided that she wanted to breastfeed. Mrs. S. started reading books about breastfeeding relatively early in her pregnancy and was looking forward to the experience. At 34 weeks gestation, she ruptured her membranes prematurely, went into labor, and delivered a premature baby girl. She was disappointed about not being able to

breastfeed right away and inquired whether she would be able to breastfeed at all. The nursing staff helped Mrs. S. by teaching her how to pump and store breast milk, which was fed to her baby by gavage feedings. Outcomes and interventions from the standardized care plan, in relation to pumping the breasts and maintaining safety of expressed milk, were relevant. When the baby was able, breastfeeding was initiated.

PLAN OF CARE FOR MRS. MONICA S.

Nursing Diagnosis: *Interrupted Breastfeeding Related to Prematurity*

Expected Patient Outcomes	**Nursing Interventions**
• Mrs. S. initiates breastfeeding at appropriate time.	• Assess Mrs. S.'s infant for ability to initiate breastfeeding (organized suck and swallow, clinical stability, maintenance of body temperature outside incubator).
	• Inform Mrs. S. of the infant's progress related to factors influencing readiness to breastfeed: infant gains weight; suck organized into bursts of 4-5 with ability to swallow secretions; clinical stability (absence of ventilatory support, parenteral fluids, neurologic problems); tolerates enteral feedings; maintains body temperature outside incubator.

II

Nursing Diagnosis: *Interrupted Breastfeeding Related to Prematurity*

Expected Patient Outcomes	Nursing Interventions
• Mrs. S. maintains breastfeeding of her infant.	• Provide an environment that is comfortable and private. • Assist Mrs. S. to assume comfortable position for breastfeeding. • Assist Mrs. S. in positioning baby at breast. • Instruct to initiate let-down by using a pump before starting baby at breast. • Instruct to allow baby to do licking and nonnutritive sucking which is helpful for conditioning milk ejection. • Assist by exerting gentle downward pressure on baby's mandible as baby opens mouth. • Help Mrs. S. move baby's head onto nipple when baby opens mouth; maintain gentle pressure behind head. • Help Mrs. S. recognize signs of satiety to know when to terminate feeding. • If breast is not empty, have mother pump breasts to completely empty them.
• Mrs. S.'s infant will exhibit adaptive responses to initiation of breastfeeding, i.e., maintains adaptive temperature and exhibits adaptive indices of oxygenation; lengthens nutritive suck at each feeding; terminates feeding when tired or satiated; can be fed on demand by breast.	• Assess/monitor temperature and oxygenation; terminate feeding if any become abnormal. • Assess for signs of satiety (falling asleep or ceasing to suck), and then terminate feeding.
• Mrs. S.'s infant receives adequate nutrition and fluid intake for premature.	• Test weighed at each feeding (weighed before and after feeding); subtract prefed from postfeed weight to obtain amount of breast milk obtained by baby at that feeding. • Supplement with nasogastric tube as needed to maintain intake at amount it was when exclusively tube fed. • Monitor baby's weight gain. • Monitor feeding patterns, demand schedule, sleep-wake cycle, fussiness. • Monitor infant's output (at least six wet diapers/day and regular bowel movements). • Monitor for signs of dehydration.

REFERENCES

1. Amspacher KA: Necrotizing enterocolitis: The never-ending challenge, *J Perin Neonat Nurs* 3(2):58-68, 1989.
2. Asselin BL and Lawrence RA: Maternal diseases as a consideration in lactation management, *Clin Perinatol* 14(1):71-87, 1987.
3. Auerbach KG: Assisting the employed breastfeeding mother, *J Nurse-Midwifery* 35(1):26-34, 1990.
4. Auerbach KG and Gartner LM: Breast feeding and human milk: Their association with jaundice in the neonate, *Clin Perinatol* 14(1):89-107, 1987.
5. Ballard P: Breast-feeding for the working mother, *Issues in Comp Pediatr Nurs* 6:249-259, 1983.
6. Boyce KM: Case Study: Breast-feeding following mastectomy, *Midwives Chronicle* June: 173-174, 1991.
7. Bronner YL and Paige DM: Current concepts in infant nutrition, *J of Nurse-Midwifery* 37(2):435-585, 1992.
8. Curtin G: The infant with cleft lip or palate: More than a surgical problem, *J Perin Neonat Nurs* 3(3):80-89, 1990.
9. Day NL and Richardson GA: Prenatal marijuana use: Epidemiology, methodologic issues, and infant outcome, *Clinics in Perinatology* 18(1):77-89, 1991.

II

10. de Steuben C: Breast-feeding and jaundice, *Journal of Nurse-Midwifery* 37(2):59S-66S, 1992.

11. Eliason MJ and Williams JK: Fetal alcohol syndrome and the neonate, *J Perin Neonat Nurs* 3(4):64-72, 1990.

12. Gerdes JS: Clinicopathologic approach to the diagnosis of neonatal sepsis, *Clin Perinatol* 18(2):361-379, 1991.

13. Gosse G: Neonatal abstinence syndrome, *Canadian Nurse* May: 17-22, 1992.

14. Graves BW: Differential diagnosis of respiratory distress, *J Nurse-Midwifery* 37(2):27S-35S, 1992.

15. Greenberg CS and Smith K: Anticipatory guidance for the employed breast-feeding mother, *J Pediatr Health Care* 5(4):204-209, 1991.

16. Jensen MD and Bobak IM: *Maternity and Gynecologic Care,* St. Louis, 1985, Mosby–Year Book.

17. Kaufman KJ and Hall LA: Influences of the social network on choice and duration of breast-feeding in mothers of preterm infants, *Research Nursing Health* 12:149-159, 1989.

18. Kennard MJ: Cocaine use during pregnancy: Fetal and neonatal effects, *J Perin Neonat Nurs* 3(4):53-63, 1990.

19. Lawrence RA: The management of lactation as a physiologic process, *Clin Perinatol* 14(1):1-10, 1987.

20. Lemons P and Stuart M and Lemons JA: Breast-feeding the premature infant, *Clin Perinatol* 13(1):111-122, 1986.

21. Lewis KD: Pathophysiology of prenatal drug-exposure: In utero, in the newborn, in childhood, and in agencies, *J Pediatr Nurs* 6(3):185-190, 1991.

22. McBride MC and Danner SC: Sucking disorders in neurologically impaired infants: assessment and facilitation of breast feeding, *Clin Perinatol* 14(1):109-130, 1987.

23. McCoy R and Kadowaki C and Wilks S and Engstrom J and Meier P: Nursing management of breast feeding for preterm infants, *J Perin Neonat Nurs* 2(1):42-55, 1988.

24. Minchin MK: Positioning for breast feeding, *Birth* 16(2):67-80, 1989.

25. Neifert M and DeMarzo S and Seacat J and Young D and Leff M and Orleans M: The influence of breast surgery, breast appearance, and pregnancy-induced breast changes on lactation sufficiency as measured by infant weight gain, *Birth* 17(1):31-38, 1990.

26. Neifert MR and Seacat JM: Lactation insufficiency: A rational approach, *Birth* 14(4):182-190, 1987.

27. North American Nursing Diagnosis Association (NANDA): Description of proposed diagnoses, distributed with ballot following the Tenth Conference on the Classification of Nursing Diagnoses, St. Louis, May 1992.

28. Olds SB and London ML and Ladewig PW: *Maternal-Newborn Nursing,* ed 4, Menlo Park, 1992, Addison-Wesley.

29. Rivera-Calimlin L: The significance of drugs in breast milk, *Clin Perinato* 14(1):51-70, 1987.

30. Shaw N: Common surgical problems in the newborn, *J Perin Neonat Nursing* 3(3):50-64, 1990.

31. Sollid DT and Evans BT and McClowry SG and Garrett A: Breastfeeding multiples, *J Perin Neonat Nursing* 3(1):46-65, 1989.

32. Steichen JJ and Krug-Wispe SK and Tsang RC: Breast feeding the low birth weight preterm infant, *Clin Perinatol* 14(1):131-171, 1987.

33. Tan KL: Phototherapy for neonatal jaundice, *Clin Perinatol* 18(3):423-439, 1991.

34. Turnage CS: Meconium aspiration syndrome, *J Perin Neonat Nurs* 3(2):69-80, 1989.

35. Walker M: Functional assessment of infant breastfeeding patterns, *Birth* 16(3):140-147, 1989.

36. Walker M: Management of selected early breastfeeding problems seen in clinical practice, *Birth* 16(3):148-157, 1989.

Ineffective Infant Feeding Pattern

Ineffective Infant Feeding Pattern is a state in which an infant demonstrates an impaired ability to suck or coordinate the suck/swallow response.

OVERVIEW

The development of functional feeding for the infant is an intricate physiologic process compounded by neurologic maturation and learned behaviors. Essential to the process of normal feeding and swallowing is adequate nutrition and airway competence.[14] The infant who demonstrates dysfunctional feeding or swallowing is often malnourished and experiences respiratory symptoms with significant risk of aspiration. Clinical manifestations of aspiration can include apnea and bradycardia in the young infant, choking and coughing, chronic congestion, recurrent wheezing, atelectasis, and overt pneumonia.[8] Infant feeding problems can be the result of a physical or medical condition, inappropriate food choice, maladaptive parent-infant feeding interaction, or any combination of these origins.[13]

Providing nourishment and caring for the infant is central to the parent-infant relationship. Our society views the well-nourished infant as the well-nurtured infant. It is important to note that not only do parents influence infant feeding behavior but that the infant exerts a substantial influence on the parent and surrounding family members.

Classic studies by Ainsworth and Bell[1] suggest that infant feeding is most successful when parents are sensitive to the infant's cues. Important to note are the timing, amount, preference, pacing, and eating capabilities of the infant. Parents and infants reciprocally refine the feeding process, aquiring skill and regulating their adaptability. Feeding begins with the reflexive suck, swallow, breathing response in the newborn. The newborn's anatomy commands that the infant's tongue move in an in and out pattern (referred to as suckling) because of the circumscribed space within the oral cavity.[9] The suck consists of an up and down motion, the dorsum of the tongue in harmony with the mandible. The lips are tightly closed around the nipple to draw out liquid from breast or bottle. The suckle/suck swallow response continues in the infant until approximately 4 to 6 months of age.[14]

The infant's breathing pattern is coordinated with swallowing. Respiration ceases during the pharyngeal stage of swallowing.[5] The young infant sucks two or more times from the breast or bottle before taking a breath or swallowing.[8,9] The presence of a nipple coupled with the infant's small oropharynx require him to nose breath. The infant who experiences any type of respiratory difficulty does not feed well. Infants with prematurity, neurologic impairment, central nervous system dysfunction, severe gastrointestinal disease, and congenital anomalies (cleft lip, cleft palate) may demonstrate uncoordinated suck/swallow and require prolonged enteral and or parenteral feedings.

Literature supports the concept of a critical period related to feeding development.[1,7,15,16] Orr and Allen[11] support that non-oral feedings prevent the infant from experiencing rhythmic sucking and satiety. Infants can become defensive and resistant to oral feeding even after the period of enteral and parenteral feedings has been resolved.[15] Defensive and resistant oral feeding behaviors can include persistent head turning, tongue thrusting, gagging, and vomiting.[6] Infants at risk for an ineffective feeding pattern require a plan of care that includes an oral stimulation program to prevent feeding resistance and to acquire positive oral feeding skills.

ASSESSMENT

Each infant must be assessed individually as to their ability to initiate, sustain, and coordinate sucking with swallowing and breathing. The appropriate feeding schedule and method are an essential part of nutritional management for the infant. Feeding times and methods may have to be changed or adjusted several times before the correct combination can prove to be adaptive.

Chatoor and associates[4] report that feeding disturbances occuring during the first three months of life may be due to the infant's physical limitations, such as poor coordination of the oropharyngeal musculature, congenital anomalies of the gastrointestinal tract (e.g., cleft lip, cleft palate, esophageal atresia, and tracheoesophageal fistula), or a labile autonomic nervous system (oral hypersensitivity in an infant difficult to calm). These problems may be further compounded by limited parental sensitivity and responsiveness to the infant's feeding cues.

The assessment of infant feeding interactions can be readily attained with the use of the Chatoor Observational Scale for mother-infant toddler interaction during feeding,[5] the Barnard Nursing Child Assessment Feeding Scale,[2] or the Price AMIS Scale of sensitivity in mother-infant interactions.[12]

The premature infant presents a particular challenge in feeding for the nurse. Gestational age, physical condition, and neurologic status must be assessed. Conditions frequently encountered by the preterm infant, such as asphyxia, sepsis, and intraventricular hemorrhage, may impair the infants ability to suck.[10] Severe mental retardation presents risk of aspiration to the infant who has difficulty sucking or an uncoordinated suck, swallow, breathing response. Apnea during feeding may occur in the premature infant when milk or formula flows too quickly for his swallow or when continuing bottle feeding with a premature nipple when the infant's suck has progressively

improved.[3] Other signs and symptoms of difficulty during feeding include tachypnea, coughing, choking, cyanosis, bradycardia, and sleepiness.[10]

Intermittent gavage feeding is the method of choice for the infant with an uncoordinated suck swallow or who tires easily when nippling.[3,10,16] The infant who experiences apnea with intermittent gavage or who sustains neurologic insult such as asphyxia and can not nipple receives continual gavage feedings.[3] One complication of long term gavage feeding is that the infant is deprived of the pleasures and comforts of sucking. Literature supports that infants who experience sucking during gavage feedings are better prepared for nutritive sucking.[3,7,9,10,16]

The nursing process is of particular importance in the management of ineffective infant feeding, because of the amount of time the nurse is engaged in the observation, handling, and feeding of the infant.[3] The nurse continually revises and modifies the plan of care until the infant is tolerating feedings and thriving.

❖ Defining Characteristics

The presence of the following defining characteristics indicates that the patient may be experiencing Ineffective Infant Feeding Pattern.
- Inability to initiate or sustain an effective suck
- Inability to coordinate sucking, swallowing and breathing

❖ Related Factors

The following related factors are associated with Ineffective Infant Feeding Pattern:
- Prematurity
- Poor coordination of the oropharyngeal musculature
- Congenital anomaly
- Surgery of the gastrointestinal tract
- Prolonged NPO status
- Weight loss
- Neurological impairment/delay
- Hyper-irritability
- Oral hypersensitivity
- Lethargy
- Sedation
- Force feeding
- Delay feeding
- Failing to feed to satiety

❖ Related Medical/Psychiatric Diagnoses

The following are examples of related medical/psychiatric diagnoses for Ineffective Infant Feeding Pattern.

- Asphyxia
- Aspiration
- Atelectasis
- Cardiac defect/disease
- Cleft lip/cleft palate
- Down's syndrome
- Esophageal atresia
- Failure to thrive
- Hydrocephalus
- Inflammatory bowel disease
- Intraventricular hemorrhage
- Mental retardation
- Pneumonia
- Respiratory distress syndrome
- Sepsis
- Small for gestational age
- Sudden infant death syndrome
- Tracheoesophageal fistula

NURSING DIAGNOSES

Examples of *specific* nursing diagnoses for Ineffective Infant Feeding Pattern are:

- Ineffective infant feeding pattern related to hyperirritability.
- Ineffective infant feeding pattern related to lethargy.
- Ineffective infant feeding pattern related to force feeding.

PLANNING AND IMPLEMENTATION WITH RATIONALE

Nursing care for the infant with an ineffective feeding pattern fosters normal growth and development for the infant and encourages positive parental interaction. Nursing goals ensure the prevention of fatigue and aspiration with feedings and provide for adequate nutrition.[10] Research indicates that optimizing parent-infant interaction facilitates effective feeding.[13]

❖ *NURSING CARE GUIDELINES*

Nursing Diagnosis: *Ineffective Infant Feeding Pattern*

Expected Patient Outcomes	Nursing Interventions
The infant will ingest adequate amounts of breast milk/formula by nipple and/or gavage feeding to meet growth needs.	• Perform a.m. daily weights and document infant weight gain. • Weigh all diapers and record urine specific gravity • Supplement nipple or gavage feedings with intravenous therapy as ordered. • Measure abdominal circumferences, note distention and aspirate for gasteric residuals prior to feedings.
The infant will tolerate nipple and/or gavage feedings without evidence of fatigue, respiratory difficulties, or emesis.	• Feed infant in a semi-sitting position. • Observe and document evidence of feeding difficulty (tachypnea, choking, coughing, cyanosis, apnea, bradycardia, sleepiness). • Gently burp infant after nipple or gavage feedings and position on right side with support.
The infant will experience oral gratification and other emotional satiety during feeding times.	• Hold infant and provide with pacifier during feedings as tolerated • Initiate nipple feedings with a smaller more pliable nipple until suck reflex becomes strong. • Increase nipple feedings slowly and progressively as tolerated. • Monitor infant strength and ability to tolerate a regular sized nipple. • Involve parents in infant feeding and teach appropriate goals, techniques and behaviors as necessary.

Gavage feeding is the method of choice for the ill or premature infant. *This allows the infant to rest, thus conserving energy and calories for growth.* Eventually, as the infant demonstrates consistent weight gain and tolerance of gavage feedings (without apneic spells or the presence of residuals), an oral stimulation program is begun. The infant is offered a pacifier with gavage feedings. *This not only strengthens the infant's ability to suck but also provides the infant with pleasure. The infant is soothed and comforted and relaxes and the gavage feedings flow is facilitated.*[10,11]

As the infant grows and matures as evidenced by weight gain, length increase, and other increases in body measurements (such as head circumference and chest circumference) and continues to tolerate gavage feeding with non-nutritive sucking, a nipple feeding program is instituted. *Daily weights are carefully monitored and the baby is placed on the right side after feeding with support to enhance gastric emptying and lessen the risk of aspiration if regurgitation occurs.*[10,16] During feedings the infant is fed in a semisitting position and observed for possible respiratory difficulty and the presence of exhaustion or fatigue.

The neonatal and pediatric nurse can lend guidance and support to unsure parents learning to feed their ill or premature infant. Unlike more primitive societies our culture provides only limited support to parents during the infant's early months.[13] Parents need nursing assistance to learn and appropriately execute effective feeding techniques that are pleasurable to the infant. The primary goal of infant feeding is to provide the infant with congenial and satisfying feedings. Effective feeding is a dynamic process that depends upon the abilities of the infant and caretaker, requiring much more than getting nutrition into the infant. *Feeding the infant is highly successful when the caretaker is sensitive and responsive to the infant's illicited cues.*[13] *The infant indicates the desire to feed, and should be allowed to determine the timing, amount, preference and method of feeding.*[1]

EVALUATION

The nursing care plan for the infant with an ineffective feeding pattern is successful when the infant demonstrates adequate and consistent weight gain for growth and an improved or normal suck, swallow response during feedings times. The need for gavage feedings will be eliminated, and the infant tolerates nipple feedings without evidence of exhaustion or fatigue. Parents will have an understanding of feeding dynamics and feel confident in their abilities to provide for the infant's emotional needs during feeding. Together, the nurse and the infant's parents address goals, interventions, and modifications for the plan of care to benefit both the infant and the family.

❖ CASE STUDY WITH PLAN OF CARE

Baby girl Bernice, born at 37 weeks by maternal dates and confirmed by gestational age assessment, weighed only 1250 grams (2 pounds, 12 ounces)—below the tenth percentile. Bernice's mother is a 28-year-old gravida 1, para 1 and was diagnosed with pregnancy-induced hypertension (PIH) at 34 weeks gestation. Because of poor uterine growth, a series of sonograms were obtained and a sonogram at 36 weeks gestation indicated that fetal head circumference remained larger than fetal abdominal circumference. Apgar scores were 6 at 1 minute after birth and 8 at 5 minutes. Bernice had a vigorous cry and alert appearance. Physical examination revealed no obvious congenital anomalies but indicated the presence of a heart murmur. Infant pulses were normal with no evidence of CHF. A cardiology follow-up and echocardiogram gave evidence to a small atrial septal defect.

The primary nurse noted that baby Bernice was tiring easily when given formula by nipple and losing more weight than 2% per day. Bernice's parents were involved in her care and had many concerns about their infant's heart defect and ability to tolerate nippling. They stated, "We don't want to push her if she's too tired to finish her feeding, we'll just let her rest awhile."

PLAN OF CARE FOR BABY BERNICE

Nursing Diagnosis: *Ineffective Infant Feeding Pattern Related to Decreased Birth Weight, Heart Defect, and Delayed Feeding.*

Expected Patient Outcomes	Nursing Interventions
Baby Bernice will tolerate adequate amounts of formula for growth through intermittant nipple/gavage feedings.	• Maintain Bernice in a neutral thermal environment. • Decrease environmental stress and sensory overload during feedings. • Perform daily weights and document weight gain. • Weigh all diapers and record urine specific gravity. • Supplement nipple feedings with intravenous therapy as ordered. • Measure abdominal girths, note the presence of distension and aspirate for gastric residuals prior to feeds.
Baby Bernice will demonstrate an improved tolerance of nipple feedings without fatigue.	• Monitor Bernice's strength and ability to tolerate a regular sized nipple with feedings. • Observe and report any evidence of exhaustion, respiratory distress or emesis during feeding times.
Bernice's parents will feel confident in their ability to feed her.	• Teach parents to feed Bernice in a semi-sitting position. • Encourage parents to avoid overbundling and excessive cuddling during baby's feedings. • Gently burp Bernice after feeding and position her on her right side with support. • Encourage, praise and reassure Bernice's parents as to their feeding techniques and efforts and reteach appropriate feeding goals and behaviors as necessary. • Provide Bernice's parents with additional educational materials as desired.

REFERENCES

1. Ainsworth MDS Bell SM: Some contemporary patterns of mother-infant interaction in the feeding situation. In Ambrose A, editor: *Stimulation in early infancy,* New York, 1969, Academic Press.
2. Barnard KE, et al: Measurement and meaning of parent-child interaction. In Morrison F, Lora C, Keating D, eds. *Applied developmental psychology;* vol 3. New York: Academic Press 1991.
3. Bragdon, D: A basis for the nursing management of feeding the premature infant, *JOGN Nursing* Suppl, May/June 51-57, 1983.
4. Chatoor I, Dickson L, Schaefer S: A developmental classification of feeding disorders associated with failure to thrive: diagnosis and treatment. In Drotar D, ed. *New directions in failure to thrive: implications for research and practice.* New York: Plenum, 1986.
5. Chatoor I, Menville E, Getson P, O'Donnell R: Observational Scale for mother infant-toddler interaction during feeding. Washington D.C., Children's Hospital Medical Center, 1989.
6. Geerstma, MA and others: Feeding resistance after parental hyperalimentation, *Am J Dis Child,* 139:225-226, 1985.
7. Illingsworth RS, Lister, J: The critical or sensitive period with special reference to certain feeding problems in infants and children. *J Pediatr* 65:839, 1964.
8. Loughlin, GM: Respiratory consequences of dysfunctional swallowing and aspiration. *Dysphagia* 3:126, 1989.
9. Morris SE, Klein M: *Pre-Feeding Skills.* Tuscon, Therapy Skill Builders, 1987, p 13.
10. Olds, SB, London, ML, Ladewig, PA: *Maternal newborn nursing: a family centered approach,* ed 3, Menlo Park, 1988, Addison-Wesley Publishing Co.
11. Orr, MJ, and Allen SS: Optimal oral experiences for infants on long term total parenteral nutrition, *Nutr Clin Pract,* 9:288-295, 1986.
12. Price GM: Sensitivity in mother-infant interactions: the AMS Scale. *Infant Behav Dev,* 6:353-360, 1983.
13. Satter, EM: The feeding relationship: problems and interventions, *J Pediatr* 117:184, 1990.
14. Stevenson, RD and Allaire, JH: The development of normal feeding and swallowing, *Pediatr Clin of North Am,* 38:1450, 1991.
15. Tuchman DN: Dysfunctional swallowing in the pediatric patient: Clinical considerations. *Dysphagia* 2:203, 1988.
16. Whaley, LF, and Wong, DL: *Nursing care of infants and children,* ed 4, St. Louis, 1990, Mosby Year Book.

ELIMINATION PATTERN

Constipation

Perceived Constipation

Colonic Constipation

Diarrhea

Bowel Incontinence

Constipation is the state in which an individual has a decreased frequency in the passage of stool and/or passage of hard, dry stool.[11]

Perceived Constipation is the state in which an individual makes a self-diagnosis of constipation and consequently ensures a daily bowel movement through the abuse of laxatives, enemas, or suppositories.[2]

Colonic Constipation is the state in which an individual's pattern of elimination is characterized by hard, dry stool, which results from a delay in the passage of food residue.[2]

Diarrhea is the state in which an individual has a change in normal bowel patterns, characterized by the frequent passage of loose, liquid, and unformed stool.[11]

Bowel Incontinence is the state in which an individual has a change in bowel patterns, characterized by the involuntary passage of stool.[11]

OVERVIEW: ALTERED BOWEL ELIMINATION

An alteration in bowel elimination can be manifested in the following ways: Diarrhea, Constipation (both Perceived and Colonic), and Incontinence. The normal pattern of bowel elimination varies widely among individuals and is influenced by many factors, including age, gender, activity level, emotional state, and the presence of disease. To understand alterations in bowel elimination, one must review the normal processes of stool formation and elimination.

Stool is formed when waste products and fluid pass through the gastrointestinal (GI) tract from the mouth to the anus. Shortly after food is ingested, it enters the stomach, where the combined action of digestive juices and mixing actions convert the food bolus into a hypertonic substance called chyme. Small quantities of chyme pass from the stomach into the duodenum with each peristaltic wave in the antrum. The rate at which chyme leaves the stomach and enters the duodenum is determined by the degree of fluidity of chyme in the stomach, the quantity of chyme in the duodenum, the presence of fats in the duodenum, and the acidity of duodenal contents.[8] Chyme that is more liquid enters the duodenum rapidly, but fats, increased acidity, and increased quantity of chyme in the duodenum decrease the rate of gastric emptying. Any condition that obstructs the stomach outlet, such as tumors, ulcers, edema, or fibrosis, will also interfere with gastric emptying.[7] Normally, the stomach will empty in 2 to 4 hours. Within 6 to 9 hours after the meal is ingested, the chyme passes through the duodenum, jejunum, and ileum into the cecum. By the time it reaches the ileum, chyme has been converted into an isotonic solution that is easily reabsorbed. The time required for the food bolus to pass from the cecum to the sigmoid colon ranges from hours to days.

The GI tract receives up to 9 to 10 L of fluid every day. The source of this fluid is both endogenous, that is, from within the individual (from salivary, billiary, and intestinal bodily secretions), and exogenous, that is, from outside of the body's confines (for example, dietary intake). The largest amount of fluid, approximately 8 L, is from endogenous sources, and the remaining quantity is from exogenous sources. Normally, all of the fluid except 100 to 150 ml is reabsorbed in the large and the small intestine. The small intestine absorbs the largest quantity of fluid (approximately 8 L), and the remaining fluid is absorbed in the large intestine. The small amount of fluid that is not reabsorbed is excreted in the feces.

Defecation is the process of eliminating wastes and undigested food from the body in the form of feces (stool). The normal defecation pattern in the United States varies widely among individuals and is influenced by a number of factors. A survey of young adults by Sandler, Jordan, and Shelton[18] indicated that 90% of respondents reported a stool frequency of two to seven stools per week, with the passage of one stool per day as the most common bowel elimination pattern.

Patterns of stool frequency vary by gender, age, race, activity level, and diet.[4,5] Men tend to report more frequent defecation patterns than women, whites tend to defecate more often than

African-Americans, young people defecate more often than older adults, and persons who consume more fruits and vegetables defecate more often than those whose diets contain less fiber. Cultural factors also influence the pattern of defecation. For example, Senegalese people normally defecate twice a day and consider themselves constipated if they pass only one stool a day.[18] Among Americans the pattern of bowel elimination is at least three stools per week. Most Americans have a fecal mass that is intact, deep brown in color, with a slight odor, weighing from 100 to 200 g, and containing approximately 70% water.[4] The color, odor, and consistency of stool depends on factors such as the individual's diet and emotional state, the presence of microorganisms or intestinal disease, a deficiency of digestive enzymes, or an autonomic nervous system (ANS) dysfunction.

Defecation is a voluntarily controlled act that occurs in response to the defecation reflex. The defecation reflex is stimulated when fecal matter is pushed into the rectum in response to mass movements of the colon. Mass movements are modified peristaltic movements of the colon that occur infrequently, usually within the first hour after eating breakfast, and last approximately 10 to 30 minutes.[8] They are facilitated by the gastrocolic and duodenocolic reflexes that develop in response to distention of the stomach and duodenum. When a mass movement forces feces into the rectum, the rectal wall distends. This distention initiates afferent signals, which in turn initiate peristaltic waves to the descending colon, sigmoid, and rectum. The peristaltic waves force the feces toward the anus, and the urge to defecate is then felt. Afferent signals also initiate effects such as the taking a deep breath, closure of the glottis, and contraction of the abdominal muscles, which assist in the passage of fecal matter into the anal canal. Straightening of the anorectal angle is another factor involved in the act of defecation. The anorectal angle is created by the forward pull of the puborectalis muscle. If the urge to defecate is acknowledged, the puborectalis muscle relaxes, the anorectal angle straightens, the internal and external sphincters relax, and feces are evacuated.

III

If the urge to defecate is ignored, it subsides until more feces enter the rectum. Individuals delay defecation for several reasons: childhood training practices, the urge to defecate occurring at a socially unacceptable time, uncomfortable or unclean toilet facilities, and confinement to bed because of illness or other disability. When defecation becomes convenient,[8] the individual can stimulate the defecation reflex by taking a deep breath and contracting the abdominal muscles. This action forces feces into the rectum, eliciting new reflexes. Individuals who consistently ignore the urge to defecate often develop chronic constipation, because voluntarily stimulated reflexes are not as effective as those that occur naturally.[6] Feces that remain in the colon and rectum become increasingly dry, hard and difficult to pass as water continues to be reabsorbed.

Constipation

Constipation is a symptom that may indicate a number of diseases, including irritable bowel syndrome (IBS), Hirschsprung's disease, and diabetes mellitus. The outcomes of Constipation include fecal impaction, hemorrhoids, and anal fissure. Constipation has also been associated with cancer of the colon and rectum, especially in women.[4]

The term *constipation* has a variety of meanings, and a standard definition is lacking. Physicians and researchers tend to define Constipation according to stool frequencies that fall below the normal range of three stools per week. Patients, on the other hand, are more likely to define Constipation according to the amount of straining associated with defecation and the consistency of stools, that is, dry or hard.[17] Others describe themselves as constipated when they have a feeling of incomplete stool evacuation.

Studies have indicated that the size of fecal matter is not a reliable measure of Constipation, because stool size is influenced by anorectal structures and the forces of gravity during defecation.[4] The weight of the fecal mass is an unreliable measure, because fecal mass weight varies according to geographical location and age of the

individual.[4] In addition, both normal stool consistency and subjective ratings vary widely. Consequently, stool frequency is the easiest parameter to quantify.

Most cases of Constipation result from habitual neglect of the urge to defecate. Constipation may also be associated with psychogenic, neurogenic, muscular, or mechanical disorders. Transient constipation often follows diagnostic procedures that include the use of barium.

Psychogenic or psychological causes of Constipation are characterized by the voluntary delay of defecation. Voluntary delay of defecation may occur for several reasons: emotional disturbances, childhood training practices, unacceptable time or location for defecation, unacceptable or unavailable toilet facilities, confinement to bed because of illness or other disability, or pain on defecation because of hemorrhoids or other anal disorders. If the delay occurs repeatedly, the defecation reflex may cease to function.

The relationship between emotions and bowel habits is not well understood.[4] Findings that have been documented indicate a relationship between personality and quantity of stool produced. For example, healthy, outgoing individuals with positive self-esteem tend to have an increased frequency of stool production, and their stools tend to be heavier than the stool of those with low self-esteem. The increased intestinal tone that accompanies stressful situations is believed to interfere with peristalsis, resulting in Constipation. Stressful situations can range from physical pain to difficult situations. In addition, a depressed individual may develop Constipation because of anorexia, which results in a decrease in the intake of dietary fiber and fluids.

Neurogenic causes of Constipation involve the spinal cord. Central nervous system lesions above the first lumbar vertebral segment and trauma to the cauda equina are associated with Constipation.[4] Hirschsprung's disease is a neurogenic disorder that causes Constipation resulting from absent neurons in a segment of the colon. Lesions on the spinal cord can destroy efferent or afferent nerves, interfering with the defecation reflex. The afferent (sensory) stimulus is initiated by accumulations of stool in the rectum. If the afferent stimulus does not reach the brain or if there is no efferent (motor) response, defecation will not occur.

Muscle weakness occurs secondary to a number of conditions, including emphysema, pregnancy, obesity, and ascites. As a result, the rectum is constantly distended with feces, and the individual becomes less aware of the rectal fullness. Bowel movements are less frequent and require more downward pressure, leading to the development of hemorrhoids or anal fissures. The individual then avoids defecation because of the fear of pain, initiating a vicious circle.

Mechanical causes of constipation are related to a physically abnormal bowel content or to an obstructed bowel lumen. Narrowing of the lumen results from neoplasms, inflammatory lesions, and specific disorders affecting the colon, such as intussusception, volvulus, or hernia. Occasionally, the individual may avoid defecation because of painful hemorrhoids, fissures, or abscesses. Constipated persons have been found to have a more acute anorectal angle, which may increase resistance to defecation.[19]

In addition to psychogenic, neurogenic, muscular, and mechanical causes, certain drugs are known to contribute to the development of Constipation. Opiates and meperidine compounds increase the tone of the small intestine and colon. Anticholinergic drugs, such as atropine, decrease motility in the colon through their effect on the parasympathetic nerves. Antacids containing aluminum are also implicated. Laxative abuse can lead to muscular atony and subsequent difficulty with defecation, leading to further laxative abuse. The seriousness of laxative abuse is evident when one realizes that laxative consumption in the United States cost an estimated $368 million in 1982.[4] Additional causes of Constipation include limited fluid intake, insufficient dietary roughage, lack of exercise, inadequate time for complete defecation, pregnancy, the luteal phase of menstruation, and long-distance travel.

Inadequate fluid intake results in stools that are hard and dry. When the body lacks fluid (because of lack of intake or increased losses), the colon compensates by increasing the amount of water absorbed from stool. Dietary fiber helps to increase the water content of stool, resulting in stool that is softer and easier to pass. Insufficient dietary roughage will produce a fecal mass that is dry and difficult to pass. Physical activity helps stimulate peristalsis in the colon. Therefore decreased exercise levels will increase the time between bowel movements. Inadequate time for defecation may result in unnecessary straining, with resultant hemorrhoids and fissures, and incomplete evacuation of stool. Elevated progesterone levels during pregnancy and the luteal phase of menstruation contribute to constipation by prolonging the transit time of gastrointestinal contents.

Perceived and Colonic Constipation

Perceived Constipation and Colonic Constipation are two recently developed diagnoses under the nursing diagnosis category Elimination Pattern. These new diagnoses were adopted at the Eighth National Conference of the North American Nursing Diagnosis Association (NANDA) held in March, 1988.[2]

The patient with Perceived Constipation may have a normal bowel elimination pattern, but he or she perceives it as abnormal. The factors contributing to this diagnosis may be a lack of knowledge about normal bowel function and variations in bowel elimination patterns. Other factors contributing to Perceived Constipation are cultural and family health beliefs and impaired thought processes. The effects of the overuse of laxatives are discussed earlier in this section.

Colonic Constipation results from the lack of dietary intake of fluids and fiber, inadequate physical activity, the lack of privacy during defecation, a change in daily routine, chronic use of medication and enemas, or stress and metabolic problems (for instance, hypothyroidism, hypocalcemia, or hypokalemia).

III

Diarrhea

Definitions of Diarrhea are numerous and varied, but most focus on the consistency of stool (watery or semisolid), the frequency of stool, increased stool weight, or a combination of these. Although most cases are mild and self-limiting, diarrhea can be a serious health problem. It is the leading cause of death for children under 4 years of age.[15] Diarrhea is also a serious problem for adults, because the loss of fluids and electrolytes can result in life-threatening hypovolemic shock.

Diarrhea occurs when the absorptive capacity of the colon is exceeded,[1] resulting in stool that is less formed and more liquid. The maximum quantity of fluid that can be absorbed by the colon daily ranges from 4.5 to 5 liters.[1] The absorptive capacity of the colon may be exceeded for several reasons: increased fluid load from the ileum because of inflammation or infection such as regional enteritis; deficiency of a digestive enzyme, such as lactase, leading to increased concentration of osmotically active lactose, which pulls fluid into the bowel lumen; ingestion of a solute that cannot be absorbed, such as magnesium sulfate (Epsom salts); increased secretion resulting from bacterial or viral toxins; an ANS dysfunction, which causes a disruption in intestinal motility and absorption; and emotional stress.

There are several approaches to the categorization of Diarrhea. A convenient and common approach is to use the categories *acute* and *chronic*. Each of the causes of Diarrhea previously mentioned can be subsumed under these two categories. Some disorders, such as salmonellosis, amebiasis, and ulcerative colitis, may cause both acute and chronic diarrhea.

Acute Diarrhea has a sudden onset, is self-limiting, and is usually of short duration, lasting from 24 to 48 hours. Etiological factors include infectious agents (viruses, bacteria and parasites), drug reactions, dietary intake, and spices, e.g., MSG. Heavy metal poisoning and fecal impaction are other etiologic factors. Most cases of acute diarrhea are caused by enterotoxins from microorganisms such as viruses, noninvasive bacteria, and protozoa. The viral agents most commonly associated with Diarrhea are the rotavirus and the Norwalk virus. In young children, the rotavirus is implicated, but adults and older children are commonly affected by either the rotavirus or the Norwalk virus. Bacteria-induced Diarrhea may occur secondary to ingestion of food that is not maintained at the proper temperature or is improperly prepared. The protozoan *Giardia lamblia* is spread through ingestion of water contaminated by the organism.

Drug-induced diarrhea most commonly results from antibiotic therapy. Antibiotics such as ampicillin, cephalosporins, or tetracyclines produce an inflammation of the colon, because the bacterium *Clostridium difficile* proliferates in the colon when the normal bacterial flora are destroyed by the antibiotic. Other drugs that can produce acute diarrhea include colchicine, quinidine, antacids containing magnesium, and antimetabolites used in cancer chemotherapy; cathartic abuse may also cause acute diarrhea.[6]

Diarrhea is considered chronic when it has persisted for several weeks or months regardless of the pattern (that is, constant or intermittent).[6] There are three categories for the etiologies of chronic diarrhea: decreased absorption, increased secretion, and motor disturbances. In some disorders, such as Crohn's disease, all three problems exist. The location of the problem can be either the small intestine (for instance, celiac disease or pancreatic insufficiency) or the colon (such as ulcerative colitis or amebiasis). The individual with chronic diarrhea often has accompanying findings that may help confirm the diagnosis. Associated findings can include weight loss from conditions that cause anorexia; intestinal obstruction resulting in postprandial pain and decreased food intake; malabsorption; arthritis, which may accompany Crohn's disease; systemic lupus erythematosus (SLE); ulcerative colitis; skin manifestations; fistulas; and nausea, vomiting, chills, and fever.

Anything that interferes with the absorption of fluids and other contents in the small intestine can result in excessive stool production. Malabsorption primarily involves water, fat, protein, carbohydrates, or a combination of these. There may also be problems in uptake and losses of certain vitamins and other trace elements. Decreased absorption may result in osmotic diarrhea, a type of diarrhea caused by an overabundance of water-soluble molecules in the lumen. Etiologic factors include lactose or sucrose intolerance, or the individual may ingest a poorly absorbed solute, such as magnesium sulfate (Epsom salts) or lactulose. If the patient receives nothing by mouth or avoids the offending solute, osmotic diarrhea ceases.

Secretory diarrhea occurs secondary to secretions in the lumen that interfere with water absorption. Fasting has no effect on secretory diarrhea. Many infectious diarrheas are secretory. The presence of excess bile acids or fatty acids in the chyme entering the colon can also cause secretory diarrhea. Because bile salts are absorbed in the ileum, excess bile salts are found when disease affects the ileum or when bacterial overgrowth occurs in the small bowel.

Diarrhea that occurs secondary to motor disturbances is usually related to dysfunction of the ANS. Alterations in muscular innervation and transit time may result in hypomotility and subsequent bacterial overgrowth.[16] Irritable bowel syndrome (IBS) is a disorder of intestinal motility in which increased contractility of both muscular layers of the colon creates Diarrhea and Constipation. It is more common in women than in men, with its onset during the second and third decades of life. IBS rarely begins after the age of 35. Manifestations of IBS usually begin after meals through the initiation of the gastrocolic reflex. The individual experiences low-volume diarrhea with mucus in the stools, alternating with constipation. The individual often complains of pain in the lower left quadrant, abdominal distention, and a feeling of incomplete evacuation of the bowels. IBS is episodic and is often associated with emotional or physical stress.

Bowel Incontinence

Bowel Incontinence is an embarrassing disorder that may be difficult to identify without a thorough patient history. Continence is maintained by a balance between neurological and muscular activity of the lower bowel. It requires the ability to sense rectal filling and distinguish the nature of rectal contents, the ability of the rectum and distal colon to store feces, and the ability of the internal and external anal sphincters to control defecation.

Two common causes of fecal incontinence are fecal impaction and neurogenic factors. Other causes include neoplasms, inflammatory bowel disease, diverticular disease, gastroenteritis, weakness of the pelvic floor, rectal prolapse, anorectal procedures, and injuries sustained during childbirth.

Fecal impaction is a common, treatable cause of fecal incontinence, especially in the elderly. Constant overdistention of the rectum with feces eventually results in a decreased awareness of the urge to defecate. The stool becomes dry and hard and accumulates in the rectum. The resulting incontinence is caused by liquid stool that makes its way around the impacted fecal mass. This type of incontinence may also be termed paradoxical diarrhea.[6]

Neurogenic influences on the bowel are similar to those affecting the bladder. A neurogenic bowel occurs in persons with a damaged cerebral cortex caused by dementia or focal lesions. Injury of spinal cord segments T1 to T12 results in incontinence because voluntary control of abdominal muscle contraction and the subsequent contraction of the rectal wall may be lost. If the injury involves cord segments S3 to S5, incontinence will result because of the loss of sphincter tone and reflex activity.

Dementia accompanied by personality changes or altered mental functions may result in temporary or chronic Bowel Incontinence. Focal lesions, such as cerebral hemorrhage or infarct that leads to cerebrovascular accident (CVA) with aphasia, predispose some patients to incontinence. In this instance, incontinence results because the patient is unable to communicate his or her need to defecate. An unconscious patient will also be incontinent because he or she is unable to recognize the urge to defecate and has no muscular control.

ASSESSMENT: ALTERED BOWEL ELIMINATION

The manifestations of altered bowel elimination (Constipation, Diarrhea, and Incontinence) are related to numerous medical diagnoses and can have profound physiological and psychological effects. Each manifestation affects the body differently, depending on the subsystems involved.

Constipation does not commonly result in life-threatening complications, but chronic constipation may eventually progress to fecal impaction and other anorectal disorders, such as hemorrhoids, fissures, and rectal prolapse. Fecal impaction develops over time. As feces continue to enter the rectum, the fecal mass increases in size. Subsequent changes in reabsorption of fluid from the GI tract occur, depending on the extent of the fecal accumulation. The end result is a dry, hard fecal mass that cannot be passed. Hemorrhoids and fissures result from the constant downward pressure exerted against fecal accumulations in the rectum. Rectal prolapse occurs secondary to decreased sensitivity to rectal distention, decreased contractility of the pelvic muscles involved in defecation, diminished muscular tone, and the reduced sphincteric tone that results from prolonged distention of the anal canal. Pruritus ani (rectal itching) is an uncomfortable symptom associated with chronic constipation. Pruritus ani results from poor anal hygiene, perspiration and maceration of perianal tissue, or infection with pinworms or fungi.

Diarrhea can result in a serious loss of body fluids and electrolytes. GI secretions are rich in sodium, potassium, chloride, and bicarbonate. Decreased levels of these electrolytes result in altered cardiovascular function, altered neurological function, and fluid imbalance. Cardiac dysrhythmias, hypotension, dehydration, and flaccid paralysis can also result from decreased electrolyte levels. Alterations in fluid balance result when large quantities of fluid are lost from the body and not reabsorbed. Metabolic acidosis can result from severe diarrhea because of the loss of bicarbonate. Rapid fluid loss from severe diarrhea can lead to hypovolemic shock and finally death if the fluid loss occurs over a short time.

The effects of incontinence are both physiological and psychological. If the patient is aware of his or her environment, then it is extremely embarrassing to find that he/she has no control over bowel elimination. In fact, many patients with incontinence originally complain of diarrhea because they are ashamed to admit their incontinence. The fecal soiling that occurs with incontinence is demeaning, often causing the patient to lose self-esteem and feel ashamed. In addition to the psychological effect, physiological problems can result from fecal incontinence. The major concern is skin irritation and breakdown. The consequences of skin breakdown are numerous, including pain and discomfort for the patient and an increased work load for the nurse. In addition, female patients may develop urinary tract infections because of the proximity of the urethra to the anus.

Data collected during the assessment serves as the basis for identifying etiological factors, formulating nursing diagnoses, and planning interventions. Defining characteristics of altered bowel elimination can be indicated by both subjective and objective data. A thorough history of the patient's past and present bowel elimination pattern provides subjective data. Objective data are obtained during the physical examination and from diagnostic tests. Obtaining an accurate history is crucial because treatment measures are determined by the cause of the problem. Some patients may only need education, whereas others will require more extensive interventions.

Results of the physical examination and diagnostic tests are the source of objective data. Privacy must be maintained to minimize embarrassment and ensure patient cooperation. The physical examination should begin with the vital signs. An increased temperature and heart rate may indicate infection, whereas a decreased blood pressure may signal fluid losses. The abdomen should be assessed for bowel sounds, distention, ascites, or the presence of a mass. A rectal examination is also important, because many rectal cancers and other lesions lie low in the rectum and may be missed by a barium enema. A rectal examination may also reveal a common cause of diarrhea: fecal impaction. Normally the rectum is free of stool. The presence of stool in the rectum indicates constipation. At the time of the rectal examination, the perianal region should be examined for fissures, abscesses, fistulas, and hemorrhoids. Any stool that remains on the examiner's glove should be assessed for blood (including occult blood), color, odor, and consistency. Diagnostic tests and procedures include stool examination, measurement of serum electrolytes, proctosigmoidoscopy, barium enema, and colonoscopy.

Assessment of the patient with an alteration in elimination can be organized using the 11 functional health patterns as a guide. A review of assessment data will be discussed within this framework.

Health Perception—Health Management Pattern. The first step in assessing the patient with altered bowel elimination (Constipation, Diarrhea, and Incontinence) is to have the patient describe the symptoms in his/her own words. This gives the clinician an accurate picture of the patient's perception of the problem. If a change in the pattern of elimination has occurred, it should be described in terms of what has happened, that is, how the pattern has changed. Is there more frequent or less frequent stool? More liquid or harder stool? Stool that is difficult to pass?

The nurse should determine what self-treatment measures have been implemented, such as taking medications or modifying the diet. Use of laxatives and prescription drugs such as quinidine or codeine can lead to Constipation, while antimetabolites used in cancer chemotherapy, antibiotics, and antacids may cause Diarrhea.

It is also important to assess the presence of risk factors and previous illnesses that may influence the current findings. A history of disorders such as Crohn's disease, ulcerative colitis, diabetes mellitus, adrenal insufficiency, hypoparathyroidism, or trauma to the spinal cord should be identified.

Nutritional—Metabolic Pattern. Alterations in the pattern of bowel elimination are often associated with changes in the patient's diet. Therefore, it is important to assess the patient's dietary intake to identify possible etiological factors. Di-

arrhea that develops within 12 hours after a meal is often caused by ingestion of food contaminated with staphylococcal exotoxins.[6] Alcohol consumption is also associated with diarrhea. Constipation results from a lack of dietary fiber (e.g., fruits and vegetables) and fluids in the diet and may result in a decreased appetite. Older adults are at risk for Constipation because improperly fitted dentures or lack of dentures make chewing high-fiber foods difficult. They may also lack sufficient income to purchase appropriate foods. Older adults are also at risk for Diarrhea because of intolerance of certain nutrients, such as lactose, or inability to digest foods, including fruits and vegetables.[21]

Elimination Pattern. Because diarrhea and constipation are individually defined, the patient's normal pattern of elimination must be determined in order to evaluate the presence of an actual alteration. The number of stools passed daily and the presence of associated symptoms such as pain, abdominal cramping, urgency, and frequency should be assessed. Patients with diarrhea should be asked to estimate the volume of stool passed at each movement or for each day.

Requesting the patient to describe the amount of stool passed in terms such as a teaspoon, tablespoon, or cup may help to quantify the amount of stool output. The ability to control bowel elimination should be assessed carefully. Incontinence is embarrassing and difficult to discuss, and many patients do not share this information without encouragement. Whenever possible a stool sample should be observed.

Activity—Exercise Pattern. The patient's ability to control defecation is related to his/her activity level, exercise pattern, and muscle strength. The nurse must assess the patient's ability to get to and use the toilet or commode and determine whether bedridden patients can use the bedpan. Patients who cannot get to the toilet or commode are at risk for constipation and incontinence. Because colonic motility increases with physical activity, it is important to determine the patient's level of physical activity. Individuals experiencing prolonged periods of immobility are at increased risk for constipation. The nurse must also assess the usual activity pattern, including recreational and leisure activities of the patient. Travel to countries with poor sanitation may be a factor in the development of diarrhea and constipation.

Sleep-Rest Pattern. Alterations in elimination may interfere with the sleep-rest pattern of patients. In addition, the use of sedatives to promote sleep may be associated with constipation.

Cognitive—Perceptual Pattern. Lack of sensation in the rectal area may be associated with incontinence. Individuals with hemorrhoids or anal fissures may delay defecation to avoid pain. The patient's knowledge of normal variations in patterns of bowel elimination must be determined. Confused patients may ignore the urge to defecate. Patients with Alzheimer's disease and organic brain disorders will have difficulty learning new information to change bowel elimination behaviors.

Self-Perception–Self-Concept Pattern. Anxiety, depression, and stress are related to altered bowel elimination. Persons who are constipated or incontinent may feel ashamed, causing them to limit their interaction with others. They may not talk about these alterations without encouragement.

Role-Relationship Pattern. Altered elimination may interfere with role performance, especially incontinence. The nurse should assess the level of interference with role performance.

Sexuality-Reproductive Pattern. Constipation is associated with pregnancy and certain stages of the menstrual cycle. All three altered elimination patterns may interfere with intimacy. The patient should be asked about the effect of the problem on intimacy with his/her partner.

Coping-Stress Tolerance Pattern. The emotional sate of the patient influences the pattern of elimination. McLane and McShane[14] reported that respondents identified being upset or worried as precipitating the onset of constipation. Therefore the nurse should determine the presence of recent psychological stressful events. Older adults are particularly at risk because of the increased likelihood of experiencing stressful events such as widowhood, loss of independence, or retirement. Irritable bowel syndrome (IBS) is a disorder characterized by alternating constipation and diarrhea that is thought to be associated with stressful life situations.

Value-Belief Pattern. Attitudes about what constitutes a normal pattern of elimination are culturally based. If the patient equates the passage of one stool per day with health and normalcy, this will affect his/her definition of constipation and will guide the patient's response to it. Therefore it is important to determine the value attached to defecation.

Constipation, Perceived Constipation, and Colonic Constipation

Collecting objective data for the patient with Constipation includes stool examination, rectal examination, sigmoidoscopy, and bowel transit studies. Stool examination reveals a small and dry fecal mass. The stool should be examined for the presence of blood or mucus. A digital examination of the rectum will reveal fecal impaction or a rectal or pelvic tumor. The rectum may contain large amounts of stool, even immediately after defecation. During the rectal examination, the perianal region is examined for any fissure, abscess, fistula formation, or hemorrhoids.

The sigmoidoscopy and barium enema usually reveal no abnormalities. The presence of blood or mucus or a mucosal abnormality should be investigated further. A barium enema is indicated for individuals with intractable symptoms, older patients, or those with a recent change in bowel habits.

Bowel transit studies are indicated if there is no response to a high-fiber diet. Radiopaque markers are administered with breakfast, and an abdominal x-ray examination follows within 2 to 5 days. Normal subjects excrete some of the markers within 2 days and at least 80% of the markers in 5 days.

The patient with perceived constipation may have normal results for these diagnostic procedures, depending on the duration of the problem. The nurse must review the patient's diary of food intake, fluid intake, and bowel movements to identify potential causes. Prolonged use of laxatives may necessitate bowel retraining along with dietary modification.

CONSTIPATION
❖ Defining Characteristics

The presence of the following defining characteristics indicates that the patient may be experiencing Constipation:
- Decreased frequency of stool passage
- Hard, dry, small stools
- Decreased weight of stools
- Difficulty passing stools
- Straining to defecate
- Abdominal distention
- Pain with defecation
- Pruritis ani
- Feeling of incomplete bowel evacuation
- Feeling of rectal fullness
- Weak abdominal muscles
- Failure to respond to the urge to defecate
- Decreased appetite

❖ Related Factors

The following related factors are associated with Constipation:
- Pregnancy, menstruation
- Prolonged immobility
- Impaired neuromuscular function
- Medications (e.g., opiates, aluminum-based antacids, anticholinergics)
- History of poor eating habits
- Lack of or inadequate dietary fiber
- Inadequate fluid intake
- Inability to chew high-fiber foods
- Inattention to the defecation reflex
- Laxative abuse
- Overuse of enemas
- Lack of physical exercise
- Travel
- Lack of acceptable toilet facilities
- Lack of privacy for defecation
- Childhood training practices
- Anorexia
- Stress
- Grief or anger

❖ Related Medical/Psychiatric Diagnoses

The following are examples of related medical/psychiatric diagnoses for Constipation:
- Cerebrovascular accident
- Depression
- Diabetes mellitus
- Hirschsprung's disease
- Hypothyroidism
- Paralytic ileus
- Intestinal obstruction (mechanical or neurogenic)
- Spinal cord injury

PERCEIVED CONSTIPATION
❖ Defining Characteristics

The presence of the following defining characteristics indicates that the patient may be experiencing Perceived Constipation:
- Overuse of laxatives, enemas, or suppositories
- Expectation of a daily bowel movement
- Expectation of stool passage at the same time every day

❖ Related Factors

The following related factors are associated with Perceived Constipation:
- Lack of knowledge of normal bowel function
- Faulty appraisal of bowel elimination pattern
- Cultural and family health beliefs
- Impaired thought processes

❖ Related Medical/Psychiatric Diagnoses

The following are examples of related medical/psychiatric diagnoses for Perceived Constipation:
- Dementia
- Depression
- Laxative abuse

COLONIC CONSTIPATION
❖ Defining Characteristics

The presence of the following defining characteristics indicates that the patient may be experiencing Colonic Constipation:
- Decreased frequency of stool passage
- Hard and dry stool
- Straining to defecate
- Painful defecation
- Abdominal distention
- Palpable mass
- Rectal pressure
- Headache
- Abdominal pain
- Appetite impairment

III

❖ **Related Factors**

The following related factors are associated with Colonic Constipation:

- Inadequate fluid, dietary, or fiber intake
- Inadequate physical activity
- Metabolic problems (hypothyroidism, hypocalcemia, or hypokalemia)
- Immobility
- Lack of privacy for defecation
- Emotional disturbances
- Chronic use of medication and enemas (e.g., cathartics, iron)
- Stress
- Change in daily routine

❖ **Related Medical/Psychiatric Diagnoses**

The following are examples of related medical/psychiatric diagnoses for Colonic Constipation:

- Cerebrovascular accident
- Diabetes mellitus
- Hypocalcemia
- Hypokalemia
- Hypothyroidism
- Spinal cord injury

DIARRHEA

A stool examination should be done using a fresh stool specimen. The goal is to identify the causative agent so that an appropriate plan of intervention can be developed. Stool is analyzed for the presence of bacteria, ova, parasites, blood, leukocytes, fat, and meat fibers. In addition, a stool smear may be completed using Wright's stain to identify the presence of leukocytes, which indicates inflammation. Stool should also be tested for the presence of occult blood on at least three samples. (This is referred to as "stool for guaiac.")

Serum electrolytes (sodium, potassium, chloride, and bicarbonate) are assessed to determine the presence of fluid and electrolyte imbalances. A complete blood count, including levels of hemoglobin, hematocrit, white blood cells, differential white blood cells, red blood cells, and platelets, helps to identify inflammation and anemia. Evaluation of calcium, total protein, blood sugar,

and prothrombin time are also recommended.

A proctosigmoidoscopy is recommended to identify the presence of Crohn's disease, ulcerative colitis, rectal neoplasms, or laxative abuse. Stool specimens can be obtained and biopsies completed during the proctosigmoidoscopy. A biopsy identifies the presence of inflammatory disease and neoplasms. It is recommended that the proctosigmoidoscopy be completed before radiological studies and without special preparation so that the most accurate results can be obtained. Enemas may produce edema and excessive secretions or wash away the organisms causing the diarrhea.

A barium enema assists in the identification of mucosal abnormalities, such as ulcerations and edema; abnormalities of the bowel lumen, such as narrowing or dilation; and the presence of masses, diverticula, and fistulas. Colonoscopy allows for the visualization of the colon, proximal to the area reached by sigmoidoscopy. Finally, abdominal x-ray examinations identify the presence of distention and bowel obstruction.

❖ **Defining Characteristics**

The presence of the following defining characteristics indicates that the patient may be experiencing Diarrhea:

- Increased urgency and frequency of stools
- Increased frequency of stool passage and bowel sounds
- Loose liquid stools
- Change in color and odor of stools
- Anal irritation
- Abdominal pain or cramping
- Fluid and electrolyte imbalance

❖ **Related Factors**

The following related factors are associated with Diarrhea:

- Change in dietary intake
- Fecal impaction
- Tube feedings
- Antibiotic treatment
- Magnesium-based antacids
- Cathartic abuse
- Ingestion of contaminants
- Heavy metal ingestion

- Inflammation, irritation, or malabsorption of bowel
- Bacterial or viral toxins
- Protozoa
- Stress and anxiety

❖ **Related Medical/Psychiatric Diagnoses**

The following are examples of related medical/psychiatric diagnoses for Diarrhea:

Acute Diarrhea
- Diverticulitis
- Drug reaction
- Lactose intolerance
- Lead poisoning
- Infection with *Shigella, Salmonella, Campylobacter,* or *Giardia lamblia*

Chronic Diarrhea
- Acquired Immune Deficiency Syndrome
- Alcohol abuse
- Colon cancer
- Crohn's disease
- Hyperthyroidism
- Irritable bowel syndrome
- Lactase deficiency
- Ulcerative colitis

BOWEL INCONTINENCE

Obtaining objective data related to bowel incontinence begins with a rectal examination. During the digital examination, muscle strength (or weakness) can be assessed. To test muscle strength, the patient is asked to cough while the examiner observes the anal area. If stool leakage occurs during coughing, the problem is related to weak muscles. An electromyogram (EMG) is useful in locating specific areas of anal muscle weakness.

Loss of sensation in the anal area is another etiological factor of fecal incontinence. Stroking the skin near the anus with a piece of cotton should result in local contraction (the anal wink). If contraction does not occur, the defecation reflex is damaged. In addition, the presence of surgical scars in the anal area may provide clues to sphincter abnormalities. Assessment of the neurological system can also provide valuable information if the patient has a generalized neurological disorder or a disorder affecting the central spinal cord or brain. A barium enema is indicated to determine whether the incontinence is linked to inflammatory bowel disease.

❖ **Defining Characteristics**

The presence of the following defining characteristics indicates that the patient may be experiencing Bowel Incontinence:
- Fecal soiling of underwear
- Involuntary passage of stool
- Lack of awareness of urge to defecate
- Decreased sensation below spinal level of T1

❖ **Related Factors**

The following related factors are associated with Bowel Incontinence:
- Anal surgery
- Neuromuscular impairment
- Anal-rectal muscle weakness
- Laxative abuse
- Stress, anxiety
- Cognitive impairment

❖ **Related Medical/Psychiatric Diagnoses**

The following are examples of related medical/psychiatric diagnoses for Bowel Incontinence:
- Anorectal surgery
- Cerebrovascular accident
- Dementia
- Depression
- Diabetic neuropathy
- Rectal cancer
- Rectal prolapse
- Spinal cord injury/disease
- Ulcerative colitis

NURSING DIAGNOSES

Examples of *specific* nursing diagnoses for Constipation are:
- Constipation related to lack of privacy in work setting restroom
- Constipation related to immobility secondary to hip fracture

III

III

- Constipation related to inattention to defecation reflex secondary to overscheduling appointments at work during morning
- Constipation related to inability to chew high-fiber foods secondary to poorly fitted dentures

Examples of *specific* nursing diagnoses for Perceived Constipation are:

- Percieved Constipation related to belief that lack of a daily bowel movement is a sign of constipation
- Perceived Constipation related to impaired thought processes resulting in inability to recall recent bowel defecation pattern

Examples of *specific* nursing diagnoses for Colonic Constipation are:

- Colonic Constipation related to inadequate daily fluid intake
- Colonic Constipation related to decrease in usual physical activity routine secondary to hypothyroidism

Examples of *specific* nursing diagnoses for Diarrhea are:

- Diarrhea related to antibiotic treatment with ampicillin
- Diarrhea related to ingestion of sauce with milk base secondary to lactose intolerance
- Diarrhea related to intake of poultry contaminated with salmonella

Examples of *specific* nursing diagnoses for Bowel Incontinence are:

- Bowel Incontinence related to anal-rectal muscle weakness secondary to recent anorectal surgery.
- Bowel Incontinence related to neuromuscular impairment secondary to spinal cord injury.

PLANNING AND IMPLEMENTATION WITH RATIONALE

The overall goals of nursing interventions for the individual with altered bowel elimination are to help the patient regain his/her normal pattern of bowel elimination and to treat any accompanying psychological or physiological problems. The most effective treatment is the correction of the underlying cause.

Constipation, Perceived Constipation, and Colonic Constipation

The initial expected outcome for the patient with constipation is the identification of his/her normal pattern of bowel elimination. This outcome is accomplished by explaining the wide variations in normal patterns of bowel elimination and encouraging the patient to keep a diary describing the day and time for each bowel movement for 1 week. It is also helpful to include a description of the color, odor, and consistency of stool, whether straining occurred during defecation, whether there was complete or incomplete evacuation of stool, whether defecation was achieved through the use of laxatives or enemas, and the dietary intake. *These actions will help in determining whether the constipation is actual or perceived by providing a visual record of the bowel elimination pattern and the factors influencing it.*

The patient should spend at least 10 minutes after one meal daily, preferably breakfast, seated on the toilet. The nurse should explain the importance of responding to the urge to defecate, provide privacy, and allow adequate time for defecation. *Mass movements, which push fecal material into the rectum, frequently occur after breakfast. Sitting on the toilet (or commode) after a meal helps stimulate the gastrocolic reflex, which assists with defecation. When the urge to defecate is ignored, water is reabsorbed from the fecal mass, resulting in stool that is dry, hard, and difficult to pass. Attention to privacy creates a more relaxed atmosphere for the normal process of stool elimination. Lack of privacy may result in avoidance of defecation and persistent Constipation, especially in older adults.*

The patient with Constipation must modify his/her diet to include adequate amounts of bulk and fluids. Bulk can be added to the diet by increasing dietary fiber. Fiber is the unabsorbable element of food, found most abundantly in plants. Bacterial degradation of fiber enhances colonic motility. Fiber can be obtained by ingesting raw fruits and vegetables, and whole-grain cereals and bread.

❖ *NURSING CARE GUIDELINES: CONSTIPATION*

Nursing Diagnosis: Constipation

Expected Patient Outcomes	Nursing Interventions
The patient will identify his/her normal pattern of bowel elimination.	• Explain to the patient the wide variations of normal bowel elimination among individuals. • Encourage the patient to keep a diary of his/her bowel elimination pattern.
The patient will spend 10 minutes after one meal each day seated on the toilet.	• Explain to the patient the importance of responding to the urge to defecate when it occurs. • Provide privacy to the patient during defecation. • Allow adequate time for defecation
The patient will alter his/her diet to include adequate amounts of fiber and fluids.	• Encourage daily intake of foods high in fiber (e.g., whole-grain cereal and bread, fresh fruits and vegetables). • Encourage patient to take at least eight glasses of water daily. • Teach the patient to avoid highly refined cereals and breads (e.g., pastries and pasta). • Encourage the patient to keep a diary of foods eaten each day. • Caution the patient against the overuse of bran.
The patient will avoid straining to defecate.	• Explain the hazards of straining to defecate: hemorrhoids, anal fissures, and cardiac irregularities. • Administer stool softener as ordered.
The patient will engage in physical exercise for at least 15-20 minutes daily.	• Explain the importance of maintaining muscle tone. • Explain the relationship between exercise and intestinal motility. • Encourage the patient to walk at least 15 to 20 minutes daily.
The patient will identify the importance of avoiding laxative use.	• Teach the patient the hazards of laxatives (e.g., that constipation worsens because of muscular atony).
The patient will achieve a normal pattern of bowel elimination with normal consistency of stools.	• Monitor the pattern of bowel elimination. • Monitor the consistency of stool. • Maintain dietary and exercise modifications.

Bran is another recommended source of dietary bulk. Bran can be mixed with applesauce, juice, yogurt, or other food to make it more palatable. Highly refined foods such as pastries and "fast foods" should be avoided. In addition to bulk, an adequate fluid intake is necessary for proper bowel function. Fluid intake should be increased to one to two quarts per day. *The addition of fluids assists in reestablishing fluid and electrolyte balance. Bulk, in the form of bran, whole-grain cereals and breads, fresh fruits and vegetables, helps to increase the fluid content in stool, decrease the transit time in the colon, increase the weight of stool, normalize stool consistency, and increase frequency of defecation.*

Straining at stool must be avoided. The nurse should explain the hazards of straining at stool and reinforce the importance of allowing adequate time for defecation, dietary modification, and responding to the urge to defecate. *Straining at stool may result in hemorrhoids, anal fissures, and cardiac irregularities.*

The patient with Constipation should increase the time allotted for physical activity to at least 15 to 20 minutes daily. The nurse should explain the importance of muscle tone for defecation and the relationship between exercise and intestinal motility. Walking is a good exercise that most individuals can do. Activity levels should be increased gradually, and the nurse should encourage the patient to focus on strengthening the abdominal muscles. *Physical exercise increases colonic motor activity and speeds transit time.[19] It also increases circulation to the bowel and promotes digestion and peristalsis. Physical exercise may also assist in stimulating the gastrocolic reflex, increase the appetite, and enhance general feelings of well-being. Increased colonic motility facilitates the passage of stool.*

The overuse of laxatives has an adverse effect on the bowel elimination pattern. *Laxatives may aggravate Constipation because they may damage the myenteric plexus, resulting in muscular atony and interfering with defecation.*

The final expected outcome for the patient with Constipation is the achievement of a normal bowel elimination pattern with normal consistency of stools. The nurse monitors the pattern of elimination and the consistency of stools. Previous interventions such as dietary modification and exercise are maintained. Achievement of a normal pattern of elimination improves the patient's well-being and diminishes the complications and discomfort associated with Constipation.

Patients who are constipated because of stool impaction may need to be disimpacted if other approaches (such as enemas and laxatives) are not successful. Some individuals may benefit from stool softeners such as docusate sodium (Colace) and docusate calcium (Surfak). These products are surface-wetting agents that soften stool for easier passage by allowing water to penetrate the fecal mass. Persons receiving stool softeners should be encouraged to maintain their fluid intake and continue with a high-fiber diet. Kallman[10] reported that 86% of institutionalized elders with Constipation responded to this regimen.

Diarrhea

The goals of care for the patient with Diarrhea are to decrease the number and frequency of stools passed and to prevent or correct fluid and electrolyte imbalances. Although most cases of Diarrhea are mild,[20] the patient with Diarrhea is at risk for the development of dehydration, cardiac dysrhythmias, hypovolemic shock, and eventually death. Expert nursing care is required to avoid these life-threatening complications.

The first expected outcome for the patient with Diarrhea is a decreased frequency of bowel elimination. This can be accomplished through oral intake of glucose and electrolytes. Oral rehydration therapy (ORT) is becoming the preferred method of treating fluid and electrolyte losses.[20] The nurse should encourage oral intake of up to 2000 ml daily, even in patients experiencing nausea and vomiting.[9] Patients with fever should increase their fluid intake to 3000 ml. Small, frequent sips of cool liquids are recommended. The type of fluid administered is determined by the severity of the diarrhea and the age of the patient. Adults respond to Gatorade or nondiet, decaffeinated soft drinks alternated with nonfat chicken broth. Children may respond to lemonade or fruit punch. Prune juice, milk, milk products, and concentrated sweets should be avoided. When Diarrhea subsides, soft foods such as bananas, rice, potatoes, skinless chicken, cooked carrots, toast, and soda crackers may be introduced. *Glucose and electrolyte intake is necessary to replace fluids and electrolytes lost in the diarrhea stool. Cool liquids are preferred because cold liquids stimulate the bowel and could exacerbate the Diarrhea. Gatorade and other recommended liquids are a good source of sodium and potassium. Liquids are taken in small amounts to assure their*

❖ *NURSING CARE GUIDELINES: DIARRHEA*
Nursing Diagnosis: *Diarrhea*

Expected Patient Outcomes	Nursing Interventions
The patient will have decreased frequency of bowel elimination and will evacuate stools of normal consistency.	• Encourage oral intake of liquids high in glucose and electrolytes. • Provide chilled, but not cold, liquids. • Gradually introduce nonstimulating foods (e.g., toast, crackers) • Eliminate milk, caffeine, alcohol, and raw vegetables from the patient's diet.
The patient's fluids and electrolytes will be maintained within normal limits: sodium (Na): 135-145 mEq/L, potassium (K): 3.5-5.0 mEq/L, chloride (Cl): 23-30 mEq/L, and bicarbonate (HCO_3): 97-107 mEq/L.	• Assess serum electrolytes, skin turgor, and mucous membranes. • Weigh the patient daily. • When able, increase the fluids that the patient receives by mouth to 2500 ml daily.
The patient's skin will be intact without redness or breakdown.	• Practice meticulous skin care with mild soap and water. • Use commercial skin cleansing products as indicated. • Apply petroleum jelly or A&D ointment to protect the skin. • Keep the bedside commode within easy reach. • Apply Tucks wipes as ordered for comfort.
The patient will establish effective patterns of coping.	• Assist patient in identifying stressful life situations. • Teach the patient stress-reducing techniques (e.g., deep breathing, getting adequate rest, meditating, or taking medication as needed).

absorption. Large quantities of fluid may exacerbate Diarrhea.

A second expected outcome for the patient with Diarrhea is to maintain the fluid and electrolyte values within normal ranges. The nurse must monitor serum electrolyte values, assess skin turgor and mucous membranes for signs of dehydration, and monitor the patient for altered vital signs, particularly heart rate and rhythm. Daily weights assist in determining fluid gains and losses. *Monitoring fluid and electrolyte values is crucial because alterations in fluids and electrolytes can lead to life-threatening disorders. For example, hypokalemia may lead to cardiac dysrythmias, and fluid volume deficit may result in* *hypovolemic shock and hyponatremia.*

The patient with Diarrhea should have skin that is intact, clean, dry, and without redness. This outcome can be accomplished by implementing a skin-care regimen that includes frequent observation and prompt cleansing with mild soap and water after each loose stool. Commercial skin cleansers such as PeriWash or Hollister skin Cleanser emulsify stool for easier removal.[12] The skin should be patted dry and protective ointments or creams such as petroleum jelly or A&D ointment applied. A diet that is nutritionally sound with adequate amounts of protein will facilitate maintenance of intact skin. It is also important to avoid immobility, which will add to skin break-

III

❖ *NURSING CARE GUIDELINES BOWEL INCONTINENCE*
Nursing Diagnosis: Bowel Incontinence

Expected Patient Outcomes	Nursing Interventions
The patent patient will regain sphincter control.	• If appropriate, teach the patient strengthening exercises for abdominal and rectal muscles. • Begin bowel retraining program.
The patient will have decreased episodes of soiling.	• Encourage the patient to use abdominal and rectal muscle-strengthening exercises. • Offer the patient the bedpan or bedside commode after each meal.
The patient's stool will be of normal consistency.	• Encourage daily intake of dietary bulk and adequate fluid intake; psyllium products (Metamucil) may be indicated.
The patient's skin will remain intact.	• Cleanse the patient's skin after each bowel movement with warm, soapy water and dry carefully. • Maintain adequate nutritional intake. • Turn and position the patient every 2 hours. • Inspect the skin after each bowel movement. • Apply petroleum jelly or A&D ointment to protect the skin after each bowel movement.
The patient will regain a regular pattern of bowel elimination.	• Assess the usual pattern of bowel elimination. • Provide privacy to the patient during toileting.

down. *Skin care for the patient with Diarrhea is important because digestive enzymes and other substances in diarrheal stool can cause skin breakdown, placing the patient at risk for local and systemic infection. The very young and very old are particularly susceptible to infection. Keeping a bedside commode nearby assists in preventing accidents. Tucks wipes assist in cleaning the rectal area and are also soothing to irritated rectal skin.*

Patients who have an emotional basis for their Diarrhea must establish an effective pattern of coping. The nurse should assist the patient in identifying stressful life situations. The patient can then be taught stress-reduction techniques such as deep breathing exercises, meditation, and participating in diversional, relaxing activities. *Emotional stress increases intestinal motility, thereby contributing to diarrhea.*[3]

Bowel Incontinence

The nursing goal for the patient with Bowel Incontinence is to achieve control over bowel elimination. This goal will be unrealistic in cases where the patient is unconscious or mentally incompetent.

The first expected outcome for the incontinent patient is to regain sphincter control. This can be accomplished by implementing a bowel training program that should be maintained for at least 10 to 15 days.[13] A bowel training program includes increased fluid intake, warm or hot liquids meals, high-fiber foods, low-fat or fat-free foods, increased physical activity, abdominal and rectal strengthening exercises, establishing a regular time for defecation, and biofeedback. Laxatives and suppositories may be indicated for persons with spinal cord injury. The patient should be encouraged to keep a daily record of bowel elimination and dietary intake. *Increasing fluid intake helps normalize the consistency of stool, warm liquids stimulate the gastrocolic reflex, and fat is avoided because it delays the gastrocolic reflex and slows digestion. Abdominal exercises increase muscle strength and facilitate fecal evacuation. Rectal muscle strength enhances external sphincter control. Biofeedback provides sensory and visual feedback regarding anal sphincter activity and increases awareness of rectal distention. Laxatives and suppositories stimulate the gastrocolic reflex and relax the anal sphincters.*[13]

The next expected outcome is for the patient to have decreased episodes of soiling. The bedpan should be offered after each meal and adequate time and privacy should be provided for defecation. Patients who are ambulatory may have a commode near the bed. The patient should be encouraged to continue the abdominal and rectal muscle exercises and maintain the bowel elimination diary. *Placing the bedpan or commode nearby helps prevent accidental soiling resulting from inability to hold stool for extended periods of time. It also facilitates toileting for patients with limited mobility and serves as a visual reminder to the patient. Placing the patient on the bedpan or commode after meals stimulates the gastrocolic reflex.*

The patient who is incontinent should have stool that is of normal consistency. This outcome is accomplished by dietary modification as discussed for the patient with constipation.

The patient's skin should remain intact, dry, and without redness. Nursing interventions for this outcome include proper skin care, adequate nutritional intake, and frequent position changes. All of these interventions have been discussed under Diarrhea.

The final outcome for the patient with Bowel Incontinence is the achievement of a regular pattern of elimination. It is important to assess the usual pattern of bowel elimination and to allow the patient privacy during toileting.

EVALUATION

The long-term goal of nursing interventions for the patient with any alteration in bowel elimination is to return to a normal pattern of bowel elimination. The stool should be normal in color, odor, frequency, and consistency. Associated symptoms should also be resolved. The patient should understand normal bowel function; he/she

---

❖ CASE STUDY WITH PLAN OF CARE: CONSTIPATION

Mrs. Audrey S. is an 82-year-old widow who lives alone. She regularly attends the health clinic for treatment of a long-standing case of coronary artery disease (CAD) and compensated congestive heart failure (CHF). She is complaining of pain on defecation, anal itching, and passage of a hard, dry stool once a week. She admits to using laxatives to stimulate her bowel movements. A medical history reveals that Mrs. S. has had degenerative arthritis for several years. Last year she underwent a successful left total hip replacement. She is a nonsmoker. She has had a long history of hypertension along with CAD and CHF. Both of Mrs. S.'s parents are deceased. Her mother died of heart disease, and her father died at the age of 95 of complications from a fractured hip. Mrs. S. has two daughters who live nearby, and a son who lives in another city.

She has four grandchildren whom she sees often. Mrs. S. sees her daughters at least two or three times a week. She is active in her church and in the local senior citizens' center. At home, Mrs. S. spends most of her time watching television, sewing, and working with her plants. She eats lunch at the senior citizens' center every weekday. She travels to the center by bus. She eats a small breakfast and has a light snack for dinner. She usually eats dinner with one of her daughters on Sunday. Mrs. S. has dyspnea on exertion when she "works too much." Her blood pressure is 170/86 mm Hg, pulse is 88/min, respiratory rate is 24/min, and her temperature is 98° F. Her heart rate is irregular. Her abdomen is slightly distended, and she is complaining of a feeling of fullness.

Continued.

III

PLAN OF CARE FOR MRS. AUDREY S.

Nursing Diagnosis: *Constipation Related to Laxative Abuse*

Expected Patient Outcomes	Nursing Interventions
Mrs. S. will identify her normal pattern of bowel elimination.	• Explain to Mrs. S. the wide variations in normal patterns of bowel elimination. • Assist Mrs. S. in identifying her usual pattern of bowel elimination.
Mrs. S. will spend 10 minutes after one meal each day seated on the toilet.	• Explain the importance of responding to the urge to defecate when it occurs. • Ensure that Mrs. S. has privacy during defecation.
Mrs. S. will alter her diet to include adequate amounts of fiber and fluids.	• Explain the importance of fiber in the maintenance of a regular bowel elimination pattern. • Encourage Mrs. S. to eat foods high in fiber (e.g., whole-grain cereal and bread, fresh fruits and vegetables, nuts, and seeds). • Explain the importance of avoiding highly refined cereals and breads (e.g., pastries and pasta). • Caution Mrs. S. against the overuse of bran. • Encourage Mrs. S. to drink 2500 ml of fluids daily.
Mrs. S.'s skin near the anal area will be intact and without pruritis.	• Stress the importance of cleansing the skin near the anus after each bowel movement, using warm, soapy water and patting dry carefully. • Teach Mrs. S. to inspect the anal area daily.
Mrs. S. will regain a regular pattern of bowel elimination.	• Assess Mrs. S.'s usual pattern of bowel elimination. • Encourage Mrs. S. to drink something warm at the same time each day. (Determine this time according to the usual bowel elimination pattern). • Stress the importance of maintaining adequate nutritional intake. • Encourage Mrs. S. to keep a record of each bowel movement (including time of day, consistency of stool, and whether the "full" feeling is resolved).
Mrs. S. will eliminate the use of laxatives.	• Explain to Mrs. S. the hazards of laxative abuse (e.g., muscle atony and increased difficulty with elimination). • Reinforce the importance of responding to the urge to defecate and the importance of adequate fiber and fluids in the diet.

should also understand that patterns of bowel elimination vary among individuals.

The nurse and the patient together will determine whether the goals of care have been met. Goals that have not been met must be revised. The patient should be reassessed to determine barriers to meeting the goals. Interventions will then be planned to remove those barriers. The nursing diagnosis may need revision, the patient may require reinforcement of previous education, or the goal may need to be revised. The nurse must remember that any of these conclusions may be reached through collaboration with the patient. The patient must acknowledge that the goal is important and attainable or the plan will be ineffective.

REFERENCES

1. Binder HJ: Pathophysiology of acute diarrhea, *Am J Med* 88:(Suppl)6a-4s, 1990.
2. Carroll-Johnson RM: *Classification of nursing diagnoses: proceedings of the Eighth Conference,* Philadelphia, 1989, JB Lippincott.
3. Cohen S, Snape WJ: Movement of the small and large intestine. In Sleisenger MH, Fordtran JS, editors: *Gastroin-*

testinal disease pathophysiology, diagnosis, and management, ed 4, vol 2, pp 1088-1105, Philadelphia, 1989, WB Saunders.

4. DeVroede G: Constipation. In Sleisenger MH, Fordtran JS, editors: *Gastrointestinal disease: pathophysiology, diagnosis and management,* ed 4, vol 1, pp 331-368, Philadelphia, 1989, WB Saunders.

5. Everhart JE and others: A longitudinal survey of self-reported bowel habits in the United States, *Digest Dis Sci* 34:1153-1162, 1989.

6. Goldfinger SE: (1991). Constipation and diarrhea. In Wilson J and others, editors: *Harrison's principles of internal medicine,* pp 256-259, New York, 1991, McGraw-Hill.

7. Groer MW, Shekleton ME: *Basic pathophysiology: a holistic approach,* ed 3, St Louis, 1989, Mosby–Year Book.

8. Guyton AC: *Textbook of medical physiology,* ed 8, Philadelphia, 1991, WB Saunders.

9. Harig JM, Ramaswamy K: Acute diarrhea in adults, *Postgrad Med* 86(8):131-140, 1989.

10. Kallman H: Constipation in the elderly, *Am Fam Phys* 27:179-184, 1983.

11. Kim MJ, McFarland GK, and McLane AM: *Pocket guide to nursing diagnosis,* ed 4, St Louis, 1991, Mosby–Year Book.

12. Lincoln R, Roberts R: Continence issues in acute care, *Nurs Clin North Am* 24:741-754, 1989.

13. Maas M, Specht J: Bowel incontinence. In Maas M, Buckwalter KC, and Hardy M, editors: *Nursing diagnosis and interventions for the elderly,* Menlo Park, Calif, 1991, Addison-Wesley Publishing.

14. McLane AM, McShane RE: Constipation. In Maas M, Buckwalter KC, and Hardy M, editors: *Nursing diagnosis and interventions for the elderly,* Menlo-Park, Calif, 1991, Addison-Wesley Publishing.

15. Porth CM: *Pathophysiology concepts of altered health states,* ed 3, Philadelphia, 1990, JB Lippincott.

16. Rogers AI: Answers to questions on diarrhea, *Hosp Med* 19:267, 1983.

17. Sandler RS, Drossman DA: Bowel habits in young adults not seeking health care, *Digest Dis Sci* 32:841-845, 1987.

18. Sandler RS, Jordan MC, and Shelton BJ: Demographic and dietary determinants of constipation in the U. S. population, *Am J Public Health* 80:185-189, 1990.

19. Sarna SK: Physiology and pathophysiology of colonic motor activity, part 2, *Digest Dis Sci* 36:998-1018, 1991.

20. Wadle KA: Diarrhea, *Nurs Clin North Am* 25(4):901-908, 1990.

21. Wadle KA: Diarrhea. In Maas M, Buckwalter KC, and Hardy M, editors: *Nursing diagnosis and interventions for the elderly,* Menlo Park, Calif, 1991, Addison-Wesley Publishing.

III

Altered Patterns of Urinary Elimination

Functional Incontinence

Stress Incontinence

Reflex Incontinence

Urge Incontinence

Total Incontinence

Urinary Retention

Altered Patterns of Urinary Elimination *is the state in which the individual experiences a disturbance in urine elimination.*[15]

Functional Incontinence *is the state in which an individual experiences an involuntary, unpredictable passage of urine. This occurs because of a nonurinary problem.*[15]

Stress Incontinence *is the state in which an individual experiences a loss of urine of less than 50 ml with increased abdominal pressure.*[15]

Reflex Incontinence *is the state in which an individual experiences an involuntary loss of urine, occurring at somewhat predictable intervals when a specific bladder volume is reached.*[15]

Urge Incontinence *is the state in which an individual experiences involuntary passage of urine soon after a strong sense of urgency to void.*[15]

Total Incontinence *is the state in which an individual experiences a continuous and unpredictable loss of urine.*[15]

Urinary Retention *is the state in which the individual experiences incomplete emptying of the bladder.*[15]

OVERVIEW
Altered Patterns Of Urinary Elimination

Urinary elimination starts with the complex blood-filtering and regulatory system of the kidneys. In this system, the water, electrolytes, and nonelectrolytes (such as glucose, amino acids, urea, uric acid, and creatinine) from blood plasma combine to form urine. Tubes (ureters) then convey the urine from the kidneys to the bladder. The lower urinary tract is composed of a storage receptacle (the bladder) and a drainage mechanism (the urethra and two sphincters).

Structurally, the bladder is composed of mucous membranes, connective tissue, and the detrusor muscle, which has the ability to expand and contract. Two sphincters, one internal and involuntary and the other external and voluntary, control the expulsion of urine into and through the urethra. The muscles of the pelvic floor surround part of the external sphincter. When the detrusor is relaxed and the sphincter closed, urine is stored. When the detrusor contracts and the sphincter relaxes, urine is eliminated.

This reciprocal relaxation and contraction relationship is controlled by a complex system of nerves. In an infant, voiding is a reflex action—stretch receptors in the bladder stimulate a sacral reflex that causes detrusor contraction. This is coordinated with sphincter relaxation through a micturition center that is speculated to be in the pons area of the brain.[25,34] As an infant develops, so does a parietal recognition center in the brain that allows for recognition of bladder fullness. Later the cerebral cortex develops an inhibitory center that allows for voluntary control of voiding. Therefore after toilet training, and given no unusual circumstances, a person can maintain voluntary control over urinary elimination.

Normal voiding is a cyclical event. As the bladder fills, tension increases on the walls. Threshold stretch receptors in the bladder wall and the proximal urethra send a signal to the sacral spinal cord micturition center. Parasympathetic impulses are sent back to the detrusor muscle, causing it to contract and the internal sphincter to relax. Meanwhile, this contraction causes nerve impulses to move up the spinal cord to the brain, alerting the person to a need to void. If the person is in an acceptable circumstance to void, the external sphincter is relaxed to allow the expulsion of urine; if not, the urge to void is suppressed. In the latter case, the external sphincter remains closed and, if the bladder is not overly full, the contractions may cease and the basal bladder tone pattern returns. If voiding does not occur, this cycle is repeated anytime from a few minutes to an hour later. With each round of the cycle, the urge becomes more powerful.

Normal urine output varies with the amount of input over any given time period. On the average, most persons urinate five or six times per day for a total of 1,500 ml. However, many factors influence urination, so wide variations from these numbers may be seen and may be within normal range. The term oliguria is used to describe urine output of less than 400 ml per day. Anuria refers to urine output of 100 ml or less over 24 hours. Polyuria describes a large volume of urine voided in a specified time.

On the average, urine is acidic with a pH of 6.0, although it can range from 4.5 to 8.0 in the normal adult. Concentration of urine or its specific gravity depends on fluid intake and the amount of solutes in the urine; on the average it is 1.010, but it can vary widely. Small amounts of protein may be excreted in the urine, but excess protein is not an expected finding in normal urine. Glucose and ketones are also not normally found in the urine.[3]

Normal urination is a painless process that is first stimulated when a person feels the urge to void. Then the stream of urine begins easily, flows with a steady pressure, and finally ends with the nearly complete emptying of the bladder. The voided urine is clear yellow with only a slight ammonia odor. After normal childhood toilet training, urination becomes voluntary. Any deviation from this set average is a suspected problem until some normal set of events, such as fluid depletion or excess, can explain the deviation.

Men and women differ slightly in urinary structures and voiding styles. The urethra is much

III

shorter in women. The prostate gland in men, while not directly part of urinary structures, is posterior to the bladder neck and, when enlarged, can exert pressure against the internal sphincter and urethra. In women the uterus, located above and behind the bladder, can exert pressure on the bladder. Men usually urinate standing up, whereas women squat or sit. In women the urethral meatus is located in proximity to the anus, sometimes making the migration of bacteria a problem.

Of the seven urinary elimination diagnoses, Altered Patterns of Urinary Elimination is the least specific. Because most of the urinary elimination problems for which nurses provide care relate to incontinence or retention, the more general diagnosis of Altered Patterns of Urinary Elimination will be made less frequently. When a patient's signs and symptoms correlate with one of the more specific nursing diagnoses, such as Urge Incontinence or Urinary Retention, that label would apply rather than the more general diagnosis of Altered Pattern of Urinary Elimination. However, instances may arise when a patient exhibits a urinary problem that is neither incontinence nor retention. In this event, the nurse should consider either labeling it with a diagnosis not yet on the NANDA list or using the diagnostic category of Altered Patterns of Urinary Elimination until a more specific diagnosis can be made.

Many problems could fall into the broad category of Altered Patterns of Urinary Elimination. Some patients with commonly experienced problems that might indicate an altered urinary pattern include pregnant women, who generally urinate frequently or feel the urge to urinate frequently because of uterine pressure on the bladder; men who have difficulty urinating unless they are in a standing position and have had a medical or surgical problem requiring them to be supine or prone; and children who are being toilet-trained and hold urine for long periods, urinate more frequently, resist wearing a diaper, or try to wait to urinate until they are wearing a diaper at night.

The clusters of data related to each problem would be classified as Altered Patterns of Urinary Elimination. In each of these cases, no concrete label on the NANDA nursing diagnosis list would describe the phenomenon observed. In these instances, some nurses would devise a concrete diagnostic label; others would refer to these problems as Altered Patterns of Urinary Elimination. Either approach would be acceptable at this time because the nursing diagnosis classification system is incomplete and continually developing to include more specific diagnoses.

Nurses must also be alert to situations in which a factor that may indicate an obvious alteration in elimination might actually be the result of another type of problem. For example, patients who have indwelling urinary catheters may experience discomfort, embarrassment, or a knowledge deficit. Such patients always have the potential to develop a urinary tract infection. Although this situation clearly indicates an alteration in urinary elimination, the overall problem is often better described using accepted nursing diagnoses such as High Risk for Infection, for Injury, Knowledge Deficit, or Body Image Disturbance. In such cases the indwelling catheter, rather than being the problem, causes other problems.

Beginning nurses may find it easier to use the broader diagnosis of Altered Patterns of Urinary Elimination, but with increasing expertise they will be able to discriminate between specific urinary problems and describe them concretely using more specific diagnoses.

All Types Of Incontinence

Incontinence is a very common problem, especially among elderly patients. There are wide differences in the reported figures on the prevalence of this problem. Most figures show that 40% to 60% of institutionalized patients and 15% to 30% of community-dwelling persons are incontinent.[28,35,41,45] One reason cited for differences in these figures is the various definitions of incontinence used by researchers.[45] Regardless of the diverse figures, however, it is clear that incontinence is a psychologically distressing, socially disruptive problem, especially for the elderly.

Incontinence has been studied extensively in recent years. The surge of interest in the topic is prompted by many factors, not the least of which is that incontinence is a common reason for nursing home admission.[31,43] Another factor is the cost of incontinence care, which is said to be approximately $10 billion per year[29,41] with the federal government paying $8 billion of that bill.[1]

So much attention is being paid to this costly problem that the federal government is placing importance on devising new policies. Federal guidelines now require standards of incontinence care for nursing home facilities. These guidelines specify assessment time and require retraining programs or other care be set up for incontinent patients.[51] Urinary incontinence in the adult continues to gain attention and has been the focus for development of one of the sets of guidelines being developed by a multidisciplinary group as an outgrowth of the 1989 Omnibus Budget reconciliation Act (OBRA). OBRA established the Agency for Health Care Policy and Research (AHCPR), which directs the development of guidelines for selected conditions, including incontinence.[36]

Incontinence is a complex problem. The accepted standard definition for this problem is "a condition in which involuntary loss of urine is a social or hygienic problem and is objectively demonstrable."[3] However, many different types of incontinence have been described. You will recall from the preceding discussion on normal voiding that when the detrusor muscle of the bladder is relaxed and the sphincters are closed, urine is stored in the bladder. When the detrusor contracts and the sphincters relax, urine is eliminated. This relaxation and contraction relationship is governed by the pressure changes of the filling, full, and empty bladder. Simply stated, continence depends on pressure in the urethra being higher than pressure within the bladder. Conversely, incontinence can occur when pressure in the urethra is lower than pressure within the bladder. Several factors can influence these pressures. Bladder pressure depends on bladder volume, intraabdominal pressure, and detrusor muscle tone. Urethral pressure depends on pelvic muscle tone, intraab-

dominal pressure, urethral and bladder neck muscle condition, and the thickness of urethral mucosa. Each of these factors depends on an intact nervous system and a functional environment that allows for toileting.

In the cycle of (1) a felt need to void, (2) holding urine, and (3) an increasing need to void, voiding is the inevitable outcome. Eventually, if voiding is not allowed, the bladder will distend so far that the intravesicular (bladder) pressure will overcome the intraurethral pressure and the external sphincter will relax; incontinence will result. In the normal person who is past toilet-training age, voiding is voluntary so that urine is expelled only at appropriate times in appropriate receptacles. When this does not occur and voiding becomes involuntary, incontinence occurs.

There are many classifications of incontinence, a variety of labels for each type, and lack of agreement on terms. Voith[55] proposed a set of labels useful for nursing, and these influenced the accepted North American Nursing Diagnosis Association (NANDA) classification. The five types of incontinence presently in the NANDA taxonomy are Functional, Stress, Reflex, Urge, and Total.

The essential differences among the five types of incontinence are presented in Table 8. This table can serve as a tool for determining which type of incontinence is present; it includes defining characteristics and related factors for the five types of incontinence. It should be noted that some patients have a combination of types of incontinence; for example, persons with urge incontinence also may have functional incontinence if their mobility is decreased.

Urinary Retention

Urinary Retention is diagnosed when a person has problems with bladder emptying. It may be manifested by a total inability to void, difficulty with starting a stream of urine, or incomplete bladder emptying. The difficulty may be transient, lasting for hours or days; long-term, lasting weeks or months; or permanent. Urinary Retention is potentially very serious: when the bladder

III

III

TABLE 8 Comparison of Characteristics of Five Types of Incontinence*

Characteristic	Functional	Stress	Reflex	Urge	Total
Character of voiding urge	Usually strong	Sudden and associated with increased abdominal pressure	None	Very strong	None
Amount voided	Moderate to large	Small	Moderate	Small, moderate, to large	Constant leakage
Nocturia	May be present	Possible, not usual	Always	Common	Always
Precipitating factors	Inability to reach receptacle	Increased intraabdominal pressure	Full bladder, unhibited bladder contraction/spasm	Sensation of full bladder, inability to reach toilet in time	Unpredictable
Awareness of incontinence	Aware	Aware	Unaware	Aware	Unaware
Frequency of urination	Variable	Increased	Regular intervals related to volume	Increased	Unpredictable and constant
Anatomical problem	Not urinary, but sensory, cognitive, mobility, or environmental defects	Increased urethrovesicular angle, sagging support structures, weak sphincter tone	Nerve pathway problems	Stretch receptor changes, reduced bladder capacity, detrusor overactivity	Sensorimotor nerve damage, no neuron control, fistulas
Related factors/causes	Altered environment, sensory deficits. cognitive deficits. mobility deficits, drug use, stool impaction, closed head injury, emotional illness	Obesity, gravid uterus, increased age, incompetent bladder outlet, weak pelvic muscles, over distention between voiding, jolting exercise (for instance, jogging)	Spinal cord injury, multiple sclerosis, spinal cord tumors, spondylosis, cerebral lesions	Abdominal surgery, catheter use, bladder infections, alcohol intake, caffeine use, increased fluid intake, increased urine concentration, overdistention of bladder, neurological disorders (cerebrovascular accident, incomplete supraspinal cord injury, multiple sclerosis, Parkinson's disease, brain tumors, trauma), Alzheimer's disease, cancer of bladder, urethritis	Neuropathy, neurological misfiring, surgery, trauma, spinal cord diseases, anatomical problems (fistula), severe neurological diseases

*References 15, 30, 34, 42, 49, 55.

III

is overdistended, urine may reflux through the ureters into the kidneys, causing renal damage. Persistent bladder overdistention also causes the detrusor muscle to decompensate. Incomplete bladder emptying allows urine to stagnate in the bladder, which predisposes to urinary tract infections and stone formation.

Urinary Retention is often described as a type of incontinence, because when the bladder does not empty completely urine may eventually overflow without control. Other terms used to describe patterns associated with Urinary Retention include obstructive incontinence, overflow incontinence, paradoxical incontinence, flaccid bladder, atonic bladder, detrusor hyporeflexia, and lower motor neuron incontinence.[30,56] Neurogenic bladder is a term often used to describe a variety of neurological dysfunctions of the bladder, including incontinence and retention. Voith and Smith,[56] who surveyed nurses in an effort to identify the signs and symptoms of Urinary Retention, concluded that Urinary Retention was a better term than overflow incontinence because the incontinence was actually a sign of the retention. Their data influenced the NANDA decision to use the term Urinary Retention as a nursing diagnosis accepted for testing and clinical use.[39]

Nurses should be aware of the various terms used to describe Urinary Retention and its associated phenomena. They need to evaluate their clinical practice and literature on the subject with openness to these variations. It is also important to have a clear idea of the definition of Urinary Retention so as not to confuse it with other urinary disorders. For example, in oliguria the kidneys produce less than normal urine volume, and in anuria no urine; therefore there is no urine in the bladder to be retained. When retention occurs, urine cannot be expelled because the bladder, the urethra, or surrounding structures are malfunctioning.

It is difficult to determine the actual incidence of Urinary Retention in the general population. Voiding difficulties or bladder emptying problems seem to be more common in elderly men than in women.[19,38] However, retention can be a problem for many patients, especially those with neurological or muscular problems or those who have undergone surgery. The onset of urinary retention may occur suddenly or may develop gradually over time. It may or may not be linked to a specific event such as surgery.

ASSESSMENT
Altered Patterns of Urinary Elimination

Because normal urinary elimination encompasses varied individual patterns, an assessment should begin with baseline data on the patient's usual urinary elimination pattern. Ask the patient about usual urinary patterns, including timing and frequency of voiding; the amount, color, and odor of urine; usual position during voiding; and any discomfort with voiding. Combine this description with patient data on usual fluid intake, including type, amount, and timing of input. All forthcoming data about the present or future situation can then be compared with this normal urinary pattern.

After this baseline has been established, ask the patient whether any changes in this pattern have occurred and, if so, what may have caused them. Very often the patient's own perspective will guide the nurse into logical areas of assessment, therefore saving time in data collection. Sometimes patients have perfectly simple reasons for Altered Patterns of Urinary Elimination. For example, a decreased urinary output with more concentrated urine may be the result of the patient's not drinking cola because the vending machine at work was out of order. When there is no such simple explanation, ask for descriptions of the change by prompting the patient to consider the following areas: pain or discomfort, frequency, hesitancy, urgency, incontinence, retention, amount, color, odor, concentration, or edema in any part of the body.

For a complete assessment, the nurse must consider family and patient history of urinary problems. Inquire about a history of renal disease, hypertension, diabetes, infectious diseases, congenital disorders, connective tissue diseases (such as lupus erythematosus), urinary or renal calculi, gout, urinary tract infections, or trauma. Ask women about their history of pregnancies and any associated urinary problems. A history of any of these can indicate risk factors or problems in urinary elimination. Because sexual and urinary structures are anatomically combined, one must also obtain a sexual profile of the patient, including amount and type of sexual activity and any discomfort or vaginal/penile infections. A significant question for women patients is whether they have any difficulty voiding after sexual intercourse.

Hygiene measures must also be considered. Women should be asked about their method of wiping after urination and bowel movements. A front-to-back wiping technique decreases the likelihood of fecal bacteria entering the urinary tract. Drug intake is another important assessment parameter. Ask the patient about all drug intake, including over-the-counter medications. Some drugs are toxic to the kidneys; others can change the characteristics of urine.

After the nurse assesses subjective data from the patient the nurse should collect objective data on the person's urination pattern. Percuss and palpate the abdomen to determine abdominal muscle tone and to check for bladder distention. Observe the patient voiding to determine the necessity of any special positions, appliances, or procedures and to note the patient's ability to use these things appropriately. Note fluid intake including the amount, timing, and type of intake. Compare this intake with output. Check the patient for edema, especially in dependent body parts. Finally, the urine itself should be examined for amount, color, odor, specific gravity, and pH. When laboratory urinalysis and cultures are available or indicated, check those results.

The box on p. 243 provides a summary of these assessment parameters. It should be used as a guide for a broad, baseline assessment of urinary elimination patterns.

❖ **Defining Characteristics**

The presence of the following defining characteristics indicates that the patient may be experiencing Altered Patterns of Urinary Elimination*:

- Dysuria
- Hesitancy
- Nocturia
- Urgency
- Edema
- Bladder distention
- Inability to urinate without special assists
- Frequency
- Incontinence
- Retention
- Change in amount, color, or odor of urine
- Decreased/increased force of stream

❖ **Related Factors**

The following related factors are associated with Altered Patterns of Urinary Elimination:

- Changes in fluid intake
- Anatomical obstruction
- Fecal impaction
- Indwelling urinary catheters
- Use of commode, bedpan or urinals
- Mechanical trauma
- Immobility
- Pregnancy
- Drug therapies
- Motor impairment
- General or spinal anesthesia
- Psychological disorders
- Age-related or developmental factors
- Cognitive or sensory impairments
- Emotional stress
- Lack of privacy
- Strange environment

❖ **Related Medical/Psychiatric Diagnoses**

The following are examples of related medical/psychiatric diagnoses for Altered Patterns of Urinary Elimination:

- Cerebral vascular accidents
- Circulatory disorders
- Connective tissue diseases
- Diabetes mellitus
- Infectious diseases
- Neuromuscular diseases
- Prostatic hypertrophy
- Renal disease
- Spinal cord injuries
- Urinary tract infections

NOTE: Altered Patterns of Urinary Elimination is a broad category. As such, the defining characteristics are broad. Whenever possible, the nurse should further check for specific signs and symptoms to see if a more specific diagnostic label could be applied.

❖ *GUIDELINES FOR ASSESSING URINARY ELIMINATION*

Subjective data

Usual urinary elimination pattern
  Timing, frequency
  Amount, color, odor of urine
  Position during voiding
  Discomfort with voiding
  Special assists (commode, bedpan, catheters, etc.)
Usual fluid intake
  Timing, amount, type of fluids
Recent changes in pattern
  Known related factors
  Pain, discomfort
  Frequency, hesitancy, urgency
  Incontinence, retention
  Urine amount, color, odor, concentration
  Edema
Family and personal history
  Renal disease, hypertension, diabetes
  Infectious diseases
  Congenital disorders
  Connective tissue diseases (e.g., lupus erythematosus)
  Neurological diseases (e.g., multiple sclerosis)
  Urinary or renal calculi, gout
  Urinary tract infections
Personal history
  Trauma
  Sexual problems, related infections, discomfort
  Drug intake (over-the-counter and prescription)
  Women: history of pregnancies and associated urinary problems, hygiene practices, method of wiping perineal area
  Men: history of prostate problems

Objective data

Abdominal muscle tone
Bladder distention
Amount, color, odor, specific gravity, pH or urine
Force of stream
Timing, frequency
Position during voiding
Special assists, ability to use
Fluid intake, amount, timing, type
Edema
Laboratory data: urinalysis, cultures

All Types of Incontinence

The nurse's goal in assessing patients for incontinence is to identify the specific signs or symptoms that are critical to differentiating the type of incontinence. The general guidelines for assessing urinary elimination patterns presented in the section on Altered Patterns of Urinary Elimination should be used. If incontinence is found, then this more specific assessment is in order. The nurse must first assess how long the incontinence has existed and consider any obvious change in the patient's health that correlates with the onset. If there is no clear correlation, such as a spinal cord injury, the next set of questions or observations should be directed at assessing for obvious characteristics of one or two types of incontinence. Stress Incontinence is perhaps one of the easiest to rule out. Does the incontinence occur only with an increase in intraabdominal pressure, such as sneezing, coughing, or strenuous exercise? If so, then Stress Incontinence is very likely. If not, the second easiest characteristic to eliminate is the patient's sense of urgency to void. If the urge is very strong, sudden, and usually uncontrollable, Urge Incontinence can be suspected. If there is no strong urge, Reflex or Total Incontinence can be suspected.

The nurse also must assess the voiding intervals. If urine is expelled at regular intervals with dry periods interspersed, without the patient's awareness, incontinence is of the reflex type. If urine is leaked constantly, Total Incontinence is likely. If there is no clear-cut pattern to the incontinence, a Functional Incontinence should be suspected. In that case look for answers to such questions as why the patient is not able to reach a receptacle appropriate for voiding. If there are problems associated with more than one type of incontinence, the nurse must consider the possibility that a combination of types exists. This is not uncommon. These key initial assessment parameters are summarized in Table 9.

After the possibilities are narrowed down, a more detailed assessment is needed. Most authors and clinicians advocate the use of a voiding record or an incontinence chart that can be kept either by the patient who is cognitively able or by the nurse.[22,41,46] This record allows for documentation of voiding times, indication of incontinent or continent episodes, the amount of urine (large, medium, small, dribbling), the nature of the urge before voiding, and what the person was doing at the time the incontinence occurred. Autry and others[2] (1985) developed a voiding record that would be kept for 7 days with a system of colored adhesive dots to be used hourly to indicate if the patient was wet or dry and if voiding occurred when toileting was offered. Although these types of records provide a good picture of incontinence patterns, Robb[50] cautioned that such records may

TABLE 9   Key Initial Assessment Parameters and Suspected Type of Incontinence

Assessment Parameter	Suspected Type of Incontinence
Does incontinence occur only with an increase in intraabdominal pressure?	Stress Incontinence
Is the urge to void before an incontinent episode always extremely strong and uncontrollable?	Urge Incontinence
Is urine expelled at regular intervals, with dry periods between, without the patient's awareness?	Reflex Incontinence
Is urine leaked continuously?	Total Incontinence
Is there no clear pattern of response to the questions presented above?	Functional Incontinence or combined types of incontinence

call attention to the problem and change behaviors of patients or nurses before a true picture of the usual pattern is obtained. This is less a problem for the clinician than for a researcher. Therefore, in clinical situations the voiding record is definitely a valuable tool for assessment. It should be kept around the clock for several days until a clear pattern is established. From data on a voiding record the nurse will know the pattern of incontinent episodes, the frequency, time of day, amount of urine, nature of the urge, and the environmental circumstances or activity at the time of episodes. A sample of how this record could be organized is presented in the box on p. 245.

Although nurses may diagnose types of incontinence independently, in many cases the definitive diagnosis is made in collaboration with others, usually the physician. Ideally, after incontinence is identified, a thorough urologic, gynecologic, neurologic and medical history and physical exam

Sample Voiding and Incontinence Record

Date	Time	Voiding		Amount 1. Very strong 2. Medium 3. Small 4. Dribbling	Urge 1. Very strong 2. Strong 3. Normal 4. Minimal 5. None	Activity at Time
		Continent	Incontinent			

III

are done. Cystometry, urethral pressure profilometry, uroflowmetry, and pressure flow studies are examples of specific tests that physicians typically use to differentiate types of incontinence.[18] There is not yet a consensus as to which patients should have these detailed medical assessments for incontinence.[48] Therefore, nurses, who often are the first to notice incontinence, should see thorough assessments and differentiation of the types of incontinence as part of their role.

Functional Incontinence

With the nursing diagnosis of Functional Incontinence, the line between defining characteristics and related factors is not clear-cut because of the fact that the related factors help to define the "functional" part of the label or problem. In medicine a functional disease is defined as "any derangement of an organ in which there is no apparent degeneration, damage, impairment, or structural change."[58]

Therefore, in assessing for Functional Incontinence, one is assuming there is no apparent impairment of the urinary system itself; rather, some other problem is causing incontinence in a potentially continent person. Functional Incontinence usually is diagnosed initially by the elimination of factors that would point to other types of incontinence. After the nurse has established that no overt urinary problem is causing the incontinence, the nurse focuses on secondary problems that might be interfering with normal voiding and toileting practices. What is it that keeps the patient from reaching a toilet, bedpan, commode, or urinal in time to void? Therefore the assessment of Functional Incontinence is focused largely on related factors or causes.

To narrow down the possible related factors the nurse should look for obvious problems not related to urinary function. Williams and Gaylord[61] advocated a functional assessment of the following areas: (1) physical functional ability (transfer ability, mobility, balance, arm strength, torso flexibility, manual dexterity, toileting, and vision), (2) mental functional ability, (3) social functional considerations, and (4) environmental considerations (access from bed, chair, or sofa, toileting distance, availability of bedside commode, lighting, supports such as grab bars and rails, access to bathroom, and toilet height). Any of these could prevent timely voiding. It also is important to look at data collected in other functional patterns. Bowel elimination often is a problem area, because a stool impaction can exert enough pressure on the bladder and urethra to prevent normal urinary elimination.

Drug treatments always should be assessed in an incontinent patient. Many drugs have incontinence as a potential side effect. Anticholinergic drugs (for example, atropine and some cold rem-

III

edies) may cause relaxation of the detrusor muscle; this results in urinary retention and overflow of urine. Alpha-sympathetic blockers (antihypertensives such as methyldopa and phenoxybenzamine) may cause relaxation of the internal sphincter. Drugs that are beta sympathetic in action (such as isoproterenol and metaproterenol) may cause relaxation of the detrusor muscle. Skeletal muscle relaxants (for instance, baclofen and diazepam) also can cause relaxation of the external urinary sphincter. Diuretics (furosemide and hydrochlorothiazide) obviously increase urine output.[22,41]

Nothing should be overlooked in an attempt to identify functional or environmental problems that could cause incontinence. Sometimes the simplest of things, such as a new garment with complicated fasteners or a cluttered room, can prevent normal toileting. Many times in institutional settings a major factor contributing to functional incontinence is a nurse's busy schedule. If a patient's call for toileting is delayed, incontinence can result from this lack of available assistance.

❖ Defining Characteristics

The presence of the following defining characteristics indicates the patient may be experiencing Functional Incontinence:
- Variable frequency of incontinent episodes
- No overt urinary problem found (other types of incontinence ruled out)
- Presence of some obstacle to normal voiding pattern (see related factors)

❖ Related Factors

The following related factors are associated with Functional Incontinence:
- Stool impaction
- Sensory deficits
- Mobility deficits
- Drug use
- Cognitive deficits
- Emotional problems (e.g., anger or hostility)
- Altered environment
- Lack of available assistance for voiding

❖ Related Medical/Psychiatric Diagnoses

The following are examples of related medical/psychiatric diagnoses for Functional Incontinence:
- Dementia
- Depression
- Traumatic brain injuries

Stress Incontinence

The classic characteristic of Stress Incontinence, which is much more common in women than in men, is that urine is involuntarily leaked when there is an increase in intraabdominal pressure. This may occur consistently or in varying degrees depending on the degree of pressure exerted. The severity of this problem initially can be assessed from a voiding record. A complete assessment of stress incontinence to determine severity would be a collaborative effort of the physician and nurse. The nurse often is the first person to identify this problem. A nursing assessment would identify the frequency of the incontinence, circumstances precipitating the incontinence, and timing of the episodes.

Objective assessment measures include direct observation of the urinary meatus to check for leakage. The patient should be instructed to cough with a full bladder while in the lithotomy position. If there is no leakage, raise the head of the bed or examination table to 45 degrees, and repeat the process. If there is still no leakage, have the patient stand with feet apart and cough again. This procedure gives the nurse an idea of the severity of the problem. Leakage while in the lithotomy position generally indicates a more severe Stress Incontinence than that seen only in a standing position.

With these data a diagnosis of Stress Incontinence can be made. The patient's physician should be consulted to determine if further diagnostic tests are in order. There are several tests that physicians may use to determine the severity and causes of Stress Incontinence. A pelvic examination will rule out a cystocele or rectocele and establish the size and position of the uterus. A cystoscopic examination and a urethral pressure profile may be done. A Marshall or Bonney test may be performed; these involve lifting the anterior wall of the vagina with a finger against one side of the urethra while having the patient exert pressure.[25,42] Various laboratory tests may be ordered to rule out precipitating factors.

Assessment of related factors should begin with a look for weakened pelvic floor muscles. When these muscles are weakened or traumatized, a misalignment of the bladder and urethra can occur and can cause stress incontinence.[4,42] Weakened pelvic floor muscles can be caused by multiple or traumatic pregnancies and births, obesity, increased age, menopause, or neurological problems. Therefore the nurse should assess for a history of pregnancies, pelvic trauma or surgery, patient age, and weight.

Stress Incontinence in women also can be caused by an estrogen deficiency. Estrogen is important for urethral tissue tone; if there is a deficiency, urethral tissue is flaccid and loses its contractility. Such a problem may be a suspected condition in elderly, postmenopausal women or in women whose uterus and ovaries have been removed surgically. Women should be questioned about menopause, hysterectomies, and any felt changes in vaginal tissue that might indicate estrogen deficiency.

Another category of related factors is damage to the sphincter, which can occur after fractures of the pelvis, transurethral resection of the prostate, or other genitourinary surgical procedures. The nurse should assess for a history of any such problems.

Other functional variables in a person with Stress Incontinence may make the problem even worse. An overdistended bladder will increase the ratio of bladder pressure to urethral pressure. Therefore it is important to assess how often the patient voids and the usual amounts voided.

❖ **Defining Characteristics**

The presence of the following defining characteristics indicates the patient may be experiencing Stress Incontinence:

- Urine leakage associated with activities that cause increased intraabdominal pressure (such as coughing, laughing, lifting, and jogging)
- Small volume of urine loss
- Little or no nocturia

❖ **Related Factors**

The following related factors are associated with Stress Incontinence:

- Chronic increase in intraabdominal pressure
- Weak pelvic muscles
- Multiple pregnancies
- Traumatic infant deliveries
- Bladder overdistention between voidings
- Obesity
- Estrogen deficiency
- Weak sphincter tone
- Increased urethrovesicular angle
- Sphincter damage caused by transurethral resection of the prostate, other genitourinary surgeries, or pelvic trauma

❖ **Related Medical/Psychiatric Diagnoses**

The following are examples of related medical/psychiatric diagnoses for Stress Incontinence:

- Diabetes mellitus
- Multiple sclerosis
- Parkinson's disease
- Stroke

Reflex Incontinence

Reflex Incontinence is a voiding pattern much like that seen in an infant whose bladder emptying occurs at regular intervals without any inhibitions. It occurs in individuals who have damage to spinal nerve pathways to and from the brain but have intact sacral spinal reflexes. The spinal reflex arc allows for voiding, but there is no mechanism to inactivate the reflex. This type of incontinence is sometimes called *automatic, spastic, hypertonic, upper motor neuron,* or *suprasacral bladder.*[20]

Assessment for this type of incontinence involves looking for a pattern of regular voiding without the patient having a sensation of voiding.

III

This pattern usually will occur equally day and night. Percussion over the bladder area will reveal a distended bladder before incontinence. After the patient voids the nurse can check for urine still in the bladder by catheterizing the patient. Generally persons with Reflex Incontinence have increased residual urine after voiding.[20] This is important in assessing for the problem and also for planning interventions. A large postvoiding residual urine volume can indicate a second problem, Urinary Retention, and predispose the patient to urinary tract infections (see discussion for the nursing diagnosis Urinary Retention).

Even though a sensation of a full bladder is not felt before voiding, some patients may report other body sensations. Often, especially with spinal cord injuries, a full bladder may trigger a sympathetic response that the patient can identify. These responses are different from person to person. Therefore the nurse should ask the patient to identify sensations felt before voiding. These responses often can be seen objectively. In mild forms the sympathetic response may produce diaphoresis, flushing, pilomotor responses (gooseflesh), or nausea. In an extreme form such a response can be life-threatening and is called *autonomic dysreflexia* or *hyperreflexia*. This is seen most commonly in patients with high thoracic and cervical cord lesions and can occur when a distended bladder or bowel triggers an exaggerated automatic/sympathetic nervous system response. Signs of hyperreflexia include severe hypertension, severe throbbing headache, bradycardia, profuse diaphoresis, blurred vision, nausea, flushing of the skin above the lesion level, severe pilomotor spasms, shortness of breath, and anxiety.[6]

The causes of Reflex Incontinence are always medical problems. Because of this, Reflex Incontinence usually is diagnosed by the physician and the nurse. Reflex Incontinence often is seen in patients with spinal cord injuries that result from such things as auto accidents, sports accidents, or trauma from bullet wounds. Spinal cord tumors or degenerative changes in the spine (spondylosis) also can result in Reflex Incontinence.[49] It is

sometimes seen with multiple sclerosis and certain cerebral lesions.

❖ **Defining Characteristics**

The presence of the following defining characteristics indicates the patient may be experiencing Reflex Incontinence:
- Voiding occurs without urge being felt
- Regular intervals between incontinent episodes
- Nocturia
- Probable increased postvoiding urine residual
- Sympathetic response (such as diaphoresis, flushing, or nausea) before voiding

❖ **Related Factors**

Because related factors for Reflex Incontinence are always medical problems, the related medical diagnoses become the related factors.

❖ **Related Medical/Psychiatric Diagnoses**

The following are examples of related medical/psychiatric diagnoses for Reflex Incontinence:
- Multiple sclerosis
- Spinal cord injury
- Spinal cord tumors
- Spondylosis

Urge Incontinence

Urge Incontinence is the most common type of incontinence in elderly patients.[42,44] It is characterized by a sudden uncontrolled loss of urine preceded by a strong urge to void. Because patients are aware of the need to urinate but cannot hold urine long enough to reach a toilet or appropriate receptacle, it sometimes can be misdiagnosed as Functional Incontinence. Also, because it frequently is seen in elderly patients who may have other mobility or sensory deficits, Urge Incontinence and Functional Incontinence often are seen simultaneously. Therefore, in patients who seem to have Functional Incontinence, the nurse should assess other signs and symptoms indicating Urge Incontinence. These signs and symptoms are frequent periodic voiding, nocturia, loss of urine in any position (standing, sitting, lying), low postvoiding residual volumes, and suprapubic discomfort with voiding.

Much of these data come from a voiding or incontinence record (see discussion under All Types of Incontinence, p. 245). Along with that information the nurse looks for the classic symptom of the strong urge to void that precedes the incontinent episodes. In addition, to make sure that Urinary Retention is not being masked by these symptoms, the nurse should check postvoiding residual volumes through catheterization.

Assessment of related factors or causes will tell the nurse if this problem can be cured or only managed for symptoms. In some patients no cause is evident. More frequently the cause is detrusor overactivity, also termed *detrusor instability* or *hyperreflexia*. With this condition the bladder contracts reflexively while the central nervous system inhibitory mechanism malfunctions. The bladder contracts but cannot be controlled adequately. Disorders of the central nervous system, such as strokes, Alzheimer's disease, Parkinson's disease, or brain tumors, are common causes of this problem. Reduced bladder capacity is another related factor; it may be caused by abdominal surgery, bladder tumors, or long-term use of an indwelling catheter. Other related factors are those that directly cause the bladder to be overactive or irritable, such as cystitis (bladder infection) or urethritis. Less severe irritants to the bladder are alcohol, caffeine, or increased urine concentration. Overdistention of the bladder caused by increased fluid intake, decreased voiding frequency, or use of diuretics also can cause Urge Incontinence.

From this long list of related factors one can see that this assessment often is a collaborative effort of physicians and nurses. Physicians who assess for medical problems may diagnose the Urge Incontinence and its related factors. Nurses who focus on patient responses to illness may diagnose Urge Incontinence and its related factors. Often the diagnosis is made collaboratively.

Nurses should be especially aware of related factors such as overdistention of the bladder, decreased voiding frequency, increased urine concentration, intake of bladder-irritating substances, and patient responses after removal of indwelling catheters. A thorough assessment will involve a search for any of these related factors, even in the presence of an obvious medical cause.

❖ Defining Characteristics

The presence of the following defining characteristics indicates the patient may be experiencing Urge Incontinence:

- Sudden uncontrolled loss of urine preceded by strong urge to void
- Increased frequency of voiding
- Nocturia
- Loss of urine in any position (standing, lying, sitting)
- Suprapubic discomfort with urination
- Small, moderate, or large amount of urine voided
- Low postvoiding residual volumes

❖ Related Factors

The following related factors are associated with Urge Incontinence:

- Decreased bladder capacity after long-term indwelling catheter use or from bladder tumors or abdominal surgery
- Increased bladder irritability from cystitis, urethritis, use of alcohol or caffeine, or increased urine concentration
- Overdistention of bladder from increased fluid intake, decreased voiding frequency, or use of diuretics

❖ Related Medical/Psychiatric Diagnoses

The following examples of are related medical/ psychiatric diagnoses for Urge Incontinence:

- Alzheimer's disease
- Bladder tumors
- Brain tumors
- Cerebrovascular accident
- Parkinson's disease
- Spinal cord injuries
- Spondylosis
- Urinary tract infections

III

Total Incontinence

Total Incontinence is a rarity. It is sometimes referred to as *true incontinence* or *constant incontinence* because of its characteristic of a nearly continuous flow of urine without a predictable cycle of bladder filling and emptying. Total Incontinence also is used to describe incontinence that does not respond to treatments. It often is diagnosed by ruling out all other types of incontinence.

The key assessment finding for this diagnosis is the unpredictable, constant leakage of urine that occurs day and night. The nurse should collect other data to validate this diagnosis and rule out other possible problems. Sometimes urinary retention with urine overflow initially can appear to be Total Incontinence because there is frequent leakage of small amounts of urine (see discussion of Urinary Retention). Therefore the bladder area should be palpated and percussed to check for distention, and the patient should be catheterized to check for urine in the bladder. If there is a large volume of urine in the bladder, other assessment directed toward Urinary Retention, not Total Incontinence, is needed.

It also is important to check the patient's awareness of incontinence. Most patients with Total Incontinence have no sensation of bladder filling and emptying. Cognitively aware patients will, of course, feel the wetness of the leaked urine but may not feel it being expelled. Patients with severe neurological deficits may be aware of nothing.

Total Incontinence is caused by a disease process, anatomical problems, or damage resulting from surgery, trauma, or radiation treatments. The most common related factor in male patients is prostate surgery where damage may be done to the external sphincter or to the nerves of the bladder. Other surgeries, such as abdominoperineal resection for rectal cancer, may result in Total Incontinence. Other related factors are fistulas that develop from trauma, radiation treatments to the pelvis, obstetrical injuries, or surgery. There also are rare congenital anomalies (such as exstrophy of the bladder, where the bladder is exposed on the abdomen, or ectopic ureters that are misplaced into the vagina) that cause total incontinence.[24] Disease processes that produce Total Incontinence usually are those that destroy nerves, such as spinal cord infarction or demyelinating diseases. Neurological diseases may prevent the bladder reflex transmission or may cause misfiring of nerve signals, resulting in voiding at unpredictable times.

Some surgical procedures are done to produce Total Incontinence when normal bladder emptying must be bypassed. Ileal conduits (urinary diversion where ureters are attached to a segment of ileum that is brought through the abdominal wall) or cystostomies (urinary diversion where bladder is opened and drained through an abdominal opening) are examples where the normal cyclic emptying of the bladder is replaced by a constant, uncontrolled flow of urine. Although patients with these urinary diversions technically have Total Incontinence, it does not usually warrant the nurse making this diagnosis, because, in itself the diversion is a treatment, not a problem. Other nursing diagnoses, such as Impaired Skin Integrity, might well be made with the Total Incontinence as a related factor.

❖ Defining Characteristics

The presence of the following defining characteristics indicates the patient may be experiencing Total Incontinence:

- Continuous or nearly continuous flow of urine No predictable cycle of bladder filling and emptying
- Nocturia
- Little or no residual urine in the bladder
- No patient awareness of incontinence

❖ Related Factors

The following related factors are associated with Total Incontinence:

- Surgical procedures that damage nerves or sphincter, such as transurethral resection of the prostate and abdominoperineal resection
- Fistulas developed from trauma, radiation treatments, obstetrical injuries, or surgery

- Congenital anatomical anomalies such as exstrophy of bladder and ectopic ureters

❖ Related Medical/Psychiatric Diagnoses

The following are examples of related medical/psychiatric diagnoses for Total Incontinence:
- Congenital anomalies (e.g., exstrophy of bladder, ectopic ureters)
- Multiple sclerosis
- Neuropathy
- Spinal cord tumors or infarction
- Vesicovaginal or urethrovaginal fistulas

Urinary Retention

Any decrease in urine output should be considered a diagnostic cue for Urinary Retention. If the patient can communicate, difficulty with voiding may be reported. This difficulty may be expressed as a problem in starting a stream of urine, a decrease in the force or interruptions of the stream, a sensation of bladder fullness after voiding, painful voiding, or actual inability to void at all. Even without a patient report of symptoms, the nurse should suspect Urinary Retention when a patient voids frequently in small amounts or has frequent dribbling of incontinent urine. Frequent dribbling is easily misdiagnosed as incontinence rather than retention. Further assessment is needed when frequent dribbling of urine occurs.

A most critical sign is a distended bladder. Percuss and palpate the lower abdominal area to detect bladder fullness. Percussion of a full bladder will produce a dull or nonresonant sound in the suprapubic area that is different from the somewhat hollow sound found in the normal intestine-filled lower abdomen. A full bladder may be felt during palpation of the lower abdomen. Pressure over the bladder area may cause discomfort or dribbling of urine when the bladder is very full.

Catheterization is usually performed to determine the amount of urine in the bladder. This is best done after the patient voids to determine the amount of residual urine in the bladder. A large postvoiding residual urine volume (generally more than 100 ml) is indicative of retention.[44] Patients with severe retention may have very large amounts of urine in the bladder. Before catheterization in a patient with suspected urinary retention the nurse should know if there is an institutional policy or a physician's order to clamp the catheter before completely emptying the bladder. It was thought that no more than 1000 ml should be drained at one time; the rapid decrease in pressure on the surrounding pelvic blood vessels may cause shock. However, a recent study showed no actual risk.[8] If there are no guidelines the nurse should use judgment and observe the patient closely during the procedure. If the nurse is in doubt, the catheter may be clamped for 30 minutes and then unclamped to allow the bladder to empty fully.

The nurse should suspect Urinary Retention when a patient is restless or diaphoretic. In this case, the amount of recent urine output should be checked immediately. Patients with any risk for Urinary Retention or those who have some signs of retention should be monitored for intake and output. If the patient is receiving a regular diet, fluid intake is usually about equal to output. Nonmeasurable fluids in foods will usually balance out the insensible fluid loss through the lungs, skin, and intestines. If the patient is receiving fluids only, urine output will be somewhat less than intake. If output is significantly less than intake, Urinary Retention should be suspected.

Many factors may contribute to Urinary Retention. Postoperative urinary retention is fairly common, especially in elderly patients and in those who have had spinal anesthesia. Postoperative assessment should always include assessment of urine output. After delivery women should also be assessed for Urinary Retention caused by swelling of the meatus or the perineal area or by hemorrhoids. Sometimes there are postpartum spasms of the perineal muscles. Women who have had traumatic vaginal deliveries may fear pain with voiding and may have difficulty relaxing the external sphincter.

Another group of related factors are bladder outlet obstructions, for example, prostatic hypertrophy, urethral strictures, fecal impactions, hemorrhoids, tumors, or perineal edema. Obstructions

III

are more common in men than in women.[42,48] Many obstructions, such as fecal impactions, hemorrhoids, or edema, may be detected through nursing assessment; others are detected by medical examination.

Resnick[48] reported a newly discovered common phenomenon—detrusor hyperactivity with impaired contractility (DHIC) that was associated with Urinary Retention. With DHIC the bladder contracts slowly and inefficiently, resulting in urinary retention.

Neuromuscular disorders may affect the bladder contractility or the sphincter muscle, causing urinary retention. Examples of these disease processes include autonomic neuropathy associated with diabetes or alcoholism; tabes dorsalis; spinal cord injuries, lesions, or tumors or herniated disks, especially in S2-4 spaces; multiple sclerosis; and cerebral lesions.[22,25,42] Patients with these and similar conditions should be assessed for urinary retention.

Side effects of some medications produce Urinary Retention. Anticholinergic medications such as atropine, propantheline bromide, or belladonna preparations, cold remedies such as pseudoephedrine, tranquilizers such as the phenothiazines or butyrophenone calcium channel blockers, and narcotic analgesics are but a few examples of such medications.[17,22,25] All medications, including over-the-counter products such as cold remedies, should be evaluated for this side effect before they are administered to a patient with Urinary Retention.

Environmental or psychosocial problems may also contribute to urinary retention. Events that cause anxiety or muscle tension may produce temporary retention. Lack of privacy, inability to assume a usual voiding position, timing difficulties, or use of different receptacles (bedpans, urinals, commodes) are potential contributors to this problem and are easily overlooked in an assessment that is focused too narrowly on the urinary system. As with any assessment, the patient's total response must be considered in searching for related factors to problems.

❖ Defining Characteristics

The presence of the following defining characteristics indicates the patient may be experiencing Urinary Retention:

- Cessation or decrease in urinary output
- Reported difficulty with starting urine stream
- Inability to start stream of urine
- Decrease in force of stream
- Interruptions in urine stream
- Sensation of bladder fullness
- Painful voiding
- Frequent voiding of small amounts
- Dribbling incontinence
- Distended bladder
- Pressure, discomfort in lower abdomen
- Postvoiding residual urine volume more than 100 ml
- Restlessness
- Diaphoresis
- Output less than input

❖ Related Factors

The following related factors are associated with Urinary Retention:

- General or spinal anesthesia
- Postpartum condition such as swelling of meatus or perineum, hemorrhoids, perineal muscle spasms, or fear of discomfort with voiding
- Bladder outlet obstruction such as urethral strictures, fecal impactions, hemorrhoids, or perineal edema
- Medication side effects, especially anticholinergic drugs, cold remedies, and tranquilizers
- Environmental or psychosocial factors such as anxiety, muscle tension, lack of privacy, inability to assume usual voiding position, timing difficulties, and use of different toileting receptacles

❖ Related Medical/Psychiatric Diagnoses

The following are examples of related medical/psychiatric diagnoses for Urinary Retention:

- Bladder tumors or stones
- Cauda equina syndrome
- Cystitis or urethritis

- Herniated disks
- Multiple sclerosis
- Myelomeningocele
- Neuropathy secondary to diabetes mellitus or alcoholism
- Prostatic hypertrophy
- Spinal cord injuries, tumors, or infarction
- Tabes dorsalis

NURSING DIAGNOSES

Examples of *specific* nursing diagnoses for Altered Patterns of Urinary Elimination are:
- Altered Patterns of Urinary Elimination related to lack of privacy
- Altered Patterns of Urinary Elimination related to motor impairment
- Altered Patterns of Urinary Elimination related to pregnancy
- Altered Patterns of Urinary Elimination related to emotional stress

Examples of *specific* nursing diagnoses for Functional Incontinence are:
- Functional Incontinence related to mobility deficits
- Functional Incontinence related to lack of available assistance for voiding
- Functional Incontinence related to use of skeletal muscle relaxants
- Functional Incontinence related to cognitive deficits secondary to dementia

Examples of *specific* nursing diagnoses for Stress Incontinence are:
- Stress Incontinence related to weak pelvic muscles secondary to multiple pregnancies
- Stress Incontinence related to obesity
- Stress Incontinence related to bladder overdistention between voidings
- Stress Incontinence related to chronic increase in intraabdominal pressure secondary to chronic cough

Examples of *specific* nursing diagnoses for Reflex Incontinence are:
- Reflex Incontinence related to spinal cord injury
- Reflex Incontinence related to multiple sclerosis
- Reflex Incontinence related to spinal cord tumor

- Reflex Incontinence related to spondylosis

Examples of *specific* nursing diagnoses for Urge Incontinence are:
- Urge Incontinence related to decreased bladder capacity secondary to long-term use of indwelling catheter
- Urge Incontinence related to bladder irritability secondary to urinary tract infection
- Urge Incontinence related to bladder irritability secondary to excessive caffeine intake
- Urge Incontinence related to chronic overdistention of bladder

Examples of *specific* nursing diagnoses for Total Incontinence are:
- Total Incontinence related to vesicovaginal fistula after surgery
- Total Incontinence related to spinal cord infarction
- Total Incontinence related to neurological damage secondary to multiple sclerosis
- Total Incontinence related to congenital exstrophy of bladder

Examples of *specific* nursing diagnoses for Urinary Retention are:
- Urinary Retention related to bladder outlet obstruction secondary to chronic fecal impactions
- Urinary Retention related to side effects of over-the-counter cold remedy medications
- Urinary Retention related to inability to void in usual standing position and unfamiliar environment
- Urinary Retention related to postpartum perineal edema

PLANNING AND IMPLEMENTATION WITH RATIONALE
Altered Patterns of Urinary Elimination

Because the diagnostic label "Altered Patterns of Urinary Elimination" is so broad, a standard plan of care is difficult to determine. As noted earlier, this diagnostic label should not be used when one of the more specific types of incontinence or urinary retention is applicable. Ideally, if a cluster of data does not fit with one of the incontinence or retention diagnoses the nurse should devise a label that is more specific than Altered Patterns of Urinary Elimination. Care planning will then flow from the specified nursing diagnosis.

There are some general approaches to care for urinary problems. Most persons find urinary problems embarrassing. They are reluctant to discuss such problems and often look for ways to take care of the problem themselves. Nurses must establish rapport with patients to promote ease and open communication about urinary concerns.

Another general rule for care of urinary problems is to debunk the myth that urinary problems are a natural result of aging. Patients, families, and health care providers often believe this myth. Any urinary problem should be seen as an abnormal phenomenon for which care approaches should be planned.

Urinary elimination is a complex physiological phenomenon, about which lay persons are often confused. Nurses must take care to use language that can be understood by patients when care, especially teaching, is provided.

When the urinary problem is incontinence, nurses often focus on managing the soiling rather than on managing the incontinence. Nurses often view patients with incontinence in a negative light. Health care providers often reflect society's stereotypical beliefs about incontinence. Nurses must focus care on eliminating or controlling incontinence rather than accepting the incontinence and soiling as inevitable.

Incontinence care needs an interdisciplinary approach. It is a problem that crosses disciplines and cannot be treated in a multidisciplinary manner when each provider does a piece of the care. Many care approaches to incontinence require consistency and collaboration from several providers.

Functional Incontinence

The obvious focus of care for patients with Functional Incontinence is to eliminate or compensate for the causative factors. The expected outcome for the patient is continence or a reduction in episodes of incontinence. In most cases

this is a realistic outcome because the incontinence is functional in nature. The overall rationale for nursing interventions is that *removing or decreasing obstacles to voiding will allow for normal or adapted voiding.*

The approaches taken will vary greatly depending on the identified related factor. The voiding or incontinence record (discussed earlier in the assessment of incontinence) should be the basis of the plan *because that will show where, when, and under what conditions incontinent episodes occur.* For instance, it may be found that incontinence occurs only at night. In that case strategies are aimed at nighttime patterns. The patient may be unable to get out of bed because side rails are up. A patient may have poor night vision. Another patient may drink the bulk of daily fluids in the evening.

If the environment can be adapted to a patient's needs, that strategy should be tried first. *Environmental changes are usually easiest to implement and the least disruptive to the patient.* Examples of some environmental adaptations that have been successful follow: (1) leave side rails down if safety factors allow, (2) place phosphorescent tape on the floor from the bed to the bathroom, (3) leave bathroom doors ajar with the light on, (4) move all unnecessary items away from the path to the bathroom, and (5) install support bars by the toilet. The patient should be advised to discontinue wearing clothing that requires much effort to remove. Velcro closures applied to clothing will make for easy removal. Bedpans, urinals, and call lights should be placed within easy reach. Nurses themselves may be part of the environmental problems. If call lights are not being answered promptly, staffing changes should be made so that this problem is eliminated.

When the environment is as conducive to normal voiding as possible, other strategies are directed toward the patient. If the secondary problem causing the incontinence can be eliminated, that should be done first. *Further strategies may be unnecessary if the secondary problem is eliminated.* If there is a stool impaction, a bowel evacuation plan is needed. The impaction may be re-

❖ *NURSING CARE GUIDELINES: FUNCTIONAL INCONTINENCE*

Nursing Diagnosis: *Functional Incontinence*

Expected Patient Outcomes	Nursing Interventions

The patient will be continent at all times or at a specified percentage of times (indicate realistic percentage).	• Identify incontinence pattern.
	• Remove environmental obstacles.
	• Remove or control secondary patient problems.
	    Begin bowel management program.
	    Maximize mobility.
	    Assess drug use to identify any incontinence-related side effects.
	    Change drug regimens if possible.
	• Institute bladder training, habit retraining, timed voiding, or prompted voiding regimen based on patient characteristics.
	• Adjust times of fluid intake to coincide with optimal voiding times.
	• Provide reinforcement for continence.
	• Maintain voiding record.

III

moved digitally or with enemas, and a program to prevent future impactions should be started. Such a program may involve increasing fiber and fluids in the patient's diet, exercise, monitoring bowel movements, giving enemas as needed, giving laxatives, and bowel habit training. Habit training involves the patient trying to have a bowel movement at the same time each day and, if 2 consecutive days go by with no bowel movement, using an enema to stimulate one. Enemas should be used with caution because routine use could cause the patient to become dependent on them.

If the patient has a mobility problem that can be treated, then that should be addressed. For example, if the person has morning stiffness from arthritis that makes movement difficult, pain medications may need to be given more frequently or earlier in the morning. Adaptive devices, such as a trapeze on the bed, may assist with mobility. If drug use is affecting urinary elimination, the nurse in collaboration with the physician should consider if alternate drugs can be given or if schedules may be changed so that the drug's peak action time coincides with optimal toileting time.

Habit training, *bladder training,* or *timed voiding,* are frequently used behavioral interventions. *The rationale for these interventions is that old habits can be changed through behavior modification and reinforcement.* In Godec's (1984) study of 20 patients who had Functional Incontinence, 79% were cured with timed voiding. Similar success rates were noted in many reports.[37,47] Several methods can be used in this type of intervention; one is the classification of behavioral interventions developed by Hadley.[26] Bladder training encourages the patient to suppress the voiding urge while intervals between voiding are gradually increased to every 3 or 4 hours. Habit retraining encourages suppression of voiding while intervals between voiding are adapted to the person's voiding pattern. Timed voiding involves a fixed schedule of voiding, such as the every-2-hour schedule used by Godec.[23] Prompted voiding depends on asking patients at regular intervals if they need to void and assisting them if the answer is yes. A study by Schnelle and others[51] showed promoted voiding to be effective in reducing functional incontinence. The choice of one of these interventions largely depends on the pattern of incontinence found on the voiding or incontinence record used for assessment, and on the underlying related factors for the individual patient. Those who have cognitive deficits might respond best to timed voiding or prompted voiding.

Those with mobility or sensory deficits might respond better to habit retraining.[21]

Patients with psychological or emotional problems and some with neurological or cognitive problems may respond to other behavioral therapies. Also called *contingency management,* this intervention uses *reinforcers to promote continence.* Verbal or social rewards are given when the patient is continent in voiding.[16,37] This intervention must be well coordinated so that all staff are taking a similar approach. *Behavioral therapies are ineffective if consistency is not maintained.*

The care plan for a patient with Functional Incontinence provides a general guide to interventions. It is general in nature because specific approaches very much depend on the identified related factors. These general guidelines should be individualized and specified to a patient's unique situation.

Stress Incontinence

Some interventions for Stress Incontinence are within the realm of nursing, especially if the severity of the problem is minimal and if the related factor is poor tone of pelvic floor muscle. When the problem is more severe and related to structural defects or estrogen deficiency, medical or surgical interventions are needed. Medical interventions may be needed if the patient with mild Stress Incontinence also has cognitive deficits. In these cases the problem becomes a medical diagnosis. Sometimes the care is collaborative and is planned and implemented by a physician and a nurse.

With mild Stress Incontinence in an alert patient, a realistic patient outcome is the elimination or significant reduction of incontinent episodes over a period of several weeks to several months, with a progressive decrease in the number of episodes in that time period. In that time period patients can learn to minimize the discomfort and embarrassment of incontinent episodes with planning aimed at maintaining dryness.

These patient outcomes can be achieved with exercises to increase pelvic and abdominal muscle

tone and with weight loss if needed. Kegel exercises are a time-honored and research-supported intervention for stress incontinence.* These exercises, first introduced in the late 1940s by Kegel, focus on *strengthening the pubococcygeal muscle, which is the main support for the pelvic floor.* This muscle surrounds the urethra, vagina, and rectum. Many women are unaware of these muscles and how to exercise them, so they must be taught these exercises. Wells[59] suggested using the description "pelvic muscle exercise" because some women thought "pelvic floor exercises" had to be done on the floor. One simple method of teaching is to have the patient sit with legs apart and urinate. Ask her to squeeze the muscles to stop the stream of urine. If this can be done then the pubococcygeal muscle has been contracted. Another method is for the nurse to place a finger at least three quarters of the way into the patient's vagina and ask the patient to squeeze the finger. The patient also can do this herself and feel the contracting muscle. Some studies have shown that a greater reduction in incontinence is achieved when biofeedback is used with Kegel exercises.† Biofeedback is achieved with a device called a perineometer placed in the vagina that can register on a gauge the pressure exerted with the muscle so that the patient can see how well she is doing with the exercises. If a perineometer is available, it should be used for optimal teaching and evaluation of exercises.

After it is established that the patient can contract the pubococcygeal muscle, she should be instructed to tighten the muscle, hold it for the count of 10, relax it, and then repeat the procedure 100 times per day.[53] Another method, called *quick Kegels,* is to tighten and relax this muscle repeatedly as rapidly as possible.[11] Whatever exercise is used, the patient should accept that these should be done for the rest of her life to maintain that muscle tone.

It is also helpful to teach patients to strengthen

---

*References 4,5,10,32,59
†References 9,10,12,53,54

❖ *NURSING CARE GUIDELINES STRESS INCONTINENCE*
Nursing Diagnosis: *Stress Incontinence*

Expected Patient Outcomes	Nursing Interventions
The patient will achieve continence (or significantly decrease incontinent episodes) within 2 to 6 months.	• Have the patient identify pubococcygeal muscle, and instruct on how to contract muscle by successfully stopping a stream of urine during voiding while sitting with legs apart; squeezing vaginal muscles against examiner's finger; and observing a biofeedback instrument activated by squeezing a perineometer in vagina. • Describe how to do Kegel exercises: *slow Kegels,* squeeze muscle, hold to count of 10, relax, and repeat 100 times daily; and *quick Kegels,* repeatedly contract and relax muscle as rapidly as possible. • Teach abdominal muscle exercises: "pull in–push out," pull up pelvic floor as though trying to suck water into the vagina, then push out as though trying to push water out; then repeat exercise. • Discuss a total body exercise program that is conducive to the patient's lifestyle. • If the patient is obese, plan weight-reduction and exercise plan.
The patient will maintain optimal dryness at all times.	• Encourage the patient to wear a pad, especially during strenuous activity or when there is an increased likelihood of coughing or sneezing. • Have the patient assess fluid intake, decrease intake of caffeine drinks, and schedule least intake before periods of strenuous activity. • Advocate that the patient carry "incontinent episode bag" with change of underwear and stockings. • Encourage the patient to empty bladder more often if overdistention is a problem. • Advise obese or pregnant patients to avoid long periods of standing.

abdominal muscles so that *these muscles can help in supporting the bladder in its correct anatomical position.* Some nurses teach "pull in–push out" exercises along with Kegel exercises. Patients are taught to pull up the pelvic floor as though trying to suck water into the vagina and then to push out as though trying to push water out.[11]

If the patient has generalized poor body muscle tone, a complete exercise program to strengthen muscles should be planned. If the patient is obese, a diet and exercise plan should also be included in care.

Another focus of care is to assess the patient in managing the incontinent episodes until the incontinence is cured through nursing, medical, or surgical treatment. Although many patients develop such strategies, some suggestions may be helpful. Instruct the patient to wear a menstrual pad, especially during strenuous exercise or when she has a cold and is coughing and sneezing. Encourage the patient to carry an "incontinence episode bag" (a bag containing an extra pair of underwear and stockings).

The patient should also be taught to avoid caffeine drinks that are *irritable to the bladder* and to empty the bladder more frequently *so that there is less pressure on the sphincter*. Patients also may be able to change their schedule of fluid intake so that the *bladder is not overdistended during periods of peak stress*. Patients who are obese or pregnant should avoid long periods of standing, which *increase intraabdominal pressure*.

It is important that nurses understand the medical and surgical interventions available for more severe stress incontinence, although these are outside the realm of nursing. If the bladder has descended in the pelvis, a surgical bladder suspension can be done. This is often done after pelvic floor exercises have failed.[27] For patients who have damaged sphincters, artificial urinary sphincters can be implanted. Vaginal pessaries have been used in the past, but because they are uncomfortable and impractical, they have limited use today.[42]

Medication treatments are effective for some patients. For estrogen deficiency with accompanying atrophic vaginitis, oral or intravaginal estrogen may be administered.[14] Alpha-adrenergic agonists, such as pseudephedrine and phenylpropanolamine, are useful to increase sphincter contractions. Imipramine, an antidepressant anticholinergic drug, has been used to decrease bladder contractility and increase the sphincter resistance.[4,22] Interestingly, although acknowledging the need for further study, Wells and others[60] found that pelvic exercises were as effective as phenylpropanolamine.

Reflex Incontinence

Because of the nature of the diseases that cause Reflex Incontinence, it usually is not possible to cure this problem. It is, however, possible to control the voiding so that the patient can remain dry most of the time and use a voiding stimulus to urinate into an appropriate receptacle at appropriate intervals. Because of the risk of autonomic dysreflexia another important patient outcome is the avoidance of an overdistended bladder. To achieve that outcome the patient needs to coordinate voiding times with fluid intake. It also is im-

portant for the patient to empty the bladder enough so that residual urine volume is low. Limits for acceptable residual volume range from 50 to 150 ml.[20,42] This outcome often is set by the nurse and physician collaboratively or is set by protocol guidelines. *Residual urine increases the risk of infection, stone formation, and overdistention*. Patients need to be able to recognize signs of overdistention and infection so that cures can be sought. Patients also need to have a plan of action for unscheduled voiding or incontinent episodes, because reflex voiding can be triggered at unpredictable times.

To achieve these outcomes nursing interventions must be tailored to the individual patient's unique characteristics. Many patients with reflex incontinence have gone through an acute stage of their illness when an indwelling catheter was in place. Long-term indwelling catheters are now used as a last resort treatment because of the associated dangers of infection. Once the catheter is out, patients can begin to explore triggering mechanisms that will initiate reflex voiding. *The rational for such stimulation is that sacral-lumbar dermatomes are stimulated and the micturition reflex is activated*. Different mechanisms work for different people. Some possibilities are stroking the inner thigh, pulling lightly on pubic hairs, tapping or jabbing over the bladder area, digital stimulation of anal sphincter, stroking the glans penis or vulva, or even flexing the toes. Any or all of these can be explored, although there is some evidence that tapping or jabbing works best.[13] While exploring these mechanisms, the patient should be sitting on a commode or toilet if possible so that the *normal voiding position is promoted*. If the patient has functioning abdominal muscles, the Valsalva maneuver should be used during voiding to increase emptying. After the patient has voided, a straight catheter should be inserted to check for residual urine in the bladder. If residual volumes are consistently lower than the limit set, then this type of patient-stimulated reflex voiding may be adequate. If residual volumes are too high, other interventions may be necessary.

❖ *NURSING CARE GUIDELINES: REFLEX INCONTINENCE*

Nursing Diagnosis: *Reflex Incontinence*

Expected Patient Outcomes	Nursing Interventions
The patient will participate in a planned voiding schedule, using a voiding stimulus or intermittent catheterization, until a regular pattern of bladder emptying is achieved.	• Explain mechanics of bladder reflex to the patient. • Explore various triggering mechanisms (stimuli) to initiate voiding, such as stroking inner thigh, pulling lightly on the pubic hairs, tapping or jabbing lower abdomen, digital stimulation of anal sphincter, stroking glans penis or vulva, and flexing toes. • Have the patient practice these mechanisms in optimal voiding positions using the Valsalva maneuver during voiding if possible. • If the triggering mechanism is effective, catheterize the patient after voiding to check for residual urine. Continue checking postvoiding residual volumes until they are less than 75 ml. • If the triggering mechanism is ineffective or if postvoiding residual volumes are too high, teach intermittent self-catheterization technique to the patient (or significant other, if the patient is unable to do it). Instruct the patient to use the following regimen: (1) gather equipment; (2) wash hands; (3) get in a comfortable position— sitting up in bed or chair or standing; (4) lubricate 1 inch of catheter tip with water soluble lubricant; (5) wash perineal area or penis; (6) for women (after practice viewing meatus with mirror and feeling it), spread labia with nondominant hand and insert catheter until urine flows; (7) for men, hold penis at about 60 degree angle from body and insert catheter until urine flows; (8) allow urine to flow until stream stops; (9) rotate catheter and check for further urine flow; (10) remove catheter slowly; (11) wash catheter inside and out; and (12) store catheter in clean, dry place.
The patient will coordinate voiding times with fluid intake schedule.	• Monitor fluid intake and urine output to determine optimal times for voiding or catheterization to keep urine volumes lower than 300 ml. • Plan a schedule for amount and timing of fluid intake. • Start timing of voiding or catheterization at 3- to 4-hour intervals, and extend time to 5- to 7-hour intervals until desired volume is reached.
The patient will identify the signs of autonomic dysreflexia.	• Discuss with the patient any signs of sympathetic nervous system response to full bladder. • Teach the patient and significant others signs of autonomic dysreflexia: throbbing headache, profuse perspiration, blurred vision, nausea, flushing of skin, severe pilomotor spasms, hypertension, bradycardia, shortness of breath, and anxiety. • Urge patient to empty bladder at any hint of these signs of autonomic dysreflexia.

Continued.

❖ *NURSING CARE GUIDELINES: REFLEX INCONTINENCE—cont'd*

***Nursing Diagnosis:** Reflex Incontinence*

Expected Patient Outcomes	**Nursing Interventions**
The patient will identify the signs of urinary tract infection.	• Teach patient to recognize signs of urinary tract infection: increased temperature, malodorous or cloudy urine, change in color, sediment, or blood in urine, or increasing bladder irritability.
The patient will devise a plan for dealing with unexpected incontinent episodes.	• Discuss with the patient a plan that fits with his/her lifestyle for preventing and dealing with unexpected incontinent episodes. • Urge the patient to carry a catheter at all times, carry extra clothing, empty bladder earlier if lack of opportunity to void on schedule is anticipated, and empty bladder before sexual activity. • Consider need for incontinence underwear depending on frequency of unexpected incontinence.

Intermittent catheterization is used widely today. The patient or a significant other may do this. Initially, while the patient is learning the procedure, the nurse does the catheterization. A catheter is inserted through the meatus into the bladder, the bladder is emptied, and the catheter is removed. This procedure may be done as a sterile or as a clean technique. A sterile procedure is sometimes used in the hospital where a new catheter is used for each catheterization. Patients who do this procedure at home usually use a clean technique in which the catheter is cleaned after each use and reused. The care plan for the patient with Reflex Incontinence describes the steps in teaching intermittent self-catheterization.

For either a trigger-stimulated voiding or an intermittent catheterization, a schedule for voiding is imperative. This schedule is initiated by first setting the times at fixed intervals, then recording the amounts voided or released by the catheter. *The object is to keep the bladder from filling beyond a 300 to 400 ml limit.*[42] Times between voiding or catheterizations are adapted until this goal is reached. At the same time, a fluid intake schedule is set up, and the patient is urged to maintain this schedule so that a regular pattern of intake and output can be established. *Overdistention of the bladder is thought to contribute to urinary tract infection.*[40]

To *avoid the risk of autonomic dysreflexia as a result of an overdistended bladder,* the patient must be taught to recognize any signs of this problem and to empty the bladder immediately if signs appear. It also is important that the patient know to shorten the interval between voidings or catheterizations if there has been an increase in fluid consumption. Patients who can void successfully using a trigger mechanism also need to know how to catheterize themselves in case of overdistention. Patients should carry a catheter with them at all times.

Because of the *increased risk of urinary tract infections from residual urine and intermittent catheterization,* patients must be taught to observe and smell the urine so that any abnormalities can be reported to their physician or nurse. Any cloudiness, blood, or sediment in the urine or a change in the color or odor of urine may indicate an infection. Sometimes an infection can increase bladder irritability, which can cause unexpected incontinent episodes or difficulty with voiding.

One other area of intervention is aimed at helping the patient be prepared for "accidents." A *reflex bladder may be triggered at unscheduled times.* It may be triggered by odd kinds of activities such as scratching a leg. Fondling or stroking, especially in the genital or leg area, may trigger voiding. *Strict adherence to the set voiding schedule will minimize the number of accidents,* but other actions can help the patient and significant others cope with accidents if and when they do occur. Patients should be encouraged to carry extra underwear and pants or skirts with them. If they are going to be some place where voiding is going to be difficult at their scheduled voiding time, they should empty the bladder before the activity. Sexual activity should be planned if possible so that the patient can empty the bladder first. Some patients who have frequent accidents may choose to wear incontinence underpants.

Urge Incontinence

Depending on the related factors for Urge Incontinence, care may be focused on eliminating the problem or on management of the problem. Care may be within the realm of nursing or medicine or a combination of both. If the cause is a medical problem, medical treatment may lead to a cure of the incontinence when the medical problem is cured. However, many of the medical problems that cause Urge Incontinence cannot be cured. Then, because the related factor cannot be eliminated, the incontinence must be managed through medical treatments or nursing measures.

The expected patient outcome will be either an elimination of incontinent episodes (cure) or a reduction in episodes of incontinence (management). The outcome chosen as a realistic goal of care will depend on the nature of the related factors. Other secondary expected patient outcomes will flow from one of these two primary outcomes.

Nursing care plans with elimination of incontinent episodes as a goal will likely apply to patients with these types of related factors: (1) decreased bladder capacity; (2) previous use of an indwelling catheter; (3) increased bladder irritability from alcohol or caffeine intake and increased urine concentrations; and (4) overdistention of the bladder from increased fluid intake, decreased voiding frequency, and use of diuretics. Secondary patient outcomes then will be to increase bladder capacity, to decrease bladder irritability, or to decrease bladder distention.

Nursing care plans aimed at reduction of the number of incontinent episodes will apply to patients with these types of related factors: (1) increased bladder irritability from chronic cystitis and urethritis and (2) incurable neurological disorders such as cerebrovascular accident, Alzheimer's disease, Parkinson's disease, and spinal cord injuries. Secondary patient outcomes will relate to a reduction in bladder irritability or participation in a set voiding schedule that allows for voiding before the bladder is full enough to stimulate the strong urge to void.

Nursing interventions aimed at eliminating incontinent episodes focus on eliminating causative factors. For example, decreased bladder capacity is caused by the extended use of an indwelling catheter. A plan for progressively lengthening the intervals between voiding will cause a *gradual increase in the bladder stretch receptor threshold.*[25,42] With data on the incontinence record, the initial interval for voiding can be set at a time before the incontinence usually happens. Then, with careful recording, that interval should be increased gradually. The patient should be reminded to continue to void at these optimal intervals to *avoid overdistention and to allow the bladder to reach a full capacity.*

If increased bladder irritability caused by alcohol or caffeine intake is the related factor, the patient should be educated about the effect of these irritants, and alternate fluids should be consumed. If increased urine concentration is causing bladder irritability, patients should be encouraged to increase their fluid intake. Patients with Urge Incontinence from other causes sometimes will decrease their fluid intake to decrease incontinent episodes; they should be taught that this makes the situation worse, because the *urine becomes more concentrated.* Diabetic patients whose disease is not well controlled may have concentrated urine; if so, these patients should be assisted in adjusting their diet and fluid intake.

If overdistention of the bladder is the related factor, patients should be encouraged and helped to void more frequently. Those taking diuretics should be taught to recognize peak action times

III

❖ *NURSING CARE GUIDELINES: URGE INCONTINENCE*
Nursing Diagnosis: Urge Incontinence

Expected Patient Outcomes	Nursing Interventions
The patient will experience either an elimination of incontinent episodes or a reduction in the number of incontinent episodes.	• Assess related factors to determine choice of realistic outcome and reasonable time frames for meeting outcomes. • Monitor patient for side effects of medications used to treat incontinence. • Maintain voiding record.
Depending on related factors, the patient will have increased bladder capacity (increased urine volume and lengthened voiding intervals), decreased bladder irritability (lengthened voiding intervals), or decreased bladder distention (shortened voiding intervals and decreased urine volumes).	• To increase bladder capacity plan the voiding schedule: start the voiding schedule at intervals shorter than intervals between incontinent episodes; progressively increase time between voidings until incontinence is decreased or eliminated; teach the patient to maintain the schedule; and coordinate fluid intake with the voiding schedule. • To decrease bladder irritability eliminate the patient's intake of irritants such as alcohol or caffeine, increase the patient's fluid intake to maintain dilute urine, and educate the patient on the irritating effects of concentrated urine and how to counteract this with increased fluid intake. • To decrease bladder overdistention encourage and assist the patient to void more frequently; set up a voiding schedule that balances with fluid intake, being careful not to increase voiding intervals so much as to promote decreased bladder capacity; have call light, bedpan, urinal, and commode within easy reach; and for the patient taking diuretics, teach peak action times, and plan increased voiding at that time.
The patient will participate in a set voiding schedule.	• If equipment is available and if the patient is cognitively intact, attempt use of biofeedback to assist in patient control of bladder and sphincter.

for these diuretics *so that they can plan to void more frequently at that time.* If patients who need assistance with toileting are experiencing Urge Incontinence, they should be put on a voiding schedule *so that help is available more frequently.* Call lights should be answered promptly. Bedpans, urinals, and commodes should be made readily accessible to such patients.

It is vital that the nurse study the voiding or incontinence record before initiating these interventions. It would be counterproductive to use an in-

tervention aimed at reducing overdistention with a patient who has reduced bladder capacity. Choice of interventions, therefore, critically depends on an accurate identification of the related factors for the Urge Incontinence.

Nursing interventions directed toward managing incurable Urge Incontinence focus on helping the patient to reduce the number of incontinent episodes. Patients with increased bladder irritability from chronic cystitis or urethritis need interventions to decrease the irritability. These patients often are helped with medication. In addition, nurses should focus on keeping the urine dilute *(dilute urine is less irritating)* by seeing that the patient increases fluid intake. These patients also may respond to a toileting schedule aimed at emptying the bladder before it gets full enough to trigger incontinence. Choosing this approach depends on the bladder capacity of individual patients, and the decision should be made jointly by the patient's nurse and physician.

For patients with neurological disorders, bladder training and toileting regimens seem to be the most widely used intervention.[34a,42] Some authors note that this technique is successful in up to 80% of patients.[30,51a] Bladder training and habit retraining are discussed in more detail under the Functional Incontinence diagnosis. Generally, the patient with Urge Incontinence is put on a schedule of fluid intake, and a voiding schedule is set up. After a schedule is established the intervals between voidings are progressively increased. Merely toileting these patients more often is not recommended; *with a too-frequent voiding schedule there is a risk of decreasing bladder capacity. A decreased bladder capacity will only compound the Urge Incontinence problem.*

Biofeedback may be another treatment option for patients with Urge Incontinence. A method of recording bladder pressure, abdominal pressure, and anal sphincter activity (with innervation identical to that of the urinary sphincter) is made visible to the patient. *This allows the patient to try to control the sphincter, detrusor, and abdominal muscles.*[34,41,42] This type of intervention has produced improvement in incontinence in some patients, but biofeedback is not practical for patients with severe cognitive impairments.

Because medical interventions often are used along with nursing measures to eliminate or reduce Urge Incontinence, a short overview of these measures is important to the nurse's full understanding of care.

Corrective surgery of the genitourinary system, bladder denervation (selected central or peripheral nerves are cut), and hydrostatic dilatation (bladder is distended while patient is anesthetized) are some of the medical treatments used for Urge Incontinence.[25,37]

Some medications can reduce detrusor instability or overactivity. Imipramine, oxybutynin, and propantheline bromide are examples of drugs that are sometimes effective for treatment of Urge Incontinence.[22,37] These drugs relax the bladder and expand its capacity, but they have potentially serious side effects, especially when used by elderly patients. Dry mouth, decreased sweating, constipation, and urinary retention are but a few of the noted side effects. Nurses must monitor patients closely for any such side effects.

For nurses and physicians Urge Incontinence continues to be a frequently encountered treatment challenge. Some new treatments are being explored, such as electrical stimulation of selected nerves.[52] However, at present these are still under study. Cure or management care requires creativity and a controlled set of interventions tailored to each patient. As evident from the care plan, there are few interventions that work with all patients.

Total Incontinence

Patients with Total Incontinence whose problem cannot be corrected medically or surgically are a real nursing challenge. Very often the care for these patients is directed toward other nursing diagnoses that have been caused by the Total Incontinence. High risk for Infection and Actual or High Risk for Impaired Skin Integrity related to Total Incontinence often become the priority nursing diagnoses. Planning and implementation for these problems should include nursing actions aimed at managing Total Incontinence.

The nursing care focus directed toward managing Total Incontinence shifts when caring for patients whose Total Incontinence can be corrected through medical or surgical procedures. Fistulas, especially those caused by trauma or obstetrical injuries, often can be closed surgically or with electrodes. Congenital anomalies such as bladder exstrophy often may be corrected surgically. Patients with sphincter damage can have artificial sphincters implanted. Artificial sphincters allow patients to deflate a cuff, which, when inflated,

III

acts to keep urine in the bladder.[20] The bladder sometimes can be totally bypassed when an "artificial bladder" is made, into which the ureters are transplanted. An ileal conduit is a pouch of resected ileum with an opening to the abdominal wall. A ureterosigmoidostomy transplants the ureters into the sigmoid colon. A continent ureterostomy via a Koch pouch is an ileal conduit with two valves: One keeps urine in the pouch until released by the patient by catheterization, and one prevents reflux of urine into the kidneys.[33] Patients who have these procedures need nursing care to help them adapt to these new methods of urinating. However, their problems would be identified by other diagnostic categories.

Unfortunately many diseases that cause Total Incontinence cannot be corrected medically or surgically. In these cases a urine collection device is needed. For men, this can be either a condom catheter or an indwelling urethral catheter. For women, indwelling catheters are used more often, because external devices are difficult to apply and not always successful. Such devices are still quite new and need further testing.[31,57] Most men can wear an external condom catheter attached to a collection bag. These should be changed on a regular schedule, and the penis should be checked for any skin breakdown or constriction. *Bacteria can build up inside an external catheter and, if it is applied tightly, blood supply can be restricted.* Therefore these catheters should be checked for twisting, which can restrict the flow of urine.

Indwelling Foley catheters generally are used only as a last resort; long-term catheter use has many risks, the greatest being infections that can be life-threatening. Diligent nursing care often can prevent the need for indwelling catheters; patients without catheters have nursing care focused toward managing Total Incontinence. These patients need creative and time-consuming nursing care. Approaches that work for one patient often will not work for another, so care must be individualized.

Determining expected outcomes is therefore difficult. Often, maintaining optimal dryness is the only realistic outcome. For some patients it may be possible to reduce the number of incontinent episodes. Patients who have intact verbal or non-verbal communication skills may be able to identify their needs for assistance in keeping dry. Those who have motor ability may be able to participate in an incontinence management regimen.

Nursing actions will depend on the expected outcome, so these too will be highly individualized. It is helpful to place these patients on a set schedule of fluid intake so *that urine output is predictable.* There is sometimes a temptation to restrict fluid. This should never be done because this *increases the already present risk of urinary tract infection.* A fluid intake of at least 2,000 ml per day should be maintained.

Containment garments, such as incontinence underpants, usually are necessary. Sometimes large menstrual pads may be used. These can be changed on a regular schedule.

Disposable, waterproof pads on beds are often used to keep patients dry. Unfortunately they often wrinkle and stay wet. They also are very expensive. If they are used, they should be straightened and changed frequently *so that they do not cause skin breakdown.*

Recently, however, alternatives to these "blue pads" have become available. These include disposable diapers and pads, and washable pants with removable pads.[7]

Whether containment garments or disposable pads are used, the nursing plan should have a set schedule for changing them. Strict adherence to a preset schedule, such as every 2 hours day and evening and every 3 hours at night, will *minimize the risks of skin problems and infections.* It also will *ensure comfort for the patient and decrease undesirable odor.*

It also is important that family members are aware of the plan for managing incontinence. They need to be educated as to the options for maintaining dryness so they understand that their family member is not being left wet for long periods of time through lack of care. If patients are able to communicate their needs, they should be involved in the incontinence management schedule.

❖ *NURSING CARE GUIDELINES: TOTAL INCONTINENCE*
Nursing Diagnosis: Total Incontinence

Expected Patient Outcomes	Nursing Interventions
The patient will maintain optimal dryness.	• Use containment garment and change garment on regular schedule, such as every 1 to 2 hours during the day and every 2 to 3 hours at night. • Set up a schedule for linen and pad changes; use checklist to record times.
The patient will reduce the number of incontinent episodes (if realistic).	• Set up fluid intake schedule so that at least 2,000 ml is taken in per day at regular intervals; do not restrict fluids unless medically ordered. • For men, apply condom catheter and drainage bag, check penis regularly for constriction and excoriation, and check condom regularly for twisting. • Use waterproof pads or special bed sheets as needed, and check these frequently for wrinkles. • Perform intermittent catheterization if enough urine is stored in bladder to make procedure worthwhile.
The patient will identify need for assistance with keeping dry (if realistic).	• If patient can communicate needs, set up message system for indication of wetness. • Encourage patient not to remain wet for long periods.
The patient and family will participate in incontinence management regimen (if realistic).	• Discuss incontinence care with family members, and encourage their participation in changing garments and pads. • If the patient can move well enough, have supplies readily available for self-changing of garments, pads, and linens.

III

Because patients may feel embarrassed about incontinence, they should be made to feel free to ask for clothing or for changes of bed linen. They may be able to indicate a linen changing schedule that works best for them. Patients who are adequately mobile should have undergarments, linens, or incontinent pads for their own care. These should be available in sufficient quantities to allow for frequent changes.

Intermittent catheterization (discussed under Reflex Incontinence, p. 260) is not appropriate for patients who have true Total Incontinence with constant leakage of urine. It may be helpful to patients who have some urine storage capabilities

that reduce the quantity of leaked urine. The potential risks would need to be weighed against the benefits of intermittent catheterization for each patient.

Ultimately some patients with Total Incontinence may need to be managed with indwelling catheters. Technically the maintenance of dryness for these patients is being treated medically by the catheter, and nursing care is supportive of the medical treatment. The patient's response to the use of the catheter must be assessed, and other diagnoses should be made. The reader should refer to diagnoses such as High Risk for Infection and devise plans that aim to reduce the risk of infection in patients with indwelling catheters.

III

Urinary Retention

Realistic patient outcomes will depend on the severity of Urinary Retention, factors contributing to retention, and whether the patient has difficulty starting a stream of urine. Several outcomes are possible but may not all apply to any one patient. The ideal general outcome is for the patient to achieve complete emptying of the bladder. This may be met by interventions aimed at aiding the patient to void or through an intermittent catheterization program. Therefore secondary outcomes may be that the patient will participate in an augmented voiding program or will perform intermittent catheterization. Complete emptying of the bladder may be measured by a criterion such as postvoiding residual urine volume of 75 to 100 ml or an amount deemed safe by the patient's physician or according to the patient's condition.

Interventions will stem from whichever patient outcome is reasonably expected. If the patient has postoperative urinary retention, strategies oriented toward initiating a stream of urine are often effective. Getting the patient into as near a normal voiding position as possible is helpful to initiate patterned responses. *Patterned responses will occur most easily when the circumstances surrounding the usual pattern of voiding are replicated.* Many nurses use "tricks" that help trigger the micturition reflex, such as running water near the patient, putting the patient's hands in water, stroking the lower abdomen with ice, or pouring water over the perineal area. *These maneuvers will stimulate the micturition reflex.*

Many of these strategies also work for postpartum patients. In addition, if swelling of the perineal area is contributing to Urinary Retention, application of ice to the perineum will *decrease swelling* and *remove this obstruction.* If fear of discomfort with voiding is a factor, giving pain medication before initiation of voiding and providing calming communication and support will help. For postoperative or postpartum patients the nurse must assess fluid intake and fluid loss *to determine a probable expected urine volume in the bladder.* In addition, the bladder area should be palpated and percussed to check for distention.

These *data will help determine how long a patient can safely go without voiding.* If patients cannot void and the bladder is not overdistended, it is helpful to have them rest and then try again. If none of these strategies is effective, catheterization will be needed to empty the bladder. A patient should never be "threatened" with catheterization; this *merely causes more tension.*

A bladder obstruction that is causing incontinence should be removed if possible. Nurses can remove fecal impactions and start bowel regimens when constipation is causing urinary retention. Hemorrhoids causing obstructive pressure on the bladder outlet may be treated medically or may be reduced with sitz baths and bed rest. *Sitz baths will increase circulation to the hemorrhoid area, and bed rest will decrease the downward pressure on the rectal area.*

Other obstructive problems, such as prostatic hypertrophy, tumors or urethral strictures, are treated medically or surgically. Prostate gland surgery or the insertion of a suprapubic catheter are common treatments for prostatic hypertrophy. Strictures are sometimes treated by dilating the urethra. In these cases nursing care is supportive to the medical treatment, and other nursing diagnoses may apply.

Patients with neuromuscular conditions causing Urinary Retention may respond to an augmented voiding regimen, but often intermittent catheterization is needed to empty the bladder completely. Augmented voiding regimens include setting a schedule for voiding that is correlated with fluid intake; double voiding (having the patient void and then try to void again); using the Valsalva maneuver (bearing down on with abdominal muscles); Credé's method (pressing down on bladder area); and using an optimal voiding position and receptacle. In addition, *because the innervation of the anal and urinary sphincter muscles is identical,* stretching the anal sphincter may cause the urinary sphincter to relax.[42] Such procedures *compensate for weak bladder muscles and maximize the natural voiding reflex patterns.* These tactics should not be used when there is an obstruction; the extra pressure will not help open

❖ *NURSING CARE GUIDELINES: URINARY RETENTION*
Nursing Diagnosis: Urinary Retention

Expected Patient Outcomes	Nursing Interventions
The patient will achieve complete emptying of the bladder or will maintain postvoiding residual urine volume of less than 75 ml (or amount deemed safe by patient's physician).	• Assure privacy for patient. • Help patient into voiding position as near normal as possible. • Encourage relaxation: deep breathing, loosening muscles, closing eyes. • Assist with initiating voiding reflex by trying techniques such as running water near patient, placing patient's hands in water, stroking lower abdomen with ice, pouring water over perineum. • Alleviate constrictions or obstructions: for perineal edema, apply ice; for fecal impactions, remove impaction or give enema; for constipation, start bowel regimen; for hemorrhoids, give sitz baths and bed rest. • Reduce discomfort or fear of discomfort with pain medications before voiding attempts; use calming communication and support. • Determine safe duration for patient to go without voiding by comparing intake and output and palpating for bladder distention. • If bladder is not overdistended, have patient rest, then try above strategies again. • If above strategies are ineffective and bladder is overdistended, catheterize and wait for bladder fullness; then repeat interventions. • Check postvoiding residual urine volume if voiding is accomplished. • If voiding is repeatedly unsuccessful, go to next part of plan.
The patient will participate in an augmented voiding regimen.	• Set up voiding schedule correlated with fluid intake. • Position patient in optimal voiding position, preferably on toilet or commode. Women should sit, leaning slightly forward with feet and legs apart. Men who usually stand to void should stand if possible. • Teach double-voiding technique. • Encourage patient to use Valsalva maneuver (check with physician first; this may be contraindicated in patients with some health problems). • Use Credé's method over bladder area (use only if no obstruction). • Teach patient and assist with anal sphincter stimulation while the patient bears down to void (insert finger into anus and pull slightly). • If voiding is successful, check postvoiding residual urine volume. • If voiding is repeatedly unsuccessful, catheterize and go to next part of plan.
The patient will perform (or participate in) intermittent catheterization.	• Assess patient's or significant other's ability to learn technique. • See care plan under Reflex Incontinence for intermittent self-catheterization procedure.

a blocked urethra and may cause reflux of urine into the kidneys. The Valsalva maneuver is contraindicated in patients with certain conditions such as myocardial infarction, aneurysms, eye surgery, and glaucoma.

When augmented voiding regimens are used, postvoiding residual urine volume should be monitored *to determine if the bladder is being adequately emptied.* If there is a high residual urine volume, intermittent catheterization may be indicated. This procedure is usually a clean technique when done by the patient at home but is sometimes done as a sterile technique in hospitals, where there are many sources for infection (Intermittent catheterization is discussed under interventions for Reflex Incontinence.)

Medications producing Urinary Retention should be changed if possible. Nursing interventions are usually limited to detection of medication side effects and notifying the patient's physician of the problem.

When environmental or psychosocial factors contribute to Urinary Retention, care should be focused on alleviating those that inhibit sphincter relaxation. Maintaining complete privacy and setting up near-normal voiding conditions will promote reflex voiding. If the patient is anxious or tense, contributing factors should be addressed and relaxation-promoting interventions implemented.

EVALUATION
Functional Incontinence

Because the expected patient outcome is complete continence or at least continence for a given percentage of times, the first step in evaluation is to compare the new voiding record with the one kept before treatment to determine if this goal was achieved. Depending on the severity of the related factors and the unique characteristics of the patient, complete continence or a reduction in incontinent episodes should occur. If not, the nurse must evaluate interventions to determine which were effective and which were not. If interventions are ineffective, alternate ones should be tried, and the related factors should be reevalu-

ated. Often, as a plan is being implemented, additional related factors surface; these must then be addressed, and the care plan must be amended.

Stress Incontinence

Patients should be asked to keep a voiding record, noting incontinent episodes and precipitating factors so that evaluation of the first outcome is possible. Comparing the posttreatment voiding record with the pretreatment voiding record will determine if the incontinent episodes have decreased. The time frame for achieving the outcome will vary from one patient to another. If the patient is not overweight and has mild incontinence, positive results should be achieved more quickly than if the patient is obese and needs time to lose weight.

The patient's ability to do the Kegel exercises correctly should be evaluated. If a perineometer is available, this is the most objective instrument to show if the pubococcygeal muscles are being contracted and how the muscle tone is increasing. If such an instrument is unavailable, the nurse can check the muscle contractions by inserting a finger into the vagina and having the patient do the Kegel exercise. Deciding how often this should be evaluated will depend on how well the patient is meeting the first outcome. If the incontinent episodes are decreasing quickly, it is likely that the patient is doing the exercise correctly. If not, more frequent checks of the patient's ability to do the exercises will be needed.

The second outcome is an ongoing one. With each patient encounter the nurse can check on what the patient is doing to maintain dryness.

Reflex Incontinence

A great deal of time and effort are needed to implement the plan of care for a patient with Reflex Incontinence. The time needed for achievement of the stated outcomes will vary from patient to patient depending on the patient's manual dexterity, education level, age, and intake and output patterns.

The first outcome can be evaluated at intervals until it is fully achieved (for instance, when a regular pattern of bladder emptying is achieved); this may take several weeks. The patient will need constant encouragement and reteaching over this period of time. The postvoiding residual amount will determine whether to use a voiding triggering mechanism or implement a plan for catheterization. If postvoiding residual volumes are greater than the set amount, the intermittent selfcatheterization plan must be initiated. The second outcome is evaluated along with the first one, because a fluid intake schedule is critical to a successful voiding schedule. It may be easier to achieve a set fluid intake schedule for patients in the hospital than for those at home. Therefore the nurse can expect need for adaptations of schedule on discharge of the patient from the hospital. Follow-up by a home care nurse or at an outpatient clinic is critical to the continued achievement of the second outcome.

The third and fourth outcomes are critical to the patient's safety while he/she manages bladder emptying. The nurse needs positive evidence that the patient understands the signs of infection and autonomic dysreflexia so that these problems can be corrected immediately.

The last outcome should be evaluated in the hospital and after the patient goes home. Each patient's individual lifestyle will affect the frequency of unexpected incontinent episodes and will dictate the best interventions.

Urge Incontinence

To determine if the expected patient outcomes have been met, the nurse, the patient, or both need to maintain a voiding record that notes the number of incontinent episodes, each interval between voidings, the amount of urine voided, and the nature of the urge to void. From such a record the nurse will know if the number of incontinent episodes has decreased. Data from this record also will indicate if changes in bladder capacity, irritability, and distention are occurring.

Evaluation of these patients must be part of a cycle of looking at results and adapting interventions to changes that occur. Some patients will show changes very quickly; others will need more

time. Schedules for evaluation will need to be set for each patient.

Total Incontinence

The expected outcome, optimal dryness, must be defined for each patient. Each patient's tolerance for wet skin is different. What is critical for evaluation is that optimal dryness is defined from the patient's perspective and not from a staff's perspective of how often a patient's clothing, linen, or pads must be changed. Whereas nurses may feel they can change clothing and linen only every 2 or 3 hours, this may not be sufficient to maintain adequate dryness for some patients.

The other expected outcomes in the plan should be stated only if they are truly realistic. If it seems possible to reduce the number of incontinent episodes, this can be measured with a voiding record. For patients who have constant leakage with no ability to store urine in the bladder, it is unlikely that this outcome would apply. For patients who are potentially communicative, the expectation that they will identify their needs may apply. Evaluation of this outcome may be possible through use of the voiding record or from direct interaction with the patient. The fourth outcome depends on the patient having some mobility. All patients should be urged to participate in care at any level possible. Evaluation of this outcome depends on the patient being involved in self-care.

Urinary Retention

The time needed for meeting expected outcomes will vary greatly depending on the factors contributing to the Urinary Retention. Some patients will meet the first outcome quickly after a few interventions and the problem will be resolved; others will need all of the interventions just to reach a level of control of Urinary Retention.

The three parts of the care plan can be implemented sequentially and evaluated accordingly. If the first outcome is unrealistic, the next one can be attempted. If augmented voiding is unsuccess-

III

❖ *CASE STUDY WITH PLAN OF CARE: FUNCTIONAL INCONTINENCE*

Mrs. Jolynn F., a 78-year-old Hispanic woman, has been a resident of a nursing home for 6 years. She is 5'2" tall and weighs 192 pounds, which she says has been her usual weight all her life. She resides in a nursing home because she is wheelchair-bound as a result of severe osteoarthritis and degenerative joint disease that have greatly decreased her hip and knee mobility. She also has mild congestive heart failure with dependent edema. She is a quiet woman who spends much of her day sitting in her wheelchair in the main floor lounge, in the chapel, or in the crafts room working on a hooked rug. She likes to get out of bed early in the morning and stay downstairs until after lunch time. After lunch she returns to her unit until about 3 PM, after which she returns to the main floor until supper time. Until a month ago, Mrs. F. was continent. She was able to stand and pivot onto the toilet with the help of two aides. Then her arthritis progressively worsened and she could not stand. So that she would not fall, three aides were needed to lift her onto the toilet. With each toileting Mrs. F. apologized for taking up so much of their time. The aides privately complained about how difficult it was to toilet her. Soon Mrs. F.

was remaining off the unit all day, returning only to get her 1 PM medication and after supper. Each evening her clothing and chair were very wet with urine. At night she was continent; she could get on and off a bedpan with the assistance of one person. Her medications were aspirin, two tablets at 9 AM, 1 PM, and 5 PM; Lasix, 40 mg at 9 AM; and digoxin, 0.125 mg at 9 AM.

At first the nurses thought Mrs. F. had Stress Incontinence because she was obese and had delivered five children, including one set of twins. They considered that she might have Urge Incontinence because she couldn't hold urine long enough to get to the toilet. When questioned, Mrs. F. said she didn't necessarily void when she moved or coughed. She also said she could hold her urine for a while. She held it at night until help arrived to get her on the bedpan. She admitted that she felt very bad about wetting herself, but she felt even worse having to take up the time of three people to help her to the toilet. Saying "I've never been such a bother to anyone in my whole life," she conceded that she would rather be wet than to be a bother. The nurse made the diagnosis of Functional Incontinence related to mobility deficits, avoidance behavior, and medication effects.

PLAN OF CARE FOR MRS. JOLYNN F.

Nursing Diagnosis: *Functional Incontinence related to mobility deficits, avoidance behavior, and medication effects*

Expected Patient Outcomes	Nursing Interventions
Mrs. F. will be continent at all times	• Change time of Lasix to 6 AM (peak action 1 to 2 hours). • Assist Mrs. F. to toilet before she leaves unit (by 8 AM). • Consult with physician to consider an increase in pain medication. • Provide positive reinforcement for continent behavior. • Consult with nutritionist to plan a weight-loss program. • Maintain voiding record to evaluate plan.
Mrs. F. will participate in a set toileting regimen.	• Contract with Mrs. F. for specific times, at least once in morning and once in afternoon, when she will return to unit for toileting. • Assure her that three staff members will be available at contracted times. • Instruct Mrs. F. to increase her fluid consumption in the late afternoon and decrease it early in the afternoon.

ful in maintaining a low postvoiding residual, then the final outcome, intermittent catheterization, is the focus of care.

In evaluating this care it is important that all possible attempts are made to get the patient to void without the invasive catheter. Therefore it is vital that nurses continuously evaluate both the outcomes and all attempted nursing interventions.

REFERENCES

1. Abdellah FG: Incontinence implications for health care policy, *Nurs Clin North Am* 23(1):291-297, 1988.
2. Autry D, Lauzon F, and Holliday P: The voiding record, an aid in decreasing incontinence, *Geriatr Nurs* 5(1):22-25, 1984.
3. Bates P and others: The standardization of terminology of lower urinary tract function, *J Urol* 121:551, 1979.
4. Bavendam TG: Stress urinary incontinence in women, *J Enterostom Ther* 17:57-66, 1990.
5. Benvenuti F, and others: Reeducative treatment of female genuine stress incontinence, *Am J Phys Med Rehabil* 66:155-168, 1987.
6. Braddom RL, Rocco JF: Autonomic dysreflexia: a survey of current treatment, *Am J Phys Med Rehabil* 70:234-241, 1991.
7. Brink CA: Absorbent pads, garments, and management strategies, *J Am Geriatr Soc* 38:368-373, 1990.
8. Bristoll SL, and others: The mythical danger of rapid urinary drainage, *Am J Nurs* 89:344-345, 1989.
9. Burgio KL, Engel BT: Biofeedback-assisted behavioral training for elderly men and women, *J Am Geriatr Soc* 38:338-340, 1990.
10. Burgio KL, Robinson JC, and Engel BT : The role of biofeedback in Kegel exercise training for stress incontinence, *Am J Obstet Gynecol* 154:58-64, 1986.
11. Burns PA, Mareck MA, Dittmar SS, and Bullough B: Kegel's exercise with biofeedback therapy for treatment of stress incontinence, *Nurs Pract* 10(2):28-34, 46, 1985.
12. Burns PA, and others: Treatment of stress incontinence with pelvic floor exercises and biofeedback, *J Am Geriatr Soc* 38:341-344, 1990.
13. Cardenas DD, Mayo ME: Manual stimulation of reflex voiding after spinal cord injury, *Arch Phys Med Rehabil* 66:459-462, 1985.
14. Cardozo L: Role of estrogen in the treatment of female urinary incontinence, *J Am Geriatr Soc* 38:326-328, 1990.
15. Carroll-Johnson RM, editor: *Classification of nursing diagnosis: proceedings of the Eighth Conference*, Philadelphia, 1989, JB Lippincott.
16. Cohen RE: Behavioral treatment of incontinence in a profoundly neurologically impaired adult, *Arch Phys Med Rehabil* 67:883, 1986.
17. DeRidder PA, Vallerand HG: Medication: its role in the cause and treatment of urinary incontinence, *J Enterostom Ther* 13:187-189, 1986.
18. Diokno AC: Diagnostic categories of incontinence and the role of urodynamic testing, *J Am Geriatr Soc* 38:300-305, 1990.
19. Diokno AC, Brodk BM, Brown MB, and Herzog R: Prevalence of urinary incontinence and other urological symptoms in the noninstitutionalized elderly, *J Urol* 136:1022-1025, 1986.
20. Dittmar SS: *Rehabilitation nursing: process and application,* St Louis, 1989, Mosby–Year Book.
21. Fantl JA, Wyman JF, Harkins SW, and Hadley EC: Bladder training in the management of lower urinary tract dysfunction in women, *J Am Geriatr Soc* 38:329-332, 1990.
22. Fowler EM, Ouslander J, and Papen J: Managing incontinence in the nursing home population, *J Enterostom Ther* 17(2):77-86, 1990.
23. Godec CJ: Timed voiding: a useful tool in the treatment of urinary incontinence, *Urology* 23:97-100, 1984.
24. Gray M: Congenital causes of incontinence in childhood: presentation and treatment, *J Enterostom Ther* 17(2):47-53, 1990.
25. Gray M, Dougherty MC: Urinary incontinence—pathophysiology and treatment, *J Enterostom Ther* 14:152-162, 1987.
26. Hadley EC: Bladder training and related therapies for urinary incontinence in older people, *JAMA* 256:372, 1986.
27. Heaton JPW and others: Bladder neck suspension for stress incontinence as an out patient procedure, *Urol Clin North Am* 14:209, 1987.
28. Herzog AR, Fultz NH: Prevalence and incidence of urinary incontinence in community-dwelling populations, *J Am Geriatr Soc* 38:273-281, 1990.
29. Hu T-W: Impact of urinary incontinence on health care costs, *J Am Geriatr Soc* 38:292-295, 1990.
30. Irrgang SJ: Classification of urinary incontinence, *J Enterostom Ther* 13(2):62-65, 1986.
31. Johnson DE, Muncie HL, O'Reilly JL, and Warren JW: An external urine collection device for incontinent women, *J Am Geriatr Soc* 38:1016-1022, 1990.
32. Kegel AH: Progressive resistance exercises in the functional restoration of the perineal muscles, *Am J Obstet Gynecol* 56:238-248, 1948.
33. LaFollette SS: A continent urostomy: a case history, *AORN J* 40:207-215, 1984.
34. Lockhart-Pretti P: Urinary incontinence, *J Enterostom Ther* 17:112-119, 1990.
34a. Long ML: Incontinence: defining the nursing role, *J Gerontol Nurs* 11:30, 1985.
35. McCormick KA: From clinical trial to health policy—research on urinary incontinence in the adult, part I, *J Prof Nurs* 7:147, 1991.
36. McCormick KA: From clinical trial to health policy—research on urinary incontinence in the adult, part II, *J Prof Nurs* 7:202, 1991.

III

III

37. McCormick KA, Scheve AAS, and Leahy E: Nursing management of urinary incontinence in geriatric patients, *Nurs Clin North Am* 23(1):231-264, 1988.
38. McGrother CW, Castleden CM, Duffin H, and Clark M: A profile of disordered micturition in the elderly at home, *Age Ageing* 16:105-110, 1987.
39. McLane AM, editor: *Classification of nursing diagnoses: proceedings of the Seventh Conference, North American nursing diagnosis association,* St Louis, 1987, Mosby–Year Book.
40. Moore KN: Intermittant catheterization: sterile or clean? *Rehabil Nurs* 16(1):15-18, 33, 1991.
41. National Institutes of Health: *Urinary incontinence in adults: National Institutes of Health consensus development conference statement,* 7(5), Bethesda, Md, 1988, National Institutes of Health.
42. Orzeck S, Ouslander JG: Urinary incontinence: an overview of causes and treatment, *J Enterostom Ther* 14:20-27, 1987.
43. Ouslander JG: Urinary incontinence in nursing homes, *J Am Geriatr Soc* 38:289-291, 1990.
44. Ouslander J, and others: Prospective evaluation of an assessment strategy for geriatric urinary incontinence, *J Am Geriatr Soc* 37:715-724, 1989.
45. Palmer MH: Incontinence: the magnitude of the problem, *Nurs Clin North Am* 23(1):139-157, 1988.
46. Petrilli CO, Traughber B, and Schnelle JF: Behavioral management in the inpatient geriatric population, *Nurs Clin North Am* 23(1):265-277, 1988.
47. Ramphal M: Urinary incontinence among nursing home patients: issues in research, *Geriatr Nurs* 8:249, 1987.
48. Resnick NM: Initial evaluation of the incontinent patient, *J Am Geriatr Soc* 38:311-316, 1990.
49. Resnick NM, Yalla SV: Management of urinary incontinence in the elderly, *N Engl J Med* 313:800-805, 1985.
50. Robb SS: Urinary incontinence: verification in elderly men, *Nurs Res* 34:278-282, 1985.
51. Schnelle JF, and others: Assessment and quality control of incontinence care in long term nursing facilities, *J Am Geriatr Soc* 39:165-171, 1991.
51a. Sunstad DG and Rosenthal T: Urinary incontinence in the elderly, N Engl J Med 313(13):800, 1985.
52. Tanagho EA: Electrical stimulation, *J Am Geriatr Soc* 38:352-355, 1990.
53. Taylor K, Henderson J: Effects of biofeedback and urinary stress incontinence in older women, *J Gerontol Nurs* 12(9):25-30, 1986.
54. Tries J: Kegel exercises enhanced by biofeedback, *J Enterostom Ther* 17:67-76, 1990
55. Voith AM: A conceptual framework for nursing diagnosis: alteration in urinary elimination, *Rehabil Nurs* 11:18-20, 1986.
56. Voith AM, Smith DA: Validation of the nursing diagnosis of urinary retention, *Nurs Clin North Am* 20(4):723, 1985.
57. Warren JW: Urine-collection devices for use in adults with urinary incontinence, *J Am Geriatr Soc* 38:364-367, 1990.
58. *Webster's new universal unabridged dictionary,* ed 2, New York, 1983, Simon and Schuster.
59. Wells TJ: Pelvic (floor) muscle exercise, *J Am Geriatr Soc* 38:333-337, 1990.
60. Wells TJ, and others: Pelvic muscle exercises for stress urinary incontinence in elderly women, *J Am Geriatr Soc* 39:785-791, 1991.
61. Williams ME, Gaylord SA: Role of functional assessment in the evaluation of urinary incontinence, *J Am Geriatr Soc* 38:296-299, 1990.

ACTIVITY-EXERCISE PATTERN
Altered Growth and Development

Altered Growth and Development is the state in which an individual demonstrates deviations from norms from his/her age group.[21]

OVERVIEW

The developmental process in humans is continuous and dynamic throughout the entire life span. Until the twentieth century, the study of growth and development, particularly that of children, was based largely on myths and folklore. During the past century, however, research-based theory has expanded into a large body of knowledge from which we can now draw many valid nursing implications.[20,25] Developmental theorists have focused on different aspects of the process of growth and development. For example, Gesell focused on maturation and heredity as the the basis of development. The learning theorists, such as Pavlov and Skinner, emphasized the importance of reward, punishment, and learned responses in development. Erickson's theory of psychosocial development describes age-related stages, each with a critical problem or conflict that must be resolved for normal development to occur. This theory is an outgrowth of Freud's theory of psychosexual development, which deals with the influence of sexual and aggressive instincts on development. Theories of cognitive development and the development of logical thinking were proposed by Piaget and others.[25,37]

The study of Altered Growth and Development encompasses the physical, cognitive, psychosocial, and spiritual aspects of a person. Causative factors of Altered Growth and Development fall into four broad categories: heredity, which includes genetic and metabolic abnormalities; problems that occur during pregnancy or in the perinatal period; acquired diseases; and ecological and behavioral problems.[11,29] The dysfunction that causes Altered Growth and Development can occur before a child's birth, during delivery, or after birth. An infant who is normal at birth can later develop a dysfunction as a result of maladaptive family relationships or other harmful environmental conditions. A person of any age can experience an injury or acquire a chronic illness that adversely affects development.

Children with Altered Growth and Development are often labeled dysfunctional, developmentally delayed, at risk, or disabled. These children can generally be identified as having a disability that interferes with the development of motor, adaptive, communication, and/or social skills, causing them to progress at a significantly slower rate than normal children in their peer group.[11,32] The Rehabilitation, Comprehensive Services and Developmental Disabilities Amendments of 1978 (P.L. 95-602) states that the mental or physical dysfunction that causes a developmental disability "is manifested before the person attains the age twenty-two" and "is likely to continue indefinitely."

Several general principles relate to the nursing diagnosis of Altered Growth and Development. Although the timetable is unique for each person, normal growth and development follow a predict-

IV

able pattern that progress in an orderly fashion. Any disruption or interference in the specific sequence of the stages may result in Altered Growth and Development.

Growth and development begin as a general response to the environment and progress to a more specific, refined, and skilled response. As development progresses, skills and behaviors become integrated, and new skills and behaviors are built on previously acquired ones. Growth and development continues to be influenced by a wide variety of factors. There are critical or sensitive periods during which the person is more vulnerable to both beneficial and harmful influence. Children who lack appropriate resources to cope with and adapt to these critical periods may exhibit Altered Growth and Development.[25,36,37]

ASSESSMENT

The nursing diagnosis of Altered Growth and Development can be identified in patients who have a broad spectrum of medical diagnoses and conditions. Vaughan[36] defines growth as "changes in size of the body as a whole or of its separate parts" and development as "changes of function, including those largely shaped by interaction with the structural, emotional, or social environment." Altered Growth and Development therefore describes a deviation from accepted norms in both the quality and quantity of maturational changes. The nursing diagnosis Altered Growth and Development can be assigned to an individual who has failed to progress at a normal rate in acquiring certain developmental skills in the areas of motor, adaptive, communication, and social functioning.[30,32]

Altered development of motor skills includes abnormal body movement, for example, spasticity and athetoid movement, and the lack of coordination and balance necessary for such developmental milestones as rolling over, standing up, walking, and running. This also includes the inappropriate presence or absence of primitive reflexes.

Altered development of adaptive skills encompasses deficits in problem-solving abilities and in the skills of hand control necessary for self-suffi-

ciency and effective interaction with the environment, such as feeding, dressing, and toileting.

Altered development of communication skills involves some degree of inability to understand and/or express oneself verbally and non-verbally. This includes the entire range of communication, from expressing oneself by gesture only to being unable to construct a complex sentence. Deficits in comprehension are exhibited by the inability to follow simple or complex instructions.

An alteration in the acquisition of social skills would involve a delay in the development of or a deficit in those abilities that a person needs to interact with others (for example, social smiling and the ability to engage in appropriate peer relations).

Vaughan[36] conceptualizes growth and development as "a continuum of interaction" between innate genetic potential (stored in the genetic substance of the fertilized ovum) and the environment. The extent to which each person realizes his/her biologic potential is determined by the interrelation of many factors. In many cases, the environment influences genetic factors to determine the extent to which one's biological potential will be realized. For example, the injurious effects of the abnormal genes in phenylketonuria may be halted if the newborn's diet restricts phenylalanine intake.

The presence of trauma, either prenatally or postnatally, compromises the genetic potential for growth and development. This may include chemical trauma, as in the effects of teratogenic drugs; physical trauma, such as birth injury or child abuse; the effects of an infection; exposure to radiation; or reaction to an immunological agent such as pertussis vaccine.

Both prenatal and postnatal nutritional factors are basic to optimal growth and development, but provision of adequate nutrition largely depends on socioeconomic factors that also determine the extent to which adequate health care, education, and housing are available to the child. Socioeconomic factors modify growth potential by influencing the child-rearing environment and the interaction between a parent and child. These factors shape the parents' personal needs and concerns that are then conveyed to the child either subconsciously or consciously, thereby having a profound effect on the child's ability to achieve self-realization. Diverse issues such as birth order and maternal age at the time of birth also influence self-realization. Finally, cultural factors establish norms and expectations against which the acquisition of developmental milestones is measured.

Medical diagnoses related to the nursing diagnosis Altered Growth and Development include all of the disabling conditions that involve every body system. These include deficits in cardiac formation and structure, such as, tetralogy of Fallot, and metabolic dysfunction that affects the chemical processes in the body, such as galactosemia and Tay-Sachs disease, and causes abnormal growth patterns, for example, hypothyroidism. Also included are congenital malformations of the nervous system, such as spina bifida and myelomeningocele; chromosomal abnormalities, such as Down syndrome; chronic diseases, such as cancer; and an array of systemic disorders affecting the child's physical development, such as cystic fibrosis, diabetes, muscular dystrophy and dwarfism. Prematurity also frequently causes altered patterns of growth and development.

In addition, a group of conditions result in the abnormal structure, maturation, and function of the brain that causes a child to fail to progress or to progress at a delayed rate. Such diagnoses are known as developmental disorders and include mental retardation, language delay, learning disabilities, microcephaly, autism, cerebral palsy, sensory deficits, and seizure disorders. Though they have great variation in their cause and how they symptomatically appear in each individual, the common thread in these disorders is a dysfunctional brain—one that does not operate at the appropriate level for the child's age.[33]

Developmental assessment can confirm normal development or can identify developmental delays. A nurse is frequently the first professional to identify a child as having abnormal development in one or more areas. The use of standardized screening tests enables early recognition of delay or dysfunction, referral for further testing, and treatment of disabling conditions. The nurse also uses assessment tools to discern functional levels in a patient and to facilitate anticipatory guidance that enhances the parents' ability to encourage and participate in the evolving process of development.

The nursing diagnosis Altered Growth and Development is usually made after a comprehensive developmental evaluation by a multidisciplinary team that includes a nurse. Gross and fine motor, cognitive, language, and social development as well as health, physical growth, familial relationships, and environmental factors are assessed.

The nurse also evaluates the family's knowledge about the condition and its management, the home setting, family structure, support network, coping skills, and family adaptation and uses these observations to plan and implement teaching and individualized home care. Family assessment should be nonintrusive and geared toward the practical concerns and needs of the family that the nurse is willing and able to address.[3] Nursing assessment for Altered Growth and Development involves the use of an array of screening methods and tools, some of which are described in Table 10.

❖ Defining Characteristics

The presence of the following defining characteristics indicate that the patient may be experiencing Altered Growth and Development:[11,33,35]

- Impaired physical growth
- Impaired sensory function
- Delayed, altered, or compromised development of motor skills
- Abnormal movement patterns
- Abnormal neurologic function
- Abnormal muscle tone
- Deficient in following instructions
- Delayed, altered, or compromised development of social skills
- Impaired ability to interact with others
- Deficient in modulating behavior
- Limitation in ability for self-direction
- Limited capacity for independent living

IV

IV

Table 10 Screening and Assessment Tools for Nursing Diagnosis Altered Growth and Development*

Tool	Applicable Age	Areas Assessed	Procedure	Additional Information	Source
Brazelton Neonatal Behavioral Assessment Scale	3 days to 4 weeks	Motor, social, and neurological functioning	Direct observation	Special training required; valuable for demonstration to parents to increase awareness of infant cues	Neonatal Behavioral Assessment Scale, J.B. Lippincott Co., East Washington Square, Philadelphia, PA 19105
Alpern-Boll Developmental Profile II (DPII)	Birth to 9½ years functional age	Physical development and self-help; social, academic, and communication skills	Direct observation interview	Self-instructional manual available; developmental screening tool	Western Psychological Services, 12031 Wilshire Blvd., Los Angeles, CA 90025
McCarthy Scales of Children's Abilities	2½-8½ years	Motor development, cognitive function, memory, and verbal skills	Direct observation	Self-instructional manual available; developmental assessment tool with manipulative items, gross motor tests and verbal response items	McCarthy Scales of Children's Abilities, The Psychological Corp., 555 Academic Court, San Antonio, TX 78204-2498
Denver II	1 month to 6 years	Personal-social, fine motor-adaptive, language, and gross motor skills	Observation/parent report	Instructional manual, kit, proficiency test available; updated version of Denver Developmental Screening Test (DDST)	Denver Developmental Material, Inc., P.O. Box 6919, Denver, CO 80206-0919
Milani-Comparetti Motor Development Screening Test	Birth to 24 months	Motor development, primitive reflexes, mature patterns of movement, and postural control	Direct observation	Manual and film available for instruction in administration and scoring	Milani-Comparetti Motor Development Screening Test, Meyer Children's Rehabilitation Institute, University of Nebraska, Medical Center Omaha, NE 68131

Test	Age range	Measures	Method	Comments	Source
AAMD Adaptive Behavior Scale	3 to 69+ years	Adaptive behavior in the following domains: independent functioning, physical development, economic activity, language development, numbers and time, domestic and vocational activity, self-direction, responsibility, and socialization	Direct observation/parent or caretaker interview	Administration manual available; training not required; evaluates and describes effectiveness of coping with demands of environment; also includes maladaptive behavior scale	AAMD Adaptive Behavior Scale, ProEd, 8700 Shoal Creek Blvd., Austin, TX 78758
Home Observation and Measurement of the Environment (HOME)	Birth to 3 years 3 to 6 years 6 to 10 years	Home environment and support for emotional, social, and cognitive development	Parent interview/structured observation	Administration manual available; training desirable; can be used to plan interventions	R.H. Bradley, PhD B.M. Caldwell, PhD Center for Research on Teaching and Learning, College of Education University of Arkansas at Little Rock, 2801 S. University Ave., Little Rock, AR 72204
Adapted HOME for children with moderate handicaps	Infant Preschool Elementary	Home environment and support for emotional, social, and cognitive development	Parent interview/structured observation	Administration manual available; training desirable; modified for mental retardation, orthopedic, hearing, and vision impairment	Same as above
Extended HOME for children with severe handicaps	Same as above	Same as above	Same as above	Same as above	Same as above
Early Language Milestone Scale (ELM Scale)	0-36 months	Expressive and receptive language functioning	Interactive test/parent interview	Manual and test kit available; training not required; screening tool	ELM Scale, Modern Education Corp., P.O. Box 721, Tulsa, OK 74107

IV

Continued.

Table 10 Screening and Assessment Tools for Nursing Diagnosis Altered Growth and Development—cont'd

Tool	Applicable Age	Areas Assessed	Procedure	Additional Information	Source
Family Needs Survey (Revised)	Parents	Perceived needs and extent of each need	Questionnaire	Helps family become aware of available services	D.B. Bailey, Jr., PhD R.J. Simeonsson, PhD, Frank Porter Graham Child Development Center, CB# 8180, University of North Carolina, Chapel Hill, NC 27599
Parent Perception Inventory (PPI)	Parents	Concerns, beliefs, and feelings, coping, general information, siblings and spouse concerns and coping	Questionnaire	Modification of Chronicity Impact and Coping Instrument: Parent Questionnaire (CICI:PG); training not required; entire inventory or individual scales can be used; for use with families of individuals with long-term disabilities or chronic illness	D.P. Hymovich, PhD, RN, FAAN, College of Nursing, University of South Florida, Health Sciences Center, MDC Box 22, 12901 Bruce B. Downs Blvd., Tampa, FL 33612-4799

*References 1, 3-8, 10, 15, 17-20, 23, 24, 27, 29, 32, 37.

- Decreased coordination
- Decreased balance
- Unable to perform age-appropriately in activities of daily living
- Cognitive development inappropriate for age

- Limited capacity for economic self-sufficiency
- Delayed, altered, or compromised development of receptive and/or expressive communication skills

❖ Related Factors

The following related factors are associated with Altered Growth and Development:[11,29,32]

- Prenatal-maternal chronic or acute disease
- Inadequate prenatal care
- Maternal age
- Exposure to teratogens
- Fetal distress
- Prolonged or precipitous labor
- Interruption of oxygen intrapartally
- Prematurity
- Low birthweight
- Asphyxia in neonatal period
- Low Apgar score
- Birth injury
- Significant blood loss
- Kernicterus
- Congenital defect(s)
- Genetic abnormality
- Metabolic disorder
- Familial history: mental retardation, genetic disorders
- Unknown mechanism
- Neonatal disease

- Trauma: physical, chemical, infection, radiation, immunological, psychological, or emotional
- Difficult infant temperament
- Inadequate caretaking
- Poor support system
- Disadvantaged social environment: poverty
- Suboptimal infant-parent attachment
- Separation from significant others
- Lack of stimulation in the environment
- Overstimulation from the environment
- Neonatal infection
- Chronic illness
- Serious illness
- Malnutrition: maternal, infant

❖ Related Medical/Psychiatric Diagnoses

The following are examples of related medical diagnoses for Altered Growth and Development:[11]

- Autism
- Blindness
- Cancer
- Cerebral palsy
- Congenital rubella
- Deafness
- Down syndrome
- Duchenne muscular dystrophy
- Fetal alcohol syndrome
- Fragile X syndrome
- Galactosemia
- Head trauma
- Hurler syndrome
- Hypothyroidism
- Intraventricular hemorrhage
- Kernicterus
- Language disorder
- Lead poisoning
- Learning disability
- Low birth weight

- Maple syrup urine disease
- Maternal cytomegalovirus
- Maternal diabetes mellitus
- Maternal rubella
- Maternal substance abuse
- Meningitis
- Mental retardation
- Neural tube defects
- Neurofibromatosis
- Placental insufficiency
- Prematurity
- Seizure disorder
- Tay-Sachs disease
- Use of teratogenic prescription drugs

NURSING DIAGNOSES

Examples of *specific* nursing diagnoses for Altered Growth and Development are:

- Altered Growth and Development related to cognitive difficulties
- Altered Growth and Development related to prolonged illness and disability that exhausts coping abilities
- Altered Growth and Development related to poor support system

PLANNING AND IMPLEMENTATION WITH RATIONALE

There are three major areas of nursing intervention for patients with Altered Growth and Development: (1) those involving education or nursing functions related to the ongoing health needs of the patient, (2) those involving coordination of services with other professionals, and (3) those relating to the provision of family support. All interventions should be family-centered, recognizing and supporting the family's role as the primary and constant caretaker, educator, and advocate. The family's ultimate responsibility for making decisions about care must be acknowledged.[31,35,37]

Nursing interventions may take place at any stage in the family's process of adapting to the disability. Each family has a unique way of adapting to the stress of a long-term disability. Although some families adapt poorly and become dysfunctional, others function at a high level and make a positive adjustment.[16,26,34,37] Assisting the family as they adapt to the challenges and lifestyle changes brought about by a disability is an important aspect of the nursing role in the diagnosis Altered Growth and Development.[29] This process evolves throughout the life of the individual with Altered Growth and Development, and the nurse must be sensitive to all family members, who may be in different stages of the process.[16] The nurse has the ongoing responsibility to assist the family in understanding and coping with the unique and changing needs at various stages of development of the individual with Altered Growth and Development.

Families must have sensitively and appropriately delivered information to enable them to actively participate in setting therapeutic goals. All goals and interventions should be based on existing abilities and strengths, and reflect the extent of the disability and functional or developmental age. Professional recommendations must be balanced with family needs, goals, and priorities. *Unrealistic goals and unmet expectations frustrate the family and patient, disrupting the family's coping ability and interfering with the family-patient relationship.*[31] *Challenges should closely approximate abilities so that the goals are attainable and the family can experience success.* The patient should participate in formulating goals to the best of his/her ability. Functional, not chronological, age is the determining factor in deciding

to what extent an individual with Altered Growth and Development can be included in goal setting,

When there is a minor delay or disability, the health concerns of an individual with Altered Growth and Development may be practically the same as his/her "normal" counterpart. However, a major delay or multiple disabilities tend to complicate these concerns. The nurse will usually supervise a medical regimen that supports and teaches the family until they become comfortable and proficient in using the equipment, administering the medication, and performing the procedures necessary to maintain health and functional abilities at the optimal level and, in some cases, to sustain life. The family may have to use monitoring equipment such as an apnea monitor, life-support equipment such as a ventilator or a suction machine, feeding equipment such as a continuous infusion pump, and adaptive equipment to facilitate home care such as a bath seat or a lift. The nurse may also have to teach the family to monitor the patient's response to medications, as with a seizure disorder or cardiac dysfunction. Frequently, families must learn to perform medical procedures that will enable the family member with Altered Growth and Development to live at home. *The nurse must plan for initial teaching and ongoing supervision of these procedures to ensure that they are performed safely and effectively.*

Because of the complex medical needs of many individuals with Altered Growth and Development, basic health and safety issues can be easily overlooked. The nurse must be aware of the need for regular medical and dental care and be able to assist the family in locating appropriate resources for this care. Safety should be integrated into any care plan. This involves such diverse concerns as adaptive seating for automobile transportation, child-proofing for poisons, and fire safety.

The nurse must also address the behaviors known collectively as activities of daily living. Teaching the family to deal with feeding, sleeping, bathing, dressing, toileting, and handling difficult or inappropriate behavior is critical and requires much insight into the family's coping strategies, the family's personal and group goals, and the practical limitations and realities of the situation. *These activities of daily living evolve as the patient grows in size and attains or does not attain new levels of development. The family dynamics and the family's ability to cope are not static, and the nurse must be sensitive to the family's needs at different stages of development.*

The planning and implementation of care for the individual with Altered Growth and Development usually involve coordination of services with many other professionals. The individual with Altered Growth and Development is often seen by many specialists who may not always communicate effectively with each other, causing confusion for the family and resulting in gaps in the child's health care. The nurse can facilitate communication between physicians and other professionals and can clarify information for the family. *Improved communication will help ensure that the family has access to all necessary professional services and equipment, such as physical, occupational, and speech therapy; nutrition counseling; social work intervention; and financial resources.* Coordination of professional services is frequently required after a hospitalization to ensure a smooth transition from hospital to home. Interaction with school personnel is another aspect of providing care for the disabled. Often this involves interpretation of health needs as they relate to the educational or vocational program. Because of improved medical care in recent years, developmentally disabled individuals are able to live longer. Collaboration is necessary to prevent discontinuity as an individual makes the shift between service delivery systems that are geared to certain age groups, especially during the major transition from pediatric to adult services.[11,22] Coordination of the many professionals who are involved with an individual experiencing Altered Growth and Development can overwhelm a family, but its importance to the overall success of the plan of care should not be overlooked.

By establishing a trusting relationship and conveying an attitude of acceptance and concern, the nurse can support the individual with Altered

Growth and Development as he/she accepts and adapts to the diagnosis. Frequent contact with the patient allows the nurse to observe the individual's response to the disability, his/her functional ability within the individual's own environment, and his/her relationships with family members and significant others. The nurse can assist the family in meeting the emotional needs of the patient by encouraging his/her expression of fears and concerns and by helping the individual with Altered Growth and Development to cope with those things that make him/her different from others in the peer group. The information the nurse shares with the patient depends on the patient's age and cognitive ability. For instance, an adolescent with cognitive abilities in the normal range and a motor deficiency would probably have the same questions and concerns about sexuality as other adolescents, in addition to the special concerns related to his/her disability. A young adult with cystic fibrosis needs to know how this condition affects the choices he/she must make about his/her future. Encouraging the patient to discuss the condition facilitates clarification of misinformation. The nurse can be instrumental in enhancing self-esteem and a positive self-concept and in encouraging self-care behaviors that lead to independence from the family.[2] Normalization of activities within the family and community should be encouraged at all times, helping the individual with Altered Growth and Development to achieve normal developmental tasks whenever possible.[28,37]

The family of an individual with Altered Growth and Development needs many types of support. A delicate balance must be reached between the family's need for support and their need to remain autonomous.[35] The nurse can act as an advocate for the family while at the same time support the parents as they develop and refine their own advocacy skills. Emotional support must be offered to all family members, including siblings, as they try to understand the disabling condition and deal with feelings of guilt, inadequacy, anger, and sorrow. These feelings are not only present in the early stages of a child's life,

IV

❖ NURSING GUIDELINES
Nursing Diagnosis: Altered Growth and Development

Expected Patient/Family Outcomes

Nursing Interventions

The family will demonstrate an understanding of the nature and etiology of the disability, the recommended interventions, and the possible complications and demonstrate their ability to participate in formulating realistic goals.

- Using assessment data and feedback from the family, determine each family member's level of knowledge.
- Teach family by sharing information (verbal, written, drawings, printed booklets) at appropriate level with patient, siblings, and other family members.

The family will demonstrate increased confidence and competence as caregivers by seeking independence from health care providers, assuming increased responsibility for care, and successfully incorporating all therapy and treatments into the daily routine of the family.

- Teach family (by modeling, use of posters, charts, pamphlets) to use necessary equipment, medications, and procedures to maintain health and functional abilities.
- Encourage appropriate stimulation and compliance with therapeutic regimen.
- Clarify information, willingly repeat terminology, explanations, and information as often as necessary.

The patient with Altered Growth and Development will have access to and use appropriately all necessary health services as evidenced by the maintenance of optimal health and adequate respiration, elimination, and nutrition, as well as the absence of secondary disabilities.

- Support medical regimen by providing direct care to child and planning and implementing individualized health care within the family context.
- Promote safety (assist the family in obtaining an adapted car safety seat) and maintenance of health and wellness (refer to physicians and dentists who are familiar with the special health care needs of individuals with Altered Growth and Development).

The patient with Altered Growth and Development will attain maximal level of functioning as evidenced by the highest possible degree of independence in activities of daily living.

- Assist family in dealing with difficulties in behavior, feeding, sleeping, dressing, bathing, and toileting. (Assist family to implement behavior modification program.)

❖ *NURSING GUIDELINES—CONT'D*

Nursing Diagnosis: *Altered Growth and Development*

The patient with Altered Growth and Development will receive comprehensive, developmentally appropriate education and habilitative interventions, including physical, occupational, and speech therapy in addition to prescribed prosthetic or orthotic devices, and the family will demonstrate appropriate use of community resources.

- Act as liaison to coordinate program of care.
- Work collaboratively with family and interdisciplinary team to identify and meet health, psychological, social, and emotional needs.
- Identify appropriate community resources and assist the family in gaining access to all needed professional services, equipment, and financial resources.

The patient with Altered Growth and Development will achieve a positive and supportive relationship with the nurse as evidenced by: (to the extent of his/her ability) compliance with therapy; behavior that indicates a positive self-concept, improved self-esteem, and positive adaptation; increased understanding of his/her disability, treatment, and the effect of the disability; and involvement in goal setting and the management of his/her own care.

- Establish caring and trusting relationship with individual with Altered Growth and Development
- Encourage verbalization of questions, fears, and concerns.
- Reinforce positive adaptation and behavior.
- Share information about disability and its effect; correct misinformation.
- To the extent possible, encourage normalization of activities.

IV

Continued.

IV

❖ *NURSING GUIDELINES—CONT'D*
Nursing Diagnosis: *Altered Growth and Development*

The family members will constructively deal with emotions about the diagnosis as evidenced by the integration of the individual with Altered Growth and Development into the family, development of a relationship with the nurse based on mutual trust and respect (as evidenced by decreased anxiety, increased confidence, increased ability to discuss fears and concerns, and increased information seeking), and increased willingness and ability to assume the advocacy role.	• Support family through crisis of diagnosis and later critical periods or developmental crises periods or development crises (emotional support, telephone calls, home visits, information about parent-to-parent support). • Advocate the rights and needs of the family, e.g., assist in obtaining respite care or placement in the most appropriate educational program. • Teach advocacy skills. • Model attitudes and acceptance. • Encourage expression of feelings, fears. • Assist with identification and solution of problems. • Support positive relationships within the family (emphasize family's strengths, skills).

but also resurface periodically, especially at important transitions, such as the start of formal education. Anticipatory guidance can be offered before and during stressful periods to prevent the problems from becoming a crisis.[9,14] Some of these stressful periods are: the assessment and diagnosis of the condition; emerging sexuality in an adolescent; and the time when parents face their own aging and thus deal with issues of guardianship and life-long care. Nonjudgemental listening helps to clarify concerns and lets the family know that their ideas and concerns are valid. The nurse can recommend appropriate literature, community resources, and support groups for parents, siblings, and in some cases the individual with Altered Growth and Development. The nurse supports decision-making as alternatives in care or residential placement are identified and examined and goals are reevaluated and clarified. Most important, by providing support in whatever form the family needs and by building on the family's

strengths, the *nurse enables and empowers the family and helps to develop competence and instill confidence in the family* as members of the health care team.[12,28,37]

EVALUATION

Parents and other caregivers should regularly evaluate preventive, maintenance, rehabilitative, and curative aspects of the care plan. The optimal level of health will vary in each patient with Altered Growth and Development and will depend on many complex variables, including the response of the disability to the treatment, the family situation, and the ability of the family to obtain recommended health, therapy, education, and social services.

Evaluation of services should determine to what extent the parents and family successfully use social and emotional support systems, deal with crisis situations and strong emotions, and integrate the disabled child into the family with

❖ CASE STUDY WITH PLAN OF CARE

Kurt H. is a 10-year-old boy with spina bifida. He was referred to the community health nurse for assistance with intermittent self-catheterization training. Born with a myelomeningocele at the L-4 level of his spine, Kurt was treated by surgical closure of the defect shortly thereafter. A ventriculoperitoneal (VP) shunt was placed to prevent hydrocephalus. Kurt's most recent shunt revision was 1 year ago. He has had frequent urinary tract infections. Physical findings include a height of 4'4", which is in the 25th percentile, and a weight of 72.5 pounds, which is in the 50th percentile. Kurt has lower extremity motor paralysis that has resulted in musculoskeletal deformities (hip flexion and adduction and knee flexion). He can ambulate with the aid of crutches and braces. Kurt receives regular physical therapy but is inconsistent and unmotivated to perform his self-exercise program as recommended. Kurt is independent in feeding and bathing, but he requires assistance with dressing. Kurt has a neurogenic bladder and bowel and has been taught clean, intermittent self-catheterization but is not yet fully compliant or independent in performing the procedure. A bowel management program has also been established. His intellectual functioning was found to be close to normal for his age, but Kurt performs poorly in school. Poor management of urinary incontinence has led to difficulties with socialization and poor self-esteem. Kurt lives with his mother and older sister. His parents are divorced, and Kurt's father does not have contact with the family. His mother reports that his father could not accept Kurt's disability. He does not contribute financially to the family. Kurt's mother is employed and has a moderate income, but high medical expenses cause financial stress. No relatives live in the area. The mother has one or two close friends from her church who have been very supportive, but otherwise she is fairly isolated. She has little free time for pleasurable activities and spends little time with her daughter. The mother has difficulty managing Kurt's care and has not been successful in motivating Kurt to assume more responsibility for his self-care activities. The mother reports feeling overwhelmed and unable to cope.

PLAN OF CARE FOR KURT H. AND HIS MOTHER

Nursing Diagnosis Altered Growth and Development related to disadvantaged social environment and poor support system

Expected Patient/Family Outcomes	Nursing Interventions
Kurt's mother will improve her understanding of Kurt's disability and the therapeutic goals as evidenced by improved compliance with the treatment plan.	• Ascertain Kurt's mother's understanding of basic shunt mechanics and signs of shunt malfunction and infection. • Assist Kurt's mother in developing a behavioral program to encourage compliance with self-catheterization and self-exercise program. • Assist Kurt's mother in using resources for well-child care (medical and dental) as needed.
Kurt's mother will use available support system as evidenced by improved coping ability and decreased isolation.	• Help Kurt's mother deal with ambivalent feelings and negative emotions. • Coordinate with social worker to assist Kurt's mother in using community resources for financial assistance. • Assist Kurt's mother in obtaining respite services and using other support services within the community (e.g., support group for parents of handicapped children).

Continued.

IV

Expected Patient/Family Outcomes — cont'd	Nursing Interventions — cont'd
Kurt's mother will develop realistic goals and expectations as evidenced by improved problem-solving ability.	• Teach Kurt's mother to differentiate normal child behavior from problems resulting from the disability.
Kurt will improve compliance with self-catheterization program and consequently remain dry and free of odor and urinary tract infections, while retaining intact skin that has no pressure sores.	• Assess Kurt's level of comfort with self-catheterization program and monitor and encourage compliance with self-catheterization program. • Coordinate with school nurse to assure school support and cooperation with self-catheterization program. • Teach Kurt skin care, emphasizing the importance of good hygiene routines, changing position frequently, and an awareness of potential problems resulting from decreased sensation.
Kurt will improve compliance with self-exercise program to avoid contractures and osteoporosis and increase upper extremity strength.	• Coordinate with physical therapist in encouraging Kurt to ambulate and to exercise on a regular schedule.
Kurt will maintain body weight and avoid obesity.	• Teach dietary and nutritional management to prevent obesity and constipation.
Kurt will have increased self-esteem as evidenced by improved attitude and outlook.	• Provide Kurt with positive feedback. • Explore the relationship of incontinence to social problems. • Encourage greatest possible independence and positive outlook.

minimal disruption to family functioning. Evaluation of the plan of care should also measure the extent to which the patient with Altered Growth and Development can obtain and use recommended health and educational services, is able to attain optimal physical and psychological independence, is accepted and valued by others, and can achieve a positive sense of self-worth.

REFERENCES

1. Alpern G, Boll T, and Shearer M: *Developmental profile II manual,* Los Angeles, Calif, 1985, Western Psychological Services.
2. Austin JK: Assessment of coping mechanisms used by parents and children with chronic illness, *MCN* 15:98-102, 1990.
3. Bailey DB: Issues and perspectives on family assessment, *Infants Young Child* 4:26-34, 1991.
4. Bradley RH, Caldwell BM: *Home observation for measurement of the environment,* Little Rock, Ark, 1984, University of Arkansas at Little Rock.
5. Bradley RH, Caldwell BM: Using the HOME inventory to assess the family environment, *Pediatr Nurs* 14:97-102, 1988.
6. Bradley RH, and others: *Addendum to HOME manual: use of the HOME inventory with children with handicaps,* Little Rock, Ark, 1987, University of Arkansas at Little Rock.
7. Bradley RH, Rock SL, Caldwell BM, and Brisby JA: Uses of the HOME inventory for families with handicapped children, *Am J Ment Retard* 94:313-330, 1989.
8. Brazelton TB: *Neonatal behavioral assessment scale,* Philadelphia, Penn, 1973, JB Lippincott.
9. Clements DB, Copeland LG, and Loftus, M: Critical times for families with a chronically ill child, *Pediatr Nurs* 16:157-161, 1990.
10. Coplan J: *Early language milestone scale,* Tulsa, Okla, 1987, Modern Education Corp.
11. Crocker AC: The spectrum of medical care for developmental disabilities. In Rubin IL, Crocker AC, editors: *Developmental disabilities: delivery of medical care for children and adults,* Philadelphia, 1989, Lea & Febiger.
12. Dunst C, Trivette C, and Deal A: *Enabling and empowering families: principles and guidelines for practice,* Cambridge, Mass, 1988, Brookline Books.

13. Elder DS, Feetham SL: Patterns of impairment: myelome-ningocele. In Rose MH, Thomas RB, editors: *Children with chronic conditions: nursing in a family and community context,* Orlando, Fla, 1987, Grune & Stratton.
14. Fraley AM: Chronic sorrow: a parental response, *J Pediatr Nurs* 5:268-273, 1990.
15. Frankenburg WK, Dodds JB: *Denver II,* Denver, Colo, 1990, Denver Developmental Materials.
16. Futcher AJ: Chronic illness and family dynamics, *Pediatr Nurs* 14:381-385, 1988.
17. Glascoe FP: Developmental screening: rationale, methods and application, *Infants Young Child* 4:1-10, 1991.
18. Hymovich DP: Development of the chronicity impact and coping instrument: parent questionnaire (CICI:PQ), *Nurs Res* 33:218-222, 1984.
19. Hymovich DP: Measuring parental coping when a child is chronically ill. In Strickland OL, Waltz CF, editors: *Measurement of nursing outcome vol. IV. Measuring client self-care and coping skills,* New York, 1990, Springer.
20. Illingworth R: *The development of the infant and young child, normal and abnormal,* ed 9, Edinburgh, 1987, Churchill Livingstone.
21. Kim M, McFarland G, and McLane A: *Pocket guide to nursing diagnoses,* ed 4, St Louis, 1991, Mosby–Year Book.
22. Matson JL, Marchetti A, editors: *Developmental disabilities: a life-span perspective,* Philadelphia, 1988, Grune & Stratton.
23. McCarthy D: *McCarthy scales of children's abilities,* Chicago, 1972, The Psychological Corp.
24. Milani-Comparetti A, Gidoni EA: *Milani-Comparetti developmental scale,* Omaha, Neb, 1973, University of Nebraska Medical Center.
25. Mott SR: Developmental theories: how the child grows. In Mott SR, James SR, and Sperhac AM, editors: *Nursing care of children and families,* ed 2, Redwood City, Calif, 1990, Addison Wesley Nursing.
26. Mott SR, James SR, and Sperhac AM, editors: *Nursing care of children and families,* ed 2, Redwood City, Calif, 1990, Addison Wesley Nursing.
27. Nihira K, Foster R, Shellhaas M, and Leland H: *AAMD adaptive behavior scale,* Washington, DC, 1974, American Association on Mental Deficiency.
28. Patterson JM, Geber G: Preventing mental health problems in children with chronic illness or disability, *Children's Health Care* 20:150-161, 1991.
29. Rossetti LM: *Infant-toddler assessment: an interdisciplinary approach,* Boston, 1990, Little, Brown.
30. Shapiro BK, Palmer FB, and Capute AJ: Diagnosis and management of developmental disabilities, *Comp Ther* 13:17-25, 1987.
31. Shelton TL, Jeppson ES, and Johnson B: *Family centered care for children with special health care needs,* ed 2, Washington, DC, 1987, Association for the Care of Children's Health.
32. Sperhac AM: Developmental assessment. In Mott SR, James SR, and Sperhac AM, editors: *Nursing care of children and families,* ed 2, Redwood City, Calif, 1990, Addison Wesley Nursing.
33. Starrett AL: Early recognition of and intervention in developmental disorders, *Semin Neurol* 8:61-70, 1988.
34. Stone D: Professional perceptions of parental adaptation to a child with special needs, *Children's Health Care* 18:174-177, 1989.
35. Thomas RB, Wicks K: Nursing assessment of chronic conditions in children. In Rose MH, Thomas RB, editors: *Children with chronic conditions: nursing in a family and community context,* Orlando, Fla, 1987, Grune & Stratton.
36. Vaughan V: Developmental pediatrics. In Nelson W, Behrman R, Vaughn V, editors: *Nelson's textbook of pediatrics,* ed 13, Philadelphia, 1987, WB Saunders.
37. Whaley LF, Wong DL: *Nursing care of infants and children,* ed 4, St Louis, 1991, Mosby–Year Book.

IV

Fatigue

Fatigue is an overwhelming, sustained sense of exhaustion and decreased capacity for physical and mental work.[2]

OVERVIEW

Fatigue is a universal complaint that occurs with almost every illness, mental or physical.[5] The prevalence of Fatigue complaints ranges from 4% to 9% of all physician office visits in the United States and Canada. Complaints of chronic fatigue are responsible for more than 10 million office visits and $1 billion in direct costs in the United States alone.[9] It has been cited as the most common, yet least understood and most neglected symptom in medicine.[3]

Identification of the specific cause of Fatigue may not always be possible. Often its source is an interplay of several concomitant factors. Fatigue may be a precursor of disease, and in some diseases, Fatigue can remain for the duration of the illness. Chronic fatigue, which is not reversible by rest and recuperation, is a pervasive problem for patients with a number of illnesses.

In the 1980s chronic mononucleosis, or chronic Epstein-Barr virus (EBV), infection drew media attention. Patients who suffered unexplained fatigue and a prolonged attack of acute mononucleosis often received the diagnosis of chronic EBV infection. Despite the role of EBV in the acute illness, studies have been unable to substantiate its role in subsequent chronic fatigue.[4]

The controversy about the causes of chronic fatigue continues. Some believe that psychological disturbance is the basis for the complaint. Another longstanding theory claims that chronic fatigue is the result of an infection or inflammatory process.[10]

In one study, investigators assessed the psychiatric status of patients with chronic fatigue syndrome. The subjects chosen for the study met the CDC case definition of chronic fatigue syndrome and had unusual EBV serologic profiles. The findings concluded that the high lifetime prevalence of psychiatric disorders as well as the increased likelihood of psychiatric illness predating the chronic fatigue suggested that psychiatric factors contributed to the pathogenesis of chronic fatigue syndrome. However, psychiatric illness was an incomplete explanation because many of the physical and immunologic features of the chronic fatigue syndrome were not clearly attributable to psychiatric illness.[8]

Despite the lack of consensus about its cause, chronic fatigue is a widely pervasive phenomenon that robs quality from the lives of millions of people. In renal patients, chronic fatigue is so common that it is often identified by dialysis nurses as something that can't be changed.[12] Cardenas and Kutner[1] studied Fatigue in patients undergoing maintenance hemodialysis for end stage renal disease. They examined the relationships between fatigue and age, diagnosis, length of time on dialysis, depression, activity level, and laboratory data. Fatigue was found to be significantly associated with both depression and the diagnosis of systemic lupus erythematosus (SLE). Fatigue in multiple sclerosis is related to the level of the patient's disability, meaning that patients with greater disability reported more fatigue.[5] In systemic lupus erythematosus, fatigue is associated with not only disease activity and depression, but also the patient's perception of disease. That is, patients who perceived their disease to be more active also felt more fatigued.[7]

Fatigue has also been associated with radiation therapy. In one study, patients undergoing a two-week course of localized radiation were found to be significantly less fatigued on Sundays because no therapy was performed on weekends.[6]

Fatigue can have a profound effect on patients' lives. Fatigue reportedly affected one group of chronically ill patients most frequently in maintaining full-time employment and performing acceptably on the job. Fatigue also affected family relationships, making it virtually impossible for women to fulfill many of the roles expected of contemporary women in our society. Moreover, the number and types of social activities and commitments were greatly reduced because of Fatigue. One patient stated, "Limiting activities is an effective mechanism against fatigue, but it can also be a defense mechanism resulting in reclusiveness. I have not developed many friendships so I'm not asked out and don't have to deal with saying no."[7]

Because Fatigue is subjective, its presence and magnitude may not be readily apparent. It may precede or coexist with depression and is usually not reversible by a night's sleep. The pathognomonic processes of fatigue in illness are unclear. Whether disease triggers the production of fatigue-causing chemicals and somehow accelerates energy consumption is not known. Likewise, the beneficial effects of fatigue are not known. Unlike the warning that pain gives an individual, the potential protection that fatigue may provide is not understood. Despite the unclear etiology of fatigue, its presence with chronic illness can substantially complicate patients' lives.

Fatigue can accompany both acute and chronic illness. In acute illness, Fatigue is usually self-limiting and will abate when the acute phases of illness pass. In chronic illness, however, Fatigue may be ubiquitous and distress the patient as much as the disease itself.

Most patients with chronic fatigue are anxious to discuss the problem with the nurse. They are relieved to know that the severe fatigue is not unique to them and that their lack of energy is real and not just imagined.

ASSESSMENT

The diagnosis of Fatigue is usually not attributable to one sole cause but involves a constellation of related factors. Because Fatigue is subjective, its identification, extent, and effect must come from the patient. Some of the related factors associated with fatigue should be explored, including illness, emotional stress and depression, medications, anemia, sleep disorders, and nutrition.

The relationship between Fatigue and illness must be determined before planning care. Whether to encourage rest or physical activity will depend largely on the nature and extent of illness. The nurse can determine this by considering the following questions: Is the illness acute or chronic? Is it inflammatory or degenerative, or is it a viral infection? In the patient's view, how does the Fatigue relate temporally to the illness? Is the Fatigue constant or does it wax and wane?

The nurse must also assess emotional stress and depression because the diagnosis of a chronic illness can be both physically and emotionally traumatic. In many cases, trying to cope with an illness that can disrupt virtually all aspects of one's life can cause situational depression. Allowing the patient to explain the meaning that this illness has for him/her may provide some insight into emotional stress or depression.

Various medications have been known to cause fatigue. Propranolol, a beta blocker used to control hypertension, causes fatigue in men.[11] Tranquilizers, alcohol, muscle relaxants, and soporifics should be considered potential contributors. Corticosteroids taken in high doses over long periods of time can cause myopathies and muscle wasting, making physical activity more difficult.

Iron deficiency anemia, deficiencies of certain vitamins such as folate and B_{12}, and anemia related to chronic disease will readily cause fatigue. Assess the laboratory data to determine if anemia is present. The nurse should also ask about the patient's sleep patterns, keeping in mind that people generally evaluate the quality of their sleep based on (1) how long it takes to fall asleep, (2) subjective feelings of how "soundly" or "deeply" they sleep, and (3) how rested they feel on awakening.

IV

The nurse should also do a nutritional assessment because symptoms such as lethargy, irritability, insomnia, and difficulty concentrating may reflect an underlying marginal nutritional deficiency. The nurse must also evaluate the patient's energy requirements and demands. The patient may state that daily tasks seem to require more energy. The nurse should assess any changes in psychological, social, and role demands. Have new or more expansive demands been placed on the patient? If so, the nurse should determine the patient's ability to cope with these demands.

❖ Defining Characteristics

The presence of the following defining characteristics indicates that the patient may be experiencing Fatigue:

- Verbalization of an unremitting and overwhelming lack of energy
- Inability to maintain usual routine
- Increase in rest requirements
- Inability to restore energy, even after sleeping
- Decreased performance
- Lethargy or listlessness
- Disinterest in surroundings
- Impaired ability to concentrate
- Noninvolvement in social activities
- Decreased libido
- Perceived need for additional energy to finish required tasks
- Feelings of guilt for not keeping up with responsibilities

❖ Related Factors

The following related factors are associated with Fatigue:

- Acute or chronic illness
- Anemias
- Nutritional deficiencies
- Sleep disorders
- Certain medications
- Increased energy requirements
- Depression
- Overwhelming psychological, social, or role demands
- Lack of social support

❖ Related Medical/Psychiatric Diagnoses

The following are examples of related medical/psychiatric diagnoses for Fatigue:
- Acquired immunodeficiency syndrome (AIDS)
- Anemia
- Chronic obstructive pulmonary disease (COPD)
- Depression
- Epstein-Barr virus
- Guillain-Barré syndrome
- Hepatitis
- Lupus erythematosus
- Multiple sclerosis
- Rheumatoid arthritis

NURSING DIAGNOSES

Examples of *specific* nursing diagnoses for Fatigue are:
- Fatigue related to the effects of a recent viral infection
- Fatigue related to altered sleep pattern resulting from changing work shifts
- Fatigue related to increase in familial role demands caused by spouse's illness
- Fatigue related to effects of COPD.

PLANNING AND IMPLEMENTATION WITH RATIONALE

The nursing interventions for Fatigue are aimed at *assisting patients to live their lives as normally as possible*. It is important for patients to identify how they can conserve energy to accomplish those activities and tasks that they see as important to maintaining an independent lifestyle. This means helping patients to assign priorities to tasks and allow less important tasks to remain undone or to be delegated to someone else. For example, household chores should be broken down into discrete, manageable entities to be performed throughout the week. Only one or two rooms should be vacuumed each day, and a rest period may be required between rooms. Shopping for groceries or clothes should be carefully planned because both can be physically tiring. *Perhaps the most important thought to keep in mind is the that overexertion can exacerbate disease.*

In planning and implementing strategies to help patients with Fatigue, the nurse must remember the importance of ongoing assessment. *Because the plan of care will vary with the individual patient's home and work schedule, the nurse must periodically monitor progress within the particular care plan.* It may be helpful to have the patient keep a daily log of times when Fatigue seems to worsen and the activities that exacerbate it. Together the nurse and patient can review these data and make revisions as needed.

Developing nursing interventions for Fatigue will tap the nurse's acumen and ingenuity. The nurse may have to test several interventions before finding one that is workable. *The success of an intervention outcome will undoubtedly depend on close cooperation and collaboration with the patient and family because modifications to the patient's usual routine can best be identified by the patient and those able to support such changes.*

EVALUATION

Evaluation of the effectiveness of most interventions for fatigue should be corroborated with the patient. The success of most interventions will greatly depend on how well the patient was able to make modifications in his/her life and adhere to them. These modifications should be realistic and achievable if patient compliance is expected. Friends or family members may also provide insights into whether patient outcomes were achieved.

IV

❖ NURSING CARE GUIDELINES

Nursing Diagnosis: Fatigue

Expected Patient Outcomes	Nursing Interventions
The patient will use at least one energy conservation technique.	• Help the patient understand energy conservation principles. • Discuss with the patient techniques that may assist in conserving energy. • With the patient, monitor the effectiveness of the identified technique.
The patient will incorporate a rest period into daily activity.	• Discuss with the patient any arrangements that will accommodate rest periods. • Review with the patient his/her daily routine. • Assist the patient in assigning priority to activities to accommodate specific rest periods.
The patient will ask for help and delegate tasks when necessary.	• Assess the understanding of both family and friends about the reasons the patient is fatigued. • Assist the patient in identifying tasks that family and friends can perform.

❖ CASE STUDY WITH PLAN OF CARE

Mrs. Alice Z. is a 35-year-old woman with a 7-year history of systemic lupus erythematosus. She is married and has an 8-year-old daughter. She works part-time (3 days per week) as a secretary at a publishing firm, where her main duties include typing manuscripts and updating files. During the assessment of Mrs. Z. in the outpatient clinic, she stated that her Fatigue has become constant throughout the day and she's been unable to keep up with her house or her child.

Mrs. Z.'s medical history shows that flares of her

Continued.

disease have been predominantly manifested by rash, alopecia, and migratory joint pains. She is currently taking 15 mg of prednisone every other day, indomethacin 25 mg three times a day, and hydrochlorothiazide 50 mg every day for mild hypertension.

Her parents live in a midwestern city about 800 miles away. Her maternal grandmother had rheumatoid arthritis and died when Mrs. Z. was 8 years old. She has no relatives living in the area. Her husband works as a plumber's apprentice and, according to Mrs. Z., "doesn't understand my disease." A physical exam re-

veals a blood pressure of 140/90 mm Hg, pulse of 86/min, respirations of 20/min, temperature of 98.4° F, height 5′4″, and weight 128 pounds. Mrs. Z. is also slightly cushingoid with an erythematous malar rash. When asked about her support system, Mrs. Z. identifies members of her church and neighbors as people she can count on to help her when disease flares and she is unable to do much. Her daughter, although only 8 years old, is a tremendous help to her mother around the house. Mrs. Z. feels guilty for having to rely so heavily on her daughter.

PLAN OF CARE FOR MRS. ALICE Z.

Nursing Diagnosis: *Fatigue related to chronic illness*

Expected Patient Outcomes	Nursing Interventions
Mrs. Z. will assign priority to tasks and arrange for their completion.	• Assist Mrs. Z. in identifying priorities and arranging for completion of tasks.
Mrs. Z. will ask for help and delegate tasks when necessary.	• Determine the level of Mrs. Z.'s understanding spouse and family members have about her illness and fatigue. • Discuss feasibility of having family or friends assume selected chores.
Mrs. Z. will establish regular rest periods each day.	• Review activities of a typical day. • Help Mrs. Z. to decide the best time for daily rest periods.
Mrs. Z. will participate in social activities.	• Discuss with Mrs. Z. the importance of remaining active socially. • Assist Mrs. Z. in identifying activities in which she would like to participate.
Mrs. Z. will verbalize increased energy and improved well-being.	• Provide Mrs. Z. and her family information about energy conservation. • Evaluate Mrs. Z.'s activity/rest schedule and her satisfaction with the schedule. • Recommend changes in activity/rest schedule as appropriate.

REFERENCES

1. Cardenas DD, Kutner NG: The problem of fatigue in dialysis patients, *Nephron* 30:336-340, 1985.
2. Carroll-Johnson RM: *Classification of nursing diagnosis: proceedings of the Eighth Conference,* Philadelphia, 1989, JB Lippincott.
3. Eidleman D: Fatigue: towards an analysis and unified definition, *Med Hypotheses* 6:517-526, 1980.
4. Greenberg DB: Neurasthenia in the 1980s, *Psychosomatics* 31(2):129-137, 1990.
5. Hart LK: Fatigue in the patient with multiple sclerosis, *Res Nurs Health* 1(4):147-157, 1978.
6. Haylock PJ, Hart LK: Fatigue in patients receiving radiation, *Cancer Nurs* 2(4):122-126, 1979.
7. Knippen MA: *The relationship among selected variables associated with fatigue in women with systemic lupus erythematosus.* (Doctoral dissertation, The Catholic University of America, 1988) University Microfilms International Dissertation Information Service, Order Number 8919391.
8. Kruesi MJP, Dale J, and Straus S: Psychiatric diagnoses in patients who have chronic fatigue syndrome, *J Clin Psych* 50(2):53-56, 1989.
9. Manu P, Lane TJ, and Matthews DA: Somatization disorder in patients with chronic fatigue, *Psychosomatics* 30(4):388-395, 1989.
10. Moldofsky H: Nonrestorative sleep and symptoms after a febrile illness in patients with fibrositis and chronic fatigue syndrome, *J Rheumatol* 16(suppl 19):150-153, 1989.
11. Potempa K, Lopez M, Reid C, and Lawson L: Chronic fatigue, *Image* 18(4):165-169, 1986.
12. Srivastavi RH: Fatigue in the renal patient, *ANNA* 13(5):246-249, 1986.

Self-Care Deficit: Feeding

Self-Care Deficit: Bathing/Hygiene

Self-Care Deficit: Dressing/Grooming

Self-Care Deficit: Toileting

Self-Care Deficit: Feeding, Bathing/Hygiene, Dressing/Grooming, Toileting is the state in which the individual experiences impaired ability to perform or complete any or all of these activities for himself/herself.[9]

OVERVIEW

Feeding, bathing/hygiene, dressing/grooming, and toileting are considered activities of daily living (ADLs). These activities necessary to meet daily needs are learned activities. Children begin practicing them in their first year of life and are expected to assume responsibility for their performance as soon as they become developmentally mature. Self-care is learned over time and is influenced by parents, family, and peers and by environmental factors, especially sociocultural factors. These activities develop into lifelong habits. Habitual activities have value not only with respect to what is done but how it is done, when, where, and with whom. When for any reason the ability of the individual to perform these self-care activities is disrupted, there is a threat to the sense of control. This in turn may be a threat to self-concept. The person may respond with fear and anxiety related to becoming dependent on others. Indeed, the ability to perform self-care, or the lack thereof, affects the quality of life.

ASSESSMENT

Self-care deficits are related to impaired musculoskeletal function or impaired cognitive/perceptual function. Assessment for these deficits will include a history of any pathology or medical treatment that might be associated with such changes. Upon initial interview and physical examination, the patient should be questioned with respect to the ability to feed, bathe, dress, and toilet. If any of the defining characteristics are present, a further focused assessment should be done to determine the extent of the deficit and the related factors. Numerous interview guides and assessment instruments are available to guide in the collection of such data and to assist in making

293

a nursing diagnosis.[1-3,5,8] Each of these guides takes into account the functional health patterns of the individual and asks questions related to age, developmental status, patient-environment interactions (including other individuals), and disease and its treatment because these factors significantly affect patterns of behavior.

Treatment may also be a contributing factor in self-care deficits. For example, a cast for a fracture, intravenous feedings, and monitoring equipment may restrict self-care ability. These are temporary; long-lasting problems may develop related to surgically created diversions to normal activities, such as tracheotomies and colostomies. Typically patients in critical care settings are unable to provide much self-care.

Age and related biological factors must be assessed and compared with normal values. With the increasing number of older persons in the population, there will be an associated increase in chronic disease. For this large group, most of whom will reside in the community, self-care will become an issue. Self-care deficits will arise not only from disease but from age-related changes. Visual and hearing acuity may lessen, changes may occur in dentition, and musculoskeletal changes may alter the older person's ability for self-care. These changes may only slow the person, but slowing or decreased activity are significant factors to consider in living with or caring for the elderly.

The degree of independence in self-care is also affected by environmental resources. These include household arrangement, neighborhood and community services, availability of transportation, professional services, and family and social support systems.

The loss of ability to perform self-care may range from minimal impairment to complete loss. Different levels of impairment require different nursing interventions. Thus it is recommended that a scale or code be used to indicate the level of dependency when identifying the presence of a particular self-care deficit. Patients may be dependent in some activities but independent in others. It is also important, especially in patients with

neuromuscular impairment, that changes in the level of dependency over time be documented. Such changes could indicate the effectiveness or lack of effectiveness of exercises or rehabilitation therapy.

The following scale for classifying functional (working) ability is a modification from the national resident assessment instrument for nursing homes:[8] 0 = independent; 1 = supervision or oversight needed, including encouragement, reminders, cueing; 2 = limited assistance needed, highly involved in activity but needs some physical assistance from others; 3 = extensive assistance, contribution to the activity is minor and needs extensive physical assistance from others; 4 = total dependence, does not participate in activity and requires total care by caregivers.

❖ Defining Characteristics

The presence of the following defining characteristics indicates that the patient may be experiencing one or more of the following Self-Care Deficits: Feeding, Bathing/Hygiene, Dressing/Grooming, or Toileting[4,6,9]:

Feeding (specify level)
- Inability to bring food from a receptacle to mouth
- Inability to cut food

Bathing/hygiene (specify level)
- Inability to wash body or body parts
- Inability to obtain water or get to water source
- Inability to regulate temperature or flow of water

Dressing/grooming (specify level)
- Impaired ability to put on or take off necessary items of clothing
- Impaired ability to obtain or replace articles of clothing
- Impaired ability to fasten clothing
- Inability to maintain satisfactory appearance

Toileting (specify level)
- Unable to get to toilet or commode
- Unable to sit on or rise from toilet or commode
- Unable to manipulate clothing for toileting
- Unable to carry out proper toilet hygiene
- Unable to flush toilet or empty commode

❖ Related Factors

The following related factors are associated with Self-Care Deficit: Feeding, Bathing/Hygiene, Dressing/Grooming, or Toileting[4,6,9]:

- Intolerance to activity
- Decreased strength and endurance
- Pain, discomfort
- Perceptual or cognitive impairment
- Neuromuscular impairment
- Musculoskeletal impairment
- Depression
- Severe anxiety

❖ Related Medical/Psychiatric Diagnoses

The following are examples of related medical/psychiatric diagnoses for Self-Care Deficit: Feeding, Bathing/Hygiene, Dressing/Grooming, or Toileting[11]:

- Alcohol abuse/dependence
- Alzheimer's disease
- Arthritis
- Cancer
- Cerebrovascular accident
- Chronic obstructive pulmonary disease
- CNS injury
- CNS tumors
- Congestive heart failure
- Coronary artery disease
- Fractures
- Mood disorders
- Multiple sclerosis
- Muscular dystrophy
- Parkinson's disease
- Schizophrenia
- Visual disorders

NURSING DIAGNOSES

- An example of a *specific* nursing diagnosis for Self-Care Deficit is:
  - Self-Care Deficit: Feeding, Bathing/Hygiene, Dressing/Grooming, Toileting related to immobility
- An example of a *specific* nursing diagnosis for Self-Care Deficit: Feeding is:
  - Self-Care Deficit: Feeding related to lack of desire to eat secondary to major depression
- An example of a *specific* nursing diagnosis for Self-Care Deficit: Bathing/Hygiene is:
  - Self-Care Deficit: Bathing/Hygiene related to pain and shortness of breath secondary to coronary artery disease
- An example of a *specific* nursing diagnosis for Self-Care Deficit: Dressing/Grooming is:
  - Self-Care Deficit: Dressing/Grooming related to visual perceptual disorder (left-sided hemianopsia) secondary to CVA
- An example of a *specific* nursing diagnosis for Self-Care Deficit: Toileting is:
  - Self-Care Deficit: Toileting related to inability to transfer to toilet secondary to severe arthritic contractures

PLANNING AND IMPLEMENTATION WITH RATIONALE

Planning care for patients with Self-Care Deficit: Feeding, Bathing/Hygiene, Dressing/Grooming, and Toileting must address the specific deficit, the related factor, and the functional level of performance. The expected outcome will be affected by whether the deficit is temporary or long-term, whether progressive deficits may occur, and whether a partial or full return of function can be anticipated. Changes in the level of self-care should be documented. If assistive devices are used the patient should be instructed in their use and observed for skill in accomplishing the tasks. The nurse should encourage the patient in self-care and should minimize setbacks.

The patient outcomes expected as a result of nursing intervention in the treatment of all four self-care deficits can be described under three major headings: maintenance (by the patient) of as much situational control as possible, satisfactory completion of self-care activities such that basic human needs are met, and the avoidance of complications.

In addressing the issue of control, the nurse must determine the significance or meaning of the loss of function to the patient. *Being dependent on others for the basic activities of daily living signifies loss of control, and with this loss of control there is likely a decline in self-esteem and morale.* The patient may perceive a threatened, or

IV

real, loss of respect from others. In these situations the care and attitude of nurses and caregivers are vital in determining the responses and outcomes of interventions. The maintenance of situational control involves behavioral, cognitive, and decisional control.[7] Behavioral control makes it possible for the patient to directly influence or modify an event, such as the time for bathing. Cognitive control relates to informing the patient and interpreting activities so there is understanding. Decisional control provides the patient the opportunity to select among alternatives.

Fulfillment of the basic activities of daily living: feeding, bathing/hygiene, dressing/grooming, and toileting is necessary for adequate nutrition, elimination, cleanliness, appearance, comfort, and satisfaction with oneself. Patients should be supervised or assisted, depending on their level of self-care ability, in these activities.

Finally, complications should be avoided. Obvious complications such as nutritional deficits and problems of elimination should be avoided with observation and attendance to food and fluid intake and output. Powerlessness or loss of control should be avoided or minimized. Physical hazards that may lead to slipping and falls should be eliminated. Activity tolerance should be monitored to decrease fatigue and frustration.

Specific rationales for nursing interventions for all self-care deficits include the following:

1. *A sense of control is necessary for a healthy self-esteem. Activities designed to maximize the amount of control by the patient should maintain or improve self-esteem.*
2. *Performance of self-care activities is necessary to meet the basic needs and demands of daily living. Being clean, adequately fed, clothed, and toileted are necessary for health, comfort, and self-respect.*
3. *Regardless of the deficit, patients should be offered desired privacy and treated with dignity and respect in performing self-care rituals.*
4. *For effective patient education determine the needs and goals mutually with the patient. Use praise and encouragement and provide the needed support in a timely fashion.*
5. *The energy level of the patient should be assessed so that he/she is not overtaxed when performing self-care and fails as a result.*

EVALUATION

Each expected outcome should be evaluated to determine whether it has been achieved as evidenced by the given behavioral indicators. If not, the plan of care should be modified. In some instances the goals may be overly optimistic; in others the intervention strategy will need to be changed. If the functional level has changed, that must be considered.

❖ *NURSING CARE GUIDELINES*

Nursing Diagnosis: *Self-Care Deficit: Feeding, Bathing/Hygiene, Dressing/Grooming, Toileting*

Expected Patient Outcomes	**Nursing Interventions**
The patient will achieve or maintain as much situational control as physically and cognitively capable as evidenced by: stating realistic appraisal of own strengths and limitations; verbal participation in plan of care; able	• Monitor and discuss changes in situation with patient and how and what activities can be performed—giving the patient the opportunity to take an active part in the assessment and plan of care acknowledges patient rights and increases self-esteem. • Plan care and validate conclusions with patient to add to sense of situational control necessary for morale. • Discuss changes in condition with patient and inform of any anticipated effects of therapy to improve sense of trust and security in situation and with caregivers.

References 3, 10, 11.   *Continued.*

❖ *NURSING CARE GUIDELINES—cont'd*

Expected Patient Outcomes	**Nursing Interventions**
to discuss and express feelings concerning limitations and progress.	• Assist in relating concerns to physician—overcoming fear of not knowing the "right language" or overcoming reluctance and hesitancy in addressing physician or having concerns made known contributes to security and likely improves self-care options. • Discuss daily routine with patient to allow opportunity for voice in scheduling and sequencing activities. • Consult with patient in making choices about his/her treatment to allow opportunity for expressing preferences. • Evaluate outcomes of care with patient—shared evaluation is natural outcome of shared decision-making process and is patient's right.
Self-care is completed with participation of patient to fullest extent as evidenced by satisfactory fulfillment of basic human needs for cleanliness, grooming, nutrition, and toileting; expressions of comfort; satisfaction with mastery of skill.	• Provide prescribed treatment for underlying disease conditions or disruptive symptoms, such as pain, to decrease effects of impairment on self-care performance. • Encourage or allow patient to do as much as possible for himself/herself to support and/or help restore independence. • Initiate exercises to strengthen weakened limbs, improve balance and dexterity. • Provide help, supervision, and teaching as necessary to improve self-care. • Explore the use of assistive devices that can help the patient become more self-sufficient. • Monitor interest and motivation for increasing level of participation in care; offer cues and encouragement, to maximize readiness to relearn or participate in a skill. • Make changes in the environment (moving furniture, placing objects within reach, etc.) to improve opportunity for self-care. • For discharge planning, assess factors in home and work setting that support or hinder self-care—physical arrangements (stairs, narrow traffic ways, clutter, access to transportation etc.) can influence self-care activities.
Complications are avoided as evidenced by absence of or minimal signs or symptoms of: powerlessness (perceived lack of situational control with decreased self-esteem, sense of worthlessness, etc.), physical harm, and deterioration of abilities.	• Evaluate success of nursing interventions designed to increase behavioral, cognitive, and decisional control. • Evaluate risks and take safety precautions to minimize physical hazards and prevent injury. • Monitor self-care activities to determine energy expenditure and tolerance level to decrease fatigue, reduce frustration, and enhance compliance. • Increase level of support resources, if necessary, to decrease or reduce rate of further disability and maintain patient involvement.

IV

IV

❖ *NURSING CARE GUIDELINES*
Nursing Diagnosis: Self-Care Deficit: Feeding

Expected Client Outcomes	Nursing Interventions
The patient, independently or with assistance, satisfactorily completes feeding activity as evidenced by: consuming adequate food and drink, maintaining appropriate weight, and showing interest in overcoming feeding limitations.	• Consider cognitive or perceptual dysfunctions, oral-motor impairment, or ability to control arms and hands in prescribing intervention, selecting assistive devices and utensils, and choosing and preparing food and drink to facilitate independence and safety. • Monitor feeding activity at each meal to determine progress, identify problems, and offer reinforcement. • In concert with patient or family identify food preferences, preferred time for eating, preferred place, and with whom to provide as nearly customary pattern as possible. • Provide ample time for eating, cut up food as necessary, arrange utensils within reach, place in comfortable position for eating and swallowing to decrease frustration, to aid chewing and swallowing, and to reduce risk of choking or aspiration. • Have suction equipment available for emergencies.

❖ *NURSING CARE GUIDELINES*
Nursing Diagnosis: Self-Care Deficit: Bathing/Hygiene

Expected Client Outcomes	Nursing Interventions
The patient, independently or with assistance, completes bath and hygiene care as evidenced by clean body, hair, nails, teeth; no offensive odors; expressions of satisfaction with resulting accomplishment.	• Provide teaching, supervision, and assistance as necessary; offer praise and encouragement as reinforcement and reward. • Provide bath at time desirable to patient and afford maximum privacy to encourage more active participation. • Use tub or shower if possible (seat in chair for safety), place equipment within easy reach, check water temperature, and place call bell within reach as measures to increase safety.

❖ *NURSING CARE GUIDELINES*
Nursing Diagnosis: Self-Care Deficit: Dressing/Grooming

Expected Client Outcomes	Nursing Interventions
The patient, independently or with assistance, completes dressing and grooming activities as evidenced by being appropriately clothed and neat in appearance.	• Provide loose-fitting clothing with simple fasteners and give ample time to complete dressing, both of which decrease frustration and improve likelihood of success. • Monitor dressing and grooming activity (combing hair, applying makeup, shaving) and offer assistance as necessary to ensure satisfactory completion of task so that patient's appearance is neat, clean.

❖ NURSING CARE GUIDELINES

Nursing Diagnosis: Self-Care Deficit: Toileting

Expected Client Outcomes	Nursing Interventions
The patient, independently or with assistance, completes toileting activity as evidenced by adequate intake and output and satisfactory management of toileting and cleaning.	• Monitor toileting activity and provide supervision and assistance as needed to determine progress, identify problems, and offer praise and encouragement in self-care. • Identify pattern or help to establish program of urination and defecation; respond promptly to patient's request for assistance to help achieve control and avoid "accidents." • Provide privacy when toileting, be nonjudgmental in case of incontinence, to avoid embarrassment and withholding need to toilet. • Provide assistive devices if needed, e.g., raised commode and grab bars. Have call bell within reach. Have adequate assistance in lifting and transferring patient to avoid risk of accidental physical harm. • Assist patient with cleaning, rearranging clothes as necessary to assure cleanliness, comfort, neat appearance.

IV

❖ CASE STUDY WITH PLAN OF CARE

Ms. Joan J., a 50-year-old teacher, was admitted to a step-down unit from the hospital shock trauma unit after a car accident. She was conscious, complaining of pain across her chest, which she related to her seatbelt, and had a small laceration of her right knee. Multiple x-ray studies, an ECG, and blood tests were done. The medical diagnosis was blunt chest trauma, fractured rib (ninth right), and neck strain. Intravenous fluids were started, as well as telemetry to observe for possible cardiac complications. Medication was ordered for pain, and Ms. J. was instructed to remain in bed. When Ms. J. was admitted to the unit the nurse questioned and observed her to determine those diagnoses known highly likely to accompany such an accident. (Patients in critical care may not have the energy, capacity, or attention span to provide a complete history; thus a selected review is done at admission. Data may have to be collected from family members or friends.) Ms. J.'s functional level was as follows: feeding, 0; bathing/hygiene, 1, in bed; dressing/grooming, 0; toileting, 1, in bed.

PLAN OF CARE FOR MS. JOAN J.

Nursing Diagnosis: Partial Self-Care Deficit related to prescribed bed rest

Expected Patient Outcomes	Nursing Interventions
Feeding: Ms. J. will maintain complete control over feeding activity as evidenced by: (1) Adequate food and fluid intake (2) No expressed problems with feeding.	• Encourage Ms. J. to maintain fluid intake because fluid and electrolyte balance may be altered related to stress. • Provide Ms. J. the opportunity to make choices about food selections.

PLAN OF CARE FOR MS. JOAN J.—cont'd

Expected Patient Outcomes	Nursing Interventions
Bathing/hygiene: Ms. J. will give own bath with minimal assistance as evidenced by: (1) Completion of bathing/hygiene (2) Expressed satisfaction.	• Because of prescribed bed rest, hygiene must be done in bed. • Provide bathing equipment. • Offer to assist Ms. J. if pain interferes with bathing back and lower extremities. • Allow Ms. J. to control the amount of time needed. • Provide privacy.
Dressing/grooming: Ms. J. will maintain optimal dressing and grooming as evidenced by: (1) Neat appearance (2) Expressed comfort, satisfaction.	• Ms. J. is on bed rest and will be wearing hospital gowns while under observation for cardiac complications. • Provide Ms. J. with clean gowns, make-up, and hairbrush. • Encourage and praise Ms. J.'s efforts to maintain her appearance.
Toileting: Ms. J. will voice no complaints related to toileting.	• Ms. J. will need minimal assistance with toileting because of bed rest. • Provide bedpan, toilet tissue, and washcloth. • Provide privacy. • Make equipment available when needed and attend to disposal promptly.

REFERENCES

1. Carnevali DL: Daily living and functional health status: a perspective for nursing diagnosis and treatment, *Arch Psychiatr Nurs* 2:330, 1988.
2. Carnevali DL, Reiner AC: *The cancer experience, nursing diagnosis and management,* Philadelphia, 1990, JB Lippincott.
3. Carpenito LJ: *Handbook of nursing diagnosis,* ed 4, Philadelphia, 1991, JB Lippincott.
4. Chang BL, Hirsch M, Brazal-Villanueva E, and Iverson DWR: Self-care deficit with etiologies: reliability of measurement, Nurs Diagn, 1:31, 1990.
5. Gordon M: *Nursing diagnosis: process and application,* ed 2, New York, 1987, McGraw-Hill Book Co.
6. McKeighen RJ, Mehmert PA, and Dickel CA: Bathing/hygiene self-care deficit: defining characteristics and related factors across age groups and diagnosis-related groups in an acute care setting, Nurs Diagn, 1:155, 1990.
7. Miller JM: *Coping with chronic illness: overcoming powerlessness,* ed 2, Philadelphia, 1991, FA Davis.
8. Morris JN, and others: Designing the resident assessment instrument for nursing homes, Gerontologist 30:293, 1990.
9. NANDA: *Taxonomy I revised,* St Louis, 1990, North American Nursing Diagnosis Association.
10. Sparks SM, Taylor CM: Nursing diagnosis reference manual, Springhouse, Penn, 1991, Springhouse.
11. Thompson J, and others: *Clinical nursing,* ed 2, St Louis, 1989, CV Mosby.

Diversional Activity Deficit

Diversional Activity Deficit is the state in which an individual experiences decreased stimulation from or interest or engagement in recreational or leisure activities.[1] *Another definition focuses on the highly personal nature of this phenomenon: A Diversional Activity Deficit is a personally defined dissatisfaction with a lack of sufficient leisure-time recreational activities.*[11] *This second definition serves to rule out patients who, while not engaging is such activities, may not have a deficit because they do not perceive a need for such activity.*

OVERVIEW

Thoughts of diversional activities conjure up images of children at play, skiing on weekends, going to movies or parties, painting, or lounging around in a bathrobe doing crossword puzzles. These images are highly personal, and many special favorite activities could be added to the list. The significance of these activities has not yet been studied fully, but some themes about leisure and recreation are emerging. It has been suggested that leisure activities should be studied qualitatively to determine their personal meaning.[5] There is evidence that one's past play experiences are important to the formation of attitudes toward leisure.[14] Ethnic differences in leisure activities have been considered.[2]

Leisure was linked to quality of life and life satisfaction in Ferrans and Powers' Quality of Life Index.[3] Another nurse-researcher, studying loneliness, found that recreational activities were cited as the most frequently missed thing by hospitalized elderly.[10] Smith[12] found that healthy persons confined to bed felt more rested in the environment with sequences of music, quiet, and narration than did those in a quiet room with no such structured diversions.

Diversional activities for elderly populations are increasingly acknowledged as important.[9] Putnam[8] pointed to the dilemma of elderly persons filling their leisure time in a meaningful manner. In early life boredom or aimlessness is usually transitory, but time can drag on for elders whom society has ill-prepared for meaningful leisure time. Vogel and Mercier[13] emphasized the need in nursing homes for diversional activities that are tailored to individual interests. Group interests, the usual focus of standard recreational programs, although important, do not necessarily fill the clients' individual diversional activity needs.

From studies such as these, it can be seen that, while Diversional Activity Deficit as a nursing diagnosis has received little empirical study, there is support for the importance of diversional activities in relation to the quality of life. There is also ample evidence of the need to define diversional activities for each individual.

Diversional activities are determined by individuals' use of time, their environmental opportunities, and their functional abilities. Innate in all of these factors is a person's individual perceptions and interests. Individuals define for themselves what they can or want to do with their available time and opportunities for diversion.

Use of time combines work, rest, self-care, and leisure.[6] Leisure is time free of obligations. However, the spectrum of available leisure time is highly variable. Many persons have little leisure time, either by choice or circumstances. Others have too much.

Environment dictates cultural patterns, available space, resources, and social opportunities for leisure activities. For example, persons with limited finances are unlikely to pursue expensive hobbies. Those who live in northern climates are more likely to be skiers than are their southern counterparts. Persons who live in one room are unlikely to collect large objects.

Functional ability defines what one is capable of doing and the energy available for diversional activities. Someone with a mobility deficit is unlikely to be a jogger. A person with a physically demanding occupation is more likely to have a sedentary, energy-conserving hobby.

Perhaps the most important aspect of diversional activities, however, is the person's individual interests. There is a freedom in choosing leisure activities that is not always available in work, rest, or self-care choices. The overriding purpose of diversional activities is personal satisfaction. A satisfying balance of time, environmental factors, and personal abilities and interests varies greatly from person to person.

When there is a deficit in diversional activities, part of the very essence of a person's self-concept and fulfillment is affected. From a review of the above components of diversional activities, we can see that a deficit may exist when there is an excess or a lack of unobligated time. A deficit can also occur when the environment is changed so that usual activities or resources are unavailable. Likewise, a deficit can occur when functional ability changes. Any one or a combination of these factors will lead to a situation in which a person cannot achieve the personal satisfaction of chosen diversional pursuits.

Nurses in almost any work setting come in contact with persons of all ages who have Diversional Activity Deficits. Patients with too little leisure time may be seen with stress-related illnesses in clinics, homes, or treatment centers. Patients with too much leisure time may be seen in those settings also. For example, patients receiving lengthy, passive treatments, such as dialysis, may get bored without diversional activities. Being hospitalized, except with acute illness, can leave a person with excess unobligated time with no diversional activity.

ASSESSMENT

Because diversional activities have meaning, purpose, and value to the patient, the nurse must be persistent in focusing assessment not only on objective data but also on the patient's perception of the situation. It is important to ascertain the patient's usual pattern of diversional activities before illness or whatever change brought him/her to the health care system. This assessment data may be categorized as (1) amount of leisure time, (2) environmental factors related to activities, (3) personal functional abilities, (4) description of usual activities, and (5) satisfaction with those activities.

The baseline assessment, in some instances, can serve as predictor of the severity of the patient's diversional activity deficit. Jongbloed and Morgan,[4] studying leisure activities after stroke, found that persons with multiple interests before illness were better able to continue an activity after illness than those who had limited activities before illness.

The baseline assessment can be contrasted with data from the present situation. The following questions related to time, environment, functional abilities, and interest in activities can help to focus data gathering. How much unobligated time does the patient have? Does this time seem to pass slowly or too fast? What are the environmental constraints in terms of space or resources? What is the patient's functional ability or constraints, actual and perceived? What activities has the patient attempted? Have these been successful? Are preillness (or prechange) activities possible? What would the patient like to do?

Finally, answers to these questions should be combined with an objective assessment of the patient's behavior. Look for signs of boredom, such as flat affect, frequent yawning, daytime napping, or inattentiveness. Pay attention to seemingly unwarranted hostility or restlessness. To test time perception, ask the patient to let you know when a specific amount of time, such as 15 minutes, has elapsed, without checking a clock. Those for whom time is dragging will usually indicate that the time has elapsed in less time than actual clock time; those with very busy obligated schedules often feel that time goes by too fast, so they will tend to indicate their perception of the time passage as being longer than actual clock time.

Related factors contributing to Diversional Activity Deficits can also be assessed within the categories of time, environment, functional abilities, and interest in activities. Time factors may be either too little or too much leisure time. Persons who have too little time may have problems with time management or an excess of obligations on their time. Those with too much time may have recently undergone a major change, such as retirement, grown children moving out of their home, or an illness that curtailed their usual obligations and increased free time.

Environmental factors tend to be different for home-based patients than for patients in treatment centers (e.g., hospitals, long-term care settings, dialysis centers, clinics). Home environmental factors that contribute to diversional activity deficits may be limited finances, lack of transportation, social isolation, or fear of crime. A thorough assessment of a person's living conditions will reveal these types of factors. A treatment center environment may have space and resource constraints that are actual or perceived by the patient. Very often patients assume they cannot do certain things in a hospital when in reality they may be able to. Also, patients may be unfamiliar with routines or expectations of them so that they are unsure of when or how they would engage in some self-chosen diversional activity.

Assessing functional abilities will reveal personal obstacles that may be preventing individuals from pursuing their usual activities or starting new ones. Some of these deficits are impaired mobility and sensory or cardiopulmonary malfunctions. If the person is fatigued, what would be leisure time becomes needed rest time. Depression has been shown to affect time perception.[7] It exerts a negative effect on diversional activities. Likewise, a person with many problems may become apathetic about diversional activities.

Finally, assessing interest in activities may show that some people have a deficit because

something is interfering with their desire or interest in diversional activity. Some persons lack exposure or an orientation toward diversional activities. They have a strong work orientation and think that leisure activities are not desirable, and may have difficulty defining what to do with leisure time. Others lack knowledge of options and therefore have no interest in those things.

❖ Defining Characteristics

The presence of the following defining characteristics indicates that the patient may be experiencing Diversional Activity Deficit:
- Frequent yawning
- Flat affect
- Overeating or eating too little
- Inattentiveness
- Restlessness
- Daytime napping (seemingly unwarranted)
- Hostility/irritation
- Perception of time passing slowly
- Perception of time passing too quickly
- Statement of boredom
- Statement of missing recreational activity
- Statement of frustration
- Little or no unobligated time
- Increase in unobligated time
- No pattern of leisure activities
- Preillness (or before life change) leisure activities impossible since illness
- No postillness (or after life change) substitute activities defined
- Statement of desire for something to do
- Unavailability (actual or perceived) of resources for desired activity
- Confined space
- Disinterest in television
- Refusal to attend planned recreational programs
- Selective attendance at planned recreational programs

❖ Related Factors

The following related factors are associated with Diversional Activity Deficit:
Time factors
- Problematic time management

- Excess obligations on time
- Decrease in obligated time (increase in available unobligated time)
- Major life change such as retirement, children leaving home, long-term illness

Environmental factors

- Home-based patients: limited finances, lack of transportation, social isolation, fear of crime
- Treatment-center-based patients: space constraints, lack of resources, unfamiliarity with routines or expectations

Functional abilities

- Impaired mobility
- Activity intolerance
- Impaired senses, pain
- Impaired cardiopulmonary functions
- Fatigue
- Depression/lack of motivation
- Apathy
- Loneliness
- Maturational factors (e.g., child—no toys)

Interest in activities

- Lack of exposure or orientation to diversional activities
- Lack of knowledge of options
- Personal preference at odds with available options

❖ **Related Medical/Psychiatric Diagnoses**

The following are examples of related medical/psychiatric diagnoses for Diversional Activity Deficit:

- Blindness
- Cancer
- Chronic obstructive pulmonary disease
- Chronic renal failure
- Congestive heart failure
- Cystic fibrosis
- Depression
- Multiple sclerosis
- Osteoarthritis
- Spinal cord injury

NURSING DIAGNOSES

Examples of *specific* nursing diagnoses for Diversional Activity Deficit are:

- Diversional Activity Deficit related to activity intolerance secondary to COPD
- Diversional Activity Deficit related to retirement and limited finances
- Diversional Activity Deficit related to impaired mobility and space constraints of treatment center
- Diversional Activity Deficit related to problematic time management and excess obligations on time

PLANNING AND IMPLEMENTATION WITH RATIONALE

The essential principle underlying care for patients with Diversional Activity Deficits is that *interventions to correct the deficit must be personally meaningful. The patient's perception of the deficit in relation to usual patterns of activity must provide the groundwork for planning a new or adapted activity.* Turning on television for a patient who is bored is not enough. Telling the person with the busy schedule to relax more is not enough. An expected outcome for the patient should be to explore the personal meaning of usual or desirable diversional activities. The patient can be helped to break down usual activities into meaningful components by prompting. The patient can be asked, "What is it about [the activity] that you like?" For the skier, is it the movement, the speed, the outdoors, the solitary challenge, or the hot chocolate afterward? For the antique collector, is it the history, the hunt, or the contemplation of the object itself? *Such analysis will help broaden the options that the person has in choosing a new or adapted activity, because it focuses on the components that are truly gratifying more than on the activity itself.* Similar or related activities may then be chosen and still be personally meaningful.

Another expected outcome is that the patient is able to choose a desired diversional activity that can be engaged in now. To meet this outcome the nurse should focus on the positive, or what the patient is able to do. *Patients may tend to focus on what they cannot do, especially if an illness has radically changed their functional ability.* The nurse can prompt thinking without actually making a choice for the patient. This can be accomplished by asking questions such as, "What other activities might meet the need that you met

❖ *NURSING CARE GUIDELINES*
Nursing Diagnosis: Diversional Activity Deficit

Expected Patient Outcomes	Nursing Interventions
The patient will identify the personal meaning of diversional activities.	• Encourage the patient to discuss usual or desired diversional activities. • Prompt the patient to analyze usual activities into components that are meaningful (e.g., ask "What is it about this activity that you like?").
The patient will choose a desired diversional activity to engage in.	• Focus on the positive more than the negative (e.g., say "You can do this" rather than "You can't do that"). • Encourage the patient to choose an activity related to usual activities whenever possible. • Use prompting rather than actually suggesting a specific activity (e.g., ask "What other activities might meet the need that you met with your usual activity?"). • If necessary, prompt thinking by suggesting activities, such as music, games, arts, crafts, physical exercise, toys, reading, writing, change of scene or routine, companionship, video or audio programs, talking, productive chores (e.g., sorting, cleaning). • For overstressed patients with little leisure time, assist in setting activity priorities. • Orient patients to routines of care and let them know what areas are within their control and which routines can be adapted for their use.
The patient will satisfactorily engage in chosen diversional activity.	• Have the patient identify needed resources. • Assist in obtaining resources. • Adapt environment as necessary. • If needed, teach time management or stress management strategies to optimize the opportunity for diversional activities for those with little leisure time. • Allow for change of plans if activity is unsatisfactory.

with your usual activity?" Further prompting may be needed. The nurse can avoid suggesting an actual activity by listing possible categories of activities, such as music, games, arts, and crafts. Whenever possible, it *is best if the patient can choose an activity related to one that has been enjoyed in the past.*

All too often, especially in hospitals, *patients think they cannot engage in chosen activities because they have little say in the daily routine.* It is imperative that nurses orient patients to routines and let them know what areas are within their control and what aspects of the environment can be adapted for their use. Allowing patients to control the environment means that nurses must be willing to be flexible and to acknowledge the value of diversional activities. Nurses must be willing to allow patients to choose "odd" things, such as painting a watercolor during the morning when the light is best in the room, even if this

IV

means a bath must be rescheduled for afternoon. Or the nurse may allow the patient to set up Tibetan bells in a private area and to have an hour of uninterrupted time to chant daily.

After the patient chooses an activity, the nurse may help obtain resources or adapt the environment to the activity. Again, *to promote personally meaningful activities,* the nurse should encourage the patient to identify needed resources and, if possible, ways to obtain them. Getting resources may be simple or complex. If a patient has little leisure time but would like to have a quiet half-hour each day for listening to music, counseling on time management may be needed to provide that resource of time.

Finally, the nurse must not assume the problem is resolved once the patient is busy with a project. The patient must be allowed to have a change of mind if other or additional activities are desired. *Remembering the principle that diversional activities must be personally meaningful means allowing for the patient's evaluation of the success of the activity.*

EVALUATION

Evaluation of care centers on the three patient outcomes. Has the patient been able to identify the personal meaning of diversional activities? Has an activity been chosen? Was it successfully implemented by the patient?

More than the actual pursuit of an activity, the personal meaning of the pursued activity is the key to successful interventions. The patient who seemed bored but who is now watching television may still be bored, because TV is not a personally meaningful diversion. However, the patient who identified carpentry as a usual leisure activity and who is watching a program on renovating old houses may indeed be experiencing a meaningful diversion. That same person, even in a hospital bed, may try small-scale wood carving to round out a set of activities, all of which relate to the usual meaningful activity of carpentry.

The important component of evaluation is to ask the patient about satisfaction with the diversional activity and not merely to focus on the fact that the patient is doing something. If the patient is not satisfied, planning for other diversional activities is needed.

❖ CASE STUDY WITH PLAN OF CARE

Mr. Frank F. is a 46-year-old black construction foreman who recently started outpatient hemodialysis treatments three times a week because of chronic renal failure secondary to diabetic nephropathy. An internal arteriovenous fistula in his left arm is used as access for dialysis. Physically he has been tolerating the dialysis treatments well, with only mild dizziness at the end of each session. The nurses noted, however, that increasingly Mr. F. gets irritated about an hour into the treatment. He calls to the nurses often to check the machine or his blood pressure, both of which are normal. He frequently turns the channel selector on his TV set but doesn't seem to watch anything for long. Because he doesn't feel well enough to drive after dialysis, Mr. F.'s wife brings him to the dialysis center during her lunch hour at noon on Monday, Wednesday, and Friday; she returns after work to pick him up at 6:00 PM. His treatment is scheduled from 1:00 to 6:00 PM. When asked about his usual routines Mr. F. reported that his greatest joy is fishing with his 13-year-old son. Because his job is stressful (he still works 30 hours per week) he likes the quiet of this sport. Between fishing trips he designs and ties flies. He doesn't watch much TV except for old movies at night, and doesn't read much except for sporting magazines. When asked how he felt about the dialysis treatments he replied, "It's better than dying, so I'm adjusting. It's just that these 5 hours seem to drag on and on. I just can't read magazines and watch TV that long."

Continued.

PLAN OF CARE FOR MR. FRANK F.

Nursing Diagnosis: *Diversional Activity Deficit related to long hours of treatment and relative immobility during treatment*

Expected Patient Outcomes	Nursing Interventions
Mr. F. will identify the personal meaning of his usual diversional activities, fishing and tying flies.	• Encourage Mr. F. to discuss fishing and fly tying in detail. • Ask Mr. F. to list what parts of these activities are most meaningful to him. • Prompt Mr. F.'s thinking if necessary with reminders of fishing (e.g., the solitude, nature watching, the fish, the beauty of the surroundings, the timing of the catch, the testing of various flies, and the creativity of the flies).
Mr. F. will choose a desired diversional activity he can engage.	• Focus on what Mr. F. can do with one hand and his other senses while sitting for 5 hours rather than on what he cannot do. • Encourage Mr. F. to use his analysis of the meaningful aspects of fishing and fly tying to find something related to these activities. • If necessary, prompt with ideas related to Mr. F.'s analysis, such as listening to a tape of water sounds, playing a magnetic fishing game, drawing plans for flies with colored pencils, tying flies with the assistance of a clamp on a table, writing fishing stories, watching a fish tank. (Use specific suggestions sparingly until he begins to list possibilities.) • Let Mr. F. know what areas of the environment could be adapted for his use, for example, moving a larger table close by, allowing him time to set up before hooking up the machine, providing periods of uninterrupted time.
Mr. F. will satisfactorily engage in a chosen diversional activity.	• Have Mr. F. identify needed resources and plan together how to obtain them. • Adapt environment as needed for the chosen activity. • Observe for initial frustrations with attempts to adapt the environment and assist as possible. • Let Mr. F. know that changes in plans for diversional activities or adding new activities are possible.

REFERENCES

1. Carroll-Johnson RM, editor: *Classification of nursing diagnoses: proceedings of the Eighth Conference,* Philadelphia, 1989, JB Lippincott.
2. Chin-Sang V, Allen KR: Leisure and the older black woman, *J Gerontol Nurs* 17:30-34, 1991.
3. Ferrans CE, Powers MJ: Quality of life index: development and psychometric properties, *Adv Nurs Sci* 8(1):15-24, 1985.
4. Jongbloed L, Morgan D: An investigation of involvement in leisure activities after a stroke, *Am J Occupat Ther* 45:420-427, 1991.
5. Krefting L, Krefting D: Lesiure activities after a stroke: an ethnogaphic approach, *Am J Occupat Ther* 45:439-436, 1991.
6. McConnell ES: Nursing diagnosis influenced by settings of care. In Matteson MA, McConnell ES, editors: *Gerontological nursing: concepts and practice,* Philadelphia, 1988, WB Saunders.
7. Newman MA, Gaudiano JK: Depression as an explanation for decreased subjective time in the elderly, *Nurs Res* 33:137-139, 1984.
8. Putnam PA: Coping in later years: the reconciliation of opposites, *Image* 19(2):67-69, 1987.
9. Rantz M: Diversional activity deficit. In Maas M, Buckwalter UC, and Hardy M, editors: *Nursing diagnoses and interventions for the elderly,* Redwood City, Calif, 1991, Addison-Wesley Nursing.
10. Rodgers BL: Loneliness: easing the pain of the hospitalized elderly, *J Gerontol Nurs* 15(8):16-21, 1989.
11. Rubenfeld MG: Diversional activity deficit. In Thompson J and others, editors: *Mosby's manual of clinical nursing,* ed 2, St Louis, 1989, CV Mosby.
12. Smith MJ: Human-environment process: a test of Rogers' principle of integrality, *Adv Nurs Sci* 9(1):21-28, 1986.
13. Vogel CH, Mercier J: The effect of institutionalization on nursing home populations, *J Gerontol Nurs* 17(3):30-34, 1991.
14. Zoerink DA: Attitudes toward leisure: persons with congenital orthopedic disabilities versus able-bodied persons, *J Rehabil* 54(2):60-64 1988.

Impaired Home Maintenance Management

Impaired Home Maintenance Management is the state in which an individual or family is unable to independently maintain a safe, hygienic growth-promoting environment.

OVERVIEW

Home is a special place for Americans. Personal privacy and personal property are valued so much that they are protected by the Constitution. Living in a private home is believed to provide a higher quality of life than institutional care because it supports independence and individuality. Private home life facilitates self-care, which is associated with self-esteem.[18] The current trend to support community-based living for high-risk populations and to discharge stable acutely ill patients has led to a dramatic increase in home health care services.

These trends are an outgrowth of three separate social movements that have occurred since the 1960s. The first is the deprofessionalization of health care. In the 1950s Americans had come to expect the physician and other health care providers to cure their health problems through accurate diagnosis and intervention that included pharmacologic agents and high technology. Americans viewed the hospital as a place to go to be cured. By 1960 health professionals realized America's major health problems were long term and required active participation by the public for prevention and treatment. Disease was multicausal and related to lifestyle patterns. The patient and family were recognized as important members of the health team.

Up to the 1960s home health care had been done by the family, physician, and nurse. Then home health care agencies began to employ licensed professional nurses, community aides, and trained homemakers to use a nursing team approach to provide home care. Agencies also began to hire professionals from other disciplines, such as social workers, physical therapists, speech therapists, and nutritionists, to broaden the scope of home care. Home care then involved a multidisciplinary team with various levels of preparation that included family caregivers and the patient.[8]

The second social movement was the medical self-care or consumer movement. It is related to the deprofessionalization of health care. As Americans became more aware that they had a role in health care they also sought a more active role in planning, evaluating, and controlling care decisions. Health care knowledge no longer belonged exclusively to professionals such as physicians and nurses. New courses were developed in schools and the community in response to the public's interest in health promotion and the evaluation of professional health care. One example is the courses given by the Health Action Network in Reston, Virginia, sponsored by a health maintenance organization.

The third social movement was cost containment. With the advent of the Social Security Act of 1963, Medicare paid for acute skilled nursing care in the home but not custodial care.[11,12] Each year health care costs have escalated at a higher rate than the consumer price index. This has resulted in several attempts by the federal government to control costs. The most recent has been to change payment for hospital services from retrospective payment for services rendered to a prospective payment system (PPS) by medical diagnosis (DRG). One outcome of this change has been shorter hospitalizations, resulting in a growth of home-based health care.

Also associated with cost containment has been the increase in ambulatory surgical treatment and decrease in long-term institutionalization of the infirm, mentally ill, mentally retarded, and other high-risk disabled populations. State and federal funding has been structured to provide incentives for the development of community-based treatment programs.[11,12]

Today the community health nurse provides home-based care for the patient by working with the family unit to provide skilled nursing care; coordinate care provided by the family, paraprofessionals, social agencies, and other health professionals; and assist them in behavioral changes that will increase their level of self-care and home maintenance management. Home health care nursing is now recognized as a specialized field of community health nursing, with separate standards of practice established by the American Nurses' Association.[1]

In providing care the nurse, in cooperation with the patient, must assess not only the health care demands of the patient and family but also the home and community environment. The nurse's documentation of services must include these activities. Mundinger[11] found that community health nurses do routinely provide both health promotion and maintenance services to the entire family unit. She also found that nurses assessed and intervened at the environmental level but only recorded direct care given the patient. Documentation must reflect all nursing activities performed to ensure demonstration of the scope of nursing practice and justification of adequate compensation. In a recent study, Impaired Home Maintenance Management was found to be the eighth most common nursing diagnosis used by nurses in one health department.[3]

ASSESSMENT

Impaired Home Maintenance Management is rarely the reason that a patient seeks nursing care in the home. However, in the nursing assessment of the patient, family, supports, dwelling, and community, the nurse may identify current home maintenance management as a barrier to either healthful living or to providing nursing care. Necessary adaptations of the structure or furnishings for home care may be missing. Aids that could increase the patient's independence may be missing. Knowledge of how to obtain necessary durable medical equipment for treatment or how to operate it safely may be needed. Intervention for this diagnosis may take precedence over others to create a workplace for safe care or to prevent injury to the patient and family. The home maintenance practices and facilities may be adequate for a family with healthy members but be hazardous for a patient.

A number of excellent tools developed for the assessment of the family and the home environment are printed in the community health literature. A home assessment tool for use with all families is illustrated in the box on pp. 310-311. It demonstrates the importance of assessing a home from room to room for safety and hygiene. When conducting a home assessment, the nurse may find that personal standards or values of cleanliness are different from the patient's. For example, the home might seem dirty to the nurse but not necessarily affect the resident's health.[10] Impaired Home Maintenance Management applies only when the home environment presents an actual or potential risk to the resident's health.[4]

Two high-risk populations needing specific home assessments are children and the elderly. Several tools are available to assess the home environment with regard to both safety and developmental stimulation of children at several stages.[6]

When planning home health care for the elderly the nurse needs to include a safety assessment that is sensitive to their special needs. One tool written to be used by professionals or by the elderly patient or family is the *Home Safety Checklist* published by the U.S. Consumer Product Safety

IV

❖ HOME ASSESSMENT CHECKLIST

Type of dwelling

Apt.————Rowhouse————House————Owned————
Rented————
No. of rooms in dwelling————No. of persons in the home————
Water: Public————Well————
Sewer: Public————Septic————
Plumbing: Indoor————Outdoor————

Home exterior and environment	Yes	No	Comments
Are there any pollutants in external environment?	——	——	
Are sidewalks/steps in good condition?	——	——	
Do steps have railings?	——	——	
Are handrails adequately fastened?	——	——	
Are there barriers to accessing this home for any household member (e.g., need ramp)?	——	——	
Is entrance adequately lighted?	——	——	
Has the home been tested for radon?	——	——	

Home interior: general			
Are emergency numbers posted by the phone?	——	——	
Are smoke detectors available and working?	——	——	
Is there an emergency exit plan?	——	——	
Are electric cords in good condition?	——	——	
Are there pests (e.g., vermin, roaches)?	——	——	
Are rooms uncluttered to permit easy mobility?	——	——	
Are doorways wide enough to permit assistive devices?	——	——	
Are carpets, rugs, flooring in good condition?	——	——	
Are scatter rugs secured by two-way tape or have rubber backing?	——	——	
Is the water heater thermostat set at 110° F or lower?	——	——	
Is lighting adequate?	——	——	
Is temperature kept within healthful range (68° to 75° F)?	——	——	
Are medications stored safely and properly?	——	——	
Are chemicals stored safely and properly?	——	——	

Continued.

Commission.[20] If the elderly person depends on a caregiver, the nurse needs to assess both the burden of care and the environment. Worcester[21] has developed a caregiver assessment guide, and Tynon and Cardea[19] report on a tested hazard assessment tool.

When assessing for the nursing diagnosis of Impaired Home Maintenance Management the nurse must consider the individual, family, dwelling, and community. The key observation is of the dwelling and its organization, cleanliness, and safety for both daily living and patient care. Observation for signs of provision for personal growth and individuality of family members is also necessary. The following parameters should be considered:

❖ *HOME ASSESSMENT CHECKLIST*—*cont'd*

Stairs and halls

Are stairways and halls well illuminated, with light switches at top and   ____ ____
  bottom?
Are steps in good condition and free of objects?   ____ ____
Do steps have nonskid strips or securely fastened carpet?   ____ ____
Are handrails sturdy and securely fastened?   ____ ____

Kitchen

Is there adequate light around the stove and sink?   ____ ____
Is a gas stove pilot light equipped with automatic cutoff if flame fails?   ____ ____
Are small appliances unplugged when not in use?   ____ ____
When working in the kitchen, does worker   ____ ____
  Turn pan handles away from edge of stove?   ____ ____
  Avoid wearing garments with loose, long sleeves?   ____ ____

Bathroom

Are there skidproof strips or mat in tub/shower?   ____ ____
Are there grab bars on tub, shower, and toilet?   ____ ____
Is medication cabinet well illuminated?   ____ ____
Is medication safely stored?   ____ ____

Bedroom

Are bed and chairs adequate height to allow getting one and off easily   ____ ____
  (e.g., elderly)?
Are night lights available?   ____ ____
Is there a flashlight or lamp within easy reach of bed?   ____ ____
Other comments/observations

---

1. What is the individual patient's physical or mental status?
   a. Is there a disease or disability present that may impede home maintenance?
2. What is the home situation?
   a. Type of housing unit.
   b. Location of housing unit.
   c. Condition of housing unit.
   d. Numbers of occupants in unit.
3. What is the patient's "standard" of home maintenance?
   a. Does the individual require care supported by "high-tech" durable medical equipment?
4. What is the patient's perception of his/her ability to maintain the home?
5. What support system is available and what are its capabilities?
6. What community resources are available to enable the patient to remain in the home situation?
7. Are financial resources adequate to maintain the home?
8. What equipment is needed to facilitate adaptation?
9. Are there structural deficits or barriers that make home maintenance difficult?
10. What effect does the neighborhood or

community have on the patient's ability to maintain the home?

11. Is the pollution or other other environmental hazards requiring adaptation for healthful living?

❖ **Defining Characteristics**

The presence of the following defining characteristics indicates that the patient may be experiencing Impaired Home Maintenance Management.*

Objective factors (nurse observed)

- Presence of disease or disability necessitating adaptation of home maintenance
- Overtaxed family members (e.g., exhausted, anxious)
- Repeated hygienic disorders, infestations, or infections
- Accumulation of dirt, food waste, or hygienic waste
- Insufficient supply of or unwashed cooking utensils, linens, or clothes
- Inappropriate household temperature or ventilation
- Inadequate or contaminated water supply or sewage
- Presence of vermin or rodents
- Lack of necessary equipment or aids
- Home structure needs adaptation to facilitate safe use of equipment (e.g., wiring outlets)
- Lack of durable medical equipment
- Offensive odors
- Overcrowding of available space
- Inadequate lighting
- Presence of structural barriers (e.g., a family member must use wheelchair, but home has thick carpeting and doorways are narrow)
- Presence of indoor pets that are not housebroken
- Disorderly surroundings
- Unrepaired defects in structure or utilities
- Home lacks personal items and attempts at decoration
- Lack of knowledge of caregiver

- Apparent lack of economic resources
- Knowledge of home maintenance inconsistent with current environment (e.g., family moving from one country or culture to another may not know how to maintain a home in the new environment)
- Inadequate support system
- Characteristics of neighborhood make effective home maintenance difficult

Subjective factors (patient or household member stated)

- Expresses ignorance in providing environment conducive to patient care
- Expresses exhaustion or inability to keep up the home
- Expresses difficulty in maintaining home in a comfortable, safe, and hygienic manner
- Expresses dissatisfaction related to overcrowding or lack of personal space
- Complains that furnishings are inadequate to support healthful living patterns
- Expresses inability to have apparent defects in structure repaired
- Requests assistance with home maintenance management
- Describes outstanding debts or financial crises that impeded home maintenance management
- Expresses difficulty in supporting personal growth of family members
- Expresses lack of knowledge about community resources
- Expresses that environmental factors negatively affect ability to maintain the home
- Expresses frustration that known resources are unavailable or insufficient in the community

❖ **Related Factors**

The following related factors are associated with Impaired Home Maintenance Management:

Individual/Family Characteristics

- Disabled by acute illness, injury, or congenital anomaly (e.g., temporarily restricted mobility after surgery)
- Chronic debilitating disease (e.g., diabetes, chronic obstructive pulmonary disease, cancer, multiple sclerosis, arthritis, congestive heart failure)

*References 2, 4, 5, 8, 9.

- Impaired sensory functioning
- Impaired cognitive or emotional functioning (e.g., Alzheimer's disease, mental retardation, mental illness, substance abuse)
- Change in family composition (e.g., newborn, elderly, death, "empty nest")

Insufficient knowledge

- Lack of training in adaptation of home maintenance skills and use of durable medical equipment
- Unfamiliarity with neighborhood resources
- Lack of socialization (role model or emigration)

Insufficient family organization and planning

- Insufficient finances
- Dysfunctional grieving

Inadequate social support system

- Insufficient amount
- Insufficient quality
- Impaired family member

Inadequate dwelling or furnishings

- Overcrowding
- Lack of adaptation of home structure or furnishings
- Structural defects
- Lack of equipment or aids for home care by disabled individual

Inadequate community resources

- Insufficient community environmental sanitation or control of environmental contaminants or pollutants
- Lack of community professional and paraprofessional home care services

❖ **Related Medical/Psychiatric Diagnoses**

The following are examples of related medical/psychiatric diagnoses for Impaired Home Maintenance Management:

- AIDS
- Alzheimer's disease
- Amputation
- Bipolar disorder
- Cerebral palsy
- Cerebrovascular accident
- Chronic obstructive pulmonary disease
- Cystic fibrosis
- Fractured hip
- Major depression
- Mental retardation
- Multiple sclerosis
- Rheumatiod arthritis
- Schizophrenia
- Spinal cord injury
- Substance abuse

NURSING DIAGNOSES

Examples of *specific* nursing diagnoses for Impaired Home Maintenance Management are:

- Impaired Home Maintenance Management related to impaired cognition
- Impaired Home Maintenance Management related to immobility
- Impaired Home Maintenance Management related to fatigue
- Impaired Home Maintenance Management related to financial constraints

PLANNING AND IMPLEMENTATION WITH RATIONALE

Discharge planning has become more important in this era of shorter hospitalizations. Patients now commonly require complex care at home while they convalesce. Whether the patient is chronically ill, newly disabled, terminally ill, or recovering from an acute illness, the family will be the principal caregivers.[14] The multidisciplinary team needs to include the family for information on the home and feasibility of adapting their lifestyles to include caregiving activities.[7] The goal of the care plan is to maintain the patient at home with maximal independence as long as is feasible and desirable.

The patient and family need to discuss capacity for home maintenance with the health care team to develop a plan of care that is realistic for the patient. The nurse assists the client to identify potential supportive resources available from friendship networks, work associations, the neighborhood, extended family, and community-based professional services. Constraints such as neighborhood safety, lack of community services, environmental pollution, age of home, or social isolation must also be explored as cogent factors to develop a feasible and realistic plan.[16]

The patient's functional capacity is diminished, often requiring lifestyle changes and role adaptations or reversal for family members. Thus it is important that, jointly with the nurse, families and patients explore the meaning of these lifestyle changes and potential reinforcement of new behaviors.[13]

The nurse assists the client to determine a realistic standard of cleanliness and safety.[15] To ac-

IV

❖ *NURSING CARE GUIDELINES*

Nursing Diagnosis: Impaired Home Maintenance Management

Expected Patient Outcomes	Nursing Interventions
The patient will participate with the family and nurse in the development of a feasible discharge plan as evidenced by actual development of a realistic discharge plan that is satisfactory to patient.	• Establish realistic plan for home management involving patient and family members. • Systematically identify factors that impede meeting the household standard. • Have members state what factors in their home environment affect their health and how. • Compare the patient's perceptions with the nurse's observations. Share the nurse's observations. • Identify factors in the community that negatively affect the family's ability to maintain their home. • Identify local resources that work to promote changes. • Encourage family participation. • Assist family in completing a home safety assessment; follow up on identified deficits. • Make appropriate referrals utilizing the multidisciplinary team. • Order necessary durable medical equipment for home treatment. • Establish necessary adaptations to the home to facilitate use of durable medical equipment. • Teach the patient and family as appropriate.
The patient will be aware of own capacity for daily maintenance and provide for appropriate support as evidenced by identification of factors associated with home maintenance, making needed changes, and/or seeking appropriate community resources.	• Discuss what each member now does and how often; if necessary discuss possible role changes. • Differentiate aesthetic hygienic factors from those that negatively affect health. • Listen (without judging) to realities of the home situation. • Have patient or caregivers demonstrate use of durable medical equipment. • Identify members of current support system and assess their capabilities. • Discuss community resources for daily home maintenance. • Mutually develop a plan of care to increase supports consistent with family values. • Initiate referrals for supplementation of daily home maintenance. • Investigate community resources for long-term maintenance. • Review with support system members how to utilize nurse as continuing resource.

Continued.

❖ *NURSING GUIDELINES —cont'd*

Expected Patient Outcomes	Nursing Interventions
The patient will adapt home and lifestyle to promote health as evidenced by removing unsafe objects and participating in activities of daily living as much as possible.	• Discuss specific lifestyle and home changes that will promote health. • Discuss rearranging furnishings for cleanliness and safety. • Teach universal precautions for infection control. • Encourage removal of clutter that may endanger patient and caregiver safety. • Reinforce changes by discussing positive effect and praise attempts at adaptation. • Review with family a plan to respond to emergencies. • Assist family to complete a home safety assessment and follow up on deficits found. • Discuss relationship of deficits to health. • Discuss possible disease caused by defects.
The patient will accomplish adequate home maintenance management as evidenced by a clean, safe, and growth-promoting environment.	• Investigate alternative ways to have repairs made within financial capabilities of family. • Support attempts to obtain repairs. • Determine equipment and supplies needed, identify sources, obtain. • Teach appropriate use and maintenance of equipment. • Review means of maintaining sufficient supplies. • Arrange for additional support on a regular or periodic basis for caregiver respite. • Have caregiver and family establish a mutually agreeable standard of cleanliness and order that is safe. • Teach caregiver to support maximum independence of patient. • Observe for increased level of health secondary to cleaner home environment, and when observed, compliment on changes.

complish adequate home maintenance management and achieve optimal health, discussions should include periodic maintenance, respite provision, structural adaptations, safety measures, general cleanliness, and acquisition of appropriate durable medical equipment and supplies. Before discharge, provision for training, use of durable medical equipment, and the prescribed treatment regime is arranged[17] to familiarize the patient with adjustments needed and learn required skills. The home care nurse should evaluate family patterns for support of maximum independence and self-care by the patient and praise successful adaptations.

EVALUATION

The next step in the nursing process is to evaluate whether the expected patient outcomes have occurred. For the nursing diagnosis of Impaired Home Maintenance Management, outcomes focus on comprehensive assessment that involves the patient and family sharing their perceptions and plans. Many changes can be directly observed, such as obtaining safety aids or home repairs. Other outcomes are reported to the nurse, such as arrangements for respite care or shopping support or changes in daily routines. In devising the care plan the nurse must keep in mind what is both realistic and measurable to ensure that the plan is feasible.

❖ CASE STUDY WITH PLAN OF CARE

Mrs. Sarah S. is a 72-year-old widow who lives alone in a three-bedroom house in which she has resided for the last 35 years. Mrs. S. was discharged from the community hospital yesterday after hospitalization because of a cerebrovascular accident with right-side hemiplegia. She has been referred to the home health agency, and a home health nurse will make the initial home visit. The referral indicates that Mrs. S. was discharged with medications, a splint for her right arm, a quad cane, wheelchair, and orders and supplies for dressing change of a decubitus on her coccyx. Physical therapy, registered nurse, and home health services were requested. On the nurses's first visit Mrs. S. is alert, oriented, and adamant about staying in her home. She says, "I'm going to do everything I can to stay here. I don't know how, but I'll manage!" Her daughter is visiting from out of state and plans to stay "until I can get Mom situated." She says, "I feel so helpless. I don't know what to do or who to call. I was so relieved when the social worker at the hospital told me a nurse would come to visit." The nurse observes that (1) Mrs. S. has a decubitus on her coccyx, which neither she nor her daughter knows how to care for; (2) she needs assistance with personal care; (3) she can transfer by pivoting from bed to wheelchair with minimal assistance; (4) the wheelchair cannot fit through the narrow doorway to the bathroom; (5) the bathroom has no assistive devices such as railings on tub or commode; and (6) Mrs. S. can ambulate with a quad cane with a great deal of assistance.

PLAN OF CARE FOR MRS. SARAH S.

Nursing Diagnosis: *Impaired Home Maintenance Management related to restricted mobility*

Expected Patient Outcomes	Nursing Interventions
Mrs. S. and daughter will make an accurate assessment of factors associated with home maintenance, as evidenced by Mrs. S. and daughter stating personal home maintenance standard and identifying factors that maintain or impede this standard.	• Observe limitations on mobility. • Make a home assessment using a tool as a guide. • Have Mrs. S. and her daughter state home factors that negatively affect recovery.
Mrs. S. will learn to use community resources as evidenced by remaining in own home as long as desirable and feasible.	• Discuss need for home health aide and daughter to assist with cleaning, shopping, and laundry, and method of payment. • Devise and review plans for handling emergencies.
Mrs. S. will adapt her home and life style to accommodate her restrictions as evidenced by remaining in own home as long as desirable and feasible.	• Discuss need for and how to obtain safety aids for bathroom, bedroom, and kitchen. • Assess likelihood of resuming social activities engaged in before cerebrovascular accident.

IV

Expected Patient Outcomes	Nursing Interventions
Mrs. S. will arrange to have structural defects of her home repaired as evidenced by observation of repaired defects.	• Make plans for repairs identified in home assessment.
Mrs. S. will have increased awareness of effect of neighborhood on home maintenance as evidenced by identifying neighbor hood improvement resources.	• Discuss with Mrs. S. how she arranged for home maintenance in the past and whether she can continue. • Point out community programs to assist with utility bills, if appropriate. • Observe immediate neighborhood for level of danger for an immobilized resident.

REFERENCES

1. American Nurses Association: Standards of home health nursing practice, Kansas City, Mo, 1986, The Association.
2. Carpenito L: *Nursing diagnosis: application to clinical practice,* Philadelphia, 1987, JB Lippincott.
3. Carroll-Johnson RM editor: *Classification of nursing diagnosis,* Philadelphia, 1989, JB Lippincott.
4. Cox H, and others: *Clinical applications of nursing diagnosis,* Baltimore, 1989, Williams and Wilkins.
5. Dienemann J, Trotter J: Home maintenance management, impaired. In Thompson J, and others, editors: *Clinical nursing,* St Louis, 1992, Mosby–Year Book.
6. Ell K, Narthen H: *Families and health care: psychosocial practice,* New York, 1990, Aldene de Gruyter.
7. Jackson J, Johnson E: *Patient education in home care,* Rockville, Md, 1988, Aspen Publishers.
8. Keating S, Kelmon G: *Home health nursing: concepts and practice,* Philadelphia, 1988, JB Lippincott.
9. Kim MJ, McFarland G, and McLane A: *A pocket guide to nursing diagnosis,* ed 4, St Louis, 1991, Mosby–Year Book.
10. Lentz J, Meyer E: The dirty house, *Nurs Outlook* September, 300-303, 1979.
11. Mundinger M: *The relationship between policy and practice in the delivery of medicare home health services,* doctoral dissertation. New York, 1981, Columbia University.
12. Mundinger M: *Home care controversy,* Rockville, Md, 1983, Aspen Systems Publishing.
13. Perry G, Roades de Menenses M: Cancer patients at home: needs and coping styles of primary caregivers, *Home Health Nurs* 7(6):27-30, 1989.
14. Popovich B, Grubba C, and Jirovec M: Functional assessments and home care, *Home Health Nurs* 8(6):16-19, 1990.
15. Schlapmon N: Elderly women and falls in the home, *Home Health Nurs* 8(4):20-24, 1990.
16. Stanhope M, Lancaster J: *Community health nursing,* ed 2, St Louis, 1988, CV Mosby.
17. Stephenson M: Discharge criteria in day surgery, *J Adv Nurs* 15(5):601-13, 1990.
18. Stuart G, Sundeen S: *Principles and practice of psychiatric nursing,* St Louis, 1987, CV Mosby.
19. Tynon C, Cardea J: Home health hazard assessment, *J Gerontol Nurs* 13(10):25-27, 1987.
20. U.S. Consumer Product Safety Commission: *Home safety checklist. Publication No. 1985-475981; 32202,* Washington, DC, 1985, US Government Printing Office.
21. Worcester M: Family coping: caring for the elderly in home care. In Horn B, editor: *Facilitating self care practices in the elderly,* New York, 1990, The Haworth Press.

High Risk For Activity Intolerance

Activity Intolerance

IV

High Risk For Activity Intolerance is the state in which an individual is at risk of having insufficient physiological or psychological energy to endure or complete required or desired daily activities.[4]

Activity Intolerance is a state in which an individual has insufficient physiological or psychological energy to endure or complete required or desired daily activities.[4]

OVERVIEW

Activity in which individuals engage reflects their physical capacity, structural and functional abilities, interests, and desires. Activity is a basic human need. It contributes to physical and emotional well-being. Activity is action; it requires intent and expenditure of energy. Activity is purposeful; it is required to maintain self-care, to accomplish occupational tasks, and to engage in physical exercise.

Unrestricted choice of activities contributes to one's sense of autonomy and independence. When an individual has no physiological or psychological constraints on the activities in which he chooses to engage, he or she feels a sense of control. But when limitations are imposed on an individual's usual activity pattern, this sense of control can be altered. White and associates,[28] in their discussion of the effects of the prolonged inactivity that was recommended for myocardial infarction patients in the 1950s, confirmed this ef-

fect. They stated: "The end of the ability to engage in constructive, purposeful activity is, for most persons, a tragedy—it symbolizes the end of independence and purpose in life."

Yura and Walsh[29] define the human need for activity as "a behavior or action requiring an expenditure of energy by the person with volition and intent." The need is further described as one that contributes to a person's survival. The potential inability to tolerate activity can threaten a person's well-being. The consequences of inactivity, imposed or assumed, affect the individual's total well-being—physiological, psychological, social, cultural, and spiritual. Any alteration in an individual's activity pattern that occurs in response to a potential or actual health problem is of concern to professional nurses. When a potential or actual health problem interferes with the individual's ability to tolerate physical activity, the response is labeled Activity Intolerance; if the problem puts the individual at risk for becoming intolerant of activity, the response is labeled High Risk for Activity Intolerance.

The diagnoses of Activity Tolerance and Potential for Activity Intolerance were accepted for clinical testing in 1982 at the Fifth National Conference on the Classification of Nursing Diagnoses.[17] Although definitions for these diagnostic labels were not presented at the conference, various authors have provided relevant definitions. Campbell's definition[2] is presented in terms of the degree of activity that can be tolerated, that is, minimum, mild, and moderate activity tolerance. Her definitions are as follows:

Minimum activity tolerance: the inability to tolerate any physical activity without the presence of discomforts. . . . Mild activity tolerance: the ability to tolerate only a very limited amount of physical activity without the presence of discomforts. . . . Moderate activity tolerance: the ability to tolerate a moderate, but not a full day of physical activity without the presence of discomfort. Campbell identified six possible etiologies of these three levels of altered activity tolerance: endocrine disturbances, tissue toxicity, inadequate tissue oxygenation, recovery from surgical procedures, poor nutrition, and depression.

Gordon[11] offered a similar diagnostic label in 1982—activity tolerance, decreased—that implies a change (decrease) in the level of tolerance for activity. It was defined as "insufficient energy to complete required or desired daily activities due to physiological or therapeutic limitations." The physiological and therapeutic limitations addressed by Gordon in this definition could be related to etiologies that are functional, structural, or situational in nature.

In 1985, Gordon[12] adopted the diagnostic labels of Activity Intolerance and Potential for Activity Intolerance and provided definitions for the labels in the *Manual of Nursing Diagnoses:* Activity Intolerance was defined as "abnormal responses to energy-consuming body movements involved in required or desired activities"; Potential activity intolerance was defined as "presence of risk factors for abnormal responses to energy-consuming body movements." Gordon[13] continues to use these definitions in the latest edition of her manual but has changed the label of Potential for Activity Intolerance to High Risk for Activity Intolerance in accordance with the guidelines for labeling high-risk diagnoses that were issued at the Ninth Conference for the Classification of Nursing Diagnoses.[5]

The North American Nursing Diagnosis Association included definitions for the actual and potential for activity intolerance labels in the 1987 publication of the *Proceedings of the Seventh Conference.* [23] Activity intolerance was defined as "a state in which an individual has insufficient physiological or psychological energy to endure or complete required or desired daily activities." The definition for Potential (now termed High Risk for) Activity Intolerance was the same as that for Activity Intolerance except for identifying that the individual was "at risk of experiencing" insufficient energy to endure or complete activities. These definitions imply that a response of High Risk for or actual Activity Intolerance would be identified in patients whose physiological and psychological resources necessary to carry out daily activities have the potential of being or are actually diminished. A comprehensive assessment will assist the nurse in determining a patient's status as it relates to activity intolerance.

ASSESSMENT

Activity Intolerance, actual or High Risk for, is a diagnosis that is frequently made in critical care[14] and acute care[15] settings as well as in long-term care,[20] ambulatory care,[8] home care,[26] and rehabilitation settings.[24]

The initial nursing assessment provides the opportunity to collect data relevant to the patient's ability to engage in activity and his/her response to activity. Review of the patient's usual lifestyle and current physiological and psychological status is incorporated into a thorough health assessment.[9,25] Patients with cardiovascular, respiratory, musculoskeletal, and neurological alterations are especially at risk for experiencing Activity Intolerance[6,16,19] Treatments for a particular physical alteration may in themselves make a patient more vulnerable to Activity Intolerance, for example, prolonged bed rest. Therefore ongoing assessment is critical and should focus on changes in a patient's level of activity as well as the patient's response to activity in terms of cardiovascular and respiratory changes and feelings of fatigue and weakness.[10]

The following parameters provide a general guide for gathering data relative to assessing an individual's tolerance for or intolerance to activity. The type, intensity, duration, and frequency

IV

of each activity in which an individual engages also must be considered when evaluating response to activity.

1. Activity pattern, past and present
   a. What activities (self-care, exercise, and leisure) were engaged in in the past? How were these activities tolerated?
   b. What activities are now engaged in? How are these activities tolerated?
2. Physical impediments
   a. Are there physical impediments that restrict participation in particular activities?
   b. Are there physical impediments that prevent active participation in activities?
3. Physiological status
   a. Is there a change in physiological status when engaging in activity?
   b. Cardiovascular response: note heart rate and rhythm, pulse strength, and blood pressure.
   c. Respiratory response: note rate, depth, and rhythm of respirations.
   d. Skin: note color, temperature, and moistness.
   e. Posture: note signs of muscle fatigue.
   f. Equilibrium: note gait and fine and gross movements.
4. Emotional status
   a. Is there a change in emotional status before or while engaging in activity?
   b. Is the individual fearful of harming himself/herself?

In using this assessment guide, the nurse will collect data that may indicate the patient is at risk for or is experiencing Activity Intolerance. The nurse should seek additional data to determine whether the diagnosis of High Risk for Activity Intolerance or Activity Intolerance can be made.

High Risk For Activity Intolerance

The data from the health history and initial assessment should provide cues that indicate whether a patient may be at High Risk for Activity Intolerance. The nurse should review specific assessment data to determine whether any of the

risk factors for Activity Intolerance are present, and the nurse should answer specific questions. The nurse must determine whether the patient has a history of intolerance to activity. If so, what type of intolerance did the patient have? What was the reason for the intolerance? Was there a related medical condition?

During the review of data related to the patient's current physical condition, the nurse should address the following questions: What is the current status of the patient's circulatory system? For example, does the patient have bradycardia or tachycardia? Has he/she had a decrease in pulse strength, a decrease in systolic pressure, or an excessive increase in systolic or diastolic pressure? Does the patient have respiratory problems, such as dyspnea or an irregular respiratory rhythm? Does the patient have arthritis or any other condition that would lead to functional limitations?

The nurse should also consider the mental and emotional status of the patient. The nurse should determine whether the patient has emotional or mental stress that would lead to his/her refusal to participate in prescribed activities.

Finally, the nurse should evaluate the overall condition of the patient. Does the patient have a sedentary lifestyle? Is the patient overweight? The presence of any or all risk factors listed below could lead to the formulation of the nursing diagnosis of High Risk for Activity Intolerance.

❖ Risk Factors

The presence of the following behaviors, conditions, or circumstances* render the patient more vulnerable to High Risk for Activity Intolerance.
- History of intolerance to activity
- Fatigue or weakness
- Sedentary lifestyle
- Deconditioned status (such as prolonged bed rest or inactivity)
- Climate extremes affect tolerance of activity
- Chronic or progressive disease (e.g., chronic obstructive pulmonary disease, multiple sclero-

*References 3, 4, 13, 18, 19, 22.

sis, coronary artery disease, arthritis, depression)
- Circulatory or respiratory problems
- Weight more than 15% over acceptable standard
- Pain
- Inexperience with activity
- Expressions of concern about ability to perform an activity
- Expressions of disinterest in an activity
- Refusal to participate in prescribed activities

❖ Related Medical/Psychiatric Diagnoses

The following are examples of related medical/psychiatric diagnoses for High Risk for Activity Intolerance:
- Acute glomerulonephritis
- Alzheimer's disease
- Cardiovascular diseases
- Cerebrovascular accident
- Chronic fatigue syndrome
- Depression
- Multiple sclerosis
- Musculoskeletal injuries
- Neurological disorders affecting balance, muscle tone and strength, and movement

Activity Intolerance

After completing the initial health assessment and assessing the patient's tolerance for engaging in activity, the nurse identifies the specific signs and symptoms (defining characteristics) that indicate that the patient may be experiencing Activity Intolerance. The defining characteristics may be vague, as in the patient making a single report of feeling exhausted after taking a shower, or obvious, as in the patient experiencing dysrhythmia, dyspnea, and profuse diaphoresis after walking up a flight of stairs.

The assessment data is analyzed further to determine a specified etiology or related factor that is limiting the patient's ability to tolerate activity. The limitations that can contribute to an intolerance of activity can be classified as functional, structural, or situational.

Functional limitations include those factors reflecting altered or impaired physiological func-

tioning. The required energy expenditure to perform the activity may be more than the individual has to expend. For an individual with cardiac disease, the required myocardial oxygen consumption during various activities may exceed the amount of oxygen available. Pulmonary diseases are often characterized by alterations of the oxygen and carbon dioxide transport process, which compromise the supply of oxygen available to support the performance of activities.

Diseases causing endocrine disturbances (such as hypothyroidism), fluid-electrolyte imbalances (such as chronic renal disease), neurological alterations (such as multiple sclerosis and Guillain-Barré syndrome), hepatic dysfunction (such as hepatitis), and circulatory and hematological disorders (such as Raynaud's disease and anemia) also present functional limitations that can cause discomfort during activity. These disease-related functional limitations include generalized weakness, decreased mobility or immobility, and an imbalance between oxygen supply and demand.

Structural limitations that can lead to activity intolerance are associated with an impairment or alteration of the anatomical structure. A structural impairment is related to a congenital or acquired anatomical deficit (for example, an individual whose right leg is shorter than the left leg) that limits mobility. A structural alteration can be caused by a therapeutic intervention (for example, a surgical incision that is painful or a cast applied to a leg rendering the leg immobile) or to the use of therapeutic equipment (such as a leg or back brace). The intervention or the use of equipment, although therapeutic in nature, can temporarily or permanently impose constraints (for example, the pain from an incision or fatigue from the weight of a cast or brace) that decrease an individual's willingness or ability to be mobile and active. The extent of the structural impairment or alteration influences the degree to which the individual's mobility is restricted and the consequent effect on his or her ability to tolerate activity.

Situational limitations that can alter an individual's tolerance for activity include factors relevant to the individual's cognitive and emotional status and environment. These limitations include lack of knowledge, lack of motivation, deconditioning, lack of support, and climate extremes (e.g., living in high altitudes or in areas where inclement weather impedes activity). The individual may lack the knowledge necessary to engage in a particular activity in a manner that would provide for conservation of energy. An example of this is an individual with chronic obstructive pulmonary disease who avoids all activity to prevent shortness of breath. The individual becomes more and more deconditioned and experiences an increasing resting oxygen consumption. Although the disease imposes functional constraints, the individual's avoidance of all activity because of a lack of knowledge imposes unnecessary restrictions on certain activities in which he/she could participate comfortably and safely. With proper instruction the individual can be made aware of the importance of specific conditioning exercises tailored to meet his/her physiological needs.

Even though an individual may be knowledgeable of the importance of physical activity and how to engage in it so as to conserve energy, he/she may avoid activity because of depression. Consequently the individual lacks the motivation required to endure physical activity. Even when the cognitive and emotional status of the individual is such that he/she is encouraged to participate in activity, the environment can contribute to his/her reluctance in becoming involved. A sedentary lifestyle that promotes deconditioning also promotes intolerance of activity. The diagnosis of Activity Intolerance is made in relation to a specified etiology or causative factor. This cause can be a functional, structural, or situational limitation that an individual experiences.

❖ Defining Characteristics

The presence of the following defining characteristics* indicates that the patient may be experiencing Activity Intolerance:
- Decrease in activity (self-care, exercise, or leisure)

*References 1, 4, 7, 13, 18, 21.

- Avoidance of activity
- Verbal report of fatigue or weakness
- Cardiovascular response to activity: bradycardia, inappropriate tachycardia, dysrhythmia, decrease in pulse strength, or inappropriate increases or decreases in blood pressure
- Respiratory response to activity: dyspnea, tachypnea, or irregular rhythm
- Skin in response to activity: pallor, cyanosis, flushing, profuse diaphoresis, or dryness with strenuous activity
- Posture: drooping of shoulders or head or decrease in muscle tone and strength
- Equilibrium (e.g., ataxia, dizziness, vertigo, syncope)
- Emotional status (e.g., lack of interest in activity or fearful of activity)

❖ Related Factors

The following related factors* are associated with Activity Intolerance:
Functional limitations
- Generalized weakness
- Decreased mobility or immobility
- Imbalance between oxygen supply and demand
- Obesity
- Pain
Structural limitation
- Decreased mobility or immobility
Situational limitations
- Lack of knowledge, motivation, or support
- Deconditioning (related to lifestyle)
- Climate extremes

❖ Related Medical/Psychiatric Diagnoses

The following are examples of related medical/psychiatric diagnoses for Activity Intolerance:
- Anemia
- Chronic renal disease
- Coronary artery disease
- Degenerative dementia of the Alz-
- heimer type, senile type with depression
- Depression, major
- Guillain-Barré syndrome
- Hepatitis

*References 1, 4, 13, 22, 26.

- Hypersomnia disorder
- Hypothyroidism
- Lupus erythematosus
- Myasthenia gravis

- Peripheral vascular disease
- Pneumonia
- Rheumatoid arthritis
- Schizo affective disorder, depressive type

NURSING DIAGNOSES

Examples of *specific* nursing diagnoses for High Risk for Activity Intolerance are:

- High Risk for Activity Intolerance related to history of periodic intolerance to activity secondary to multiple sclerosis
- High Risk for Activity Intolerance related to pain secondary to sprain of back muscles
- High Risk for Activity Intolerance related to refusal to participate in prescribed activities secondary to depression.

Examples of *specific* nursing diagnoses for Activity Intolerance are:

- Activity Intolerance related to imbalance between oxygen supply and demand secondary to chronic obstructive pulmonary disease
- Activity Intolerance related to decreased mobility secondary to prescribed bed rest
- Activity Intolerance related to lack of support of family in providing assistance needed to ambulate each day.

PLANNING AND IMPLEMENTATION WITH RATIONALE
High Risk for Activity Intolerance

The person who is at **High Risk** for **Activity Intolerance** requires support and guidance in choosing activities that promote optimal well-being. Most important, *the nurse must consider the patient's physiological response to particular activities when she/he develops an appropriate plan for the patient's participation in required or desired activities*. The patient should be given information that will assist him/her in identifying activities that are therapeutic, enjoyable, and within the patient's physiological capabilities. *It is important that the prescribed exercise program is of appropriate duration and frequency*. The nurse

should instruct the patient on the performance of unfamiliar activities and on alternative ways of performing familiar activities. Patients should be informed about factors that might interfere with their ability to tolerate activity so that they can make appropriate changes that will help promote activity tolerance. For example, factors that may aggravate Activity Intolerance include inadequate sleep or diet, inappropriate use of medications, excessive alcohol intake, noncompliance with treatment regimen, and stressful environmental conditions.

The nurse should also consider the patient's psychological response to particular activities. The nurse should assess the patient's own values about health-promoting activities by encouraging the patient to describe his/her thoughts about engaging in an exercise program. If the patient lacks the motivation to participate in required or desired activities on a regular basis, the nurse should elicit support from significant others or through organized activities or exercise programs. Finally, the nurse should encourage the patient to seek consultation with appropriate health professionals (for example, a physician, physical therapist, or occupational therapist) to achieve optimal health.

Activity Intolerance

The expected outcomes for a patient with **Activity Intolerance** are that the patient will (1) participate in activities that enhance his/her physiological well-being, (2) develop an activity and rest pattern that supports increased tolerance of activity, and (3) use the support of family, friends, and health care providers in adjusting the activity and rest pattern to meet the need for activity.

Although the expected patient outcomes and interventions are presented in general terms, these should be adapted and expanded according to the needs of each patient. *The activity-exercise prescription must be tailored to each patient's needs and abilities.* Primary considerations in planning nursing care include the general physiological and

IV

IV

❖ *NURSING CARE GUIDELINES*

Nursing Diagnosis: High Risk for Activity Intolerance

Expected Patient Outcome	Nursing Interventions
The patient will participate in activities that promote optimal well-being.	• Assess the patient's past and present activity pattern. • Assess type, intensity, duration, and frequency of each patient activity. • Determine the patient's physiological and psychological response to activity. • Assess risk factors for potential activity intolerance. • Provide the patient with information about desired or required daily activities. • Assist the patient in selecting enjoyable activities that can be integrated into his/her lifestyle. • Assist the patient in identifying risk factors that reduce activity tolerance. • Encourage the patient to participate in activities that promote an increase in activity tolerance within therapeutic limits. • Identify organized activities and exercise programs in which the patient might participate. • Encourage family and significant others to support the patient and to participate in activities and exercise programs with the patient.

*References 6, 10, 22, 27, 29.

emotional status of the individual and the optimal therapeutic level of activity that should be attained.

The data gathered in the assessment phase of the nursing process and the consequent development of the patient goals should be validated with the patient. The nurse should review the patient's past and present activity pattern and his/her physiological and emotional response to participation in activity and exercise. The nurse should determine whether the patient's physiological status changes when the patient engages in activity. For example, the nurse should assess the cardiovascular response for changes in heart rate and rhythm, pulse strength, and blood pressure. The nurse should assess the respiratory response for changes in rate, depth, and rhythm of respirations. In addition, the nurse should note the color, temperature, and moistness of the skin, as well as signs of muscle fatigue and changes in gait and fine and gross movements. The nurse should also note the emotional response to activity. Is the patient fearful of harming himself/herself when engaging in certain activities?

The nurse should share information with the patient *to assist in the identification of activities that will enhance the patient's physiological well-being.* In the same manner, the nurse should assist the patient in identifying factors that reduce activity tolerance (for example, inadequate sleep, medication, or stressful environmental conditions). The nurse should encourage independence in the patient's performance of activities, but also provide assistance as necessary. *To ensure a patient's adherence to a recommended activity-exercise pattern, it is important that the pattern be integrated into the patient's lifestyle.* The patient should be assisted in developing and implementing an activity and rest schedule that supports an increased tolerance of activity. The schedule

❖ *NURSING CARE GUIDELINES*

Nursing Diagnosis: Activity Intolerance

Expected Patient Outcomes	Nursing Interventions
The patient will participate in activities that enhance his/her physiological well-being.	• Assess the patient's past and present activity pattern. • Determine past self-care, exercise, and leisure activities in which the patient engaged; the intensity, duration, and frequency of each activity; and how the patient tolerated these activities. • Determine present activities and how the patient tolerates these. • Determine whether any physical impediments restrict or prevent active participation in particular activities. • Determine whether there is any change in the patient's physiological status when engaging in activity. • Determine whether there is any change in emotional status before or when engaging in activity. • Provide the patient with information about activities in which to participate. • Seek consultation with a physician, exercise physiologist, or occupational and physical therapists as necessary. • Aid the patient in identifying factors that reduce activity tolerance. • Engage immobile patient in passive exercise regimen. • Assist the patient in adapting self-care, exercise, and leisure activities to circumvent any structural limitations. • Provide assistance to the patient as needed, encouraging independence in the patient's performance of activities. • Encourage the patient to engage in self-care, exercise, and leisure activities that he/she can tolerate.
The patient will develop an activity and rest pattern that supports the increased tolerance of activity.	• Discuss with the patient his/her usual activity and rest pattern; suggest ways to modify an ineffective pattern. • Discuss the importance of increasing activity tolerance. • Adjust medication and treatment schedule to support adequate rest. • Teach the patient to monitor his/her response to activity and to alter activity when signs and symptoms of anoxia or excessive fatigue are present. • Encourage the patient to gradually increase active participation in self-care, exercise, and leisure activities. • Encourage the patient to adhere to the activity and rest schedule that best promotes an increase in activity tolerance.

Continued.

IV

❖ NURSING CARE GUIDELINES—cont'd

Expected Patient Outcomes	Nursing Interventions
The patient will use the support of family, friends, and health care providers in adjusting his/her activity and rest pattern to meet the need for activity.	• Provide the patient and significant others with information about the importance of establishing a therapeutic activity and rest pattern. • Encourage the patient and significant others to participate in planning a mutually agreeable daily schedule of activity and rest periods. • Encourage the patient and significant others to express their concerns about the proposed schedule. • Identify support available from health care providers, if the need arises to revise or alter schedule. • Encourage family and friends to support the patient in efforts to meet the need for activity.

References 1, 6, 8, 21, 27.

should incorporate the patient's requirements for medications and treatments, as well as participation in self-care and leisure activities. The patient should be taught to monitor responses to activity and to adjust the activity-exercise schedule as needed.

The patient's lifestyle incorporates the lifestyles of family, friends, and significant others. Family members may be required to alter or revise their daily activities to support a therapeutic activity and rest schedule for the patient. The support of family and friends can be essential in assisting the patient to adhere to an activity and rest pattern that will promote optimal participation in therapeutic activities and exercise. Willingness of family members and friends to schedule meals, group activities, and time for personal activities around the patient's activity needs contributes to the patient's tolerance of and adherence to therapeutic activities. Encouragement and guidance from health care professionals can further enhance the patient's motivation and willingness to engage in activity.

EVALUATION

The effectiveness of the nursing interventions is determined by the patient's achievement of the expected outcomes. Each identified outcome reflects the elimination or reduction of a specific etiology, which enhances the patient's tolerance to activity. The effectiveness of the nursing interventions for High Risk for Activity Intolerance and Activity Intolerance is evidenced by the following:

1. The patient demonstrates increased participation in self-care, exercise, and leisure activities.
2. The patient does not report fatigue or weakness after engaging in activity, and there is evidence of a balance between oxygen supply and demand.
3. The patient describes the benefits of engaging in activity, and he/she participates in the prescribed activity and exercise as recommended.
4. The patient seeks and uses the support of significant others and health care professionals to maintain a therapeutic activity schedule.

❖ CASE STUDY WITH PLAN OF CARE

Mr. John R., an 85-year-old man, was admitted to the medical unit for treatment of a fracture of the right tibia and fibula and compression of L3 (the third lumbar vertebra). Mr. R. reported that over the past 6 months he has been experiencing a decrease in mobility and a generalized lack of energy. He has also been ex-periencing bradycardia and dysrhythmia and has been treated with digoxin and furosemide (Lasix). His appe-tite has been poor, and he is mildly depressed. One of the nursing diagnoses formulated was Activity Intoler-ance related to functional and situational limitations.

PLAN OF CARE FOR MR. JOHN R.

Nursing Diagnosis: Activity Intolerance related to functional and situational limitations

Expected Patient Outcome	Nursing Interventions
Mr. R. will regain optimal activity tolerance.	• Ensure balanced diet, including sufficient protein and calcium intake. • Monitor cardiovascular status and administer digoxin as ordered. • Encourage participation in self-care as tolerated by Mr. R. • Perform passive range-of-motion exercises and encourage active range-of-motion exercises as tolerated. • Refer for physical therapy follow-up. • Maintain proper body positioning at all times. • Assess Mr. R.'s hobbies and interests, and provide diversional activities as tolerated. • Establish a therapeutic sleep-rest pattern. • Reassure Mr. R. that increasing tolerance for activity is a slow process so that he does not become discouraged. • Teach Mr. R. to monitor his response to activity and to alter the activity when signs and symptoms of fatigue are present. • Encourage Mr. R. to gradually increase his participation in activities. • Encourage active participation of the family and significant others in Mr. R.'s care.

IV

REFERENCES

1. American Association of Critical-Care Nurses: *Outcome standards for nursing care of the critically ill,* Laguna Niguel, Calif, 1990, The Association.
2. Campbell C: *Nursing diagnosis and intervention in nursing practice,* New York, 1978, John Wiley & Sons.
3. Carrieri VK, Lindsey AM, and West CM, editors: *Pathophysiological phenomena in nursing: human responses to illness,* Philadelphia, 1986, WB Saunders.
4. Carroll-Johnson RM, editor: *Classification of nursing diagnoses: proceedings of the Eighth Conference,* Philadelphia, 1989, JB Lippincott.
5. Carroll-Johnson RM, editor: *Classification of nursing diagnoses: proceedings of the Ninth Conference,* Philadelphia, 1991, JB Lippincott.
6. Chyun D, Ford CF, and Yursha-Johnston M: Silent myocardial ischemia, *Focus Crit Care* 18(4):295-302, 1991.
7. Fitzmaurice JB: A comparison of statistical and subjective weights in judgments of activity intolerance in simulated cardiac patients. In Carroll-Johnson RM, editor: *Classification of nursing diagnoses: proceedings of the Eighth Conference,* Philadelphia, 1989, JB Lippincott.
8. Fukuda N: Outcome standards for the client with chronic congestive heart failure, *J Cardiovasc Nurs* 4(3):59-70, 1990.
9. Fuller J, Schaller-Ayers J: *Health assessment: a nursing approach,* Philadelphia, 1990, JB Lippincott.
10. Gordon M: Assessing activity intolerance, *Am J Nurs* 76:72-75, 1976.
11. Gordon M: *Nursing diagnosis: process and application,* New York, 1982, McGraw-Hill Book Co.
12. Gordon M: *Manual of nursing diagnosis: 1984-1985,* St Louis, 1985, McGraw-Hill Book Co.
13. Gordon M: *Manual of nursing diagnosis: 1991-1992,* St Louis, 1991, Mosby–Year Book.

14. Greenlee KK: The effects of implementation of an operational definition and guidelines for the formulation of nursing diagnoses in a critical care setting. In Carroll-Johnson RM, editor: *Classification of nursing diagnoses: proceedings of the Ninth Conference,* Philadelphia, 1991, JB Lippincott.

15. Henning M: Comparison of nursing diagnostic statements using a functional health pattern and a health history/body systems format. In Carroll-Johnson RM, editor: *Classification of nursing diagnoses: proceedings of the Ninth Conference,* Philadelphia, 1991, JB Lippincott.

16. Ignatavicius DD, Bayne MV: *Medical-surgical nursing: a nursing process approach,* Philadelphia, 1991, WB Saunders.

17. Kim MJ, McFarland GK, and McLane AM, editors: *Classification of nursing diagnoses: proceedings of the Fifth National Conference,* St Louis, 1984, CV Mosby.

18. Kim MJ, McFarland GK, and McLane AM: *Pocket guide to nursing diagnoses,* ed 4, St Louis, 1991, Mosby–Year Book.

19. Lancaster LE, Rice V: Nursing care planning: overview and application to the patient in shock, *Crit Care Nurs Clin North Am* 2(2):279-286, 1990.

20. Matheny ML, Wolff LM: Critical dimensions of chronic care, *J Cardiovasc Nurs* 4(3):71-78, 1990.

21. McFarlane EA: Activity intolerance. In Thompson JM, McFarland G, Hirsch J, Tucker SM, editors: *Mosby's manual of clinical nursing,* St Louis, 1989, CV Mosby.

22. McFarlane EA: Potential activity intolerance. In Thompson JM, McFarland G, Hirsch J, Tucker SM, editors: *Mosby's manual of clinical nursing,* St Louis, 1989, CV Mosby.

23. McLane AM, editor: *Classification of nursing diagnoses: proceedings of the Seventh Conference,* St Louis, 1987, CV Mosby.

24. Miers LJ, Arnold R: The cardiovascular response to exercise in the patient with congestive heart failure, *J Cardiovasc Nurs* 4(3):47-58, 1990.

25. Rubenfeld MG, McFarlane EA: Health assessment. In Flynn JM, Heffron PB, editors: *Nursing from concept to practice,* ed 2, Norwalk, Conn, 1988, Appleton & Lange.

26. Tack BB, Gilliss CL: Nurse-monitored cardiac recovery: a description of the first 8 weeks, *Heart Lung* 19(5):491-499, 1990.

27. Wesorick B: *Standards of nursing care: a model for clinical practice,* Philadelphia, 1990, JB Lippincott.

28. White PD and others: *Rehabilitation of the cardiovascular patient,* New York, 1958, McGraw-Hill Book Co.

29. Yura H, Walsh MB: *The nursing process: assessing, planning, implementing, evaluating,* ed 5, Norwalk, Conn, 1988, Appleton & Lange.

Impaired physical mobility

Impaired Physical Mobility is the state in which the individual experiences a limitation of ability for independent physical movement.[8]

OVERVIEW

The nursing diagnosis of Impaired Physical Mobility is one of the most frequent and most important that nurses encounter in their practice. Impaired Physical Mobility is found in conjunction with numerous medical-surgical conditions. In addition, this nursing diagnosis can occur as a result of prescribed medical-surgical treatments. Impaired physical mobility affects patients across the life span in a variety of health care settings.

"For people to be mobile, three essential elements must be present: (1) the ability to move (an intact neuromuscular system or compensated movement), (2) the motivation to move, and (3) a free nonrestrictive environment in which to move."[6] It has been emphasized that "Impaired Physical Mobility describes an individual with limited use of arm(s) or leg(s) or limited muscle strength. Impaired Physical Mobility should not be used to describe complete immobility; instead, Potential for Disuse Syndrome is more applicable."[1] Much of the theoretical and research literature basic to an understanding of the nursing diagnosis of Impaired Physical Mobility is found in such subspecialty areas as neuroscience nursing, orthopedic nursing, rehabilitation nursing, and geriatric nursing.

"Nursing interventions for Impaired Physical Mobility would focus on strengthening and restoring function and preventing deterioration."[1]

ASSESSMENT

Thorough assessment of Impaired Physical Mobility begins with data collection and culminates in the identification of specific nursing diagnoses. The following assessment parameters should be included: gait, balance, symmetry and strength of muscle movements, presence of involuntary muscle movements, ability to perform activities of daily living, presence of structural deformities, range of joint motion, muscle strength, and overall physical fitness. In addition, the need for equipment and/or prostheses for activity and/or ambulation is an important assessment factor.[13] The following functional levels have been described relative to Impaired Physical Mobility[4]:

Level I: Requires use of equipment or device

Level II: Requires help from another person(s): assistance, supervision, or teaching

Level III: Requires help from another person(s) and equipment device

Level IV: Is dependent and does not participate in movement

❖ Defining Characteristics

The presence of the following defining characteristics indicates that the patient may be experiencing Impaired Physical Mobility[1,4,7,8]:

- Inability to purposefully move within the physical environment, including bed mobility, transfer, and ambulation
- Decreased muscle strength, control, or mass
- Impaired coordination
- Imposed restrictions of movement, including mechanical or medical protocol restrictions
- Range-of-motion limitations
- Reluctance to attempt movement

IV

❖ **Related Factors**

The following related factors are associated with Impaired Physical Mobility[1,4,7,8]:

- Intolerance to activity
- Decreased strength or endurance
- Pain or discomfort
- Neuromuscular impairment
- Musculoskeletal impairment
- External devices such as casts, splints, braces, or intravenous tubing

- Advanced age
- Trauma
- Surgical procedures such as amputation
- Nonfunctioning or missing limbs
- Perceptual or cognitive impairment
- Depression
- Severe anxiety

❖ **Related Medical/Psychiatric Diagnoses**

The following are examples of related medical/psychiatric diagnoses for Impaired Physical Mobility[1,4,8,10]:

Musculoskeletal impairment
- Connective tissue disease (e.g., systemic lupus erythematosus)
- Flaccidity, atrophy, weakness
- Fractures
- Gout
- Osteoporosis
- Spasms

Neuromuscular impairment
- Autoimmune alterations (e.g., multiple sclerosis, arthritis)
- Central nervous system tumor
- Increased intracranial pressure
- Muscular dystrophy
- Nervous system diseases (e.g., Parkinson's, myasthenia gravis)
- Partial or total paralysis (e.g., spinal cord injury, stroke)

Perceptual or cognitive impairment
- Altered perception of position/presence of limbs (unilateral neglect)
- Sensory impairment (e.g., blindness)

Psychiatric impairment
- Depression
- Severe anxiety

Miscellaneous
- Burns
- Edema
- Trauma

NURSING DIAGNOSES

Examples of *specific* nursing diagnoses for Impaired Physical Mobility are:
- Impaired Physical Mobility related to arthritic pain.
- Impaired Physical Mobility related to cast on right leg.
- Impaired Physical Mobility related to multiple sclerosis.
- Impaired Physical Mobility related to depression.

PLANNING AND IMPLEMENTATION WITH RATIONALE[1,12]

The planning of care for the patient with Impaired Physical Mobility is influenced by several factors. First, the results of the nursing assessment will provide the nurse with an understanding of the level of Impaired Physical Mobility present and the related factors. Another element that influences the planning of nursing care for patients with Impaired Physical Mobility is an understanding of the principles and rationales that serve to guide the development of outcomes and to direct the nursing interventions.

Following are rationales for the nursing interventions related to the expected patient outcomes in the Nursing Care Guidelines: (1) For the interventions related to the expected patient outcome that the patient will demonstrate measures to increase mobility, the rationale is that *the use of such approaches will improve the functional abilities of the patient.*

(2) For the interventions related to the expected patient outcome that the patient will demonstrate maximum range of motion in all joints, the rationale is that although *active range-of-motion exercises increase muscle mass, tone, and strength, passive range-of-motion exercises improve joint mobility.*

Text continued on p. 332.

❖ NURSING CARE GUIDELINES*

Nursing Diagnosis: Impaired Physical Mobility

Expected Patient Outcomes	Nursing Interventions
The patient will demonstrate measures to increase mobility as evidenced by the performance of progressive mobilization and functional activities.	• Provide for progressive mobilization. • Assist the patient to progress from active range of motion exercises to functional activities, as indicated. • Teach transfer techniques.
The patient will demonstrate maximum range of motion in all joints as evidenced by maintenance of strength in the unaffected limbs and maintenance of joint mobility in the affected limbs.	• Teach patient to perform active range-of-motion exercises on unaffected limbs at least four times a day. • Perform passive range-of-motion exercises on affected limbs at least four times a day.
The patient will demonstrate the use of adaptive devices to increase mobility.	• Teach and observe proper use of appropriate adaptive devices: crutches, walkers, wheelchairs, prostheses, slings, ace bandages. • Teach and observe use of appropriate adaptive equipment to enhance use of arms.
The patient will utilize safety measures to minimize potential for injury.	• Teach and observe safety precautions such as: protecting areas of decreased sensation from extremes of heat and cold, instructing patients confined to wheelchairs to shift position and lift up buttocks every 15 minutes, and instructing patients with decreased perception of lower extremity to check where limb is placed when changing positions.
The patient will participate in a plan for integrating the mobility impairment into established lifestyle patterns.	• Explore patient perceptions of mobility impairment in terms of previous lifestyle patterns, chance to resume prior patterns, and willingness to accept limitations. • Discuss alternatives (i.e., substitutions or modifications) for activities that are unachievable (either temporarily or permanently). • Identify resources, special equipment, devices, and environmental modifications necessary to permit functioning despite physical limitations.
The patient will identify and use institutional or community resources to manage altered mobility.	• Provide patient with information about available resources. • Facilitate access to available resources by means of printed materials, telephone contacts, introductions, or written referral. • Mobilize resources existing within the patient's support network. • Refer to support services according to need: physical therapy, occupational therapy, and social services.

*References 1, 2, 3, 5, 9, 11, 12, 14.

IV

IV

(3) For the interventions related to the expected patient outcome that the patient will demonstrate the use of adaptive devices to increase mobility, the rationale is that *the use of adaptive devices can significantly improve mobility and independent functioning.*

(4) For the interventions related to the expected patient outcome that the patient will use safety measures to minimize potential for injury, the rationale is that *these approaches will serve to decrease the possibility of physical dangers associated with Impaired Physical Mobility.*

(5) For the interventions related to the expected patient outcome that the patient will participate in a plan for integrating the mobility impairment into established lifestyle patterns, the rationale is that *these approaches will enhance the patient's sense of control and actual control.*

(6) For the interventions related to the expected patient outcome that the patient will identify and utilize institutional or community resources to manage altered mobility, the rationale is that the use of *these approaches will assist the patient to achieve the highest level of independence possible.*

EVALUATION

Evaluation is the process of comparing actual patient status with expected patient outcomes. The outcome of demonstrating measures to increase mobility can be measured by the performance of progressive mobilization, the performance of functional activities, and the use of appropriate transfer techniques by the patient.

The outcome of demonstrating maximum range of motion in all joints can be measured by the maintenance of range of motion, muscle mass, and strength in unaffected limbs at the patient's usual level. Measurement of the outcome for affected limbs is based on the maintenance of joint mobility.

The outcome of demonstrating the use of adaptive devices to increase mobility can be measured by the proper use by the patient of whatever adaptive devices are appropriate for use in his/her particular situation.

The outcome of utilizing safety measures to minimize potential for injury can be measured by observing the patient's compliance with whatever safety precautions are appropriate for use in his/her particular situation.

The outcome of participating in a plan for integrating the mobility impairment into established lifestyle patterns can be measured by the patient's active participation in discussions about and positive responses to possible alternatives and modifications necessary in his/her lifestyle patterns.

The outcome of identifying and utilizing institutional or community resources to manage altered mobility can be measured by the patient's acceptance of and use of whatever support services are appropriate in his/her particular situation.

If expected patient outcomes are not achieved, this could be due to several factors. One factor could be an incomplete or inaccurate data base leading to inappropriate expected patient outcomes. Another factor could be inappropriate nursing interventions. Often a reassessment of the patient's situation leads to the establishment of more realistic outcomes. Also, improved clarity about the patient's situation can lead to more individualized nursing interventions with a higher probability of bringing about the expected patient outcomes.

❖ CASE STUDY WITH PLAN OF CARE

Mrs. Florence C. is 76 years old. Mrs. C. has lived alone since the death of her husband 7 years ago. She has two daughters, one of whom lives in the same small town. Three weeks ago Mrs. C. sustained a vertebral compression fracture of L-1 secondary to spinal osteoporosis. She was hospitalized for 1 week on bedrest, then she spent 2 weeks at the home of her daughter. Now she is returning to her own home. She is still experiencing pain caused by the fracture and associated muscle spasms. She has a prescription for a mild analgesic and is permitted to have activity as tolerated.

PLAN OF CARE FOR MRS. FLORENCE C.

Nursing Diagnosis: *Impaired Physical Mobility related to back pain resulting from vertebral compression fracture and muscle spasms.*

Expected Patient Outcomes	Nursing Interventions
Mrs. C. will demonstrate increasing mobility as evidenced by a return to previous level of functional activities within 1 month.	• Negotiate with Mrs. C. a plan that allows a gradual return to previous level of activities (including for example, increasing number of hours out of bed, increasing amounts of walking, standing, and sitting, increasing independence in personal care, increasing independence in home maintenance activities). Facilitate pain management (analgesic use as ordered and periodic rest periods).
Mrs. C. will utilize safety measures to minimize potential for injury as evidenced by adherence to specified precautions.	• Teach Mrs. C. to avoid sudden jarring movements and to avoid heavy lifting to help prevent another vertebral fracture.
Mrs. C. will identify and utilize resources to manage altered mobility as evidenced by the use of existing support networks.	• Negotiate with Mrs. C. a plan that allows for input from all available and willing support network members. Tasks to be shared include items such as food preparation, house cleaning, shopping, errands, and companionship until Mrs. C. is fully functional.

IV

REFERENCES

1. Carpenito LJ: *Handbook of nursing diagnosis,* ed 4, Philadelphia, 1991, JB Lippincott.
2. Carpenito LJ: *Nursing care plans and documentation: nursing diagnoses and collaborative problems,* Philadelphia, 1991, JB Lippincott.
3. Engelking CH, Lestz PW: Impaired physical mobility. In Daeffler RJ, Petrosino BM, editors: *Manual of oncology nursing practice: nursing diagnoses and care,* Rockville, Md, 1990, Aspen Publishers.
4. Gordon M: *Manual of nursing diagnosis: 1991-1992,* St Louis, 1991, Mosby–Year Book.
5. Halar EM, Bell KR: Rehabilitation's relationship to inactivity. In Kottke FJ, Lehmann JF, editors: *Krusen's handbook of physical medicine and rehabilitation,* ed 4, Philadelphia, 1990, WB Saunders.
6. Hodges LC, Callihan C: Human mobility: an overview. In Mitchell PM, Hodges, LC, Muwaswes M, and Walleck CA, editors: *AANN's neuroscience nursing,* Norwalk, Conn, 1988, Appleton and Lange.
7. Keenan K: Clinical validation of the etiologies and defining characteristics of the nursing diagnosis impaired mobility. In Carroll-Johnson RM, editor: *Classification of nursing diagnoses: proceedings of the Eighth Conference,* Philadelphia, 1989, JB Lippincott.
8. Kim MJ, McFarland GK, and McLane AM: *Pocket guide to nursing diagnoses,* ed 4, St Louis, 1991, Mosby–Year Book.
9. Kulp CS: Changes in mobility and daily living skills. In Sands JK, Matthews JH, editors: *A guide to arthritis home health care,* New York, 1988, John Wiley & Sons.
10. Maylen N: Impaired physical mobility. In Wesorick B, editor: *Standards of nursing care: a model for clinical practice,* Philadelphia, 1990, JB Lippincott.
11. Milde FK: Impaired physical mobility, *J Gerontol Nurs* 14(3):20-24, 1988.
12. Neal MC, Paquette M, and Mirch M: *Nursing diagnosis care plans for diagnosis-related groups,* Boston, 1990, Jones & Bartlett Publishers.
13. Robinson KL: Activity/sleep assessment. In Bellack JP, Bamford PA, editors: *Nursing assessment: a multidimensional approach,* Monterey, Calif, 1984, Wadsworth Health Sciences Division.
14. Sullivan M: Atrophy and exercise, *J Gerontol Nurs 13* (7):26-30, 1987.

High Risk for Disuse Syndrome

High Risk for Disuse Syndrome is a state in which an individual is at risk for deterioration of body systems as the result of prescribed or unavoidable musculoskeletal inactivity.[2]

OVERVIEW

The diagnosis High Risk for Disuse Syndrome focuses on inactivity that is necessary, desired, and prescribed to prevent other health problems or to promote wellness. Prescribed or unavoidable musculoskeletal inactivity can range from immobilization of the extremities, such as occurs in bilateral leg casting, to total bed rest, as in the case of threatened spontaneous abortion.

Disuse Syndrome is a potential condition that involves complex human responses, including cardiovascular and musculoskeletal deterioration, psychosocial disequilibrium, and homeostatic complications. These responses often appear in combination and can threaten wellness or result in a future disability. The nurse must understand each facet of this potential syndrome to intervene and prevent permanent complications.

ASSESSMENT

The assessment must be thorough. It should involve the patient's history of body system function, present health problems, and prescribed treatment plan. The nurse must be aware of possible resultant complications from the patient's particular prescribed inactivity. The nurse should emphasize assessing the potential for cardiovascular and musculoskeletal deterioration, psychosocial disequilibrium, and homeostatic complications.

Assess the cardiovascular system for the presence of cardiovascular deterioration especially during prolonged inactivity. Inactivity causes decreased venous flow, blood pooling, thrombus formation, orthostatic hypotension, and decreased work capacity.[4] In this state, the body cannot maintain an effective blood pressure in the upright position, and the following orthostatic problems are evident: hypotension, weakness, dizziness, giddiness, pallor, and at times, confusion.[7] Decreased work capacity results from deconditioning, and minor levels of activity produce shortness of breath, tachycardia, fatigue, and other defining characteristics of activity intolerance.[7]

Musculoskeletal deterioration can be a direct result of disuse.[5] Muscle atrophy, bone mass loss, joint dysfunction, and decubitus ulcers can occur. Muscle atrophy can delay the patient's return to normal function or result in a permanent disability. Reduced bone stress predisposes the individual to calcium loss, and osteoporosis bone resorption. This increases the risk of fractures and nonfunctional bone remodeling. When joints are not fully ranged, the surrounding tissues increase in density, causing joint contractures. Joint contractures are abnormal limb positions that may become permanent, and are characterized by extremes in flexion and fixation. Other joint dysfunctions can result from any incorrect ligament stretching or relaxing that results from positioning. In this case, the joint will be flaccid, lax, unstable, or nonfunctional.

Decubitus ulcers are another musculoskeletal concern. They are caused by ischemic hypoxia of the tissues that results from prolonged pressure between tissue and prominent bones. They are typically found on the sacrum, hips, heels, elbows, ankles, knees, shoulder blades, and ears of inactive, bedridden patients. Severity of the condition can extend from a reddened skin area to a deep, open sore involving skin and subcutaneous tissues with potential damage to underlying muscle, fascia, and bone.

Psychosocial disequilibrium is also a facet of High Risk for Disuse Syndrome. This disequilibrium is caused by the patient's inability to fulfill emotional, intellectual, and social functions.[1] Each patient differs in his/her ability to cope adaptively and maintain emotional equilibrium. Inactive patients may perceive their condition as a threat to self and feel powerless, or as if they have lost control. They may fear the outcomes of their condition. All perceptions can result in maladaptive or ineffective individual coping. The patient may be tearful, angry, withdrawn, indecisive, and maladaptively unable to take action. These behaviors all indicate emotional disequilibrium.

Intellectual functions can be hampered by the patient's inability to participate in intellectually stimulating and satisfying behaviors in which he/she previously engaged. For instance, the patient can become deficient in reading because of an inability to hold a book or turn the book's pages. Intellectual processes can be repressed by prescribed pharmacological agents or disease processes. The patient may be isolated from events outside of the treatment facility and therefore be unaware of the outside world and community situations.

Social function can be impaired by (1) the illness itself, (2) the nature of the treatment, (3) the location of the treatment facility in relation to the social community, and (4) the patient's emotional and intellectual functional capabilities. The patient may feel socially isolated and react by not communicating, stating feelings or voicing complaints of loneliness and rejection acting disinterested, withdrawing, rejecting support, and refusing treatment.

There are many homeostatic complications of inactivity. They may include pulmonary emboli from thrombus formation, as discussed in cardiovascular deterioration; compromised respiration from ineffective or positional respiratory efforts;

kidney stones from calcium resorption, as described in musculoskeletal deterioration; and often gastric ulcers from increased pepsin secretion. Complications can also include urinary retention from voiding in the supine position or from using bedpans. Constipation and impaction can result from decreased peristalsis caused by inactivity or toileting difficulties. This list of homeostatic complications is not all-inclusive. All body systems are affected by inactivity. To counteract the maladaptive changes resulting from inactivity and the Disuse Syndrome, the nurse must know about all normal body systems and processes.

After the assessment data are collected and analyzed, the nurse must identify the patient's responses by assigning a nursing diagnosis such as High Risk for Disuse Syndrome. The etiological factors of this diagnosis, as is the case of all nursing diagnoses, are to be treatable by nursing interventions. In the case of diagnoses that involve the potential development of an actual diagnosis, the nurse must identify and analyze potential rather than actual human responses.

The nurse must be careful not to prematurely cluster risk factors or label an observed condition. The High Risk for Disuse Syndrome involves patient responses that occur simultaneously. The nurse must view the responses as a whole and not isolate them into singular components and nursing diagnoses, such as High Risk for Activity Intolerance, Impaired Physical Mobility, Self-Care Deficit, Unilateral Neglect, and Ineffective Individual Coping. Identifying different nursing diagnoses when one would be more appropriate complicates the care plan by separating interventions that should occur simultaneously.

❖ Risk Factors

The presence of the following behaviors, conditions, or circumstances renders the patient more vulnerable to High Risk for Disuse Syndrome[2]:

- Prescribed immobilization
- Mechanical immobilization
- Paralysis
- Severe pain
- Altered states of consciousness

IV

❖ **Related Medical/Psychiatric Diagnoses**

The following are examples of related medical/psychiatric diagnoses for High Risk for Disuse Syndrome:

- Cerebrovascular accident
- Degenerative joint disease
- Guillain-Barré syndrome
- Major depression
- Neuromuscular diseases, e.g., amyotrophic lateral sclerosis

- Rheumatoid arthritis
- Spinal cord injury
- Systemic sclerosis
- Trauma

NURSING DIAGNOSES

Examples of *specific* nursing diagnoses for High Risk for Disuse Syndrome are:

- High Risk for Disuse Syndrome related to impaired physical mobility resulting from splint
- High Risk for Disuse Syndrome related to pain from trauma
- High Risk for Disuse Syndrome related to impaired cognition and musculoskeletal activity caused by head trauma
- High Risk for Disuse Syndrome related to severe depression

PLANNING AND IMPLEMENTATION WITH RATIONALE

Nursing interventions center on resolving the cause of the nursing diagnosis and the potential effects of disuse syndrome. Expected patient outcomes should focus on mobility, self-care, self-control, psychosocial interaction, and complication prevention within the confines of the prescribed inactivity.

Cardiovascular and Musculoskeletal Function

To maintain cardiovascular and musculoskeletal function, the patient needs to be as passively or actively mobile as possible within the confines of the prescribed inactivity. *Active participation in daily living skills such as bathing, eating, turning, relieving pressure, and wheelchair propelling can produce aerobic exercise and musculoskeletal stabilization.*

Exercise plans can also maximize mobility and prevent joint contractures. Plans can include both active and passive range-of-motion exercises. Arm or leg lifts without resistance and weight lifting can increase cardiovascular and musculoskeletal tone. Hand and arm weight lifting can be used as a weight-bearing technique for the upper torso. Weight bearing is essential for the patient's production of bone stress and maintenance of muscle and bone mass. Small and light weights are used and gauged to the individual's ability and status.[8] Lower extremity weight bearing is essential for maintaining leg and lower torso muscle and bone mass. If weight bearing is feasible, the patient should attempt short intervals of standing or sitting upright. Mobility and exercise are essential for the prevention of deconditioning and orthostatic hypotension. The exercise plan does not need to be extreme, but it can include activities the patient can easily achieve, such as bathing or folding clothes.

Cardiovascular interventions include position changes. Position changes can be as simple as progressing from the supine to high Fowler's position or moving from the bed to a chair. *Changes in position can assist venous return and prevent orthostatic hypotension by altering muscle tensions.*

Prevention of Thrombi

Thrombus formation must be prevented. Preventive measures include active or passive leg movements and range-of-motion exercises, correct positioning, application of antiembolus stockings, and the correction of factors that increase the risk for venous stasis, such as clothing constriction and leg crossing. Although thrombus prevention is ideal, the nurse must still assess for its presence. Thrombus can lead to homeostatic threats such as a pulmonary embolus, cerebral embolus, or myocardial infarction.[4] The assessment parameters should include leg measurements, palpation, and thermal checks. Legs should be measured daily. The point of measurement on the legs is marked with an indelible ink marker; this provides a consistent measurement point. *Increase in leg circumference may suggest a deep vein thrombus*. Palpation along the legs can reveal a lump, indicating a clot formation. Touch can reveal the heat and erythema of thrombophlebitis. The legs should also be tested for a positive Homan's sign, which can indicate a thrombus formation, and is present when the patient complains of calf pain while the foot is being dorsiflexed.[4]

The patient needs to maintain musculoskeletal activity. To achieve this, the nurse must maintain patient mobility. Recommended mobility techniques are discussed earlier in this section. The patient should also be assisted in maintaining joint movement, alignment, and function. Range-of-motion exercises assist in ensuring joint flexibility. Extremities must be kept in functional positions. While the patient is sitting or lying, extremities should be supported in a slightly flexed, non-extended position. Pillows or foam wedges can be used to assist in this process. Splints may be employed to maintain joint alignment and counteract contractures. Night splinting for hand support is especially advantageous and does not interfere with the fulfillment of other mobility and skill activities. Overextension or lack of extension can produce a nonfunctional joint.[6] Constant passive range-of-motion machines may be ordered to assist in maintaining joint mobility.[3]

Prevention of Decubiti

The patient must remain free of decubitus ulcers. Decubitus ulcers can lead to sepsis and threaten the entire body system. To prevent these ulcers, the nurse must promote normal tissue perfusion and limit prolonged inactivity in one position. Position changes, pressure reliefs, and skin massages must be as frequent as the patient requires. Patient needs are determined by any evidence of redness or breakdown. Any positive findings indicate that more aggressive treatment is needed. For example, the patient may require a more frequent turning schedule. The patient can be taught pressure relief exercises such as lifting buttocks up off the bed or wheelchair or performing weight shifts. It is essential that the skin remain dry, clean, intact, and free of infection.

Skin inspection is the key to ensuring skin integrity. Check bony prominences for redness, edema, or tenderness. If any of these symptoms exist, the nurse may need to increase pressure relief schedules or adjust preventive equipment. The patient's bed and chair may need to be padded to reduce tension on the tissues.[9] Specialty beds may need to be ordered.

Homeostatic Equilibrium

Homeostatic equilibrium and maintenance are essential for the patient. The nurse intervenes to maintain function and prevent complications. Additional systems affected by inactivity are respiratory, renal and urinary, and gastrointestinal and elimination.

The patient's respiratory system must be intact and uncompromised. Respiratory treatments focus on preventing homeostatic threat from disorders such as atelectasis and pneumonia. Breathing exercises should be included in the patient's care plan. This may involve deep breathing, coughing, or incentive spirometry. The nurse must be aware of the patient's position. Positioning must support maximal ventilation and respiratory effort. The patient should be in an erect position, and he/she should not slouch or roll his/her shoulders.

Concerns of the renal and urinary system focus on emptying the bladder and preventing stones. Fluid intake must be increased to dilute free-floating calcium and prevent stone formation. Bladder emptying is facilitated by maintaining patency of urinary adjunctive equipment. Discomfort from bedpan use can be decreased and bladder emptying ensured if the patient is able to sit upright on the bedpan and privacy is provided. If the patient must void in a supine or prone position, facilitation techniques such as running warm water over the perineum can help prevent urinary retention.

The patient's gastrointestinal tract is greatly affected by inactivity. Peristalsis decreases and gastric pepsin secretion increases. This leads to gastric distress and discomfort. The patient needs to maintain normal peristalsis, digestion, and elimination. *By supporting mobility, the nurse can also help facilitate peristalsis.* Other interventions include controlling the patient's fluid and fi-

❖ NURSING CARE GUIDELINES

Nursing Diagnosis: *High Risk for Disuse Syndrome related to altered level of consciousness*

Expected Patient Outcomes	Nursing Interventions
The patient will maintain optimal cardiovascular and musculoskeletal function.	• Assess cardiovascular and musculoskeletal status. • Change the patient's position frequently. • Institute a program of passive and active range-of-motion exercises. Arm and leg lifts with and without resistance should be included. • Consult with physical therapist as needed.
The patient will maintain homeostatic equilibrium.	• Assess additional body systems affected by inactivity (e.g., respiratory, renal, and gastrointestinal). • Position the patient to support maximal ventilation and respiratory effort. • Keep record of the patient's intake and output. • Maintain patency of urinary adjunctive equipment. • Maintain adequate fluid intake. • Consult with physician regarding the need to administer antacids. • As appropriate, encourage family and friends to become involved with the patient's care. • Encourage family and friends to speak with the patient even if he/she is unable to respond. • Provide auditory stimulation, such as soft music.
The patient will maintain psychosocial equilibrium.	• With the patient, evaluate the effectiveness of coping strategies and discuss other strategies that may be helpful. • Encourage patient to engage in activities that are mentally stimulating, such as reading, writing, or tape recording letters to friends. • Encourage patient to engage in activities with others.

IV

ber intake and providing medications such as stool softeners and laxatives. The patient may require antacids to control heartburn or secretion-reducing medication for gastric ulcer prevention.

The patient and his/her family are important components of the care plan. *Patient motivation is mandatory in preventive and maintenance interventions.* Family members can assist in providing range-of-motion exercises and psychosocial stimuli. All this can be accomplished by developing a patient-family education plan. The more the patient and the family understand treatment rationale and how to perform treatment modalities, the more likely the treatment plan will be imple-

mented. *Active patient-family participation in the care plan maximizes the preventive aspects of treatment.*

Psychosocial Equilibrium

The patient must be supported in maintaining psychosocial equilibrium. To do this, the nurse must promote emotional, intellectual, and social functioning. The patient should be taught effective and adaptive coping mechanisms. The patient should test different coping strategies and evaluate them with his/her nurse and significant others. *The patient should feel free of anxiety, fear, and frustration.*

Intellectual stimulation can be promoted through conversation, reading, television, and tape recordings. The patient may be encouraged to record his/her feelings by keeping a journal.

Social interaction can be provided by inviting the patient to participate in group activities within the confines of his/her room or the treatment facility. Activities can include group card games, puzzles, conversation, or watching television. The inability to participate in outside community events can be less stressful if family and friends videotape major events such as weddings or school dances. Friends who are unable to visit can be encouraged to video-record or tape-record personal messages. *This type of interaction is not only social in nature, but can be emotionally therapeutic as well.*

EVALUATION

In evaluating the care plan for the patient with a diagnosis of High Risk for Disuse Syndrome, the patient's achievement of the expected outcomes is assessed. Patients should be able to return to or regain their previous level of functioning, regardless of a prolonged and prescribed period of inactivity. When a patient's disease process limits functional return, he/she should not experience any preventable disability, deconditioning, or deterioration of body systems. The patient with this diagnosis should maintain optimal cardiovascular, musculoskeletal, and psychosocial functioning. High Risk for Disuse Syndrome requires comprehensive care with various levels of functional evaluation. For each patient, the nurse must develop an integrated plan with key objective evaluation criteria, such as the expected degree of joint mobility or achievement of specific tasks by the patient.

IV

❖ CASE STUDY WITH PLAN OF CARE

Mr. Dan G. is a 41-year-old male who was in a motor vehicle accident. He arrives at the medical/surgical unit 4 days after his stay in the acute trauma center. He has a cast on his right leg, and his left leg is in skeletal traction with 5 pounds of resistance. He has an indwelling Foley catheter. He is on a regular diet. Mr. G.'s intravenous line is at 60 ml/hr but is to be discontinued today. He complains of overall pain from his multiple contusions. His health has been excellent to this point; this is his first hospital admission.

PLAN OF CARE FOR MR. DAN G.

Nursing Diagnosis: *High Risk for Disuse Syndrome related to impaired physical mobility secondary to application of skeletal traction*

Expected Patient Outcomes	Nursing Interventions
Mr. G. will maintain an optimal level of mobility.	• With Mr. G., assess all avenues to maximize his ability to follow through on directions for active and passive movements. • Maximize Mr. G.'s upper body movement by allowing independence in self-care (e.g., washing, eating, and reaching).
Mr. G. will maintain cardiovascular and musculoskeletal fitness.	• Support upper torso fitness by planning arm exercises that promote maximum joint range of motion. • Encourage Mr. G. to perform upper torso exercises that promote aerobic conditioning, such as lifting 5-pound weights, arm lifts, and arm extensions.
Mr. G. will not experience the complications of joint contractures.	• Promote passive and active range-of-motion exercises. • Support Mr. G. in independent arm activities.

Continued.

Expected Patient Outcomes	Nursing Interventions
Mr. G. will be free of decubitus ulcers.	• Pad bed with egg crate mattress or air mattress. • Develop schedule of pressure lifts and reliefs. • Assist Mr. G. with repositioning at least every 2-4 hours while maintaining functional traction. • Assess skin integrity with repositioning. • Massage skin with special attention to bony prominences.
Mr. G. will have normal bowel elimination at least every 3 days.	• Promote fluid intake by providing access to fluid of Mr. G.'s preference. • Request and administer stool softeners. • Promote fiber intake. • If patient has not eliminated, obtain order for laxative or enema and administer every 3 days.
Mr. G. will not complain of discomfort.	• Administer pain analgesics as ordered. • Relieve Mr. G.'s anxiety by explaining treatment modalities and pain control measures. • Investigate with Mr. G. the use of relaxation techniques.
Mr. G. will use effective coping techniques.	• Provide an atmosphere of trust and caring. • Assist Mr. G. in identifying and testing new coping mechanisms that are adaptive and effective. • Assist Mr. G. in setting realistic goals. • Provide information to Mr. G. on his condition and progress.
Mr. G. will maintain intellectual function.	• Provide information to Mr. G. so that he can make independent decisions. • Provide materials for intellectual absorption. • Keep Mr. G. aware of outside events by providing newspapers, television, and discussion.
Mr. G. will participate in social activities.	• With Mr. G.'s permission, invite other patients to visit. • Develop a recreational plan for group leisure activities such as cards, games, and puzzles. • Plan group meals with other patients or with Mr. G.'s friends.
Mr. G. will be free of homeostatic complications.	• Assess leg measurements daily. • Assess patient's legs for Homan's sign. • Assess and maintain bowel elimination. • Maintain patency of indwelling catheter system. • Assess and support fluid intake of at least 2000 ml per day. • Assess and alter skin care regimen as needed. • Observe for signs of gastric complications, assess for complaints of heartburn or nausea, and perform stool checks for occult blood. • Perform cast and neurovascular checks to rule out compartment syndrome and poor cast fit. • Provide skeletal pin and wound care as ordered.

REFERENCES

1. Carnevali D, Brueckner S: Immobilization—reassessment of a concept, *Am J Nurs* 70:1502-1507, 1970.
2. Carroll-Johnson RM, editor: *Classification of nursing diagnoses: proceedings of the Eighth Conference,* Philadelphia, 1989, JB Lippincott.
3. Cronan T: Effects of immobilization and mobilization on cartilaginous, bony and soft tissue structure: review of the literature, *JBCR* 7:52-56, 1986.
4. Guyton AC: *Textbook of medical physiology,* ed 7, Philadelphia, 1986, WB Saunders.
5. Lentz M: Selected aspects of deconditioning secondary to immobilization, *Nurs Clin North Am* 16:729-737, 1981.
6. Mumma CM and others: *Rehabilitation nursing: concepts and practice,* ed 2, Evanston, Ill, 1987, Rehabilitation Nursing Foundation.
7. Olson E and others: The hazards of immobility, *Am J Nurs* 67:780-797, 1967.
8. Tompkins E: Effects of restricted mobility and dominance on perceived duration, *Nurs Res* 29:333-338, 1980.
9. Weinberg LK, Babicki C, and McIntyre KM: *Rehabilitation nursing care plan stimulators,* Washington, DC, 1988, National Rehabilitation Hospital.

Dysreflexia

Dysreflexia is the state in which an individual with a spinal cord injury at the sixth thoracic vertebra (T_6) or higher experiences a life-threatening, uninhibited sympathetic nervous system reflex in reaction to a noxious stimulus.[2] The sympathetic reflex occurs typically in response to visceral distention of the bowel or bladder and/or in response to a skin stimulus. The term autonomic dysreflexia is commonly used to refer to this response or syndrome.

OVERVIEW

To understand autonomic dysreflexia one must understand the basic components and mechanisms of the autonomic nervous system. In the normal mechanisms of the autonomic nervous system, its two divisions, the sympathetic and parasympathetic, react to noxious stimuli. The sympathetic system accelerates the human system toward the "fight or flight" reflex. The parasympathetic system assists the body by counteracting the sympathetic response and returning the body to homeostasis.[6]

The sympathetic nervous system controls the chemical neurotransmitters that accelerate the heart rate, constrict blood vessels, increase blood pressure and muscle blood volume, shunt blood from nonvital areas, increase energy by liver glycolysis, and increase mental activity. The parasympathetic nervous system works toward body relaxation rather than the stress reflex. It slows the heart rate, increases intestinal peristalsis and gland activity, and relaxes sphincter control.

In individuals whose spinal cord has been injured at T_6 or higher, this mechanism is no longer intact. Basically the spinal cord lesion presents a mechanical obstruction or severance of neurotransmission from below T_6 up to the vasomotor centers of the nervous system. The parasympathetic neurons are located in the gray matter of the sacral cord and in the brain stem. Therefore there are neurotransmitters above and below the level of injury; whereas, in the sympathetic system, neurons are located only below the level of injury.[6]

This is a simplistic description of the anatomy and physiological process of the nervous system. The major concept in autonomic dysreflexia is that the sympathetic system information goes virtually undetected in an individual with spinal cord injury, whereas the parasympathetic system and its response provide observable and detectable signs and symptoms. Therefore the human system works without its normal protective checks and balances for maintaining homeostasis.

This is particularly crucial when considering the autonomic reflexes. These reflexes are homeostatic and involuntary neurological processes. Such sympathetic reflexes regulate the body's cardiovascular, gastrointestinal, and bladder systems. These visceral functions are also the major concerns in autonomic dysreflexia. If problems arise in any of the reflex areas, the normal sympathetic reflex occurs along with its parasympathetic counterpart. The result is the symptoms and problems of autonomic dysreflexia in individuals with spinal cord injury.[1]

ASSESSMENT

The nurse's first role in the assessment process is to determine which patients will experience autonomic dysreflexia. Individuals with spinal cord injuries at or above the T_6 level are the most likely to be affected. This is true in approximately 85% of that population.[3] These individuals typically have symptoms 3 months after the acute injury, but the onset of symptoms can be delayed as long as 6 years.[1] This is an important factor because patients may or may not be hospitalized at the time of their first and potentially critical episode of autonomic dysreflexia. Therefore it is essential that patients be instructed in symptom recognition, causative factors, and treatment before discharge.

The nurse also needs to know if the patient has experienced the signs and symptoms of autonomic dysreflexia in the past. If such is the case, the patient may be aware of his own unique set of symptoms, the factors that may have triggered the episode, and the preventive and actual treatment plan. Patients with a new injury or a first episode of Dysreflexia will need the nurse to place relevance to the signs and symptoms they might experience and help identify the cause. These symptoms, if prolonged, can lead to a hypertensive crisis that can result in seizures, cerebral hemorrhage, myocardial infarction, renal or retinal hemorrhage, and death.[3] Therefore it is crucial that while the nurse assesses the patient, intervention occurs simultaneously. An important aspect of the nursing assessment is to determine the cause of the Dysreflexia. Autonomic dysreflexia can be accurately diagnosed by assessing for the presence of the defining characteristics and related factors, alleviating the causative factor, and returning the patient to homeostatic baseline.

❖ **Defining Characteristics**

The presence of the following defining characteristics indicates that the patient may be experiencing Dysreflexia:[1-5,7]

- Diaphoresis, typically above the level of injury
- Pilomotor erection (gooseflesh)
- Bradycardia initially; reflex tachycardia if the episode if prolonged
- Paroxysmal hypertension
- Cold, clammy skin
- Nausea
- Chills without fever
- Throbbing headache
- Conjunctival congestion
- Nasal congestion
- Horner's syndrome—miotic pupils, ptosis, facial anhidrosis
- Parasthesia
- Blurred vision
- Flushed, pale, or blotchy skin above the level of injury
- Pallor below the level of injury
- Chest pain
- Metallic taste in mouth
- Seizures

❖ **Related Factors**

The following related factors are associated with Dysreflexia:

Injury
- Spinal cord injury at or above the T_6 level
- Injury present for 3 months or longer

Bladder factors
- Unregulated bladder program
- Urinary adjunctive equipment and tubing
- Excessive fluid intake and intermittent catheterization program
- Urinary tract manipulations or infections

Bowel factors
- Unregulated bowel program
- Constipation or impaction

Skin factors
- Restrictive clothing or tubings
- Skin insults—decubitus ulcers, burns, abrasions
- Infrequent pressure reliefs

Other visceral factors
- Menstrual cramps or uterine contractions
- Disease processes with visceral symptoms, as in gastrointestinal bleed, gallbladder and pancreatic disease, or abdominal insult

❖ **Related Medical/Psychiatric Diagnosis**

The following is the related medical/psychiatric diagnosis for Dysreflexia:
- Spinal cord injury at the sixth thoracic vertebra (T_6) or above

NURSING DIAGNOSES

Examples of *specific* nursing diagnoses for Dysreflexia are:
- Dysreflexia related to unregulated bladder program
- Dysreflexia related to unregulated bowel program
- Dysreflexia related to infrequent pressure reliefs

PLANNING AND IMPLEMENTATION WITH RATIONALE

Nursing interventions for autonomic dysreflexia fall into the three facets of nursing practice: independent, interdependent, and dependent practice. The independent practice facet includes assessment of symptoms and causative factors, the nursing diagnosis, relief interventions, patient/family education, prevention, and wellness planning. In the interdependent facet the nurse practices with the physician in pharmacological management (administration and regulation of stool softeners and laxatives). In the dependent facet the nurse acts with the physician as change agent and clinician in the management of life-threatening seizures or in addressing causative clinical concerns such as gastrointestinal bleeds or urinary tract infections. The differences in the three nursing practice roles should become more apparent as interventions and rationale are presented in this chapter.

The autonomic dysreflexic state creates a hypertensive crisis that can produce seizures, cerebral hemorrhage, and possibly death. The patient must not reach this climactic point. *The patient must be free of any complications resulting from autonomic dysreflexia.* When dysreflexia symptoms are first seen, the nurse's first and most essential intervention is to support reversing the hypertensive state and to lower cerebral pressures. The nurse can achieve this by elevating the patient's head at least 45 degrees or, if possible, by placing the patient in an upright sitting position. The patient's vital signs are monitored at least every 5 minutes until the cause of the dysreflexia has been determined and alleviated, and the patient's vital signs have returned to baseline. The nurse notifies the physician of the hypertensive emergency, administers ordered medications, and assists with prevention of complications. After the patient's safety has been assured, *nursing interventions are directed toward identifying and resolving the causative source of Dysreflexia.*[8]

Visceral stimuli that may prompt the occurrence of Dysreflexia are classified and prioritized according to the most common causative factors: (1) bladder distention, (2) bowel distention, (3) skin irritation, and (4) visceral stimulation related to clinical problems or diseases. The bladder is the prime causative factor of Dysreflexia; it is also the easiest to resolve. Bladder *distention is the visceral reflex trigger producing the symptoms of Dysreflexia.* Therefore all nursing interventions are focused on emptying the bladder. The patient should not experience any episodes of bladder distention.

Patients with spinal cord injury are on bladder treatment regimens. *The ability to void and empty the bladder is a limitation in this population.* Treatment may include an indwelling Foley or suprapubic catheter, a condom catheter, and an intermittent catheterization program. The nurse must verify the patency of any urinary adjunctive system the patient is using. All tubing must be checked for twisting, kinks, or any other obstructions to urinary flow. Even a twisted condom catheter can prevent urinary flow; not all patients have forceful urethral flow pressures to override such an obstruction.[8]

Next, check the patency of the catheter. Catheter irrigation can validate tube patency. If the catheter is obstructed, it must be removed and replaced immediately and the bladder emptied. Whereas irrigation of an obstructed catheter may facilitate flow and bladder emptying, the catheter should be replaced with a new one to prevent recurrence of an obstruction and Dysreflexia.

For a patient on an intermittent catheterization program, the nurse must initially catheterize the patient to determine the bladder volume. *A large bladder volume will produce bladder distention, and the patient's program may need modification.* The catheterization frequency may need to be increased and schedules changed (for instance, from every 6 hours to every 4), or the patient may require a restriction of oral fluid intake to prevent excess urinary volumes and potential bladder distention.

The patient must not experience any additional bladder stimulation during bladder catheterization and interventions. To prevent this the nurse applies lidocaine jelly 2% as a lubricant for tube insertion;

the jelly will act to anesthetize the urethra and reduce stimulation caused by manipulation.

If the bladder assessment and interventions do not resolve the Dysreflexia symptoms, then the next potential source of irritation must be assessed: the bowel. The nurse may anticipate bowel distention as the visceral stimulus in patients with a history of constipation or hard stools and in patients who are not on a regulated bowel program. *It is essential that patients with spinal cord injury have a regulated scheme for bowel care, because this is a limitation of the disability.* The patient's bowel should be empty and not distended with stool.

The nurse can physically assess the bowel during dysreflexic episodes through a digital examination of the rectum and lower colon. Nupercainal ointment should be ordered, placed around the rectum, and used as a lubricant for the examining finger. Nupercainal ointment acts as an anesthetic and reduces any further stimulation of the bowel during the examination process. If the bowel is distended and stool is present, the nurse digitally removes any impaction. If the patient's vital signs are stable, digital rectal stimulation may be done to facilitate bowel emptying. After the acute dysreflexic episode, enemas for cleansing and stool softening may be administered. The bowel program then needs to be modified and adjusted in relation to frequency of defecation, administration of oral stool softeners, and diet control.

If the bladder and bowel are not the cause of Dysreflexia, the nurse then seeks to rule out skin stimulation as the causative factor. Skin stimulation can result from constrictive clothing, lack of pressure relief from infrequent position changes, presence of skin insults such as decubitus ulcers or abrasions, and thermal exposure. The patient's skin should be free of any adverse stimulation to the skin.[4]

To assess bowel and bladder status, the nurse would have already removed the patient's clothing and would have noted clothing fit and skin condition. The nurse should observe for any skin redness or indentations, sores, burns, or early signs of skin breakdown. The nurse should also assess the fit and placement of catheter straps, limb splints, casts, or any item that can result in pain or skin insult.[7] *The nurse's role in intervention is treatment and prevention of further painful stimuli to the skin.* Wounds are to be kept clean, dry, and free of infection. Analgesics should be administered to prevent pain and potential visceral stimulation. *Because thermoregulation is altered in the individual with spinal cord injury, the patient will be sensitive to extremes of hot and cold.* Such exposure can result in visceral stimulation caused by shivering or the body's response to any sudden temperature change.

If the bladder, bowel, and skin assessment do not reveal a cause of visceral stimulation, the cause may be an underlying disease or medical problem. *It is essential that the patient with spinal cord injury remain free of any type of visceral stimulation, because this type of stimulation produces autonomic dysreflexia.*[5] The physician needs to be aware of episodes of autonomic dysreflexia as well as any changes in the cause, nature, or frequency of episodes. Such changes can indicate a new problem for the patient.

Any disease that produces visceral stimulation, such as pain and increased peristalsis or gastric secretion, can produce autonomic dysreflexia and affect severity of the episode. This is a clinical problem that may be treated interdependently or dependently by the nurse with the physician.

For instance, patients with urinary tract infections will have bladder-related dysreflexic episodes. After the bladder is empty, the Dysreflexia resolves, but the patient may start to have Dysreflexia symptoms with progressively reduced urine volumes. Outcomes for this problem will be physician regulated; that is, an indwelling catheter and antibiotics will be ordered until the infection is controlled.

Emergency episodes of autonomic dysreflexia are managed by physicians. As previously stated, the patient's condition should not deteriorate to this drastic point; *however, if the episode does occur, the primary aim is to resolve the hypertensive crisis and prevent related complications.*

Text continued on p. 346.

❖ *NURSING CARE GUIDELINES*

Nursing Diagnosis: Dysreflexia

Expected Patient Outcomes	Nursing Interventions
The patient's blood pressure will be stabilized.	• Elevate the head of the patient's bed at least 45 degrees or, if possible, place the patient in an upright sitting position. • Notify physician of the patient's hypertensive emergency and administer prescribed medications. • Assure patient's safety; institute seizure precautions. • Monitor vital signs until the cause of the dysreflexia has been determined and alleviated and the patient's vital signs have returned to baseline. • Assess the patient for presence of visceral stimulation and institute interventions directed toward relieving such stimulation.
Bladder distention will be eliminated.	• Assess for bladder fullness. • Assess patency of the urinary adjunctive system the patient is using; correct problems that may be interfering with bladder emptying and free urinary flow. • If the patient does not have an indwelling catheter in place and if bladder is distended, the patient should be catheterized. *After the acute episode* • Monitor fluid intake and output. • Assess for signs and symptoms of urinary tract infection. • With the patient, develop an individualized and regulated bladder program; frequently assess and evaluate the effectiveness of the program.
Bowel distention will be eliminated.	• Review the patient's bowel history and assess for bowel distention or presence of impaction. • If the patient has a rectal impaction, remove stool. • An ointment such as Nupercainal should be ordered for patients at risk for developing stool impactions. • The ointment should be used when examining the rectum or removing the impaction. • Assess need for a change in diet; discuss possible changes with the patient and dietitian. • Assess need for a cleansing enema; if needed, obtain an order and administer the enema. • Assess need for use of stool softeners; if needed, obtain an order and administer. • With the patient, develop an individualized and regulated bowel elimination program; frequently assess and evaluate the effectiveness of the program.

Continued.

IV

❖ *NURSING CARE GUIDELINES—cont'd*

Expected Patient Outcomes	Nursing Interventions
The patient's skin will be free of pressure and irritation.	• Inspect the patient's skin and the fit of clothing. • Remove any restrictive clothing or appliances. • Control the patient's exposure to extremes in room temperature. *After the acute episode* • Keep wounds clean and dry. • Assess skin for any breakdown and assess potential for infection. • Teach the patient to monitor fit of clothing and appliances.
Visceral stimulation related to a clinical problem or disease process will be eliminated or controlled.	• Assess for visceral stimulation that may be related to a particular disease process (such as gastrointestinal ulcers and gallbladder and pancreatic disease) or clinical problem (such as pain). • Administer medications prescribed to reduce visceral stimulation; administer medications prescribed to control pain. • Monitor the patient's response to treatments and prescribed medications. *After the acute episode* • Teach the patient to monitor for symptoms that precede Dysreflexia.

Pharmacological agents may be ordered on a single-episode basis or for permanent prophylaxis. Hydralazine hydrochloride (Apresoline) may be injected for life-threatening hypertension. Nifedipine (Procardia) may be used sublingually in urgent hypertension or orally to prevent further occurrences. Mecamylamine HCl, MSD (Inversine) is another preferred oral agent.

The nurse's major role in autonomic dysreflexia is to prevent its recurrence. Thus it is important to develop patient/family educational programs. The patient must be able to state, demonstrate, and independently problem solve any aspect in the care and prevention of autonomic dysreflexia. Programs should incorporate information on the signs/symptoms and treatment of Dysreflexia, as well as bowel, bladder, and skin care specific to patients with spinal cord injuries. *Programs need to be specific yet flexible to match lifestyles and allow self-maintenance and self-control* (that is,

the timing of the bowel program needs to match the individual's work and social schedule).

EVALUATION

The clinical evaluation of autonomic dysreflexia is based on the resolution of the crisis episode and prevention of its recurrence. The key evaluation criterion is the patient's performance in recognizing and independently resolving any acute events and, more important, in preventing future episodes. The long-term goal is that the patient maintains wellness and achieves it independently.

Short-term evaluation is based on the effectiveness of the teaching plan and achievement of its goals. Patients need to demonstrate an understanding of the signs and symptoms of autonomic dysreflexia, the steps to resolve and prevent episodes, bowel and bladder programs, fluid restriction, catheterization and defecation techniques, and complications.

IV

❖ *CASE STUDY WITH PLAN OF CARE*

Mr. Virgil W. is admitted to the rehabilitation center daily for living and wheelchair skill training. He is 41 years old. He works as a computer operator but has not been employed since his car accident 4 months ago. He owns an inaccessible two-story dwelling, where he lives alone. Medical history includes an injury at the T_3 level of the spinal column. The patient also has a history of hayfever. Physical examination reveals a flushed face and warm skin. The patient complains of nasal congestion and throbbing headache. An indwelling Foley catheter leads to a leg bag. Mr. W.'s blood pressure is 200/100 mm Hg; pulse is 60 beats/min and regular; respirations are 14/min; and oral temperature is 98.6° F. The patient passed one small, hard formed stool 3 days earlier. His diet consists of large portions at meals and snacks in the afternoon and evening.

PLAN OF CARE FOR MR. VIRGIL W.

Nursing Diagnosis: *Dysreflexia related to visceral stimulation*

Expected Patient Outcomes	Nursing Interventions
Mr. W.'s blood pressure will be within normal limits.	• Place Mr. W. in upright, sitting position. • Assess and monitor vital signs every 5 minutes until episode resolves. • Notify physician of assessment findings. • Administer medications as ordered.
Mr. W.'s bladder will be empty and his urinary equipment will be functional.	• Assess Mr. W.'s catheter and tubing for patency. • Have Mr. W. empty his bladder. • Reassess Mr. W. for status of symptoms.
Mr. W.'s bowel will be empty and nondistended.	• Assess bowel for distention. • Digitally remove any impaction and promote bowel emptying.
Mr. W. will follow a regulated bowel program.	• Develop, with Mr. W., an individualized program of bowel regulation and self-care. • Assist and support Mr. W. with the implementation of the program.
Mr. W. will experience a decrease in the frequency of episodes of autonomic dysreflexia.	• Assist Mr. W. in developing an individualized program to eliminate any causative factors of dysreflexia. • With Mr. W., monitor his progress related to adhering to the program and make revisions to the program as needed.
Mr. W. will describe the symptoms and treatment measures of autonomic dysreflexia.	• Teach Mr. W. signs and treatment measures of autonomic dysreflexia. • Encourage Mr. W. to ask questions. • Provide written material providing a summary of the verbal information given to Mr. W. • Ask Mr. W. to describe the signs and symptoms of dysreflexia. • Have Mr. W. demonstrate interventions he may use to prevent or control an episode of dysreflexia.

Autonomic dysreflexia is a lifelong concern for the individual with spinal cord injury. It is a complex health issue. The nurse plays a major role in assisting these individuals in maintaining wellness and independence in a disabled state.

REFERENCES

1. Bell J, Hannon K: Pathophysiology involved in autonomic dysreflexia, *J Neurosci Nurs* 18:86-88, 1986.
2. Carroll-Johnson RM, editor: *Classification of nursing diagnoses: proceedings of the Eighth Conference*, Philadelphia, 1989, JB Lippincott.
3. Ceron G, Rakowski-Reinhardt A: Action stat! autonomic dysreflexia, *Nursing* 21:33, 1991.
4. Chadwick A, Oesting H: Caring for patients with spinal cord injuries, *Nursing* 11:53-56, 1989.
5. Craig D: The adaptation to pregnancy of spinal cord injured women, *Rehabil Nurs* 15:6-9, 1990.
6. Guyton AC: *Textbook of medical physiology* , Philadelphia, 1986, WB Saunders.
7. Metcalf J: Acute phase management of persons with spinal cord injury: a nursing diagnosis perspective, *Nurs Clin North Am* 21:589-598, 1986.
8. Weinberg L, Babicki C, and McIntyre KM: Rehabilitation nursing care plan stimulators, Washington, DC, 1988, National Rehabilitation Hospital.

IV,

Ineffective Airway Clearance

Ineffective Airway Clearance is the state in which an individual is unable to clear secretions or obstructions from the respiratory tract to maintain airway patency.[5]

OVERVIEW

Normally, the upper and lower airways possess distinct defense mechanisms that act to maintain airway patency. The upper airway consists of the nose, pharynx, larynx, and extrathoracic trachea. The defense mechanisms of these structures include heating, humidifying, and filtering foreign matter from inspired air. After contact with the nasal mucous membrane, air becomes humidified with water vapor to 100% saturation, and its temperature regulates to body temperature. The nasal passage also filters and traps foreign particles that will then be expelled through sneezing or blowing the nose. Ciliated epithelium entrap particles that pass through the nasal passage and propel them into the pharynx to be swallowed.

The lower airway consists of the trachea, main stem bronchi, segmented bronchi, subsegmental bronchi, terminal bronchioles, and gas exchange units. The defense mechanisms of the lower airway include mucociliary clearance, macrophage clearance, and coughing.[4] Of these, mucociliary clearance is the most active and effective. Mucus is secreted by goblet cells that line the airway tract to the terminal bronchioles. Foreign particles are trapped by this mucus and are propelled by ciliary action toward the mouth, where they will be expelled from the body. The macrophage clearance system works in the terminal lung unit, where foreign matter is ingested by the macrophages and transported to be swallowed. The cough reflex is initiated to expel the foreign matter when these mechanisms are ineffective.

ASSESSMENT

Under normal circumstances, the breathing pattern of an adult is quiet and smooth, the respiratory rate ranges from 12 to 20 breaths per minute, the skin appears well oxygenated, and quiet breathing is heard throughout all lung fields. The defining characteristics of Ineffective Airway Clearance include abnormal breath sounds, changes in rate or in depth of respiration, tachypnea, cough, cyanosis, dyspnea, and fever.[5]

Abnormal or adventitious breath sounds generally consist of rales (crackles) and rhonchi (sonorous wheezes) and indicate an alteration in normal function. Various forms of rales and rhonchi can be found. In general, rales are heard as crackles, mostly during inspiration as air passes through small, congested airways. The sounds are noncontinuous and usually do not clear through coughing. Crackles may be heard in patients with congestive heart failure, pulmonary edema, consolidation, pulmonary fibrosis, atelectasis, and bronchitis.[4] Rhonchi are continuous sounds produced as air passes through narrowed airways. Wheezes are musical, squeaking noises that are known as rhonchi when they are low pitched and resemble loud snoring. Sonorous wheezes or rhonchi indicate the presence of secretions in the airway. The rhonchi usually clear with a cough or by suctioning. A narrowing of the airway results from secretions, tumors, foreign bodies, bronchial stenosis, bronchospasm, or a swelling of mucosa.[4] Changes in the rate or the depth of respiration, such as hyperpnea (an increase in the number of breaths), may indicate an obstruction of the air flow. The respiratory rate increases to maintain oxygenation and increase air flow around a partially obstructed airway. Coughing is a normal

IV

defense mechanism of the airway, but a persistent cough can indicate abnormal function or underlying processes. Some causes of persistent cough are excessive mucus, foreign particles, irritation from erosive lesions, or airway hyperreactivity.[9] The presence of cough, with or without sputum production, is associated specifically with many diseases, such as acute sinusitis, bacterial pneumonia, aspiration, inhaled irritants, asthma, cystic fibrosis, lung abscess, bronchiectasis, bronchitis, and left ventricular failure.[2]

Cyanosis is a bluish discoloration of the skin and mucous membranes resulting from excessive concentration of reduced hemoglobin in the blood. Cyanosis may indicate hypoxemia (deficient oxygenation of the blood); however, it is a late indicator. Also, if cyanosis is located in the nail beds, it may only represent stagnant blood flow.[4]

Dyspnea (breathing difficulty) is a subjective complaint of breathlessness and may be caused by a number of conditions that can increase ventilatory requirements, decrease ventilatory capacity, or increase resistance to breathing. Some examples are exercise, anemia, fever, weak respiratory muscles, pleural effusion, asthma, emphysema, and chronic bronchitis.[3,4] Dyspnea probably results from the work of breathing against an obstruction that inhibits adequate oxygenation.

A number of related factors may affect an individual's ability to maintain airway clearance. Decreased energy and fatigue may influence an individual's ability to cough effectively. Furthermore, the adequacy of food and fluid intake and an individual's mobility status will directly affect airway stability. Tracheobronchial factors such as infection and irritation cause the goblet cells to secrete large amounts of mucus, possibly leading to airway obstruction, especially when the cough reflex is weak or ineffective.[9] Normally loose mucus can cause obstruction when it becomes thick because of dehydration. Individuals with perceptual or cognitive impairments are likely to develop airway obstruction resulting from noncompliance or resistance to therapy. For instance, these patients may refuse to use humidified oxygen or follow

coughing and deep breathing exercises. Furthermore, neurologically impaired individuals may have a diminished cough, and patients affected by trauma may not be able to cough effectively because of injury, pain, or sedation.

Developmental factors such as those associated with aging may have an effect on maintaining airway clearance. Specifically, in the elderly there is a general decline in the lung or host defense, which may lead to an increase in infections. Furthermore, the cough mechanism is impaired, ciliary function is less effective, there is a decrease in immunoglobulin A, and there is defective activity of alveolar macrophages. Also, the elderly may experience a reduction in exercise tolerance because the muscles of breathing weaken with age, thereby increasing the work of breathing.[6]

❖ Defining Characteristics

The presence of the following defining characteristics indicates that the patient may be experiencing Ineffective Airway Clearance:
- Abnormal breath sounds: rales (crackles) and rhonchi (wheezes)
- Changes in rate or in depth of respiration
- Tachypnea
- Cough, effective or ineffective, with or without sputum
- Cyanosis
- Dyspnea
- Fever

❖ Related Factors

The following related factors are associated with Ineffective Airway Clearance:
- Decreased energy and fatigue
- Tracheobronchial infection, obstruction, or increased secretions
- Perceptual or cognitive impairment
- Trauma

❖ Related Medical/Psychiatric Diagnoses

The following are examples of related medical/psychiatric diagnoses for Ineffective Airway Clearance:
- Asthma
- Cerebrovascular accident (CVA)

IV

❖ *NURSING CARE GUIDELINES*

Nursing Diagnosis: *Ineffective Airway Clearance*

Expected Patient Outcomes	Nursing Interventions
• The patient will develop and maintain a patent airway.	• Assess respiratory status, documenting respiratory rate and rhythm, breath sounds, and cough and sputum characteristics. • Teach the patient to cough effectively after he/she takes deep breaths. • Assist the patient into high Fowler's position. • Splint incisions if applicable. • Suction airway if necessary. • Preoxygenate and hyperinflate before and after suctioning if patient is intubated. • Limit each pass to 15 seconds. • Perform chest physiotherapy, e.g., percussion and postural drainage as ordered. • Monitor finger oximetry and ABG as ordered. • Instruct patient to take deep breaths to increase chest expansion. • Stay with patient during acute periods of shortness of breath.
The patient will maintain adequate ventilation and oxygenation status.	• Provide the patient with adequate hydration status—encourage intake of oral fluids and maintain IV fluids as ordered. • Administer humidified oxygen as ordered, especially if patient has an artificial airway. • Administer medications as ordered, e.g., bronchodilators, expectorants, steroids, and antibiotics. • Position patient to maximize oxygenation status; e.g., position patients with unilateral lung disease with unaffected lung down as tolerated. (Considerations during positioning include lung pathophysiology, comfort, medical problems, and related factors such as obesity, fractures, and surgeries.) • Monitor respiratory status as above as the patient responds to treatment.

• Chronic obstructive pulmonary disease
• Coma
• Pneumonia
• Spinal cord injury

NURSING DIAGNOSES

Examples of *specific* nursing diagnoses for Ineffective Airway Clearance are:
• Ineffective Airway Clearance related to incisional pain with respiratory splinting.
• Ineffective Airway Clearance related to fatigue as evidenced by diminished coughing ability.
• Ineffective Airway Clearance related to comatose state with decreased ventilation.

PLANNING AND IMPLEMENTATION WITH RATIONALE

The nursing goals for the individual with Ineffective Airway Clearance are to establish and maintain airway patency and adequate ventilation. The nurse achieves these goals by enhancing the patient's defense mechanisms or supplementing them through nursing interventions. The effectiveness of the interventions can be measured in the patient by the alleviation of the defining characteristics.[10]

First, the nurse should assess the patient's respiratory status to establish a baseline from which to develop interventions. The nurse should document the breathing pattern, rate of respirations, presence of cyanosis, ability to cough and breathe deeply, adventitious breath sounds, body position, ability to change body position, secretions expectorated, presence of dyspnea, and condition and color of the skin. Arterial blood gas analysis will reveal oxygenation and ventilation status as well as patient response to pulmonary interventions. Pulse oximetry has become a popular method of assessing oxygen saturation at the bedside. It is commonly used in the medical/surgical population for a quick assessment of the development of respiratory problems or as a means to monitor oxygenation status when weaning patients from oxygen.[1] *A thorough assessment is performed so appropriate interventions can be devised and the plan can be evaluated.*

Second, if partial airway obstruction is assessed, the patient should be instructed to cough productively to clear the airway. Secretions should be suctioned if coughing is ineffective or if rales or adventitious breath sounds are heard over lung fields. Suctioning is a potentially deleterious maneuver and therefore should only be performed when necessary, in contrast to suctioning at regularly scheduled intervals.[7] Side effects such as dysrhythmia, vagal stimulation, and cardiac arrest can result from severe hypoxia induced by suctioning. Therefore the patient should be hyperoxygenated with 100% oxygen and hyperin-

flated before and after each suction attempt.[9] Patients should be encouraged to perform deep breathing exercises to prevent closure of the airways resulting from obstruction. *These are necessary components in pulmonary management to limit airway obstruction, which can lead to atelectasis or airway collapse.*

Third, to enhance mucociliary clearance, provide adequate hydration and continuous humidified oxygen. In conjunction with the respiratory therapist, perform chest physiotherapy and postural drainage to mobilize the secretions and enhance expectoration of them as the patient's general status allows.[9] Position the patient according to the lung pathology present[8] and maximize mobility status as tolerated. *Excessive secretions can lead to obstruction of the alveoli.*

Fourth, administer prescribed medications that decrease air flow obstruction, such as bronchodilators, expectorants, proteolytic enzymes, mucolytic agents, and heated aerosols used for treatment of acute episodes and for maintenance therapy. The nurse should continually evaluate the patient's response to the treatment plan to achieve maximum ventilatory capacity. *Medical management can increase airflow and maintain an adequate oxygenation status.*

EVALUATION

The expected patient outcome is the establishment and maintenance of airway patency for adequate ventilation. Data indicating improvement in this condition will reveal an alleviation of the defining characteristics that support the diagnosis. The patient will demonstrate clear breath sounds bilaterally; normal respiratory rate for the particular patient; effective cough expectorating loose,

---

❖ CASE STUDY WITH PLAN OF CARE

Mr. Peter C. is a 75-year-old widowed nursing home resident admitted to a medical unit with a diagnosis of left lower lobe pneumonia and dehydration. The patient had suffered a left hip fracture 2 weeks before and had been in traction since the fall. On admission, Mr. C. had a rectal temperature of 102.4° F and a respiratory rate of 36/min. Further examination revealed sonorous rhonchi over the left lung field, dry and pale skin, poor oral intake, and concentrated urine. The nursing diagnosis was Ineffective Airway Clearance related to the presence of thick secretions.

PLAN OF CARE FOR MR. PETER C.

Nursing Diagnosis: *Ineffective Airway Clearance related to presence of thick secretions*

Expected Patient Outcomes	Nursing Interventions
Mr. C. will be able to cough up secretions.	• Assess respiratory status for baseline. • Provide hydrating IV fluid as ordered. • Encourage oral intake of fluids. • Provide humidified O_2 as ordered. • Monitor secretions. • Send sputum for culture, cytology, and sensitivity as ordered.
Mr. C. will manifest a patent airway.	• Assist Mr. C. in coughing and deep breathing.
Mr. C. will achieve and maintain adequate ventilation.	• Change Mr. C.'s position to mobilize secretions: use the right lateral position for maximum oxygenation. • Monitor arterial blood gases and pulse oximetry as ordered and report. • Have suction apparatus available and suction if needed. • Administer medications as ordered and evaluate therapeutic and adverse effects. • Document the effects of interventions.

thin secretions; and adequate oxygenation status evidenced by the presence of natural skin color and the absence of cyanosis.

REFERENCES

1. Ehrhardt BS, Grahm MV: Pulse oximetry, *Nurse 90,* 20(3):50-54, 1990.
2. Hanley MV, Tyler ML: Ineffective airway clearance related to airway infection, *Nurs Clin North Am* 22(1):135-150, 1987.
3. Ingersoll GL: Respiratory muscle fatigue research: implications for clinical practice, *Appl Nurs Res 2* 6-15, 1989.
4. Kerston LD: *Comprehensive respiratory nursing: a decision making approach,* Philadelphia, 1989, WB Saunders.
5. Kim MJ, McFarland GK, and McLane AM: *Pocket guide to nursing diagnoses,* ed 4, St Louis, 1991, CV Mosby.
6. Matteson MA, McConnell ES: 1989, *Gerontological nursing: concepts to practice,* Philadelphia, 1989, WB Saunders.
7. Phipps WJ, Long BC, Woods NF, and Cassmyer VL: *Medical surgical nursing concepts and clinical practice,* ed 4, St Louis, 1991, CV Mosby.
8. Robichaud A: Alteration in gas exchange related to body position, *Crit Care Nurse* 10(1):56-59, 1990.
9. Sheklton ME, Nield M: Ineffective airway clearance related to artificial airway, *Nurs Clin North Am* 22(1):167-177, 1987.
10. Siskind MM: A standard of care for the nursing diagnosis of ineffective airway clearance, *Heart Lung* 18(5):477-482, 1989.

IV

Ineffective Breathing Pattern

Ineffective Breathing Pattern is the state in which an individual's inhalation and/or exhalation pattern does not enable adequate ventilation.[4]

OVERVIEW

The breathing control center is located in the medulla of the brainstem. This center receives input from various subcenters in the body that interact to regulate breathing in a rhythmical pattern. An increase in the concentration of carbon dioxide in the blood causes an alteration in pH level, thereby stimulating ventilation. Numerous conditions can result in the development of Ineffective Breathing Patterns. For example, the development of chronic obstructive pulmonary disease, the response of the respiratory system to changes in the pH level of the blood, and the response of the pulmonary system to irritants will influence breathing patterns.

Effective ventilation is influenced by many factors, including adequate muscle strength and energy. Three main centers regulate respiration: the medullary center controls the cyclic pattern of respiration, and the apneustic and pneumotaxic centers located in the lower and upper pons, respectively, both maintain a normal, coordinated pattern of respiration. The diaphragm is the main muscle involved in the ventilation process. From the medulla, phrenic nerves carry impulses to the diaphragm, causing a downward contraction of the muscle. This process is known as inhalation.[8] Along with the diaphragm, the external intercostal muscles are involved in inhalation, acting primarily by stabilizing the chest wall. These muscles are innervated by the thoracic intercostal nerves acting on command from the medulla. In contrast, exhalation is a more passive process that depends on the recoil properties of the lung for easy, effective exhalation and relaxation of the muscles. This requires little energy expenditure.[8] The muscles involved are the internal intercostal muscles and the abdominal respiratory muscles, also known as the rectus abdominis and transversus abdominis and the internal and external oblique muscles.

Overall, ventilatory control is regulated by the cortical centers, mechanical factors, central chemoreceptors, and peripheral chemoreceptors.[8] The cerebral cortex can provide input into ventilation patterns, thereby allowing the process of breathing to be partially under voluntary control. During lung inflation, the stretching causes mechanical factors located in the skeletal muscle spindles of the pulmonary vessels and tissues to activate. Changes in the formation of receptors, which occur in restrictive diseases, may increase ventilation.[8] Central chemoreceptors near the medulla react to changes in the pH of the extracellular fluid in the brain. The stimuli for these changes in pH usually arise from changes in the pH of the arterial blood caused by an increase in carbon dioxide (CO_2). In this case, ventilation will increase to lower the concentration of carbon dioxide in the blood. Peripheral chemoreceptors in the carotid arteries and along the arch of the aorta respond to changes in both the partial pressure of oxygen (P_{O_2}) and the partial pressure of carbon dioxide (P_{CO_2}) concentrations in the blood by changing the ventilation pattern.[8]

ASSESSMENT

The related factors associated with the diagnosis Ineffective Breathing Pattern are neuromuscular impairment, pain, musculoskeletal impairment, perception or cognitive impairment, anxiety, decreased energy and fatigue, inflammatory process, decreased lung expansion, and tracheobronchial obstruction.[4] In general, breathing (inhalation and exhalation) is a natural, involuntary process that can be interrupted by a number of causes. The nurse must make an accurate assessment, and also note the medical diagnoses to determine the etiology of the breathing impairment. In doing so, the nurse can implement preventive measures when possible and also develop accurate care plans based on observable clinical data.

A number of neuromuscular and musculoskeletal impairments can adversely affect an individual's breathing pattern. Generally, the problems result from the inability to innervate the proper muscles because of nerve damage, myelin degeneration, spinal cord and brain damage, and inconsistent impulses from the phrenic and intercostal nerves.[3,6] The location of the damage or degeneration and the extent of the disease usually determine the potential adverse effects on breathing patterns. For instance, spinal cord problems may interfere with the normal breathing pattern, depending on the site of damage and whether the phrenic nerve is involved. Specific diseases such as myasthenia gravis, muscular dystrophy, poliomyelitis, multiple sclerosis, and Guillain-Barré syndrome may cause altered breathing patterns resulting from the physiological destruction involved.[3] Furthermore, sedation and drug overdoses may depress the respiratory center and cause Ineffective Breathing Patterns such as hypoventilation.

Conditions that decrease lung expansion will interfere with normal breathing patterns.[2] The presence of pain may limit lung expansion because of existing injuries to the chest or other body structures. The limitation can be the result of anatomical injuries. Rib fractures will limit lung expansion and may produce paradoxical (uneven) breathing. Kyphoscoliosis, a disabling disease characterized by abnormal curvature of the spine, results in an uneven, limited breathing pattern because of the inability of the lung to properly expand. Conditions that add pressure on the lung, such as pneumothorax and hemothorax, will cause altered breathing patterns. Specific problems within the lung itself, which are associated with tracheobronchial obstruction and inflammation, may cause alterations in breathing patterns, especially in the individual who is already compromised. An example is the individual who suffers from asthma. The pathophysiology is as follows: the airway narrows from the constriction of the bronchial walls, the production of mucus increases, the bronchial walls may thicken, and airways narrow further from the presence of secretions. This course of events may lead to altered breathing patterns depending on the extent of the symptoms.

Furthermore, conditions that affect the individual's ability to inhale adequately and consistently, such as decreased energy and fatigue, will result in altered breathing patterns stemming from alveolar hypoventilation. Effective muscle contraction and ventilation require energy and adequate nutrition. Emotional problems such as anxiety are primarily responsible for hyperventilatory breathing patterns.

The defining characteristics for a nursing diagnosis of Ineffective Breathing Pattern are dyspnea, shortness of breath, tachypnea, fremitus, abnormal arterial blood gas levels, cyanosis, cough, nasal flaring, respiratory depth changes, assumption of the three-point position, pursed lip breathing, prolonged expiratory phase, increased anteroposterior diameter, use of accessory muscles, and altered chest excursion.[4]

Many of the defining characteristics of Ineffective Breathing Pattern generally are found in patients with chronic obstructive pulmonary diseases (COPD). COPD is a classifying term used for a number of respiratory diseases that manifest common characteristics.[8] Bronchial asthma, chronic bronchitis, and emphysema are diseases frequently encompassed in the COPD classification, although each disease has a distinct pathophysiological course. The common clinical link among these obstructive pulmonary diseases is the pathological change in the airway or lungs that results in chronic airflow limitation (CAL).[5] The clinical manifestations of CAL and interventions used to treat CAL involve the pathophysiological processes of the trapping of air and the collapse of the airways on expiration.

To improve ventilation and force air out of the lungs, the accessory muscles of respiration are recruited involuntarily by patients with obstructive diseases. The scalene muscles, which elevate the first two ribs; the sternocleidomastoid muscles, which raise the sternum; and the trapezius muscles, which fix the shoulder,[8] are used and will often become pronounced and enlarged as a result of the excessive demands placed on them.

The affected individual often breathes through pursed lips to increase or slow exhalation. This process helps create a back pressure, which lessens the collapse of the airway and improves exhalation.[5] The three-point position—sitting forward, hands on knees, and shoulders elevated—is the position many patients with COPD choose because it allows for easier elevation of the diaphragm, leading to better airflow. The anteroposterior diameter of the chest will become enlarged over time because of the trapping and pulmonary overdistention of air. Diaphragmatic movement becomes greatly depressed or absent as the movement of the rib cage becomes taut resulting from changes in the chest wall. A chronic cough, with or without the expectoration of sputum, frequently accompanies an obstructive disease and will potentiate fatigue and inspiratory muscle weakness. Patients with obstructive diseases must undergo abnormal pulmonary function tests such as a decreased forced expiratory volume (FEV1) in 1 second or a decreased forced vital capacity (FVC), which measures the maximum amount of air expired on expiration. Altered chest excursion refers to either visual or palpable asymmetry of the chest cage.

Dyspnea is the subjective complaint of breathlessness or difficult breathing. The patient may appear to be short of breath. Dyspnea is a complex concept that describes the feeling that ventilatory requirements are not being met by the current ventilation pattern. Typically, the respiratory rate increases to meet the increased demands. Nasal flaring often shows distress and may be present during dyspnea. An intolerance for activity frequently accompanies dyspnea especially in patients with CAL. Lareau and Larson[5] can provide the reader with a description of assessment tools commonly used to document dyspnea and activity intolerances in the clinical setting.

An arterial blood gas analysis will determine the efficiency of ventilation and gas exchange. The gas analysis measures the concentration of oxygen and carbon dioxide and the percent of oxygen saturation, bicarbonate, and pH of the arterial blood. The normal values for arterial blood gases at sea level are Po_2: 90+/− 10 mm Hg; O_2 saturation: 96% +/− 1%; Pco_2: 40 +/− 3 mm Hg; pH: 7.4 +/− 0.03; and bicarbonate: 22 to 26 mEq/L.[8]

Pulse oximetry can be used at the bedside to assess oxygenation through assessment of oxygen saturation (Sao_2). About 97% of oxygen in the blood binds with hemoglobin. Saturation is a measure of the percentage of hemoglobin that is saturated by oxygen. An Sao_2 of 90% to 100% is needed to adequately replenish plasma. Problems occur when Sao_2 goes below 85%, and a saturation under 70% is considered life threatening.[1] Pulse oximetry gives the practitioner a quick means to assess impending hypoxemia. It must be remembered that this test does not measure ventilation status.

The lungs function as a buffer system to maintain the close balance of pH in the blood by regulating the ratio of bicarbonate to carbon dioxide (CO_2). Alterations in blood gases, especially the pH, will result in changes in the respiratory pattern.[8] For instance, respiratory acidosis (a decrease in the pH and increase in carbon dioxide), which results from alveolar hypoventilation, will cause hyperventilation in an individual with intact compensatory mechanisms. This response decreases the concentration of carbon dioxide in the blood and restores balance.

❖ Defining Characteristics

The presence of the following defining characteristics indicates that the person may be experi-

encing Ineffective Breathing Pattern:
- Dyspnea
- Shortness of breath
- Tachypnea
- Fremitus
- Abnormal arterial blood gas
- Cyanosis
- Cough
- Flaring of nostrils
- Respiratory depth changes
- Assumption of three-point position
- Lips pursed when breathing
- Prolonged expiratory phase
- Increased anteroposterior diameter
- Use of accessory muscles
- Altered chest excursion

❖ Related Factors

The following related factors are associated with Ineffective Breathing Pattern:
- Neuromuscular impairment
- Pain
- Musculoskeletal impairment
- Perceptual or cognitive impairment
- Decreased energy or fatigue
- Inflammatory process
- Decreased lung expansion
- Tracheobronchial obstruction
- Anxiety

❖ Related Medical/Psychiatric Diagnoses

The following are examples of related medical/psychiatric diagnoses for Ineffective Breathing Pattern:
- Cerebral injury
- Chest trauma
- Drug overdose
- Rib fracture
- Pneumothorax
- Pulmonary embolus
- Thoracic surgery

NURSING DIAGNOSES

Examples of *specific* nursing diagnoses for Ineffective Breathing Pattern are:
- Ineffective breathing pattern related to excessive secretions and airway obstruction as evidenced by rapid respiratory rate and presence of adventitious breath sounds.
- Ineffective breathing pattern related to airflow limitation as evidenced by altered respiratory rate.
- Ineffective breathing pattern related to narrowing of airways as evidenced by the presence of wheezing and stridor and an increased respiratory rate.
- Ineffective breathing pattern related to decreased lung expansion as evidenced by decreased breath sounds in affected area and increased respiratory rate.

PLANNING AND IMPLEMENTATION WITH RATIONALE

The nursing goals for the patient with ineffective breathing pattern are to maximize ventilation and improve airflow. The effectiveness of the interventions is measured by the alleviation of existing defining characteristics and the reduction of dyspnea.

First, the effectiveness of the patient's respiratory status should be assessed to establish a baseline and to develop appropriate interventions.[8] A complete health history should be obtained, including questions about exposure to environmental irritants, present and past occupations and use of cigarettes. Assess the patient's current breathing pattern for rate, rhythm, and regularity. Document the patient's overall appearance, including color of skin and body position. If the patient is breathing abnormally, document the pattern, the events preceding the alteration, and the patient's emotional state. Assess and document the presence of any defining characteristics, such as use of accessory muscles, chest expansion, dyspnea, pursed lip breathing, and so on, to determine the etiology of the breathing alteration. *Assessment of baseline respiratory status is essential for developing an appropriate plan of care and assists in evaluation of therapy.*

Second, instruct and position the patient to facilitate breathing and maximize ventilation. This process is sometimes termed "breathing retraining" and involves (1) teaching and assisting the patient in breathing through pursed lips, (2) assisting the patient in assuming a position of maximum ventilation—often the three-point position, (3) teaching the patient diaphragmatic and abdominal breathing techniques, and (4) assisting the patient with progressive relaxation techniques

IV

IV

❖ NURSING CARE GUIDELINES

Nursing Diagnosis: *Ineffective Breathing Pattern related to physiological alterations*

Expected Patient Outcome	Nursing Interventions
The patient will experience adequate airflow in and out of lungs.	• Assess and document the patient's respiratory status, including a complete health history. • Assess and document the patient's breathing pattern (rate, rhythm, chest expansion, breath sounds, use of accessory muscles, pursed lip breathing, arterial blood gases, and color). • Instruct and assist the patient in using the most effective respiratory position, e.g., the three-point position, if patient experiences pursed lip breathing. • Administer medications as ordered to increase airflow and evaluate effectiveness (e.g., bronchodilators, anticholinergics, and antiinflammatory medications). • Assist the patient with activities of daily living. Assess the patient's level of activity intolerance and provide the patient with adequate rest periods to conserve energy. • Maintain adequate nutritional intake to support the respiratory muscles and supply the energy required for breathing. • Teach the patient to avoid airway irritants (e.g., cigarette smoke). • Teach the patient to prevent respiratory infections. • Monitor the patient's respiratory status in response to the above treatments. • Monitor pulse oximetry every shift and as ordered/as needed. • Assess for improvements in arterial blood gases, pulmonary function tests, and the total clinical picture.

and biofeedback. These interventions should increase the exhalation phase and reduce airway collapse. During pursed-lip breathing, the patient is coached to exhale through pursed lips, thereby slowing expiration and stabilizing the airway through the prevention of collapse. Diaphragmatic breathing incorporates the abdominal muscle group for improved ventilation, because these muscles are close to the diaphragm. To encourage full expansion of the diaphragm, patients are taught to relax abdominal muscles during inspiration and to tighten them slightly during expiration. Many positions can facilitate ventilation, including the forward-leaning position, the head-down position, and the supine position.[5] In general, patients usually assume the position of maximum ventilation and comfort. *Available interventions may improve dyspnea and lead to effective breathing patterns.*

Third, administer bronchodilators, anticholinergics, and antiinflammatory medications ordered to improve airflow.[7] Nurses should clearly evaluate the effectiveness of these medications. Improvements in respiratory status are supported clinically by improvements in arterial blood gases, pulmonary function tests, and the patient's overall clinical picture, including a reduction in symptoms. *These agents may improve airflow.*

Fourth, a comprehensive plan should be directed at (1) reducing the work of breathing, (2) minimizing the expenditure of energy by assisting the patient with daily activities as needed,[9] (3) providing rest periods as necessary if activity intolerance is assessed, (4) maintaining adequate nutritional stores to support the respiratory muscles and supply the energy required for breathing, and (5) teaching the patient to avoid airway irritants such as cigarette smoke and prevent respiratory infections. *A comprehensive plan facilitates long-term maintenance of breathing patterns.*

EVALUATION

The overall patient outcome is the preservation and improvement of ventilation. Data indicating improvement in this condition will reveal the alleviation of the defining characteristics that support the diagnosis. The patient will demonstrate bilateral breath sounds, a less labored breathing pattern, normal blood gas levels for the patient, an increase in FEV1 and FVC, and a general decrease in symptoms.

❖ *CASE STUDY WITH PLAN OF CARE*

Mrs. Shirley S. is a 75-year-old woman admitted to the medical unit with a chief complaint of breathing difficulty. A physical examination revealed a thin, elderly woman in mild respiratory distress. Her respiratory rate was 36/min with decreased breath sounds and some wheezes, especially on expiration; skin was cold and clammy; face appeared flushed; pulse was 126 beats/min; and blood pressure was 180/90 mm Hg. Arterial blood gas revealed a Po_2 of 55 mm Hg, a Pco_2 of 50 mm Hg, and a pH of 7.32. The patient admitted that she had expectorated yellow sputum for the previous 3 days. The patient's history also included smoking two packs of cigarettes per day for 30 years until she stopped smoking 2 years before. A chest x-ray examination revealed consolidation of the right middle lobe. The diagnosis was COPD exacerbation related to respiratory infection. One of the nursing diagnoses formulated was Ineffective Breathing Pattern related to decreased airflow.

PLAN OF CARE FOR MRS. SHIRLEY S.

Nursing Diagnosis: Ineffective Breathing Pattern related to decreased airflow

Expected Patient Outcomes	Nursing Interventions
Mrs. S.'s airflow will be maximized.	• Assess and document Mrs. S.'s breathing pattern and the associated parameters. • Administer continuous intravenous bronchodilator therapy as ordered. • Administer other medical agents as ordered, such as antibiotics, steroids to decrease inflammation, and aerosol treatments.
Mrs. S. will experience an absence of respiratory distress.	• Assist Mrs. S. into a position of maximum ventilation and comfort, e.g., sitting upright or alternating with left lateral position. • Administer oxygen cautiously at low flow rate of 1 L/min, and evaluate Mrs. S.'s response closely. • Monitor vital signs and pulse oximetry and report arterial blood gas levels to physician. • Conserve Mrs. S.'s energy by assisting with activities of daily living. • Provide Mrs. S. with adequate rest periods.
Mrs. S. will return to baseline respiration.	• Encourage Mrs. S. to expectorate secretions. • Encourage adequate nutritional intake; monitor and report status to physician. Maintain hydrating IV as ordered. • Stay with Mrs. S. and provide emotional support and reassurance during periods of acute shortness of breath. • Continually assess and document the effectiveness of interventions on Mrs. S.'s respiratory status and breathing pattern.

IV

REFERENCES

1. Ehrhardt BS, Grahm M: Pulse oximetry, *Nurs 90* 3:50-54, 1990.
2. Hopp LJ, Williams M: Ineffective breathing pattern related to decreased lung expansion, *Nurs Clin North Am* 22(1):193-206, 1987.
3. Kim MJ, Larson JL: Ineffective airway clearance and ineffective breathing patterns: theoretical and research base for nursing diagnoses, *Nurs Clin North Am* 22(1):125-133, 1987.
4. Kim MJ, McFarland GK, and McLane AM: *A pocket guide to nursing diagnoses,* ed 4, St Louis, 1991, CV Mosby.
5. Lareau S, Larson JL: Ineffective breathing pattern related to airflow limitation, *Nurs Clin North Am* 22(1):179-191, 1987.
6. Larson JL, Kim MJ: Ineffective breathing pattern related to respiratory muscle fatigue, *Nurs Clin North Am* 22(1):207-223, 1987.
7. Petty TL: Drug strategies for airflow obstruction, *Am J Nurs* 2:180-184, 1987.
8. Phipps WJ, Long BC, Woods NF, and Cassmyer VL: *Medical surgical nursing concepts and clinical practice,* ed 4, St Louis, 1991, CV Mosby.
9. Sheklton ME: Coping with chronic respiratory difficulty, *Nurs Clin North Am* 22(1):569-581, 1987.

IV

Impaired Gas Exchange

Impaired Gas Exchange is the state in which an individual experiences an imbalance between oxygen uptake and carbon dioxide elimination at the alveolar-capillary membrane gas exchange area.[3]

OVERVIEW

Impaired Gas Exchange is a complicated diagnosis that obviously requires medical corroboration of clinical information for support. The arterial blood gas analysis is the most accurate indicator of oxygenation and gas exchange status. However, other clinical signs such as respiratory rate and rhythm, cardiac dysrhythmias, breath sounds, tidal volume, heart rate, body position, and skin color can indirectly measure gas exchange.[5] The symptoms of impaired gas exchange generally result from interference with cellular metabolism.

The overall purpose of respiration is the exchange of oxygen and carbon dioxide at the alveolar level. In normal gas exchange, the following processes occur; (1) oxygen is delivered into the system so that adequate alveolar ventilation takes place (ventilation), (2) alveoli become adequately perfused with blood for the transport of oxygen and carbon dioxide (distribution), (3) the alveolar-capillary membrane diffuses the gases (diffusion), and (4) hemoglobin in the red blood cells picks up and delivers the oxygen to the tissues (perfusion).[5] Therefore Impaired Gas Exchange usually results from clinical disease states that alter these four processes.

Hypoxia is most frequently caused by ventilation and perfusion (V/Q) imbalances.[5] Overall, the adequate matching of ventilation to perfusion results in an adequate oxygenation status. In the normal lung, ventilation to perfusion is unevenly distributed. The location of the pulmonary artery branches affects the amount of blood flowing to the bases of the lung. Similarly, ventilation is unevenly distributed throughout the lung. The actions of the diaphragm and the rib cage during inspiration and the heavy concentration of blood flow cause the bases of the lung to receive more ventilation than the apices in the gravity-dependent areas of the lungs.[5] Certain pathological conditions, such as hypovolemic shock or emphysema, can cause the mismatching of ventilation to perfusion, resulting in symptoms of hypoxia.

ASSESSMENT

The defining characteristics for Impaired Gas Exchange include confusion, somnolence, restlessness, irritability, inability to move secretions, hypercapnia, and hypoxia.[3] In general, the clinical characteristics result from the effects of hypoxia and hypercapnia on the individual. Hypoxia refers to a general deficiency of oxygen in body tissues. Signs and symptoms vary, depending on the extent and nature of the hypoxia. Mild hypoxia stimulates the peripheral chemoreceptors, increasing heart rate and respiratory rate to compensate for decreased oxygen. Other symptoms such as confusion, somnolence, restlessness, and irritability demonstrate altered mentation resulting from decreased oxygen delivery to the tissues of the brain.[5] Hypercapnia refers to an abnormal increase of carbon dioxide in the blood that may be caused by many factors, including the presence of thick secretions that can cause airway obstruction and obstructive diseases such as chronic obstructive pulmonary diseases (COPD) that lead to chronic retention of carbon dioxide.

The related factors (etiologies) of Impaired Gas Exchange are an altered oxygen supply, alveolar-capillary membrane changes, an altered blood flow, and the altered capacity of blood to carry oxygen.[3] An altered oxygen supply representing a low V/Q ratio occurs when perfusion to the alveoli is adequate, but ventilation is less than adequate. In this case, oxygen is not available to the cells, and carbon dioxide is not properly eliminated. Some clinical examples that can cause this are an airway obstruction, muscle weakness, central nervous system depression, chest trauma, emphysema, and high altitudes (low oxygen concentration).[5]

Changes in the alveolar capillary membrane may impair the diffusion of gases. Some examples include the reduction of the gas exchange area caused by lung resection; the thickening of alveolar membrane, as occurs with adult respiratory distress syndrome; and the interference from the displacement of interstitial fluids, as occurs with pulmonary edema. Altered blood flow results in a high V/Q ratio; the alveoli are adequately ventilated but poorly perfused. Therefore ventilation is wasted, and hypoxia and hypercapnia result because blood is not available to pick up or remove the gases. Some causes of decreased perfusion are circulatory or hypovolemic shock, pulmonary embolism, cardiac dysrhythmia, myocardial depression, and the destruction of the capillary bed.

Any alteration in hemoglobin, the blood's primary transporter of oxygen, results in an altered level of oxygen transported to the tissues. Some causes for this are (1) inadequate hemoglobin, such as in anemia, (2) inadequate force to pump the cells, such as with congestive heart failure, and (3) vessel patency that does not allow for the normal flow of blood.[5]

Developmentally, the elderly exhibit physiological changes that render them at risk for Impaired Gas Exchange. There is a reduction of alveolar surface area, so gas exchange and saturation are reduced. Furthermore, the signs of hypoxia that are manifested in the younger population, such as increased heart rate, increased blood pressure, and increased respiratory rate, are often blunted in the elderly. Sometimes the only early sign of hypoxia in the elderly is a change in mentation.[4]

❖ Defining Characteristics

The presence of the following defining characteristics indicates that the patient may be experiencing Impaired Gas Exchange:
- Inability to move secretions
- Hypercapnia
- Hypoxia
- Confusion
- Somnolence
- Restlessness
- Irritability

❖ Related Factors

The following related factors are associated with Impaired Gas Exchange:
- Altered oxygen supply
- Alveolar capillary membrane changes
- Altered blood flow
- Altered capacity of the blood to carry oxygen

❖ Related Medical/Psychiatric Diagnoses

The following are examples of related medical/psychiatric diagnoses for Impaired Gas Exchange[6]:

- Anemias
- Atelectasis
- COPD
- Leukemia
- Pneumothorax
- Pulmonary embolism

NURSING DIAGNOSES

Examples of *specific* nursing diagnoses for Impaired Gas Exchange are:
- Impaired Gas Exchange related to collapsed lung (atelectasis) as evidenced by decreased or absent lung sounds on affected side
- Impaired Gas Exchange related to alveolar hypoventilation as evidenced by abnormal arterial blood gas analysis
- Impaired Gas Exchange related to inflammation of the visceral and parietal pleura as evidenced by adventitious breath sounds and abnormal arterial blood gas analysis

PLANNING AND IMPLEMENTATION WITH RATIONALE

The nursing goal for the individual with Impaired Gas Exchange is to maintain adequate

❖ *NURSING CARE GUIDELINES*

Nursing Diagnosis: *Impaired Gas Exchange*

Expected Patient Outcome	Nursing Interventions
The patient will experience adequate gas exchange as evidenced by normal ABGs and the absence of hypoxia.	• Monitor patient for signs of hypoxia: changes in mental status, tachycardia, irritability, and abnormal breath sounds and report to physician. • Monitor vital signs, arterial blood gas levels, EKG, and pulse oximetry every shift and prn. • Position patient to maximize ventilation and perfusion matching. • Administer oxygen as ordered. • Maintain patient airway by facilitating cough and encouraging deep breaths. • Administer medications as indicated, including bronchodilators, expectorants, inhalants, and antibiotics. • Encourage rest periods. • Provide ongoing assessment of the effectiveness of interventions. • Monitor and assist the patient requiring mechanical ventilation in the maintenance of adequate gas exchange.

IV

ventilation and oxygenation status. The nurse achieves this by assisting in the identification of the etiology designating Impaired Gas Exchange and by performing interventions to improve overall gas exchange. The effectiveness of the interventions can be measured by the alleviation of the defining characteristics that support the diagnosis. One must collaborate with the physician to accurately assess gas exchange through the analysis of arterial blood gas (ABG) levels.

First, assess the patient's respiratory status to establish a baseline and plan interventions. Document breath sounds, respiratory rate and rhythm, sputum production, skin color, body position, alterations in mental status, heart rate, and dysrhythmias. Also note the medical diagnoses. Assist the physician in obtaining the arterial blood gas sample and report other laboratory values that affect oxygenation status, such as hemoglobin level. Monitor pulse oximetry to determine oxygen saturation.[1] *A thorough assessment is performed so appropriate interventions can be devised and an evaluation of the plan can*

occur.

Second, perform nursing interventions that maximize and coordinate the ventilation and perfusion relationship. If partial airway obstruction is determined, instruct and assist the patient in coughing and expectorating secretions. Suction the patient if the cough is ineffective. Provide supplemental oxygen if the patient is hypoxemic. *These measures have a positive effect on oxygenation status by improving the ventilation and perfusion relationship.* Depending on the specific lung pathology, place the patient in a position that will facilitate ventilation and perfusion matching. Although clinical nursing research in this area is just developing presently, some support for therapeutic positioning is noted. The individual with unilateral lung disease exhibits the most noted effect. The lateral position with the "good" (unaffected) lung down (dependent) will improve oxygenation by increasing perfusion to the healthy tissue.[2,7] This research reveals evidence opposing the idea that patients should be repositioned frequently and arbitrarily and suggests the development of a more, specific plan based on the patient's lung pathology. However, only future study can answer the many remaining questions about the effects of other positions on oxygenation and the frequency and duration of therapeutic position changes.

Third, provide maintenance and supportive treatment to facilitate gas exchange and adequate ventilation. Encourage and provide rest periods before and after physical activity to prevent exacerbations of hypoxia. Assist the patient with activities of daily living to conserve energy and oxygen requirements. Administer medications as ordered and evaluate effectiveness; these may include bron-

chodilators, expectorants, corticosteroids, antibiotics, and antihistamines to improve pulmonary function. *Measures to decrease oxygen consumption and demand may improve gas exchange by preventing the development of hypoxia.*

EVALUATION

The overall patient outcome is the achievement and maintenance of adequate gas exchange. Data indicating improvement reveal the eradication of the defining characteristics that supported the diagnosis. The patient will demonstrate an arterial blood gas level within normal limits for the patient and the absence of hypoxia.

❖ CASE STUDY WITH PLAN OF CARE

Mr. Barry H. is an 80-year-old male who underwent hip surgery 1 week before, and while resting, he developed sudden, severe substernal chest pain. His color deteriorated, he became apprehensive, and he complained of breathing difficulty (dyspnea). After a phys-

ical examination, the pain was attributed to pleurisy; arterial blood gas levels revealed hypoxia (PaO_2 was 60 mm Hg); pulse was tachycardic; and rales were present in the left upper field.[6] A diagnosis of pulmonary embolism resulted.

PLAN OF CARE FOR MR. BARRY H.

Nursing Diagnosis: *Impaired Gas Exchange related to altered blood flow*

Expected Patient Outcomes	Nursing Interventions
Mr. H. will maintain adequate oxygenation.	• Monitor Mr. H. for signs and symptoms of hypoxia: restlessness, apprehension, abnormal breath sounds, cyanosis, and headache. • Monitor vital signs, including heart rhythm via EKG, arterial blood gases, and pulse oximetry; report abnormalities.
Mr. H. will maintain adequate oxygenation/ventilation status.	• Administer oxygen as ordered. • Assess respiratory status in response to therapy: inspect the chest for respiratory rate, rhythm, and regularity; auscultate breathing for abnormal or diminished sounds; and assess color of skin and anxiety level. • Assist in bronchial hygiene measures if necessary, such as coughing and deep breathing, chest physical therapy, suctioning, and aerosol therapy. • Position Mr. H. to maximize ventilation and perfusion coordination.

REFERENCES

1. Ehrhardt BS, Grahm M: Pulse oximetry, *Nurs 90* 20(3):50-54, 1990.
2. Gillespie D, Rehder K: Body position and ventilation-perfusion relationships in unilateral pulmonary disease, *Chest* 90:91, 1987.
3. Kim MJ, McFarland GK, and McLane AM: *Pocket guide to nursing diagnoses,* ed 4, St Louis, 1991, CV Mosby.
4. Matteson MA, McConnell ES: *Gerontological nursing: concepts to practice,* Philadelphia, 1989, WB Saunders.
5. Phipps WJ, Long BC, Woods NF, and Cassmyer VL: *Medical surgical nursing concepts and clinical practice,* ed 4, St Louis, 1991, CV Mosby.
6. Roberts SL: Pulmonary tissue perfusion altered: emboli, *Heart Lung* 16(2):128-137, 1987.
7. Robichaud A: Alteration in gas exchange related to body position, *Crit Care Nurse* 10(1):56-59, 1990.

Decreased Cardiac Output

Decreased Cardiac Output is the state in which the amount of blood pumped by the heart is insufficient to meet the needs of the body's tissue.[14]

OVERVIEW

Since the 1970s, mortality from cardiovascular disease has declined as the result of the development of sophisticated emergency medical systems in coronary care units, advances in antidysrhythmic and fibrinolytic therapy, development of techniques for recanalization of coronary arteries via a percutaneous approach, and the advance in cardiac surgery.[13] Because of the increasing level of acuity in today's long-term case population, interventions previously found only in acute care are now commonplace in the chronic-care setting. These changes result from health care and reimbursement legislation, advances in medical technology, and the overall increased life expectancy of the population at large. To meet these challenges, nursing leaders are making efforts to identify and anticipate patient care needs and to implement educational programs for staff to meet these needs.[23]

Decreased Cardiac Output is one of the most complex and frequently encountered problems among patients. Frequently, the patients experiencing this condition present life-threatening situations that require critical nursing judgments and immediate interventions.[3] It is important that nurses be knowledgeable and skilled in the diagnosis of this disorder.

Cardiac output is the volume of blood pumped by each heart beat (or stroke volume) times the number of beats per minute. Normal cardiac output averages about 5 L/min in an adult human being at rest.[7] The cardiac output of an individual may vary with activity, postural changes, and metabolic rate. If heart rate and stroke volume decrease, cardiac output decreases. Hemostatic mechanisms regulating cardiac output involve not only factors controlling performance of the pump, but also factors affecting the peripheral vascular system and resistance. Normally the heart can vary its cardiac output up to five to six times the resting level, depending on the age and physical condition of the patient. There are two basic methods by which the heart regulates cardiac output in response to stress or diseases: (1) changes in heart rate and (2) changes in stroke volume.[6]

Numerous systemic and cardiac factors affect the ability of the heart to pump blood and thereby alter cardiac output.[2,10] Cardiac failure results from any condition that reduces the heart's ability to pump.[24] The most common cause of low cardiac output, at rest, is diminished myocardial function resulting from myrocardial infarction with coronary artery disease.[5] The only peripheral factor that usually decreases cardiac output is decreased mean systemic pressure, most often caused by decreased blood volume. Rapid bleeding (25% to 30% of total blood volume) will reduce the cardiac output to zero; and slow bleeding (40% to 50% over a period of an hour) will do the same thing.[10] With deterioration of left ventricular function, left ventricular dilation may occur as a compensatory mechanism to maintain cardiac output.[7] When cardiac output is significantly diminished, heart failure can occur.

It is estimated that three million people in the United States have congestive heart failure and that this disorder affects nearly 15 million people worldwide. In 1985, hospital discharge records listed congestive heart failure as a secondary diagnosis for 1.7 million patients.[4] The incidence of congestive heart failure is escalating. Congestive

Table 11 New York Heart Association functional classification

Functional Class	Definition	Manifestation
I	Patients with cardiac disease but without resulting limitations of physical activity.	Ordinary physical activity does not cause undue fatigue, palpitations, dyspnea, or angina.
II	Patients with cardiac disease resulting in slight limitation of physical activity, but comfortable at rest.	Ordinary physical activity results in fatigue, palpitations, dyspnea, or angina.
III	Patients with cardiac disease resulting in marked limitation of physical activity, but comfortable at rest.	Less than ordinary physical activity causes fatigue, palpitations, dyspnea, or angina.
IV	Patients with cardiac disease resulting in an inability to carry out any physical activity without discomfort.	Symptoms of cardiac insufficiency or of angina may be present even at rest.

From Wright SM: Pathophysiology of congestive heart failure, *J Cardiovasc Nurs* 4(3):12, 1990.

heart failure has been the objective of extensive research yet still prevails as the leading cause of death.[18] The Framingham Study[16] revealed a 40% 5-year survival rate. The New York Heart Association has categorized heart failure into four classes based on cardiac reserve or functional capacity, as shown in Table 11.[24] One-year mortality rates have been correlated with functional class and increased from 0% to 5% for class I, to 10% to 20% for class II, to 35% to 45% for class III, and to 85% to 95% for class IV.[14]

Decreased cardiac output resulting from heart failure may be caused by mechanical, electrical, or structural factors. Mechanical factors include alterations in preload, alterations in afterload, and alterations in inotropic changes of the heart. *Preload* is the pressure exerted by the blood volume and venous return to the heart.[1] Preload is related primarily to contractility; a reduction in contractility results in a decreased cardiac output. *Afterload* is the resistance against which the heart pumps, arterial pressure.[1] An increase in afterload decreases stroke volume. If stroke volume decreases, cardiac output decreases.

Noncardiac factors, as noted earlier, influence preload and afterload, resulting in a decreased cardiac output. Invasive hemodynamic monitoring, such as balloon-tipped pulmonary artery catheters, is the measurement of factors affecting preload and afterload and of the stimuli that affect the inotropic state of the heart. Inotropic changes occur in the normal heart during exercise. During exercise catecholamines, tachycardia, and an increase in sympathetic nerve impulses augment myocardial contractility and stroke volume, resulting in an increase in cardiac output. In patients with heart failure the heart does not respond to exercise in the same way. The normal increase in cardiac output does not occur. The compromised myocardium is incapable of meeting the increased demands of exercise. As a result cardiac output is decreased.

Electrical factors that decrease cardiac output include alterations in heart rate, rhythm, and conduction. Pacemaker therapy may be beneficial. Cardiac output may be optimized by increasing or decreasing the rate of the pacemaker.[12,19] Nursing responsibilities include (1) knowledge of the type and functional capabilities of the pacemaker, (2) early identification of changes in electrical factors affecting cardiac output, and (3) knowledge regarding appropriate interventions to correct electrical abnormalities (for instance, use of medications and reprogramming parameters).

Structural factors that decrease cardiac output include papillary muscle dysfunction and ventricular abnormalities. These structural problems interfere with the normal functioning of the heart. Conditions such as papillary muscle dysfunction, ventricular aneurysm, rupture of the interventricular septum, and rupture of the ventricle can lead to a decline in cardiac output.

The patient with low output failure shows clinical evidence of impaired peripheral circulation and peripheral vasoconstriction. The extremities are usually cold, pale, and cyanotic. In late stages the stroke volume decreases and the pulse pressure narrows. Low output failure occurs in patients with congenital or rheumatic, valvular, coronary, hypertensive, and cardiomyopathic heart disease.[7] It is the responsibility of the nurse to (1) attempt to understand the cause underlying the symptoms of decreased cardiac output, (2) initiate the appropriate nursing interventions, and (3) recognize the necessity for early medical intervention.

ASSESSMENT

The 11 functional health patterns can provide conceptual direction for the initial assessment of the patient. Because of their apparent relevance to clinical practice, the functional health patterns are useful in categorizing the NANDA nursing diagnoses.[9]

Defining characteristics of Decreased Cardiac Output are obtained from a complete biopsychosocial patient history. Subjective data from the history provide information about the disease process and the patient's lifestyle, family structure, and preexisting health problems. Health problems may include conditions such as heart enlargement, elevated cholesterol or triglyceride levels, diabetes, heart murmurs, heart attacks, rheumatic fever, or hypertension. In addition the patient's family history may reveal pertinent information of certain familial disease (for instance, hypertension, rheumatic fever, stroke, blood disease, asthma, glaucoma, and gout).

Objective data are obtained by assessing the patient's mental status, cardiovascular system, peripheral vascular system, respiratory system, and urinary output. The signs and symptoms of de-creased cardiac output may differ depending on the etiology of the associated health problem. The four techniques of inspection, palpation, percussion, and auscultation are used to complete the assessment.[21]

The nurse begins the assessment by monitoring the patient's heart rate, blood pressure, and respirations. A low blood pressure may indicate low cardiac output. The nurse assesses respiratory status and notes any productive or nonproductive cough. The patient is observed for the signs of fear or anxiety that may appear in decreased cardiac output. Signs of dyspnea and orthopnea may be apparent in a patient with left ventricular failure. Distention of external jugular veins may be seen in right-sided heart failure. Cyanosis of the lips and nail beds indicates venous distention and inadequate oxygenation of blood. Another characteristic of this diagnosis is pale, cool, diaphoretic skin. The patient may appear tired and weak because of sleep disturbances and poor perfusion of skeletal muscles caused by a decrease in cardiac output. Edema and ascites resulting from right ventricular failure may be noted. Dependent edema may be observed in the patient's ankles, feet, and hands. The nurse inspects the patient for impression marks from socks, rings, and shoes. If the patient has been confined to bed rest, the nurse should observe the sacrum for dependent edema. Urine output is observed for signs of oliguria and anuria, which may indicate decreased cardiac output and subsequent decreased renal blood flow.

The nurse auscultates the heart for rate and rhythm. Tachycardia and other dysrhythmias often reflect an attempt by the heart to compensate for decreased cardiac output.[17] The nurse should document any noted dysrhythmias in the patient's medical record and report them to the physician for immediate treatment.

Alterations in hemodynamic parameters indicate early left ventricular failure, often preceding other signs and symptoms of failure; therefore noting such alterations is an essential part of nursing assessment.[17] It is important for the nurse to realize that even in hemodynamically stable patients, results may vary as a result of (1) errors in measurements or (2) physiological alterations occurring within the patient.[5,8,17]

The nurse should palpate the carotid, brachial, femoral, popliteal, dorsalis pedis, and posterior tibial pulses. These are evaluated for patency, rate, rhythm, and character.[1] Lungs are auscultated for rales and decreased breath sounds caused by excess fluid in lung fields. Percussion is an especially useful tool in assessing the pulmonary and abdominal systems.[21] Dull sounds are noted when abnormal fluid is present in the lungs or abdomen. The nurse should carefully record assessment data in the patient's medical record. A chest film will confirm pulmonary congestion. Evaluation of the results of the assessment will provide information from which the nurse can develop an effective plan of care.

Blood pool imaging can help determine the pumping ability of the myocardium. This test may be done at rest or during exercise. The patient is given an intravenous bolus of a radionuclide substance (such as technetium pertechnetate or technetium-tagged albumin or red blood cells). Wall-motion abnormalities will be reflected by a decreased ejection fraction. The *ejection fraction* is the ratio of blood expelled from the ventricle in one contraction to the ventricle's total capacity. At rest the healthy heart has an ejection fraction of 60% to 70%. The ejection fraction provides important information about stroke volume during periods of stress and increased cardiac output.

If the blood pool imaging is to be done only at rest, a single ejection fraction will be reported. If the blood pool imaging is to be done during an exercise–gated-blood pool study, two ejection fractions will be reported: one at rest and one during exercise. If the resting ejection fraction is low or if the ejection fraction decreases with exercise, cardiac pumping has decreased and has compromised cardiac output. The nurse should be aware of the ejection fraction reported in the summary of the gated-blood pool study. The patient should know the test is quite accurate and involves little risk. The patient should be instructed regarding preparations and protocol of the testing proce-

dures. The nurse should emphasize that there is no danger of harmful radiation.[7]

An echocardiogram, at rest or during exercise, will provide information regarding chamber hypertrophy, wall motion, or stenosis.

Laboratory tests will reflect changes caused by impaired tissue perfusion, diuretic therapy, or renal insufficiency (e.g., elevated blood urea nitrogen, elevated serum potassium).

❖ Defining Characteristics

The presence of the following defining characteristics indicates the patient may be experiencing Decreased Cardiac Output:

- Variations in hemodynamic readings
- Dysrhythmias, electrocardiographic changes
- Fatigue
- Rales, dullness percussed in lungs
- Dyspnea, orthopnea, nonproductive cough
- Cyanosis—pallor of skin and mucous membranes
- Altered arterial blood gases
- Weakness
- Hypotension
- Cold, clammy skin
- Edema, ascites
- Decreased urinary output
- Decreased peripheral pulses
- Jugular vein distention
- Anxiety
- Confusion
- Restlessness

❖ Related Factors

The following related factors are associated with Decreased Cardiac Output:

Mechanical factors
- Alteration in preload
- Alteration in afterload
- Alteration in inotropic changes in the heart

Electrical factors
- Alterations in rate
- Alterations in rhythm
- Alterations in conduction

Structural factors
- Papillary muscle dysfunction
- Ventricular abnormalities[11]

❖ Related Medical/Psychiatric Diagnoses

The following are examples of related medical/psychiatric diagnoses for Decreased Cardiac Output:

- Cardiomyopathy
- Congestive heart failure
- Myocardial infarction
- Rheumatic heart disease
- Valvular heart disease

NURSING DIAGNOSIS

Examples of *specific* nursing diagnoses for Decreased Cardiac Output are:

- Decreased Cardiac Output related to ventricular tachycardia
- Decreased Cardiac Output related to failure of permanent pacemaker
- Decreased Cardiac Output related to left ventricular aneurysm

PLANNING AND IMPLEMENTATION WITH RATIONALE

Nursing interventions for patients with Decreased Cardiac Output are based on measures to (1) improve cardiac pump performance, (2) reduce cardiac work load, and (3) control salt and water retention.[7] Independent nursing actions to achieve these measures are primarily monitoring functions and health teaching. Direct treatment of Decreased Cardiac Output requires collaboration of the nurse with the physician to institute appropriate interventions.

Nursing actions to improve pump performance are based on the administration of medications and their subsequent action. Digitalis and inotropic agents are commonly prescribed. Digitalis is given to patients with heart failure to improve the depressed myocardial contractility, increase cardiac output, and promote diuresis.[7,20] Inotropic agents are given to augment heart rate, stroke volume, and myocardial contractility. Nursing intervention involves observation for side effects of the drugs, especially dysrhythmias. Any abnormality in cardiac rate and rhythm can result in a decrease in cardiac output. Patients who experience severe bradycardia or atrial or ventricular dysrhythmias may require a temporary pacemaker to restore heart rate to normal. Because drug therapy plays a major role in the management of heart failure, patient and family education is imperative to promote adherence with the overall plan of care.

Reduction in work load is accomplished with the administration of vasodilators in conjunction with physical and emotional rest. Restrictions in activity depend on the degree and severity of heart failure. Nursing interventions focus on observations for possible side effects, such as hypotension, bradycardia, headaches, and drug interactions. If needed, circulation may be assisted by use of intraaortic balloon counterpulsation or ventricular assist devices. With cardiac output assistance, blood can be circulated through the body at a physiologically acceptable rate, relieving cardiac work and increasing oxygen supply to the failing ventricle, yet augmenting cardiac output and systemic coronary perfusion.[22] The nurse should encourage obese patients to participate in a weight-reduction program with dietary supervision.

Excess salt intake and water retention increase cardiac work load. Sodium restriction should be managed through dietary supervision. Diuretics are administered to correct fluid volume overload. Accurate daily weights will reflect changes in fluid status. A gain or loss of 1 kg (2.2 pounds) of body weight approximates the gain or loss of 1 L of fluid.[17] The nurse should maintain accurate intake and output records as they are essential to assess effectiveness of treatment with diuretics. Monitoring electrolyte levels daily is essential to patient care. The nurse should report and document any change in the patient's heart rate, heart rhythm, respirations, blood pressure, skin temperature, skin color, mental status, or urine output. Any changes in these may indicate electrical factors corresponding to a decreased cardiac output. Nursing interventions should initiate actions to correct abnormalities.

EVALUATION

Encourage the patient to participate in evaluation of his or her progress as much as possible.

The nurse should instruct the patient regarding observable signs of Decreased Cardiac Output. Appropriate questions to ask the patient are as follows: Are you still having difficulty breathing? Are your feet, ankles, hands, and abdomen still swollen? Do you still have difficulty breathing at night? Do you sleep on more than one pillow? Do you still have a cough and how often? Have you gained any weight rapidly? Have you decreased your intake and how? If your urine output normal for you? How have you modified your activities?

❖ *NURSING CARE GUIDELINES*

Nursing Diagnosis: *Decreased Cardiac Output*

Expected Patient Outcomes

The patient will have improved cardiac pump performance as evidenced by the following: normal blood pressure; normal pulse; normal sinus rhythm; normal breath sounds without rales or wheezes; warm and dry skin without cyanosis; normal urine output; no cough, dyspnea, or orthopnea; no diaphoresis; no jugular vein distention; no peripheral or sacral edema; no ascites; normal hemodynamic status (cardiac output resting range, 4 to 8 L/min[8]; cardiac index, 2.5 to 4 L/min/m^2; pulmonary artery wedge pressure, <13 mm Hg; mean right atrial pressure, 4±2 mm Hg; central venous pressure, 4 to 15 cm H_2O or 3 to 11 mm Hg).

The patient will have a reduction in cardiac work load as evidenced by outcomes noted above.

Nursing Interventions

• Monitor blood pressure.
• Auscultate and monitor heart rate and rhythm.
• Auscultate the lungs.
• Assess skin temperature and color.
• Maintain accurate intake/output records.
• Note respiratory rate and pattern.
• Assess jugular veins for distention.
• Observe for peripheral edema, and report daily weight gain to physician.
• Monitor hemodynamic status; consult physician if values exceed normal ranges.
• Assess effects of prescribed medications.

• Instruct the patient in ways to reduce energy expenditure, such as bed rest with bedside commode (as indicated); semi-Fowler's or high Fowler's position; frequent rest periods; possible need to restrict fluids as directed; need to take prescribed medication; and need to reduce salt intake as directed.
• Promote calm environment.

Continued.

❖ NURSING CARE GUIDELINES—*cont'd*

Expected Patient Outcomes	Nursing Interventions

The patient will maintain normal fluid and electrolyte balance as evidenced by the following: intake equal to output; normal electrolyte values (Na, 135 to 145 mEq/L; K, 3.5 to 5.5 mEq/L; Ca, 4 to 5 mEq/L or 8.6 to 10.5 mg/dl); no weight gain; no peripheral edema; no peripheral venous distention; no orthopnea or paroxysmal nocturnal dyspnea; no cough; no frothy sputum; normal hemodynamic readings (as noted); and no tachypnea.

- Maintain accurate intake records.
- Monitor electrolyte values; consult physician if values are not within normal range.
- Encourage the patient to adhere to low-sodium diet.
- Encourage the patient to adhere to fluid restrictions as ordered.
- Instruct the patient in proper administration of diuretics and inform the patient of potential side effects of diuretics and need for adequate dietary intake.
- Assess for effectiveness of prescribed medication.
- Weigh the patient daily (same clothes, same scales, same time each day).
- Monitor changes in vital signs (compare with baseline signs).

IV

❖ CASE STUDY WITH PLAN OF CARE

Mr. M., aged 72, is a retired architect. He occasionally does consultant work with the firm he established. He is married and has one son. He enjoys playing golf twice a week and walks one mile daily. He is active in civic affairs and volunteers at the local community college as a teacher to students interested in an architectural career. He is 5'9" tall and weight 180 pounds. He eats moderately and works diligently to maintain his normal weight. He does not smoke. Other than his golfing, he has few hobbies. He prefers staying "busy," often maintaining 10 to 12 hours of daily activities.

Over a 2-week period, Mr. M. noticed swelling in his hands and feet progressively increasing. His weight rose to 185 pounds. His wedding ring felt tight. His belts felt snug and had to be increased in size. He developed a nonproductive cough. At night, he required two pillows to breath comfortably. He resorted to sleeping in a chair. He became increasingly anxious and fatigued from lack of sleep. His shortness of breath worsened. After a night of minimal sleep his wife insisted he go to the emergency room. Physical findings were as follows: Mr. M. was anxious and short of breath. Lips and nailbeds appeared dusky. His skin was cool and clammy. Bilateral jugular vein distention was present. Blood pressure was 102/60 mm Hg, heart rate was 118/min with frequent irregularities, and respirations were 29/min and labored. Bilateral rales were present. A chest x-ray revealed marked pulmonary congestion. The abdomen was distended. Edema of the hands was noted with pressure marks from his rings noted. Edema of both feet was observed with indentations from his socks present. Pedal pulses were difficult to palpate.

Continued.

PLAN OF CARE FOR MR. M.

Nursing Diagnosis: Decreased Cardiac Output related to electrical, mechanical, or structural factors

Expected Patient Outcomes	Nursing Interventions
Mr. M. will have normal breath sounds without rales or wheezes and no cough.	• Note respiratory rate and pattern. • Auscultate lungs. • Administer oxygen as ordered. • Administer medications as ordered (for instance, diuretics). • Reduce Mr. M.'s fluid intake if ordered.
Mr. M. will express no complaints of dyspnea, orthopnea, or paroxysmal nocturnal dyspnea.	• Instruct Mr. M. regarding need for lung assessment, fluid restriction, and pacemaker therapy (when applicable).
Mr. M. will maintain normal blood pressure, pulse, and sinus rhythm.	• Monitor blood pressure. • Auscultate and monitor heart rate and rhythm.
Mr. M. will have no jugular vein distention.	• Assess jugular veins for distention.
Mr. M.'s urine output will be normal.	• Maintain accurate intake/output records. • Observe for peripheral edema; examine sacrum for dependent edema. • Note ascites. • Weigh Mr. M. daily, and instruct him on the need to weigh daily (same time of day, same clothes) after voiding and to report weight gain. • Teach Mr. M. to observe for and report edema.
Mr. M. will experience reduced anxiety and fear.	• Teach Mr. M. about the disease process, including the following: medications—actions and potential side effects; correct way to take pulse; purpose of cardiac monitoring; and purpose of cardiac testing.
Mr. M. will maintain normal hemodynamic status as evidenced by mean right atrial pressure of 4 ± 2 mm Hg, cardiac output resting rate of 4 to 8 L/min, cardiac index of 2.5 to 4 L/min/m^2, mean pulmonary artery pressure < 13 mm Hg, and central venous pressure of 4 to 15 cm H_2O or 3 to 11 mm Hg.	• Monitor hemodynamic status; consult physician if values exceed normal ranges. • Instruct Mr. M. in need and procedure for hemodynamic monitoring. • Assess skin color and temperature: skin pink, warm, and dry; no cyanosis, decrease in temperature, or diaphoresis.
Mr. M. will demonstrate a reduction in cardiac work load: maintains bed rest with bedside commode; uses semi-Fowler's or Fowler's position; takes rest periods; demonstrates no anxiety or fear; has no daily weight gain; adheres to fluid restriction if indicated; has positive reaction to medications, without side effects; and is normothermic.	• Encourage bed rest with bedside commode. • Maintain Mr. M. in semi-Fowler's or high Fowler's position. • Encourage frequent rest periods. • Instruct Mr. M. in need to reduce fluid intake, take prescribed medications (instruct regarding action and potential side effects), monitor temperature, and use stress-management techniques.

IV

Expected Patient Outcomes

Mr. M. will maintain normal fluid balance as evidenced by the following: normal electrolyte values; Na, 135 to 145 mEq/L; K, 3.5 to 5.5 mEq/L; Ca, 4 to 5 mEq/L or 8.6 to 10.5 mg/dl; no rapid weight gain; no peripheral edema; adherence to sodium-restricted diet as indicated; adherence to fluid restriction as indicated; and no side effects from prescribed medications.

Nursing Interventions

• Instruct Mr. M. in importance of maintaining accurate intake/output records; monitoring electrolyte levels (consult physician if levels are not within normal range); monitoring sodium intake as directed; following dietitian's sodium-restricted diet; lifelong dietary restrictions; medications and side effects; exercise (limitations and potential complications); and assessing for effectiveness of prescribed medications.

IV

REFERENCES

1. Andreoli KG, and others: *Comprehensive cardiac care,* ed 6, St Louis, 1987, CV Mosby.
2. Berne RM, Levy MN: *Physiology,* ed 2, St Louis, 1987, CV Mosby.
3. Bumann R, Speltz M: Decreased cardiac output: a nursing diagnoses, *Dimen Crit Care Nurs* 8(1):6-15, 1989.
4. Chesebro J: Cardiac failure. In. Brandeburg RO, Fuster V, Giuliani ER, and McDoon DC, editors: *Cardiology: fundamentals and practice,* Chicago, 1987, Year Book.
5. Daily EK, Mersch J: Thermodilution cardiac outputs using room and ice temperature injectate: comparison with the Fick method, *Heart Lung* 16:294, 1987.
6. Daily EK, Schroeder JS: *Techniques in bedside hemodynamic monitoring,* ed 4, St Louis, 1989, CV Mosby.
7. Dossey BM, Guzzetta CE, and Kenner CV: *Essentials of critical car nursing,* Philadelphia, 1990, JB Lippincott.
8. Gardner PE, Monat LA, and Woods SL: Accuracy of the injectate delivery system in measuring thermodilution cardiac output, *Heart Lung* 16:552, 1987.
9. Gordon M: *Nursing diagnosis: process and application,* New York, 1987, McGraw-Hill Book Co.
10. Guyton AC: *Textbook of medical physiology,* ed 8, Philadelphia, 1990, WB Saunders.
11. Guzzetta CE, Dossey BM: *Cardiovascular nursing: body mind tapestry,* St. Louis, 1984, CV Mosby.
12. Iskandrian AS, Mintz GS: Pacemaker therapy in congestive heart failure: a new concept based on excessive utilization of Frank-Starling mechanism, *Am Heart J* 112:867, 1986.
13. Jaffe A, Albarran-Sotelo R, and Athins J: *Textbook of advanced cardiac life support,* ed 2, Dallas, 1987, American Heart Association.
14. Killip T: Epidemiology of congestive heart failure, *Am J Cardiol* 56:2A-7A, 1985.
15. Kim MJ, McFarland GK, and McLane AM: *Pocket guide to nursing diagnoses,* ed 4, St Louis, 1991, CV Mosby.
16. McKee P, Castell W: The natural history of congestive heart failure: the Framingham study, *N Engl J Med* 285:1441-1446, 1971.
17. Metheny NM: *Fluid and electrolyte balance: nursing considerations,* Philadelphia, 1987, JB Lippincott.
18. Michaelson C: *Congestive heart failure,* St Louis, 1983, CV Mosby.
19. Miura DS: Indications and guidelines for cardiac pacing in the 1980s, *Cardiovasc Rev Rep* 8:51, 1987.
20. Packer M: Prolonging life in patients with congestive heart failure: the next frontier, *Circulation* 75(suppl IV):1, 1987.
21. Reuther MA, Hansen CB: *Cardiovascular nursing* 1-24, New York, 1985, Medical Examination Publishing.
22. Teplitz L: An algorithm for ventricular assist devices, *Dimen Crit Care Nurs* 9(5):256-265, 1990.
23. Wengate S: Nursing grand rounds, *J Cardiovasc Nurs* 4(3):71, 1990.
24. Wright S: Pathophysiology of congestive heart failure, *J Cardiovasc Nurs* 4(13):1-15, 1990.

Altered Tissue Perfusion (Specify Type) (Renal, Cerebral, Cardiopulmonary, Gastrointestinal, Peripheral)

Altered Tissue Perfusion (Specify Type) (Renal, Cerebral, Cardiopulmonary, Gastrointestinal, Peripheral) *is the state in which an individual experiences a decrease in nutrition and oxygenation at the cellular level as a result of a deficit in capillary blood supply.*[9]

OVERVIEW

Adequate tissue perfusion is essential to the life and functioning of each body organ and tissue. It depends on a competent circulatory system that will continually deliver oxygen and nutrients to the cells. Cells are the basic living unit of the body.[6] Their proper functioning depends on the energy they derive from the oxygen and nutrients that are delivered continuously by the circulation. The circulation also is responsible for removing the metabolic waste products from the tissues and cells that result when energy is released from the oxygen and nutrients.

An alteration in tissue perfusion will ensue if there is an interruption of any of these functions of the circulation causing a decrease in the delivery of oxygen and nutrients to the cells, and thus a decrease in cellular function, energy metabolism, and removal of waste products.[22] A local decrease in tissue perfusion is referred to as ischemia, and a systemic decrease is referred to as shock.

Tissue ischemia disrupts the cells' natural ability to obtain energy through aerobic metabolism because of the decrease in the supply of oxygen and nutrients. When this occurs the cells obtain their energy from anaerobic glycolysis.[6,22] This process results in release of excess quantities of lactic acid. The decreased blood flow also prevents the normal removal of carbon dioxide. This excess carbon dioxide will react locally with water to produce carbonic acid. Both of these waste products result in a decrease in the cell's pH. The acidosis activates lysosomal enzymes, which destroy the cellular membranes and digest the cellular contents. This disruption of the cellular membranes causes intracellular enzymes and fluid to leak into the tissues.

A positive feedback system may develop and lead to further progression of the ischemia. According to Rice[14] the inadequate supply of oxygen and nutrients causes a functional impairment of cells, tissues, organs, and eventually body systems. It is characterized by an increase in swelling of the tissues, compression of the vessels, and a further decrease in blood flow. Eventually, the tissue deteriorates and organ failure will follow.

Conditions that can result in an alteration in tissue perfusion are occlusion or constriction of a vessel, and a decrease in cardiac putput or systemic vascular resistance resulting in hypotension.[21] Clinical manifestations can occur in any of the following tissues: renal, cerebral, cardiopulmonary, gastrointestinal, and peripheral. The extent of the effects of the decrease in tissue perfusion depends on the duration of the deficit and the metabolic needs of the tissues.[22] Its cause may be related to an interruption of arterial flow, an interruption of venous flow, exchange problems, hypervolemia, or hypovolemia.

Renal

An alteration in renal tissue perfusion is initially manifested by a decrease in urine output and signs of excess fluid volume. If the alteration is prolonged, the result may be ischemia, tissue death, and renal failure. The etiology is based on any condition that results in an interruption of circulatory flow to the kidneys. Some of these conditions include hypovolemia resulting from blood loss, plasma loss, or sodium and water loss, prolonged hypotension as in septic shock, and reflex vasoconstriction.[6,22] It also may be the result of myocardial insufficiency caused by infarction, dysrhythmias, or congestive heart failure.

No matter what the cause of the ischemia, it will evoke the same compensatory response in an effort to improve flow to the kidney. A reflex vasoconstriction in both the arterial and venous systems will occur.[6] An increase in the formation of angiotensin will constrict peripheral arteries, resulting in an increase in the retention of sodium and water by the kidneys. There also is an increase in the release of vasopressin, or antidiuretic hormone, which further constricts arteries and veins, causing an increase in water retention by the kidneys.

This vasoconstriction may improve venous return to the heart, but it will further impair blood flow through the kidneys, denying them the oxygen and nutrients they need for metabolism.[6,22] Ischemia will increase, and anaerobic metabolism will become the cells' source of energy. Urine output will cease with prolonged ischemia, and renal failure will occur.

Any condition that interferes with an adequate flow of oxygen and nutrients to the kidneys can result in permanent damage if it is not corrected. Along with the etiologies listed above, other clinical conditions that are associated with renal tissue ischemia include diabetic nephropathy,[18] Rhabdomyolysis,[7] renal trauma,[19] and HIV infection.[13] Once permanent damage occurs, the patient requires an artificial means of dialysis to remove excess waste products and fluid volume and to sustain life. Because the kidneys control these functions in addition to maintaining acid-base balance, nurses must attempt to preserve the kidneys' proper functioning.

Cerebral

An alteration in cerebral tissue perfusion often is manifested by a change in mental status or a loss of consciousness, because there is a decrease in flow to the cerebral vessels. The cause may be physiological inadequacy of the cerebral vessels, compression of surrounding tissues, or infection.[10,22]

A cerebrovascular accident and a transient ischemic attack are the result of an interruption of blood flow to certain areas of the brain as a result of a pathological process.[23] This interruption may be due to an occlusion by a thrombus or embolus, rupture of a vessel wall, hypotension, or vasospasm. It also can be the result of a vascular disorder such as atherosclerosis, trauma, arteritis, and hypertensive arteriosclerosis.

Orthostatic hypotension can result in decreased cerebral tissue perfusion caused by an autonomic dysfunction resulting in defective postural reflexes.[11,23] The expected compensatory mechanism of peripheral vasoconstriction in response to position changes will be diminished or absent. Other factors associated with orthostatic hypotension include a decrease in intravascular volume, hypokalemia, anesthesia, immobility, and medications (sedatives, hypnotics, antianxieties, antiemetics, analgesics, and antihistamines). Chronic orthostatic hypotension can result from degenerative neurologic diseases such as Parkinson's, Addison's, diabetic neuropathy, or neurogenic tumors. Regardless of the etiology, the result is a rapid drop in arterial pressure and syncope.

Memmer[11] indicates that orthostatic hypotension due to immobility can occur after only 2 to 3 days of bedrest. The etiology includes decreased use of the baroreceptors, reducing their ability to

IV

cause peripheral vasoconstriction. Other related factors include decreased muscle tone and incompetent vein valves, which impair venous return.

Syncope and falls in the elderly are often attributed to orthostatic hypotension.[11] Etiologies in this group include degenerative changes in both the central and peripheral nervous system, endocrine system, and vascular system. It may be complicated by chronic disease, medications, decreased mobility, and confusion.

A cerebral aneurysm and an arteriovenous malformation also may interfere with the circulation of the cerebral system, with the result being an interruption of flow. An aneurysm is a small, saccular protrusion that weakens the arterial wall of a major cerebral vessel.[23] Patients may have no symptoms until the vessel ruptures and bleeds. An arteriovenous malformation is a group of arteries and veins with deficient muscle coats that is often dilated and twisted and that interferes with the flow of blood.[22]

Head injuries, both open and closed, can result in either rupture of cerebral vessels or compression of the vessels by the surrounding tissues as a result of edema or hemorrhage.[23] The result is an impedance or cessation of flow. In the case of edema the vessels are compressed by the surrounding tissues resulting in brain ischemia.[6] The ischemia is accompanied by hypoxemia and hypercarbia and initiates a positive feedback mechanism that can be fatal. It causes arteriolar dilation with increased capillary pressure. There is an increase in edema fluid and intracranial pressure (ICP), and a more severe alteration in cerebral tissue perfusion. Extraordinary measures must be instituted to prevent total destruction of tissues.

Compression of cerebral vessels and impedance of blood flow also can be the result of tumors, both benign and malignant, or hydrocephalus.[22] Central nervous system tumors can cause progressive, irreversible damage to the vasomotor center and/or sypathetic responses.[11] As a tumor increases in size it affects the circulatory system of the brain and can be fatal.[10] The result is an increase in intracranial pressure (ICP). When hydrocephalus is present there is an excessive amount of cerebrospinal fluid, which increases ICP; this results in compression of cerebral blood vessels and interference with normal circulation.[22]

Neurological deficits may result from an infection within the nervous system.[10] The patient may have an altered level of consciousness accompanied by hyperthermia. The signs and symptoms present will differ depending on the area of involvement within the nervous system. The main cause of the deficits usually is an increase in ICP because of inflammation and swelling of the meninges, or the brain, which can affect blood supply.

All of these abnormal physiological processes may interfere with the delivery of oxygen and nutrients to the brain. This interruption can result in either temporary or permanent alterations in brain functions as a result of ischemia. A nurse caring for a patient experiencing any of the aforementioned conditions must assess for neurological deficits that would indicate an alteration in tissue perfusion.

Cardiopulmonary

An alteration in cardiopulmonary tissue perfusion is often manifested by cardiac ischemia or problems with oxygenation caused by a decrease in flow to the coronary vessels or in the pulmonary blood supply.[22] The cause may be atherosclerotic heart disease, cardiac spasm, pulmonary infarction or emboli, chronic obstructive pulmonary disease (COPD), or any condition that predisposes a patient to a decrease in cardiac output or interferes with the exchange of oxygen and carbon dioxide within the system. Other possible etiologies include pulmonary edema, shock, atelectasis, pneumothorax, congestive heart failure (CHF), and anemia. Patients with an alteration in cardiopulmonary tissue perfusion will exhibit signs of tachypnea, tachycardia, angina, and dyspnea.

Atherosclerosis refers to a plaque that develops along the intima of coronary arteries and comes in contact with coronary blood flow.[6] Platelets and fibrin adhere to the plaque, and a thrombus is formed that slowly occludes the vessel. A spasm causes an acute occlusion of a coronary vessel that results in a contraction of the coronary artery and a sudden cessation of flow. The cardiac dysfunction that ensues as a result of the decrease in perfusion to the myocardium will interfere with the normal functioning of the heart. This ischemia may result in a decrease in cardiac output or a myocardial infarction.

Pulmonary emboli are large clots that lodge in the pulmonary circulation and interrupt the blood supply to the pulmonary capillaries.[22] Because this is where gas exchange occurs, the result will be a decrease in the amount of oxygen available to all body tissues. Without blood supply to an area of the lung, a pulmonary infarct will occur, resulting in tissue necrosis and possibly hemorrhage. If the clot lodges in both of the major branches of the pulmonary artery, it becomes fatal.[6]

COPD, as well as other obstructive lung diseases, will interfere with the ability of the lung to adequately exchange oxygen and carbon dioxide with the blood supply.[6] It destroys the walls of the alveoli, which is where gas exchange occurs. It also may destroy some of the small blood vessels of the pulmonary system and thereby cause an increase in resistance in the pulmonary vasculature. An impedance of oxygen exchange also can occur in patients with fibrotic lung disease and atelectasis.

Each of the conditions discussed interferes either with the flow of blood or with the exchange of oxygen and carbon dioxide within the circulatory or pulmonary systems. The result is an alteration in cardiopulmonary tissue perfusion. If it is prolonged, there may be permanent damage to the other body systems and tissues that are so highly dependent on the supply of oxygen and nutrients, which are normally available when there is an adequately functioning cardiopulmonary system.

Gastrointestinal

An alteration in gastrointestinal tissue perfusion often is manifested by constipation, weight loss, and nausea and vomiting because there is a decrease in flow to the gastrointestinal system. The cause may be vascular disease, a postoperative complication or shock.[14,22] The gastrointestinal system includes the bowel, liver, and pancreas.

Vascular disease, such as atherosclerosis, can interfere with the mesenteric vessels that supply blood to the intestines.[10] People may have no symptoms for some time, but as atherosclerosis progresses they will begin to experience abdominal cramping after meals. This is referred to as abdominal angina. It occurs at this time, because the process of digestion increases the need for oxygenation and the compromised arterial system cannot accommodate this increased need.

As this vascular insufficiency progresses the function of the bowel may be compromised, resulting in a decrease in peristalsis. Bowel function will stop if there is a complete occlusion of the arterial blood supply. The patient will experience severe abdominal pain accompanied by nausea and vomiting caused by ischemia of the tissues that follows an interruption of the blood supply. It is a surgical emergency that, if not treated, will result in infarction and necrosis of the tissue.

As with other body systems, the gastrointestinal tract is affected by the prolonged vasoconstriction associated with shock.[15] The resulting ischemia can lead to ulceration of the stomach and intestines, allowing bacteria to invade the circulation. Another potential complication is gastrointestinal hemorrhage.

Bowel ischemia and obstruction also may occur after abdominal surgery.[10] It is referred to as a paralytic ileus and occurs because of a lack of peristalsis during abdominal surgery. Paralytic ileus may last from hours to days, and if not treated with gastric suction, it will cause the patient to experience nausea and vomiting.

A decrease in tissue perfusion to the liver and pancreas also will result in ischemia and an alteration in function.[22] During acute stages of shock there may be ischemic damage to the liver, because the decrease in circulation does not provide enough nutrients to support the liver's high rate of metabolism.[6] If the deterioration continues, liver function is depressed, and cellular metabolism

IV

and detoxification of materials are reduced.

The ischemia that develops in the pancreas causes the arterioles to constrict, thus activating pancreatic enzymes.[6] As the pancreatic tissue degenerates it releases toxic factors into the blood. One of these is myocardial toxic factor, which has a depressant effect on the contractility of the heart. This potentiates the progression of the shock syndrome.

Each of the conditions presented represents some type of an alteration in gastrointestinal tissue perfusion, which results from a decrease in blood flow to the organs because of vascular disease, shock, or postoperative complications. The alteration can be a slowly progressive problem, acute in onset, or the result of abdominal surgery. If it is prolonged, there may be permanent damage that results in necrosis and death of the tissues.

Peripheral

An alteration in peripheral tissue perfusion often is manifested by cold extremities that are blue or purple when they are in a dependent position and pale when they are elevated. Arterial pulses are either diminished or absent. The cause may be arteriosclerosis, atherosclerosis, inflammation, spasm, shock, hypothermia, emboli, or thrombophlebitis.[22]

Arteriosclerosis is a hardening and calcification of arterial vessel walls, and atherosclerosis is characterized by a buildup of plaque lesions that adhere to the intima of vessel walls.[22] Each of these conditions interferes with blood flow in the peripheral vessels and thereby prevents the tissues from receiving amounts of nutrients and oxygen adequate to meet their needs.[10] Along with inadequate nourishment to the tissues, waste products are not removed efficiently, with the result being stasis of blood and damage to the tissues.

These types of disturbances in blood flow are characteristic of peripheral vascular disease.[10] Symptoms may be present at rest in a patient with severe peripheral vascular disease, whereas others with less advanced stages may exhibit problems only when the metabolic demands of the body in-

crease. An increased need for oxygen and nutrients by the tissues occurs during increased physical activity, with the direct application of heat, and during infection.

The normal response of the arterial vessels is to dilate and allow increased blood flow to the tissues.[10] Because of the alterations in the vessel walls caused by peripheral vascular disease, the vascular system is unable to compensate. The patients may therefore experience pain in their extremities with increased activity and tissue damage from direct heat. They will have difficulty with healing and may have leg ulcers or a cellulitis, because the tissues are not supplied with the nutrients and oxygen needed to fight infection.

An alteration in peripheral tissue perfusion can be the result of inflammation and occlusion of a vessel caused by thrombophlebitis, emboli, or thromboangiitis obliterans.[22] Thrombophlebitis is characterized by an inflammation and clot formation in a vein where there is decreased blood flow, hypercoagulability, or disruption of the vessel wall.[10] Emboli are an aggregation of platelets floating within the arterial system; these can adhere to a vessel wall and cause a narrowing or an occlusion of blood flow to the area.

Thromboangiitis obliterans, also called Buerger's disease, may be characterized by acute inflammatory lesions and eventual occlusive thrombosis of arteries and veins.[10] There is a progressive narrowing of the peripheral vessel walls as a result of inflammation and thrombus formation.[22,23] There is fibrosis, thickening, and scarring, which many times lead to a complete occlusion of the artery.

Vasospastic disorders also interfere with tissue perfusion, especially if coupled with an already underlying arterial or venous insufficiency. Raynaud's disease is characterized by intermittent episodes of constriction of small arteries in the extremities, usually caused by a cold environment or emotional stimuli.[10,23]

Hypothermia, whether accidental or induced, can result in damage to body organs and tissues if it is not carefully controlled. It decreases the rate of metabolism, oxygen consumption, and circulation time.[10] As hypothermia becomes more profound, cerebral, renal, pulmonary, and cardiovascular functions become impaired. There can be permanent damage to peripheral tissues from frostbite. If the hypothermia is not controlled and corrected, death will ensue.

The decrease in cardiac output and perfusion caused by shock results in a powerful sympathetic nervous system response in an attempt to maintain circulatory flow to vital organs.[6,15] The arterioles constrict, and thus flow to the periphery is decreased. The veins also constrict to maintain an adequate venous return. The skin will become cool and pale. If prolonged, shock can result in permanent damage and even death to the peripheral tissues.

Each of the conditions discussed can result in an alteration in peripheral tissue perfusion because of a decrease in blood flow. It may be a structural problem such as vascular disease or a functional problem such as vasospasm, or it may be induced by other physiological conditions such as shock and hypothermia. The signs and symptoms may occur abruptly or can be gradual in onset.

Regardless of the cause, if tissue ischemia is prolonged, the cells will revert from aerobic metabolism to anaerobic metabolism for energy. The buildup in lactic acid will set off a positive feedback mechanism that will cause an increase in tissue swelling and further compression of the vessels. If blood supply to the tissues is inhibited completely and if the problem is not corrected, tissue necrosis and death will occur.

ASSESSMENT

Assessing the patient with an alteration in tissue perfusion is an important nursing function. Once Altered Tissue Perfusion is identified, steps must be taken to improve tissue perfusion and prevent permanent damage. The causes stem from five basic factors: an interruption of arterial flow, an interruption of venous flow, exchange problems, hypervolemia, or hypovolemia.[9]

Each of these impairs the ability of the cells to obtain the oxygen and nutrients needed for proper functioning and to rid themselves of the metabolic waste products. All of the medical diagnoses previously discussed can be associated with at least one of these factors. Therefore the presence of any of these related factors should alert the nurse that an alteration in tissue perfusion may be present.

Each of the body systems must be assessed individually for an alteration in tissue perfusion. Included in the assessment must be both subjective and objective data before a diagnosis can be made. It is important to recall that once an alteration in tissue perfusion is identified, along with its cause, the nurse also should identify the adverse effects it will have on life processes. The plan of care developed for the patient must address these adverse effects as well as the alteration in tissue perfusion.[2]

There are many defining characteristics for an alteration in tissue perfusion. Those related to individual tissues and organs are still in the process of being developed. They are sometimes more difficult to identify, because they may differ from patient to patient, depending on the underlying disease. Therefore, if an alteration in tissue perfusion is suspected, a thorough assessment of each system is vital.

Renal

When assessing a patient with an alteration in renal tissue perfusion, the nurse can acquire subjective data through an assessment, including the patient's tolerance to activity, and by obtaining a history. A patient with renal failure may exhibit thirst, anorexia, and fatigue.[10] The patient should be assessed for an excessive urine output followed by a decrease in output. Other important symptoms include vomiting, headaches, fatigue, and lethargy.

If renal insufficiency or failure is suspected, the nurse should monitor the patient's urine output and inquire about any recent weight gain.[3,10] Is the patient taking any medications that are nephrotoxic? What are the blood urea nitrogen, creatinine, and serum electrolyte levels? Is the patient's mentation good, or are there problems maintaining concentration?

IV

Objective data can be obtained through physical examination and blood values. Besides BUN, creatinine, and electrolytes, monitoring of serum pH and hemoglobin becomes important.[10] Acidosis commonly is associated with renal failure because of the inability of the kidneys to excrete waste products. If severe, it may be treated with oral sodium bicarbonate as prescribed. Hyperkalemia can be a life-threatening complication because of its effect on the cardiovascular system. Serial electrocardiograms (ECG) will assist the nurse in identifying changes related to hyperkalemia. These ECG changes include peaked T waves, prolonged P-R intervals, and depressed ST segments.[18]

Kidneys also are responsible for the production of erythropoietin.[10] This substance stimulates the bone marrow to produce red blood cells. Because erythropoietin decreases in patients with renal failure, these patients have a chronic anemia. Because oxygen is carried through the bloodstream by hemoglobin, these patients will have a decrease in their oxygen-carrying capacity. Therefore it is important to assess the patient's tolerance to activity. The inability to compensate for the increased oxygen demand with activity may be exhibited by an increase in shortness of breath, weakness, palpitations, and fatigue.

As an alteration in renal tissue perfusion becomes more severe and as renal failure progresses, salt and water retention gradually increases.[6] The fluid will be both intracellular and extracellular. Patients usually exhibit chronic edema in dependent areas. If the edema is excessive, these areas must be monitored closely to maintain skin integrity. The nurse must assess the patient's breath sounds for signs of fluid overload and congestive heart failure.

Increased jugular vein distension (JVD) is another indication of excessive fluid volume. Under normal circumstances jugular veins cannot be seen more than 3 cm above the sternal angle when the patient is at a 30 to 45-degree angle.[12]

Monitoring the blood pressure also becomes important, because as glomerular filtration rate of the kidney decreases, release of renin increases.[3,6] This, in turn, raises the blood pressure in an attempt to increase perfusion to the kidney. Patients with renal failure often require antihypertensive medications to control this increase in blood pressure.

Cerebral

When a patient is assessed for an alteration in cerebral tissue perfusion, subjective data can be obtained by performing a nursing assessment that includes normal daily functioning. First, the nurse should assess the patient for any alteration in mental status or loss of consciousness.[2,3] Does the patient black out, have problems remembering things, have periods of confusion, or have fainting spells or complaints of dizziness? Is the patient oriented to time, person, and place? Is there a problem with restlessness?

A pertinent history includes problems with numbness and tingling as well as complaints of headaches, dizziness or weakness.[3] The patient may have a history of cerebrovascular accidents, transient ischemic attacks, head injuries, orthostatic hypotension, or a seizure disorder. What medications are being taken? Can the medications cause alterations in blood pressure or alter thought processes? Does the patient become lightheaded when moving from lying to sitting positions and then to standing?

Objective data can be obtained through physical examination. The nurse must assess the patient's blood pressure and pulse in the lying, sitting, and standing positions. An increase in heart rate greater than 20 beats per minute when position is changed from supine to vertical is a significant sign of orthostatic hypotension.[11]

If the patient has orthostatic hypotension, the nurse should assist in determining if it is due to medications, cardiac dysrhythmias, or hypovolemia or if it is an idiopathic problem. Temperature is important, because hypothermia will alter cerebral flow. Pupils should be assessed for equality, size, and reaction to light.[2]

If any of the above alterations are found in the history or physical examination, it is a clue to the nurse that the patient may have an acute or chronic neurological problem that can interfere with cerebral function. The nursing assessment then becomes one of the most important indicators of a potential or actual interruption of cerebral blood flow. Whether the patient has a head injury or an acute stroke, one of the most important functions of the nurse is to assess the patient for signs of progressive neurological deficit resulting from an increase in ICP.[5] This would include monitoring for headaches, nausea, vomiting, restlessness, confusion, hemiplegia, visual deficits, conjugate deviation of the eyes, sensory loss, nuchal rigidity, otorrhea, or rhinorrhea.[4] Accurate identification of these early signs of increased ICP will aid in preventing further increases in ICP and interruptions of blood flow. If not prevented, tissue ischemia will progress, and the tissue eventually will cease to function.[5]

Late signs of progressive increased ICP include poor cognitive function with a continuous deterioration of the level of consciousness, sometimes accompanied by decorticate and decerebrate posturing, aphasia, and seizures.[4,10] Pupils may be unequal in size and may react sluggishly to light. Fixed and dilated pupils indicate a medical emergency that must be reported promptly; irreversible damage to the cerebral tissue has probably occurred. Wide changes in temperature can also be attributed to progressive increases in ICP.

A slowly falling pulse accompanied by a rise in blood pressure also is an abnormal finding associated with an increase in ICP.[4,10] Along with assessing for changes in vital signs, the nurse should closely monitor the patient's pulmonary status. As ICP rises it will interfere with the normal functioning of the respiratory center, and the respiratory rate will decrease. The patient's breath sounds, chest expansion, gag and cough reflex, and ability to clear secretions may be impaired. If the ICP continues to rise, these functions will cease, and respirations will become irregular, with longer and longer periods of apnea. There will be irreversible tissue damage and death.

Cardiopulmonary

When a patient is being assessed for an alteration in cardiopulmonary tissue perfusion, information about current health perceptions and symptomatology, as well as a health history, will provide the nurse with valuable information. Has the patient had a myocardial infarction, problems with congestive heart failure (CHF), or respiratory failure? Is the patient taking any medications that can affect either the cardiovascular or pulmonary system? Is there a history of smoking, obesity, or a high-stress lifestyle? Does the patient have hypertension or hypercholesterolemia? Is there a family history of cardiovascular disease?

Subjective information can be obtained by a careful evaluation of symptoms presented. Chest pain, or other types of related discomfort, are often due to inadequate amounts of oxygen available to meet the needs of the myocardium, and are often associated with some type of cardiovascular disease.[8] It should be evaluated for characteristics, location, radiation, severity, duration, precipitating and aggravating factors, accompanying symptoms, and alleviating factors. Complaints of palpitations and/or syncope may indicate the presence of a compromising dysrhythmia. Weight changes and ankle swelling are associated with the sodium and water retention that occurs with CHF and hypertension.

Both fatigue and dyspnea are important symptoms that can be present with either a cardiac or pulmonary problem.[8,20] Assess the activity level of the patient for a day. Determine when the patient first began to feel short of breath and whether it is associated with activity. How much activity can the patient tolerate without feeling fatigued? Does the patient have paroxysmal nocturnal dyspnea (PND)? Sleep with one, two, or three pillows? These findings may indicate how advanced the cardiopulmonary disease is. Does the patient have an increase or decrease in sputum production? An increase may be associated with infection, whereas a decrease may be a sign of impending respiratory failure as the patient is too weak to cough.

While obtaining this subjective data it is important to observe the patient's behavior as well as to evaluate his support systems.[8] Respiratory patients often appear anxious because they focus on their breathing and fear they will not get enough air.[20] Cardiac patients usually exhibit early anxiety, especially when they consider the effect of their disease on their lifestyle and their family or significant other.[8] These feelings may progress to denial, anger, depression, dependence, aggressive sexual behavior, and hypochondriasis.

More objective data can be obtained through physical examination and monitoring laboratory values. It is important to assess baseline electrolyte, BUN, and creatinine values, because if cardiac output is not adequate, there will be a decrease in blood flow to the kidneys.[3,6] This results in an inadequate ability to excrete metabolic waste products.

Monitoring of cardiac enzymes and isoenzymes is important, especially when trying to confirm a diagnosis of myocardial infarction (MI).[8] When a patient has chest pain or other salient features of cardiac disease, along with electrocardiogram (ECG) changes, enzyme levels will help to confirm a diagnosis of MI. When the patient exhibits less characteristic clinical symptoms and nonspecific ECG changes, then a finding of CPK-MB and flipped LDH isoenzymes are indicative of myocardial damage.

A baseline cholesterol level should be documented, because an elevated level is one of the risk factors of cardiovascular disease.[6,22] The hematocrit also must be checked, because anemia will increase a patient's susceptibility to developing an alteration in cardiopulmonary tissue perfusion subsequent to hypoxemia. This can result in chest pain or dyspnea. Baseline measurements of arterial blood gases should be obtained to determine if the patient's oxygenation is adequate, especially in the presence of anemia.

If an alteration in cardiopulmonary tissue perfusion is suspected, it is important to conduct a thorough physical exam of the cardiopulmonary system. Cardiac rate and rhythm should be documented, because dysrhythmias can alter cardiac output, which will result in an alteration in tissue perfusion. The patient also should be assessed for abnormal or extra heart sounds, because these may indicate an alteration in cardiac function.[8]

Blood pressure should be checked, because hypertension is an important risk factor in cardiovascular disease that should not be overlooked.

The presence of jugular vein distension (JVD), hepatojugular reflux, and peripheral edema indicate problems with CHF.

Respirations should be monitored for rate, depth, and character.[20] Breath sounds should be auscultated for both normal sounds and any indication of adventitious breath sounds. Conditions that cause a narrowing of the airway, such as bronchospasm or tumor, may be exhibited by wheezing. Rales, or crackles, may indicate an increase in fluid in the lung. Rhonchi, which make a bubbly sound, may indicate an increase in fluid or mucus within the pulmonary system, which can impair ventilation. Peripheral edema and peripheral cyanosis also are signs of an alteration in cardiopulmonary function.

Any medical condition that interferes with the ability of the pulmonary system to exchange oxygen and carbon dioxide with the circulation can precipitate an alteration in tissue perfusion.[6,22] This will be exhibited by a decrease in oxygen and an increase in carbon dioxide on an arterial blood gas measurement. Therefore the nurse should assess the patient for a history of pulmonary emboli, pneumonia, obstructive or restrictive lung disease, lung abscesses, pleural effusions, and any disease that interferes with the muscles of respiration.

The nurse should monitor the patient's respiratory effort for use of accessory muscles and for symmetrical expansion of the chest. Signs of respiratory muscle fatigue and impending respiratory arrest include an elevated respiratory rate accompanied by an abdominal paradox or respiratory alternans breathing pattern.[20] Skeletal deformities such as scoliosis should be noted, because they could impede respirations. Patients with a history of COPD may exhibit an increase in the anteroposterior diameter of the chest wall, referred to as a barrel chest. It is imperative that an alteration in cardiopulmonary tissue perfusion be identified, because this system plays a vital role in the functioning of all other body systems.

Gastrointestinal

When assessing a patient for an alteration in gastrointestinal tissue perfusion, the nurse can obtain subjective data by performing a nursing assessment that focuses on changes in bowel habits and complaints of nausea and vomiting.[2,3] Are there problems with constipation or diarrhea? Is there blood in the stool? Has the patient had any recent surgical procedure? Is there abdominal distention?

If there has been vomiting, the nurse should determine whether there was any blood and the consistency of it. Has the patient had any recent abdominal pain, and does it increase in intensity after meals? Where is the pain located, and when is it most severe? Has there been any significant weight loss or weight gain? Is there a medical history of gastrointestinal disorders, such as ulcer disease or colitis? Is the patient taking any medication that could affect the normal functioning of the gastrointestinal tract?

Objective data can be obtained through physical examination. The nurse could begin by assessing the patient's blood pressure, because a decrease in blood pressure will result in a decrease in flow to the gastrointestinal tract.[6] The nurse should auscultate bowel sounds and document their presence or absence in all four quadrants.[3] Abdominal girth should be recorded at least daily. Palpating the abdomen may elicit guarding if any acute abdominal process is present. Intake and output should be monitored to determine if intake is adequate to meet the patient's needs. All stool and emesis should be tested for occult blood, and results should be recorded on the patient's flow sheets.

Peripheral

When a patient is assessed for an alteration in peripheral tissue perfusion, subjective data can be obtained by paying particular attention to complaints of pain, numbness, cramping, burning, or tingling.[2,3] The nurse should determine if any of these are associated with particular activities, time of day, or temperature changes. Are they associated with pallor, cyanosis, or coolness of the skin? Is there any loss of motor or sensory function?

A pertinent medical history might include a history of arteriosclerotic heart disease, Raynaud's disease, diabetes, or peripheral vascular disease.[2] Is there any history of phlebitis or deep vein thrombosis? Are there problems with intermittent claudication, peripheral edema, leg ulcers, or even gangrene? Are hematocrit and hemoglobin levels and blood pressure sufficient to supply adequate nutrition to peripheral tissues?[3] Have there been any problems with hypothermia or shock? Is the patient on any medications that cause vasoconstriction, thereby decreasing the flow of blood to the periphery?

More objective data that may indicate an actual or a high risk for an alteration in peripheral tissue perfusion can be obtained by physical examination. The nurse should assess the extremities for both color and temperature as well as for the presence and equality of arterial pulses. Is edema or ulcerations present? Is there erythema or swelling associated with calf tenderness? A positive Homans' sign may indicate the presence of a thrombophlebitis. This is elicited by having the patient bend the knee and dorsiflex the foot at the same time. Calf pain is considered a positive sign for thrombophlebitis.

Pressure changes in the extremities or the presence of bruits may indicate an alteration in tissue perfusion.[9] Skin texture and turgor also should be noted. Is there shiny skin with a lack of lanugo hair? Does the patient report dry, thick, slow-growing nails? Is there a decrease in capillary filling? Does the patient have problems with paresthesias or trophic skin changes (these include calluses or fissures and often are more prevalent on the toes, soles, and heels)? Physical examination also may reveal atrophy of leg muscles along with a loss of tone. All of these findings are important defining characteristics of an alteration in peripheral tissue perfusion.

Assessing a patient for an alteration in tissue perfusion is an important nursing function. When a health history and physical examination are performed, the presence of any of the signs, symptoms, or complaints discussed should alert the nurse to further investigate the possibility that an alteration in tissue perfusion exists. Because the causes are so widespread, identifying that a problem is present often depends on determining if any of the related factors are evident or if any of the defining characteristics have evolved.

If the nurse does identify an alteration in tissue perfusion, regardless of the organ involved, she/he should report it to the physician. The nurse and physician in collaboration can develop a plan of care for the patient. It is then the nurse's responsibility to help the patient and family learn ways to minimize symptoms and complications. This is done by developing a nursing care plan based on the etiology of the problem. The plan will include teaching the patient ways to minimize the causative factors and to improve tissue perfusion to the affected organs and tissues.

❖ Defining Characteristics

The presence of any of the following defining characteristics indicates that the patient may be experiencing an Altered Tissue Perfusion (Specify Type) (Renal, Cerebral, Cardiopulmonary, Gastrointestinal, Peripheral):

Renal
- Decrease in urine output
- Complaints of thirst, anorexia, and fatigue
- Elevated BUN and creatinine levels
- Weight gain
- Peripheral edema
- Hypertension

Cerebral
- Orthostatic hypotension
- Fainting spells
- Restlessness
- Alteration in mental status
- Alteration in cognitive function
- Alteration in level of consciousness
- Memory loss
- Confusion
- Disorientation

Cardiopulmonary
- Shortness of breath
- Tachycardia or palpitations
- Abnormal breath sounds—rales and rhonchi
- Peripheral edema and cyanosis
- Slow capillary filling
- Chest pain
- Tachypnea
- Dysrhythmias
- Hypotension
- Cold, clammy skin

Gastrointestinal
- Nausea and/or vomiting
- Lack of bowel sounds
- Abdominal pain that increases after meals
- Constipation
- Diarrhea
- Abdominal distention

Peripheral
- Decreased or absent arterial pulses
- Cyanosis of extremities in a dependent position
- Pale extremities on elevation; color does not return on lowering leg
- Round scars covered with atrophied skin
- Slow-growing, dry, thick, brittle nails
- Blood pressure changes in extremities
- Numbness and tingling of extremities
- Loss of motor and/or sensory function
- Decreased capillary filling
- Slow healing of lesions
- Intermittent claudication
- Cold extremities
- Gangrene
- Lack of lanugo
- Shiny skin
- Peripheral edema
- Bruits

❖ Related Factors

The following related factors are associated with Altered Tissue Perfusion (Specify Type) (Renal, Cerebral, Cardiopulmonary, Gastrointestinal, Peripheral):

- Interruption of arterial flow
- Interruption of venous flow
- Exchange problems
- Hypervolemia
- Hypovolemia

❖ Related Medical/Psychiatric Diagnoses

The following are examples of related medical/psychiatric diagnoses for Altered Tissue Perfusion (Specify Type) (Renal, Cerebral, Cardiopulmonary, Gastrointestinal, Peripheral):

- Aneurysm
- Atherosclerosis
- Buerger's disease
- Cerebrovascular accident
- Congestive heart failure
- Deep venous thrombosis
- Hypovolemic shock
- Myocardial infarction
- Paralytic ileus
- Pulmonary embolism
- Raynaud's phenomenon
- Renal failure

NURSING DIAGNOSES

Examples of *specific* nursing diagnoses for Altered Tissue Perfusion (Specify Type) (Renal, Cerebral, Cardiopulmonary, Gastrointestinal, Peripheral) are:

- Altered Renal Tissue Perfusion related to prolonged hypotension as indicated by urine output less than 10 ml/hr, elevated BUN and creatinine, specific gravity greater than 1.030, and decreased glomerular filtration rate.
- Altered Cerebral Tissue Perfusion related to increased intracranial pressure secondary to a ruptured aneurysm as indicated by comatose state, widened pulse pressure, wide sluggishly reactive pupils, negative corneal reflexes, and negative doll's eyes.
- Altered Cardiopulmonary Tissue Perfusion related to decreased right ventricular function as indicated by tachypnea, dyspnea, PND, crackles, increased peripheral edema, and tachycardia.
- Altered Gastrointestinal Tissue Perfusion related to use of narcotics as indicated by decreased bowel sounds, nausea, vomiting, and constipation.
- Altered Peripheral Tissue Perfusion related to swelling after a traumatic leg injury as indicated by increased leg pain, tenderness accompanied by increased redness and warmth, muscle weakness, numbness, cool foot, and decreased peripheral pulses and capillary refill.

PLANNING AND IMPLEMENTATION WITH RATIONALE

The specific nursing goals and interventions for patients with an alteration in tissue perfusion depend on the tissue involved, but the desired patient outcomes are the same. These outcomes can be grouped into three major areas: (1) There will be adequate blood flow in the affected vessels, and tissue perfusion and cellular oxygenation will be maximized; the result will be maintenance of the integrity of the tissue or organ. (2) The metabolic needs of the tissue or organ will be reduced or maintained. (3) The patient and family will understand the cause of the problem and will modify their lifestyle to minimize the causative factors or side effects related to the decrease in tissue perfusion.

To ensure adequate blood flow to the affected vessels and maximize tissue perfusion, nursing goals should include maintaining cardiac output and blood pressure as well as enhancing blood flow. By the time a decrease in blood pressure is evident, compensatory mechanisms to maintain cardiac output and blood pressure have been triggered and changes may be occurring at the cellular level. *Therefore any situation or medical condition that causes prolonged hypotension will put many of the vital tissues and organs at risk of permanent damage because of the decreased delivery of oxygen and nutrients.* [6] It is an important nursing function to monitor and document vital signs as well as to notify the physician of any changes.[14]

Cardiac output and blood pressure are influenced by venous return.[6] All forms of shock will result in a decrease in circulating blood volume and in venous return. Eventually the tissues will be compromised. *If intravascular volume is not maintained in these patients, the decrease in flow will result in death of the tissues.* It is important that nurses monitor intake and output in these patients. Hemodynamic pressures, such as pulmonary artery and wedge pressures, also are important indicators of circulating blood volume. Daily weights will be helpful in assessing overall fluid balance.

After blood flow has been assessed sufficiently and has been maximized, the nurse should focus interventions on attempting to reduce, or at least maintain, the metabolic needs of the tissues.[22] Again, adequate arterial blood pressure is the first necessity, because if the blood pressure drops, the compensatory response of the body is vasoconstriction and a decreased flow to the less vital organs and tissues.[6]

Temperature also is an important parameter that can affect each of the body systems. *Hyperthermia increases the cellular rate of metabolism; this results in an increase in metabolic needs of the tissues.*[10] So regardless of the cause of hyperthermia, an attempt should be made to maintain body temperature at its baseline.

IV

Because hypothermia, whether induced or accidental, can impair the functions of other organs, an accurate nursing assessment is necessary. Hypothermia may be induced for surgical procedures, especially cardiac surgery.[10] As the rate of metabolism decreases, the heart rate and respiratory rate also begin to fall, and an impairment of neurological function and an eventual loss of consciousness will follow.

Arterial blood gases are another important parameter that can be monitored to help to ensure that the metabolic needs of the tissues are being maintained or reduced. Although adequate blood flow will provide the nutrients necessary for metabolism, oxygen also must be readily available.[6] *Pulmonary function must be sufficient to supply the blood with adequate amounts of oxygen to deliver to the tissues.*[16]

The nurse should monitor a patient's hematocrit and hemoglobin and notify the physician if they drop. Under normal conditions hemoglobin carries most of the oxygen to the tissues.[6] A decrease in circulating blood volume will inhibit the ability of the blood to bring adequate amounts of oxygen to the tissues. *Therefore, even if adequate oxygen is available, it will not be delivered to the tissues and organs if the overall circulating volume is decreased.*

Teaching the patient and family about medication is an important aspect of nursing care that should be incorporated into the nursing care plan of each patient.[3] If a drug's metabolic effects are more severe than the symptoms for which it was instituted, the physician may want to discontinue it. Careful questioning and assessment of patients will elicit these untoward side effects. For example, if an alteration in tissue perfusion already exists because of some type of vascular disease, then a medication with vasoconstrictive properties may cause more harm than good.

Once adequate tissue perfusion is attained and the metabolic needs of the tissues are met, the nurse should help the patient and family to understand the cause of the problem. *This should include teaching about the present disease process if the problem is chronic as well as teaching ways to adapt and modify lifestyles to minimize the presence of the causative factors.*[3] The dietary modifications that must be taught will vary depending on the cause of the underlying decrease in tissue perfusion and the organs affected.

In all cases, if the indicated treatment is surgery, then the nurse should prepare and support both the patient and the family.[3] Nursing supports include preoperative teaching to help patients and their families understand the postoperative course of events. If the treatment is to be medical, then they will need more information on the diagnostic tests, including their interpretation, and the procedure.

Several other risk factors may be present in a patient with an alteration in tissue perfusion caused by atherosclerosis and/or peripheral arterial occlusive disease; these should be modified in an effort to prevent progression of the underlying disease process. These factors include smoking, dietary indiscretions, and a sedentary lifestyle. The nurse should inform the patient and family of the adverse effects of smoking and encourage the patient to stop. Teaching about diet and exercise may be indicated.

Along with all of the aforementioned plans, several other factors, more specific to the tissue or organ involved, should be included in the plan of care for a patient with an alteration in tissue perfusion.

Renal

A patient with an alteration in renal tissue perfusion should be monitored for a decrease in urine output.[17,21] This assessment becomes particularly important after a prolonged period of hypotension. Normal urine specific gravity is 1.010 to 1.030. *When the kidney loses its ability to concentrate or dilute urine, the specific gravity will remain low.*

Serum laboratory values also provide important diagnostic information.[3]*An alteration in electrolytes and an elevation in BUN and creatinine are indicative of an alteration in renal function. As blood flow through the kidney decreases, there*

❖ NURSING CARE GUIDELINES

Nursing Diagnosis: *Altered Tissue Perfusion: Renal*

Expected Patient Outcomes	Nursing Interventions
The patient will have adequate tissue perfusion and cellular oxygenation of renal system as evidenced by a urine output ≥ 30 ml/hr; normal BUN, creatinine, and glomerular filtration rate; and absence of excess fluid volume.	• Monitor and document vital signs; notify the physician of any changes. • Monitor urine output every 1 to 2 hours. • Monitor urine specific gravity. • Monitor BUN, creatinine, and electrolytes. • Monitor results of glomerular filtration rate if ordered. • Monitor serum pH and hematocrit. • Monitor medications and identify those with nephrotoxic effects. • Monitor intake and output. • Weigh the patient daily. • Assess for peripheral edema. • Assess breath sounds at least once a shift and with any complaints of dyspnea.
The patient will have control of metabolic needs of the kidney.	• Monitor for hyperthermia, and institute measures to decrease an elevated temperature. • Monitor hematocrit and hemoglobin. • Administer low-dose dopamine, if ordered.
The patient will modify lifestyle to minimize the causative factors and/or side effects of a decrease in renal tissue perfusion.	• Provide dietary teaching to the patient will have an adequate caloric intake despite anorexia and decreased oral intake. • If anorexia is severe, instruct the patient to eat small meals. • Help the patient and family to understand the need to restrict protein intake and foods high in potassium. • Teach the patient to base sodium intake on weight. • If antihypertensives are used, instruct the patient on indications as well as side effects. • Instruct the patient on the need for exercise and rest periods to increase tolerance to activity. • Teach the patient skin care measures to decrease the occurrence of injury to areas where dependent edema is present. • Provide the patient and family with psychological support if the outcome is chronic renal failure. • Teach the patient about dialysis, whether hemodialysis or peritoneal dialysis.

will be a decrease in glomerular filtration rate. [6] *Arterial blood gases will reveal a metabolic acidosis caused by the retention of metabolic waste products.* In the case of permanent renal damage the nurse will see a gradual decrease in the hematocrit caused by the decrease in the amount of erythropoietin produced by the kidney.

If a renal insufficiency is noted at any time, it is important to note if any of the medications the patient is receiving have nephrotoxic effects. These types of medications can even be the cause of the renal problem, and if discontinued normal renal function may resume. If peak and trough levels of medications are ordered, it is important for the nurse to monitor the results and notify the physician of any abnormalities.

Because a patient with an alteration in renal function may experience an increase in fluid volume, it is vital to monitor daily weights and intake and output. A positive fluid balance and an increase in weight, accompanied by peripheral edema, indicate an overall increase in fluid volume and venous pooling, which is often indicative of an alteration in renal function. If dyspnea is present, assessing breath sounds for crackles becomes important in order to prevent the complications associated with the pulmonary edema that can accompany renal failure.

Along with controlling hyperthermia to decrease metabolic needs of tissues, some physicians may elect to use low dose intravenous dopamine to treat patients with a renal insufficiency. *In doses of 2 to 5 mcg/kg/min dopamine acts on the dopaminergic receptors in the renal vessels to cause vasodilitation.* In some patients this is a very effective way to increase renal blood flow and urine output.

Teaching plans for patients with an alteration in renal function related to a decrease in tissue perfusion should emphasize frequent periods of rest.[3] *The anemia associated with renal failure contributes to these patients' decrease in activity tolerance.* They also should be taught to check with their physicians before taking any over-the-counter medications. *Many medications are metabolized in the kidneys and may cause further impairment of renal function.*

Dietary teaching for patients with an alteration in renal function is often a big challenge, because their disease process is associated with nausea, vomiting, and anorexia.[3]*They may need to be taught to eat small meals more frequently in order to provide a calorie intake that will meet their daily needs.* In teaching the patient about diet, the nurse should include the importance of eating foods that are low in protein and potassium, because with inadequate renal function the patient will be unable to excrete either the end products of protein metabolism or the potassium.[10]*Patients also must learn how to base their sodium intake on their weight so that they do not become hyponatremic or have problems with fluid overload.*

If the outcome of the decrease in renal tissue perfusion is chronic renal failure, the patient and family will need support. After the decision is made for the patient to receive hemodialysis or peritoneal dialysis, the nurse also should provide information regarding the procedure and the need to modify lifestyle further.

Cerebral

Monitoring the neurological status, especially level of consciousness, will assist the nurse in detecting an alteration in cerebral function. *Increasing restlessness and confusion is an early sign of an increase in intracranial pressure.*[4]

Changes in systolic blood pressure have a direct effect on perfusion to the brain. As the blood pressure decreases, blood flow to the cerebral tissue will not be adequate to prevent ischemia. Cerebral perfusion pressure (CPP) is an indirect assessment of cerebral blood flow.[4] It is calculated by subtracting the intracranial pressure (ICP) from the mean arterial blood pressure. *It is generally believed that if the CPP falls below 50 mm Hg, then the cerebral tissue will not receive adequate amounts of oxygen and nutrients.* Because of this, vasopressors are sometimes used to maintain arterial blood pressure.

Positioning is an important aspect of care for a patient with an alteration in cerebral tissue perfusion.[2] If the cause of the decrease in tissue perfusion is orthostatic hypotension, patients should be positioned flat. Unless contraindicated, they should be taught to wear waist-high elastic stockings when they are out of bed. This will promote venous return. They should learn to move slowly from a recumbent position to a sitting position and to dangle their feet before standing.

On the other hand, patients with increased ICP associated with craniocerebral trauma should have the head of the bed elevated to promote venous return.[4] These patients must be monitored closely and accurately, because prompt treatment is needed to preserve cerebral function. Other types of treatment that may be utilized to maintain

❖ *NURSING CARE GUIDELINES*

Nursing Diagnosis: *Altered Tissue Perfusion: Cerebral*

Expected Patient Outcomes	Nursing Interventions
The patient will have maintenance of adequate tissue perfusion and cellular oxygenation of the cerebral system as evidenced by a level of consciousness of wakefulness and alertness, a systolic blood pressure greater than 100 mm Hg, a cerebral perfusion pressure (CPP) of 60 to 90 mm Hg, and an ICP of 0 to 15 mm Hg.	• Monitor and document the patient's mental status and level of consciousness; establish baseline and ongoing neurological assessment. • Monitor and document vital signs; promptly report changes in vital signs or neurological status to the physician. • Monitor orthostatic vital signs, and notify the physician if the difference is greater than 10 mm Hg. • Administer medications as ordered; patients may require anticoagulants if the cause is related to emboli. • Administer vasopressors as ordered by the physician to maintain blood pressure. • Monitor for signs of increased ICP: decrease in consciousness; headache; vomiting, seizures, and hypertension; bradycardia; papilledema; pupillary changes; loss of motor and sensory function; and irregular respiratory function (Cheyne-Stokes respirations). • Monitor arterial blood gases for a decrease in Po_2 and an increase in Pco_2.
The patient will have control of metabolic needs of the cerebral tissue.	• Monitor temperature, and induce hypothermia if ordered. • Monitor arterial blood gases, and maintain adequate oxygenation through artificial ventilatory support, if needed. • If increased ICP is present, the following may be included in the plan of care: elevate the head of the bed; maintain controlled hyperventilation, with $Paco_2$ between 25 and 35 mm Hg; maintain fluid restriction; maintain a quiet environment, and space nursing activities; administer osmotic diuretics as ordered; institute seizure precautions; and maintain barbiturate coma, if indicated.
The patient will modify lifestyle to minimize causative factors and/or side effects of a decrease in cerebral tissue perfusion.	• Prepare the patient for surgery, and do preoperative teaching, if indicated. • Identify medications that may contribute to an alteration in cerebral tissue perfusion, such as antihypertensives, diuretics, barbiturates, and phenothiazines. • Discuss necessary dietary changes (for instance, if the cause is atherosclerosis). • Teach the patient to change position slowly when rising from a recumbent position. • Teach the patient to use elastic stockings and to apply and remove them when supine. • Encourage the patient to exercise daily.

IV

cerebral function and decrease ICP include os-motic diuretics, hyperventilation via a mechanical ventilator, barbiturate-induced coma, steroids, neuromuscular blockers, and invasive intracranial pressure monitoring with cerebral drains. To ac-company these medical treatments, the nurse should space out nursing activities, institute sei-zure precautions, and monitor the patient's re-sponse to medical therapy.

Temperature control is an important aspect of care in a patient with craniocerebral trauma.[4] *Hy-perthermia and the shivering associated with fe-vers will result in a further increase in ICP.* In some cases treatment of these patients will include inducing hypothermia to further decrease the meta-bolic needs and oxygen consumption of the tis-sues. The nurse, in collaboration with the physi-cian, can accomplish this by using a cooling blan-ket and ice packs, instilling cool intravenous flu-ids, or lavaging body orifices with cool fluids.

Patients and families should be taught the side effects of medications that may contribute to an alteration in cerebral tissue perfusion.[3] Antihyper-tensives and diuretics often have vasodilatory ef-fects. Therefore their use in patients with ortho-static hypotension should be avoided.

Cardiopulmonary

Planning the care of a patient with an alteration in cardiopulmonary function includes thorough monitoring of both the cardiac and pulmonary systems. *Abnormalities in heart sounds and breath sounds are important indicators of func-tion.*[10] All complaints of chest pain and shortness of breath must be investigated. *Systolic blood pressure and cardiac output are important indica-tors of tissue perfusion to all organs.* Normal car-diac output is 4 to 8 L/min. According to Rice,[15] cardiac output and blood pressure will fall during the early phases of shock. The compensatory re-sponse is stimulation of the sympathetic nervous system, causing vasoconstriction, resulting in a redistribution of blood to the heart and brain.

When intrinsic compensatory mechanisms do not maintain blood pressure adequately the doc-tor may order a vasopressor, such as dopamine, which in high doses will vasoconstrict the vessels to improve venous return. This increased venous

---

❖ NURSING CARE GUIDELINES

Nursing Diagnosis: *Altered Tissue Perfusion: Cardiopulmonary*

Expected Patient Outcomes	Nursing Interventions
The patient will have ade-quate tissue perfusion and cellular oxygenation of the cardiopulmonary system: as evidenced by a cardiac output $\geq$ 4 L/min; a sys-tolic blood pressure $\geq$ 90 mm Hg; hemodynamic parameters within normal range, absence of dys-rhythmias, chest pain, and shortness of breath; and a $Pao_2 > 80$ with a satura-tion > 90%.	• Monitor and document vital signs. • Administer and monitor effects of vasopressors if ordered. • Administer and monitor the effects of inotropic agents as ordered. • Monitor hemodynamics: central venous pressure, pulmonary artery pressure, wedge pressure, and cardiac output. • Assess for JVD. • Titrate vasoactive and inotropic agents to maintain hemodynamics within normal range as ordered. • Administer diuretics or fluids as ordered. • Monitor heart sounds, and notify the physician of any abnormali-ties. • Assess cardiac rhythm, and administer antidysrhythmics, if or-dered. • If hemodynamically compromising dysrhythmias are present, assess need for restricting activity level.

❖ *NURSING CARE GUIDELINES—cont'd*

Expected Patient Outcomes	Nursing Interventions
	• Assess electrocardiogram for ischemia.
	• Administer and monitor effects of nitrates if ordered.
	• Assess medications for adverse cardiopulmonary effects.
	• Assess the cause of chest pain or shortness of breath.
	• Assess breath sounds, and notify the physician of any abnormalities.
	• Maintain oxygen if ordered. Monitor pulse oximetry if indicated.
	• Assist with activities as needed.
	• Perform chest physiotherapy if indicated.
	• Encourage the patient to perform active and passive range-of-motion exercises and to become ambulatory as soon as the condition permits.
	• Monitor hemoglobin.
	• Monitor creatine phosphokinase, lactic dehydrogenase, and arterial blood gases.
The patient will have control of metabolic needs of the cardiopulmonary tissues.	• Assess the metabolic effects of any medications administered.
	• Monitor for hyperthermia and institute measures to decrease an elevated temperature.
	• Teach the patient to avoid stress and to begin stress-reducing activities.
	• Encourage frequent periods of rest.
	• Teach the patient to avoid straining with bowel movement.
	• Teach the patient to eliminate activities that result in chest pain and/or shortness of breath.
The patient will modify lifestyle to minimize the causative factors and/or side effects of an alteration in cardiopulmonary tissue perfusion.	• Prepare the patient and family for surgery if indicated.
	• Instruct the patient on indications and side effects of medications.
	• Instruct the patient on dietary restrictions (such as low-sodium or low-cholesterol diets).
	• Teach the patient to increase activity slowly and to take frequent rest periods.
	• Teach the patient to take nitroglycerin before activities that usually cause chest pain (e.g., taking a shower).
	• Encourage the patient to quit smoking.
	• Teach the patient and family the risk factors of heart and lung disease.
	• Provide the patient and family with psychological support if the outcome is cardiogenic shock or respiratory failure.

IV

IV

return may improve overall cardiac output. *In some circumstances a physician may order an inotropic agent, such as dobutamine, which may improve contractility and hence cardiac output.*[16]

Hemodynamic parameters, such as CVP, PA, and PCW should be monitored for abnormalities. *These parameters are important indicators of fluid volume and pumping effectivenes of the heart.* Diuretics may be needed if the patient exhibits signs of congestive heart failure. Vasoactive drugs can also be useful in treating congestive heart failure. *The vasodilatory response to the medication allows excess fluid to pool in the periphery, decreasing the workload on the heart and improving overall pumping function.*

An electrocardiogram should be monitored for alterations in rate and rhythm. *Dysrythmias can affect cardiac output and result in hypotension.* These patients should be placed on a cardiac monitor. The nurse should document the patient's cardiac rhythm as well as the effects of any antidysrhythmics given. These patients may also require a limitation in their activity to prevent falling if the dysrythmia occurred while ambulating.

An electrocardiogram obtained during chest pain will assist in determining which part of the myocardium is at risk for damage or has sustained damage resulting from ischemia. A patient with an alteration in cardiac tissue perfusion who experiences chest pain with common daily activities, such as taking a shower, can be taught how to use nitroglycerin prophylactically to prevent the chest pain. In any case, patients should be told the indications of each medication as well as any common or untoward side effects. They should be taught to modify their intake of cholesterol and sodium.[3]

Nurses should assess the quality of the ventilatory effort of their patients, including rate, rhythm, use of accessory muscles, air movement, and breath sounds.[10] If respiratory function is inadequate and hypoxemia or hypercarbia develops, the patient may require artificial ventilatory support to supply the tissues and organs with adequate oxygen; this is especially important in the patient who has a known alteration in pulmonary function, such as COPD.

Patients with inadequate ventilatory function will need to have their activities spaced to conserve energy. They may need assistance with activities of daily living. Active and passive range-of-motion exercises will assist them in gradually increasing their activity. They can be taught to eat several small high-calorie meals spread over the day.

Arterial blood gases will give a clear indication of whether or not adequate oxygen is being supplied to the bloodstream. A hematocrit determination will indicate a decrease in circulating blood volume and the amount of hemoglobin available for delivery of oxygen to the tissues.

To control the metabolic needs of cardiopulmonary tissue, the patient will need to begin stress-reducing activities and take frequent rest periods. All medications should be evaluated to determine if their benefit outweighs any cardiopulmonary side effects. As with other organs, temperature control will reduce the metabolic needs of the tissue. Indications for modification of lifestyle will vary with the underlying cardiopulmonary problem. Some of these modifications may be making dietary changes, decreasing activity, carrying medications such as nitroglycerin, stopping smoking, and losing weight.

Gastrointestinal

The decrease in perfusion associated with hypotension can result in a shutdown of the gastrointestinal system.[22] Vascular disease and postoperative complications also can compromise the system. Postoperatively the nurse should assist in maintaining gastric decompression until bowel function is restored. The plan of care also should include assessing bowel sounds in all four quadrants and monitoring patients for abdominal pain accompanied by nausea and vomiting, especially after meals. *A decrease in gastrointestinal tissue perfusion also can be manifested by constipation, so changes in bowel habits become an important indicator of function.*[2] A bowel program may need to be incorporated into the care plan.

Intake and output should be monitored; from this information the nurse should anticipate the need for intravenous fluids. *Gastric secretions*

❖ *NURSING CARE GUIDELINES*

Nursing Diagnosis: *Altered Tissue Perfusion: Gastrointestinal*

Expected Patient Outcomes	Nursing Interventions
The patient will have adequate tissue perfusion and cellular oxygenation of the gastrointestinal system as evidenced by normal bowel sounds in all four quadrants, and absence of nausea and vomiting.	• Assess blood pressure. • Monitor bowel sounds in all four quadrants, and document any changes. • Monitor the patient for alterations in bowel habits such as constipation. • Maintain gastric decompression postoperatively. • Maintain intake and output. • Maintain a record of any episodes of nausea and/or vomiting. • Guiac any emesis.
The patient will have control of metabolic needs of the gastrointestinal tissue.	• Encourage rest periods after meals. • Provide small meals that are easily digested. • If tube feedings are used, provide an elemental product. • Assess medications, and try to minimize those that decrease peristalsis and gastrointestinal function. • Administer intravenous fluids as ordered. • Test all gastrointestinal secretions and excretions for the presence of blood.
The patient will modify lifestyle to minimize the causative factors and/or side effects of the decrease in gastrointestinal tissue perfusion.	• Prepare the patient for surgery if indicated. • Discuss necessary dietary changes. • Teach the patient the importance of rest periods after meals. • Instruct the patient to notify the physician of frequent problems with nausea, vomiting, diarrhea, and abdominal pain.

IV

should be tested for the presence of blood. The patient should be taught to avoid medications that decrease peristalsis. *Those medications that can irritate gastric mucosa should be given with meals or milk,* if they are not contraindicated for this patient.

The plan of care also should include careful documentation of nutritional intake. The patient may be taught to eat several small meals that are easily digested.[3] *If tube feedings are used, an elemental product may be chosen to decrease the metabolic needs of the tissues during digestion.*

Abdominal angina can be reduced if the patient is encouraged to rest after meals to allow for the maximum amount of blood flow to the stomach. The nurse should space the activities over the day so that the patient does not become fatigued. Stress-reducing activities also may help the patient to relax, which will decrease his metabolic needs.

Peripheral

Planning the care for a patient with an alteration in peripheral tissue perfusion includes frequent assessments of the overt signs and symptoms. Along with vital signs, the quality of arterial pulses will help to indicate adequacy of flow. *A patient with an actual alteration in peripheral*

IV

❖ *NURSING CARE GUIDELINES*

Nursing Diagnosis: *Altered Tissue Perfusion: Peripheral*

Expected Patient Outcomes	Nursing Interventions
The patient will have adequate tissue perfusion and cellular oxygenation of the peripheral system as evidenced by palpable pulses; warm, dry skin; an ankle-arm index of 1.0 to 1.2; and normal motor function, sensation, and skin integrity in extremities.	• Monitor and document vital signs. • Assess quality of arterial pulses. • Assess skin temperature, color, and texture. • Encourage active and passive range-of-motion exercises. • Maintain oxygen if needed. • Avoid long periods of exposure to cold environments. • Assess for peripheral edema. • Auscultate for bruit or murmer over the lower abdomen or groin. • Assess ankle-arm index on admission. • Monitor at least every 4 hours for patients at risk for arterial insufficiency. • Notify the physician of any change in ankle-arm index. • Assess skin surface for any alteration in its integrity or longstanding ulcers that have not healed. • Evaluate motor function and skin sensation at least every 4 hours for a patient at high risk for arterial insufficiency. • Assess capillary refill. • Assess for muscle asymmetry.
The patient will have control of metabolic needs of organs and tissues by reduction or by maintenance at current level.	• Monitor temperature; encourage frequent periods of rest and early ambulation if possible. • Assess metabolic effects of any medications, especially those with vasoconstrictive side effects. • Avoid long periods of pressure to extremities. • If there is a problem with arterial blood flow, maintain extremities in a dependent position to facilitate flow. • If there is a problem with venous blood flow, elevate the extremities to facilitate venous return.
The patient will modify lifestyle to minimize the causative factors and/or side effects related to the decrease in peripheral tissue perfusion.	• Teach the patient and family about the importance of diet. • Instruct the patient to avoid standing for long periods of time or crossing the legs. • Encourage use of elastic stockings to prevent venous stasis. • Instruct the patient to avoid the use of hot water bottles or heating pads. • Have the patient wear warm clothing in cold weather, especially protective shoes and warm gloves. • Instruct the patient to use foot cradles, water mattress, egg-crate mattress, and other appliances that decrease pressure to extremities. • Teach the importance of good foot care and keeping the skin well lubricated. • Instruct the patient to avoid wearing tight or occlusive clothing.

tissue perfusion resulting from inadequate arterial flow may have color changes, loss of hair, irregular nail growth, ulcerations, and muscle atrophy.[1] Different pressures in each arm are also a sign of arterial disease. If capillary refill is checked, a finding of less than 3 seconds is normal.

Arm-ankle index should be assessed on admission in any situation where a patient is at risk for arterial insufficiency. A doppler flow systolic pressure is taken in both the dorsalis pedis and posterior tibial.[1] This number is divided by the higher of the two brachial systolic pressures. *The normal is 1.0 to 1.2; anything less indicates a vascular problem.*

If the patient has an alteration in peripheral tissue perfusion, activities should be encouraged that will not interfere with blood flow to the area.[2,3] *Patients in bed should be turned frequently to avoid long periods of pressure to the extremities.* The use of protective devices also may help to decrease pressure and prevent damage to these areas.

Extremities that have an impedance in arterial flow should be positioned in a dependent position to facilitate blood flow.[1,24] *If the problem is with the venous system, then the extremity should be elevated to enhance return to the heart.* In either case the extremity should be assessed carefully to be certain that delivery of oxygen and nutrients is adequate to maintain the skin integrity and function of the extremity.

Many over-the-counter medications, such as antihistamines, have vasoconstrictive properties. Patients should be taught to avoid these, because they can perpetuate vascular insufficiency and further decrease blood flow to the compromised extremities of patients with peripheral vascular disease.

The dietary teaching will depend on the cause of the underlying decrease in tissue perfusion and the organs that are affected. Patients with peripheral arterial occlusive disease may need to make dietary modifications to decrease their intake of cholesterol.[24] Those with atherosclerotic heart disease may need to decrease both cholesterol and sodium intake.[3]

Some changes may be required in activities of daily living, and the patient should be taught the importance of daily exercise. *Exercise will help to enlarge the involved vessels and also to promote the development of collateral circulation.* Exercise includes active and passive range of motion and early ambulation for the hospitalized patient. Frequent rest periods become important to prevent ischemia to the involved area. All exercise should be increased gradually over time, provided the patient does not have signs and symptoms of fatigue or ischemia.[2]

Several preventive measures can be shared with a patient that can help to decrease the side effects associated with an alteration in tissue perfusion.[2,3] First, the patient should be taught to inspect the skin daily for breaks and pressure points. Frequent foot care should include washing and thoroughly drying the feet as well as massaging them and keeping them well lubricated. Clean, warm footwear that fits comfortably should be worn.

Second, the patient should be discouraged from sitting or standing for long periods of time and from crossing the legs.[2,3] *Flexion of the hips and knees can impede blood flow and venous return.* The patient should be taught to avoid constrictive clothing but also to wear warm clothes to prevent further damage from exposure to cold weather. Hot water bottles should be avoided, because the patient may have a decrease in the sensitivity of peripheral tissues. In addition, heat increases tissue metabolism and the need for oxygen. *Last, foot cradles, sheepskins, water mattresses, egg crate mattresses, and other such appliances can be used to decrease pressure on certain areas and prevent damage.*

Evaluation

The first indicator of the effectiveness of nursing interventions, and therefore the attainment of expected patient outcomes, is maintenance of adequate tissue perfusion and cellular oxygenation of the involved tissues or organs. This can be determined by the absence of the defining characteristics that first alerted the nurse that an abnormality was present. Cardiac output and blood pres-

IV

IV

sure, coupled with effective ventilation, will be adequate to maintain tissue perfusion and cellular oxygenation. Body systems will receive adequate circulation to prevent ischemia of the tissues or organs. Extremities will be warm, with palpable pulses. The gastrointestinal and renal systems will function properly so that food is digested, energy is available to the cells, and waste products are excreted. Patients will not experience chest pain, dyspnea, or an alteration in mental status.

A second important indicator of the effectiveness of nursing interventions is that the metabolic needs of the tissues and organs are being met. Body temperature and oxygenation will be maintained within normal limits. The patient will alternate activity with frequent periods of rest to minimize the possibility of increasing the metabolic needs of the tissues. The patient will protect his/her extremities from long periods of pressure to

the involved area and exposure to cold environments. The patient will become involved in stress-reducing activities, because the metabolic needs of the tissues can be increased because of fear, worry, and anxiety.[22]

A third indicator that patients have achieved expected outcomes is that they understand the cause of their problem and have begun to modify their lifestyle in an effort to minimize complications. The patient and family can explain the uses and side effects of medications, the need for safety precautions and clothing, and the importance of both regular activity and rest periods. They should understand the rationale for, and be able to perform, any specialized skin care regimens. Modifications in dietary habits and verbalization of any further learning needs also are indicative of effective nursing interventions.

❖ *CASE STUDY WITH PLAN OF CARE*

Mr. Terry T. is a 70-year-old retired electrician who was admitted to the emergency room with complaints of fever, a superficial left leg ulcer of 2 weeks' duration, pain on walking, and some decreased sensation in his legs. The patient stated, "I haven't been sick a day in my life, but about 10 or 15 years ago my doctor told me that I had high blood pressure and diabetes. Since I never had problems, I never went back." Social history revealed that his wife died about 7 years ago, and he has since lived alone and cooked for himself. His three children are married and live some distance away, so he sees them mainly on holidays. Since he retired about 5 years ago, he spends many afternoons playing cards with his friends and many evenings relaxing and watching television, in the recliner chair his children bought him when he retired. Most recently he and his friends developed a plan to help them "stay in shape." He bought new high-top sneakers, and each evening, after dinner, they walk for at least a mile. He attributed his leg ulcer to a blister from the rubbing of his new sneakers on his shin. On questioning it was determined that he frequently has calf pain that goes away with rest.

This, he felt, was due to the increased use of his leg muscles. Physical examination revealed a well-groomed man who is slightly overweight. His lungs were clear, and his heart sounds were normal. His abdominal examination was benign. His neurological examination was normal except for a decrease in sensation in his lower extremities. Pulses were equal bilaterally but barely palpable in the feet. Ankle-arm index was 0.9. His vital signs were temperature, 101° F; blood pressure, 154/86 mm Hg; pulse, 110/min and regular; and respiratory rate, 20/min. Electrolyte, BUN, creatinine, hematocrit, and hemoglobin values were all within normal limits. His white blood cell count was 15,000/mm,[3] and his blood glucose level was 264 mg/dl. Lower extremities were without hair and cool to touch. The color was somewhat dusky, and vascular filling was poor. The ulcer was about the size of a quarter and superficial. It was located on the lower portion of his shin, and the area around it was slightly swollen and erythematosus. The medical diagnosis is peripheral vascular disease, diabetes mellitus, and ulcer of the left leg.

PLAN OF CARE FOR MR. TERRY T.

Nursing Diagnosis: *Altered Tissue Perfusion: Peripheral, secondary to peripheral arterial disease and diabetes mellitus*

Expected Patient Outcomes	Nursing Interventions
Tissue perfusion to the lower extremities will be maximized for Mr. T. as evidenced by palpable pulses, warm, dry skin, an ankle-arm index ≥ 0.9, and normal motor function, sensation, and evidence of wound healing.	• Monitor vital signs, and notify the physician if systolic blood pressure falls below normal. • Place Mr. T.'s lower extremities in a dependent position. • Assess quality of arterial pulses and the color and temperature of extremities. • Monitor ankle-arm index at least once a shift, and notify the physician of any change. • Encourage active and passive range-of-motion exercises. • Instruct Mr. T. to maintain a warm environment and avoid excessive exposure to cold and pressure.
Metabolic needs of the tissues will be minimized for Mr. T. as evidenced by a normal temperature, denial of leg pain, and a normal blood glucose level.	• Monitor temperature; administer acetaminophen as ordered to decrease Mr. T.'s fever. • Administer antibiotics as ordered to fight infection. • Encourage frequent periods of rest. • Provide local skin care to aid in healing. • Follow medical regimen to maintain Mr. T.'s blood glucose within normal limits.
Mr. T. will verbalize understanding of the cause of the leg pain and take action to minimize it.	• Explain to Mr. T. that the pain occurs because the narrowed arteries cause inadequate blood flow to the vessels during exercise. • Help Mr. T. to develop an exercise plan that increases slowly, based on his tolerance. • Explain the importance of frequent rest periods alternating with activity to prevent ischemia to the tissues. • Encourage Mr. T. to stop activity and rest at the first sign of leg pain. • Teach Mr. T. to avoid activity in cold environments.
Mr. T. will perform good foot care, and the ulcer will show signs of healing.	• Provide local cleansing and topical treatments to the wound as ordered. • Assess and document changes in the appearance of the wound. • Explain to Mr. T. the importance of keeping the skin clean and dry. • Ask Mr. T. to demonstrate foot care. • Teach Mr. T. the importance of adequate hydration and maintaining good lubrication of the skin. • Explain to Mr. T. the importance of wearing comfortable shoes that fit properly.
Mr. T. will verbalize the importance of any dietary modifications that must be made.	• Explain the relationship between a high-fat diet and vascular disease. • Help Mr. T. to develop a diet plan that is low in fat. • Explain the importance of following the prescribed diabetic diet, and help Mr. T. to incorporate this into his diet plan.

Continued.

Expected Patient Outcomes	Nursing Interventions
Mr. T. will verbalize the safety precautions that can be taken to minimize the potential for injury to the affected tissues.	• Instruct Mr. T. to avoid standing or sitting for long periods of time, as well as crossing his legs. • Teach Mr. T. to avoid the use of hot water bottles or heating pads. • Help Mr. T. to understand the importance of wearing warm protective clothing and of avoiding long periods of exposure to cold environments. • Instruct Mr. T. to keep the temperature in his home above 70° F. • Introduce Mr. T. to the following safety devices that can help decrease pressure to the affected areas: foot cradles, water mattresses, egg crate mattresses, sheepskins, and padding. • Teach Mr. T. why it is important that his legs be below the level of his heart when he is sitting in his recliner.

IV

REFERENCES

1. Baker JD: Assessment of peripheral arterial occlusive disease, *Crit Care Nurs Clin North Am* 3(3):493-498, 1991.
2. Carpenito LJ: *Nursing diagnosis: application to clinical practice,* ed 4, Philadelphia, 1992, JB Lippincott.
3. Doenges ME, Moorhouse MF: *Nurse's pocket guide: nursing diagnosis with interventions,* ed 3, Philadelphia, 1991, FA Davis.
4. Drummond BL: Preventing increased intracranial pressure, *Focus Crit Care* 17(2):116-122, 1990.
5. Goetter W: Nursing diagnosis and interventions with the acute stroke patient, *Nurs Clin North Am* 21(2):309-319, 1986.
6. Guyton AC: *Textbook of medical physiology,* ed 8, Philadelphia, 1990, WB Saunders.
7. Harper J: Rhabdomyolysis and myoglobinuric renal failure, *Crit Care Nurse* 10(3):32-36, 1990.
8. Huang SH, Kessler C, McCulloch C, and Dasher LA: *Coronary care nursing,* ed 2, Philadelphia, 1989, WB Saunders.
9. Kim MJ, McFarland GK, and McLane AM: *Pocket guide to nursing diagnosis,* ed 4, St Louis, 1990, CV Mosby.
10. Luckmann J, Sorensen KC: *Medical-surgical nursing: a psychophysiologic approach,* ed 3, Philadelphia, Penn, 1987, WB Saunders.
11. Memmer MK: Acute orthostatic hypotension, *Heart Lung* 17(2):134-141, 1988.
12. Nelson DP: Congestive heart failure. In *Cardiopulmonary nursing,* Springhouse, Penn, 1991, Springhouse.
13. Pearlstein G: Renal system complications in HIV infection, *Crit Care Nurs Clin North Am* 2(1):79-88, 1990.
14. Rice V: Shock, a clinical syndrome: an update. Part 1, an overview of shock, *Crit Care Nurs* 11(4):20-27, 1991.
15. Rice V: Shock, a clinical syndrome: an update. Part 2, the stages of shock, *Crit Care Nurs* 11(5):74-82, 1991.
16. Rice V: Shock, a clinical syndrome: an update. Part 3, therapeutic management, *Crit Care Nurs* 11(6):34-39, 1991.
17. Rice V: Shock, a clinical syndrome: an update. Part 4, nursing care of the shock patient, *Crit Care Nurs* 11(7):28-40, 1991.
18. Roberto PL: Diabetic nephropathy: causes, complications, and considerations, *Crit Care Nurs Clin North Am* 2(1):55-66, 1990.
19. Smith MF: Renal trauma: adult and pediatric considerations, *Crit Care Clin North Am* 2(1):67-78, 1990.
20. St Onge D: Acute respiratory failure. In *Cardiopulmonary nursing,* Springhouse, Penn, 1991, Springhouse.
21. Thelan LA, Davie JK, and Urden LD: *Textbook of critical care nursing: diagnosis and management,* St Louis, 1990, CV Mosby.
22. Thompson JM, McFarland GK, Hirsch J, Tucker S, and Bowers A: *Clinical nursing,* ed 2. St Louis, 1989, CV Mosby.
23. Thorn GW, and others: *Harrison's principles of internal medicine,* ed 12, New York, 1991, McGraw-Hill Book Company.
24. Turner J: Nursing intervention in patients with peripheral vascular disease, *Nurs Clin North Am* 21(2):233-240, 1986.

Inability to Sustain Spontaneous Ventilation

Dysfunctional Ventilatory Weaning Response

Inability to Sustain Spontaneous Ventilation (ISSV) is a response pattern of decreased energy reserves in which a patient is unable to maintain adequate breathing to support life.[24]

Dysfunctional Ventilatory Weaning Response (DVWR) is the state in which a patient's inability to adjust to lowered levels of mechanical ventilatory support interrupts and prolongs the weaning process.[13,18,19,24]

OVERVIEW

Spontaneous ventilation (breathing), the ability of an individual to perform the necessary ventilatory work to maintain adequate gas exchange,[16] occurs as a result of interactions among the pulmonary, cardiovascular, renal, musculoskeletal, and neurologic systems. Deterioration of these systems places certain categories of patients at risk for mechanical ventilatory dependency. Successful weaning and extubation from mechanical ventilation may occur effortlessly or it may become a prolonged and complicated process for both the patient and the health care team.[11,23] Although much progress has been made with mechanical ventilation, disagreements, controversies, and challenges continue to exist regarding the best ways in which to systematically and successfully wean patients from mechanical ventilation.* The process of weaning consists of three phases: preweaning, weaning, and extubation.[16] Weaning readiness is a state in which the patient has the necessary physical and emotional resources to engage in the work of weaning.[8,16,18] For example, the patient must have adequate respiratory muscle function to maintain a sufficient tidal volume, to be able to cough effectively, and to breathe deeply. The patient's lungs must be able to ventilate sufficiently to maintain baseline arterial blood gases.[11] Caloric intake must be sufficient and specific to the individual's requirements to ensure appropriate nutritional support to meet the patient's energy needs.[2,27] Psychological readiness is influenced by emotionally charged events that can cause feelings such as anxiety, fear, frustration, and hopelessness. Reactions to emotionally charged events can precipitate physiological responses that increase shortness of breath, exacerbate the emotional response, and create a cycle of increased inability to breathe.[10,11]

Inability to sustain spontaneous ventilation (ISSV) occurs when the patient's hypermetabolic energy needs, increased oxygen consumption, or depletion of energy reserves are unable to sustain the workload of spontaneous breathing.[2,5,10,28] The diagnosis of ISSV is based on deterioration of arterial blood gases, increased work of breathing, and decreasing energy. Patients with ISSV may present with outward manifestations of increased restlessness, increased use of accessory

---

*References 8, 13, 16, 23, 25, 32.

muscles, and compromised ability to cooperate.[24] Interpretations of findings from monitoring equipment may reveal other indications of ISSV, such as cardiac arrhythmias and decreased SaO_2.[10,11] Mechanically ventilated patients recovering from surgery, cachectic patients with COPD, and patients with head injuries may present with hypermetabolic energy requirements that impair their ability to sustain spontaneous ventilation.

Dysfunctional Ventilatory Weaning Response (DVWR) refers to a patient state or response to a health problem, ventilator dependency.[13] DVWR is a temporary state when a patient is not ready to mobilize the required physical and emotional resources for adjusting to lowered levels of mechanical ventilatory support. This inability to adjust to lowered levels of mechanical ventilatory support interrupts and prolongs the weaning process.[18,19] DVWR represents more than a failure to meet goals or the inability of the patient to maintain comfort. It encompasses any specific behaviors that are associated with the failure to wean, such as dyspnea, anxiety, or increased muscle tension that increase metabolic energy expenditure and exacerbate respiratory muscle fatigue, and an overall perception by the patient of a loss of control.[13]

Jenny and Logan,[13] who conducted research on DVWR, found in their literature review that up to 20% of patients who are mechanically ventilated are unable to tolerate discontinuation. Patients with severe, complicated acute or chronic lung disease, patients with multisystem extra pulmonary disease or neuromuscular disease who are on mechanical ventilation, as well as patients who have been on the ventilator more than 30 days, often experience difficulties that interfere with and may prolong successful weaning.*

ASSESSMENT

Although the nursing diagnoses Dysfunctional Ventilatory Weaning Response and Inability to Sustain Spontaneous Ventilation are interrelated in many respects, they, nevertheless, refer to two distinct patient responses. However, the initial physiological assessment of patients with ISSV or DVWR is the same. Assessment of pulmonary, cardiac, musculoskeletal, and neurologic systems is essential for diagnosing patients with ISSV during the preweaning phase of mechanical ventilation as well as patients with DVWR during the weaning and extubation phases.

Because the patient with ISSV is usually unable to provide historical data, it is important for the nurse to obtain information from the patient's family, other members of the health care team who know the patient, and medical records. The nurse also conducts a thorough baseline physical assessment to identify organs at risk due to pulmonary insufficiency. For example, assess measures of oxygen carrying capacity, e.g., arterial blood gases: ph 7.35-7.45, paO_2 greater than 50 mm Hg, pCO_2 less than 60 mm Hg, or variation less than 33% from baseline; hemoglobin: 12-15 gm/100 ml; cardiac status: heart rate, arrhythmias, blood pressure, SaO_2, CVP, pulmonary artery pressures, SVO_2 when available. Assess renal function, e.g., electrolytes: K 3.5-5.9 mEq/L, Mg 1.8-3 mg/dl, PO_4 2.4-4.8 mg/dl, ph 7.35-7.45; hydration: Hct 40-50/100 ml, plasma proteins (normals per institution), urinary output 30 ml/hour or greater, and bowel function. The presence of diarrhea and constipation can be indicative of ileus. Evaluate for the presence of processes that increase metabolic needs, such as systemic or local infection: elevated white blood cell count and configuration, malnutrition: decreased visceral proteins, and decreased albumin.[16,17,25,27]

Nursing assessment of the patient's pulmonary status includes observation of physical parameters and the patient's response to mechanical ventilation. Physical parameters to evaluate the patient's work of breathing include: tachypnea, dyspnea, abdominal paradox/asynchrony, spontaneous tidal volume, skin color and turgor, diaphoresis, chest wall expansion, deviation of trachea, auscultation of adventitious breath sounds, arterial blood gases, appearance of the chest x-ray.[3,4,16,23,31] Parameters for assessing the patient's response to

---

*References 11, 12, 16, 28, 29, 31.

mechanical ventilation include: patient comfort, bilateral breath sounds, tidal volume, minute ventilation, ability to breathe "with" the ventilator, position of the endotracheal tube.[30,31] A complication of mechanical ventilation is an increase of intrathoracic pressure with subsequent decreased venous return and possible liver congestion. Liver function, e.g., LDH, SGOT, SGGT, is assessed to identify the presence of this complication. Observe for indicators of airway obstruction that can increase the work of breathing, such as pulmonary secretions.[17,22] Review the patient's pulmonary medical history to identify diseases such as COPD, ARDS, and atelectasis, that reduce pulmonary compliance. The neurologic exam and a review of the patient's medication history provide the nurse with data for assessment of ventilatory drive.

Assessment of the severity of DVWR (mild, moderate, severe) determines the patient's ability to progress to the next step in the plan for weaning. Severe dysfunctional ventilatory weaning response is indicative of physiological factors that will cause inability to sustain spontaneous ventilation. Unlike the patient with ISSV, the patient with DVWR is able to interact with the nurse and is expected to be an active participant in the weaning and extubation phases of mechanical ventilation. Additional assessment parameters focus on the patient's ability to interact with the health care team. The nurse must determine the most effective mechanism for communicating with the patient, e.g., writing, sign language, communication board. In some instances, the nurse must collaborate with the multidisciplinary team to assess if a tracheostomy is necessary to facilitate communication.[6,9,10,12,28] Assess for negative environmental factors that trigger emotional responses and can cause shortness of breath, e.g., the patient's perception of the absence of health care members from the bedside or excessive distractional noise. Evaluate the patient's circadian rhythm and identify factors that contribute to sleep deprivation, e.g., unnecessary monitoring during normal sleep hours.[11,13,18]

Determine the patient's baseline mental status.

Assess the patient's cognitive ability e.g., attention, concentration and short term memory, to understand and to remember information about the weaning process and plan. It is important to use the same assessment criteria for ongoing monitoring of mental status and reporting of findings. The presence of altered thought processes (acute confusion), such as fluctuations in attention, concentration, and ability to follow commands, is often indicative of underlying physiologic abnormalities that can interfere with the weaning process.[10,21] Assessment of the patient's psychologic readiness for weaning includes: the patient's goals, concerns, and beliefs about the weaning process; the impact of previous attempts to wean; the patient's perception of a support system. Evaluate for behaviors that are indicative of psychologic dependence on the ventilator, such as anticipatory anxiety, expressions of fear of dying, "tuning out" or blocking discussion of weaning. Find out the patient's past coping techniques for stress reduction that can be incorporated into the weaning process.[10,11]

❖ Defining Characteristics

The presence of the following defining characteristics indicates that the patient may be experiencing inability to Sustain Spontaneous Ventilation*:

- Dyspnea
- Tachypnea
- Increased restlessness
- Increased use of accessory muscles
- Decreased spontaneous tidal volume
- Increased heart rate
- Cardiac arrhythmias
- Apprehension
- Compromised ability to cooperate
- Decreased SaO_2
- Decreased pO_2
- Increased pCO_2
- Increased metabolic rate

---

*References 2, 4, 10, 16, 17, 24, 31.

❖ **Related Factors**

The following related factors are associated with Inability to Sustain Spontaneous Ventilation*:

- Anemia
- Infection
- Increased metabolic requirements to resist nosocomial infections
- Hyperthermia
- Electrolyte imbalance
- Left ventricular dysfunction
- Increased intrathoracic pressure
- Pulmonary edema
- Atelectasis
- Carbohydrate overfeeding
- Abdominal distension (e.g., bowel, obesity)
- Uncontrolled pain
- Activity greater than available energy
- Respiratory muscle fatigue

❖ **Related Medical/Psychiatric Diagnoses**

The following are examples of related medical/psychiatric diagnoses for Inability to Sustain Spontaneous Ventilation:

- Abdominal surgery
- Adult respiratory distress syndrome
- Chronic obstructive pulmonary disease
- Delirium
- Generalized organic anxiety syndrome
- Infection
- Malnutrition
- Multisystem organ failure
- Pneumonia
- Reactive airway disease
- Thoracic surgery

❖ **Defining Characteristics**

The presence of the following defining characteristics indicates that the patient may be experiencing Dysfunctional Ventilatory Weaning Response†:

Mild DVWR

- Restlessness
- Slight increased respiratory rate from baseline

- Responses to lowered levels of mechanical ventilator support may include:

  conveying increased need for oxygen, experiencing breathing discomfort, complaining of fatigue, feeling warm, questioning about possible machine malfunction, exhibiting undue concentration on breathing

Moderate DVWR

- Responses to lowered levels of mechanical ventilatory support include:

  slight increase from baseline blood pressure, increase from baseline heart rate, baseline increase in respiratory rate

- Hypervigilence to activities
- Inability to respond to coaching
- Inability to cooperate
- Apprehension
- Diaphoresis
- Eye widening "wide-eyed look"
- Decreased air entry on auscultation
- Color changes (e.g., pale, slight cyanosis)
- Slight respiratory accessory muscle use

Severe DVWR

- Responses to lowered levels of mechanical ventilatory support include:

  agitation, deterioration in arterial blood gases from current baseline, increase from baseline blood pressure, increase from baseline heart rate, significant increase in respiratory rate from baseline

- Profuse diaphoresis
- Full respiratory accessory muscle use
- Shallow, gasping breaths
- Paradoxical abdominal breathing
- Discoordinated breathing with the ventilator
- Decreased level of consciousness
- Adventitious breath sounds, audible airway secretion
- Cyanosis

❖ **Related Factors**

The following related factors are associated with Dysfunctional Ventilatory Weaning Response*:

---

*References 2, 4, 5, 10, 11, 15, 16, 17, 20, 24, 28.
†References 2-5, 8-11, 13, 16, 18, 19, 28, 32.

*References 8, 10-12, 16, 18, 19, 23, 24, 28, 31.

- Ineffective airway clearance
- Respiratory muscle fatigue
- Multisystem disease
- Neuromuscular chronic disability
- Cardiac failure
- Acute or chronic lung disease
- Electrolyte disorders (e.g., hypophosphatemia)
- Anemia
- Sleep pattern disturbance
- Malnutrition, less than or more than body requirements
- History of multiple unsuccessful weaning attempts
- Inability to effectively communicate
- Adverse environment (e.g., noisy, overly active)
- Negative events in patient's room
- Moderate to severe anxiety
- State anxiety
- Low nurse-patient ratio
- Extended absence of nurse from bedside
- Pharmacologic therapy
- Obesity
- Infection
- Uncontrolled pain or discomfort
- Uncontrolled episodic energy demands or problems
- Inappropriate pacing of diminished ventilatory support
- History of ventilatory dependence greater than one week
- Unfamiliar nursing staff
- Lack of trust in nurse
- Decreased motivation
- Terminal illness
- Inadequate information about role in weaning process
- Perception of futility regarding own ability to be weaned
- Fear
- Clinical depression or prolonged depressed state
- Hopelessness
- Powerlessness
- Decreased self-esteem

❖ Related Medical/Psychiatric Diagnoses

The following are examples of related medical/psychiatric diagnoses for Dysfunctional Ventilatory Weaning Response:

- Adjustment disorder with anxious mood
- Adjustment disorder with depressed mood
- Chronic obstructive pulmonary disease
- Congestive heart failure
- Delirium
- Generalized anxiety disorder
- Major depression
- Malnutrition
- Multisystem organ failure
- Organic anxiety syndrome
- Reactive airway disease
- Thoracic or abdominal surgery

NURSING DIAGNOSES

Examples of *specific* nursing diagnoses for Inability to Sustain Spontaneous Ventilation are:

- Inability to sustain spontaneous ventilation related to left ventricular dysfunction
- Inability to sustain spontaneous ventilation related to pneumonia

Examples of *specific* nursing diagnoses for Dysfunctional Ventilatory Weaning Response are:

- Dysfunctional ventilatory weaning response related to multisystem disease
- Dysfunctional ventilatory weaning response related to malnutrition, less than body requirements

PLANNING AND IMPLEMENTATION WITH RATIONALE
Inability to Sustain Spontaneous Ventilation

The desired outcome for patients with ISSV is: to breathe without the assistance of mechanical ventilation. The primary nurse or registered nurse case manager plays a pivotal role in the coordination of multidisciplinary care and evaluating progress toward outcomes.[29] Nursing interventions focus on correcting physiologic conditions that deplete energy reserves, prevent ventilator-induced complications, and regulate the work of breathing. Observation for the presence of dia-

❖ NURSING CARE GUIDELINES

Nursing Diagnosis: *Inability to Sustain Spontaneous Ventilation*

IV

Expected Patient Outcomes	**Nursing Interventions***
Sustain spontaneous ventilation as evidenced by: oxygenation of tissues; synchronous use of respiratory muscles.	• Monitor for complications related to mechanical ventilation such as, increased cardiothoracic pressure, decreased venous return, and pulmonary infection. • Observe for presence of diaphragm/respiratory muscle fatigue, increased respiratory rate, minute ventilation, hypercarbia with respiratory acidosis. • Check for correct initial placement of endotracheal tube and monitor placement according to unit protocols. • Collaborate with the multidisciplinary team to determine ventilation parameters (e.g., FIO_2, mode of ventilatory assistance, tidal volume frequency). • Collaborate with multidisciplinary team to develop a suction protocol that incorporates parameters for hyperoxygenation, hyperinflation, and length of stabilization period between suction catheter passes. • Observe for trends in the patient's cardiac, renal, and neurologic status. • Initiate passive and/or active exercise (e.g., turning, postural drainage, range of motion exercises, induced coughing and deep breathing). • Use sterile technique when removing secretions. • Position patient comfortably in a manner that allows for full lung expansion. • Use negative inspiratory pressure, positive expiratory pressure, and tidal volume as parameters to regulate activity. • Establish a schedule for muscle reconditioning such as mechanically assisted muscle training and/or graded manual diaphragmatic muscle exercises.
Meet metabolic energy requirements as evidenced by maintaining nutritional intake equal to calculated requirements for nutrition	• Collaborate with dietician and/or physician to maintain adequate nutrition (e.g., 25-35 k cal/kg with appropriate carbohydrate, fat, and protein). • Monitor daily weight, intake and output. • Monitor bowel function (e.g., constipation, diarrhea) • Monitor levels of serum phosphate, potassium, calcium, and magnesium, and collaborate with physician, dietician, and or pharmacist to provide replacement therapy as necessary. • Regulate environmental activity. • Establish a regular schedule for muscle reconditioning that incorporates adequate rest periods. • Schedule rest periods that are congruent with patient's circadian rhythm. • Revise activity schedule on a daily basis, according to patient's tolerance.

*References 1, 2, 4-7, 10, 11, 14, 15, 17, 18, 20-23, 27, 30-32.

phragm/respiratory muscle fatigue *to identify organs at risk because of decreased oxygen and to evaluate adequacy of oxygen therapy parameters* is an essential intervention for patients with ISSV.[10,14,22,28] Diaphragmatic rest in the presence of respiratory muscle fatigue requires twelve to twenty-four hours for recovery.[4] Negative inspiratory pressure, positive expiratory pressure, and tidal volume are measures that are used *to determine the presence of diaphragm fatigue.* The use of methylxanthines can prevent diaphragm fatigue by improving diaphragm contractility.[4,28] Even though these patients are usually too sick to interact with the health care team, it is important for the nurse to call the patient by the patient's preferred name and to introduce himself/herself during each patient contact. It is also important to offer a brief explanation of the purpose for being with the patient during each contact *to decrease the patient's anxiety that is associated with an unfamiliar environment.*[11,18,21]

Monitoring the patient's nutritional status and collaborating with the dietician and physician *facilitate meeting the patient's metabolic energy requirements.*[2,27] Appropriate nutrition is especially important, *because carbohydrate overfeeding increases the production of carbon dioxide resulting in increased work of breathing.*[2] Adequate nutrition from proteins and fats *reduces the potential for muscle wasting.*[2,27] Interventions that ensure oral hygiene, teach visitors to report exposure to infections, emphasize the importance of universal precautions to all health care team members, and monitor the sterility of equipment *conserve the patient's energy expenditure by minimizing exposure to infection.*[27,28]

Dysfunctional Ventilatory Weaning Response

Nursing interventions that optimize the likelihood of the patient's ability to tolerate lowered levels of mechanical ventilation include preparing the patient physically and psychologically. The designation of a primary nurse or a registered nurse case manager to collaborate on a consistent basis with the patient and family, as well as the multidisciplinary team *facilitates successful inte-gration of treatments directed toward the outcome of resolving ventilatory problems.* Consistent explanations from all caregivers regarding the weaning process *promotes the patient's trust in the health care team.*[12,29] An essential component of the nurse's role in the weaning process is "knowing" the patient's individual response patterns to lowered levels of mechanical ventilation *to prevent setbacks.*[10,18] Because of the enormous communication constraints and social isolation associated with ventilator dependence, the establishment of an effective communication system *reduces potential patient frustration and anxiety, minimizes negative aspects of mechanical ventilation, and maximizes the patient's sense of control and energy conservation.*[6,9,26] Ongoing monitoring for the presence of altered thought processes (acute confusion), such as fluctuations in concentration, attention, and orientation is important *because these behaviors may be indicative of underlying pathology that impedes weaning.*[10]

Creating a therapeutic weaning environment is an intervention that *decreases the patient's apprehension and tension.* Using friends and family as supportive resources *helps to minimize the patient's anxiety and fears.*[26] Nursing interventions that provide family education *strengthen the family's ability to be a supportive resource for the patient.* Clarifying misconceptions and decreasing family members' anxiety about weaning *reduces the likelihood of the family member transmitting their anxiety to the patient.*[21]

The development and implementation of a weaning contract (critical pathway) *facilitates the patient's control in decision-making regarding adherence to the weaning plan.*[21,29] Consultation with clinical nurse specialists or other nurse experts provides a valuable resource to the primary nurse or case manager who is developing the weaning contract. Consistency among health care providers when communicating with the patient about the weaning plan *promotes a sense of trust in the health care team.* The use of positive reinforcements, such as touch, *conveys support and encouragement of the patient's progress and endeavors.*[6]

❖ *NURSING CARE GUIDELINES*

Nursing Diagnosis: Dysfunctional Ventilatory Weaning Response

Expected Patient Outcomes	**Nursing Interventions***
The patient tolerates lowered levels of mechanical ventilation as evidenced by maintaining baseline clinical status.	• Provide the patient with a Primary Nurse or Registered Nurse Case Manager. • Ensure that all caregivers provide consistent explanations about weaning. • Establish an effective means of communicating with the patient. • Monitor for presence of altered thought process (e.g., fluctuations in concentration, attention, orientation) prior to initiating weaning process and throughout weaning process; collaborate with patient's medical team to search for and treat underlying cause (e.g., fever, infection, drug therapy, fluid overload). • Repeat information until patient conveys understanding of explanations. • Allow patient sufficient time to respond to information and explanations. • Collaborate with multidisciplinary team to reduce ventilatory support in small increments, such as one parameter. • Use coaching during weaning process, based on prior agreement with patient, (e.g., reminding patient about correct breathing during episodes of shortness of breath). • Collaborate with resource such as psychiatric consultation/liaison clinical nurse specialist for individualized stress management techniques (e.g., relaxation, imagery, music) during weaning.

Convey a comfortable and relaxed appearance as evidenced by absence of irritability, restlessness, agitation, and/or fatigue.	• Control and minimize noise and activity level in patient's bedside area; provide privacy; allow for scheduled rest times.
	• Use family and/or friends as a supportive resource for patient.
	• Prepare family for a supportive role in weaning process by:
	    Providing information about the unit environment (e.g., alarms, monitoring equipment, nurse call system);
	    Providing information about the weaning plan;
	    Introducing all caregivers and explaining their roles in the weaning process;
	    Inviting family to share issues of concern;
	    Offering suggestions for appropriate conversation;
	    Negotiating visiting times;
	    Clarifying family's role as supportive resource.
	• Observe frequently for signs of respiratory muscle fatigue, (e.g., increased respiratory rate and minute ventilation, hypercarbia, altered breathing pattern, and increased discomfort).

*References 2, 4, 6, 9-13, 15, 16, 18, 19, 21, 25-27, 29, 32.

❖ *NURSING CARE GUIDELINES—cont'd*

Expected Patient Outcomes	**Nursing Interventions***
Adhere to the weaning plan as evidenced by participation with primary nurse or registered nurse case manager in implementation of weaning plan and ongoing regimen.	• Based on individual assessment and collaboration with the patient and the multidisciplinary team, consider use of a formal written weaning contract, mapping, or critical pathway that includes: 　Identification of specific goals; 　Timing of weaning interventions; 　Expectations regarding adherence to activity and/or exercise protocols; 　Patient's participation in self care activities; 　Role of patient and individual team members in achieving weaning goals; 　Schedule for re- evaluating, renegotiating, and revising the weaning plan. • Provide patient and caregivers with a copy of formal written plan and include a copy in patient's chart. Use clear and direct communication (e.g., short, simple sentences) to convey plans for weaning process. • Negotiate weaning process with patient. Develop a plan for positive reinforcement, such as placing gold stars on a calendar, planning activities outside of the unit, based on individual assessment. • Encourage expression of thoughts and feelings about perceptions of the weaning process. • Encourage patient to convey perceptions of physiologic changes (e.g., breathing patterns and recognition of breathing difficulties, presence of secretions). • Use touch, such as a pat on the shoulder.

EVALUATION

When the patient who has been experiencing Inability to Sustain Spontaneous Breathing is able to sustain spontaneous ventilation, parameters that measure oxygenation of tissues are within normal limits or within the limits of normal for the individual, as determined in collaboration with the multidisciplinary planning team. Synchronous use of respiratory muscles is indicative of decreased work of breathing. Does the patient have normal electrolytes, pCO_2, and visceral proteins? The presence of an elevated pCO_2 occurs with carbohydrate overfeeding. Has the patient experienced a weight gain or reversal of weight loss that is not

associated with edema? If not, the patient continues to remain dependent upon mechanical ventilation because problems with oxygenation, respiratory muscle fatigue, or malnutrition may not resolved.

The ability of the patient who has experienced Dysfunctional Ventilatory Weaning Response to maintain physiologic parameters that are consistent with his or her baseline clinical status is evidenced by physiologic and psychologic tolerance to lowered levels of mechanical ventilation. The patient's ability to adhere to the weaning plan is strengthened by early recognition of untoward physiologic or psychologic events and prompt in-

❖ CASE STUDY WITH PLAN OF CARE

Mr. Joe T., a 64-year-old widower who maintains close contact with his son and daughter who live nearby, was admitted to the surgical intensive care unit on a ventilator following a left upper lobectomy for a large cell cancerous lesion. His nursing diagnosis was ISSV, and a plan of care directed toward the outcome of meeting Mr. T.s metabolic needs without the assistance of mechanical ventilation was initiated. His preoperative medical history includes: height 6 foot 1 inch, a 15-pound weight loss over 4 months with a present weight of 70 kg; shortness of breath walking from street level to his first floor apartment; a two pack per day smoking history until the day prior to surgery;

6 to 7 cups of coffee per day; 8 to 10 beers per week. His employment history indicates that he has been a free lance writer for the past 20 years for national popular magazines, and he enjoys the traveling that is associated with his work. Mr. T. experienced three unsuccessful weaning attempts over an 8-day period. These weaning failures were characterized by cardiac arrhythmias (atrial fibrillation, PVC's, four beat run of V-Tach), shortness of breath, asynchronous breathing with the ventilator, abdominal paradox, diaphoresis, and pallor. Mr. T. is frustrated with attempts to communicate with his family and caregivers and has written that he wants to get off the ventilator or die!

PLAN OF CARE FOR MR. JOE T.

Nursing Diagnosis *Dysfunctional ventilatory weaning response related to inability to successfully wean from the ventilator after three attempts.*

Expected Interventions

Tolerate lowered levels of mechanical ventilation as evidenced by: absence of cardiac arrhythmias; shortness of breath; abdominal paradox; diaphoresis; "fighting the ventilator."

- Monitor for the presence of diaphragm/respiratory muscle fatigue (atrial and ventricular arrhythmias, shortness of breath, asynchronous breathing with the ventilator, abdominal paradox, change in concentration).
- Collaborate with multidisciplinary team:
   to determine the best method of weaning for Mr. T.,
   to minimize activities and procedures during weaning trials,
   to remove unnecessary lines (e.g., IVs, central lines, PA catheter),
   to determine the best method for feeding Mr. T.,
   to ensure that Mr. T. does not receive unnecessary medication that interferes with his ventilatory drive,
   to determine whether methylxanthines are appropriate,
   to determine parameters for discontinuation and/or continuation of Mr. T.'s weaning plan.
- Adopt a low threshold for discontinuation of activities (e.g., bathing, getting out of bed) that increase shortness of breath or reduce SaO_2 less than 90%.
- Establish a daily routine with Mr. T. that allows for his circadian rhythm.
- Coach Mr. T. during the weaning process, using a calm, low voice, to remind him about correct breathing when he experiences shortness of breath.

Adhere to the multidisciplinary plan for weaning as evidenced by participating in Activities of Daily Living and cooperating with therapeutic regimens.

- Collaborate with the psychiatric consultation/liaison clinical nurse specialist in the development of a weaning contract for Mr. T.
- Negotiate weaning plan with Mr. T.
- Arrange with Mr. T.'s son to bring in Mr. T.'s lap top computer and printer.
- Encourage Mr. T. to keep a daily log.
- Create a personal environment by encouraging Mr. T. to wear his own pajamas and robe during daytime activities, keeping his room door closed with curtain partially open for monitoring.
- Provide a poster board to hang on the wall in Mr. T.'s room and encourage him to have staff and visitors write and/or draw pictures on it.
- Provide ongoing opportunities for Mr. T. to communicate his thoughts and feelings about his physical and emotional well- being.

terventions to resolve these events. Patients who are able to wean from the ventilator convey a comfortable and relaxed appearance and no longer experience irritability, restlessness, agitation, or fatigue. Patients who are unable to tolerate lowered levels of mechanical ventilation should be evaluated for physiological and psychological factors that impede the weaning process. Some patients may never be able to breathe without mechanical assistance. Alternative interventions that address this major lifestyle change are implemented for these individuals.

REFERENCES

1. Aldrich TK et al.: Weaning from mechanical ventilation: Adjunctive use of inspiratory muscle resistive training, *Crit Care Med* 17(2):143-147, 1989.
2. Benotti PN Bistrain B: Metabolic and nutritional aspects of weaning from mechanical ventilation, *Crit Care Med* 17(2):181-185, 1989.
3. Bridges EJ: Transition from ventilatory support: Knowing when the patient is ready to wean, *Crit Care Nurs Q* 15(1):14-20, 1992.
4. Burns SM: Preventing diaphragm fatigue in the ventilated patient, *Dimens Crit Care Nurs* 10(1):13-20, 1991.
5. Cohen CA et al: Clinical manifestations of inspiratory muscle fatigue, *Am J Med* 73:308-316, 1982.
6. Connolly MA, Shekleton ME: Communicating with ventilator dependent patients *Dimensions Crit Care Nurs* 10(2):115-122, 1991.
7. Dupuis YG: *Ventilators: Theory and clinical applications,* ed. 2 St. Louis, 1992, Mosby–Year Book.
8. Geisman LK: Advances in weaning from mechanical ventilation, *Critical Care Nurs Clinics North Am* 1(4):697-705, 1989.
9. Greis ML, Fernsler J: Patient perceptions of the mechanical ventilation experience, *Focus Crit Care* 15(2):52-59, 1988.
10. Grossbach-Landis I: Successful weaning of ventilator-dependent patients, *Top Clin Nurs* 2(3):45-65, 1980.
11. Henneman EA: The art and science of weaning from mechanical ventilation, *Focus Crit Care* 18(6):490-501, 1991.
12. Jackson NC: Pulmonary rehabilitation for mechanically ventilated patients, *Crical Care Nurs Clin North Am* 3(4):591-600, 1991.
13. Jenny J, Logan J: Analyzing expert nursing practice to develop a new nursing diagnosis dysfunctional ventilatory weaning response. In Carroll-Johnson RM, ed: *Classification of nursing diagnoses, proceedings of the ninth conference.* Philadelphia, 1990, JB Lippincott.
14. Joiner JW et al: *Management of the patient-ventilator system, A team approach* ed 3, St. Louis, 1990, Mosby–Year Book.
15. Kigin CM: Breathing exercises for the medical patient: The art and the science, *Phys Ther* 70(11):700-706, 1990.
16. Knebel AR: Weaning from mechanical ventilation: Current controversies, *Heart Lung* 20(4):321-334, 1991.
17. Knipper JS, Alpen MA: Ventilatory support. In Bulechek GM, McCloskey JC: *Nursing Intervention: Essential Nursings Treatments,* ed 2, Philadelphia, 1992, WB Saunders.
18. Logan J, Jenny J: Interventions for the nursing diagnosis Dysfunctional Ventilatory Weaning Response: A qualitative study. In Carroll-Johnson RM, ed: *Classification of nursing diagnoses, proceedings of the ninth conference,* Philadelphia, 1990, JB Lippincott.
19. Logan J, Jenny J: Deriving a new nursing diagnosis through qualitative research Dysfunctional ventilatory weaning response, *Nurs Diagnosis* 1(1):37-43, 1990.
20. Lookinland S, Appel PL: Hemodynamic and oxygen transport changes following endotracheal suctioning in trauma patients, *Nurs Res* 40(3):133- 138, 1991.
21. McFarland GK, Wasli EL, Gerety EK: *Nursing Diagnoses and Process in Psychiatric Mental Health Nursing,* ed 2, Philadelphia, 1992, JB Lippincott.
22. Montenegro HD: Complications of mechanical ventilation, *Respiratory Therapy* 14(2):20-27, 1984.
23. Morganroth MI, Grum CM: Weaning from mechanical ventilation, *J Intensive Care Med* 3(2):109-120, 1988.
24. North American Nursing Diagnosis Association: Ballot, St. Louis: NANDA, March, 1992.
25. Norton LC, Neureuter A: Weaning the long-term ventilator-dependent patient: common problems and management, *Crit Care Nurs* 9(1):42-52, 1989.
26. Riggio RE, et al: Psychological issues in the care of critically-ill respirator patients: Differential perceptions of patients, relatives, and staff, *Psychol Rep* 51:363-369, 1982.
27. Spector N: Nutritional support of the ventilator-dependent patient, *Nurs Clin North Am* 24(2):407-414, 1989.
28. Sporn PHS, Morganroth MI: Discontinuation of mechanical ventilation, *Clin Chest Med* 9(1):113-126, 1988.
29. Thompson KS et al: Building a critical path for ventilator dependency, *Am J Nurs* 91(7):28-31, 1991.
30. Tobin MJ: What should the clinician do when a patient "fights the ventilator?" *Respir Care* 36(5):395-406, 1991.
31. Urden LD, Davie JK, Thelan LA: Pulmonary therapeutic management, in *Essentials of Critical Care Management,* St. Louis, 1992, Mosby–Year Book.
32. Witta K: New techniques for weaning difficult patients from mechanical ventilation, *AACN Clin Issues* 1(2):260-266, 1990.

IV

High Risk for Peripheral Neurovascular Dysfunction

High Risk for Peripheral Neurovascular Dysfunction is a state in which an individual is at risk of experiencing a disruption in circulation, sensation, or motion of an extremity.[14]

OVERVIEW

The disruption of circulation, sensation, or motion of an extremity can be related to four specific health problems: compartment syndrome; diabetes mellitus; arterial insufficiency; and venous insufficiency.

Compartment Syndrome

Muscles, nerves, and blood vessels are confined to areas called compartments which have inelastic boundaries composed of skin, epimysium, fascia, and/or bone.[17] There are 46 compartments in the human body; 38 are found in the extremities.[9] Conditions that cause an increase in pressure within a compartment compromise the circulation, viability, and function of those tissues if untreated.[12,19] The most common sites for the development of compartment syndrome are the deep posterior, superficial posterior, lateral, and anterior compartments of the lower leg and the dorsal and volar compartments of the forearm.[17]

Pressure within a compartment may increase due to (1) a decrease in size or volume of the compartment such as with premature closure of fascial defects before edema has subsided, (2) an increase in compartment contents from edema or hemorrhage, or (3) external pressure from tight casts or dressings, air splints, or pressurized antishock garments.[18] Increase in intracompartmental pressure initially results in compression of the venous capillary bed and arterioles with resultant arteriolar spasm and a subsequent decrease in capillary hydrostatic pressure.[13]

As a result of a decrease in systemic blood pressure in patients with shock, there is an increased incidence of compartment syndrome because less compartmental pressure is generated, thereby predisposing these injured areas to tissue ischemia and arteriolar spasm. Other factors which contribute to the development of compartment syndrome include reperfusion injury following replantation or reanastomosis of a major artery, decreased oncotic pressure following severe burn injuries, increased permeability of capillary beds resulting from histamine response in severe inflammatory conditions or following ischemia, and obstruction of proximal venous flow.[13]

Ischemic myositis is the end product of compartment syndrome causing muscle necrosis resulting in a severely contracted and functionally useless distal extremity. Functional changes of muscle tissue occur within 4 to 12 hours of injury with contractures developing within 12 hours of ischemia. Functional deficits of nerves occur within 12 to 24 hours of ischemia. Resorption of ischemic muscle may result in myoglobinuria with renal complications, metabolic acidosis, hyperkalemia, sepsis, or the need for amputation.[9,17]

Diabetes Mellitus

Diabetes mellitus is a genetically and clinically heterogenous group of disorders of metabolism which is manifested by carbohydrate intolerance. Long-term complications resulting from this disorder of carbohydrate metabolism may include microangiopathy and macroangiopathy. Microangiopathy is caused by the increased accumulation of glycoprotein in the capillaries and arterioles resulting in a thickening in the vessel wall and an increase in the rate of formation of the basement membrane. These small vessel changes result in the development of diabetic retinopathy, diabetic nephropathy, and diabetic neuropathy. Macroangiopathy affects large vessels and has characteristics similar to atherosclerosis. Insulin insufficiency causes accumulation of sorbitol in the vascular intima, hyperlipoproteinemia, and abnormality in blood coagulation. The combination of these biochemical disturbances eventually leads to peripheral vascular insufficiency and subsequent vascular occlusion.[16]

Diabetic neuropathy results from an increased accumulation of sorbitol and fructose and a decreased concentration of myoinositol in nerve tissue. These alterations interfere with the metabolic activity of the Schwann cells and cause axonal loss. Motor conduction velocity is diminished in the early stages of the neuropathy. Neuropathy may cause pain, paresthesia, decreased vibratory and proprioceptive sensations, motor impairment with loss of deep tendon reflexes, muscle weakness, and atrophy. It may involve the peripheral nerves as a mononeuropathy or polyneuropathy, the cranial nerves, and/or the autonomic nervous system.[16]

Arterial Insufficiency

The primary cause of arterial insufficiency is atherosclerosis. Atherosclerosis has been described as occurring in three stages. The first stage is the formation of fatty streaks, the second stage is the formation of fibroid plaques, and the third stage is characterized by necrosis, calcification, and vascularization of the plaque which can lead to the development of thrombus formation. These changes result in intimal thickening and hardening of the artery with subsequent loss of elasticity. Eventually there is a decrease in blood flow through these vessels and changes between oxygen demand and oxygen supply ensue. Com-

pensatory mechanisms including vasodilation, collateralization, and utilization of anaerobic pathways develop to meet metabolic demands. While oxygen deprived arteries quickly dilate, the long-term effect is limited. Arteriolar dilation may progress to stealing of blood from the cutaneous and peripheral nerve vessels. Ischemia to the peripheral nerves results in paresthesias, namely, coldness and "pins and needles" sensations. Over time collateral vessels develop. Ultimately cellular anaerobic metabolism attempts to meet basic oxygen requirements. Finally, lactic acid and pyruvic acid, waste products of cellular metabolism, are excreted slowly, subsequently altering the acid-base balance and resulting in gangrene.[2]

Venous Insufficiency

Venous insufficiency results from valvular incompetence secondary to venous hypertension. Increases in venous pressure cause changes which result in increased permeability of the capillary walls of the skin. Edema results from extravasation of fluid and red blood cells into the surrounding tissue. Edema prevents the exchange of oxygen, carbon dioxide, nutrients, and waste products and leads to the development of cellulitis and ulceration. Increased venous pressure can result from right heart failure, obesity, pregnancy, age, malignancy, thrombosis, or occupations that require prolonged standing.[2]

ASSESSMENT

Patients who are at high risk for the development of peripheral neurovascular dysfunction include those with a propensity for circulatory and/or neurovascular compromise. Therefore, the assessment should include examination of the skin, peripheral vascular, musculoskeletal, and neurologic systems.

Compartment Syndrome

Pain originating with passive stretching of the muscles is an early indicator of inadequate oxygenation. Deep throbbing, unrelenting pain not alleviated with narcotics and that increases with elevation of the extremity is indicative of compartment syndrome. Pain is elicited on palpation of the area and with passive movement of the distal digits. The area is tense and warm to palpation.[18]

Edema is noted at the site of injury secondary to fluid shifts to the third space of the injured muscle. Injuries causing bleeding into the muscle may also contribute to the development of edema. Progressive edema may result in circulatory and neurovascular compromise. Pulses in the extremity may be palpable; loss of pulses distal to the area is a late sign of circulatory compromise. Color changes, including mottling and cyanosis, are early signs of circulatory compromise. Pallor is a late sign of circulatory compromise and is usually indicative of major arterial occlusion. The presence of ecchymosis may obscure the evaluation of color changes.[15]

Neurovascular assessment of the injured extremity may reveal weak active movement of the distal digits. Hyperesthesia, in particular loss of two-point discrimination, may be seen early in the development of compartment syndrome. Hypoesthesia of nerves that traverse the compartment may also be noted.[12] The fingers should be assessed for active extension, flexion, abduction, and adduction when a compartment of the upper extremity is affected. It is imperative that extension and flexion of the toes and inversion and dorsiflexion of the foot be assessed when a compartment of the lower extremity is involved.[18]

Diabetes Mellitus

Assessment of the patient with diabetes mellitus as it pertains to the nursing diagnosis high risk for peripheral vascular dysfunction focuses on evaluation for arterial insufficiency, as discussed below, and peripheral neuropathy.

Diabetic neuropathy is defined as "objective evidence of neural impairment accompanied by discernible symptoms."[4] Upon diagnosis of diabetes mellitus, a baseline neurologic assessment is essential for comparison as diabetic neuropathies develop. The sensory assessment is performed before the motor assessment because pain elicited upon examination of the motor system may interfere with that of the sensory system. The nurse assesses the patient for sensation to touch (sharp and dull), discrimination between heat and cold, two-point discrimination (hyperesthesia), balance, proprioception, position sense, and vibratory sensation. These may become diminished as the disease progresses. Early manifestations of diabetic neuropathy include diminished deep tendon reflexes, particularly the Achilles tendon. The nurse assesses the patient for burns and other changes in skin integrity because the patient may not be aware of these alterations because of decreased sensation. Motor neuropathy may result in weakness; therefore, motor strength and function must be examined.[4]

Arterial Insufficiency

Patients with arterial insufficiency initially experience intermittent claudication and describe pain as a tightening pressure in the calves or buttocks, or a sharp, cramp-like sensation that occurs during walking and is alleviated with rest. The appearance of the pain is determined by the speed, incline, and surface of the walk. As arterial insufficiency progresses, episodes of intermittent claudication increase in frequency and occur with less exertion; eventually rest pain develops. Rest pain is an acute condition requiring prompt treatment. It indicates inadequate perfusion of collateral vessels.[2]

Palpation of pulses in patients with arterial insufficiency reveals the pulses to be weak or absent. Doppler evaluation can be used; however, the Doppler can pick up minimal blood flow as well as collateral blood flow. Therefore the only situation in which the reporting of a detectable Doppler flow signal is clinically relevant occurs when a signal that was present disappears.[1]

Measurement of the ankle-brachial pressure index is the most commonly used parameter for overall evaluation of extremity status. The ankle-brachial pressure index is calculated by obtaining a blood pressure reading at the dorsalis pedis artery or anterior tibial artery, the posterior tibial artery, and bilateral brachial arteries. The highest systolic blood pressure reading of the dorsalis pedis artery, anterior tibial artery, or posterior tibial artery is used and divided by the brachial artery systolic blood pressure on the same side. Should there be a greater than 20 mm Hg. difference between the brachial pressures, the higher opposite-side brachial reading is used to obtain a more accurate reading. An ankle-brachial index of greater than 0.95 to 1.0 indicates no significant reduction of blood flow, 0.70 to 0.95 denotes mild claudication, 0.40 to 0.70 signifies moderate to severe claudication, 0.30 to 0.40 implies severe claudication, and less than 0.30 indicates ischemia with impending tissue loss.[8]

Assessment of skin temperature may reveal the extremity to be cool. Capillary refill may take more than 3 seconds. Color changes vary from pallor to dependent rubor. Blanching is noted when the foot of the extremity is raised above the level of the heart; the extremity will return to its normal color when placed in a dependent position. The rapidity of color return is inversely proportional to the degree of ischemia. The presence of dependent rubor is indicative of severe ischemia and is a reflection of tissue hypoxia and reactive arteriolar and capillary dilatation. Dependent rubor is the result of ischemic tissue extracting more oxygen from arteriolar blood, with the deoxygenated blood remaining in the dilated capillaries because of low perfusion pressure.[2]

Ulcerations of the skin are associated with advanced arterial insufficiency and are most commonly found on the toes, malleoli, and heels. The ulcerations are pale with poor granulation tissue and have a cyanotic border. Hair loss, callus formation, and trophic changes of the toenails may also be seen.[2]

Venous Insufficiency

Pain is the most frequently reported symptom with venous insufficiency and is described as a dull, diffuse ache throughout the extremity which is exacerbated by long periods of standing. The pain is alleviated with elevation and worsens in the dependent position. Edema is noted toward the end of the day but resolves with elevation of the extremity. The lower extremities may be bluish in color when dependent. Hemosiderin deposits in the skin occur secondary to red cell degradation and appear as brown staining of the skin. The skin temperature is warm and capillary refill occurs in 3 seconds or less, unless perfusion is impaired by severe edema. Pulses are strong and symmetric, although it may be difficult to palpate dorsalis pedis and posterior tibial pulses because of edema.[2,10]

❖ Risk Factors

The presence of the following behaviors, conditions, or circumstances renders the patient more vulnerable to High Risk for Peripheral Vascular Dysfunction:

- Fractures
- Mechanical compression
- Orthopedic surgery
- Trauma
- Peripheral revascularization
- Hematoma
- Snake/spider bites
- Postischemic swelling
- Crush injuries
- Electrical injuries
- Prolonged use of tourniquet
- Diabetes mellitus
- Vascular injuries
- Arterial insufficiency
- Venous insufficiency
- Thermal injuries

❖ Related Medical/Psychiatric Diagnoses

The following are examples of related medical/psychiatric diagnoses for High Risk for Peripheral Vascular Dysfunction:

- Angioneuropathy
- Atherosclerosis
- Burn injuries
- Cellulitis
- Diabetes mellitus
- Hypersomnia
- Orthopedic and vascular injuries
- Obesity
- Peripheral vascular dysfunction
- Pregnancy
- Right heart failure
- Thrombophlebitis

NURSING DIAGNOSES

Examples of *specific* nursing diagnoses for high risk for peripheral neurovascular dysfunction are:

- High risk for peripheral neurovascular dysfunction secondary to compartment syndrome
- High risk for peripheral neurovascular dysfunction secondary to complications of diabetes mellitus
- High risk for peripheral neurovascular dysfunction secondary to arterial insufficiency
- High risk for peripheral neurovascular dysfunction secondary to venous insufficiency

PLANNING AND IMPLEMENTATION WITH RATIONALE
Compartment Syndrome

Nursing interventions for patients who are at high risk for peripheral neurovascular dysfunction secondary to compartment syndrome *should be directed toward decreasing tissue pressure, restoring local blood flow, and minimizing functional loss*. The injured extremity should be kept at the level of the heart *to facilitate venous return*. Ice and elevation of the extremity are contraindicated because they may impair arterial circulation and venous return. External sources of pressure are avoided. Circumferential dressings and casts must be loosened or removed; air splints should be easily indented with a finger. Excessive cycling of blood pressure monitoring machines must be avoided. When pneumatic anti-shock garments are used, the duration and degree of inflation should be at the lowest possible setting *to maintain a systolic blood pressure of 100 mm Hg*. Fasciotomy is performed if the above interventions do not resolve the symptoms. Postfasciotomy care includes continued neurologic and vascular assessments, observation for signs of infection, and maintenance of joint mobility.[20]

Diabetes Mellitus

Nursing interventions for patients who are at high risk for peripheral neurovascular dysfunction secondary to diabetes mellitus *center on slowing the development and/or progression of the diabetic complications of arterial insufficiency and peripheral neuropathy*. In order to accomplish these goals, the nurse is primarily concerned with assisting the patient to maintain the blood glucose level within normal limits through diet, exercise, insulin/oral hypoglycemic agents, and weight control. Personal hygiene measures including general cleanliness of the hair, skin, nails, teeth, and clothing, are stressed. The patient should be educated regarding factors which aggravate diabetes mellitus, such as infection, stress, obesity, and the effects of these disease processes on the arterial vascular and neurologic systems. Teaching also includes instruction in the use of home blood glucose monitoring devices and the meaning and implications of the results.[3] The patient is instructed to report any paresthesias (spontaneous uncomfortable sensations), dysesthesias (contact paresthesias), and/or pains which may be superficial, deep, burning, shooting, stabbing, aching, or tearing. The patient is advised that he/she is at risk for burns and traumatic injuries because of decreased sensation as peripheral neuropathies develop.[4]

Arterial Insufficiency

Nursing interventions for patients who are at high risk for peripheral neurovascular dysfunction secondary to arterial insufficiency *should focus on improving blood supply, promoting skin integrity, and controlling pain*. Adequate hydration is essential to sustain the patient's cardiac output and promote peripheral blood flow. Systolic blood pressure should be maintained at the high-normal range to increase the driving pressure of the blood to the affected extremity.[11] Patients are instructed to avoid cigarette smoking as *nicotine stimulates the sympathetic nervous system and causes arterial constriction*. Nicotine also increases platelet aggregation, causing platelets to adhere to each other and placing the patient at risk for clot formation. Patients are advised to follow a low cholesterol, low-fat diet to decrease hyperlipidemia and slow the atherosclerotic process. Obese patients are advised to lose weight. A regular walking exercise program is recommended *to increase collateral circulation*.[8] While in bed, the knee gatch is used and patients are instructed to avoid crossing their legs and long periods of sitting or standing.[6]

In order *to promote skin integrity,* daily skin care, with particular attention to foot care, is performed. The skin should be thoroughly dried. Tight, constricting socks or hose should not be worn. Patients are advised to wear cotton socks and well-fitting, hard-soled shoes. Ulcerations are treated as they occur. In order *to alleviate pain,* analgesics can be used and the patient is placed in the position of most comfort.[6] The pharmacologic effects of anticoagulant, anti-platelet, or vasodilator therapy are monitored when these agents are prescribed. The patient is instructed in the use of these therapies.

Text continued on p. 416.

❖ *NURSING CARE GUIDELINES*

Nursing Diagnosis: High Risk for Peripheral Neurovascular Dysfunction

Expected Patient Outcomes	Nursing Interventions
The patient will have intact or maximal peripheral circulation.	• Assess extremities for pulse amplitude, color, temperature, capillary refill, and the presence and degree of edema. Compare with contralateral extremity. • Maintain systolic blood pressure in the high-normal range without compromising cardiac function. • Monitor for signs of bleeding if on anticoagulant therapy. • Monitor effects of pharmacologic therapy (i.e., vasodilators, anticoagulants, antiplatelet agents). • Educate the patient to activate venous pumps (i.e., dorsiflex, plantarflex the foot). • Position the extremity for maximal perfusion. If the arterial circulation is impaired, maintain the extremity in a dependent position. If the venous circulation is impaired, elevate the extremity above the level of the heart. • Maintain external graduated compression for impaired venous circulation. • Encourage walking. • Avoid prolonged standing, sitting, or crossing of the legs. • Avoid use of tight or constrictive clothing.
The patient will have intact or maximal peripheral sensation.	• Assess the extremity for sensation to touch, heat and cold, and two-point discrimination (hyperesthesia). Compare with the contralateral extremity. • Instruct the patient to report sensations such as "pins and needles." • Assess extremity pain with activity, at rest, and with changes in position. • Monitor for effectiveness and side effects of analgesics. • Avoid the use of ice, hot water bottles, and heating pads.
The patient will demonstrate full range of motion for affected extremity(ies).	• Assess the extremity for motor function, i.e., complete range of motion. Compare with the contralateral extremity. • Encourage walking to activate venous pumps and to improve calf muscle tone.

Continued.

IV

❖ *NURSING CARE GUIDELINES—cont'd*

Expected Patient Outcomes	Nursing Interventions
The patient will have or maintain skin integrity in affected extremity(ies).	• Assess the skin of the affected extremity for redness, shine, discoloration, hair loss, skin breakdown, or ulcerations. Compare with the contralateral extremity. • Keep the skin clean and dry. • Inspect the skin daily. • Encourage the patient to incorporate adequate protein, vitamins (A, B, C, D, and K), and minerals (zinc and iron) into the diet to maintain skin integrity and promote wound healing.
The patient will verbalize knowledge of risk factors and demonstrate safety measures and preventive actions.	• Assess the patient's level of knowledge regarding his/her condition. • Educate the patient regarding risk factors, i.e., nicotine use, careful blood glucose control if diabetic, exposure to extremes of temperature. • Educate the patient to avoid wearing circular garters, constricting garments or devices, crossing the legs, prolonged standing, and trauma to the affected extremities. • Encourage compliance in the use of compression stockings. • Encourage health promoting behaviors such as exercise, particularly walking, to promote the development of collateral circulation. • Instruct the patient to follow a low cholesterol, low fat diet to decrease the progression of atherosclerosis.

Venous Insufficiency

Nursing interventions for patients who are at high risk for peripheral vascular dysfunction secondary to venous insufficiency *should be directed toward reducing venous hypertension*. The nurse develops a plan of care that includes exercise, leg elevation, and compression therapy. Exercises involving positive ankle movements with full dorsiflexion and plantar flexion are encouraged. *Such exercises, particularly walking, activate venous pumps, which aid venous return to the heart.* Activities involving prolonged standing should be avoided because *these increase venous pressure*. The nurse advises the patient to elevate the legs, with the feet raised above the level of the heart. *This results in a decrease in venous pressure to zero with subsequent absorption of tissue fluid.*

Finally, compression stockings are recommended to improve calf muscle tone and reduce venous hypertension.[5,7]

EVALUATION

Evaluation of outcomes for the patient with a nursing diagnosis of High Risk for Peripheral Neurovascular Dysfunction focuses upon behavior modification and changes in lifestyle that promote and maintain circulatory and neurologic integrity. The patient should be able to describe the advantages of the recommended lifestyle changes and should be willing to engage in behaviors required to enhance circulatory and neurologic function. The occurrence of compartment syndrome is an emergency situation that requires intense and frequent monitoring of nursing interventions and subsequent patient outcomes.

❖ *CASE STUDY WITH PLAN OF CARE*

Mr. Nick C. is a 55-year-old government executive who visited the employee health unit for blood pressure monitoring and help with his diet. His physician had advised him to have his blood pressure monitored because at his last visit it was "borderline." Mr. C.'s past medical history is remarkable for hyperlipidemia for the past 10 years and noninsulin dependent diabetes mellitus. His hyperlipidemia is currently being treated with medications as diet modification initially failed. His noninsulin dependent diabetes mellitus is being treated with an oral hypoglycemic agent. He has been trying to make changes in his lifestyle to decrease his health risks despite having a very stressful job requiring long hours and frequent business travel. He stopped smoking 2 years ago and subsequently gained approximately 15 pounds. He drinks at least one alcoholic beverage every evening after work and beer or wine socially on weekends. He has occasional problems with insomnia. He exercises sporadically. He attempts to modify his diet by decreasing his intake of fats and sugars and increasing his intake of foods high in fiber. He also tries to eat three regular meals daily instead of skipping meals. He is intermittently successful with this diet because of job demands and business travel.

Physical examination revealed a well-groomed slightly overweight male who appears fit. His pulse was 72 and regular. His blood pressure was 142/90 mm Hg in the right arm and 138/92 mm Hg in the left arm while sitting. No significant postural changes were noted in his blood pressure. His heart sounds were normal. His lung fields were clear to auscultation. His abdomen was benign. His neuromuscular examination was normal except for complaints of paresthesia in both feet. He stated that his lower extremities have felt "cool" for several years. He has also noted numbness in his feet, especially at night, for the past three months. He attributes this to "being on his feet" all day. Pedal pulses were weak but equal bilaterally. Both feet demonstrated decreased sensitivity to sharp and dull touch. The skin of the feet was dry and cool with anhydrosis. Dependent rubor was noted bilaterally in the lower legs and feet. He stated that edema was occasionally present at the end of the day.

A plan of care was developed for Mr. C. that focused on patient education and prevention of peripheral neurovascular complications of hyperlipidemia and diabetes mellitus.

PLAN OF CARE FOR MR. NICK C.

Nursing Diagnosis: High Risk for Peripheral Neurovascular Dysfunction secondary to complications of diabetes mellitus and arterial insufficiency

Expected Patient Outcomes	Interventions
Mr. C. will have maximal peripheral circulation in his lower extremities.	• Assess the lower extremities for pulse amplitude, color, temperature, capillary refill, and edema. • Assess the lower extremities for sensation to touch. • Encourage Mr. C. to continue his exercise program and to walk daily on his lunch hour to stimulate circulation and the venous pump.
Mr. C. will perform good foot care.	• Instruct Mr. C. to wear well fitting shoes and not to go barefoot. • Instruct Mr. C. to inspect his feet daily, looking for areas of skin breakdown or redness. • Advise Mr. C. to dry his feet thoroughly after washing and to apply moisturizing lotions daily. • Advise Mr. C. to report to his physician any increase in numbness.

Continued.

Expected Patient Outcomes	Interventions
Mr. C. will verbalize the significance of dietary modifications to his current health problems.	• Educate Mr. C. about the role of dietary fat in the development of atherosclerosis and its subsequent impairment of circulation. • Encourage Mr. C. to continue to eat regular meals with high fiber and complex carbohydrate content. • Advise Mr. C. to decrease his alcohol intake. • Instruct Mr. C. in the use of a blood glucose monitoring device. • Encourage Mr. C. to monitor his blood glucose daily before breakfast.
Mr. C. will comply with safety precautions to minimize risks for neurovascular complications.	• Advise Mr. C. to avoid activities that require prolonged sitting or standing. • Advise Mr. C. to avoid exposure to extremes of temperature. • Advise Mr. C. to avoid wearing tight fitting clothing.

REFERENCES

1. Baker JD: Assessment of peripheral arterial occlusive disease, *Crit Care Nurs Clin North Am* 3(3):493-498, 1991.
2. Blank CA, Irwin GH: Peripheral vascular disorders: Assessment and intervention, *Nurs Clin North Am* 25(4):777-794, 1990.
3. Blissitt PA: Nursing management of diabetic peripheral neuropathies, *J Neurosci Nurs* 18(2):81-85, 1986.
4. Broadstone VL et al: Diabetic peripheral neuropathy. Part I: Sensorimotor neuropathy, *Diabetes Educ* 13(1):30-35, 1987.
5. Cameron J: Compression therapy: A lifetime experience, *Nursing Standard* 5(7):32-34, 1990.
6. Canobbio MM: Cardiovascular system. In Thompson JM, McFarland GK, Hirsch JE, Tucker SM, and Bowers AC, editors: *Clinical nursing*, ed 2, St Louis, 1989, Mosby–Year Book.
7. Ertl P: Allow the ulcer to heal: Treatment of leg ulcers, *Prof Nurse* 7(6):406-412, 1992.
8. Fellows E, Jocz AM: Getting the upper hand on lower extremity arterial disease, *Nursing 91* 21(8):34-42, 1991.
9. Gamron RB: Taking the pressure out of compartment syndrome, *Am J Nurs* 88(7):1076-1080, 1988.
10. Gehring PE: Perfecting the art—vascular assessment, *RN* 55(1):40-48, 1992.
11. Hubner C: Nursing management of the patient with an ischemic limb, *Prog in Cardiovasc Nurs* 3(4):115-122, 1988.
12. Jones WG, Perry MO, and Bush HL: Changes in tibial venous blood flow in the evolving compartment syndrome, *Arch Surg* 124:801-804, 1989.
13. Lagerstrom CF et al: Early fasciotomy for acute clinically evident posttraumatic compartment syndrome, *Am J Surg* 158:36-39, 1989.
14. North American Nursing Diagnosis Association (NANDA): *Description of proposed diagnoses, distributed with ballot following the Tenth Conference on the Classification of Nursing Diagnoses,* St Louis, 1992.
15. Peck SA: Crush syndrome: Pathophysiology and management, *Orthop Nurs* 9(3):33-40, 1990.
16. Price SA, Wilson LMcC: *Pathophysiology: Clinical concepts of disease processes,* ed 4, St Louis, 1992, Mosby–Year Book.
17. Proehl JA: Compartment syndrome, *J Emerg Nurs* 14(5):283-290, 1988.
18. Ross D: Acute compartment syndrome, *Orthop Nurs* 10(2):33-38, 1991.
19. Shah PM et al: Compartment syndrome in combined arterial and venous injuries of the lower extremity, *Am J Surg,* 158:136-141, 1989.
20. Slye DA: Orthopedic complications: Compartment syndrome, fat embolism syndrome, and venous thrombosis, *Nurs Clin North Am* 26(1):113-132, 1991.

IV

SLEEP-REST PATTERN
Sleep Pattern Disturbance

Sleep Pattern Disturbance is the state in which disruption of sleep time causes discomfort or interferes with an individual's desired lifestyle.[2]

OVERVIEW

Sleep has been identified as a basic human need[5] and a survival need.[11] Bahr[1] states: "The phenomenon of sleep has the potential for relieving an individual of stress and responsibility when a break is needed to recharge the person's spirit, mind, or body; or, it can remain maddeningly aloof when it is needed the most." Henderson[4] has described the inability to rest and sleep as "one of the causes, as well as one of the accompaniments, of disease." A knowledge of sleep stages and the potential effect of illness on this most basic human need, as well as interventions to promote sleep, is essential to nursing practice in any setting.

REM and NREM Sleep

Sleep occurs in two distinct stages, rapid eye movement (REM) and non-rapid eye movement (NREM), as determined by the electroencephalogram (EEG), electro-oculogram (EOG), and electromyogram (EMG). NREM sleep is further divided into four distinct stages. Stage 1 is a transitional stage between sleep and wakefulness. During stage 2 the individual becomes progressively more relaxed. A young adult typically spends 50% to 60% of total sleep time in NREM stage 1 or 2. NREM stages 3 and 4 are characterized by slow-frequency delta waves on the EEG and are differentiated by the relative percentage of these waves. NREM stages 3 and 4, the deeper stages of sleep, constitute about 20% of total sleep time. These are the restorative stages of sleep during which much protein synthesis and energy conservation occur.

During REM sleep, or paradoxic sleep, there are bursts of eye movements seen on the EOG. The large muscles of the body become functionally paralyzed. EEG activity increases so that there is a resemblance to the waking state. REM sleep constitutes 20% to 25% of the total sleep time and is the stage during which the individual is most difficult to awaken.

Sleep is cyclic. At its onset the individual normally progresses through repetitive cycles, beginning with NREM stages 1 through 4 and then back again to stage 2. From NREM stage 2, REM sleep is entered. Stage 2 is then reentered and the cycle repeats. These cycles occur at approximately 90-minute intervals, so that four or five cycles are normally completed in the sleep period.

Illness can decrease the amount, quality, and consistency of sleep. During illness, sleep is often interrupted or fragmented, altering the normal stages and cycles and producing dysfunctional sleep. With frequent interruptions the patient spends more time in the transitional stages (NREM 1 and 2) and less time in the deeper stages of sleep (NREM 3 and 4, REM). Thus total sleep time may decrease and selective deprivation of the deeper stages of sleep can occur as well.

Sleep is normally synchronized with the circadian rhythm; thus sleep normally occurs at the low phase of the circadian cycle. Sleep that is desynchronized is rated as poor in quality. Irritability, restlessness, daytime hypersomnolence, fatigue, tiredness, depression, anxiety, and decreased accuracy of task performance are characteristic effects of desynchronized sleep.[7] Barbiturates, sedatives, hypnotics, and analgesic medications may add to sleep disorders by promoting the lighter stages of sleep (NREM 2) and further decreasing NREM stages 3 and 4 and REM sleep. Knowledge of the effects of these drugs on sleep will assist the nurse in using them more effectively in patient care.

Sleep Disorders

Sleep disorders have been classified into four major categories: (1) disorders of initiating and maintaining sleep (DIMS), (2) disorders of excessive somnolence (DOES), (3) disorders of sleep-wake schedule, and (4) dysfunctions associated with sleep, sleep stages, or partial arousals.[8] This classification scheme labels sleep disorders according to a patient's symptoms rather than the actual etiology of the sleep disorder. Sleep Pattern Disturbance is a broad nursing diagnosis that can imply any one of these four categories of sleep disorders.

A variety of health problems may result in either of the first two categories of sleep disorders, DIMS and DOES. People with affective disorders, psychophysiological illnesses, and sleep-related syndromes such as sleep apnea, myoclonus, or "restless legs" may have difficulty initiating and maintaining sleep or may exhibit excessive sleepiness. Sustained use of central nervous system (CNS) stimulants, as well as tolerance to or withdrawal from CNS depressants, can result in DIMS. Excessive sleepiness often occurs in patients who regularly use CNS depressants; it also is a symptom of narcolepsy and idiopathic CNS hypersomnolence.

The third category of sleep disorders, disorders of the sleep-wake schedule, relates to circadian desynchronization. When a person has a frequently changing sleep-wake schedule (for example, the nurse who has consistent work shift changes), a sudden change in a usual sleep-wake schedule (for example, the student who stays up all night studying for an exam), or a rapid time zone change (for example, jet lag syndrome), the usual sleep-wake pattern can be interfered with or disrupted. The fourth category, dysfunctions associated with sleep, sleep stages, or partial arousals, includes enuresis, somnambulism (sleepwalking), dream anxiety attacks (nightmares), and sleep-related headaches, seizures, and cardiovascular symptoms. Both disruptions in the sleep-wake schedule and sleep dysfunctions can result in difficulty in initiating or maintaining sleep or excessive sleepiness. By classifying disorders in separate categories, assessment and subsequent interventions focus on treating the particular disorder or dysfunction.

ASSESSMENT

Sleep is a complex physiological phenomenon influenced by pathophysiologic, physical, psychological, environmental, and maturational factors.[6] Sleep patterns are highly individual, and their natural pattern should be assessed for each individual. The cyclic pattern of sleep stages for REM and NREM sleep and the circadian rhythmic synchronization of sleep are influenced by chronic and acute illness, stress, age, pain, medications, changes in sleep environment, e.g., during hospitalization; sensory overload and deprivation, and lifestyle disruptions. Because of this complexity, assessment requires a holistic approach.

To determine whether a patient has a disturbance in his/her sleep pattern, the nurse should direct the assessment to obtain data in the following areas: the patient's perception of his/her sleep experience, the patient's past and present sleep patterns, objective characteristics indicating that the patient has a Sleep Pattern Disturbance, and the presence of factors that may be altering the patient's sleep pattern.

Patients' perception of the adequacy and effectiveness of the sleep experience is particularly important in determining whether they have a Sleep Pattern Disturbance. The nurse should question patients to obtain information about sleep duration and quality. If patients indicate that they have a sleep disturbance, the nurse should ask open-ended questions, such as "Describe your sleep problem." Although patients may be able to report sleep duration (actual time slept), they may not accurately report perceived quality of sleep unless prompted by the nurse. The nurse can ask patients about ease or delay in falling asleep, the soundness of sleep, sleep interruptions, ease or difficulty in awakening, and how they feel on awakening.[9]

When gathering the information about a patient's most recent sleep experience, the nurse should determine whether the patient's present sleep pattern differs from previous sleep patterns. If the patient reports a sleep problem of long duration, factors influencing the problem and the patient's usual manner of coping with the problem should be explored. If the sleep problem has occurred recently, the nurse and the patient should attempt to identify changes in the patient's physiological and psychological health, lifestyle, and environment that may be related to the problem. Sleep aids (such as reading material or back rubs) and sleep rituals or routines that the patient has found helpful in the past should be explored.

While asking the patient questions about his/her sleep experience, the nurse should observe the patient's appearance and behavior. Physical signs, such as dozing during the day, an expressionless face, ptosis of the eyelids, hand tremors, drooping shoulders, and mispronunciation or incorrect use of words, indicate that the patient may have a Sleep Pattern Disturbance. Behavioral signs can include restlessness, lethargy, irritability, agitation, disorientation, and listlessness.

The diagnosis of Sleep Pattern Disturbance requires the nurse and the patient to further assess for and evaluate the factors that may be contributing to the disruption in sleep duration and quality. When assessing the adequacy of a patient's sleep pattern, maturational factors must be considered. Required sleep time is greatest in infancy, decreases in childhood, stabilizes in adulthood, and then begins to decline in the older adult. Awakenings during the night are expected during infancy and childhood and tend to occur in the later adult years as well.

Physiological, psychological, and environmental factors, as well as the patient's lifestyle, must also be explored. The nurse and the patient must understand the specific factor or factors contributing to the sleep problem to determine whether to seek input from other health care providers and, consequently, plan and implement effective interventions.

❖ Defining Characteristics

The presence of the following defining characteristics indicates the patient may be experiencing Sleep Pattern Disturbance:

- Physical signs (e.g., mild, fleeting nystagmus; slight hand tremor; ptosis of eyelids; expressionless face; thick speech with mispronunciation or incorrect use of words; frequent yawning; and changes in posture—sagging or head drooping)
- Verbal complaints of difficulty sleeping
- Difficulty awakening
- Fragmented sleep
- Verbal complaints of not feeling well rested
- Daytime sleepiness
- Fatigue
- Changes in behavior and performance (e.g., increasing irritability, restlessness, agitation, decreased attention span, disorientation, lethargy, listlessness, and decreased arousal threshold)

❖ Related Factors

The following related factors are associated with Sleep Pattern Disturbance:

- Impaired oxygen transport (e.g., cardiopulmonary disease or peripheral arteriosclerosis)
- Impaired bowel or bladder elimination
- Impaired metabolism (e.g., hyperthyroidism or hepatic disorders)
- Sleep apnea
- Stress
- Anxiety
- Fear
- Depression
- Psychiatric disorders
- Change in sleep-wake pattern (e.g., change in work shift, rapid time zone change, or decrease in sleep time)
- Change in sleep routine

- Immobility (e.g., traction, casts, or restraints)
- Inadequate physical exercise
- Pain
- Pregnancy
- Effects of medications or drugs (e.g., tranquilizers, barbiturates, monoamine oxidase inhibitors, amphetamines, hypnotics, antidepressants, antihypertensives, sedatives, anesthetics, steroids, decongestants, caffeine, or alcohol)
- Change in activity pattern
- Hospitalization
- Unfamiliar or uncomfortable sleep environment
- Increased sensory stimulation (e.g., noise or bright lighting)

❖ Related Medical/Psychiatric Diagnoses

The following are examples of related medical/psychiatric diagnoses for Sleep Pattern Disturbance:

- Central sleep apnea
- Disorders of excessive somnolence (DOES)
- Disorders of initiating and maintaining sleep (DIMS)
- Disorders of sleep-wake schedule
- Insomnia
- Narcolepsy
- Obstructive sleep apnea

NURSING DIAGNOSES

Examples of *specific* nursing diagnoses for Sleep Pattern Disturbance are:

- Sleep Pattern Disturbance related to fear secondary to impending surgery for cancer.
- Sleep Pattern Disturbance related to circadian desynchronization secondary to prolonged hospitalization and critical illness.
- Sleep Pattern Disturbance related to chronic pain.
- Sleep Pattern Disturbance related to situational depression.

PLANNING AND IMPLEMENTATION WITH RATIONALE

The ultimate goal in planning care for patients with Sleep Pattern Disturbances is to eliminate or control the alteration in sleep. Patient outcomes that will help patients achieve this goal should be identified. *Most essential to eliminating or controlling the sleep alteration is the patient's knowledge of the factors that contribute to Sleep Pattern Disturbances and the factors that can contribute to correcting an altered sleep pattern.* The patient, if able, should actively participate in identifying problem areas, mutually setting goals, and implementing measures that will enhance the sleep experience.

Teaching the patient and significant others about the influence that physiological factors (for example, pain or impaired bladder function), psychological factors (for example, stress or anxiety), lifestyle factors (for example changes in activity pattern or sleep routine or rituals), and environmental factors (for example, an uncomfortable sleep environment) have on the sleep experience will assist the patient in controlling the factors that contribute to his/her sleep problem. *To assist the patient in identifying and adopting measures that will support an adequate sleep pattern,* the nurse should provide the patient with information about specific sleep-promoting techniques (such as relaxation exercises and music therapy) and recommend potential changes in lifestyle that will promote an optimal balance of rest and activity (such as low to moderate-intensity long-term exercise.[10] If the patient's sleep-wake schedule is disrupted, activities should be planned during the day to stimulate wakefulness and comfort measures employed at night to promote sleep.

The hospital and home routines and environments should be adapted *to support the patient's most effective sleep pattern.* Every effort should be made to accommodate the patient's usual sleep time. The patient should be awakened only for essential care or treatment tasks; awakenings should allow for sleep cycles of at least 90 minutes to allow for adequate NREM and REM sleep time.

Text continued on p. 424

❖ *NURSING CARE GUIDELINES*

Nursing Diagnosis: Sleep Pattern Disturbance

Expected Patient Outcomes	Nursing Interventions
The patient will describe factors that contribute to sleep pattern disturbance and factors that promote an optimal sleep pattern.	• Educate the patient and significant others about sleep and rest needs and about factors that contribute to sleep pattern disturbances (see Related Factors). • Explore with the patient and family physiological, psychological, lifestyle, and environmental factors that may be interfering with the patient's sleep. • Discuss with the patient and family comfort measures, sleep-promoting techniques, and lifestyle changes that can contribute to an optimal sleep experience. • Evaluate sleep-promoting measures to determine which may be most helpful to the patient.
The patient will demonstrate an optimal balance between sleep and activity.	• Assess the patient's past and present sleep and activity patterns. • Plan for activities during the daytime to stimulate wakefulness, and use measures to promote sleep at night. • Assist the patient to maintain normal day-night cycles by decreasing lighting, noise, and sensory stimulation at night. • Plan nap time of at least 90 minutes to assist in equilibrating normal sleep time and in promoting REM sleep.
The patient will verbalize increased satisfaction with sleep pattern.	• Implement measures that patient/family feel may promote an optimal sleep pattern. • Promote comfort, relaxation, and a sense of well-being. • Eliminate stressful situations before bedtime; use of relaxation techniques may be helpful. • Minimize awakenings; allow for sleep cycles of at least 90 minutes. • Monitor physiological parameters without awakening the patient whenever possible. • Reduce environmental stimuli at nighttime. • Assess the effects of the patient's medications on his/her sleep pattern. • Encourage the patient to carry out usual bedtime rituals and routines when possible. • Assess the effectiveness of sleep-promoting measures each day.

V

The environment, especially noise, lighting, and sensory stimulation, should be controlled to support the patient's comfort and promote sleep. The nurse should use a flashlight rather than the overhead light when possible for patient checks at night.

The medications that the patient receives should be evaluated for the effects that they have on sleep. *Many sedative and hypnotic medications decrease REM sleep.* Drugs that minimally disrupt sleep should be used to complement comfort measures and techniques that promote sleep, and, when possible, drug dosages should be reduced as the medication becomes less necessary. Diuretics may interrupt sleep by increasing the number of awakenings; therefore they should not be scheduled after 4 P.M. Fluid intake at bedtime may also cause the patient to awaken during the night. The patient can be instructed to take fluids during the day and to restrict intake 2 hours before retiring.

EVALUATION

The nurse should evaluate the care plan and its implementation on an ongoing basis. The patient's perception of the adequacy and effectiveness of the sleep experience should be assessed daily to determine the appropriateness of the interventions and changes that should be made. Because the adequacy of sleep is very difficult to evaluate clinically, nurses need to use research to guide their practice. In a study of 20 trauma patients in an ICU setting, Fontaine[3] found that nursing observation of patient wakefulness provides valid assessment data and can be used to evaluate nursing interventions that promote sleep.

The patient's perception of the duration and quality of sleep as well as his/her perception of the assistance provided by the comfort measures, sleep-promoting techniques, and lifestyle changes, are critical to evaluating care. The patient's ability to control factors that disrupt sleep and to implement measures that enhance sleep should be determined. The patient's ability and desire to participate in his/her own care through mutual goal setting are essential to maintain an adequate and effective sleep pattern on a long-term basis. In essence, the patient's sleep pattern should promote feelings of being well rested and of satisfaction with the sleep experience.

❖ *CASE STUDY WITH PLAN OF CARE*

Mrs. Wilma E., a 59-year-old widow, was admitted to the medical unit for treatment of cellulitis of the right arm. On the third hospital day, the nurse noted that Mrs. E. appeared lethargic and listless; Mrs. E. yawned frequently during the interaction with the nurse and had difficulty concentrating. Mrs. E. was responding to the intravenous antibiotics she had been receiving; over the past 3 days, her temperature had gone from 102.6° F to 99.6° F, and her respirations, pulse, and blood pressure were within normal limits. The nurse commented to Mrs. E. that she looked tired and asked whether Mrs. E. was having difficulty sleeping. Mrs. E. stated that she hadn't really slept well since she has been in the hospital. The assessment revealed that at home Mrs. E. slept 7 to 8 hours each night and maintained an active schedule during the day. She usually drank a cup of hot chocolate and read before she went to sleep, and she stated that she rarely had difficulty falling asleep or maintaining sleep. In the hospital, Mrs. E. was in a semiprivate room; she stated that she didn't read at night, because she feared that the light would keep her roommate awake. She also stated that when she was awakened at night to have her vital signs taken, she had difficulty falling back to sleep. She said that during the day she tried to take "cat naps" to catch up on her sleep and because she had little else to do.

PLAN OF CARE FOR MRS. WILMA E.

Nursing Diagnosis: Sleep Pattern Disturbance related to hospital environment and change in bedtime routine

Expected Patient Outcomes	Nursing Interventions
Mrs. E. will describe factors that contribute to her Sleep Pattern Disturbance and measures that will enhance her sleep pattern.	• Explore with Mrs. E. the factors interfering with her sleep that can be changed. • Suggest that Mrs. E. have one of her family members bring a small reading lamp or a book light so that she can feel comfortable reading at night. • Encourage Mrs. E. to ask the evening staff to prepare a cup of hot chocolate, if she feels it will help her to fall asleep. • Evaluate the need to monitor Mrs. E.'s vital signs during the night. • Inform the night staff of the importance of using minimal lighting when monitoring Mrs. E.'s vital signs and administering intravenous medications.
Mrs. E. will demonstrate an optimal balance between activity and sleep-rest pattern.	• Encourage Mrs. E. to take walks in the hospital corridors during the day. • Explore with Mrs. E. diversional activities that may interest her and occupy her time. • Provide Mrs. E. with reading material that she might enjoy. • Assist Mrs. E. in planning a specific nap time to assist in equilibrating her normal sleep and activity pattern. • Reduce the light in the room and the noise near the room during Mrs. E.'s planned nap time.
Mrs. E. will express increased satisfaction with her sleep-rest pattern.	• Evaluate the effectiveness of Mrs. E.'s attempts to implement her usual sleep routine. • Discuss with Mrs. E. and the evening and night staff the effectiveness of the measures taken to reduce stimuli during the nighttime nursing tasks. • Evaluate with Mrs. E. whether the daytime activities have contributed toward achieving an adequate and effective sleep experience. • Assess the effectiveness of the care plan, and with Mrs. E. make necessary changes.

REFERENCES

1. Bahr R: Sleep-wake patterns in the aged, *J Gerontol Nurs* 9(10):534, 1983.
2. Carroll-Johnson RM, editor: *Classification of nursing diagnoses: proceedings of the Eighth Conference,* Philadelphia, 1989, JB Lippincott Co.
3. Fontaine DK: Measurement of nocturnal sleep patterns in trauma patients, *Heart Lung* 18 (4):402-410, 1989.
4. Henderson V: *Basic principles of nursing care,* New York, 1969, Macmillan Publishing.
5. Maslow A: *Motivation and personality,* New York, 1970, Harper & Row.
6. McLane AM: *Classification of nursing diagnoses: proceedings of the seventh conference,* St Louis, 1987, CV Mosby.
7. Sanford S: Sleep and the cardiovascular patient, *Cardiovasc Nurs* 19(5):19, 1983.
8. Sleep Disorders Classification Committee, Association of Sleep Disorders Centers: Diagnostic classification of sleep and arousal disorders, *Sleep* 2:1-137, 1979.
9. Snyder-Halpern R, Verran JA: Instrumentation to describe subjective sleep characteristics in healthy subjects, *Res Nurs Health* 10:155-163, 1987.
10. Stevenson JS: Effects of moderate and low intensity long-term exercise by older adults, *Res Nurs Health* 13(4):209-281, 1990.
11. Yura H, Walsh MB: *The nursing process: assessing, planning, implementing, evaluating,* Norwalk, 1988, Appleton & Lange.

V

VI

COGNITIVE-PERCEPTUAL PATTERN

Pain

Chronic Pain

Pain *is an unpleasant sensory and emotional experience associated with actual or potential tissue damage or described in terms of such damage.[1]*

Chronic Pain *is pain that persists a month beyond the usual course of an acute disease or reasonable time for an injury to heal, or pain that reoccurs at intervals for months or years.[5]*

OVERVIEW

The North American Nursing Diagnosis Association (NANDA) includes the diagnoses of Pain and Chronic Pain on its official list of approved diagnoses. Inclusion on the list indicates that a diagnosis shows readiness for use and continuing development. The taxonomy or classification system for nursing diagnoses classifies Pain and Chronic Pain under the category of altered comfort, which is included in the human response pattern of feeling, one of the nine organizing patterns of the taxonomy.[8] Pain as a nursing diagnosis is classified on a higher level than Chronic Pain, indicating that pain is a phenomenon that is more general than Chronic Pain, and it lacks the clinical specificity inherent in the diagnosis of Chronic Pain.

Acute pain, although not yet accepted as a nursing diagnosis by NANDA, is considered by pain experts to be distinct from chronic pain in terms of definition, signs and symptoms, and management.[1,4,21] For the purpose of this chapter, the phenomenon of Pain is described in general terms, and the phenomenon is operationalized via the nursing process in terms of acute and Chronic Pain.

The Phenomenon of Pain

Pain is a complex phenomenon. Whereas it is an experience that is very real to the person who experiences it, its varying characteristics and nebulous quality often make it difficult for others to comprehend.[21] "Pain is a subjective experience that can be perceived directly only by the sufferer. It is a multidimensional phenomenon that can be described by pain location, intensity, temporal aspects, quality, impact, and meaning. Pain does not occur in isolation but in a specific human being in psychosocial, economic, and cultural contexts that influence the meaning, experience, and verbal and nonverbal expression of pain."

McCaffery offers an operational definition of Pain that is useful in the clinical setting: "Pain is whatever the experiencing person says it is, existing whenever he says it does."[17] This definition implies the personal, subjective nature of Pain and the responsibility of others to infer the presence of Pain based on the patient's communication of the experience. The patient's verbal and nonverbal behaviors, that is, what the patient says and does, become critical in determining whether the patient is experiencing Pain. The patient's communications can be used to further define and describe the specific pain experience as it relates to the patient's perception.

To increase understanding of the phenomenon of Pain and the pain experience, various theories have been proposed. Three theories are frequently found to be mentioned in the literature on Pain: specificity theory, pattern theory, and gate control theory.[6,14,20] Each of these theories addresses pain transmission and therefore could have implications for pain control. The gate control theory, which was proposed in 1965, gained wide acceptance and stimulated significant clinical research related to pain response and control. The theory suggests that the transmission of painful stimuli can be modulated through a gating mechanism located in the substantia gelatinosa in the dorsal horn of the spinal cord. It is thought that activity in the peripheral and central nervous systems could affect the opening and closing of the gate. Studies related to specific pain modulatory systems have supplemented the theory's description of pain transmission and enhanced understanding of the neural mechanisms underlying the variability of the pain experience.[11]

In addressing the variability of the experience, the patient's perception of and reaction to Pain must also be considered. Loeser[16] considers transmission, perception, and reaction in his description of the phenomenon of Pain in terms of four components: nociception, pain, suffering, and pain behavior. Nociception involves the brain's detection of tissue damage and physiological transmission of pain. The component of pain is described as the patient's perception of a nociceptive stimulus; this occurs in the brain stem. Suffering refers to the patient's affective response to pain; this involves the higher levels of the brain. Pain behavior includes "anything a person says or does or does not do that would lead one to infer that a noxious stimulus has occurred"[16] pain behaviors are influenced by environmental factors.

Classifications of Pain

Because of the multidimensional nature of Pain, clinicians find it useful to classify Pain into two major types: acute and chronic. Such a classification assists the clinician in determining an appropriate plan for pain management. Acute and Chronic Pain typically are differentiated from one another according to the onset, duration, and cause of the Pain.

Acute Pain. Bonica[6] defines acute Pain as "a constellation of unpleasant sensory, perceptual, and emotional experiences and certain associated autonomic, psychologic, emotional, and behavioral responses." Acute Pain is an event of recent onset, is usually sudden, and is limited in duration. It is associated with an acute illness/disease, operative or treatment procedures, or trauma, and the Pain subsides as healing takes place.[1] Other characteristics that distinguish acute Pain from Chronic Pain include (1) the pain area is usually identifiable, (2) suffering decreases over time, (3) defining characteristics are more obvious, and (4) there is a likelihood of eventual, complete relief.

Chronic Pain. Chronic Pain is a situation or state of existence characterized by the pain experience continuing a month after healing of an acute disease or injury should have been achieved, or recurring at intervals for months or years.[5] Although some clinicians[7,12-14] use 6 months as the time frame during which pain continues before being classified as Chronic Pain, Bonica[5] considers 6 months to be an arbitrary figure—one that can delay instituting effective therapy and may result in irreversible processes.

"Chronic pain is an ongoing experience of embodied discomfort that fails either to heal naturally or to respond to normal forms of medical intervention."[15] Arthritis, low back injury, migraine headache, neuralgia, and diabetic neuropathy are examples of conditions that can result in Chronic Pain. Characteristics distinguishing Chronic Pain from acute include (1) the pain area is less easily differentiated; (2) the pain intensity becomes more difficult to evaluate; (3) suffering usually increases over time; (4) defining characteristics are less obvious; and (5) there is little likelihood of complete relief. With Chronic Pain "pain itself becomes the patient's pathology and is considered a syndrome, the primary diagnosis and not just a symptom."[18]

Chronic Pain is frequently subdivided into two categories: chronic malignant and chronic nonmalignant pain.[21] Chronic malignant pain is described as pain associated with cancer or other progressive disorders. Chronic nonmalignant pain refers to pain in persons whose tissue injury is nonprogressive or healed. This type of pain is sometimes referred to as chronic benign pain, resistant pain, or persistent pain. The terms *intractable pain, limited pain,* and *chronic cancer pain* are often used to refer to chronic malignant pain.

The ability to distinguish between acute and Chronic Pain will assist the clinician in making a differential diagnosis that is necessary to identify realistic patient outcomes and appropriate nursing interventions.

ASSESSMENT

A thorough assessment of a patient's pain experience requires the nurse to gather subjective data that present the patient's perspective. The patient should be queried as to the location, characteristics (shooting, radiating, deep, superficial), onset/duration, frequency (constant/intermittent), quality (what the pain feels like), and intensity or severity of the pain. It is also important to determine if the patient can identify factors that precipitate or aggravate the pain. Information related to the type and effectiveness of pain control measures that have been employed in the past should also be noted. This information will assist the nurse in determining whether the Pain is acute or chronic in nature.

In addition to the patient's description of the pain experience, the nurse collects psychologic and sociocultural data that will assist the nurse in understanding the patient's interpretation of and reaction to the pain experience. Psychological determinants of pain expression can be assessed in terms of (1) affective factors (emotions such as fear, anxiety, and anger), (2) cognitive/behavioral factors (beliefs and behaviors related to the mean-

ing attributed to the pain, learned responses to pain and injury, and situational factors influencing the patient's overt expression of pain), and (3) constitutional factors (related to the personality or physiologic makeup of the patient and representing tendencies to respond to pain in normal, exaggerated, or understated ways).[10]

The patient's age, sex, religion, cultural and social background, available family and support systems, and employment responsibilities are influencing factors that can affect the patient's response to Pain.[13,18] Culture is of special interest in assessing the individual patient's interpretation of the pain experience and its concomitant emotional arousal. "Because the meaning of any given pain experience is defined by the culture in which it occurs, the total experience differs across cultures."[10]

Data specific to a patient's "pain history" provides valuable information that will contribute to a valid pain assessment and to effective pain management. The Agency for Health Care Policy and Research[1] identified seven areas that should be explored through the "pain history":

1. Significant previous and/or ongoing instances of pain and its effect on the patient;
2. Previously used methods for pain control that the patient has found either helpful or unhelpful;
3. The patient's attitude toward and use of opioid, anxiolytic, or other medications, including history of substance abuse;
4. The patient's typical coping response for stress or pain, including more broadly, the presence or absence of psychiatric disorders such as depression, anxiety, or psychosis;
5. Family expectations and beliefs concerning pain, stress, and postoperative course (or the disease process or healing of trauma);
6. Ways the patient describes or shows pain; and
7. The patient's knowledge of, expectations about, and preferences for pain management methods and for receiving information about pain management.

Assessing Pain in children requires that the assessment strategies be tailored to the child's developmental level and personality style and to the particular situation.[2] The pain history may be obtained from the child and/or the parents. Information such as the words the child uses to express Pain, previous pain experiences, the child's usual verbal and nonverbal reactions to Pain, and what works best to decrease or take away the child's Pain will be valuable to the ongoing Pain assessment as well as determining the most effective interventions.

The subjective data should be complemented by objective data gained through the nurse's careful observations of the patient's behavioral response. These data are especially crucial in assessing for the presence of Pain in infants, small children, and noncommunicative adults. Physiological signs and observed patient behaviors can indicate that a patient is experiencing Pain. These signs and behaviors may differ depending on whether the patient is experiencing acute or Chronic Pain, and they are therefore presented with the discussion of assessment as it relates to each of these types of Pain.

A variety of measures that can assist in assessing a patient's pain experience have been developed. Verbal self-reporting instruments can range from a listing of questions that require the patient to make a simple "yes" or "no" response to a list of questions that elicit descriptive responses. Pain flowcharts can be used to maintain an ongoing record of the patient's evaluation of the pain characteristics, intensity, and frequency and the nurse's observation of the patient's physiological and behavioral responses. Visual analog scales can provide a relatively simple means to measure the various dimensions of Pain. For example, to measure the intensity of the pain experience, the patient could be asked to mark a point on a horizontal line that represents a continuum of pain intensity that ranges from no pain to unbearable pain, with points in between representing various grades of intensity.

One of the better known pain assessment tools is the McGill-Melzack Pain Questionnaire. The questionnaire, a four-page tool that is recommended for use during the initial assessment, measures sensory, affective, and evaluative dimensions of Pain. Types of pain experiences, methods of pain relief, and pain patterns can be differentiated through use of the questionnaire.[19,21] One longer and three shorter versions of the questionnaire are available and used in clinical practice.[24]

McCaffery and Beebe[17] offer both an initial pain assessment tool and a pain flow sheet that are "practical in any clinical situation and easily adapted to an individual patient's needs." The initial assessment tool addresses 10 areas: location; intensity; quality; onset, duration variations, and rhythms; manner of expressing Pain; what relieves the Pain; what causes or increases the Pain; effects of pain; other comments; and the plan. The flow sheet provides a means to track frequency and intensity of Pain, the analgesic(s) used to treat Pain, changes in the patient's vital signs, the patient's level of arousal, other observations, and the plan.

Choice of a measuring tool to assess Pain will depend on the patient's physical response and pain behavior. For example, a patient experiencing intense pain may be restless and irritable and may withdraw from social contact. In such a case attempts should be made to elicit from the patient only the simplest descriptors of the pain experience. Questions requiring "yes" and "no" answers would be more appropriate than those requiring complex responses.

Acute Pain

The patient experiencing acute Pain will describe Pain that is intense and of short duration. The nurse may observe that the patient is protective of and guards the area of the body where the pain is focused. The patient's attention may be introverted, and a withdrawal from social contact may occur; thought processes may appear to be impaired, giving the impression that the patient is confused or disoriented. Distraction behaviors such as moaning, whimpering, crying, rubbing, and pacing are often observed, and irritability, restlessness, and agitation may be noted. The pa-

VI

tient may assume an unusual posture, for instance, knees drawn to abdomen.

The face of the patient experiencing acute Pain usually mirrors the pain experience. The "facial mask of pain" reflects a beaten look; facial features may appear pinched, jaw muscles tight, and teeth clenched; eyes may lack luster and be either widely open or tightly shut; and eyebrows may be knotted. The portrait of the patient experiencing acute Pain may be either vivid with well-defined characteristics or blurred with few defining characteristics.

Physiological signs that indicate the patient may be experiencing acute Pain include changes in blood pressure and pulse rate, increased or decreased respiratory rate, dilated pupils, diaphoresis, and increased muscle tension. The patient may complain of nausea.

Knowledge and understanding of the factor(s) contributing to the acute pain experience will guide the nurse and the patient in identifying realistic outcomes for the patient and nursing interventions that will support the patient in the achievement of the outcomes. The related factors for acute Pain can be classified into physiological factors and psychological factors. The physiological factors include trauma to tissue as a result of injury, disease, or surgery; invasive diagnostic tests such as venipuncture and cystoscopic examination; allergic responses that invoke painful sensations (such as "burning" skin); and untoward effects of a therapeutic treatment (such as a tight cast or dressing exerting pressure that interrupts circulation). Psychological factors include a lack of knowledge of techniques that could support pain control and anxiety. Whereas anxious behavior could be considered a defining characteristic, its role in triggering and influencing the intensity of the acute pain episode indicates inclusion as a related factor.

❖ Defining Characteristics

The presence of the following defining characteristics* indicates that the patient may be experiencing acute Pain:

- Verbal report of intense, limited pain experience
- Protective guarding behavior
- Self-focusing
- Narrowed focus
- Withdrawal from social contact
- Altered time perception
- Impaired thought process
- Distraction behaviors (e.g., moaning, whimpering, crying, rubbing, pacing)
- Irritability
- Restlessness
- Agitation
- Facial mask of pain (e.g., "beaten look," pinched features, tightened jaw muscles, clenched teeth, lackluster eyes, widely open/tightly shut eyes, knotted brows)
- Unusual posture
- Blood pressure and pulse rate change
- Increased or decreased respiratory rate
- Dilated pupils
- Diaphoresis
- Increased muscle tension

❖ Related Factors

The following related factors* are associated with acute Pain:

- Tissue trauma (e.g., injury, disease, surgery)
- Invasive diagnostic tests (e.g., venipuncture and bone marrow aspiration)
- Allergic responses
- Therapeutic treatment effects (e.g., cast causing extreme pressure or rabies vaccine)
- Lack of knowledge of pain control techniques
- Anxiety

❖ Related Medical/Psychiatric Diagnoses

The following are examples of related medical/psychiatric diagnoses for acute Pain:

- Acute Pancreatitis
- Appendicitis
- Burns
- Carpal tunnel syndrome
- Cellulitis

*References 1, 7, 12, 17, 18, 23

- Cholecystitis
- Depressive disorder with suicidal attempt (e.g., slashing wrists)
- Gastric ulcer
- Migraine headache
- Myocardial infarction
- Orthopedic injuries
- Otitis media
- Pelvic inflammatory disease
- Pulmonary emboli
- Psychoactive substance use disorders (dependence/withdrawal)
- Renal calculi
- Thrombophlebitis
- Tissue trauma (including surgical wounds and lacerations)

Chronic Pain

The patient experiencing Chronic Pain is not as likely to report the pain experience as is the patient with acute Pain. Chronic Pain has an enduring quality and becomes a stable element in the patient's daily life.[9]

Often the patient who is haunted by Chronic Pain has learned to accept the Pain as a condition of life. The nurse must be alert to the presence of defining characteristics that indicate the patient may be experiencing Chronic Pain. Some of the characteristics of Chronic Pain are the same as those listed for acute Pain; the difference rests in the more subtle and persistent nature of those characteristics as they relate to Chronic Pain.

Protective guarding behavior of the area where the Pain is concentrated often will become incorporated into the patient's manner of body positioning and movement. Chronic Pain can consume the patient's energy, and the patient may be overwhelmed by the search for pain relief or the efforts required to cope with the pain sensation. Irritability, restlessness, and depression may be noted more frequently.

The patient may experience an altered ability to maintain involvement in usual activities. As a result family and social relationships that have offered the patient support in the past may be disrupted. Weight changes related to anorexia and changes in the patient's sleep pattern often occur. The "facial mask of Chronic Pain" may reveal a "beaten," drawn look, the eyes may lack luster, and the eyebrows appear knotted.

The factors contributing to Chronic Pain include conditions in which tissue injury is nonprogressive or healed (for instance, low back pain resulting from arthritis or an injury incurred in the past). A chronic physical disability can also contribute to Chronic Pain. An example of this would be a patient who has an extreme limp as a result of a serious injury to the left leg. The patient may experience Chronic Pain in the right leg related to attempts to compensate for the limp. A deficit in knowledge of the measures that may be used to control Chronic Pain can also contribute to the chronic pain experience.

It is important to note that in the discussion of Chronic Pain, the term is used in the context of chronic nonmalignant, nonprogressive pain. Pain associated with cancer or other progressive disorders (chronic malignant pain) requires the nurse to assess for the characteristics of both acute and Chronic Pain. The patient with this type of Pain often experiences the intensity of the acute pain experience and the duration of the chronic pain experience. Assessment of psychological function is especially important, because the patient must cope with both the diagnosis of a progressive disease and the prospect of progressive intensity of Pain.

❖ Defining Characteristics

The presence of the following defining characteristics* indicates that the patient may be experiencing Chronic Pain:

- Verbal report of pain experience lasting for more than 1 month beyond usual course of acute disease or healing of an injury
- Protective guarding behavior
- Self-focusing
- Disruption of family and social relationships
- Altered ability to continue previous activities
- Irritability
- Restlessness
- Depression
- Changes in sleep pattern

---

*References 5, 7, 12, 13, 15, 23

VI

- Weight changes
- Facial mask of pain (e.g., "beaten look," lack-luster eyes, knotted brows)

❖ Related Factors

The following related factors are associated with Chronic Pain:
- Chronic condition/disease
- Chronic physical disability
- Deficit in knowledge of measures used to control Chronic Pain

❖ Related Medical/Psychiatric Diagnoses

The following are examples of related medical/psychiatric diagnoses for Chronic Pain:
- Cancer
- Chronic hepatitis
- Chronic pancreatitis
- Connective tissue diseases
- Cystitis
- Dyspareunia
- Peripheral vascular diseases
- Posttraumatic insults (e.g., phantom limb pain, low back pain)
- Rheumatoid arthritis
- Vaginismus

NURSING DIAGNOSES

Examples of *specific* nursing diagnoses for acute Pain are:
- Acute Pain related to median nerve compression secondary to carpal tunnel syndrome.
- Acute Pain related to osseous periodontal surgery.
- Acute Pain related to fear of becoming addicted to prescribed medication and lack of knowledge of effects of prescribed medication.

Examples of *specific* nursing diagnoses for Chronic Pain are:
- Chronic Pain related to rheumatoid arthritis.
- Chronic Pain related to chronic pancreatic inflammation.
- Chronic Pain related to lack of knowledge of nonpharmacologic pain control measures that can be used in conjunction with pharmacologic measures to control chronic back pain.

PLANNING AND IMPLEMENTATION WITH RATIONALE

The goal of nursing care for the patient experiencing Pain is *to assist the patient in achieving optimal control of the Pain*. Regardless of the type of pain experience, the nurse must direct attention toward working with the patient in the exploration and implementation of the pain control techniques that will be most effective. *The extent to which the nurse can support and guide the patient in the quest to control Pain depends on the depth and breadth of understanding of the patient's pain experience*. This understanding evolves from the initial and ongoing assessments of the patient's pain experience.

The nurse should be knowledgeable of the current pharmacological and nonpharmacological approaches to pain management. When assisting the patient in choosing pain control measures, the nurse must address the patient's lifestyle, support systems, daily routine, and preferences. The patient's willingness to alter his lifestyle or daily routine in order to incorporate pain control measures is critical to the success of a pain management program.

Acute Pain

An important consideration in planning care for the patient who experiences acute Pain is to *incorporate nursing interventions that address the pharmacological management of the Pain*. The nurse is responsible for administering and monitoring the effects of all medications prescribed for the patient. Often the patient in acute Pain will be receiving narcotic analgesics. The determination of when the patient will receive these medications may depend on the nurse's assessment of the patient's Pain experience and the effects that a previous dosage may have had. It is not uncommon to hear patients state that they continue to have moderate to severe Pain after receiving pain medication. This may be related to the fact that doses of narcotic analgesics are often too low or too widely spaced. *Inadequate dosing frequently is related to incorrect assessment, insufficient knowledge of the action and effects of the pre-*

Text continued on p. 434.

❖ *NURSING CARE GUIDELINES*

Nursing Diagnosis: Pain related to lack of knowledge of Pain control techniques

Expected Patient Outcomes	Nursing Interventions

The patient will describe pain control measures that reduce or eliminate Pain.	• Assess the patient's Pain and the characteristics of the pain experience.
	• Evaluate with the patient and the health care team the effectiveness of past and present pain control measures (pharmacological and nonpharmacological) that have been employed.
	• Review with the patient nonpharmacological interventions that may assist in controlling Pain.
	  1. Describe the interventions to the patient (for instance, biofeedback, transcutaneous electrical nerve stimulation (TENS), hypnosis, massage or exercise therapy, and behavioral approaches such as relaxation, guided imagery, music therapy, and desensitization).
	  2. Assess the patient's desire and willingness to use a particular intervention.
	  3. Support the patient in making a decision regarding pain control measures that should be tried.

The patient will implement pain control measures to reduce or eliminate Pain.	• Support and guide the patient in making a decision regarding choosing a particular pain control measure. • Discuss with the patient and family lifestyle modifications that may be necessary to effectively implement the measure. • Assist the patient and family in determining how lifestyle modifications may be made. • Describe the health care system and community-based resources that are available to guide the patient in using a particular pain control measure (such as physical therapy) or in modifying the lifestyle. • Evaluate the effectiveness of the pain control measure.
The patient will reduce or eliminate factors that precipitate or intensify the pain experience.	• Work with the patient to identify factors (personal, disease-related, treatment-related, environmental) that precipitate or intensify the patient's pain experience. • Encourage the patient to keep a pain diary that will assist in identifying actual and potential precipitating factors. • Discuss with the patient and family measures that may be used to control precipitating factors. • Evaluate the effectiveness of the measures used through ongoing assessment of the pain experience. • Introduce the patient to self-help groups for persons who experience Pain—such groups may provide guidance related to coping with Pain, techniques that can be used to control precipitating factors, and pain control measures.

VI

scribed drug, and personal attitudes of caregivers and patients about the drug.[1,21]

Route of drug administration should also be considered. Recent developments have added novel routes of drug administration (e.g., transdermal and transmucosal) to the more traditional routes (e.g., oral, intramuscular, and intravenous).[3] As the novel approaches to drug administration are further developed and refined, choices of the most effective and most desirable routes from the patient's perspective will expand. An obvious advantage of the transdermal and transmucosal routes of administration would be the avoidance of injections to patients who fear "needles" and whose medication cannot be taken orally.

Use of nonpharmacological measures to control Pain must also be considered for the patient experiencing acute Pain. *Often interventions that will assist the patient to relax are most effective before the intensity of pain increases.* The nurse may guide the patient in taking slow, deep breaths or in reciting a word or phrase slowly and repetitively. Imagery may be another effective technique. This can be used by guiding the patient in imagining a relaxing scene, such as a quiet beach or a forest after a rain. The scene can become the patient's "haven" when Pain becomes severe.

The nurse should assume the responsibility to explore with the patient all possible pain control measures that may provide relief from Pain. The nurse should use all members of the health care team as resources in such an exploration.

Chronic Pain

The pain experience of the patient who experiences Chronic Pain touches the family, significant others, and even social and employment contacts. Thus, when planning care the nurse must consider the patient's lifestyle, family and employment responsibilities, and daily routine.

Pharmacological agents may or may not be used in the treatment of patients with Chronic Pain. *Because of the long-term nature of this type of pain, the nurse must exert care to avoid "overtreatment" of these patients.* In an effort to control Pain that "just won't go away," the patient may take prescribed drugs or over-the-counter analgesics too often or in excessive doses. The nurse should teach the patient the expected and untoward effects of the drugs being taken, as well as the appropriate amount and frequency of dosing. If the patient has the option to vary the dose and frequency, the information the nurse provides may be critical to the patient's well-being.

Nonpharmacological pain control measures are especially helpful to the patient in Chronic Pain. Such measures can range from activities that require the patient's participation to requirements that the patient avoid certain activities that intensify the pain experience.[22] When recommending a specific pain control approach, the nurse must assess its potential effectiveness and the patient's ability and desire to use it. The effectiveness of nonpharmacological measures should be monitored as rigorously as pharmacological approaches are monitored.

The nursing care guidelines presented below list patient outcomes and nursing interventions that can be considered for any patient experiencing Pain, whether acute or chronic. The guidelines should be tailored to the individual patient and his/her pain experience.

EVALUATION

Evaluation of the effectiveness of the nursing interventions employed to assist the patient in reducing or eliminating the pain experience requires the nurse to do an ongoing assessment throughout the implementation phase of the nursing process. Measures that are used to control Pain may or may not be effective for a particular patient. If they are ineffective, the nurse and the patient should continue to seek alternative measures that would assist the patient in achieving the ultimate goal of controlling the pain experience.

Thus the effectiveness of the nursing interventions must be measured over time. Patience is required of the patient in order to feel relief and of the nurse in order to see relief through an elimination of pain behaviors that had been observed. The family or significant others can also contrib-

Text continued on p. 436.

❖ CASE STUDY WITH PLAN OF CARE

Mr. Bill T., a 55-year-old independent dry-wall contractor, sustained an injury to the lumbar spine 1 year previous to this visit. He had attempted to lift and hold a sheet of dry wall. He has come to the outpatient clinic to find out if anything can be done about the "nagging pain" he has been experiencing since the injury. The physical examination and review of Mr. T.'s health history indicate that he is in good general health except for the lower back pain he experiences. The radiographs of the lumbar spine show no abnormalities.

An assessment of Mr. T.'s pain experience reveals that the pain is "like a strong, dull ache across the lower back." He states that "the pain is worse when I'm on my feet all day," and he finds himself to be irritable at work and at home. He expressed that he was "afraid of being hooked on medicine" but that he takes aspirin "now and then" when the pain intensifies. He stated "the aspirin seems to help a little, but not much." The nurse diagnosed Mr. T. as having Chronic Pain (low back) related to back injury of 1 year's duration.

PLAN OF CARE FOR MR. BILL T.

Nursing Diagnosis: Chronic Pain (low back) related to back injury 1 year ago

Expected Patient Outcomes	Nursing Interventions
Mr. T. will describe measures that will control his low back Pain.	• Include Mr. T. and members of the health care team in determining the most appropriate measures for pain control. • Describe to Mr. T. nonpharmacological pain control measures that can reduce/eliminate his back Pain and rationale for using them: 1. Engaging in a prescribed exercise routine that strengthens the abdominal as well as the back muscles; strong abdominal muscles assist in maintaining correct posture and reduce the stress placed on back muscles. 2. Use of TENS. Use of TENS can trigger therapeutic endorphin levels (usually recommended in 1-hour cycles several times a day). 3. Use of relaxation exercises when Mr. T. is irritable or tense; relaxed muscles can decrease the pain sensation.
Mr. T. will control the factors that intensify his low back Pain.	• Work with Mr. T. to identify how he can decrease the amount of time he stands each day. • Describe and demonstrate appropriate standing, walking, sitting, sleeping, and lifting postures that Mr. T. should use; have Mr. T. return the demonstration. • Encourage Mr. T. to explore using posture aids, for instance, sacroiliac support (a support cushion that enhances spinal alignment when sitting or driving) and a firm mattress or bed board.
Mr. T. will implement pain control measures to reduce or eliminate Pain.	• Meet with Mr. and Mrs. T. to review the pain control measures that are recommended. • Discuss with Mr. and Mrs. T. the importance of familial support in promoting adherence to the proposed treatment plan. • Work with Mr. T. in incorporating a prescribed exercise plan into his daily routine. • Evaluate Mr. T.'s initial efforts in using nonpharmacological pain control measures. • Provide for regular assessment of the pain experience and effectiveness of the treatment program.

VI

ute to the evaluation of the effectiveness of the nursing care. They can provide data related to changes they observe in the patient's pain behavior, ability to resume activities and social contacts, and confidence in self that the pain experience is in his/her control.

REFERENCES

1. Agency for Health Care Policy and Research: *Acute pain management: operative or medical procedures and trauma,* Rockville, Md, 1992, Agency for Health Care Policy and Research, Public Health Service, U.S. Department of Health and Human Services (AHCPR Pub No 92-0032).
2. Agency for Health Care Policy and Research: *Acute pain management in infants, children, and adolescents: operative and medical procedures,* Rockville, Md, 1992, Agency for Health Care Policy and Research, Public Health Service, U.S. Department of Health and Human Services (AHCPR Pub No 92-0020).
3. Biddle C, Gilliland C: Transdermal and transmucosal administration of pain-relieving and anxiolytic drugs: a primer for the critical care practitioner, *Heart Lung* 21:115-124, 1992.
4. Bonica JJ: Definitions and taxonomy of pain. In Bonica JJ, editor: *The management of pain (vol I),* ed 2, Philadelphia, 1990, Lea & Febiger.
5. Bonica JJ: General considerations of chronic pain. In Bonica JJ, editor: *The management of pain (vol I), ed 2, Philadelphia, 1990, Lea & Febiger.*
6. Bonica JJ: History of pain concepts and therapies. In Bonica JJ, editor: *The management of pain (vol I),* ed 2, Philadelphia, 1990, Lea & Febiger.
7. Carroll-Johnson RM, editor: *Classification of nursing diagnoses: proceedings of the Eighth Conference,* Philadelphia, 1989, JB Lippincott.
8. Carroll-Johnson RM, editor: *Classification of nursing diagnoses: proceedings of the Ninth Conference,* Philadelphia, 1991, JB Lippincott.
9. Chapman CR, Syrjala KL: Measurement of pain. In Bonica JJ, editor: *The management of pain (vol I),* ed 2, Philadelphia, 1990, Lea & Febiger.
10. Chapman CR, Turner JA: Psychologic and psychosocial aspects of acute pain. In Bonica JJ, editor: *The management of pain (vol I), ed 2, Philadelphia, 1990, Lea & Febiger.*
11. Fields HL: Sources of variability in the sensation of pain, *Pain* 33:195-200, 1988.
12. Gordon M: *Manual of nursing diagnosis, 1991-1992,* St Louis, 1991, Mosby–Year Book.
13. Gunta KE, Schroeder PM: Pain; chronic pain. In Thompson J and others: *Clinical nursing,* St Louis, 1989, CV Mosby.
14. Ignatavicius DD, Bayne MV: *Medical-surgical nursing: a nursing process approach,* Philadelphia, 1991, WB Saunders.
15. Kotarba JA: *Chronic pain,* Beverly Hills, Calif, 1983, Sage Publications.
16. Loeser JD: *Pain and its management: an overview,* program and abstracts, NIH Consensus Development Conference on the Integrated Approach to the Management of Pain, Washington, DC, May 19-21, 1986.
17. McCaffery M, Beebe A: *Pain: clinical manual for nursing practice,* St Louis, 1989, CV Mosby.
18. Meinhart NT, McCaffery M: *Pain: a nursing approach to assessment and analysis,* Norwalk, Conn, 1983, Appleton-Century-Crofts.
19. Melzack R: The McGill Pain Questionnaire: major properties and scoring methods, *Pain* 1:277-299, 1975.
20. Melzack R: *The puzzle of pain,* New York, 1973, Basic Books.
21. National Institutes of Health: *The integrated approach to the management of pain,* National Institutes of Health Consensus Development Conference Statement, vol 6, no 3, Bethesda, Md, 1986.
22. National Institutes of Health: *Pain research,* News Features from NIH 86(3), 1987.
23. Riordan MP: Validation of the defining characteristics of the nursing diagnosis, alteration in comfort, pain. In McLane AM, editor: *Classification of nursing diagnoses: proceedings of the Seventh Conference,* St Louis, 1987, CV Mosby.
24. Wilkie DJ and others: Use of the McGill Pain Questionnaire to measure pain: a meta-analysis, *Nurs Res* 39:36-41, 1990.

Sensory/Perceptual Alterations (Specify) (Visual, Auditory, Kinesthetic, Gustatory, Tactile, Olfactory)

Sensory/Perceptual Alterations (Specify) (Visual, Auditory, Kinesthetic, Gustatory, Tactile, Olfactory) is the state in which an individual experiences a change in amount or patterning of incoming stimuli accompanied by a diminished, exaggerated, distorted, or impaired response to such stimuli.[17]

OVERVIEW

The sensory/perceptual process is the ability to receive and interpret information from the external and internal environment. It is vital for survival and essential for reflex activity, decision making, knowledge development, and behavioral change. It is necessary for cognition, that is, the process of obtaining and using knowledge about one's world. Mental status or cognitive function can affect sensory/perceptual function. A disruption or alteration in the sensory/perceptual process affects behavior and cognitive processes.

The sensory/perceptual process has physiological and psychological components.[9] The physiological or sensory component encompasses the detection of visual, auditory, kinesthetic, gustatory, tactile, and olfactory stimuli by sensory receptors and transmission of these sensations to the brain. The psychological component, perception, is a mental process of selection, integration, and the interpretation of sensory data. As such it represents an intermediate stage in the transmission of information from the sensory end organs and the process of cognition, which organizes this information and determines our actions, goals, decisions, and attainment of knowledge.[1] Because perception is an internal mental process, its presence and development are inferred from behavior. Whereas hearing seems to occur in our ears and seeing in our eyes, in actuality the impulses coming from the stimulated receptors housed in these organs are interpreted by the cortical areas of the brain. The sensory/perceptual process depends on the function of the peripheral and central nervous systems as well as the neuroendocrine system.[9]

It has been hypothesized that there is a basic need or drive for sensory stimulation and that in a waking state an individual strives to maintain an optimal level of sensory variation to the cortex. This need or drive has been labeled *sensoristasis*. The level of required stimulation is thought to vary among individuals and to be influenced by such variables as age, culture, and environment. Individuals seek additional or alternative stimuli if sensory stimulation falls below optimal levels; they will attempt to reduce sensory input when it exceeds optimal levels. Inadequate or excessive stimulation for extended periods of time results in disorganization of behavior.[9] Thus the concept of sensoristasis explains the disorganization of behavior that occurs in situations of sensory deprivation or sensory overload.

The concept of sensoristasis helps us to understand a portion of the sensory/perceptual process, but it is not sufficient to explain the entire process. Because the process is such a basic component of human functioning, it is not surprising that over the centuries theories explaining the sensory/perceptual process have been formulated by a variety of disciplines. Information-processing theories and transactional person-centered theories seem to offer the most comprehensive explanations of the process.

Information-processing theories view adaptation to the environment as a basic need.[1] Knowledge of the environment is essential to meeting that need. Knowledge is obtained from information derived from the assortment of sensory stimuli that surround the individual, and thinking and learning are used to obtain that information. This process is called *perception*. As learning and thinking modify the individual, the individual modifies perceptions of incoming stimuli. Thus the process of perception is continuously affected by experience with the environment.[2,8]

Transactional theories view perception as a uniquely individual process that is influenced by an individual's needs, goals, cognitive processes, and experiences.[23] Individuals transact with their unique environments to develop sets of ideas or precepts about the sensory stimuli they receive. From these precepts assumptions about reality are formed. Assumptions, in turn, influence perception so that perception becomes a learned behavior of constructing reality to fit a set of assumptions about it. Brunner and Postman[3] demonstrated this in a classic experiment using playing cards. Experimental subjects were asked to identify a series of playing cards. Most of the cards were normal, but some were altered: a red six of spades and a black four of hearts. Without any apparent awareness of something being different, subjects almost always identified the altered cards as if they were normal. It was proposed that the subjects expected the color and shape of the cards to be as they had previously experienced them to be: black clubs or spades and red hearts or diamonds. They distorted either the color or the shape of the altered cards to support the set of as-

sumptions that they had previously formed regarding playing cards. It might be said that our generalizations and expectations filter out and distort most of our sensory experiences to make them consistent with our expectations. Each of us creates a representation of the world around us and that representation, in turn, greatly determines our perception of that world.[1,2,4,10,23]

The preceding theoretical considerations indicate that perception is both universal and individual. The same basic anatomical structure and physiological mechanisms necessary to carry out sensory perception are possessed by all persons. However, individual physiological, psychological, and sociocultural factors affect each individual's perceptual process and interpretation of reality.[1,4,8,11,21] Drugs, physical fatigue, fever, pain, chemical imbalances, and biological variance (constitutional makeup, age, range of sensory modalities) are major physiological factors. Psychological factors include past experiences, maturation level, motivation, beliefs, values, attitudes, and emotional stress. Social class, education, customs, and ethnicity have been identified as sociocultural factors. Although none of us has exactly the same perceptual experiences, we are able to agree on certain perceptions and broad categories of sensory perception.

Perception is also affected by the variety and type of stimuli competing for our attention at any particular point in time. Intensity, size, repetition, and novelty of stimuli have been identified as characteristics that determine selection and attention during the perceptual process.[22] The sensory/perceptual process is a complex function that can be altered by any number of conditions that interfere with the reception, transmission, or interpretation of stimuli.

ASSESSMENT

Sensory/perceptual alterations affect the way reality or the world about us is viewed. Alterations may be mild or severe and acute or chronic. Acute alterations tend to occur abruptly and manifest themselves with more severe defining characteristics such as confusion, disorientation, or bizarre mood swings. Sudden sensory loss, drug intoxication, and sudden trauma are often related factors for an acute sensory/perceptual alteration. Chronic alterations usually develop gradually and tend to have related factors that are more often long-term or permanent in nature. The defining characteristics initially may be rather subtle but often become more pronounced with time. Chronic alterations are often related to such factors as socially restricted environments, progressive neurological disorders, and decline in sensory function related to aging. The critical defining characteristics for this nursing diagnosis are evidence of reality distortion.[21] This evidence is both subjective and objective in nature. The nurse obtains evidence regarding reality distortion through interviewing, observation, and examination of the patient; through consultation with other health care providers and family members; and from records and reports. The sensory status of the patient and environmental factors need to be examined.[5,7,10] The patient's level of consciousness is obviously a major determinant of the method used to obtain the needed assessment data.

While interviewing or interacting with the conscious patient, the nurse should observe and note any emotional manifestations of apathy, depression, anxiety, apprehension, listlessness, restlessness, rapid mood changes, and hostility.[5,7] Perceptual distortions such as paranoid statements, illusions, and visual or auditory hallucinations are important findings. Impaired or disorganized thought processes may also manifest themselves. Any difficulty in thinking, concentrating, reasoning, problem solving, or following the therapeutic regimen should be identified. Inappropriate or slow responses to the examiner's questions or statements should also be noted.

The patient's current medical diagnosis and health history will give the nurse information about previous and current injuries or illnesses that may affect perceptual status. The review of systems portion of the health history provides data about several of the sensory modalities and about

sensory/perceptual function. It is important to note whether the patient has or has had visual or hearing problems and if adaptive devices are used. Problems with vertigo, paresthesia, and hyperesthesia are also noted in this section of the health history. Information about the patient's personal and social history helps the nurse develop an understanding of the patient as an individual and as a member of a family and community. The personal and social history may be obtained from the patient but in many instances will be available in existing records. The history should provide information about the patient's occupation and education; leisure activities; habits, including use of drugs, over-the-counter medications, and alcohol; usual sleep patterns; and cultural background. The nurse may need to supplement recorded information with information from the patient or family members.

Objective data assessment includes a neurological and mental status examination. For a detailed presentation of the neurological examination, the reader should refer to a basic book on physical examination.[7,13] Only a brief overview of the sensory portion of the neurological and mental status examination is presented here.

The sensory system portion of the neurological examination includes tests for tactile sensation, superficial pain, vibration, and proprioception (kinesthetic sense). The patient should be told what to expect and be reassured that the examiner will not inflict pain. Each of these procedures is carried out with the patient's eyes closed. The examination should always start by examining opposite corresponding parts of the body and having the patient compare the sensations on one side with those on the other. Slight differences are not ordinarily significant. If definite differences are noted, the abnormal area should be clearly defined by further testing.

Tactile sensation is examined by lightly touching the body with a wisp of cotton. An organized but unpatterned testing of both arms, the trunk, and both legs is used. The patient is asked to indicate when and where touch is felt. The sensations on opposite sides, as well as distal and proximal parts of the body, are compared.

Pain and temperature sensations are carried in the same major pathways so that in most circumstances it is not necessary to test for temperature if the pain sensation is intact. Superficial pain is tested by determining sensitivity to a pinprick. The sharp and dull ends of a safety pin are applied with the same intensity to symmetrical areas of the body. The patient is asked to differentiate between the sharp and dull sensations. To test temperature sensation two tubes are filled with water: one with hot water and one with cold. The same pattern is followed as in testing for pain, but the patient is instructed to identify the sensation as hot or cold.

Vibration is evaluated by placing the handle of a vibrating low-frequency (128 cycles/sec) tuning fork against a bony prominence. The patient is instructed to tell the examiner when a buzz is felt and to signal when the buzz stops. If the patient does not perceive the vibrations at distal points, the examination progresses proximally until the vibrations are felt. Older patients will usually have decreased vibratory sense in the lower extremities.

Position sense is tested by holding the lateral surface of the patient's distal phalanx of the thumb, index finger, or great toe and moving it up or down. The nurse asks the patient to indicate in which direction it has been moved, and makes side-to-side comparisons. Position sense can also be tested by the Romberg test (difference between balance with the eyes open and eyes closed) or by asking the patient to touch the tip of his/her nose with eyes closed.

After peripheral sensation has been examined, integration of sensation in the brain is tested. This may be done by two-point discrimination. The patient is touched with two sharp objects simultaneously and asked to specify if one or two points are felt. If the patient is touched simultaneously on opposite sides of the body, he/she should recognize that two points have been touched. If only one point is recognized, the side where the touch is not felt is said to demonstrate extinction. This ability varies over different parts of the body. At

the tips of the fingers patients should recognize two points 2 to 3 mm apart, whereas over the back the distances between points will need to be considerably wider.

Additionally, higher cortical integration can be tested through the sensory abilities of stereognosis and graphagnosia. Stereognosis is the ability to identify familiar objects (keys, coins, paper clip) placed in one's hand. Graphagnosia is the ability to recognize numbers or letters drawn by the examiner on the palm of the hand. Again, both tests are carried out with the patient's eyes closed.

Assessment of mental status is critical to any evaluation of the sensory/perceptual process. Careful observation of the patient during history taking, during physical examination, and while providing care should give the nurse a sound basis for evaluation of the patient's mental status. A separate examination is not always indicated. For instance, memory and affect can be assessed when asking patients details about their illness and past events. Components of mental status assessment are outlined in the box on p. 441.

In some settings standardized mental status tests are routinely used. These tests can provide a fairly simple and reliable method of obtaining mental status data and can be repeated at intervals to detect in a consistent manner changes in mental status. Health assessment texts usually provide detailed examples of such tests.[7,13] However, inherent cultural biases, relevance in long-term care settings, and lack of performance norms for the elderly limit the appropriate use of these tests.[7] Current literature that provides a comparison of the parametric properties and other characteristics of such tests should be reviewed before selecting and using one on a routine basis. A recent article by McDougall[14] is an example of such literature.

Along with subjective and objective patient data, environmental data are essential to assessment. Compared with the patient's usual environment, is there sufficient stimulation in the present environment? What are the intensity, pattern, and variety of stimuli in the environment? Is the patient receiving enough social stimulation to maintain an adequate level of meaningful stimuli? Are

❖ ASSESSMENT OF MENTAL STATUS

General appearance and behavior

Motor activity, body posture, facial expression, speech, grooming

Sensorium

Level of consciousness; orientation to time, place, and person; recent and past memory; insight; judgment; problem solving; calculation

Mood and affect

Presence of agitation, anger, depression, and euphoria; appropriateness to situation

Thought content

Presence of illusions, delusions, hallucinations, and paranoia

Intellectual capacity

Ability to carry on a conversation, read, write, and copy figures

---

noise and activity in the environment creating too much stimuli? Boredom, inactivity, daydreaming, increased sleeping, lack of sleep, disorganization of thoughts, anxiety, or panic may be indicative of too few or too many stimuli in the environment.[5,6,15]

The assessment data not only provide evidence of the critical defining characteristics for the diagnosis but also identify probable related factors. Numerous factors have been identified as being related to the development of Sensory/Perceptual Alterations: Visual, Auditory, Kinesthetic, Gustatory, Tactile, and Olfactory. The North American Nursing Diagnosis Association (NANDA)[17] specified four categories of factors: altered environment; altered sensory reception, transmission, and/or integration; chemical alterations; and psychological stress. These related factors identify those at risk for Sensory/Perceptual Alterations and determine the nature, extent, and severity of the alteration when it does exist.

Altered environments result in excessive or insufficient stimuli. The use of isolation, special care units, incubators, traction, body casts, bed rest, and physical confinement results in therapeutically restricted environments. The quantity, quality, and type of stimuli available to patients in such environments are severely limited. Contact with family and friends is restricted, and familiar sights, sounds, and smells are replaced by meaningless unpatterned or monotonous sensory stimuli.[6,15] Some therapeutic environments such as intensive care units are so overloaded with sensory stimuli that are meaningless to the patient that they too affect perception. Persons confined to such environments are apt to exhibit sensory distortions, disorientation, or hallucinations.

Other environments that are not therapeutically restricted may be socially restricted because of living circumstances. Persons of any age who are confined or limited in meaningful social contact, such as the institutionalized, homebound, aged, chronically ill, terminally ill, or those stigmatized because of mental illness, retardation, or physical handicap, are apt to experience socially restricted environments. An infant or child whose home environment does not provide adequate levels of stimulation also experiences this type of restriction. Impaired emotional, intellectual, and social functioning have been attributed to such socially restricted environments.

The second major category of factors related to Sensory/Perceptual Alterations includes those that result in altered sensory reception, transmission, or integration. They may be pathophysiological, situational, or maturational. Neurological disease, trauma, or deficit; alterations in sensory organs; sleep deprivation; pain; and the inability to communicate, understand, speak, or respond are classified in this category of factors. Stroke, head injury, and spinal cord injuries are some of the medical diagnoses most often associated with neurological disease, trauma, and deficits.[22] Sensory organ alterations may be congenital and may result in malfunctioning or dysfunctional sensory organs, as occurs in congenital deafness and blindness. Alterations may also be acquired as the

VI

result of injury, surgery or other treatment. Burns that alter tactile receptors, radiation therapy that affects olfactory and taste receptors, and cataract surgery that alters the eye are examples of this. Sleep deprivation often occurs when activities involved in the care and monitoring of patients disrupt sleep patterns and deprive patients of their usual amount of sleep.[15] This is a particular problem in intensive care units. Other sensory deficits are attributable to general neurophysiological changes that occur with aging, such as decreases in vision, hearing, and gustatory and olfactory discrimination.[2,20] Patients may be unable to communicate because of a pathological condition, because of a medical intervention such as intubation or tracheostomy, or because their culture and language are different from those around them.[11]

The third category of factors related to Sensory/ Perceptual Alterations is made up of endogenous and exogenous chemical alterations. Hypoxia, electrolyte imbalances, vitamin B deficiencies, and elevated blood urea nitrogen are examples of endogenous factors. Mind-altering drugs and central nervous system stimulants and depressants are classified as exogenous factors. Both endogenous and exogenous chemical alterations affect the peripheral and central nervous systems. The visual and auditory hallucinations seen in alcohol withdrawal and color vision deficiencies with digoxin toxicity are thought to be manifestations of this.[12,19]

Psychological stress has been identified as a fourth category of factors related to Sensory/Perceptual Alterations. Such things as extreme anxiety, panic, and bereavement narrow our perceptual fields and interfere with attention to and interpretation of stimuli.[1] Misinterpretation of stimuli tends to compound a person's distress and further reduces the ability to manage stress.

❖ **Defining Characteristics**

The presence of the following defining characteristics indicates that the patient may be experiencing Sensory/Perceptual Alterations:

Reported or measured change in sensory acuity
- Diminished or distorted visual, auditory, tactile, gustatory, olfactory, and kinesthetic capabilities
- Motor incoordination
- Alteration in posture
- Changes in muscular tension

Changes in thought processes
- Disorientation in time or place or with persons
- Altered abstraction or conceptualization
- Bizarre thinking
- Decreased problem-solving ability
- Disordered thought sequencing
- Visual and auditory distortions, e.g., illusions, hallucinations

❖ **Related Factors**

The following related factors are associated with Sensory/Perceptual Alterations:

Altered sensory reception, transmission, or integration
- Neurological disease, trauma, or deficits
- Inability to communicate, understand, speak, or respond
- Sleep deprivation
- Pain

Changes in emotional lability
- Exaggerated emotional responses
- Rapid mood swings
- Anxiety
- Fear
- Apathy
- Flattened affect
- Anger
- Irritability

Decreased attention span
- Restlessness
- Boredom
- Lack of concentration
- Daydreaming
- Complaints of fatigue

Changes in usual behavior patterns
- Increased or decreased response to stimuli
- Altered communication patterns
- Noncompliance
- Altered sleep patterns

Chemical alteration
- Endogenous: hypoxia, electrolyte imbalance, or chemical imbalance (for instance, elevated blood urea nitrogen)
- Exogenous: central nervous system stimulants or depressants, mind-altering drugs

Psychological stress

- Anxiety
- Fear
- Bereavement

Altered environments

- Therapeutically restricted: isolation, special care units, bed rest, traction, or incubator
- Socially restricted: institutionalized, homebound, chronic or terminally ill, stigmatized mentally or physically ill, retarded, or handicapped

❖ Related Medical/Psychiatric Diagnosis

The following are examples of related medical/psychiatric diagnoses for Sensory/Perceptual Alterations:

- Acoustic neuroma
- AIDS
- Allergic rhinitis
- Alzheimer's disease
- Bell's palsy
- Burns
- Cataracts
- Cerebrovascular accident
- Cocaine abuse/intoxication
- Diabetic neuropathy
- Diabetic retinopathy
- Generalized anxiety disorder
- Glaucoma
- Hepatitis
- Herpes zoster
- Hip or other bone fracture
- Hypothyroidism
- Lead poisoning
- Ménière's disease
- Mood disorders
- Multiple infarct dementia
- Multiple sclerosis
- Neurosyphilis
- Organic mental disorder
- Parkinsonism
- Psychoactive substance use disorders
- Retinal detachment
- Schizophrenia
- Spinal cord compression
- Vestibular neuritis

NURSING DIAGNOSES

Examples of *specific* nursing diagnoses for Sensory/Perceptual Alterations are:

- Sensory/Perceptual Alterations (Auditory/Visual) related to sensory deprivation or sensory overload.
- Sensory/Perceptual Alterations (Gustatory) related to effects of chemotherapy and radiation.
- Sensory/Perceptual Alterations (Olfactory) related to allergic rhinitis.
- Sensory/Perceptual Alterations (Visual, Auditory, Tactile) related to alcohol withdrawal.

PLANNING AND IMPLEMENTATION WITH RATIONALE

Nursing interventions for patients with Sensory/Perceptual Alterations will depend on individual patient characteristics, identified related factors, and presenting defining characteristics for a given patient. Nursing interventions are directed toward preventing injury, modifying or eliminating the related factors and defining characteristics, and providing mechanisms to help the patient deal with related factors that cannot be modified or eliminated. The overall goal is to promote, maintain, and restore optimal sensory/perceptual function as evidenced by elimination of defining characteristics.

The nurse should institute measures to provide familiarity with the environment and prevent injury. The patient's environment should be kept uncluttered. Once patients are oriented to their surroundings, equipment and furniture should be consistently kept in the same place. Glasses, walkers, canes, or other assistive devices the patient normally uses should be within reach of the patient. Side rails should be up and the bed lowered when the patient is unattended. The call bell should be within reach. A night-light may be necessary.

The environment can be altered to increase meaningful stimuli and decrease extraneous stimuli. The patient should be given information about the routines, objects, events, sounds, and smells in his/her surroundings. Nurses who have worked in an area for a period of time become accustomed to it and need to make a conscious effort to provide the patients with information that helps give meaning to the stimuli around them. *Avoid novelty and surprise* by providing the patient with clear, concise explanations of treatments and routines.

Extraneous stimuli can be controlled through reduction of unnecessary noise, traffic, and personnel. Whereas radios and televisions are useful in providing diversional activity and stimulation to patients in restricted environments, they must be used with care. The sounds from a radio or television can contribute to extraneous noise in

VI

the environment. This may be especially true if the patient is not used to the sound of the radio or television, dislikes the station being played, or is constantly subjected to its sound. Music has been shown to be especially beneficial in reinforcing reality and providing a link to the patient's life before illness.[18] However, the type of music used should take into consideration the patient's preferences, background, and musical interests.

Orienting cues help maintain and increase orientation to reality, as well as give meaning and pattern to stimuli. The patient should be oriented to the setting. The location of the bathroom and personal belongings, how to operate the bed adjustments, the purpose and placement of equipment, and the location and use of the call bell and intercommunication systems should be included. Personnel should make frequent references to the place and time. Clocks and calendars should be placed where the patient can see them. If the patient's vision is impaired, clocks and calendars with large figures and print are used. Placing small familiar items, such as family pictures, greeting cards sent from family and friends, and other personal items, where they can be seen and touched is also helpful. When possible, patients can be encouraged to wear their own nightclothes and use toilet articles, such as powders or aftershave lotion, that have a familiar odor. Placing the patient near a window when in bed or sitting up is another useful orienting cue. If a window is not available, lighting should be changed so that there is a definite difference between day and night.

The patient should be addressed by name when being approached or spoken to. The name by which the patient prefers to be addressed should be used. Personnel should introduce themselves by name and wear name tags. When possible the same personnel should be assigned to provide care to the patient.

Before any treatments are initiated the patient should be given a description of what will be felt, heard, seen, tasted, or smelled. *Sensory information is especially helpful to patients who have not experienced a particular treatment before.*[16] Patients can also be encouraged to take an active part in their treatment. Selecting one's own menu, recording intake and output, and assisting in dressing changes *provide the patient with a sense of control and add meaning to the stimuli in the environment.*

To reduce the patient's anxiety encourage him/her to verbalize feelings about any unusual sensations. If illusions are occurring, simply clarifying the nature of any misinterpretations may be sufficient to reduce anxiety. If the patient is experiencing hallucinations, providing assurance that such experiences are not unusual for persons in this situation is often helpful.

Promotion of adequate periods of rest and sleep is essential. Dimming the lights at specified periods, controlling noise, limiting visitors, and arranging and spacing treatments and activities can ensure uninterrupted periods of time for rest and sleep.

Patients who are experiencing Sensory/Perceptual Alterations related to factors that cannot be eliminated need interventions aimed at assisting them to cope with these factors. This is particularly important for patients with visual, auditory, or kinesthetic deficits. In many instances manipulation of the environment and the use of assistive devices will promote safety and facilitate the patient's ability to compensate for the deficit.

For example, speaking slowly, articulating clearly, and using low tones are helpful when addressing the patient who is having difficulty in hearing high-frequency sounds. Shouting should be avoided, because it may actually impede hearing. Sound should be directed to the patient's better ear, and the speaker should face the patient. Lighting should be such that it illuminates the face of the speaker and does not glare in the patient's eyes. Avoid using exaggerated mouth configurations when speaking. Conversation can be supplemented with hand gestures or written information. These techniques allow the patient to take full advantage of visual cues. During conversation, background noises should be minimized so that the patient is not confronted with competing sounds. If the patient has a hearing aid, it should be in place and working properly. A hearing aid that is left on the bedside stand or has a clogged ear mold, a weak or dead battery, or switch improperly set is of little use to the patient.

To help compensate for visual deficits arrange objects in the environment consistently and inform the patient of the arrangement. Visual aids such as glasses, magnifiers, and focused lighting should be within the patient's reach. Avoid the use of small print or printed material on blue, green, or violet backgrounds with the *elderly* because they *tend to have difficulty distinguishing these colors and printed material on these colors*. Provide additional illumination for elderly clients and avoid direct fluorescent lighting, which creates glare. *Elderly clients have more visual difficulty in dim lighting and with glare.* Knock on the door and announce yourself by name before entering the patient's room. Tell the patient what you are doing in the room. Be sure to tell the patient before you touch him. When speaking to the patient stand so that your face is illuminated and back lighting doesn't glare in the patient's eyes. Tell the patient when you are leaving the room. Use verbal description and touch to provide alternate sensory information, e.g., describe the location of food items on the meal tray and, if visual impairment is severe, hold the patient's hand and move it over each item as you describe it. *These measures will help prevent startling the patient, provide the patient with a sense of control, and reduce unnecessary anxiety or misinterpretations by the patient.*

For patients with olfactory problems, identify odors for the patient. If the patient finds certain odors objectionable or noxious, try to control their presence in the environment. Serve foods hot as *hot foods tend to be more odorous*. Serve foods that are visually appealing in color and arrangement *to provide alternate visual stimulus to compensate for the olfactory deficit*. This is particularly important for elderly clients as *most olfactory ability is lost by the age of 80.*

If the patient has a gustatory deficit *compensate by stimulating other senses,* providing food that is visually appealing in color and arrangement and foods that have a variety of textures. Provide the patient with a variety of condiments and, unless contraindicated, let the patient select those that are most appealing. *A dry mouth reduces gustatory sensibility.* Have the patient rinse the mouth with normal saline several times a day. Add gravies and sauces to food to moisten them. Avoid smoking and alcoholic beverages, as well as the use of mouth washes containing *alcohol, lemon juice,* or *peroxide* as these agents *have a drying effect on mucous membranes.*

Patients with tactile and kinesthetic deficits require nursing interventions *to prevent accidental trauma and injuries.* Use assistive devices or support the client during ambulation and transfers to prevent accidental falls. Be sure that overbed tables and beds have wheel locks engaged because patients may attempt to use these as aids to ambulation, a dangerous practice that should be discouraged. Patients with severe kinesthetic problems should not transfer or ambulate unassisted. Monitor these patients frequently and leave the call bell within reach with instructions to call for assistance before transferring or ambulating. Slippers with nonskid soles should be provided. Low-heeled, sturdy shoes are often safer than slippers for ambulation. Patients with a shuffling, Parkinsonian-type gait are safer wearing shoes with a smooth sole. *Ribbed or rubberized soles tend to cause these patients to stumble.* If the patient is experiencing tactile sensations such as itching, burning, or crawling, cool compresses may relieve them. Distraction with conversation, music, or television may *stimulate other senses and temporarily alleviate the intensity of disturbing sensations.* Encourage frequent position changes and active and passive exercise, and monitor for tissue injury in patients with kinesthetic and tactile deficits. These patients *are* also *prone to tissue breakdown related to decreased movement and position changes and a diminished pain response to ischemia.*

Selective use of *touch and stimulation of intact touch receptors* through massage may *help compensate for areas of diminished tactile functioning and provide the patient with alternate tactile stim-*

Text continued on p. 447.

VI

❖ *NURSING CARE GUIDELINES*

Nursing Diagnosis: Sensory/Perceptual Alterations: Visual, Auditory, Kinesthetic, Gustatory, Tactile, Olfactory

Expected Patient Outcomes	Nursing Interventions
• The patient will have no evidence of injury.	• Institute safety precautions such as side rail up, bed in lowered position, bed and overbed table wheel locks on, call bell and assistive devices within reach, room uncluttered, furniture and equipment consistently placed, and night-light in place. • Have patient use nonskid slippers or sturdy shoes when ambulating.
• The patient will demonstrate improved orientation to time, person, and place	• Use orienting cues: identify self by name and wear name tag; address the patient by name; provide frequent reference to place and time; put clock, calendar, and familiar objects in reach of patient; position patient so he/she can see out window; dim lights at night; have the patient use personal toilet articles and nightclothes. • Keep familiar items in the patient's environment.
• The patient will accurately identify objects/events/sounds in his/her environment.	• Give meaning to stimuli and provide various and meaningful stimuli: interpret sights, smells, sounds for the patient; structure routines; give concise clear explanation of surroundings, treatments, and procedures. • Encourage patient to participate in care. • Encourage participation in familiar activities, e.g., reading, hobbies, conversation and visiting with family or friends, selective use of radio and/or television.
• The patient will sleep at least two 3 to 4-hour periods in 24 hours and have improved scores on mental status exam.	• Control extraneous stimuli and provide adequate sleep: control pain; provide for 3- to 4-hour periods of uninterrupted sleep (preferably during patient's usual hours of sleep); reduce unnecessary traffic, personnel, and noise.
• The patient will use appropriate assistive devices/mechanisms (specify) to compensate for recognized sensory/perceptual deficits.	• Use assistive devices and techniques, e.g., hearing aid, glasses, walker, touch, frequent position change, and alternative sense stimulation to compensate for sensory deficits.
• The patient will verbalize feelings regarding unusual sensory experiences.	• Encourage patient's verbalization of concerns, fear, or anxiety.
• The patient will seek clarification regarding unusual sensory experiences.	• Clarify misconceptions or misinterpretations of environmental stimuli. • Distinguish for the patient sensations that are reality-based from those that are not.

VI

ulation. Using personal clothing and blankets provides *familiar tactile experiences,* which *may be soothing to the patient.*

EVALUATION

The effectiveness of nursing interventions is determined from objective data that indicate the goals of preventing injury and promoting, maintaining, and restoring optimum contact with reality have been achieved. The absence of injury and a decrease or elimination of defining characteristics should be expected. The patient should be oriented to time, person, and place; should be able to recall past and recent events; should demonstrate appropriate responses to the environment; and should experience a stabilization of emotions. The same methods and techniques used to make the initial diagnosis will provide the needed data for evaluation. If the expected outcomes are not met or are only partially met, reassessment of the patient and environment and modification of nursing interventions may be necessary.

❖ *CASE STUDY WITH PLAN OF CARE*

VI

Mrs. Clara W. is a 69-year-old, married patient in an orthopedic unit of a general hospital. Mrs. W. had a total left hip replacement for osteoarthritis 3 days before this report. From the time of her admission she has been alert, oriented, and cooperative, but the night nurses report that Mrs. W. was confused and agitated during the night. She insisted her daughter was being held captive in the next room and that her daughter was calling for help. Health history indicates no previous hospitalizations except for childbirth. Mrs. W. has osteoarthritis and a visual acuity of 20/70 (uncorrected). However, with the use of bifocals, Mrs. W. has corrected vision of 20/30. The patient is a retired secretary and a business school graduate. Mrs. W. has been married 45 years and lives with her husband, 70 years old, a retired insurance agent, in a two-bedroom apartment in a retirement community. She has one married daughter and two teenage grandchildren who live nearby and visit frequently. She has a married son and three grandchildren in California; Mrs. W. sees them once or twice a year. The patient drives a car and does her own shopping, cleaning, and cooking. She enjoys knitting and television game shows. Mrs. W. does volunteer work with the American Red Cross and is active in a national secretaries' sorority, Polish-American club, and church. She is a nonsmoker and an occasional social drinker. Mrs. W. does not use recreational drugs.

She takes calcium supplements and Naprosyn, 400 mg three times a day, as prescribed by a physician. Mrs. W. sleeps with her husband, is usually in bed by 10:30 PM, and sleeps 8 to 9 hours a night. Vital signs, hematology, and electrolyte reports are within normal limits. The patient is conscious and responsive. She has poor recent memory and recall, but past memory is intact. She is disoriented to time, person, and place. Results of neurological and sensory examination are within normal limits except for a slight decrease in light touch and vibratory sense in the left leg. The patient is near the door in a two-bed room. The room is across from the nurses' station. Records indicate she has slept poorly the past few nights because of pain and noise. Mrs. W. was cared for by a different nurse each day of her hospitalization. She had been on bed rest until yesterday, when she was up in a chair twice, for an hour each time. She had been receiving meperidine (pethidine) hydrochloride (Demerol), 50 mg intramuscularly every 4 hours, for relief of pain. Today she starts on aspirin (Empirin) with codeine for relief of pain. Husband and daughter have not been able to visit because of a snowstorm. The following nursing diagnosis was made for Mrs. W.: Sensory/Perceptual Alterations (Auditory) related to therapeutically and socially restricted environment, noise, pain, and sleep deprivation.

Continued.

PLAN OF CARE FOR MRS. CLARA W.

Nursing Diagnosis *Sensory/Perceptual Alterations (Auditory) related to therapeutically and socially restricted environment, noise, pain, and sleep deprivation*

Expected Patient Outcomes	Nursing Interventions
Mrs. W. will have no evidence of injury.	• Institute safety precautions such as side rail up, bed in lowered position, bed and overbed table wheel locks on, call bell and glasses within reach, room uncluttered, furniture and equipment consistently placed, and night-light in place. • Have patient use nonskid slippers when transfering to chair. • Ask husband to bring low-heeled shoes with laces for use when ambulating.
Mrs. W. will demonstrate improved orientation to time, person, and place.	• Use orienting cues: identify self by name and wear name tag; address the patient by name (she prefers Clara); provide frequent reference to place and time; put clock, calendar, and personal toilet articles in reach of patient; position patient so she can see out window when up in chair; dim lights at night • Have Mrs. W. wear her own personal robe when out of bed. • Ask Mr. W. to bring Mrs. W.'s personal nightclothes and some small family pictures if available. • Put up cards from family and friends so patient can view them or place on bedside stand within reach of patient.
Mrs. W. will accurately identify objects/events/sounds in her environment.	• Give meaning to stimuli and provide varied and meaningful stimuli: interpret sights, smells, sounds for the patient; structure routine by assigning the same nurse to Mrs. W. for the next 3 days • Schedule out-of-bed periods for 11:30 AM to 12:30 PM and 4:30 to 5:30 PM • Give concise, clear explanations of surroundings, treatments, and procedures. • Encourage Mrs. W. to bathe self, comb hair, and apply usual makeup; have Mrs. W. fill out her own menu. • (Put television on for 9 AM game show and for 3 PM soap opera (Mrs. W.'s favorites). • Give Mrs. W. her knitting while up in the chair. • Have Mrs. W. speak with her husband and daughter by telephone daily until they are able to visit.
Mrs. W. will sleep at least two 3- to 4-hour periods per 24 hours and have improved scores on mental status exam.	• Control extraneous stimuli and provide adequate sleep: check for adequate analgesic control of pain every 3 to 4 hours but especially at 10 or 11 PM; if asleep do not awaken patient between 11 PM and 3 AM and between 3:30 and 4 AM; close patient's door at night to reduce noise from nurses' station.
Mrs. W. will use glasses for reading.	• Be sure Mrs. W.'s glasses are clean and within her reach.
Mrs. W. will change position with assistance every 2 hours when in bed (except for sleep periods).	• Assist Mrs. W. in position change every 2 hours while in bed except for specified sleep periods.

VI

Expected Patient Outcomes	Nursing Interventions
Mrs. W. will verbalize feelings regarding unusual sensory experiences.	• Encourage patient's verbalization of concerns, fear, or anxiety.
Mrs. W. will seek clarification regarding unusual sensory experiences.	• Clarify misconceptions or misinterpretations of environmental stimuli, e.g., if Mrs. W. is awakened by care being given to other patient in the room, explain to her what is going on. • Distinguish for Mrs. W. sensations that are reality based from those that are not. • Reorient Mrs. W. to the environment and identify any voices she hears from the next room.

REFERENCES

1. Bastick T: *Intuition: how we think and act,* Chichester, Great Britain, 1982, John Wiley & Sons.
2. Bray SA: Alterations in special senses. In Mitchel PH, Hodges LC, Murvaseves M, and Wallech CA, editors: *AANN's neuroscience nursing,* Norwalk, Conn, 1988, Appleton & Lange.
3. Brunner J, Postman L: On the perception of incongruity: a paradigm, *J Pers* 18:206, 1948.
4. Bunting S: The concept of perception in selected nursing theories, *Nurs Sci Q* 1:168, 1988.
5. Carpentino LJ: *Nursing diagnosis: application to clinical practice,* ed 4, Philadelphia, 1992, JP Lippincott.
6. Easton C, MacKenzie F: Sensory-perceptual alterations: delirium in the intensive care unit, *Heart Lung,* 17:229, 1988.
7. Fuller J, Schaller-Ayers J: *Health assessment: a nursing approach,* Philadelphia, 1990, JP Lippincott.
8. Gibson E: *Principles of perceptual learning and development,* New York, 1969, Appleton-Century-Crofts.
9. Guyton AC: *Basic neuroscience: anatomy and physiology,* Philadelphia, 1987, Saunders.
10. Kelman G: Sensory perceptual alterations. In Creasia JL, Parker B, editors: *Conceptual foundations of professional nursing practice,* St Louis, 1991, Mosby – Year Book.
11. Kloosterman N: Cultural care: the missing link in severe sensory alteration, *Nurs Sci Q* 4:119, 1991.
12. LeSage JM, Chuman MA: Color vision tests to identify elevated digoxin levels, *Res Nurs Health* 9:171, 1986.
13. Malasanos L and others: *Health assessment,* ed 4, St Louis, 1990, CV Mosby.
14. McDougall GJ: A review of screening instruments for assessing cognition and mental status in older adults, *Nurs Prac* 15:18, 1990.
15. McGonigal KS: The importance of sleep and the sensory environment to critically ill patients, *Intens Care Nurs* 2;73, 1986.
16. McHugh NG, Christman NJ, and Johnson JE: Preparatory information: what helps and why, *Am J Nurs* 82:780, 1982.
17. McLane AM, editor: *Classification of nursing diagnoses: proceeding of the Seventh Conference,* St Louis, 1987, CV Mosby.
18. Michael DE: *Music therapy,* Springfield, Ill, 1976, Charles C Thomas.
19. Squires S and others: Sensory alterations in alcohol abuse, *Top Clin Nurs* 6:51, 1985.
20. Staab AS, Lyles MF: *Manual of geriatric nursing,* Glenview, Ill, 1989, Scott, Foresman.
21. Thompson JM, McFarland GK, Hirsch J, Tucker S, and Bowers A: Mosby's *clinical nursing,* ed 2, St Louis, 1989, CV Mosby.
22. Wyness MA: Perceptual dysfunction: nursing assessment and management, *J Neurosurg Nurs* 17;105, 1985
23. Zimbardo P, Ruch F: Psychology and life, Glenview, Ill, 1974, Scott, Foresman.

VI

Unilateral Neglect

***Unilateral Neglect** is the state in which an individual is perceptually unaware of and inattentive to one side of the body.*[3]

OVERVIEW

Unilateral Neglect is one of a number of perceptual deficits that can be seen after injury to the nondominant (usually right) hemisphere[1] of the brain. Such an injury can be caused by a cerebrovascular accident (CVA or stroke), trauma, or, in rare cases, tumors, and the effect may be inattention to the affected side of the body and/or to the environment around the affected side (unilateral neglect).

Perception is the ability to integrate and interpret sensory data. Several cerebral regions provide an integrated network for the mediation of directed attention: the posterior parietal lobe, frontal eye fields, and the cingulate gyrus.[4]

If any of these areas of the brain become damaged, interpretation of data is altered and perception and attention are impaired. Perceptual deficits such as neglect can be associated with physical deficits such as hemiplegia, contralateral (opposite the side of injury) sensory deficits, or hemianopsia. These do not have to be present for neglect to occur and can be present without neglect.[2] The nondominant hemisphere is generally on the right side of the brain. Injury to the dominant parietal lobe usually correlates with problems in communication.[12] The parietal lobe is supplied by the anterior cerebral, middle cerebral, and posterior cerebral arteries. Because there is great variability in the responses of the human brain, injury or blockage of any of these arteries can cause damage to the parietal lobe, resulting in perceptual deficits.

Unilateral Neglect may appear with other perceptual deficits in combinations that are not very predictable or always related to the magnitude of injury.[6] Therefore the nurse must look for all types of perceptual deficits when assessing the patient with a lesion of the nondominant hemisphere, even when there are no physical sequelae.

Unilateral Neglect is inattention to the affected side of the body (hemi-inattention) and/or to the environment from the midline on the affected side (hemi-spatial neglect). These two types of neglect can be categorized as disorders related to perception of self and disorders related to perception of space.[10] Disorders in perception of self include anosognosia and extinction phenomenon. Agnosia and apraxia are categorized separately but are related disorders of perception. Unilateral Neglect rarely occurs in isolation and usually is associated with one or more of the other perceptual deficits listed in the following paragraph. Unilateral Neglect occurring in combination with other related perceptual deficits also is known as *neglect syndrome*.

Anosognosia is a denial phenomenon where the patient lacks insight into the presence of deficits or the significance of the deficits.[5] Anosognosia is most prominent in the acute phase after injury. *Extinction phenomenon* exists if a stimulus applied only to the affected side is perceived correctly, but when the same stimulus is applied simultaneously to both sides, it is not perceived on the affected side.[1] *Agnosia* is the inability to recognize and identify familiar objects through an otherwise intact sense. Agnosia can be visual (not recognizing an object), tactile (not recognizing a familiar object held in the hand when the eyes are closed), or auditory (not recognizing familiar sounds).[10] *Apraxia* is the inability to do a skilled motor function despite adequate muscle power, sensation, and coordination. The patient will not be able to dress if handed clothes or to brush teeth if handed a toothbrush. This is due to an inability to conceptualize and plan the task.[10] Different aspects of the neglect syndrome have been related to different regions of the brain.[4] The parietal region is linked with perceptual-sensory aspects (neglect of self, extinction, agnosia), the frontal region with exploratory-motor aspects (neglect of space, apraxias), and the cingulate region with the motivational-emotional aspects (anosognosia).

ASSESSMENT

Unilateral Neglect (and the neglect syndrome) usually is related to strokes of the right (usually nondominant) hemisphere. Neglect syndrome also can be seen after traumatic brain injury. Hemianopsia (loss of vision in half of the visual field) can compound neglect. Any form of neglect of one side of the body can affect safety and performance of activities of daily living (ADLs). If neglect is not recognized for what it is, the patient may be thought to be confused, uncooperative, or cognitively impaired.[11] Therefore the nurse caring for the patient with an injury that might cause neglect should be aware of the associated defining characteristics and of assessment parameters for Unilateral Neglect and the associated perceptual deficits.

The acute phase after a stroke or brain injury is when the neglect may be most severe. Anosognosia is most prevalent at this time. The patient with anosognosia will deny completely the stroke deficits or the significance of any effects from the stroke. The patient may state the ability to walk or confabulate reasons why walking is not possible. The patient may deny ownership of the affected limbs, asking the nurse to "Get this dead body out of my bed" or saying the limbs belong to someone else such as the doctor or a family member. To assess for anosognosia ask the patient to state what is wrong or why the patient came to the hospital. Often the patient will state something like "I fell, but now I am fine." If the

patient initially denies any deficits, ask about the strength of or the ability to use the affected limb. If the patient actively denies a deficit, ask specific questions or give simple commands regarding the affected limbs. This is when the patient may start to confabulate, saying things like "I can't move my leg because I don't have my shoes on."

The unconcern, unawareness, and/or denial associated with anosognosia sometimes is related to a general clouding of the sensorium immediately after the injury.[10] As the sensorium clears the anosognosia lessens to the point where the patient can admit to deficits but still may neglect the affected side in some fashion.

Unilateral Neglect of self or space usually is obvious. The patient experiencing an alteration in the perception (neglect) of self may roll over onto the affected arm or sit on it when assisted out of bed. The patient may not groom the affected side, leaving that side unshaved, unwashed, uncombed, or undressed. The patient may also neglect to hook eyeglasses over the affected ear, leaving them "hanging"[9] and sit with the head turned toward the unaffected side. The patient experiencing an alteration in perception (neglect) of space may not eat food on one side of the plate. The patient will not respond to stimuli on the affected side—will not respond to people, noises, or lights on that side. The patient will be unable to find objects placed on a table or nightstand on the affected side. When the patient with neglect of space starts to ambulate or self-propel around the nursing unit, he/she may bump into doorjambs or walls because of the neglect of that side of the environment. To assess more specifically for Unilateral Neglect, ask the patient to draw a stick figure or the face of a clock. The stick figure will show only the left or right side of the figure, and the numbers will be drawn on only one side of the clock face rather than distributed evenly around it. If the patient is able to read, only words on the side of the page corresponding to the unaffected side will be read, sometimes to the point of only half a word being read. This might be noticed if, when a patient is asked to fill out a form such as a daily menu, only one side of the form is filled out.

VI

Unilateral Neglect is the portion of the neglect syndrome most often associated with homonymous hemianopsia (visual field cut). Whereas the patient may need to be assessed by an ophthalmologist for the presence or absence of this visual defect, the nurse can perform a quick test to determine whether it is present. If the usual test for visual field acuity implies a field cut, the nurse should assess one side at a time, moving her hand in quickly as if about to poke the eye. If there is only a visual field cut and no neglect, the patient will not blink. If there is only neglect, the patient will blink. If both are present, all examinations will be difficult to do because of the neglect. If the patient has hemianopsia and not a cortically mediated neglect, the patient can be taught to overcome the visual defects by scanning toward the affected side. Patients with neglect will have more difficulty learning to scan toward the affected side.

A patient experiencing extinction phenomenon is able to perceive a stimulus when it is applied to the affected side alone but loses that perception when the same stimulus is applied simultaneously on both sides. To assess for this have the patient, with eyes closed, state which side of the body is being touched when one side and then the other is touched. Then touch both sides simultaneously, and have the patient state which side is being touched. This test will help finalize the diagnosis of Unilateral Neglect of self.

Agnosia is the failure to recognize and identify objects through a sense that is otherwise intact. Visual agnosia makes it difficult to recognize objects in and of themselves or as a part of a whole. Auditory agnosia is a difficulty recognizing sounds such as bells, horns, and the like. If language is involved, the patient will need to be tested for aphasia. Tactile agnosia is the inability to recognize objects by touch.

Apraxia is the inability to voluntarily carry out a previously learned activity. The patient may have the muscular and cognitive ability to carry out the task but be unable to do so when asked. At other times the patient may do the activity unconsciously. This deficit may become obvious as the patient starts to become more involved in performing ADLs. The patient may be unable to brush teeth, may put clothing on wrong or in the wrong order, or may not know how to use a razor. The patient may not sequence eating a meal correctly, as evidenced by pouring coffee in the cereal or using a fork to spread the butter. The occupational therapist can assist the nurse in assessing the exact type of apraxia that is present. Dressing apraxia is different from the dressing problems seen in Unilateral Neglect. In Unilateral Neglect the affected side is not dressed and the unaffected side is dressed properly. In dressing apraxia the patient is unable to figure out which types of clothes go on which parts of the body, and the patient may try to put a leg into a shirt sleeve or put the shirt on first, then the bra.

The defining characteristics for the nursing diagnosis Unilateral Neglect are outlined along with those of the other portions of neglect syndrome. The related factors are applicable to the entire neglect syndrome.

❖ Defining Characteristics

The presence of the following defining characteristics indicates that the patient may be experiencing Unilateral Neglect:

Unilateral Neglect
- Does not groom, dress, or wash affected side
- Ignores position of affected side (sits on hand)
- Does not eat food on one side of plate
- Ignores stimuli in the hemisphere of the affected side
- Bumps into doorway or walls on affected side

Anosognosia
- Denies deficits
- Identifies extremities as belonging to someone else
- States physical abilities that do not exist since the injury (for instance, walking)
- Demonstrates poor safety judgment

Extinction phenomenon
- Agnosia: may not recognize objects, may get lost on ward, may not recognize the sound of the telephone, alarm, or the like, does not recognize objects by feel

- Apraxia: unable to put clothes on, unable to brush teeth, unable to do previously learned tasks in proper sequence (may appear to be absentminded)

❖ Related Factors

The following related factors are associated with Unilateral Neglect:
- Effects of disturbed perceptual abilities, such as hemianopsia, one-sided blindness, or neurological trauma

❖ Related Medical/Psychiatric Diagnoses

The following are examples of related medical/psychiatric diagnoses for Unilateral Neglect:
- Cerebral aneurysm
- Cerebral neoplasia
- Cerebrovascular accident

NURSING DIAGNOSES

Examples of *specific* nursing diagnoses for Unilateral Neglect are:
- Unilateral Neglect related to right parietal cerebrovascular accident as evidenced by inattention to the left side of the body.
- Unilateral Neglect related to right frontal cerebrovascular accident as evidenced by attention only to the right side of any written material.

PLANNING AND IMPLEMENTATION WITH RATIONALE

The treatment of the patient with Unilateral Neglect varies as the patient's hospital course progresses. In the acute phase the patient may be confused as a result of the brain injury and must be supported to prevent further confusion and agitation. In the later rehabilitation stage the client must be assisted to actively include the neglected side in all ADLs. This can be stressful for the patient and family, and they all will require support from the nursing staff.

In the acute phase after the initial injury, the nurse must ensure that the patient is in a safe environment. *If the patient has anosognosia and is denying the injury altogether or grossly underestimating the effects of the injury, the nurse must ensure that the patient will not try to get out of bed unassisted.* This intervention includes keeping all four side rails in the upright position, using a safety vest as needed, reiterating the patient's deficits at all times, not overestimating or taking the patient's word for the extent of physical abilities, keeping the patient's environment simple, and keeping things such as the call light and personal items on the unaffected side so the patient can easily locate them.

As the anosognosia abates the nurse can begin to teach the patient to be aware of the neglected side by including activities that attend to both sides of the body. These include bilateral range-of-motion exercises, touching the affected side, and doing care from the affected side. The television, pictures, clock, and calendar can be kept on the affected side to promote attention to that side. If the patient is confused, reorient the patient frequently and approach from the unaffected side so as to lessen confusion and help prevent the patient from becoming frightened. The patient's family, significant others, or both must be included in these early interventions. The nurse should teach the family about the type of neglect the patient is experiencing so they will understand the need for and the rationale behind the interventions.

As the patient progresses from the acute phase to the ongoing rehabilitative phase, the interventions need to be modified to help assist the patient to attend to the neglected side of the body or the neglected environment. *If the patient recognizes to any extent the presence of the neglect, depression may occur, and the nurse will need to help the patient mobilize previously effective coping strategies.*

It is at this time the patient must start to become actively involved in ADLs. The patient should now be approached from the affected side. *This calls attention to this side on a regular basis, forcing the patient to acknowledge it.* Although the call light should remain on the unaffected side for the patient's safety, nonessential personal items should be placed on the affected side to encourage the patient to recognize that side. The patient must be taught to check the af-

Text continued on p. 455.

VI

❖ *NURSING CARE GUIDELINES*

Nursing Diagnosis Unilateral Neglect (self or space)

Expected Patient Outcomes	Nursing Interventions
The patient will display caution and prevent injury.	• Keep environment simple and well lit. • Keep the patient's call light and personal items on unaffected side. • Keep all four side rails up. • Do not overestimate the patient's abilities; anticipate the patient's needs. • Do not rely on the patient's statement of abilities. • Reorient the patient as needed.
The patient will display increased awareness of affected side.	• Include activities that attend to both sides of body. • Remind the patient to use affected extremity if able. • Have the patient position affected extremities properly after turning, sitting, and the like. • As the patient progresses, increase stimulation to affected side and encourage interaction of staff and visitors with neglected side. • Teach the patient to scan affected side on a regular basis, especially during activities involving that side.
The patient will perform ADLs at expected optimal level.	• Place food on side of tray corresponding to unaffected side so the patient will eat all the meal. (Early stages) • Assist the patient with dressing and grooming while verbally going through the steps of the activity; this is especially important for patients with apraxia, because they will need to relearn tasks. • Have the patient perform own ADLs, with verbal cuing as needed. • Teach the patient to scan affected side during ADLs. • Center meal on tray; have the patient scan tray to ensure that meal is finished. (Late stages)
The patient will use effective coping mechanisms to maintain positive self-esteem.	• Have the patient identify usual methods of coping with stress. • Have the patient use positive coping strategies that have been effective in the past. • Help the patient identify new coping strategies if past strategies were ineffective or inappropriate. • Help the patient maintain positive self-esteem through positive reinforcement of progress made.
The family and significant others will verbalize and demonstrate understanding of the patient's deficits.	• Give the family a realistic assessment of the patient's injury and deficits. • Demonstrate deficits as appropriate. • Teach the family the appropriate interventions for each stage of the patient's progress.

VI

❖ NURSING CARE GUIDELINES—*cont'd*

Expected Patient Outcomes	Nursing Interventions
The family and significant others will use coping mechanisms to provide appropriate support for the patient.	• Use interventions similar to those used for the patient. • Encourage the family to eat well and to rest. • Be an empathetic listener.
The family and significant others will assist with ADLs as needed.	• Teach the family the appropriate interventions (such as scanning and step-by-step cuing) needed to assist the patient with ADLs.

fected side during ADLs. The principles of behavior modification can be useful at this stage. The patient should not be allowed to ambulate unassisted. The neglect may cause the patient to bump into walls or door frames, and the spatial defects may make it difficult for the patient to find the route back to the room. If the neglect never resolves, the patient will remain dependent in all ADLs and will require attendant care for safety and cuing.

The family and significant others must continue to be included in the patient's care at this stage *as they will be instrumental in determining discharge needs.* They must be made aware of the rationale for the different interventions and be taught to assist the patient as needed. As the extent of the patient's permanent disabilities becomes apparent, the family must be included in planning for the patient's care at home. The patient and family should be made aware of community resources available for assistance and follow-up care.[8]

EVALUATION

The evaluation of the patient must take into account not only the type and amount of neglect that is present but also the amount of actual physical disability that is present. The amount of physical disability will determine to a great extent the patient's ability to be independent in ADLs and physical mobility. Heir and associates[7] state that "Restoration of function ('recovery') is a complex phenomenon that depends at least on four major factors: the nature of the affected function, the residual viability of damaged brain structures, the locus and extent of the injury, and the capability of other anatomic structures to assume the functions of damaged brain regions." Therefore the nurse must be aware of these factors so that list-

❖ CASE STUDY WITH PLAN OF CARE

Mrs. Faye B., a 52-year-old, right-handed woman, was transferred to the rehabilitation floor 1 month after suffering a CVA to the right side of her brain. When she was first seen, she was in a wheelchair and slumped to the left. Her hand was hanging off the side of the wheelchair. When she was approached from the left side, she did not notice. She was dressed, but her left arm was not in the sweater. The nursing staff was told that she has a dense left-sided hemiplegia as a result of the CVA, with no known visual deficits. Her eating habits have been poor (she eats only "half" her food), and she often bumps into the doorway when she propels her wheelchair. Mrs. B. has a husband and two daughters who are very attentive, but they live a 2-hour drive from the hospital. The following nursing diagnosis was made: Unilateral Neglect of self and space on the left side related to stroke involving the right cerebral hemisphere.

Continued.

PLAN OF CARE FOR MRS. FAYE B.

Nursing Diagnosis: *Unilateral Neglect of self and space related to stroke as evidenced by inattention to left side of body and environment.*

Expected Patient Outcomes	Nursing Interventions
Mrs. B. will demonstrate awareness of her left side, as evidenced by correct positioning of the left side of body after movement and use of items in the left hemispace.	• Have Mrs. B. position her left arm and leg after every change in body position. • Teach Mrs. B. to scan her left side while eating and during other activities. • Put personal items on Mrs. B.'s left side, and remind her to look to her left when trying to locate items. • Approach Mrs. B. from the left.
Mrs. B. will not injure her neglected extremities.	• Have Mrs. B. use a sling on her left arm until she is more aware of its position after activity. • Remind Mrs. B. to check the position of her affected extremities on a regular basis.
Mrs. B. will perform ADLs at expected optimal levels, (Mrs. B.'s ADLs will be affected by her hemiplegia and her Unilateral Neglect).	• Teach Mrs. B. to scan when eating to ensure all food is eaten. • Teach Mrs. B. to scan to left when grooming and bathing to ensure that the left side receives the same attention as the right. • Assist Mrs. B. with dressing at first, going through step-by-step instructions as to how to don clothing. • Have Mrs. B. recite steps for all ADLs and then try to follow the steps as they are recited.
Mrs. B. will verbalize her usual effective coping mechanisms.	• Assess Mrs. B.'s coping mechanisms, and assist her to use them. • Include social worker in interventions as needed.
Mrs. B.'s family will verbalize understanding of Mrs. B.'s deficits.	• Arrange family meeting with physician, nurse, and other appropriate team members.
Mrs. B.'s family will demonstrate effective coping mechanisms so that they are able to provide appropriate support to Mrs. B.	• Assess family's usual coping strategies; assess premorbid role of each family member. • Assess the effect that the long drive to the hospital is having on the family's ability to organize themselves, their ability to deal with daily life issues that cannot be ignored, and their eating and sleeping patterns. • Identify community resources that will be available before and after discharge.
Mrs. B.'s family will assist Mrs. B. with ADLs as needed.	• Involve the family in the nursing care of Mrs. B. as fits their comfort level; involve the family in all aspects of her rehabilitation care. • As Mrs. B.'s final needs for assistance in ADLs become clear, ensure that the family is taught how to care for her and is able to demonstrate these skills.

ing of the expected outcomes and the evaluation of these outcomes can be appropriate for the patient and will not set the patient up to fail.

Many of the effects of neglect or other perceptual deficits can be seen in the patient's ability to perform ADLs. This ability is easily monitored by the nurse and the family to assess for attainment of goals. As the awareness of the neglected side increases, the patient should be included in goal-setting and the evaluation of the expected outcomes.

REFERENCES

1. Booth K: The neglect syndrome, *J Neurosci Nurs* 14:38, 1982.
2. Burt MM: Perceptual deficits in hemiplegia, *AJN* 70:1026, 1970.
3. Carroll-Johnson RM: *Classification of nursing diagnoses: Proceedings of the Eight Conference,* Philadelphia, 1989, JB Lippincott.
4. Daffner KR and others: Dissociated neglect behavior following sequential strokes in the right hemisphere, *Ann Neurol* 28(1):97-101, 1990.
5. Hickey JV: *The clinical practice of neurologic and neurosurgical nursing,* ed 2, Philadelphia, 1986, JB Lippincott.
6. Hier D, Mondlock B, and Caplan L: Behavioral abnormalities after right hemisphere stroke, *Neurology* 33:337, 1983.
7. Hier D, Mondlock B, and Caplan L: Recovery of behavioral abnormalities after right hemisphere stroke, *Neurology* 33:345, 1983.
8. Mumma C, editor: *Rehabilitation nursing: concepts and practice, a core curriculum,* ed 2, Evanston, Ill, 1987, Rehabilitation Nursing Foundation.
9. Nicklason F, Finucane P: "Hanging spectacles" sign in stroke (letter), *Lancet* 336(8727):1380, 1990.
10. O'Brien MT, Pallett PJ: *Total care of the stroke patient,* Boston, 1978, Little, Brown.
11. Stone S, Greenwood R: Assessing neglect in stroke patients (letter), *Lancet,* 337(8733):114, 1991.
12. Wyness MA: Perceptual dysfunction: nursing assessment and management, *J Neurosci Nurs* 17:105, 1985.

VI

Altered Thought Processes

Altered Thought Processes is a state in which an individual experiences a disruption in cognitive operations and activities.[8]

OVERVIEW

Through the process of thinking, people organize their perceptions and emotions to give meaning to their lives. Thought enables one to coexist in the world through the complex structures of family, society, and culture.[10] Thought allows man not only to establish a place in the world but to create or coconstitute the world.[7]

Human thought has universal characteristic patterns of organization and sequential development that evolve and become more complex with the individual.[13] However universal these patterns, each person interprets the world in accord with a characteristic cognitive style that allows for the uniqueness and integrity of the self.[6]

Thought is not a concrete entity. It cannot be seen, only inferred. Thought occurs simultaneously with emotion and behavior. Thought takes many forms; for example, in problem solving, memory, imaging, and meditating. Thoughts may be communicated, or they may be kept private.

Thought is often conceptualized, for the sake of assessment or study, as a set of mental or cognitive processes. These processes are identified as orientation, memory, cognition, and judgment.[14] It is important to remember that just as man is more than the sum of body functions, so too is thought more than the sum of cognitive processes emanating from the central nervous system.[4]

Altered Thought Processes has been an approved nursing diagnosis since 1980. The most current definitions offered are by Gordon[5] and the North American Nursing Diagnosis Association

(NANDA).[8] Gordon's[5] definition is most succinct, defining impaired thought processes as "discrepancy between manifested cognitive operations and expected operations for chronological age" (p. 192). Kim, McFarland, and McLane,[8] who cite the NANDA definition, describe Altered Thought Processes as "a state in which an individual experiences a disruption in cognitive operations and activities" (p. 65).

Drawing from the definitions of Gordon and NANDA, alteration in thought has as its primary focus attenuated cognitive operations, resulting in the person coping ineffectively with the demands of daily living. Related factors could be organic or psychogenic in nature.

The nursing diagnosis of Altered Thought Processes is comprehensive in nature. It is hoped that identification and discussion of the related factors will provide an organizing framework for assessment and intervention. The related factors for this diagnosis can be subdivided into pathophysiological, situational, and maturational.[3]

The first category addresses pathophysiological causes of thought alterations. Nelson[12] cites major systemic problems that contribute to brain dysfunction and, therefore, to cognitive impairment. Metabolic alterations such as hypothyroidism, hyperthyroidism, hypoglycemia, hypopituitarism, and adrenal disease are identified as potential causes of cognitive impairment. Brain disorders such as stroke, tumors, and transient ischemic attack; cardiovascular alterations, renal and liver disease, vitamin deficiencies, anemias, chemical intoxications, and infections also affect brain functioning. It is important to note that the brain dysfunction caused by these conditions is often alleviated with treatment. There are several psychiatric illnesses for which Alteration in Thought

Processes is the major characteristic and for which there is evidence to support pathophysiological or genetic causative factors.

Situational limitations that are severe or chronic or that are experienced by persons with a history of coping disorder can be related to an alteration in thought processing.[3] Sensory overload or deprivation, emotionally traumatic situations, significant loss, perceived rejection or abandonment, hopelessness, and powerlessness regarding problem or conflict resolution can induce thoughts that result in destructive behaviors or life patterns. Homicidal thoughts, for example, often arise from severe situational stressors.

Maturational factors that can contribute to Alterations in Thought Processes would be those conflicts experienced by most in a particular age cohort. When these conflicts are experienced by those who are vulnerable because of an inability to cope, the ability to successfully resolve the conflict is compromised. For example, an elderly man with a long history of alcoholism and who was recently widowed would be considered likely, statistically, to successfully complete a suicide attempt.[15] This person would be very susceptible to suicide ideations and impulses if, for example, he learned he had to relocate.

ASSESSMENT

Assessment occurs when the nurse purposefully interrelates with the patient, and if possible with significant others, to collect data relevant to the patient's health care needs. The assessment process enables the nurse to discern the defining characteristics and related factors that culminate in the formulation of a nursing diagnosis. Regardless of the setting the nurse must assess the patient's cognitive functioning. Assessment of cognitive functioning will reveal subjective and objective information about the patient's level of consciousness, orientation, memory, intellect/judgment, thought flow and content, and perception.

Aside from acute observational skills, the cognitive assessment requires the nurse to have excellent interpersonal communication skills. Paramount to successfully assessing cognitive functioning is the ability to put people at ease and to establish as quickly as possible a sense of trust, empathy, and unconditional positive regard. Assessment of cognition can be quite extensive in depth and breadth, requiring the nurse to be able to decide what and how much information must be gathered during the initial interview. Otherwise the assessment can be unduly tiring and stressful for the patient.

Level of Consciousness

The first area to be assessed is level of consciousness. Consciousness is often conceptualized as a continuum ranging from alert to coma. The Glasgow Coma Scale is a tool often used to assess level of consciousness. The tool is divided into three sections, documenting the measurement of eye opening, motor response, and verbal response.[9]

Altered states of consciousness would include lethargy, stupor, semiconsciousness, and unconsciousness.[15] With lethargy the nurse will observe that the patient sleeps or dozes inappropriately but can be aroused by stimuli. The stuporous patient is slow to respond to stimuli and cannot maintain the response. Reflexes are usually present. The semiconscious patient responds overtly only to painful stimuli, a pinprick for instance. Reflexes may be present, but the plantar reflexes are often extensor. The unconscious patient displays no response to painful stimuli. Pupils are unresponsive to light. Extremities are flaccid, and reflexes are absent or minimal.[9]

Orientation

The assessment of orientation lets the nurse know the patient's level of awareness of time, place, and person. The nurse can learn a great deal about the patient's orientation to person by asking the patient to give his/her full name and address. Orientation to time can be measured by asking the patient the year, the season, the day, or even the general time of day. Assessing orientation requires that the nurse be able to validate the response as correct. Also the patient needs to

VI

have had the opportunity to learn or know (1) where he/she is at present or (2) the time of day. It is not uncommon for a patient to have been brought to the hospital or nursing home without being told of the destination and to be interviewed in a room without a window or clock.

Disorientation to time, place, and person differs significantly when the cause is psychogenic versus organic. Disorientation for the patient with a psychosis will be manifested as bizarre rather than confused. The patient with a psychosis may answer that it is the year 2010 AD and that he/she is presently reigning over the kingdom of IX13. Disorientation with an acute or organic cause will be manifested by very apparent confusion. With the acute organic type of disorientation, the patient's orientation may vary throughout the day. With a chronic organic type of disorientation, the patient may attempt to make correct responses, to cover up the disorientation, or to relate a time and place from the past. With this type of disorientation, the patient may become more disoriented toward the end of the day.

Memory

Memory is a very complex aspect of cognitive functioning. The assessment of memory includes recent memory and long-term or remote memory. Recent memory measures retention and recall of information after 2 to 5 minutes.[15] Remote memory would be the ability to recall past life events; for example, where one was raised.

The nurse should be aware that for some patients this aspect of the assessment can be quite stressful. Patients may attempt to conceal memory problems from the nurse through confabulation (making up the answer) or through refusal to comply. They may tell the nurse they are tired of all the questions or that the questions are stupid.

To determine recent memory the nurse can ask the patient to remember three numbers and then to recall them 2 to 5 minutes later. Other ways to assess recent memory would be to ask the patient who is President, what was eaten at the last meal, or his/her telephone number.[15] To assess long-term memory one could inquire as to the patient's

home state. Or, if the patient had formal education, ask where he/she went to school.

Loss of memory can be acute and temporary, or it can be chronic and progressive. Patients who have suffered head trauma may experience alterations in memory, as will patients who have had electroconvulsive therapy. In these cases the memory loss is temporary. Patients who have chronic progressive brain failure will usually experience, first, a loss in recent memory and, finally, a loss or alteration in remote memory function. As one can see, the assessment of memory is closely related to the assessment of orientation. Memory is also crucial to problem solving and learning abilities, which will be assessed in the area of judgment and intellectual functioning.

Judgment/Intellectual Functioning

Judgment can be assessed by examining the patient's decision-making ability. Is the person careless about safety, or is he/she appropriate in ways that are not characteristic or normal for the patient? The nurse needs to examine how well the patient can comprehend and problem solve. Judgment and intellectual functioning are closely associated. The ability to judge and problem solve develops throughout a lifetime. These abilities are influenced by intellectual capacity, life experiences, self-concept, and self-esteem, to name only a few factors. Knowledge of the patient's ability in these areas enables the nurse to adapt teaching plans, to set appropriate goals, and to provide needed supports for accomplishment of activities of daily living.

Assessment of intellect, in particular, tends to focus on the patient's ability to think abstractly. This is done by asking the patient to interpret the meaning of a familiar proverb.[15] Another task would be to ask the patient to touch his/her knees, close and open eyes, and then fold hands in the lap.[15] This allows the nurse to assess how well the patient can follow and recall directions. This sequence of tasks can also reflect loss of recent memory.

When one is assessing intellectual functioning, one must know if the current level of functioning is characteristic or uncharacteristic for the patient. Knowing the patient's level of education is also helpful. In-depth assessment of intellectual functioning can be done through psychological testing. The Wechsler Intelligence Scale for Children and the Wechsler Adult Intelligence Scale are the most commonly used standardized tests.[14] Most often, though, the nurse's knowledge of the patient's patterns of everyday functioning is more useful than the patient's intelligence quotient score.

Thought Flow

Thought flow can be described as how well the patient's thoughts are connected or associated. Some commonly seen alterations in thought flow are loose associations, circumstantial and tangential thinking, neologism, flight of ideas, word salad, and blocking.[11] Loose associations are poorly connected thoughts. Circumstantial thinking involves many digressions before a conclusion is reached. Tangential thinking is like circumstantial thinking except that a conclusion is not reached. A neologism is a new word that is made up and holds symbolic significance for the originator. Flight of ideas is characterized by rapid speech and quick progression from one idea to the next. Word salad is a disconnected mixture of unrelated words, and blocking is an abrupt cessation of a thought midsentence for no apparent reason.[11]

Thought Content

Delusions, obsessions, phobias, and preoccupations are types of alteration of thought content. Delusions are fixed, false beliefs that one holds to be true, contrary to evidence. Delusions can be grandiose, persecutory, or of reference. Grandiose delusions are evident in the person who, for example, believes that he/she is in control of world occurrences. The delusion is persecutory if, for instance, the person believes that all of his/her coworkers are planning to destroy his/her career. With a delusion of reference the person would believe that the two people conversing at the next table in a restaurant are talking about him/her.[1]

When a person has preoccupation of thoughts,

he/she remains focused on a particular experience or thought that holds strong emotional significance. Someone recently assaulted may become preoccupied with the incident. An obsession is an unwanted idea, feeling, or image that the person is unable to forget or suppress.[11] For example, the person may be obsessed with thoughts of being dirty.

The phobia is also a thought alteration. It entails an unrealistic or irrational fear that prevents the person from engaging in an activity important to daily functioning. When severe, all of the alterations of thought content greatly impede normal functioning. The alterations are usually a manifestation of severe anxiety, which is indicative of serious psychological conflicts.

Perception

Changes in sensorium may be the first overt sign of illness. An essential aspect to every nursing assessment is to determine if sensorial disturbances exist. All of the senses act together to influence perception. Disturbance of perception is one of the most important factors related to cognitive and behavioral dysfunction. Hallucinations are a type of perceptual dysfunction requiring close assessment; they can be auditory, visual, tactile, gustatory, and olfactory. Auditory hallucination can be sounds or voices. Command hallucinations should be assessed for level of dangerousness to the patient or others. The presence of tactile, olfactory, gustatory, and visual hallucinations, raises the possibility of a toxic or organically induced thought alteration and therefore the patient's physiological status should be assessed.

An illusion is the misinterpretation of an object in the environment. This can occur with heightened levels of anxiety, sensory overload, or sensory deprivation. Patients in intensive care units are prone to this perceptual dysfunction.[11]

Additional areas for assessment relating to Alteration in Thought Processes are general appearance and hygiene, mood, personality, sleep/rest patterns, nutritional status, past and current medical status, stressful life events, and onset and duration of symptoms.[3]

VI

❖ **Defining characteristics**

The presence of the following defining characteristics indicates that the patient may be experiencing Altered Thought Processes:

- Altered states of consciousness
- Disorientation to time, place, person
- Impaired memory, recent and remote
- Altered sleep pattern
- Suicidal/homicidal ideations
- Attention deficit
- Hyperactivity
- Wandering
- Alteration in perception (e.g., hallucination)
- Delusions
- Egocentricity
- Inappropriate/non-reality based thinking or behavior
- Disturbed thought flow (e.g., circumstantial, tangential, neologism, flight of ideas, loose associations, word salad, or blocking)
- Disturbed thought content (e.g., delusions, obsessions, preoccupations, or phobias)
- Inappropriate/labile affect
- Impaired judgment
- Impaired problem-solving
- Cognitive dissonance

❖ **Related Factors**

The following related factors are associated with Altered Thought Processes:

- Hypoxia
- Dehydration
- Hypothyroidism and hyperthyroidism
- Hypoglycemia and hyperglycemia
- Hepatic failure
- Acid-base disturbances
- Azotemia
- Hyponatremia
- Cushing's syndrome
- Hypopituitarism
- Acute myocardial infarct
- Congestive heart failure
- Vascular occlusion
- Pulmonary emboli
- Chronic liver disease
- Alzheimer's disease
- Chemical dependency, acute or chronic
- Schizophrenia
- Mood disorders
- Sensory overload or deprivation
- Physical, sexual, emotional abuse
- Dysfunctional family structure (e.g., families in which the individuals' needs for separation and individuation and also for nurturance and relatedness were not met)
- Head trauma
- Brain tumors (primary or metastatic)
- Infections (viral or bacterial)
- Chemical toxicity (e.g., lead, radiation, or medication)
- Hormonal changes seen in premenstrual syndrome and postpartum
- Traumatic situational stress (e.g., rape)
- Post-heart-lung machine
- Combat experiences
- Torture or imprisonment
- Culture shock
- Acquired immuno-deficiency syndrome
- Chronic renal disease

❖ **Related Medical/Psychiatric Diagnoses**

The following are examples of related medical/psychiatric diagnoses for Altered Thought Processes:

- Acid-base disturbances
- Acquired immunodeficiency syndrome (later stages)
- Anorexia nervosa
- Azotemia
- Bipolar disorder
- Brain injury/disease (e.g., tumor, concussion, CVA)
- Chronic renal failure
- Congestive heart failure
- Cushing's disease
- Dissociative disorders
- Endocarditis
- Hepatic failure
- Major depression
- Meningitis
- Neurosyphilis
- Organic mental disorder (e.g., primary degenerative dementia of the Alzheimer type)
- Pneumonia
- Psychoactive substance abuse disorder (e.g., alcohol, cannabis, cocaine, amphetamine, hallucinogen, sedative, hypnotic, or anxiolytic)
- Pulmonary embolus
- Schizophrenia
- Stroke

NURSING DIAGNOSES

Examples of *specific* nursing diagnoses for Altered Thought Processes are:

- Altered Thought Processes related to prolonged sensory deprivation.
- Altered Thought Processes related to posttraumatic stress.
- Altered Thought Processes related to acute alcohol intoxication.
- Altered Thought Processes related to elevated BUN.

PLANNING AND IMPLEMENTATION WITH RATIONALE

Numerous patient situations can be diagnosed as Altered Thought Processes. Consequently the nurse will find a wide range of patient self-care abilities and deficits. Subsequently *this will affect the amount, extent, and complexity of nursing interventions required to preserve biological integrity, to provide for safety and security needs, and to promote belonging, self-esteem, and self-actualization.*

It is essential for the nurse to have a sense of the patient's perspective of his/her world. In doing so, the nurse will better understand the patient's cognitive abilities, level of orientation, integrity of memory and judgment, and level of anxiety, fear, and hopelessness. It is also important for the nurse to consider the known and hypothesized causes underlying the Alteration in Thought Process. It is helpful to the nurse to know if the patient's alteration is acute or chronic, is due to physiological alterations, is reversible or progressive, or is psychogenic, situational, and/or developmental in nature. Knowing this, the nurse's estimation of outcomes and the implementation of nursing interventions will be realistic and effective.

VI

❖ *NURSING CARE GUIDELINES*

Nursing Diagnosis: Altered Thought Processes

Expected Patient Outcomes	Nursing Interventions
The patient will maintain physiological functioning within his/her normal limits.	• Take vital signs, do neurological checks, and maintain a record of intake and output. • Assist with range-of-motion exercises and ambulation. • Provide environmental stimuli as indicated by the nurse's assessment of the patient's level of functioning. • Provide reality orientation.
The patient will not inflict harm on self or others.	• Assess for suicide potential. • Assure the patient, through words and a calm and caring presence, that you will assure his/her safety; be direct and forthright in directly asking the patient about intentions to harm self. • Provide a safe and secure environment for the patient with severe agitation or impairment of judgment, memory, orientation, and cognition; this must always be done in a health-promoting way, maintaining as much freedom as possible. • Use restraints judiciously and within the policy and procedure guidelines for the institution; never use used them punitively or as a substitute for staff—to do so would inflict harm physically and psychologically

Continued.

❖ *NURSING CARE GUIDELINES—cont'd*

Expected Patient Outcomes	**Nursing Interventions**

Nursing Interventions

- Be alert to the occurrence and escalation of aggressive behavior in the patient: intervene by reducing the amount of environmental stimuli, acknowledging the patient's anger or fear; offer assistance to reduce these feelings; establish as a basic principle that physical harm to self or others will not be permitted. (To uphold this principle use seclusion or restraints but only after other nonintrusive strategies have been employed, such as verbal limit setting and redirection to an activity that the patient can then adapt as a healthy coping mechanism; relaxation, physical exercise, writing down feelings, and active problem solving may be effective strategies for the patient.)

The patient will demonstrate improved cognitive functioning, resulting in decreased anxiety, improved relations with others, increased use of adaptive coping mechanisms, and decreased use of neurotic defenses.

- Help patient to feel comfortable with sharing thoughts and feelings; be empathetic and show unconditional positive regard.
- Help the patient to examine the effect of his/her cognitive style on emotional state and ability to relate to others, achieve goals, and experience a sense of accomplishment and self-satisfaction.
- Teach the patient about stress and stress-reduction techniques.
- Provide individual, group, and family therapy opportunities.
- If the patient is prescribed psychotropic medications, educate the patient and family about the medication.
- Help the patient identify supportive community resources, for instance Alcoholics Anonymous, Overeaters Anonymous, senior citizens' groups, and community mental health center.
- If the patient is hallucinating, allow the patient to share his/her thoughts; content is very significant to the patient's intrapsychic conflict.
- Assess if the hallucinations are commanding the patient to hurt self or others.
- Confirm through direct question, if the patient is hallucinating: Are you hearing voices now? Tell me what you are seeing now.
- Express your experience to the patient: I do not hear those voices.
- Ask the patient how he/she feels about these hallucinations.
- Help the patient to focus on concrete, easy-to-accomplish tasks; help the patient to think about accomplishing activities in spite of the hallucinations.
- Limit time spent dwelling on the hallucinations.
- Encourage patient to pursue educational/vocational assistance as needed.

EVALUATION

Evaluation should focus on the abatement or improvement of the symptoms of anxiety, confusion, disorientation, self-harm, agitation, impulsiveness, acting out of aggression, dysphoria, delusions, or hallucinations. The patient should be able to resume activities of daily living, including employment and family role; should feel confident in his/her ability to care for self; and should feel hopeful about the future within an interdependent framework. The nurse must take into account the nature of the related factors. For an acute, reversible clinical situation the expectation would be a return to premorbid functioning. The outcomes for a chronic, progressive condition should be reevaluated. The patient with Alzheimer's disease would not be expected to regain premorbid level of functioning. The outcomes would need to be adjusted to reflect the patient's capabilities.

Evaluation is an integral part of the nursing process and occurs spontaneously during each patient contact. The frequency of patient contact will, of course, vary from patient to patient, in most cases tapering to no need for nursing intervention. However, termination should include an aftercare plan even if it is to reassure the patient that assistance is available when needed. The patient should always have a resource list to enable him/her to seek appropriate treatment when needed.

❖ CASE STUDY WITH PLAN OF CARE

Ms. Elaine D., age 70 years, has been a patient in a nursing home for 6 months. She was admitted to the facility by her 68-year-old sister, who was unable to continue to care for Ms. D. at her home. Ms. D. had enjoyed a 40-year career in nursing. After obtaining a master's degree in public health administration, she worked as an administrator for the Visiting Nurses Association. Ms. D. enjoyed traveling, being with friends, and caring for her two poodles. At 69 years of age Ms. D. started to experience some memory problems, but she found if she used the timer on the stove she would remember she was cooking if she happened to leave the room. She also used lists and a tape recorder to remember things to do during the day or before going to bed at night. But Ms. D. began forgetting appointments, and after she failed to pay some important bills, the bank notified her sister, who had been unaware of the extent of Ms. D.'s memory impairment. After a short visit Ms. D.'s sister realized that Ms. D. was unable to live by herself and convinced Ms. D. that she and her poodles would be welcome additions to her household. During the year that Ms. D. lived with her sister, her memory continued to deteriorate, as did her orientation to time and place. Ms. D.'s sister was unable to leave Ms. D. at home alone, since one day when left alone she had taken her dogs out for a walk and was unable to find her way home. Fortunately a neighbor brought Ms. D. back home. Ms. D. was frightened by the experience, because she realized she had been lost. Her confusion was a source of frustration and sadness for her. Toward the end of the year Ms. D.'s care became too difficult and exhausting for her sister. Ms. D. had become restless at night, was unable to dress without assistance, and was frequently incontinent. Ms. D.'s sister had expected this progressive deterioration. Her physician had diagnosed Ms. D.'s illness as Alzheimer's disease and had explained to her the nature of the illness. Although she understood the situation on an intellectual level, she was not prepared for the emotional trauma both would suffer. Ms. D. has impaired recent and remote memory and needs prompting to initiate activities of daily living and to avoid incontinence. Some activities, such as dining with others, provide enough modeling for completion of activities. Ms. D. needs assistance to complete bathing, dressing, toileting, and all newly learned activities. She responds to the presence of her sister and her dogs with joy and relief but does not recognize neighbors of her sister. Ms. D. has verbal communication deficit. She understands short concise statements and answers "yes" and "no" appropriately, but speech is characterized by halting verbalizations—Broca's expressive aphasia.[2] She will seek out the nurse and say "please" imploringly when in need of help. Her nonverbal communication expresses fear, frustration, and agitation through fast-paced wandering through the unit, sometimes pushing away other patients who approach her. Agitation increases by the end of the day.

Continued.

❖ *CASE STUDY WITH PLAN OF CARE*—*cont'd*

Ms. D. is not oriented to time and place. She will wander away from group activities that are unsupervised and is unable to return on her own. She can find her own room on the unit. Ms. D. awakens several times each night and will wander the unit, sometimes calling "sister." She enjoys group activities and will stroll hand in hand with other residents but does not initiate this activity. Ms. D. particularly enjoys the pet program and visits by young children. She also enjoys music and guided exercise. She has no interest in watching television.

PLAN OF CARE FOR MS. ELAINE D.

Nursing Diagnosis *Altered Thought Processes related to loss of memory*

Expected Patient Outcomes	Nursing Interventions
Ms. D. will maintain current level of self-care activities, accepting support and encouragement as necessary.	• Provide enough time for Ms. D. to complete as much of each task as she is able. • Provide clear directions; use short words, simple sentences, nonverbal cues, verbal repetition, and demonstration. • Break the task down into easy-to-accomplish segments; show Ms. D. you are willing to be patient. • Use nonverbal and verbal communication to convey approval and praise; display smiling, nonintrusive forms of touch, and a relaxed body posture to decrease the patient's performance anxiety. • Assist Ms. D. in establishing a routine for bowel and bladder elimination. • Schedule a routine for activities of daily living.
Ms. D. will maintain effective communication skills.	• Allow Ms. D. to convey her needs and wants, even though this is often a struggle for both patient and nurse. (It is important that the patient feel understood and that her thoughts and feelings are validated.) • Validate specific feelings such as anger, fear, sadness, and happiness, rather than ask "Are you okay today?"[2] • Acknowledge nonverbal attempts to establish closeness or a need for rest and solitude; communicate openness, empathy, and unconditional positive regard.
Ms. D. will demonstrate trust in caregivers and will seek out and accept caring from staff.	• Demonstrate genuine concern, patience, and friendliness so Ms. D. will learn that the nurse is not to be feared and avoided but rather depended on and sought out for basic and a higher level of needs. (Although memory is altered the patient's emotional system remains intact and is possibly more sensitive to environmental and interpersonal situations that are hostile and uncaring.) • Be attuned to own frustration level, which can be increased when overworked and rushed. (Realistic staffing patterns are imperative when more than custodial care is expected for a patient population that has Altered Thought Processes; patients who are confident of the nurses' caring will be secure enough to engage in self-care tasks and other activities, even though they are anxious and confused.)
Ms. D. will maintain self-esteem and pride in appearance, accomplishments, and activities of daily living.	• Direct all interactions toward promoting self-esteem and pride in Ms. D. (Patients with memory impairments rely on here-and-now contacts with staff to be oriented to themselves. Providing assistance in self-care activities, especially those that enhance pride in appearance, is a source of encouragement and reassurance.)

Expected Patient Outcomes	**Nursing Interventions**
Ms. D. will maintain interpersonal interactions with others through individual and group activities, structured and unstructured, that provide opportunities to share past and present personal experiences and to anticipate future events.	• Encourage Ms. D. to be with others in ways that will be supportive and give meaning to present-day existence. (This will promote self-esteem, security, orientation, and memory recall, and possibly direct the patient toward anticipation of future events. Patients can help each other through shared experiences in structured and unstructured groups.)
Ms. D. will maintain creative appreciation for art, music, and nature.	• Assist Ms. D. to attend to nature or the arts; use music, pictures, and tactile sensations during individual interactions to help Ms. D. maintain this outcome. (All patients have been exposed to the beauty of creation throughout their lives; appreciation of beauty integrates emotion and cognition.)
Ms. D. will maintain contact with significant others, her sister, and poodles.	• Encourage family to be with Ms. D.; provide support because families often welcome assistance in knowing how to be with the patient in ways that are helpful and satisfying. • Offer educational programs on effective patient interactions and invite Ms. D.'s family to participate in activities that are planned and conducted by staff. • Allow the patient visits from pets whenever possible. (For some patients the pet is their most significant other.)
Ms. D. will continue usual spiritual/religious activities.	• Encourage Ms. D. to engage in her usual form of worship and, if comfortable, engage in this activity with Ms. D. (This activity can also promote a sense of belonging and security as it is done within a community context, and it lets the patient use remote memory to engage in a meaningful activity of the present.)

VI

REFERENCES

1. American Psychiatric Association: *Diagnostic and statistical manual of mental disorders,* ed 3, revised, Washington, DC, 1987, Author.
2. Bartol MA: Dialogue with dementia: nonverbal communication in patients, *J Gerontol Nurs* 5:21, 1979.
3. Carpenito LJ: *Nursing diagnosis: application to clinical practice,* ed 3, Philadelphia, 1989, JB Lippincott.
4. Fischer W: Phenomenological commentary to Dr. Jones' paper. In Straus EW, Griffith RM, editors: *Phenomenology of memory,* Pittsburgh, 1970, Duquesne University Press.
5. Gordon M: *Manual of nursing diagnosis,* New York, 1987, McGraw-Hill.
6. Greene M: *Landscapes of learning,* New York, 1978, Teachers College Press.
7. Heidegger M: *Being and time,* New York, 1962, Harper & Row.
8. Kim MJ, McFarland GK, and McLane AM: *Pocket guide to nursing diagnoses,* ed 4, St Louis, 1991, Mosby–Year Book.
9. Luckman J, Sorenson KC: *Medical-surgical nursing: a psychophysiologic approach,* Philadelphia, ed 3, 1987, WB Saunders.
10. Merleau-Ponty M: *Phenomenology of perception,* New York, 1974, Humanities Press.
11. Murry RB, Huelskoetter MMW: *Psychiatric/mental health nursing: giving emotional care,* Norwalk, Conn, 1987, Appleton & Lange.
12. Nelson M: Organic mental disorders. In Hogstel MO, editor: *Geropsychiatric nursing,* St Louis, 1990, Mosby–Year Book.
13. Piaget J: *The child and reality: problems of genetic psychology,* New York, 1973, Grossman Publishers.
14. Stuart GW, Sundeen SJ: *Principles and practice of psychiatric nursing,* ed 3, St Louis, 1987, CV Mosby.
15. Yurick AG and others: *The aged person and the nursing process,* ed 3, Norwalk, Conn, 1989, Appleton & Lange.

Decisional Conflict (Specify)

Decisional Conflict (Specify) is the uncertainty about which course of action to take when choice among competing actions involves risk, loss, regret, or challenge to personal life values (specify focus of conflict, such as personal health, family relationships, career, finances, or other life events).

OVERVIEW

Every day in many clinical settings patients are faced with making choices about alternative actions. Should I have the surgery or not? Should I use condoms or birth control pills? Does my child really need to take medication for hyperactivity? Should I go to the emergency room to have this pain checked out? Should I breastfeed or bottle feed my baby? Is now the time to quit smoking (lose weight, start exercising, do something about my stressful job) or not? Should I move in with my children or go to a nursing home? Decision-making is the process of choosing between alternative courses of action (including inaction). Orem[19] describes the process of decision-making as the first phase of deliberative self-care. Effective producers of self-care understand the courses of action open to them and the effectiveness and desirability of these courses of action before making a decision about the actions they will take and those they will avoid.

Several models with which to judge the effectiveness and desirability of alternative courses of action have emerged in the fields of economics and psychology.[8] Although many theorists disagree about how individuals make or ought to make judgments and decisions, most agree that expectations and values are essential inputs into decisions.[21] These two elements correspond to Orem's concepts[19] of effectiveness and desirability. Expectations or beliefs are subjective judgments about the probability or likelihood that specific outcomes or consequences will result from a course of action. Values or utilities are the individual's preferences for or the relative desirability of these outcomes. Generally, individuals select alternatives that are likely to produce desirable outcomes and unlikely to produce undesirable outcomes. Conversely, they avoid alternatives likely to produce undesirable outcomes or unlikely to produce desirable outcomes.

Unfortunately, many important decisions have alternatives that are likely to produce both desirable and undesirable outcomes. Furthermore, the desired outcomes may occur partly with one alternative and partly with another. Thus no alternative will satisfy all of a person's personal objectives, and no alternative is without risk of undesirable outcomes. This situation is known as a *choice dilemma* or *conflicted decision*.[26] It is characterized by difficulty or uncertainty in identifying the best alternative because of the risk or uncertainty of outcomes, high stakes in terms of potential gains and losses, the need to make value trade-offs in selecting a course of action,[14] and anticipated regret over the positive aspects of rejected options.[26] Janis and Mann[11] describe Decisional Conflict as "the simultaneous opposing tendencies within the individual to accept and reject a given course of action. (p. 46)"

The authors are grateful for the advice of the following researchers whose work focuses on decision-making: Andrea Baumann, R.N., Ph.D.; Lesley Degner, R.N., Ph.D.; Hilary Llewellyn-Thomas, R.N., Ph.D.; and Marilyn L. Rothert, R.N., Ph.D.

VI

Responses to the Decisional Conflict depend on the degree of conflict inherent in the decision. Sjoberg[26] maintains that a low degree of conflict may be attractive and stimulating, a moderate degree may produce defensiveness, and a high degree may bring about hypervigilance and panic. The intensity of stress symptoms depends in part on the anticipated magnitude of losses resulting from whatever choice is made and the magnitude of the anticipated regret over the positive aspects of rejected options.

Little research has been conducted in clinical practice to examine the prevalence of Decisional Conflict experienced by patients and the variation in responses described by Janis and Mann.[11] Hiltunen's phenomenological study[9] with five clients in a home health setting supported the etiology of loss and the symptoms of uncertainty about the courses of action to take. Degner and Beaton's participant observation study[4] of life-death decisions demonstrated the complexity of decisional conflict when jointly made by clinicians, patients, and families. Disagreement in expectations, values, and decisions occurred within and between groups. These data are supported by Rostain's observations[22] Continued research in patient decision-making in clinical settings is essential, because judgment and decision processes vary with the type of decision.[21] Furthermore, concurrent medical problems, emotional distress, and the social influence of health professionals may make the difficulties patients experience with decision-making unique.

ASSESSMENT

The main characteristic manifested by persons having to make a difficult decision is verbalized concern or distress because they are uncertain about which alternative to select. While they are deliberating, they may talk about the undesirable consequences of the choice facing them and question their personal values. Individuals involved in a choice dilemma may demonstrate hesitation, vacillation, and delayed decision-making. Self-focusing behaviors and physiological signs of stress (restlessness, increased heart rate, and muscle

tension) may be manifested. During some decision-making processes, autonomic indicators of stress increase as individuals move toward a decision and gradually return to the level of the resting state after the decision is made.[11]

Responses to a difficult decision vary according to each individual's perception of the level of risk and perception of the magnitude of loss and regret. For example, people recommended for major surgery find decision-making about surgery more difficult than those recommended for minor surgery.[16] Other personal and environmental factors will also influence Decisional Conflict. In a Swedish study, women and immigrants found decisions more difficult compared with men and Swedish citizens; cancer patients also reported more difficulty in making decisions. Hesitancy about whether or not to have surgery was also associated with uncertainty about the nature, extent, and consequences of the operation and anesthesia.[16] Inexperience, past experience, poor information, and emotional distress may contribute to unclear or unrealistic perceptions about courses of action and their consequences, thereby magnifying the conflict. Hesitation in making a decision may also be influenced by a person's lack of knowledge or skill in implementing the decision once it is made. Social factors can also exacerbate the conflict. Patients may lack the social support from others to assist them in making and implementing a decision. They may also receive unwanted interference from their support network or health professionals.[11]

Often a medical diagnosis can lead to Decisional Conflict. With new information about their health, patients must usually consider how they are going to respond to the diagnosis, treatment, and lifestyle advice. Medical problems can also interfere with a person's ability to make decisions, either by reducing cognitive capacity (as sometimes results from impaired perfusion or trauma to the brain) or by producing emotional distress, which at high levels diminishes a person's ability to think clearly.[7,25] In either case, even simple decisions may generate uncertainty about which course of action to take.

Several assessment guides have been developed to identify a person's perception of a problem and the nature of the conflict, including Janis and Mann's decisional balance sheet[11] and Pender's values clarification exercise.[20] These tools assess the qualitative nature of the conflict. Important components to consider are the individual's goals, perceived alternatives and consequences, expectations, and values. From these data, the nurse can judge the source of the conflict; the clarity, comprehensiveness, and viability of alternatives; the clarity, accuracy, and realism of the expectations; and the clarity and priority of values. Other contextual data may need to be collected, depending on the situation. The depth and comprehensiveness of data collection will depend on the clinical context and time constraints. Some of the important areas for assessment are outlined below:

1. *Appearance.* Briefly note the patient's sex, race, apparent age, deportment and overt signs of distress, and composure.
2. *Patient's perception of problem.* Ask the patient to explain in his/her own words what seems to be the problem. Validate impressions.
3. *Factors contributing to difficult decision-making.* Ask the patient to explain in his/her own words what factors are making the decision difficult. As appropriate to the context, ask questions about personal and environmental factors (such as knowledge, experience, support system, other social influences, and personal resources) that are helping or hindering the decision-making.
4. *Personal goals and perceived alternatives.* What goals does the patient wish to achieve? What, in the patient's view, are the available alternatives?
5. *Expectations.* From the patient's perspective, what outcomes are possible with each alternative? How likely are these outcomes?
6. *Values and utilities.* How desirable or undesirable are these outcomes? Ask the patient to rank order.
7. *Resources to implement decisions.* Does the patient perceive difficulty in implementing

the alternatives? Does the patient have the knowledge, motivation, and resources to implement the alternatives?

Quantitative approaches to eliciting the patient's expectations and values have also been developed,[6,15] and some have been tested for reliability, validity, and suitability for clinical practice.[10,17,18] The need for quantitative assessment will depend on the need for refined judgments of the patient's expectations and values and the acceptability of the assessment to the nurse and the patient. Many studies have illustrated the difficulties encountered in eliciting patient expectations and values. Tversky and Kahneman[31] have found that individuals' expectations or judgments about the likelihood of events do not always correspond to reality. People are influenced by *representativeness;* that is, they have the tendency to ignore what is known about the likelihood of the event, and base expectations of an outcome on how similar it is to the major characteristics of the population or process from which it is generated. For example, patients may judge themselves to be less susceptible to contracting a sexually transmitted disease than the rates reported in the literature if they do not believe that they represent the type of patient who would normally contract the disease. People also tend to judge the likelihood of an outcome by the *availability* (the ease with which instances or occurrences can be brought to mind). Outcomes are often judged more likely than they really are if instances of these outcomes are frequent, recent, vivid, and easily imagined. Conversely, they are judged less likely than they really are if they are rare, remote, bland, and difficult to imagine. Depending on the initial starting point one uses in eliciting information, anchoring or adjusting biases can occur through the patient's stating expectations (such as, "Do you think your chances are greater or less than 50%?" or "Do you think your chances are greater or less than 75%?").

Methodological problems also exist when assessing the patient's values. Preference reversals have occurred, depending on whether outcomes are framed positively or negatively, whether risks involve gains or losses, how much regret was expected, and the reference point from which the person was stating a preference.[12,31] These problems make it difficult to get consistent answers about preferences. Furthermore, Fischhoff and colleagues[6] have found that people have difficulty knowing what they want in making a decision when the outcomes are unfamiliar. Values are clearer for outcomes that are familiar, simple, and directly experienced. Slovic and associates[28] have stated that in value assessment, "there may be no substitute for an interactive elicitation procedure, one that employs multiple methods and acknowledges the elicitor's role in helping the respondent to create and enunciate values." Several of these methods are reviewed by Llewellyn-Thomas and Sutherland.[17]

❖ Defining Characteristics

The presence of the following defining characteristics indicates that the patient may be experiencing Decisional Conflict:

- Physical signs of distress or tension (e.g., increased muscle tension, restlessness, and increased heart rate)
- Self-focusing
- Verbalization of distress resulting from uncertainty about choices
- Vacillation between alternative choices
- Delayed decision-making
- Examination of personal values and beliefs while attempting to make a decision
- Verbalization of undesired consequences of alternative actions

❖ Related Factors

The following related factors are associated with Decisional Conflict:

- Lack of knowledge or skills to implement decisions made
- Lack of information about alternatives and consequences
- Interference from others with decision-making
- Unclear alternatives, expectations, or values
- Lack of experience with decision-making
- Lack of an adequate support system
- Unrealistic alternatives or expectations
- Threat to values

❖ Related Medical/Psychiatric Diagnoses

For the nursing diagnosis of Decisional Conflict, any medical or psychiatric diagnosis requiring the patient to make a decision regarding treatment could be considered a related medical diagnosis.

NURSING DIAGNOSES

Examples of *specific* nursing diagnoses for Decisional Conflict are:

- Decisional Conflict (about the type of breast cancer surgery-modified radical mastectomy versus lumpectomy) related to unclear values of relative importance of conserving the breast and avoiding radiation therapy.
- Decisional Conflict (about managing child's hyperactivity with drugs) related to lack of information about other treatment options and fear of drug side effects.
- Decisional Conflict (about the nursing home placement for elder parent) related to social interference from parent's siblings.

PLANNING AND IMPLEMENTATION WITH RATIONALE

The expected outcome of Decisional Conflict is that the patient will make an effective decision. The difficulty in judging effectiveness is that there is no criterion for judging the correctness of a decision, because the decision is based, in part, on the individual's personal opinions and preferences.[21] Some theorists have imposed a mathematical or logical structure on the decision. Prescriptions for consistent behavior have been derived from expected utility theory and Bayesian decision theory, which is based on a combination of probability theory and expected utility theory.[21] These models have been applied to financial decisions[5] and more recently social and health decisions.[34] They provide a set of rules for

VI

combining the patient's expectations and values to determine the alternative with the highest expected value.

Research has demonstrated that human preferences do not correlate well with prescriptive preferences.[24] Proponents of prescriptive models argue that the processing of complex information is beyond human capacity and subsequently encourage the use of prescriptive models, because they believe that the logic of these models provides the best guide for reaching defensible decisions.[5] On the other hand, opponents of prescriptive theory maintain that a poor descriptive theory should not be used prescriptively.[24]

In spite of the difficulty in establishing criteria for effective decision-making, *some outcomes need to be specified to guide action, and they are based on the following assumptions: (1) People who have a clear understanding of the nature of the conflict make better decisions; (2) Informed decisions are better than uninformed decisions; (3) Decisions that are consistent with personal values are better than those that are inconsistent; (4) Decisions that are congruent with subsequent behavior are better than those that are not congruent.*

Therefore effective decisions will be defined as those that are informed, consistent with values, and congruent with behavior. An informed decision is one in which patients (1) are aware of relevant alternatives and their outcomes, (2) have clarified expectations of outcomes that are reasonably aligned with reality, and (3) are aware of the nature of the conflict in the decision. A decision that is consistent with personal values is one in which patients (1) are aware of the value trade-offs they need to make, (2) select the alternative consistent with their trade-off preference, and (3) express satisfaction with the decision they have made. Decisions are congruent with behavior when patients implement the action associated with the decision. The decision may change in time, but they have at least attempted to implement the operational phase of the decision.

Assisting individuals to understand and resolve a difficult decision has been compared with psychotherapy[21] and is referred to here as decision therapy. Approaches may range from unstructured counseling to the use of structured decision aids that are based on different theoretical perspectives on how decisions are or ought to be made.* Most aids provide an organized approach to examining a decision problem, and some provide methods of combining input (expectations and values) to arrive at an optimal decision. Although the latter function has been debated because of the poor correspondence to actual decision-making,[23] the former function is useful in *clarifying the individual's perception of the decision and the elements that make the decision difficult.*

The effectiveness of decision therapy and decision aids is just beginning to be explored. Pitz and Sach's review[21] identified positive benefits such as clarifying the problem, generating more alternatives through goal-oriented approaches, and recognizing the best action through the use of decision trees. Clancy, Cebul, and Williams[2] found that offering physicians a decision aid to guide their decision about whether to receive the hepatitis B vaccine increased the number of physicians who were immunized. Slimmer and Brown[27] discovered that decision therapy was no more effective than a conference control therapy in reducing parents' ambivalence about medication for their hyperactive children. However, it was effective in making parents more aware about the importance of deliberating about their decision.

In the first step of decision therapy,[14] the problem is structured through the specification of the patient's objectives and corresponding attributes and the subsequent generation of proposed alternatives. Next, the possible effect of alternatives is assessed through the determination of the magnitude and likelihood of the outcomes resulting from proposed alternatives (expectations). The third step involves identifying the preferences of decision-makers using value or utility assessment techniques. Then the alternatives are compared

---

*References 1, 8, 15, 21, 29, 35

and evaluated to determine the best choice. Finally, plans for implementing the decision are made and carried out.

This process bears a strong similarity to the assessment process, and indeed *the data obtained from the assessment are used as a first approximation of the decision problem.* It is subsequently revised through a two-way interaction wherein the nurse and patient fill gaps, clarify, and share expertise. Rothert and Talarczyk[23] have outlined the roles and expertise of the nurse and patient when making decisions about following treatment regimens. For example, nurses can provide information about the options available, the risk and probability of outcomes, and the health care resources required and available. Patients' expertise includes their preferences or values and personal, social, and economic resources available.

Control over who guides and who is involved (for example, specific significant others) in the deliberation process should depend on the patient's preference. For example, patients can be classified into one of three profiles of preference for control: those who want to keep, share, or give away control for decision-making.[3] If the patient is a "keeper," he or she may guide the deliberation, while allowing nurse input on the scientific facts. "Sharers" may prefer that the nurse begin the guidance, with input and final decision by the patient, and "givers away" may favor the nurse's adopting an advisory role, with informed consent given by the patient.

When the patient chooses to share the decision-making process with another person, the process is facilitated by the mutual (1) review and clarification of options, outcomes, expectations, values, and actions, (2) revision of elements in which patients lack information by implementing teaching strategies, and (3) the realignment of elements that are unrealistic so that they maintain consistency with current knowledge. The specific interventions depend on the data that the patient provides in the first approximation of the decision problem and the judgments that the nurse and patient make about how complete, salient, accurate, and parsimonious the first approximation is.

Goals and Alternatives

When options are unclear or patients are uninformed, nurses and patients must explore the alternatives available to meet patients' goals. When options are clear but too numerous, they need to be reduced to a few viable alternatives. When patients' range of options appears too narrow or constraining, it must be expanded to accommodate others that have the potential to meet personal objectives.

A similar process is used for identifying outcomes of the viable options. There is no need to exhaustively explore all possible outcomes of a decision. *Rather, the salient outcomes that the patient considers important should be identified. Then expectations of outcomes can be clarified and compared with known probabilities.* Unrealistic expectations need to be realigned, particularly when patients have exaggerated the chances of negative outcomes. However, the nurse must be more cautious when expectations of positive outcomes (for example, survival or remission from disease) are exaggerated. Expectations bear a conceptual resemblance to hope.[30] Most nurses would be loath to reduce patients' expectations of survival unless patients requested that they know what their chances are.

Values Clarification

Values clarification can be enhanced through qualitative[11,20] and quantitative[17] exercises. Patients are asked to rank outcomes according to relative desirability; they must also recognize the implicit trade-offs they make when selecting one alternative over the other.

In a study conducted by Ward, Heidrich, and Wolberg,[33] two competing values in the decision about modified radical mastectomy and lumpectomy were fear of radiotherapy (required after lumpectomy) and fear of losing a breast.

Decision Selection and Implementation

Once patients are aware of viable alternatives, realistic expectations, and implicit value trade-offs, they are in a better position to make an informed decision consistent with value trade-offs.

VI

❖ NURSING CARE GUIDELINES

Nursing Diagnosis: *Decisional Conflict (Specify)*

Expected Patient Outcomes	Nursing Interventions
The patient will engage in effective decision-making.	• Initiate decision therapy.
The patient will become informed and base his/her decision on this information.	• Aid the patient in clarifying goals, alternatives, and potential outcomes. • Help the patient to clarify expectations of outcomes for each alternative. • Help the patient realign unrealistic alternatives, outcomes, and expectations. • With the patient, identify viable alternatives and salient outcomes.
The patient will select a course of action that is consistent with his/her values.	• With the patient, clarify desirability of possible outcomes and priority of these outcomes. • Identify value trade-offs implicit in alternative selection. • Facilitate alternative selection.
The patient will implement the decision.	• Teach and reinforce self-help skills required for behavioral implementation of decision.

After selection, they need to act on the decision. Orem[19] refers to the operational phase of the decision as the second phase of self-care. Patients may have briefly considered resources needed before making a decision, but rarely have they worked out all of the operational details. For this part of the therapy, personal and environmental resources to aid in the implementation of the decision are evaluated. If deficits exist, the patient must acquire the self-help skills necessary for implementation and rely on external resources if necessary.

EVALUATION

Expected outcomes are achieved when the patient (1) identifies viable alternatives, (2) expresses realistic expectations of outcomes of alternatives, (3) indicates relative importance of each outcome, (4) selects a course of action consistent with expectations and values, (5) acquires and uses knowledge and skills to implement the course of action, and (6) expresses satisfaction at having made the best decision under the circumstances.

❖ CASE STUDY WITH PLAN OF CARE

Mrs. Nellie G., a 60-year-old postmenopausal patient diagnosed with breast cancer, has recently undergone a modified radical mastectomy. There was no evidence of metastasis, and her lymph nodes were negative for cancer. The hormone receptor status of the tumor was positive. The medical oncologist informed her that she would need to have adjuvant chemotherapy to reduce her chances of tumor recurrence. She was told that the usual chemotherapy was tamoxifen, an antihormone oral medication that is usually tolerated well with few side effects (such as hot flashes and mild nausea that is usually relieved if taken with milk). However,

❖ *CASE STUDY WITH PLAN OF CARE—cont'd*

there was a clinical trial in progress to establish the improvement in disease-free survival if a 6-month course of intravenous CMF (cyclophosphamide methotrexate, 5-fluorouracil) was given in addition to tamoxifen. The side effects of CMF included nausea, vomiting, fatigue, mouth sores, bladder irritation, and hair loss. Also, the white blood cell count might be depressed, thereby increasing the risk of infection, and occasionally the platelets might decrease, increasing the chances of bleeding. Therefore Mrs. G. would be monitored very closely, and treatment would be delayed or modified if platelets or white blood cell counts dropped too low. Mrs. G. was asked whether she would consider participating in the trial. If she agreed, she would have an equal chance of receiving either the tamoxifen alone or the tamoxifen plus intravenous CMF. Mrs. G. was upset that she required treatment in addition to the surgery. She became extremely agitated when intravenous chemotherapy was mentioned. She burst into tears and stated that she was unable to make any decisions at this time. The oncologist gave her the consent form and asked her to talk it over with her family and let him know at the next visit. If she agreed, Mrs. G. would have to receive treatment at that time for her to be eligible in the trial. At the next visit, Mrs. G. still appeared quite distressed. She stated that she had decided to participate in the trial because her family thought she would get more attention from the medical staff, and besides, she had a 50% chance of receiving the oral medication treatment alone. After Mrs. G. signed the consent form, the clinical trial's head office used random procedures to assign her to a treatment plan, and she was allocated to receive tamoxifen plus intravenous CMF. When she learned she would be getting CMF, she started to cry, stating that she did not know whether she could go through with the treatment. The chemotherapy nurse was asked to come and see her.

INTERACTIVE ASSESSMENT

Appearance

60-year-old, well-dressed, and well-groomed white woman in emotional state. Swollen red eyes, shaky hand movements, avoiding direct eye contact.

Patient's perception of problem

PATIENT: I know I promised I would be in the study, and my family thinks I will get more attention,

but I can't bear the thought of taking that chemotherapy. I've seen what it does to people. My mother had it, and it made her sick and miserable—and she died anyway . . . *[Stops and cries for a while.]* I used to take her to the clinic sometimes, and I saw what it did to some of the other people too. It didn't seem to do much good. I wouldn't have minded if I had been given only the pills, but the chemo . . . I don't know what to do. I've signed the form. The doctor says I have to have the treatment today to be eligible. I know how important it is to study these treatments, and he thinks it could prevent the tumor from coming back. But those side effects. I've been so upset about everything lately . . . I can't think straight.

NURSE: *[Validates.]* You don't know whether you should take the chemotherapy or not; you're finding it hard to decide.

PATIENT: Yes, that's right.

Factors contributing to difficult decision-making

NURSE: It is a hard decision to make. If you would like, we can discuss the things that make it hard for you to decide. Do you think that would be okay?

PATIENT: Yes. *[Pause.]* I'm upset, and it's hard to think straight. I wish my husband were here. He's at a meeting, so my neighbor came with me. I don't feel that I can discuss these things with her, and I need to decide now.

Goals and perceived alternatives

Patient indicated previously that decision is to take intravenous chemotherapy along with tamoxifen, or take tamoxifen and refuse intravenous chemotherapy; goals appear to be survival, quality of life, and social approval and will be validated during decision therapy.

Expectations

NURSE: Let's begin by talking about what you think the advantages and disadvantages of taking and not taking chemo are. If you took the intravenous chemotherapy, what would be the pluses and minuses of that choice?

PATIENT: Well. . . I know that I would be sick . . . nausea and vomiting and everything. My hair

Continued.

❖ *CASE STUDY WITH PLAN OF CARE—cont'd*

would fall out, and I'd get those mouth sores my mother got . . . awful . . . I would probably get more attention because they will be following me more closely. The drug may stop the tumor from coming back, but then it may not. That's why the need for the study, I suppose. It certainly didn't work for my mother.

NURSE: So from your point of view, taking the chemotherapy may get you more attention but will probably make you sick with nausea, vomiting, hair loss, and mouth sores. It may prevent the tumor from coming back, but it may not.

PATIENT: Yes, that's right.

NURSE: Have I left anything out?

PATIENT: No. I think that pretty well covers it.

NURSE: If you didn't take the intravenous chemotherapy, what would be the pluses and minuses of that choice?

PATIENT: I wouldn't have the side effects from taking just the pills. But my family will be disappointed that I didn't go through with it, and the doctor may get upset. I already signed the form, and I like to keep my word. I wouldn't get the attention, but I suppose I wouldn't need it if I didn't take those strong drugs.

NURSE: So, from your point of view, not undergoing chemotherapy will have fewer side effects, but your doctor or your family may disapprove and you may feel bad because you didn't keep your word. You'd get less attention, but maybe that isn't important.

PATIENT: Yes.

NURSE: Any other points about not undergoing chemotherapy?

PATIENT: No.

Values/Utilities

NURSE: So it would appear that, for you, taking intravenous chemotherapy means having unpleasant side effects, but not undergoing chemotherapy means having your family and doctor disapprove of your decision and you would feel bad for not keeping your word. Do you know which of these consequences would be worse for you: family and doctor disapproval, feeling bad for not keeping your word, or having side effects?

PATIENT: That's hard to say, I don't want the side effects, but I don't want my family or doctor to think badly of me. [The decision appears to involve making trade-offs between toxicity and social approval. Eliciting priorities or trade-offs is deferred until expectations are realigned with reality.]

NURSE: I've listed all the pluses and minuses of the decision you have to make. Maybe we can look these over together. I can let you know from my experience what you can realistically expect from selecting each alternative, and you can let me know how important each of these advantages and disadvantages is to you. Then maybe the best decision for you may be clearer to you.

PLAN OF CARE FOR MRS. NELLIE G.

Nursing Diagnosis: Decisional Conflict (about taking IV CMF chemotherapy) related to interference in decision-making from anxiety and time pressure and unclear values about relative importance of outcome

Expected Patient Outcomes	Nursing Interventions
Mrs. G. will engage in effective decision-making.	• Provide Mrs. G. with decision therapy.

Expected Patient Outcomes	Nursing Interventions
Mrs. G.'s expectations of side effects and social disapproval will be realigned as evidenced by her ability to make a decision.	• Reaffirm valid beliefs about alternatives and benefits of treatment. • Help Mrs. G. realign expectations of side effects (not everyone experiences difficulty). • Remind Mrs. G. that she is free to withdraw from trial at any time without influencing her care and that her family is unaware of treatment assignment and may have different advice now.
Mrs. G. will select a course of action that is consistent with her values as evidenced by her satisfaction in being able to make a difficult decision.	• Help Mrs. G. clarify priority of outcomes (e.g., toxicity, social disapproval, and keeping her word). • Facilitate alternative selection in light of new information and values clarification.
Mrs. G. will implement her decision.	• Review problems implementing decision; support decision implementation (e.g., offer to be there when she informs her family and physician of decision).

REFERENCES

1. Beach LR, Wise JA: Decision emergence: a Lewinian perspective, *Acta Psychol* 45:343-356, 1980.
2. Clancy D, Cebul R, and Williams S: Guiding individual decisions: a randomized, controlled trial of decision analysis, *Amer J Med* 84:283-288, 1988.
3. Degner LF, Aquino Russell C: Preferences for treatment control among adults with cancer, *Res Nurs Health* 11:367-374, 1988.
4. Degner LF, Beaton J: *Life-death decisions in health care,* Washington, 1987, Hemisphere Publishing.
5. Fischer G: Utility models for multiple objective decisions: do they accurately represent human preferences? *Decision Sci* 10:451-479, 1979.
6. Fischhoff B, Slovic P, and Lichtenstein S: Knowing what you want: measuring labile values. In Wallsten TS, editor: *Cognitive processes in choice and decision behavior,* Hillsdale, NJ, 1980, Lawrence Erlbaum Associates.
7. Fitten LJ, Waite MS: Impact of medical hospitalization on treatment decision-making capacity in the elderly, *Arch Intern Med* 150:1717-1721, 1990.
8. Hammond KR, McClelland GH, and Mumpower J: *Human judgment and decision making,* New York, 1980, Praeger Publishers.
9. Hiltunen E: Decisional conflict: a phenomenological description from the points of view of the nurse and client. In McLane A, editor: *Classification of nursing diagnoses: proceedings of the Seventh Conference,* St Louis, 1987, CV Mosby.
10. Holmes MM and others: Comparison of physicians vs. premenopausal women in importance ascribed to potential outcomes of estrogen replacement therapy, *Clin Res* 32:648, 1984.
11. Janis IL, Mann L: *Decision making,* New York, 1977, Free Press.
12. Kahneman D, Tversky A: The psychology of preferences, *Science* 246:160-171, 1982.
13. Kaufman DH: An interview guide for helping children make health-care decisions, *Pediatr Nurs* 11:365-367, 1985.
14. Keeney RL: Decision analysis: an overview, *Operations Res* 30:803-838, 1982.
15. Keeney RL, Raiffa H: *Decisions with multiple objectives: preferences and value tradeoffs,* New York, 1976, John Wiley & Sons.
16. Larsson US, Svardsudd K, Wedel H, and Saljo R: Patient involvement in decision making in surgical and orthopaedic practice: the project perioperative risk, *Soc Sci Med* 28:829-835, 1989.
17. Llewellyn-Thomas HA, Sutherland HJ: Procedures for value assessment. In Cahoon MC, editor: *Recent advances in nursing: research methodology,* Edinburgh, 1987, Churchill Livingstone.
18. O'Connor A: Effects of framing and level of probability on patients' preferences for cancer chemotherapy, *J Clin Epidemiol* 42:119-126, 1989.
19. Orem DE: *Nursing concepts of practice,* ed 4, St Louis, 1991, Mosby–Year Book.
20. Pender NJ, Pender AR: *Health promotion in nursing practice,* ed 2, Norwalk, Conn, 1987, Appleton & Lange.
21. Pitz GF, Sachs NJ: Judgment and decision: theory and application, *Annu Rev Psychol* 35:139-63, 1984.
22. Rostain A: Deciding to forego life-sustaining treatment in the intensive care nursery: a sociological account, *Perspect Biol Med* 30:117-134, 1986.
23. Rothert ML, Talarczyk GJ: Patient compliance and the decision making process of clinicians and patients, *J Compliance Health Care* 2:55-71, 1987.

VI

24. Schoemaker PJH: The expected utility model: its variants, purposes, evidence, and limitations. In Paelinck JHP, Vossen PH, editors: *The quest for optimality,* New York, 1984, Gower Medical Publishing.

25. Scott D: Anxiety, critical thinking and information processing during and after breast biopsy, *Nurs Res* 32:24-28, 1983.

26. Sjoberg L: To smoke or not to smoke: conflict or lack of differentiation? In Humphreys P, Svenson O, and Vari A, editors: *Analyzing and aiding decision processes,* Amsterdam, 1983, North-Holland.

27. Slimmer LW, Brown RT: Parent's decision making process in medication administration for control of hyperactivity, *J Sch Health* 55:221-225, 1985.

28. Slovic P, Fischhoff B, and Lichtenstein S: Response mode, framing, and information-processing effects in risk assessment. In Hogarth R, editor: *New directions for methodology of social and behavioral science: question, framing and response consistency,* San Francisco, 1982, Jossey-Bass.

29. Sox HC, Blatt MA, Higgins MC, and Marton KI: *Medical decision making,* Boston, 1988, Butterworths Publishers.

30. Stotland E: The psychology of hope, San Francisco, 1969, Jossey-Bass.

31. Tversky A, Kahneman D: The framing of decisions and the psychology of choice, *Science* 211:453-458, 1981.

32. Tversky A, Kahneman D: Judgment under uncertainty: heuristics and bias. In Kahneman D, Slovic P, and Tversky A, editors: *Judgment under uncertainty: heuristics and biases,* Cambridge, 1982, Cambridge University Press.

33. Wards S, Heidrich S, and Wolberg W: Factors women take into account when deciding upon type of surgery for breast cancer, *Cancer Nurs* 12:344-351, 1989.

34. Weinstein MC, Fineberg HV: *Clinical decision analysis,* Philadelphia, 1980, WB Saunders.

35. Wilson CZ, Alexis M: Basic frameworks for decisions. In Koontz H, O'Donnell C, editors: *Management: a book of readings,* ed 3, New York, 1982, McGraw-Hill.

VI

Knowledge Deficit (Specify)

Knowledge Deficit (Specify) is an individual's lack of information[15] or inability to state or explain information or demonstrate a required skill related to disease management procedures. It is also the inability to explain or use self-care practices recommended to restore health or maintain wellness.[11] It may appear as a cognitive or psychomotor deficit[6] or a combination of the two.

OVERVIEW

The nursing diagnosis of Knowledge Deficit is the nurse's judgment that the patient lacks the information needed to be an active, informed participant in his/her health care.[22] A deficit in knowledge is commonly experienced by individuals coping with new medical diagnoses, varied pharmacological and treatment regimens, and unfamiliar and often complex procedures, as well as by individuals entering developmental stages or role relationships that demand new patterns of response. Several epidemiologic studies have identified Knowledge Deficit as a high-frequency diagnosis among varied patient populations and clinical settings.*

To understand the theory of Knowledge Deficit, one must first understand the hierarchy of learning.[18] Knowledge attainment is the most basic type of cognitive learning. It entails receiving and retaining a factual statement long enough to recall it at some later moment. Attitudinal learning requires an emotional response rather than a factual one. It involves acquiring information and then personally responding to it. Psychomotor learning is the behavioral response to internalized information through neuromuscular pathways. It

*References 1, 5, 7, 9, 12, 20

represents the level of learning at which behavior change becomes possible.

The diagnosis of Knowledge Deficit is broad and can be applied to deficits in all three learning realms. It may be appropriately applied both in circumstances where a person needs increased factual information and in situations where the patient can correctly state the relevant facts but cannot incorporate them into appropriate behavior.

It should be noted that there is a difference between the patient who is unable to translate information into behavior change and the patient who elects not to do so. In the latter case the appropriate diagnosis is not Knowledge Deficit, and assessment must distinguish between the two cases. Differential diagnoses for such patients include Altered Health Maintenance, Noncompliance, Decisional Conflict, and Defensive Coping.

Taxonomy II defines *knowing* as "To recognize or acknowledge . . . to be familiar with . . . to be cognizant of something . . . to understand."[10] Several authors have discussed the broad scope and imprecision of the label and have proposed that it be revised[10] or deleted.[8,10,13,17] Jenny[13] argued that Knowledge Deficit is not a health state or a dysfunctional pattern of behavior. She postulated that Knowledge Deficit is more often a risk factor or defining characteristic of another diagnosis. Dennison and Keeling[8] found that its use fostered stereotypical interventions and failed to enhance creative nursing strategies designed to both increase information and change behavior. Rakel and Bulechek[23] argued that Knowledge Deficit is valid but too broad in scope, and is applied to situations where the problem is alteration in learning, rather than alteration in knowledge. They proposed that two additional diagnoses be included in the Knowing pattern, to describe situational learning disabilities.

Because knowledge deficit may be a symptom of another problem, the nurse must determine the appropriate clinical weight of the acquired assessment data when she formulates the differential diagnosis of every case. The diagnostician must base assessment and diagnosis on an understanding of all types of learning and must recognize that rarely is a simple increase in factual knowledge the optimal outcome of nursing care. Both diagnoses and interventions must focus on facilitating and enhancing health-promoting integration of factual knowledge. Knowledge Deficit will undoubtedly continue to be further refined and specified.

ASSESSMENT

The ability of the nurse to identify and treat a Knowledge Deficit is heavily influenced by his/her understanding of teaching and learning theories and by the scope of assessment in areas that might seem unrelated to knowledge. The impact of such variables as physiological condition, presence of anxiety, socioeconomic status, level of formal education, cultural and language barriers, and interest in learning must be weighed at each phase of the nursing process. Each of these affects the way in which each patient's Knowledge Deficit presents and the likelihood that it will be ameliorated.

Validation studies of the defining characteristics of Knowledge Deficit are limited.[8,22] Two studies found the label applied in the apparent absence of any of the published defining characteristics, which either may indicate an automatic rote application of the diagnosis to justify task-oriented patient teaching,[21] or may reflect the use of defining characteristics embedded in the art of providing skilled nursing care and yet to be adequately articulated.[3]

No critical defining characteristics for the diagnosis of Knowledge Deficit have been suggested or validated through research.[22] The patient's statements of inadequate recall or understanding of information and of inadequate knowledge are the defining characteristics best supported by the literature.[22] The defining characteristics primarily reflect the acquisition of knowledge. Defining characteristics that are behavioral include inaccurate follow-through of instructions and inadequate performance of a skill or on a test. Testing, though widely used in didactic situations and research, remains an uncommon clinical assessment tool in the acute care setting. When applied, often in ambulatory or community settings, it can provide a useful measurement of knowledge, attitude, and behavior change.[4]

Assessment must include the broad range of relevant data. These may be cultural factors, socioeconomic factors, intellectual capacity, psychological response to the existing illness or wellness under consideration, current knowledge, extent to which knowledge is incorporated into behavior, and motivation and readiness to learn. Sensory, neuromuscular, cardiopulmonary, and nutritive integrity must be considered as well. Gordon's functional patterns[11] not only organize assessment, but also address all of these areas.

Both Gordon[11] and NANDA[15] list inappropriate or exaggerated behaviors such as hysteria, apathy, agitation, and hostility among the defining characteristics of Knowledge Deficit. No other nursing literature supports this, so these behaviors have been omitted from the following list pending some support for their relevancy. Careful assessment and differential diagnosis may determine that they indicate other diagnoses, such as mild to moderate Anxiety or Ineffective Individual Coping, that may commonly occur with Knowledge Deficit.

❖ Defining Characteristics

The presence of the following defining characteristics indicates that the patient may be experiencing Knowledge Deficit:

- Verbalization of inadequate information or of inadequate recall of information
- Verbalization of misunderstanding or misconception
- Requesting information
- Inaccurate follow-through of instructions

- Inadequate performance on a test
- Inadequate demonstration of a skill

❖ **Related Factors**

The following related factors are associated with Knowledge Deficit:
- Pathophysiological states
- Sensory deficits
- Memory loss
- Intellectual limitations
- Interfering coping strategies (e.g., denial or anxiety)
- Lack of exposure to accurate information
- Lack of motivation to learn
- Lack of readiness to learn
- Inattention
- Cultural or language barriers

❖ **Related Medical/Psychiatric Diagnoses**

The following are examples of related medical/psychiatric diagnoses for Knowledge Deficit:
- Asthma
- Coronary artery disease
- Cystic fibrosis
- Diabetes
- HIV disease
- Hypertension
- Lung cancer
- Phenylketonuria

NURSING DIAGNOSES

Examples of specific nursing diagnoses for Knowledge Deficit are:
- Knowledge Deficit (hypertensive medications) related to memory loss.
- Knowledge Deficit (infant care) related to lack of exposure to accurate information.
- Knowledge Deficit (diabetic self-care) related to anxiety.

PLANNING AND IMPLEMENTATION WITH RATIONALE

Outcome criteria for the patient being treated for Knowledge Deficit can refer to any of the three types of learning: knowledge attainment, attitudinal change, and behavior change. They are described in that order in the standardized care plan on p. 483. The predominant intervention to treat Knowledge Deficit is patient education.

There is a substantial body of literature supporting that varied teaching strategies increase factual knowledge,[19,26] affect attitudinal changes,[14,25] and result in behavioral changes.[2,4,16,24]

The outcome criteria and suggested interventions in the standardized care plan represent a continuum. The full spectrum is not necessarily appropriate in all situations. At times the patient's simple demonstration of increased knowledge may be a valid end point for nursing interventions. Because the success of each outcome in the hierarchy depends on the achievement of the lower ones, the interventions identified for the lower outcomes mentioned first in the care plan also apply to the ones mentioned later, but these interventions are not repeated.

Although the categories of outcomes described in the Nursing Care Guidelines can be broadly generalized, the interventions may be quite specific to the particular type of Knowledge Deficit under consideration. These are intended to provide but a few examples of outcomes and rationales.

Simple knowledge attainment or knowledge increase is a first-stage outcome. Patient teaching or patient education is often directed at that goal. A variety of possible techniques have been used to assist the patient to increase knowledge, and there is a substantial body of literature dealing with patient education, to which the reader is referred. It is critical that the nurse weigh such variables as culture, developmental stage, acuity or chronicity of the learning need,[3] and the patient's ability and motivation to learn[23] when selecting a particular teaching approach. For the example given, the rationale for the stated intervention is that *the patient must have factual information about the adverse effect of smoking on health.*

Attitudinal change is a second-stage outcome. The patient must evaluate factual knowledge, determine its relevance to his/her own perceived circumstance, and reevaluate personal behaviors in that context. The interventions in this cluster are designed to *assist the patient to evaluate facts in the context of his/her own life.*

Behavioral change is a third-stage outcome.

VI

❖ *NURSING CARE GUIDELINES*

Nursing Diagnosis: Knowledge Deficit (hazards of smoking)

Expected Patient Outcomes	Nursing Interventions
The patient will list three adverse effects of smoking on health.	• Teach factual information about the effect of smoking on health in a 1-hour in-class format. • Use a variety of teaching techniques to meet identified learning need, such as lectures, discussions, audiovisual media, and personal presentations by former smokers. • Provide written materials (e.g., pamphlets) containing the same information to be read at home. • Involve the patient's family or significant others in learning process so they can reinforce new knowledge.
The patient will verbally express a desire to quit smoking.	• Assess recall of the factual information presented to the patient. • Provide feedback on the patient's accuracy and repeat information that was inaccurately recalled. • Maintain an accepting, nonjudgmental atmosphere. • Encourage the patient to relate adverse effects of smoking to his/her personal health. • Measure the patient's cardiopulmonary fitness and compare with the normal statistics of his/her age group. • Measure the patient's blood lipid profile and compare with desired levels. • Support the patient in identifying and expressing his/her reasons for smoking and refer to psychiatric consultant for assistance of needed. • Assist family members to share with the patient their feelings about the patient's smoking.
The patient will conduct his/her usual daily activities for 2 days without smoking a cigarette.	• Advise the patient to remove cigarettes, matches, and ashtrays from the environment to decrease behavioral stimuli. • Plan with the patient one or more techniques that will distract the patient when he/she feels an urge to smoke, e.g., chewing gum, snapping a rubber band on the wrist, or walking around the block or building. • Contact the patient by phone twice a day to offer support and access for any changed needs. • Refer the patient to a community resource that provides a support group for smoking cessation.

VI

Facts and attitudes have been internalized, and the patient is able to demonstrate the value he/she has attached to them by amending a less healthy behavior to one that is more health-enhancing. The rationale for the interventions given in the example is *to positively reinforce health-enhancing behaviors*.

EVALUATION

The measures to evaluate success will vary depending on the type of outcome criteria selected. Acquisition of factual knowledge can be readily measured by written or verbal questioning. This can be done informally as the teaching progresses or formally at the conclusion of a teaching session or series of sessions. Behavior change is best evaluated by requiring a demonstration of a skill or the attainment of a specific predetermined goal (for example, no smoking for 2 days). Attitudinal change is perhaps the most nebulous and difficult to evaluate. Verbal or written statements indicating an openness to another's viewpoint and an interest in exploring the value of behavioral change (if relevant) both indicate that the outcome criteria have been met.

❖ *CASE STUDY WITH PLAN OF CARE*

Mr. Benjamin F., a 22-year-old man, comes to the anonymous test site at the community health center for a human immunodeficiency virus (HIV) antibody test. He is worried that his work situation puts him at risk for exposure to the virus and wants to know his antibody status. He has generally good health and maintains appropriate weight. Mr. F. does not smoke or use drugs now, but he did use intravenous heroine for a 6-month period 3 years ago. He has been "clean" since then. He drinks two or three beers on weekends. His nutritional, elimination, and sleep-rest patterns are all normal and unremarkable. For exercise, he uses a stationary bicycle three times a week. He is completely independent in all activities of daily living, and he experiences occasional fatigue that he attributes to working too much overtime. Mr. F.'s vision, hearing, and memory are all excellent. After attending college for 2 years, he now works as a draftsman in an architectural firm. He describes himself as a quick learner, but he responds correctly to only three of ten questions on a quiz to measure baseline knowledge of HIV infection. Mr. F. says that he learns readily from written materials and televised programs. Mr. F. is comfortable with his body image and present life, and he hopes to complete college eventually. He lives alone in a one bedroom apartment, and his family lives in another state. His income is adequate for his needs. He has several close friends nearby. He dates two women regularly and is considering a more serious relationship with the one with whom he is sexually active twice a week. She uses oral contraceptives. Mr. F. is becoming increasingly worried about contracting the HIV infection at work. An office mate, a gay man, tested HIV positive 6 months ago. Mr. F. and this man use the same telephone, drafting implements, and bathroom facilities. Mr. F. hopes to marry within the next year and believes that it is his duty to be sure he does not "bring AIDS home from the office."

PLAN OF CARE FOR MR. BENJAMIN F.

Nursing Diagnosis: Knowledge Deficit (transmission pathways of HIV infection) related to lack of exposure to correct information as evidenced by request for information, verbalization of misconceptions, and inadequate performance on a test

Expected Patient Outcomes	Nursing Interventions
Mr. F. will state three transmission pathways for HIV infection.	• Through verbal instruction and an AIDS education video, teach Mr. F. the facts about HIV transmission. • Provide Mr. F. with pamphlets containing the same information to read at home. • Reinforce information with Mr. F. on at least two separate occasions.

Continued.

Expected Patient Outcomes	Nursing Interventions
Mr. F. will correctly state his past behavior (IV drug use) and present behavior (unprotected sex) that put him at risk for HIV infection.	• Assist Mr. F. to relate risk information to his own behaviors. • Provide Mr. F. with information to refute misconceptions. • Support Mr. F. in expressing feelings of guilt and anger. • Refer Mr. F. for psychiatric counseling if needed.
Mr. F. will correctly state the results of his antibody test and the meaning of them.	• Draw blood specimen and submit to laboratory. • Inform Mr. F. of the results of the test. • Explain the significance of the results. • Ask Mr. F. to repeat the results and the meaning of them to you.
Mr. F. will apply condoms correctly and use them when having sexual intercourse.	• Demonstrate the proper technique for condom application and removal. • Provide Mr. F. with an opportunity for return demonstration. • Instruct Mr. F. about the importance of regular use of condom. • Maintain open and nonjudgmental atmosphere.

REFERENCES

1. Aukamp V: A field study to identify nursing diagnoses for childbearing families. In McLane A, editor: *Classification of nursing diagnoses: proceedings of the Seventh Conference,* St Louis, 1987, CV Mosby Co.
2. Becker MH, Joseph JG: AIDS and behavior change to reduce risk: a review, *Am J Public Health* 78:394-410, 1988.
3. Benner P: *From novice to expert,* Menlo Park, Calif, 1984, Addison-Wesley.
4. Brailey LJ: Effects of health teaching in the workplace on women's knowledge, beliefs, and practices regarding breast self-examination, *Res Nurs Health* 9:223-231, 1986.
5. Burns CE: Field testing of a comprehensive taxonomy of diagnoses for pediatric nurse practitioners. In Carroll-Johnson RM, editor: *Classification of nursing diagnoses: proceedings of the Ninth Conference,* Philadelphia, 1991, JB Lippincott.
6. Carpenito LJ: *Nursing diagnosis: application to clinical practice,* ed 2, Philadelphia, 1987, JB Lippincott.
7. Collard AF and others: The occurrence of nursing diagnoses in ambulatory care. In McLane A, editor: *Classification of nursing diagnoses: proceedings of the Seventh Conference,* St Louis, 1987, CV Mosby Co.
8. Dennison PD, Keeling AW: Clinical support for eliminating the nursing diagnosis of knowledge deficit, *Image* 21:142-144, 1989.
9. Fitzmaurice JB, Thatcher J, and Schappler N: High-volume/high-risk nursing diagnoses as a basis for priority setting in a tertiary hospital. In Carroll-Johnson RM, editor: *Classification of nursing diagnoses: proceedings of the Ninth Conference,* Philadelphia, 1991, JB Lippincott.
10. Fitzpatrick JJ: Taxonomy II: definitions and development. In Carroll-Johnson RM, editor: *Classification of nursing diagnoses: proceedings of the Ninth Conference,* Philadelphia, 1991, JB Lippincott.
11. Gordon M: *Manual of nursing diagnosis 1986-1987,* New York, 1987, McGraw-Hill.
12. Greenlee KK: The effects of implementation of an operational definition and guidelines for the formulation of nursing diagnoses in a critical care setting. In Carroll-Johnson RM, editor: *Classification of nursing diagnoses: proceedings of the Ninth Conference,* Philadelphia, 1991, JB Lippincott.
13. Jenny J: Knowledge deficit: not a nursing diagnosis, *Image J Nurs Sch* 19:184-185, 1987.
14. Kegeles SM, Adler NE, and Irwin CE: Sexually active adolescents and condoms: changes over one year in knowledge, attitudes, and use, *Am J Public Health* 78:460-461, 1988.
15. Kim MJ, McFarland GK, and McLane A: *Pocket guide to nursing diagnoses,* ed 2, St Louis, 1987, Mosby–Year Book.
16. King I, Tarsitano B: The effect of structured and unstructured pre-operative teaching: a replication, *Nurs Res* 31:324-329, 1982.
17. Kuhn RC: American Association of Critical Care Nurses. In Carroll-Johnson RM, editor: *Classification of nursing diagnoses: proceedings of the Ninth Conference,* Philadelphia, 1991, JB Lippincott.
18. Lester PA: Teaching strategies. In Johnson SE, editor: *Nursing assessment and strategies for the family at risk: high risk parenting,* ed 2, Philadelphia, 1986, JB Lippincott.
19. Linde BJ and Janz NM: Effect of a teaching program on knowledge and compliance of cardiac patients, *Nurs Res* 28:282-286, 1979.

VI

20. Martin PA, York KA: Incidence of nursing diagnoses. In Kim MJ, McFarland GK, and McLane AM, editors: *Classification of nursing diagnoses: proceedings of the Fifth Conference,* St Louis, 1984, CV Mosby Co.

21. Nicoletti A: Nurse's Association of the American College of Obstetrics and Gynecology. In Carroll-Johnson RM, editor: *Classification of nursing diagnoses: proceedings of the Ninth Conference,* Philadelphia, 1991, JB Lippincott.

22. Pokorny BE: Validating a diagnostic label: knowledge deficit, *Nurs Clin North Am* 20(4):641-655, 1985.

23. Rakel BA, Bulechek GM: Development of alterations in learning: situational learning disabilities, *Nurs Diagn* 1:134-146, 1990.

24. Raleigh EH, Odtohan BC: The effect of a cardiac teaching program on patient rehabilitation, *Heart Lung* 16:311-317, 1987.

25. Reis J, Herz L: Young adolescents' contraceptive knowledge and attitudes: implications for anticipatory guidance, *J Pediatr Health Care* 1:247-254, 1987.

26. Steele JM, Ruzicki D: An evaluation of the effectiveness of cardiac teaching during hospitalization, *Heart Lung* 16:306-311, 1987.

VI

SELF-PERCEPTION—
SELF-CONCEPT PATTERN
Fear

Fear *is the feeling of dread related to an identifiable source that the person validates.*[6]

OVERVIEW

Fear is an uncomfortable, ominous feeling caused by conscious recognition of a source of danger. A survival mechanism, Fear is a protective emotion that mobilizes the individual for "fight or flight" to cope with a potential or actual threat.

Although similar to Anxiety, Fear occurs in response to a real and identifiable danger or threat.[13] Anxiety, on the other hand, is a vague, diffuse uneasiness occurring in response to unidentifiable threats to the individual's essential values. They are closely related, however, because underlying every fear is the anxiety of being unable to preserve one's own being.[10]

A phobia is a specific type of Fear that is exaggerated and often disabling.[8] It is characterized by an intense desire to avoid the feared object or situation—a situation that objectively poses little or no threat of danger. Acrophobia, or fear of heights, is an example of a common phobia.

As a normal, adaptive response to danger, Fear follows a specific sequence in human development.[12] The newborn infant is frightened by loud noises or by a sudden loss of support. The toddler aged 2 to 5 years—a particularly fearful period in human development—may fear ghosts, animals, the dark, or separation from significant others. These Fears are replaced in the school-aged child by more realistic fears, such as bodily injury,

war, and death. The adolescent is more often frightened of school failure, rejection by peers, pain, and disease. Generally, developmental Fears are diminished by maturation and by simple measures that reassure the child, such as a night light for fear of darkness. Elderly clients often express Fears of sensory impairment, loneliness, or poverty.

ASSESSMENT

A nursing diagnosis of Fear results from subjective and objective data obtained from three areas of observation: physiological responses, behavioral manifestations, and the subjective experiences of the patient. Neuroendocrine stress response activation signifies the physiological signs and symptoms of Fear. The resulting "fight or flight" response is initiated when a threat is perceived in the cortex of the brain. A signal via the sympathetic branch of the autonomic nervous system stimulates the adrenal glands to release epinephrine and norepinephrine. The resulting cardiovascular excitation is characterized by increased heart rate, increased blood pressure, and shunting of blood from the skin and gastrointestinal tract to the heart, central nervous system, and skeletal muscles. The nurse may observe pupil dilation, pallor, increased or irregular respiratory rate, and palmar sweating in the frightened patient. The patient may report insomnia, anorexia, and urinary frequency.

Behaviorally, the fearful individual may "flee" by withdrawing from social interaction or "fight" with aggressive or hostile actions. The patient may direct anger toward the nurse or significant others as a convenient or safe alternative to confronting the real source of Fear. The patient may exhibit increased alertness to "it, out there," as an additional behavioral manifestation. Intellectual functioning may also be affected, resulting in impaired attention, decreased learning ability, and frightening visual images.

Subjective data include reports from the fearful individual of tension, apprehension, uncertainty of self, fear, terror, panic, or jitteriness. The patient may express a desire to "run away from it all" or "pulverize" the source of the threat.

Few valid, reliable, and useful instruments are available to measure patients' Fear in clinical settings. The Fear Survey Schedule—II,[3] which is both reliable and valid, measures fear of animals, illness, death, and interpersonal events. The Fear Thermometer[12] works by having patients indicate their level of fear by placing a mark on a scale of 1 to 10. Because this instrument is simple and efficient, it can be adapted to many clinical situations for comparison measurements over time. Most often, however, a nursing diagnosis of Fear results from the nurse's observing the defining characteristics while providing care for the patient.

A variety of related factors increase the chances for a nursing diagnosis of Fear. Natural (developmental) or innate fears occur during specific developmental stages. In addition, individuals (particularly children) may learn to fear specific stimuli when they observe this response in role models or significant others. When a mother reacts in terror to spiders, her young children will likely adopt a similar response. Hospitalized patients, who are separated from their support systems in a potentially threatening situation, develop a high risk for Fear. Unfamiliarity with the hospital environment or a language barrier may compound the threat experienced by the patient. Sensory impairments, such as blindness or diminished hearing, also increase the likelihood that individuals will develop Fear, especially during hospitalization when they must depend on unfamiliar hospital

personnel for assistance in meeting basic safety needs. Although environmental stimuli may provoke a fear response in many settings, this reaction is more likely to require nursing intervention in critical care units, where sensory overload is common, familiar support systems are infrequently present, and the threat to survival is frighteningly real. Furthermore, the neuroendocrine physiological response to Fear in patients with compromised adaptive abilities can lead to cardiac dysrhythmias, fluid and electrolyte imbalances, seizures, and other serious complications.

The nursing diagnosis of Fear occurs more commonly with life-threatening illnesses, conditions requiring mechanical ventilation or other life support, situations where the patient's ability to communicate is disrupted (tracheostomy or facial trauma), and in patients with sensory losses (blindness or deafness).

❖ **Defining Characteristics**

The presence of the following defining characteristics indicates that the patient may be experiencing Fear[11]:

- Sympathetic stimulation—cardiovascular excitation, superficial vasoconstriction, pupil dilation
- Sleep disturbance
- Irritability
- Facial tension
- Terrified
- Jittery
- Scared
- Apprehension
- Increased tension
- Impulsiveness
- Increased alertness
- Wide-eyed
- Crying
- Focus on "it, out there"
- Fight behavior—aggression
- Flight behavior—withdrawal
- Persistent questioning
- Reassurance-seeking behaviors
- Decreased self-assurance
- Concentration on source

❖ **Related Factors**

The following related factors are associated with Fear:

- Sudden noise
- Loss of physical support
- Heights
- Pain
- Sensory impairment
- Threatening environmental stimuli
- Phobia (e.g., social phobia)
- Learned response (e.g., conditioning, modeling from or identification with others)

- Knowledge deficit or unfamiliarity
- Separation from support system in a potentially threatening situation (hospitalization, treatments, etc.)
- Language barrier

- Agoraphobia without history of panic disorder
- AIDS
- Blindness
- Cancer

- Multiple trauma
- Panic disorder with agoraphobia
- Social phobia

NURSING DIAGNOSES

Examples of *specific* nursing diagnoses for Fear are:
- Fear related to potential disfigurement by impending surgery
- Fear related to unfamiliar environment
- Fear related to separation from support system secondary to emergency hospitalization

PLANNING AND IMPLEMENTATION WITH RATIONALE

Once the nurse identifies a nursing diagnosis of Fear, the nurse should validate this assessment with the patient. The patient must learn to recognize and acknowledge the signs and symptoms of Fear as the "fight or flight" response to danger. At this stage, *verbalization of feelings may help the patient lessen the intensity and duration of the powerful emotions accompanying Fear.* The nurse should listen actively while encouraging the patient to discuss a fearful event or situation to assess the patient's ability to cope with fear. Together with the patient, the nurse should explore the source of the Fear and evaluate the extent to which the patient's fear is valid.

When the source of the Fear has been clearly identified, the nurse may assist the patient in avoiding the danger, decreasing the danger, or ameliorating the Fear response.[4,9] Discussing advantages and disadvantages of alternative approaches with the patient may enhance this process. Although it is often impossible to eliminate the danger, such as an uncomfortable treatment or life-threatening surgery, *providing the patient*

❖ **Related Medical/Psychiatric Diagnoses**

The following are examples of related medical/psychiatric diagnoses for Fear:

with information about what to expect (particularly on a sensory level) decreases the threat.[5] Whenever possible, allowing the patient to have some form of control over the situation also helps diminish the degree of Fear.

The nurse provides emotional support for the fearful patient by remaining with him/her, explaining the situation as indicated, touching and comforting, and assuring the patient that fear is a normal human response to danger. Instructing patients on health care or referring them to other health professionals or social service agencies may be indicated. The nurse should discuss with parents the appropriate age-related fears in children.[2]

In addition to adjusting the threatening situation to cope with Fear, patients can learn to manage the emotional distress that accompanies Fear. *Progressive muscle relaxation exercises, visual imagery, halting the fearful thoughts, and progressive desensitization to feared objects and situations all work by ameliorating the patient's fearful response.*[1] Physical exercise can serve as a healthful outlet to dissipate the tension accompanying fear. Distress may also be alleviated by the presence of significant others, as well as by music, religious objects, security blankets, or other sources of comfort.[7]

❖ NURSING CARE GUIDELINES

Nursing Diagnosis: Fear

Expected Patient Outcomes	Nursing Interventions
The patient will recognize and express feelings of Fear.	• Assist patient in recognizing sign and symptoms of fear and acknowledging them as a response to a threat.
The patient will verbalize source of Fear, realistic perception of danger, coping ability, and need for assistance.	• Using therapeutic communication, encourage patient to verbalize subjective feelings, personal perception of danger, perception of own coping skills and limitations, and the need for assistance from the nursing staff. • Reduce distorted perceptions by educating patient and encouraging specifics rather than generalizations. • Initiate teaching, as needed, to decrease lack of knowledge and unfamiliarity.
The patient will use coping mechanisms effectively to decrease Fear.	• Help patient identify resources and develop skills to cope with Fear, such as systematic desensitization or strategies to avoid or overcome danger. • Use patient's support system to increase comfort and relaxation. • Teach additional coping techniques as needed, such as progressive muscle relaxation, visual imagery, and physical exercise.
The patient will verbalize a decrease in feelings associated with Fear and display a decrease in behavioral manifestations and physiological signs of Fear.	• Continually monitor level of Fear and degree of coping.

VII

❖ CASE STUDY WITH PLAN OF CARE

Mr. Jerry S. is a 60-year-old bank manager with extensive coronary artery atherosclerosis. He is admitted to the coronary care unit for a cardiac catheterization and evaluation after repeated bouts of angina. Mr. S. has been generally healthy throughout his life, and his only previous hospitalization was for an appendectomy as a child. He remembers it as frightening. His knowledge of coronary artery disease is somewhat limited. Although he attempts to follow a low-fat, low-cholesterol diet, he admits that he has difficulty adhering to the diet during frequent business lunches. He reports anorexia since admission. Expressing fear of the anticipated cardiac catheterization procedure, he describes an acquaintance whose "heart stopped and had to be re-started" during a cardiac catheterization. Mr. S. has had some difficulty sleeping since being hospitalized and often awakes in the early morning thinking about the cardiac catheterization. Mr. S. experiences chest pain almost daily, resulting from stressful situations and physical activity. Activity more strenuous than a short walk causes angina. He expresses a concern about his future ability to support his family with a diagnosis of heart disease because his wife has moderately severe arthritis and does not work outside the home. He reports that his job is often stressful, and parenting is occasionally stressful. Mr. S. deals with stress by talking with his wife about his concerns or listening to classical music.

Continued.

PLAN OF CARE FOR MR. JERRY S.

Nursing Diagnosis: Fear related to the separation from support system in a potentially threatening situation (hospitalization and impending cardiac catheterization)

Expected Patient Outcomes	Nursing Interventions
Mr. S. will identify and discuss specific fears about cardiac catheterization.	• Encourage expression of feelings about cardiac catheterization. • Explore aspects of the procedure that threaten Mr. S. • Explain the catheterization procedure and what Mr. S. can expect—include sensory information. • Take Mr. S. to catheterization lab the day before surgery to meet the staff and ask them questions.
Mr. S. will verbalize feelings about separation from support systems.	• Encourage expression of feelings by using active listening. • Allow and encourage wife and family to visit whenever possible.
Mr. S. will use situational support to reduce Fear and increase comfort.	• Suggest visit by personal priest or hospital chaplain. • Remain with Mr. S. during catheterization procedure. • Suggest music as a diversion during hospital stay. • Teach Mr. S. other coping techniques, such as muscle relaxation and visual imagery, to use during catheterization procedure and whenever necessary.
Mr. S. will verbalize and demonstrate decreased signs and symptoms of Fear.	• Monitor Fear level and vital signs, especially cardiac rate and rhythm and chest pain, providing relief from pain if it occurs. Report and document.

EVALUATION

Evaluation involves measuring both the progress toward the expected outcomes and the reduction in the defining characteristics of Fear. Does the patient verbalize a decrease in the physical symptoms of Fear? Display a decrease in the behavioral manifestations of Fear? Verbalize recognition of the Fear response in self? Describe the source of the threat? Does the patient effectively deal with Fear and relieve the distressing effects of Fear? Are the observable defining characteristics of Fear reduced or absent? The nurse should continue to monitor the patient's level of Fear and degree of coping by assessing the patient for changes in the subjective and objective defining characteristics of fear. If the expected outcomes are not achieved in a reasonable period of time, the nurse should consider referring the patient for more intensive, specialized treatment of the Fear response.

REFERENCES

1. Bulechek G, McCloskey J, editors: *Nursing Interventions: treatments for nursing diagnosis,* Philadelphia, 1991, WB Saunders.
2. Carpenito LJ: *Nursing diagnosis: application to clinical practice,* ed 4, New York, 1992, JB Lippincott.
3. Geer JH: The development of a scale to measure fear, *Behav Res Ther* 3:45-53, 1965.
4. Grainger RD: Conquering fears and phobias, *Am J Nurs* 91(5):15-16, 1991.
5. Hartfield MT, Cason CL, and Cason GJ: Effects of information about a threatening procedure on patients' expectations and emotional distress, *Nurs Res* 31(4):202-206, 1982.
6. Kim MJ, McFarland GK, and McLane AM: *Pocket guide to nursing diagnoses,* ed 4, St Louis, 1991, Mosby–Year Book.
7. McFarland GK, Mock VL: Fear. In Kim MJ, McFarland GK, McLane AM, editors: *Pocket guide to nursing diagnoses,* ed 4, St Louis, 1991, Mosby–Year Book.
8. McFarland GK, Thomas MD: *Psychiatric mental health nursing: application of the nursing process,* Philadelphia, 1991, JB Lippincott.

VII

9. Moss RC: Overcoming fear—a review of research on patient and family instruction, *AORN J* 43(5):1107-1112, 1986.

10. Stuart GW, Sundeen SJ: *Principles and practice of psychiatric nursing,* ed 4, St Louis, 1991, Mosby–Year Book.

11. Taylor-Loughran AE, O'Brien ME, LaChapelle R, and Rangel S: Defining characteristics of the nursing diagnoses *fear* and *anxiety:* a validation study, *Appl Nurs Res* 2(4):178-186, 1989.

12. Whaley LF, Wong DL: *Nursing care of infants and children,* ed 4, St Louis, 1991, Mosby–Year Book.

13. Yocum CJ: The differentiation of fear and anxiety. In Kim MJ, McFarland GK, McLane AM, editors: *Classification of nursing diagnoses: proceedings of the Fifth National Conference,* St Louis, 1984, CV Mosby.

VII

Anxiety

Anxiety is a subjective feeling of apprehension and tension manifested by physiological arousal and varying patterns of behavior. The source of anxiety is nonspecific or unknown to the individual.

OVERVIEW

Anxiety ranks among the most commonly identified problems nurses encounter.[17] Anxiety can impair a patient's coping as well as learning,[9,23,30] quality of life,[36] immunity to disease,[1] response to medical treatment[2,26] and increase pain.[24] Anxiety has been described as a vague, uneasy sense of worry, nervousness, or anguish[21] often without an awareness of underlying feelings.[13]

Peplau, in a classic nursing work,[25] characterized Anxiety as an energy that must be defined operationally by behaviors associated with the subjective experience. She described four levels of Anxiety (mild, moderate, severe, and panic), with effects on physiological functioning, observation, awareness, learning and adaptation, and patterns of behavior.

Several conceptual models have sought to explain the phenomenon of anxiety. The psychoanalytic model, based on Freud's theories attributed Anxiety to birth trauma and separation, with subsequent Anxiety resulting from traumatic events in the life cycle. Freud distinguished realistic anxiety from neurotic anxiety which he described as a disproportionate response that required defense mechanisms for management.[20]

Neo-Freudians such as Horney[8,11,34] defined anxiety as an interpersonal phenomenon. In his model, Sullivan[34] described Anxiety as tension resulting from perceived or anticipated appraisal by others and need for social approval. Horney[11] theorized that instinctual drives were a product of

Anxiety and a defense against a hostile world. Fromm[8] interpreted Anxiety as a culturally based response to freedom and isolation.

Spielberger[32] described two types of anxiety concepts: (1) a transitory condition varying in intensity and fluctuating over time (state anxiety) and (2) a stable personality characteristic that influenced the person's perception of the environment (trait anxiety). Behaviorists and learning theorists explained anxiety as a conditioned or learned response. Mowrer[20] concluded that neurotic symptoms were reinforced because they reduced anxiety.

Using a biological model researchers have studied Anxiety in terms of genetics and brain biochemistry.[15,19] The neurobiology of Anxiety has been attributed to the $GABA_A$ benzodiazepine receptor complex, which is also the site of action for anxiolytic medications.[5] Anxiety disorders such as panic disorder and agoraphobia have been attributed to adrenergic receptor abnormalities,[6] with familial linkage.[7]

Stress and Anxiety have been linked frequently in the literature. Cognitive psychologists theorized that emotional responses are determined by the individual's cognitive appraisal of threats and coping options.[16] Robinson[28] stated that Anxiety represented a psychophysiological signal of the stress response in a person.

ASSESSMENT

Anxiety is adaptive when arousal is appropriate to the situation and the individual is able to perform activities of daily living and cope with problems. Maladaptive Anxiety occurs when an exaggerated response results in decreased levels of performance and inappropriate behavioral patterns. It may be difficult to identify when defense mechanisms function to protect the individual from the pain of Anxiety in its pure state. Anger, denial, somatic complaints, and withdrawal are some of the behavioral responses used to reduce Anxiety or avoid awareness of it.[35]

Three separate interacting response channels for emotional expression are recognized: motoric or behavioral, self-report, and physiological arousal. Responses in all channels may not be consistent; that is, behavior may indicate Anxiety but the emotion is denied by self-report, and signs of physiological arousal may or may not be present. Individual responses in the expression of Anxiety through these channels vary.

Escape from or avoidance of certain stimuli are behaviors indicating Anxiety. Self-report, measuring the degree of Anxiety usually felt (trait anxiety) or response to current specific situations (state anxiety), may be elicited by questions about current and past concerns, thoughts, and feelings. Physiological arousal may be overtly observed in muscle tension, aimless movements, tremors, or clumsiness, and may be measured by indices of autonomic nervous system activation, such as increased heart rate, blood pressure, and respiration, and changes in appetite and sleeping patterns.

Thompson[35] described a systematic approach to assessing Anxiety: first identify and describe salient patient behaviors indicating Anxiety, then ask the patient to describe related thoughts, and then concurrent emotions. The patient's ability to recall past events, analyze feelings, and project into the future will not be effective at moderate or severe levels of Anxiety. The immediate distress of Anxiety must be relieved before the patient will be able to explore the sources and dimensions of Anxiety and identify coping skills and resources.

Peplau's[25] behavioral descriptions are useful in differentiating levels of anxiety in individual patients as they affect the ability to observe, focus attention, learn, and adapt. Mild Anxiety is described as an alert aware state in which learning may readily occur. Moderate Anxiety is characterized by selective attention to relevant stimuli

that may be directed to focus on specific details when needed. Perceptions are greatly reduced and dissociative behavior may be seen with Severe Anxiety. Panic occurs with extreme arousal, resulting in dissociation or other automatic behaviors aimed at reducing anxiety, such as fight or flight.

The nurse must examine the assessment data to identify conditions or circumstances that contribute to the development of this nursing diagnosis. Environmental variations may affect the degree of Anxiety. Physical features of the environment, such as noise, space, lighting, and temperature influence Anxiety responses.[24] The experience and awareness of Anxiety may also shift depending on the social context. Observing patient responses in interactions with family, friends, and health care providers and to environmental stimuli may provide data about factors related to anxiety. Physiological responses are subject to habituation with repeated stimulation and can be affected by factors unrelated to anxiety. Determine whether other factors are present that affect autonomic responses, such as medications, drug withdrawal, delirium or acute confusional states, electrolyte imbalance, or hypoxia.[18,29]

Many medically ill populations experience significant Anxiety, which may pose diagnostic difficulties for the treatment team or exacerbate existing conditions. Uncertainty may mediate the association of Anxiety with specific diseases and the severity of illness. Mishel[22] found that the severely ill did not perceive illness-related events as highly stressful unless they perceived the events as ambiguous or unpredictable.

❖ **Defining Characteristics**

The presence of the following defining characteristics indicates that the patient may be experiencing Anxiety:

- Increased heart rate
- Increased blood pressure
- Increased respiratory rate
- Increased palmar sweating
- Insomnia
- Increased wariness
- Self-report of Apprehension Worry Nervousness

VII

- Hand tremors
- Repetitive purpose-less movements
- Increased muscle tension
- Speech pitch, rate, volume increased
- Vocal quivering
- Changes in appetite
- Urinary frequency and urgency

- Escape/avoidance behavior
- Narrowed percep-tual field
    Self-focused
    Inattentive
- Inappropriate behav-iors: anger, fear, guilt, regression
- Denial
- Withdrawal

- Inflammatory bowel disease
- Migraine headache
- Mitral valve prolapse syndrome
- Organic mental disorders
- Partial complex seizures
- Pheochromocytoma
- Psychoactive substance use disorders
- Recurrent pulmonary emboli
- Schizophrenia
- Vertigo

❖ Related Factors

The following related factors are associated with Anxiety:

- Threats to bodily health
- Threats to self-con-cept
- Threatened social losses
    Significant others
    Status
    Significant roles
- Unmet needs
    Security
    Dependency
    Power

- Conditioning
- Uncertainty
- Situational/maturational crisis
- Interpersonal trans-mission (spread of anxiety from one person to another)
- Social irresponsibil-ity, guilt or immatu-rity
- Lack of control over events

NURSING DIAGNOSES

Examples of *specific* nursing diagnoses for Anxiety are:
- Severe Anxiety related to controlled ventilation
- Panic related to being alone with threat of ter-minal illness
- Moderate Anxiety related to anticipated transfer to nursing home
- Severe Anxiety related to uncertain surgical outcome

❖ Related Medical/Psychiatric Diagnoses

The following are examples of related medical/psychiatric diagnoses for Anxiety:
- Acute labyrinthitis
- Angina
- Anxiety disorders
- Asthma
- Cardiac arrhythmias
- COPD
- Cushing's syndrome
- Delirium
- Gastric ulcer
- Hyperkinetic heart syndrome
- Hyperparathyroidism
- Hypertension
- Hyperthyroidism
- Hypoglycemia
- Hypoparathyroidism

PLANNING AND IMPLEMENTATION WITH RATIONALE

In selecting interventions the nurse needs to consider situational and patient characteristics and the degree and duration of Anxiety and self-care capacity of the patient.

In all instances the nurse's presence and empa-thy are important. Empathic understanding, the ability to go beyond the self and experience the other, can become a potent therapeutic tool to en-hance the coping abilities of patients. However, Anxiety may be transmitted interpersonally. Maintaining a calm, alert, interested presence communicates support and concern.

The goals of nursing care for the diagnosis of Anxiety include preventing severe Anxiety or panic, eliminating or reducing incapacitating Anxiety states, and identifying the sources of Anxiety and increasing effective coping skills. Specific examples of patient outcomes include at-tention to information, accurate perception and appropriate behavioral response to external stim-uli, problem solving to identify viable alternative solutions, reduced frequency or intensity of spe-cific responses (for example, nausea and vomit-

❖ NURSING CARE GUIDELINES
Nursing Diagnosis: Anxiety

Expected Patient Outcomes	Nursing Interventions
The patient will report reduced Anxiety as evidenced by relaxed state, behavior appropriate to stimuli, physiological arousal within expected parameters (heart rate, blood pressure, and respiratory rate), and ability to attend to salient details and learn.	• Develop trust and rapport by being nonjudgmental and authentic in response to the patient's behaviors; being calm, consistent, and reliable; using empathy to gain insight to the patient's perspective; using therapeutic communications; providing positive feedback; avoiding conflicts with the patient; and increasing attention to the patient as needed.
The patient will cope with Anxiety independently as evidenced by use of relaxation techniques after receiving instructions, problem solving to work through stressful periods, and identifying sources of Anxiety and underlying feelings.	• Use behavioral/cognitive strategies to teach rhythmic breathing, relaxation techniques, and imagery techniques; for stress inoculation; to provide accurate information (including orienting, temporal, and sensory content before events); and to assist the patient in reappraising the environment, gaining insight to feelings, identifying coping strengths, and developing new coping and problem-solving skills.
The patient will meet own self-care needs as evidenced by participation in care, health care seeking behaviors when appropriate, reports of rest and sleep, normal appetite, reports of satisfactory social interactions, and attention to feelings of self and others.	• Structure environment as needed by assigning consistent caregivers, decreasing stimulation, using distraction (e.g., music), attending to the patient's safety, using touch judiciously, using humor as appropriate, encouraging or supporting interactions with social network, monitoring anxiety level, and modifying interventions as indicated.

ing, sleep or eating disturbances), and the ability to comfortably participate in medical treatments.

Anticipating and preventing anxiety through patient education has proven effective.[12] Providing information before stressful situations, such as painful or threatening procedures, may *increase a patient's sense of control and decrease uncertainty*. The timing, type, and amount of information given should be varied among patients, depending on their expressed needs and preferences. Including effective coping options is important when providing information about future events.

VII

In this way patients know what to expect and how to minimize potentially distressful responses.

Actions specific for security, dependence, or power reduce anxiety by *addressing basic needs*.[4] Security measures provide structure and consistency, minimize stress, and build trust. Anticipating needs, nurturing behaviors, and increasing attention to the patient will meet dependency needs. Power needs can be addressed by offering patients choices, avoiding needless conflicts, and allowing and accepting honest emotional expressions. Acknowledging these as basic needs in all patients as a guide to care may prevent regressive behavior.[27]

Anxiety may be relieved or attenuated through strategies that are distracting or relaxing, or that change how the patient thinks about threats. These treatments have a common base in their *effects on central nervous system control of emotion and behavior*. Distraction focuses attention on nonthreatening stimuli that compete with those that elicit anxiety. This is useful when short-term intervention is needed, such as during an invasive procedure. *Relaxation is inconsistent with the muscular tension associated with Anxiety, spreading from striated (musculoskeletal system) to smooth (gastrointestinal and cardiovascular systems) muscles*.[31] *Cognitive strategies affect appraisals of threatening stimuli, primary appraisals related to the nature and severity of threats, or secondary appraisals related to the availability and effectiveness of coping options*.

Use of music,[33] touch,[14] or relaxation training[10] *elicits the relaxation response*. These methods can be especially useful as long-term therapy and can be self-administered or provided by family or friends as well as the nurse. Risks involved are usually minimal to most individuals. However, deterioration in physical or mental states is possible in individuals with a history of cardiac arrhythmias, severe depression, or psychosis with relaxation training.[31]

Imagery can be used to *potentiate relaxation techniques*. It is also an effective strategy by itself, particularly for patients experiencing fatigue or complications in multiple body systems pre-cluding use of muscle relaxation techniques.[3] Imagery may be used in conjunction with cognitive reappraisal or calming self-talk.

EVALUATION

Ongoing evaluation of patients' responses to interventions focuses on comparisons to baseline measures. Observations of behaviors and physiological arousal coupled with patients' self-reports can provide immediate data after interventions and should be repeated at critical times. Transfers between units (such as from critical care to the general ward) and discharge from the hospital may be stressful. Check on the patient after visits with family or others that the patient anticipated as potentially conflictual or when you know the patient is going to receive distressful information, such as test results.

The social learning approach to Anxiety assessment emphasizes the analysis of all relevant components, their relationships, and interactions with the environment. Those components include the stimulus class of cognitions/thoughts, images, or critical objects or events; the person's reaction in all response channels; and the immediate and long-term consequences, including social and environmental results. It may be difficult for the patient to identify significant antecedents to Anxiety, and the nurse will need to exercise caution in drawing inferences from sequential events observed. Validating conclusions with the patient is important but must be done with sensitivity.

Observations of patient Anxiety and response to interventions should be systematic and ongoing. Monitoring Anxiety levels provides critical data to guide nursing intervention. Reducing Anxiety may contribute positively to many other outcomes in the ill patient.

REFERENCES

1. Ader R, editor: *Psychoneuroimmunology*, New York, 1981, Academic Press, Inc.
2. Andrykowski MR: The role of anxiety in the development of anticipatory nausea in cancer chemotherapy: a review and synthesis, *Psychosom Med* 52:458-475, 1990.

❖ *CASE STUDY WITH PLAN OF CARE*

Mr. Karl K. is a 59-year-old man with chronic obstructive pulmonary disease and hypertension controlled by medication. He has a 3-month history of hoarseness and recent difficulty in swallowing. The patient is diagnosed as having squamous cell carcinoma of the right true vocal cord with subglottic extension. Surgical excision with partial laryngectomy is planned. Physical examination discloses that Mr. K. weighs 204 pounds and is 5'8". His heart rate is 86, and blood pressure 160/98. Respiratory rate is 22, with soft rhonchi in lung bases. The patient is somewhat barrel chested. He has a history of smoking two to three packs of cigarettes per day and drinking 8 to 10 drinks of whiskey per day. Mr. K. lives with his wife in their own home; his son and family live in the same town. He does not see old friends from work much now that he is retired because of the hypertension. He has a pension and medical insurance. He reports that he is a Methodist but has not been active in church. His father,

who is dead, and brother had prostatic cancer. Mr. K. reports eating, but without pleasurable taste, and moderate difficulty in falling asleep, with easy wakening. He reports great concern about the proposed surgical intervention, although he is unable to identify anything specific. He repeatedly asks about the possibility that he will not be able to talk after surgery. Mr. K. reports one episode of hallucinations during withdrawal from alcohol during a prior surgery. Mr. K. appears distressed. Apprehension is characterized by generalized muscular tension, alternately clenching and tremulous jaws, tightening hands into fists with jerky, restless movements, and a strained and tense facial expression. Voice pitch is elevated at times. His speech is compatible with conversational level, but volume and rate are somewhat increased. He is somewhat verbose, giving lengthy answers to questions. He makes frequent eye contact with his wife during the interview.

PLAN OF CARE FOR MR. KARL K.

Nursing Diagnosis: Severe (4^+) Anxiety related to threats to biological integrity and self-concept and uncertainty

VII

Expected Patient Outcomes	**Nursing Interventions**
Mr. K. will have reduced Anxiety as evidenced by muscular relaxation when at rest; reduced rate, pitch, and volume of speech; eupneic respirations; diastolic blood pressure <90; and facial expressions and behavior appropriate to stimuli.	• Acknowledge concerns and give assurance of close surveillance by nursing staff. • Give information on short- and long-term alternatives for communication in the postoperative period. • Offer relaxation training preoperatively. • Encourage wife's presence and support. • Facilitate communications with physician and validate understanding. • Monitor anxiety level.
Mr. K. will be able to identify sources of anxiety and ways of coping that work.	• Identify precursors of anxiety. • Clarify meaning of stimuli as needed. • Guide problem-solving or reappraisals of problems as necessary.
Mr. K. asks questions or reports satisfaction with information.	• Explain preoperative and postoperative procedures. Include expected sensations and timing and sequence of events after Anxiety level is reduced.
Mr. K. will participate in preoperative and postoperative care (especially pulmonary), and he will begin guided self-care by fourth postoperative day.	• Anticipate stressful events and plan coping strategies with patient and physician (i.e., recognize and anticipate alcohol or smoking withdrawal postoperatively).

3. Bayuk L: Relaxation techniques: an adjunct therapy for cancer patients, *Semin Oncol Nurs* 1(2):147, 1985.

4. Billings CV: Emotional first aid, *Am J Nurs* 80(11):2006, 1980.

5. Breier A, Paul SM: The GABA$_A$/benzodiazepine receptor: implications for the molecular basis of anxiety, *J Psychiatry Res* 24(suppl 2):91-104, 1990.

6. Cameron OG and others: Adrenergic status in anxiety disorders: platelet alpha-adrenergic receptor binding, blood pressure, pulse, and plasma catecholamines in panic and generalized anxiety disorder patients and in normal subjects, *Biol Psychiatry* 28:3-20, 1990.

7. Crowe RR and others: A linkage study of panic disorder, *Arch Gen Psychiatry* 44:933-937, 1987.

8. Fromm E: *Escape from freedom,* New York, 1941, Rinehart.

9. Guzzetta CE: Relationship between stress and learning, *ANS* 1(4):35, 1979.

10. Guzzetta CE: Effects of relaxation and music therapy on patients in a coronary care unit, *Heart Lung* 18(6):609-616, 1989.

11. Horney K: *The neurotic personality of our time,* New York, 1937, WW Norton.

12. Johnson J: Coping with elective surgery. In Werley HH, Fitzpatrick JJ, editors: *Annual Review of Nursing Research,* vol 2, New York, 1984, Springer Publishing.

13. Jones P, and Jakob DF: Anxiety revisited—from a practice perspective. In Kim MJ, McFarland G, and McLane AM, editors: Classification of nursing diagnoses: proceedings of the Fifth National Conference, St Louis, 1984, CV Mosby.

14. Jurgens A, Meehan TC, and Wilson HL: Therapeutic touch as a nursing intervention, *Hol Nurs Pract* 2(1):1-13, 1987.

15. Kendler KS and others: Symptoms of anxiety and symptoms of depression: same genes, different environments? *Arch Gen Psychiatry* 44:451, 1987.

16. Lazarus RS, Folkman S: *Stress, appraisal, and coping,* New York, 1984, Springer Publishing.

17. Lessow CL: Nursing diagnoses: incidence and perceived value by nurses. In McLane AM, editor: *Classification of nursing diagnoses: proceedings of the Seventh Conference,* St Louis, 1987, CV Mosby.

18. Lipowski ZJ: Delirium (acute confusional states), *JAMA* 258(13):1789-1792, 1987.

19. MacKinnon AJ, Henderson AS, and Andrews G: Genetic and environmental determinants of the lability of trait neuroticism and the symptoms of anxiety and depression, *Psychol Med* 20:581-590, 1990.

20. May R: *The meaning of anxiety,* New York, 1977, Pocket Books.

21. Metzger KL, Hiltunen EF: Diagnostic content validation of ten frequently reported nursing diagnoses. In McLane AM, editor: *Classification of nursing diagnoses: proceedings of the Seventh Conference,* St Louis, 1987, CV Mosby.

22. Mishel MH: Perceived uncertainty and stress in illness, *Res Nurs Health* 7:163, 1984.

23. Nyamathi A, Kashiwabara A: Preoperative anxiety: its effects on cognitive thinking, *AORN J* 47(1):164-170, 1988.

24. Oberle K, Wry J, Paul P, and Grace M: Environment, anxiety and postoperative pain, *West J Nurs Res* 12(6):745-757, 1990.

25. Peplau HE: A working definition of anxiety. In Burd SF, Marshall MA: *Some clinical approaches to psychiatric nursing,* New York, 1963, Macmillan Publishing.

26. Rhodes VA, Watson PM, and Johnson MH: Association of chemotherapy related nausea and vomiting with pretreatment and posttreatment anxiety, *Oncol Nurs Forum* 13(1):41, 1986.

27. Robinson L: *Psychological aspects of the care of hospitalized patients,* Philadelphia, 1984, FA Davis.

28. Robinson L: Stress and anxiety, *Nurs Clin North Am* 25(4):935-943, 1990.

29. Saravay SM and others: "Doom anxiety" and delirium in lidocaine toxicity, *Am J Psychiatry* 144(2):159, 1987.

30. Scott DW: Anxiety, critical thinking and information processing during and after breast biopsy, *Nurs Res* 32(1):24, 1983.

31. Snyder M: Progressive relaxation as a nursing intervention: an analysis, *ANS 47,* April 1981.

32. Spielberger CD: Theory and research on anxiety. In Spielberger CD, editor: *Anxiety and behavior,* New York, 1966, Academic Press.

33. Steelman VM: Intraoperative music therapy, *AORN J* 52(5):1026-1034, 1990.

34. Sullivan HS: *The interpersonal theory of psychiatry,* New York, 1953, WW Norton.

35. Thompson EA: Anxiety: a mental health vital sign. In Longo DC, Williams RA, editors: *Clinical practice in psychosocial nursing,* ed 2, Norwalk, Conn, 1986, Appleton-Century-Crofts.

36. Welch-McCaffrey D: Cancer, anxiety, and quality of life, *Cancer Nurs 151,* June 1985.

VII

Hopelessness

Hopelessness is the subjective state in which an individual sees limited or no alternatives or personal choices available and is unable to mobilize energy on own behalf.[11]

OVERVIEW

Inspiring hope in patients who feel overwhelmed and despondent because of a health crisis is a legitimate task for nurses. It is estimated that 70% of suicide victims were suffering one or more active, mostly chronic illnesses at the time of death.[10] Stressor patterns have been identified in persons who have committed suicide, with the frequency of medical illness as a stressor, that can lead to suicide increasing progressively in older populations.[15] In reviewing the psychodynamics of suicide, one can list Hopelessness and despair as two of the emotions that predominate in suicidal patients.[9] Prevalence statistics on attempted and completed suicides are probably unreliable, and official statistics are reportedly underestimated. In the United States, the number of annual deaths by suicide is reported to be 30,000.[16] The World Health Organization figures estimate that on an average day at least 1,000 people take their own lives around the world.[3] Flanders[7] states that 10 persons attempt suicide for every one who succeeds.

The nursing diagnosis of Hopelessness frequently is experienced by patients with serious chronic illnesses. The vulnerability to Hopelessness in individuals with chronic illness can be directly proportionate to the severity of their losses. The obvious losses—health status and control of bodily functions or body parts—may only be the "tip of the iceberg." Losing self-esteem, certainty, sexual attractiveness, social relationships, independence, finances, and significant roles in the family and the work setting can all cause grief in the chronically ill person that, if not resolved, can lead to Hopelessness.[13]

The elderly may be predisposed or even developmentally vulnerable for the development of Hopelessness. Aging is generally accompanied by psychosocial and physiological change, and frequently those changes involve losses. Sensory changes include diminished visual acuity, some hearing loss, and a marked decrease in the sense of taste. Body image alterations that occur with physiological changes include wrinkles in the skin, the loss or graying of hair, and reduction in muscle size with gradual replacement of these tissues with fat. Skeletal changes and calcium loss may result in posture differences and even height reduction. Energy generally diminishes, and efficiency and speed of task completion may be compromised.[2] Social roles may be dramatically revised as former caretakers become cared for by their children, as financial resources shrink, and as peers die. These losses and changes may result in feelings of powerlessness that, if not contained, may become a self-destructive cycle leading to depression and Hopelessness that could hasten death.[12,14] The nurse should be aware of the population at risk for the development of Hopelessness, as well as the nature of the feeling state and etiological factors.

Many health care professionals believe that a patient's ability to hope facilitates healing. Hope "springs" from many different sources, including an individual's faith, relationships with others, the feeling of being needed, and the sense that one has a task to accomplish.[13] The nurse must assess each individual's hope sources so that

499

hope-inspiring strategies can be planned.

Dufault and Martocchio[5] describe hope as a multidimensional, dynamic force of life characterized by a confident, yet uncertain, expectation of achieving a future good that, to the hoping person, is realistically possible and personally significant. They conceptualize that hope consists of two spheres with six dimensions. The first sphere—generalized hope—has a broad scope and a sense of a future beneficial (but presently indeterminate) development, and is characterized by the belief that things will somehow work out. Generalized hope provides a person deprived of the second sphere (particularized hope) with protection against despair and the ability to continue with life's demands. Particularized hope is described as a specific valued outcome, good, or state of being. Particularized hope is the expectation that the present can be improved, what is missing can be attained, desired circumstances will occur, and unfavorable outcomes will not happen. This sphere of hope provides incentive for coping with life's obstacles.[5]

ASSESSMENT

Hopelessness has been associated not only with suicidal behaviors in depression, alcoholism, schizophrenia, and panic disorder,[9] but also with many different medical diagnoses, including AIDS, Alzheimer's disease, burns, carcinomas, end stage renal disease, and spinal cord injuries with paralysis.[17] However, the nurse should assess each patient for behaviors reflecting defining characteristics and related factors of the nursing diagnosis rather than specific medical or psychiatric disorders.

The diagnosis should be based on observation of the patient's behavior and thematic analysis of his/her comments and described indicators of Hopelessness: (1) hypoactivation—patient reports feelings of emptiness or has difficulty identifying feelings; (2) general psychological discomfort—sense of loss, deprivation, tension, irritability, and feeling a constriction in the throat; (3) social withdrawal—emotional distance; and (4) sense of incompetence—expressions of vulnerability,

helplessness, inability to accomplish anything, or feeling overwhelmed by life.[13]

To analyze conversations with the patient, screen the conversations for words and themes that indicate despair. Miller[13] also suggests Gottschalk's system for content analysis in which the following themes represent Hopelessness: (1) not receiving good fortune, luck, or God's favor, (2) not receiving help, sustenance, or esteem from others or self, (3) pessimism, (4) discouragement from self and others, and (5) lack of ambition or interest. Other indicators include: (1) feeling at the end of one's rope or at an impasse; (2) losing gratification from roles and relationships; (3) sensing disrupted continuity between past, present, and future; and (4) recalling former incidents of helplessness.[6] The Hopelessness scale developed by Beck and others[1] can provide additional data for validation of the nursing diagnosis.

The nurse should also gather data about the patient's knowledge of his/her medical condition and prognosis; the effect of the disorder on self-care capacity; mental status, particularly mood and cognitive ability; availability of support systems; past experience with illness; frequently employed coping mechanisms; and any history of psychiatric illness.[17] Health care professionals may have difficulty acknowledging that suicidal intent is present. The nurse must be aware of his/her own feelings about suicide to develop an effective helping relationship and plan nursing interventions.

❖ Defining Characteristics

The presence of the following defining characteristics indicates that the patient may be experiencing Hopelessness:[11]

- Decreased appetite
- Increased/decreased sleep
- Decreased affect
- Lack of initiative
- Passivity
- Lack of involvement in care
- Verbal cues (indicating despondency, "I can't," sighing)
- Decreased response to stimuli
- Turning away from speaker
- Closing eyes
- Shrugging in response to speaker

❖ Related Factors

The following related factors are associated with Hopelessness:[11]

- Prolonged activity restriction creating isolation
- Failing or deteriorating physiological condition
- Stress
- Abandonment
- Loss of belief in transcendent values/God

❖ Related Medical/Psychiatric Diagnoses

The following are examples of related medical/psychiatric diagnoses for Hopelessness:[4]

- AIDS
- Alcohol dependence
- Bipolar disorder
- Burns
- Carcinoma
- Major depression
- Multiinfarct dementia
- Panic disorder
- Paralysis, second-degree spinal cord injury
- Primary degenerative dementia of the Alzheimer type
- Renal disease (end stage)
- Schizophrenia
- Stroke
- Tourette's disorder

NURSING DIAGNOSES

Examples of *specific* nursing diagnoses for Hopelessness are:

- Hopelessness related to abandonment
- Hopelessness related to long-term stress

PLANNING AND IMPLEMENTATION WITH RATIONALE

The six dimensions of hope described by Dufault and Martocchio[5] provide a framework for planning nursing strategies. Interventions in the affective dimension include encouraging the patient to express feelings and concerns about health and future and conveying empathy when the patient expresses fears, doubts, and worries. In the cognitive dimension, interventions can be used to assist the patient in clarifying or modifying reality perceptions. In the behavioral dimension, the nursing interventions focus on enabling the individual to take action, to recognize and use re-sources, and to accept support when necessary. The affiliative dimension allows the nurse to plan strategies regarding the person's sense and manner of relatedness to others. The nurse can help the patient explore ways of maintaining or strengthening relationships with others. In the temporal dimension, the patient and the nurse can review past achievements and develop correlations between past, present, and future goals. In the final dimension of hope, the contextual dimension, nursing interventions can focus on creating an environment that will provide opportunities for exploration and communication of desired goals, readjustment of plans, and reflection on the meaning of life and death.

A variety of nursing interventions and strategies can be implemented by the nurse to decrease Hopelessness.[18] *Mastery over self-care needs inspires confidence in one's personal capacity for coping.* To support maintenance of self-care, specific interventions may include providing self-care assistance when indicated; encouraging the patient's interest and curiosity in self-care; teaching to increase knowledge and competence; and creating and/or modifying the environment to facilitate active participation. *Verbalization of feelings, concerns, and goals allows for validation and catharsis, promotes the establishment of trusting relationships with caregivers, and provides an opportunity to enhance self-worth.* The nurse who provides empathic listening, conveys an understanding of the patient's affect, explores reality perceptions, and assists the patient to capitalize on achievements enhances the potential for overcoming despair.

Observation for and assessment of self-harm potential are legitimate nursing roles in providing protection for patients and relief from distress. Asking about suicidal thoughts, ideas, wishes, motives, intent, and plans will not plant the idea. Hackett and Stern[8] indicate that most patients are grateful to discuss the issue. Colt[3] stresses that caregivers should not be afraid to show the patient that they care. *The promotion of a psychosocial support system is a valid role for the nurse in*

Text continued on p. 503.

VII

❖ *NURSING CARE GUIDELINES*

Nursing Diagnosis: Hopelessness

Expected Patient Outcomes	**Nursing Interventions**
The patient will maintain adequate self-care.	• Assist the patient in meeting self-care needs. • Create or modify the environment to facilitate the patient's active participation in self-care. • Demonstrate confidence and technical competence in equipment usage. • Encourage the patient's interest and curiosity in the different aspects of care. • Provide teaching and support when indicated. • Schedule and plan with the patient to increase his/her involvement in decision-making and allow for adequate rest. • Give positive feedback for successful attempts at self-care.
The patient will identify and express feelings, concerns, and goals for self.	• Provide opportunities for the patient to express feelings about self and illness. • Facilitate expression of feelings by active listening, asking open-ended questions, and reflecting on the patient's answers. • Provide opportunities for patient to express positive emotions (e.g., hope, faith, the will to live, and a sense of purpose). • Acknowledge and accept the patient's angry feelings as a manifestation of distress. • Explore reality perceptions with patient and clarify or modify if necessary by providing information and correcting misinformation. • Convey an empathic understanding of the patient's fears, worries, and family concerns. • Assist patient to recognize and capitalize on achievements and derive meaning from past successes and failures.
The patient will demonstrate absence of suicidal intent.	• Observe for signs of suicidal intent (e.g., sudden change in mood or behavior, conversation about death, or expressing the futility of life). • Assist the patient and his/her family in valuing human strengths such as courage, endurance, and patience.
The patient will maintain relationships with significant others.	• Promote attachment ideation by active discussion of significant relationships. • Explore with patient ways to foster, maintain, and strengthen relationships with others. • Provide privacy for family visits so that intimacy needs can be met. • Provide supportive counseling for family members if indicated so that they in turn convey support to the patient. • Help patient to accept assistance from others, if needed.

VII

❖ *NURSING CARE GUIDELINES—cont'd*
Nursing Diagnosis: *Hopelessness*

Expected Patient Outcomes	Nursing Interventions
The patient will integrate therapeutic regimen into lifestyle.	• Review with the patient demonstrations that he/she is loved, cared for, and important to others. • Support the patient's use of effective coping mechanisms. • Maximize esthetic experiences. • Provide opportunities for reminiscing, renewing values, and reflecting on the meaning of life and death. • Assist patient in renewing his/her spiritual self and belief in transcendent values. • Create an environment in which patient feels free to express spiritual beliefs.

enhancing the patient's coping capabilities. Significant others can provide a source of physical and emotional assistance to the individual engaged in overcoming feelings of hopelessness.

Ultimately the goals of nursing care are to enable the patient to adapt and adjust to lifestyle changes, if necessitated by the presence of illness. The success of a nursing intervention strategy can be measured by the patient's ability to utilize the information in daily life.

EVALUATION

The success of nursing interventions to inspire hope and alleviate despondence may be apparent or subtle. Patient compliance with the therapeutic regimen and mastery of self-care demands can be readily observed by the nurse or obtained by interviewing significant others. Interviewing the patient will elicit his/her experience of the illness and capacity to employ coping mechanisms. The patient's expressions of hope for the future, acceptance of the health situation, and capacity to put the situation into perspective will also validate the nursing interventions. If successful outcome is not achieved, the nurse should consider making a referral for mental health counseling services.

❖ *CASE STUDY WITH PLAN OF CARE*

Mr. William M. is a 77-year-old male recently diagnosed with early cancer of the prostate. William's wife died approximately 1 year ago, and he lives alone, although two of his children live near him and visit regularly. William is active in several community organizations, but jokes that he "goes to more funerals than meetings" these days. He is receiving outpatient radia- tion therapy and complains of frequent urination that is especially disturbing at night. He has missed several morning radiation therapy appointments and complains about the frequent driving he must do. He states he does not believe treatment will help and that soon he will join his wife.

Continued.

PLAN OF CARE FOR MR. WILLIAM M.

Nursing Diagnosis: Hopelessness related to prostate cancer and the demands of the therapeutic regimen.

Expected Patient Outcomes	Nursing Interventions
Mr. M. will verbalize feelings about the cancer diagnosis and its effect on his life.	• Encourage expression of feelings about diagnosis and its effect on Mr. M.'s lifestyle. • Explore fears related to mortality. • Provide information on treatment outcomes, emphasizing success rate in early stage of cancer.
Mr. M. will reestablish an effective sleep-rest pattern.	• Suggest morning and afternoon nap time to promote adequate rest. • Suggest temporary use of a bed-side urinal.
Mr. M. will comply with therapeutic regimen by receiving radiation therapy as scheduled.	• Plan an afternoon schedule for radiation therapy appointments. • Encourage Mr. M. to contact his children/friends for assistance with transportation.
Mr. M. will maintain an active participation in his community organizations.	• Promote continued involvement with community organizations by expressing an interest and encouraging attendance in meetings.

VII

REFERENCES

1. Beck AT and others: The measurements of pessimism: the hopelessness scale, *J Consult Clin Psychol* 42:861-865, 1974.
2. Busse E, Pfeiffer E: *Behavior and adaption in late life,* Boston, 1969, Little, Brown.
3. Colt G: *The enigma of suicide,* New York, 1991, Simon and Schuster.
4. *Diagnostic and statistical manual of mental disorders, third edition, revised,* Washington, DC, 1987, American Psychiatric Association.
5. Dufault K, Martocchio B: Hope: its spheres and dimensions, *Nurs Clin North Am* 20(2):379, 1985.
6. Engel GL: A life setting conducive to illness: the giving up–given up complex, *Ann Intern Med* 69:293-300, 1968.
7. Flanders S: *Suicide,* New York, 1991, Oxford.
8. Hackett T, Stern T: Suicide and other disruptive states. In Cassem N, editor: *Handbook of general hospital psychiatry,* St Louis, 1991, Mosby–Year Book.
9. Hendin H: Psychodynamics of suicide with particular reference to the young, *Am J Psychiatry* 148(9):1150-1158, 1991.
10. Kaplan H, Sadock B: *Study guide and self examination review for synopsis of psychiatry,* ed 3, Baltimore, 1989, Williams & Wilkins.
11. Kim M, McFarland G, and McLane A: *Pocket guide to nursing diagnoses,* ed 4, St Louis, 1991, Mosby–Year Book.
12. Miller J: *Coping with chronic illness: overcoming powerlessness,* Philadelphia, 1983, FA Davis.
13. Miller JF: Inspiring hope, *Am J Nurs* 85(1)22, 1985.
14. Miller J, Oertel C: Powerlessness in the elderly: preventing hopelessness. In Miller J, editor: *Coping with chronic illness: overcoming powerlessness,* Philadelphia, 1983, FA Davis.
15. Rich C and others: Suicide, stressors and the life cycle, *Am J Psychiatry* 148(4):524-527, 1991.
16. *Statistical Abstract of the US 1991,* The National Data Book, Washington, DC, 1990, US Department of Commerce, Bureau of the Census.
17. Taylor C, Cress S: *Nursing diagnosis cards,* Springhouse, Penn, 1987, Springhouse.
18. Thompson J, McFarland G, Hirsch J, Tucker S, Bowers A: Mosby's *clinical nursing,* ed 2, St Louis, 1989, CV Mosby.

Powerlessness

Powerlessness is the perception that one's action will not significantly affect an outcome; a perceived lack of control over a current situation or immediate happening.[4]

OVERVIEW

The goals of nursing care frequently include patient compliance issues. How an individual perceives his/her capacity to control, master skills, and affect outcomes is an important factor for the nurse to assess. Feelings of Powerlessness may be obvious or subtle, conscious or unconscious, related to longstanding personality traits, or influenced by the immediate situation. Miller[6] describes the personal power resources available—psychological stamina, self-concept, energy, knowledge, motivation, and beliefs—and states that compromise of one or more of these resources may result in Powerlessness.

Social learning theory has contributed to the locus of control concept through the proposition that with time, relatively stable personality characteristics develop and influence the individual's perception of a given situation. Internal and external locus of control can be differentiated.[8] A person high in internal locus of control perceives that events are contingent on the individual's own behavior, actions, and characteristics. Those who believe that fate, chance, luck, powerful people, and unpredictable complex forces dictate life events are generally high in external locus of control. Confronted with illness, a person with a high internal locus of control might educate himself/herself to regain the sense of control, whereas a person high in external locus of control might be unable to perceive his/her actions affecting the outcome. An individual's general expectancy for controlling an outcome governs his/her attention to and acquisition of available information.[9] Powerlessness leads to poor learning of information that would increase the individual's control. Powerlessness is viewed as a form of alienation, as are meaninglessness, normlessness, and estrangement from culture and self.

Helplessness can be viewed as a response learned from repeated exposure to events that one cannot control.[10] This response can generalize across situations and can be unlearned. For some persons, repeated, unremitting hardships can cause Helplessness, but for others, seemingly minor mishaps may evoke the feeling.

Two types of Powerlessness have been described—trait and situational.[13] Trait powerlessness is all-encompassing, including the general affect, lifestyle, and attitude of the individual. Situational powerlessness may occur in any individual who lacks control in a specific event or circumstance.

With children, Powerlessness is related to expected or normal development, because a child progresses by gaining power and control through developmental achievements. When illness occurs in children, their coping mechanisms may be overwhelmed, and the resulting Powerlessness may be experienced as a crisis.[1]

For the elderly, vulnerability to Powerlessness increases through the often-cumulative losses and stresses that the older generation experiences.[7] Many elderly persons have fewer intact resources such as stamina, resiliency, physical strength, support systems, energy, financial resources, and the motivation to improve health and adhere to treatment regimens. Psychological stressors such as the death of loved ones, retirement, relocation, and the physiological changes that accompany aging may heighten the vulnerability of the aging person to feel powerless.

With acute illness, when the symptoms are most prevalent, when the illness is particularly debilitating, when the individual has not had much experience with illness, or when the evaluation and diagnosis are extended or intrusive, the nurse should be alert to the potential for Powerlessness. When chronic illness imposes lifelong adaptation along with a fluctuating health state, ongoing deterioration, intrusive diagnostic and treatment measures, and technology that may be unfamiliar and difficult for the patient to understand, the nurse should again be alert to the risk of increased vulnerability and Powerlessness.[6,15,17] Recent Bureau of Census[12] figures estimate that approximately 50% of the U.S. population is afflicted by one or more chronic illnesses with 9.5% of the population suffering activity limitation in major activity. Strain[14] lists eight categories of psychological reaction to chronic illness: (1) the perceived threat to self-esteem and body intactness that challenges the belief that the individual controls his/her own body; (2) fear of losing approval or love, which evolves from the patient's fears that illness and dependence on others will lead to withdrawal; (3) fear of losing control of achieved body parts and their functions with resulting loss of independence; (4) anxiety resulting from separation from loved ones and a familiar environment that provided support, gratification, and a sense of intactness; (5) fear of injury to, or complete loss of, body parts; (6) guilt and fear of retaliation for incurring the health problem or for losing control; (7) fear of pain; and (8) fear of the strangers providing intimate care.

ASSESSMENT

Most of the pertinent assessment data for Powerlessness will be obtained by interview and observation of actual care participation, but the nurse can also use medical record information for historical and medical diagnostic data. Discussion with family members may reveal additional information about the patient's coping styles and personality characteristics. The nurse should assess the patient for the presence of defining characteristics of Powerlessness (e.g., verbal expressions of having no control, passivity, etc.). Related factors have been identified that may contribute to the likelihood of a patient's developing Powerlessness, and their presence needs to be determined (e.g., lifestyle of helplessness). In the actual health care environment, technology and language may be unfamiliar to the patient. Staff members may dehumanize the patient by removing personal possessions, ignoring privacy needs, limiting access to authority figures, watching over him/her excessively, and restricting access to needed equipment. The occurrence of such interpersonal interactions must be determined because they may discourage the patient's involvement in self-care, deny the patient's participation in scheduling, reinforce previous interpersonal failures, or diminish the patient's fragile sense of control over his/her health care. Another significant related factor for which the patient must be assessed is the actual illness-related regimen, which may include progressive physical deterioration that threatens physical integrity; alteration in body appearance and/or mental status; changes in sexual, social, and occupational functioning; and constant adaptation to the demands of the illness. The patient must also be assessed for a history of Helplessness, dependence on others, and poor self-esteem. Medical illness and prognosis, as well as the patient's past experiences with illness, level of knowledge, commonly employed coping strategies, and availability of support systems, complete the assessment parameters.[16]

❖ Defining Characteristics

The presence of the following defining characteristics indicates that the patient may be experiencing Powerlessness:[4]

Severe

- Verbal expressions of having no control or influence over situation

- Verbal expressions of having no control or influence over outcome

- Verbal expressions of having no control over self-care
- Depression over physical deterioration that occurs despite patient compliance with regimens
- Apathy

Moderate

- Nonparticipation in care or decision-making when opportunities are provided
- Expressions of dissatisfaction and frustration over inability to perform previous tasks and/or activities
- Absence of monitoring of own progress

- Expression of doubt regarding role performance
- Reluctance to express true feelings, fearing alienation from caregivers
- Inability to seek information regarding care
- Dependence on others that may result in irritability, resentment, anger, and guilt
- Lack of defense of self-care practices when challenged

Low

- Passivity
- Expressions of uncertainty about fluctuating energy levels

❖ **Related Factors**

The following related factors are associated with Powerlessness:[4]

- Illness-related regimen
- State of development
- Lifestyle of helplessness

- Interpersonal interaction
- Health care environment

❖ **Related Medical/Psychiatric Diagnoses**

The following are examples of related medical/psychiatric diagnoses for Powerlessness:

- AIDS
- Alcoholism
- Alzheimer's disease
- Carcinoma
- Cardiac illness

- Schizophrenia
- Spinal cord injury with paralysis
- Stroke
- Substance abuse

NURSING DIAGNOSES

Examples of *specific* nursing diagnoses for Powerlessness are:

- Powerlessness related to health care environment
- Powerlessness related to illness-related regimen

PLANNING AND IMPLEMENTATION WITH RATIONALE

Nursing strategies for alleviating Powerlessness and enhancing aspects of patient control are basic to nursing practice and include the following: (1) modifying the environment; (2) assisting the patient in setting realistic goals and expectations; (3) increasing the patient's knowledge; (4) increasing the sensitivity of health care team members and significant others to the patient's imposed Powerlessness; and (5) encouraging verbalization of feelings.[11] The patient's power resources must also be maximized to facilitate coping. As the result of planned nursing interventions, the nurse can generally expect the patient to acknowledge and verbalize an increased sense of power and control and to recognize and identify situations that threaten the individual's sense of control. The patient will learn to engage in problem-solving behaviors to increase feelings of mastery. The long-term expected outcome, of course, is integration of the therapeutic regimen into the individual's everyday life.

The nurse employs nursing interventions and strategies to achieve expected patient outcomes. Providing information, engaging the patient in decision-making whenever possible, and modifying the environment to increase self-care involvement are nursing interventions that *enhance the potential for mastery over self-care and inspire confidence in one's personal capacity for coping.* Encouraging a sense of partnership with the health care team, reinforcing the patient's right to ask questions, and assisting the patient to develop an awareness of events over which he/she has control and to examine situations in which Powerlessness is felt *provide opportunities for reinforcing cognitive control and enhancing interpersonal relationships with health care providers.*

Nursing interventions may include the alleviation of physical discomfort, teaching self-monitoring, providing relevant learning materials,[2]

VII

❖ NURSING CARE GUIDELINES
Nursing Diagnosis: *Powerlessness*

Expected Patient Outcomes	Nursing Interventions
The patient will verbalize an increased sense of control over situation and activities.	• Provide opportunities for the patient to express feelings about self and illness. • Explore reality perceptions and clarify if necessary by providing information or correcting misinformation. • Provide information and allow time to prepare for procedures. • Provide consistent caregivers. • Modify the environment if needed to facilitate the patient's active involvement in self-care. • Engage the patient in decision-making whenever possible (e.g., the selection of roommate or wearing apparel). • Help patient anticipate sensory experiences that accompany procedures.
The patient will identify situations in which Powerlessness is felt.	• Encourage sense of partnership with health care team. • Limit incidents that may induce feeling of Powerlessness (e.g., staff use of medical jargon or focusing on unpredictability of procedural outcomes). • Reinforce the patient's right to ask questions. • Acknowledge and accept expression of angry feelings as manifestation of the patient's distress.[5] • Help patient develop awareness of care aspects that are patient controlled and separate from uncontrollable events. • Eliminate unpredictability of events by informing patient of scheduled tests and procedures. • Provide opportunities for privacy.
The patient will engage in problem-solving behaviors.	• Encourage the patient's interest and curiosity in care. • Provide positive reinforcement for increasing involvement in self-care. • Teach self-monitoring (e.g., encourage the patient to keep a diary or records). • Help patient communicate effectively with other health team members. • Provide relevant learning materials. • Alleviate physical discomfort that diminishes energy reserve.

evoking interest in mastering aspects of care, and providing positive reinforcement for increased self-care involvement. These interventions are directed toward *focusing coping capacities on specific care aspects. Enabling the patient to adapt* *to lifestyle changes imposed by illness is the ultimate goal of nursing care.* The nurse can employ strategies in involving family members and significant others, utilizing available support systems, providing opportunities for the expression of pos-

VII

❖ NURSING CARE GUIDELINES—cont'd
Nursing Diagnosis: Powerlessness

Expected Patient Outcomes	Nursing Interventions
The patient will integrate therapeutic regimen into lifestyle.	• Provide opportunities for the expression of positive emotions such as hope, faith, the will to live, and a sense of purpose. • Help patient identify strengths and improvements in condition, and the mastery of self-care, coping mechanisms, and power resources. • Facilitate continuity of significant roles that the patient fills in everyday life. • Involve family members and significant others in plan of care. • Assist patient in planning tasks that may deplete energy so that support systems are available. • If indicated, help the patient find alternative roles, interests, and use of talents. • Support involvement in self-help groups when indicated.

itive emotions (hope, faith, sense of purpose, and will to live), and supporting the patient's involvement in self-help groups when indicated.

EVALUATION

Self-reporting by the patient will provide the nurse with the most definitive evaluation of the success or failure of nursing interventions. The nurse should also be alert to patient behaviors indicating feelings of gain, mastery of knowledge, increased skill in performing technical tasks, improved capacity and willingness to meet self-care demands, development of positive relationships with health care team members, actual compliance with the treatment regimen, and capacity to state present and future goals for self. Observation of self-care and reports of coping and adaptation by significant others will enhance the nurse's ability to evaluate outcome. Failure to achieve outcome may indicate underlying personality issues that may necessitate a referral for mental health counseling.

❖ CASE STUDY WITH PLAN OF CARE

Mrs. Emma N. is a 71-year-old ambulatory female experiencing her sixth hospitalization for severe congestive heart failure. She is overweight, complains of frequent episodes of dyspnea, and has a restricted social life because of her diet. Her husband reports that she frequently does not take her medication and no longer attends her program for weight control. Mrs. N. states that weight control has been a "losing battle" since her adolescent years and denies that she does not take her medication.

Continued.

PLAN OF CARE FOR MRS. EMMA N.

Nursing Diagnosis: *Powerlessness related to illness-related regimen.*

Expected Patient Outcomes	Nursing Interventions
Mrs. N. will identify aspects of her current situation that make her feel powerless.	• Explore with Mrs. N. her concerns about the diagnosis and treatment regimen. • Encourage discussion about body image and weight control. • Explore concerns related to effect of illness on the patient's social life.
Mrs. N. will comply with medication schedules.	• Encourage self-monitoring and use of a daily pill dispenser. • Explore current daily medication schedule and suggest patient coordinate medication with daily schedule.
Mrs. N. will integrate illness into lifestyles.	• Encourage a return to the weight-control group. • Refer for nutritional counseling. • Encourage Mr. N. to support any positive gains his wife makes.

REFERENCES

1. Bauman DR: Coping behavior of children experiencing powerlessness from loss of mobility. In Miller J, editor: *Coping with chronic illness: overcoming powerlessness,* Philadelphia, 1983, FA Davis.
2. Carey N and others: Do you feel powerless when a patient refuses medication? *J Psychosoc Ment Health Serv* 10:19-25, 1990.
3. The American Psychiatric Association: *Diagnostic and statistical manual of mental disorders, third edition, revised,* Washington, DC, 1987, The Association.
4. Kim M, McFarland G, and McLane A: *Pocket guide to nursing diagnoses,* ed 4, St Louis, 1991, Mosby–Year Book.
5. Korobov L, and others: Think you're powerless? Think again, *Nursing* 19(11):103-104, 107-109, 1989.
6. Miller J: *Coping with chronic illness: overcoming powerlessness,* Philadelphia, 1983, FA Davis.
7. Miller J, Oertel C: Powerlessness in the elderly: preventing hopelessness. In Miller J, editor: *Coping with chronic illness: overcoming powerlessness,* Philadelphia, 1983, FA Davis.
8. Rotter J: Generalized expectancies for internal versus external control of reinforcement, *Psychol Monogr Gen Applied* 80(1):1-28, 1966 Whole No. 609.
9. Seeman M: Powerlessness and knowledge: a comparative study of alienation and learning, *Sociometry* 30:105-123, 1967.
10. Seligman M: *Helplessness: on depression, development and death,* San Francisco, 1975, WH Freeman.
11. Stapleton S: Decreasing powerlessness in the chronically ill: a prototype. In Miller J, editor: *Coping with chronic illness: overcoming powerlessness,* Philadelphia, 1983, FA Davis.
12. *Statistical abstract of the U.S. 1990,* The National Data Book, Washington, DC, 1990, US Department of Commerce, Bureau of the Census.
13. Stephenson C: Powerlessness and chronic illness: implications for nursing, *Baylor Nurs Educ* 1(1):17, 1979.
14. Strain J: Psychological reactions to chronic illness, *Psychiatr Q* 51:173, 1979.
15. Swanson B and others: Dementia and depression in persons with AIDS: causes and care, *J Psychosoc Ment Health Serv* 28(10):33-39, 1990.
16. Taylor C, Cress S: Nursing diagnosis cards, Springhouse, Penn, 1987, Springhouse.
17. Weisman A: Coping with illness. In Cassem N, editor: *Handbook of general hospital psychiatry,* St Louis, 1991, Mosby-Year Book.

Body Image Disturbance

Body Image Disturbance Is a Disruption in the Perceptions, Beliefs, and Knowledge Possessed About One's Own Body Structure, Function, Appearance, and Limits.[8,10]

OVERVIEW

Body image can be seen as a distinct aspect of the self-concept. It is generally known as that part of the perceived self that constitutes a personal picture or image of the appearance of the body and its functions.[18] As such, it is contained within the person and subjected to ongoing changes based on life experiences such as physical illnesses, accidents, and associated social and cultural values. Body image may overlap with other aspects of the self-concept such as personal identity, role performance, and self-esteem and is an integrated aspect of the global self-concept.[10,19] Life experiences that result in changes in body image will affect values and beliefs inherent in the self-concept and thus influence responses, performance, and thought processes. For example, a change in body structure such as the loss of a limb implies a change in body image, because appearance and functional capacity are affected. The same change also implies other possible alterations in self-concept, because beliefs and values influence self-worth and may reduce self-esteem, making the adjustment process more complex and difficult.[18]

The significance attributed to body image, the way a person sees the body and its functions, will vary according to the nature and intensity of values and related emotions invested in that image.[21] In North American society appearance, including dress and makeup, is a highly valued norm. Plastic surgery is not uncommon to alter a nose considered too large or too small or to have one's "face lifted" to eliminate the wrinkles of aging. The magnitude of the cosmetic industry and the "youth cult" seen in the advertising business are further indicators of societal values that determine what is considered desirable or undesirable in appearances. Young people in particular tend to be preoccupied with the ideal of thinness in appearance, which leads to fads in nutritional habits with possible health risks.[12] The desire to be fashionable in dress and hairstyle exerts subtle pressures for changes in appearance and reflects adjustments to changing norms. Within the context of these influences body image is dynamic and never static. Yet there is an internal consistency shaped by the developmental process and life experiences associated with emotions and social and cultural rewards that gives meaning and value to one's body image. The qualitative aspects of body image, attitudes, and feelings, whether positive or negative, tend to resist change and can lead to a discrepancy in the reality of body image as seen by self and others. The "ideal" or "undesirable" image can persist as a mental concept. This persistence can be seen when one dresses in oversized or undersized clothing based on a mental image of self and in disregard for actual changes in body size. To change one's concept of body image takes time. Further, much of "the editing of the experiences that go into making and modifying the body image is not conscious," and people have difficulty in fully describing their body image.[21]

An understanding of body image and its significance in society and therefore in health care must incorporate the developmental process of the early years.[28] Psychosocial and intellectual attributes evolve over time and shape body image in the socialization process, with ongoing associations and assimilated perceptions within the cognitive domain. The maturation process, including the integration of neuromuscular functions, allows for an increasing capacity for activities that lead to the experience of mastery and social rewards associated with body image. The ongoing changes in body size and function are valued or devalued in the social context of peers and family. Therefore early life experiences can have lasting effects on the mental perception of body image. For example, if the family shows a positive attitude to a child with a handicap, the child will gain confidence and maintain a positive body image. On the other hand, exposure to ridicule or social isolation by his peers or family will confirm a negative appearance and cause the child to form an undesirable mental image that can persist even after corrective surgery has been done.[6]

Marked changes in body structure and function take place during adolescence. Existing social and cultural norms for appearance are challenged, and peer responses develop standards for conformity in dress and behavior. Growth rates and pubertal maturation can vary considerably at a given age. Being different, or smaller or taller than the average height of the peer group, can cause ridicule or social isolation, with possible disturbances in body image.[27]

In certain areas of nursing practice attention to possible Body Image Disturbance can be significant in relation to health goals. Generally patient responses to illness and life events are in part based on the perceived threat to body image and the values and beliefs attached to it.[23] Any surgical intervention and many medical treatments or diagnostic procedures involve temporary or permanent changes in appearance and functional capacity.

In certain age ranges marked changes in appearance and function occur, and adaptation to and acceptance of these changes can be difficult and may require professional guidance and assistance. Children at the toddler and preschool stages of development exert their energies toward

autonomy and initiative in mastering locomotion and self-care tasks. Parental responses that offer positive experiences related to these developmental tasks need to be encouraged. Adolescents experience rapid growth and changes associated with puberty; they can find it difficult to cope with the imbalance and conflicts in self-perception and the need for peer approval. Anxieties and fears related to changes in body image need to be considered when working with adolescents. Similarly patients in their senior years may require assistance in making necessary adjustments to changes in body image.[15,17]

Certain life events or illnesses may cause drastic or abrupt changes in body image. Examples are accidents with severe trauma, loss of limbs, loss of hair, mutilation or physical abuse, and skin diseases. In these situations an acute disturbance in body image can be assumed, and planned nursing interventions will complement the medical/surgical treatment and assist the patient in making necessary adjustments that promote an experience of self-worth and self-acceptance.[21]

Mental illness can influence both the perception of one's body image and the care given in presenting an acceptable appearance to others. For example, in bipolar disorders grooming can be exaggerated. In the extreme situation, the patient may make little effort to present an acceptable appearance, as often is seen in depressed mental states. In such situations behaviors related to body image can guide treatment approaches and result in desired changes.[20]

Patients may come from a cultural background in which norms for body appearance or behaviors differ markedly from those generally held in the North American culture. For example, in Nigeria women strive to be obese because a corpulent appearance is valued and brings social rewards; whereas in North America obesity, especially in women, can have a negative social value.[13]

Handicaps that affect appearance and make a person different from the acceptable norm of wholeness and perfection can place considerable stress on self-perception and on the formation of a realistic body image. For example, the person with cerebral palsy lacks motor coordination. The person's grimaces and the "odd" posture, gait, and speech often cause negative social responses such as ridicule and stigmatization. The person can form a negative body image that can become the root for other problems such as social isolation, depression, or destructive violence.[4,9]

ASSESSMENT

Any patient who has experienced an illness (for example, weight loss, edema, or skin rashes) or is experiencing functional losses (for instance, immobility or limitations in self-care) will need to adjust to these alterations.[19,24] Assessment needs to focus on the patient's abilities or difficulties in making a positive adjustment. Is the patient aware of the change? Does the patient express preoccupation or distress? Does the person have the necessary knowledge to understand the change? Has the patient encountered similar changes before this experience, and how did the patient cope with these? Does the change in appearance or function have special meaning to this person?

In loss of a body part through surgical amputation or severe trauma or disfigurement, as may occur in a burn accident or in the treatment of cancer, changes are often abrupt, with long-term implications for alteration in appearance and function.[1,7,19] Adjustments in body image must take place, and ongoing assessment is necessary to determine progress or disturbances in perceptions of what is altered and the meaning of the alteration. Observations and associated exploration of feelings and perceptions are assessment strategies.[2,22] For example: "Mr. T., I noticed you keep your eyes shut when I do the dressing. Is it that you find it difficult to look at your stump?"

Disturbances in body image may occur during the various phases of growth and development. Transitional phases in which changes in body structure and function take place may present adjustment challenges or difficulties. In early childhood, parenting influences on the development of body image need ongoing assessment. How parents respond to the child's exertion of autonomy

or initiative, how they accept or reject the child's appearance and respect the child's capacity to function, or how they praise or scold behavior may indicate positive or negative factors affecting how the child learns to see himself.[1]

The nurse may observe parental responses and interactions with the child during visits to clinics, during hospitalizations, or during health counseling sessions. Observations of the child may show timidity or lack of initiative in social situations. Such behaviors can reflect insecurities related to fears of rejection. Problems adjusting to school as reported by parents or teachers may also indicate experiences of ridicule or rejection by peers, making the child feel unliked and not acceptable to others, thus contributing to a negative self-perception. Questioning the child in the following simple way will aid assessment: "How do you like school? How do you like the other boys and girls? Do you think they like you? Is there something special about you they like? Dislike? Tell me about it—what happened?"

Adolescence requires special attention in assessment of possible difficulties in adjusting to the rapid growth changes, to the appearance of secondary sex characteristics, and to the expectations of peers and adults. Observations should focus on how the individuals fit general expectations or norms for height, weight, or features of masculinity or femininity.[27] The young boy or girl who differs widely from expected norms for the age-group may avoid social contacts and peer-related activities such as games and sports. The nurse must determine whether such avoidance is based on the perceived difference in body size and associated social value.

Nutritional assessment can reveal fads related to idealized thinness or overeating resulting in obesity.[3] The nurse can explore eating habits, the frequency and nutritional value of meals, and associated attitudes, especially as these relate to actual or desired changes in body image during adolescence.[11] School health counseling sessions or visits to clinics provide opportunities for assessment.

During the adult years pregnancy may cause

VII

some women difficulties in accepting the changes in body size.[17] Although the changes are temporary, they are unavoidable. They may cause distress about the lost ideal thinness or create a sense of being less attractive to others. Expression of dislike regarding weight gain and abdominal expansion, repeated concerns about looks, and the wish to avoid others may indicate a preoccupation with body image. Negative statements about these changes during prenatal visits can offer an opportunity to explore perceptions and their associated meanings for the pregnant woman.

As the senior years bring about changes in posture, function, and general appearance, adjustments to these changes need ongoing assessment. With advancing years, contacts with health services are more frequent and offer opportunities to explore whether the person is accepting and adjusting to changes in body image. Dress and makeup may show preoccupation with a youthful appearance. Seeking remedies for normal skin changes, such as wrinkles and discolorations, may indicate a lack of knowledge about normal changes or inability to make a positive adjustment.[13]

Congenital deformities such as a clubfoot or cleft lip or birth injuries resulting in cerebral palsy present a special challenge for the development of body image. How significant others, especially the parents, respond to and learn to accept the "different" appearance or the "deficit" in function requires ongoing assessment.[14] Can they touch the deformed body part? Are they hiding the child from social exposure? Do they seek appropriate health counseling for their child? Do they experience prejudices about the deformity? As the child grows, does he/she show awareness of the difference, express dislike, or seek to avoid peer contact? Avoidance of the deformity may indicate difficulties in coping with self-perceptions. The use of figure drawings can aid assessment of body image and show avoidance, lack of inclusion, or oversized or undersized body parts.[25]

Mental illness can be based on distortions or fixations regarding perceptions of body image. Unrealistic perceptions of body size or appearance, expressed in feelings of being too tiny, too fat, or ugly, may indicate negative attitudes toward self. Lack of proper grooming, refusal to engage in self-care, sadness in facial expression, avoidance of social contacts, or open, repeated, negative complaints about body parts, functions, and appearance suggest a possible disturbance in body image affecting mental health. It is important to note that a disturbance in body image can result from a person's perceptions related to an actual change in body part or function or to a perceived change in image where no actual change in body function or part has occurred.[16,26]

Patients who come from different parts of the world may dress or behave in ways that can cause public ridicule, name-calling, or stigmatizing. Wearing head covers, such as a turban, or having the face veiled or wearing a nose ring may be seen as unusual, odd, or inappropriate. Is the patient aware of how others perceive him/her? Does the staring or name-calling cause distress or avoidance of public places? Does the patient know how to help others understand personal background or values in order to gain acceptance? Can he/she make some changes to accommodate social expectations? Assessment in this situation is directed toward finding out if the patient is experiencing difficulties with being in a different cultural environment or if the patient has the necessary knowledge and coping skills to adjust and maintain positive self-perceptions.[19]

Assessment of characteristics of disturbance in body image is ongoing and part of every encounter with patients of all ages and in any setting in which nurses offer professional services. The nurse can use some instruments, such as "draw a person" and "Disfigurement/Dysfunction Scale" to obtain measurements of body perceptions.[5] In most instances, however, nurses collect data as they observe and interact with their patients.

❖ **Defining Characteristics**

The presence of the following defining characteristics indicates that the patient may be experiencing Body Image Disturbance:

- Distress about changes in body structure
- Distress about changes in body function
- Lack of acceptance of missing body part
- Lack of acceptance of actual change in body function
- Failure to adjust to developmental changes
- Lack of self-care
- Improper grooming
- Nutritional fads
- Grieving response
- Distorted perceptions
- Hiding or inability to look at altered body site
- Depersonalization of altered body part
- Expressed fear of rejection
- Avoidance or refusal of social contact
- Perceptions of being different, unacceptable by peers
- Lack of knowledge or conflict regarding cultural or social norms
- Difficulties adjusting to cultural environment

❖ Related Factors

The following related factors are associated with Body Image Disturbance:

- Obvious body changes as a result of illness, surgery, accident, or treatment
- Functional loss (especially when loss has high personal and/or social value)
- Deviations from norms of appearance
- Inability to adjust to or integrate body changes or losses
- Eating disorders
- Mental illness
- Transitional life stages, developmental crises
- Changes in social values and role expectations
- Rigid ideas about appearance
- Negative perception of self
- Inadequate knowledge
- Social prejudices regarding handicapping conditions
- Negative parenting behaviors
- Lack of problem-solving skills in acculturation

❖ Related Medical/Psychiatric Diagnoses

The following are examples of related medical/psychiatric diagnoses for Body Image Disturbance:
- Alopecia
- Anorexia nervosa
- Bulimia nervosa
- Burns (especially second- and third-degree burns)
- Cancer (especially head and neck, breast, gastrointestinal leading to colostomy)
- Cerebral palsy
- Dermatitis (for example, eczema)
- Elephantitis
- Multiple sclerosis
- Obesity
- Paralysis (e.g., CVA)

NURSING DIAGNOSES

Examples of *specific* nursing diagnoses for Body Image Disturbance are:
- Body Image Disturbance related to loss of leg
- Body Image Disturbance related to paralysis of right arm
- Body Image Disturbance related to colostomy
- Body Image Disturbance related to dissatisfaction with weight gain

PLANNING AND IMPLEMENTATION WITH RATIONALE

The onset of a disturbance in body image can be sudden, with drastic changes induced by losses in body structure or function, such as result from accidental amputation or trauma, or it can be more insidious, occurring over a period of time, as do developmental changes, altered perceptions in mental illness, or the deformities of arthritis. Overall goals will focus on alleviating or modifying the disturbance in body image, with emphasis on the patient making a favorable adaptation and showing a return to, or development of, an integrated, realistic perception of body image. Expectations for patient outcomes are guided by a time frame that indicates a logical progression in the adaptation process.

Four successive yet interrelated phases describe the adaptation process. These are impact, retreat,

VII

❖ *NURSING CARE GUIDELINES*

Nursing Diagnosis: Body Image Disturbance

Expected Patient Outcomes	Nursing Interventions
The patient will show awareness of loss or change and express grief.	• Assist the patient to express feelings. • Assist patient through normal grieving. • Communicate acceptance of expressed feeling. • Provide privacy for expression of feelings. • Spend time with patient to show social acceptance. • Refer to altered body part with proper name.
The patient will resolve fears and anxiety.	• Assist the patient to express anger, frustration, and disappointment. • Facilitate exploration of anxiety and fears. • Accept initial need for concealment of change. • Provide gentle persuasion to explore altered body part; for example, encourage talking about it and viewing it. • Set mutual goals for progressive self-care. • Assist patient to recognize own strengths and assets in appearance and functions. • Help significant others to support and assist the patient. • Provide information to significant others.
The patient will acknowledge changes.	• Facilitate and reinforce efforts the patient makes in recognizing realities. • Offer opportunities for social contacts with persons who had similar experiences. • Introduce information about technical aids or replacements. • Introduce rehabilitative services that can assist the patient; for instance, physiotherapy and enterostomal therapy. • Teach significant others required care skills. • Offer praise and encouragement.
The patient will express constructive integration of body image.	• Provide information and guidance on how to access and use available services. • Facilitate learning of new skills. • Introduce the patient to support groups and facilitate initial contacts. • Praise and acknowledge appearance and accomplishments for even small steps of progress. • Encourage the patient to engage in normal social activities. • Discuss with the patient body image perception. • Praise constructive problem-solving to enhance appearance. • Encourage significant others in giving support and fostering independence.

VII

acknowledgment, and reconstruction.[21] The nurse can develop patient outcomes and related nursing interventions with reference to these phases as the patient experiences them.

Development of awareness of what is altered or perceived as altered is the initial goal. With a sudden change or loss the impact can be experienced as shock, disbelief, denial, and sadness. In cases of significant losses, goals for expression of grief should precede expectations for acceptance and the learning of replacement skills.[21]

Interventions focus on assisting the patient to express perceptions and feelings. *If the nurse shows acceptance and encourages expression of feelings, the patient can learn to accept his/her own responses and gain support in expressing thoughts and feelings.* Providing privacy for the expression of sadness (having a "cry") or allowing the patient to be alone for a while will *facilitate awareness and will offer the patient a sense of care and respect. Spending time with the patient and referring to the altered body aspect by naming it (for example, your stump, colostomy, rash, paralyzed arm) will convey social acceptance and provide a reality focus* for gradual awareness of the altered body part.

With awareness comes realization of what the change of body image implies; that is, how it might threaten social roles, job functions, future goals, or one's values and beliefs. These realizations characterize the retreat phase as the patient tries to sort through the inner turmoil of fears and anxieties. The goal is to support the patient and to assist in the resolution of fears and anxieties. Interventions will address showing acceptance of needs such as hiding, avoiding exposure and/or social contacts, self-care, and wishing to talk, or not talk, about experienced changes. Yet need also exists for gentle persuasion to explore the altered body site. The nurse can first give a description of what he/she sees and set goals with the patient for when the body part will be viewed or touched. *Helping the patient to realize strengths, positive efforts, or assets in appearance and function will facilitate holistic perceptions and coun-*

terbalance fears and anxieties associated with the change in body image. Assisting the patient to express and explore feelings of anger, disappointment, and frustration will help to identify underlying anxieties or misconceptions. Significant others can play a role in supporting and assisting the patient; however, they need information on what to expect and how to be helpful. They too need support and assistance to express their own thoughts and feelings. *A show of acceptance by significant others can be a trustworthy social reflection on the patient's altered body image from which a positive adjustment can develop.*

As the patient gains an understanding, he/she begins to acknowledge experienced changes in body appearance and function. The nurse can facilitate the process of acknowledgment by reinforcing efforts the patient makes in recognizing the realities of the change, such as naming the changed aspect with use of personal pronouns (my stump, my colostomy, my paralyzed side); offering opportunities for social contacts and encouraging the patient to talk with others about the changed appearance or function; introducing information regarding available technical aids for functional losses (such as crutches, makeup, or prostheses); introducing services that can assist in gaining new skills (such as physiotherapy for crutch walking, occupational therapy for managing self-care, or enterostomal therapy in case of a colostomy). *When the patient is assisted to focus on the realities of the situation and gains* a future orientation, he/she can develop readiness to invest energies and efforts toward constructive adjustments.

With readiness to learn, the reconstruction phase of adjustment can take place. Nursing interventions will now focus on providing information and guidance on possible resources; facilitating relearning such as self-care; learning of new skills in the use of appliances and technical aids or how to dress attractively; encouraging and supporting realistic goals for progress; offering praise and acknowledgment for accomplishments, even for small steps of progress; identifying available sup-

VII

port groups and supporting the initiation of contacts; and involving significant others in giving support, encouragement, and fostering independence. *Praise, support, guidance, and encouragement facilitate learning and aid acceptance and integration of changes in appearance and function into a positive perception of one's body image.*[5]

EVALUATION

As the patient is manifesting progressive adaptation to the experienced loss or change in body function or altered appearance, he/she expresses emotions of sadness and anger and names and talks about the change in function or undesired appearance. The patient is able to express feelings of frustration and disappointment; for example, This looks awful; How will I ever manage my job?; My wife/husband can never love me like this. In the nurse-patient relationship the patient expresses fears and anxieties. Similarly, significant others show acceptance of fears and encourage the patient to express these. The patient sets goals for self-care and is managing to look at or touch the changed body part, uses proper naming, and explores functional abilities. The patient gradually tolerates social exposure and seeks to resume normal social activities. The patient acknowledges the help of others and can focus on assets in appearance and abilities. He/she learns and manages new skills. Significant others are supportive and refrain from overprotection or unnecessary assistance. The patient shows pride in own efforts to manage new skills and in an attractive appearance. The patient can reflect on the total experience: the initial distress, fears, and anxieties about the altered body image, steps taken to adjust, and seeing positive and negative aspects of the body in a holistic, acceptable way. Problem-solving skills are evident in knowing how to find needed resources and how to access available health services or support groups in order to promote and maintain a positive body image.

VII

❖ *CASE STUDY WITH PLAN OF CARE*

Mrs. Susan L. is a 52-year-old widow who, 5 days ago, underwent a colon resection for a benign tumor, resulting in a permanent colostomy of the descending colon. Surgery and postoperative recovery were uncomplicated. Mrs. L. is now on a semiliquid diet and requires only occasional relief of pain. She has been fitted with a colostomy pouch that the nurse drains and cleans as needed at regular intervals during the day. Drainage has been moderate and of semiliquid consistency. The release of flatus has been necessary several times during the past day. Mrs. Susan L. shows distress about the colostomy care, stating "I wish you would go away with that tray. I never want to see you again." During appliance changes she was tearful, turning her face away and pinching her nose to avoid smelling the odor. She refused visitors, permitting only her two daughters to see her. She asked the nurse to deodorize the room before their visits. She feels discouraged and has said, "How can I live with this thing!" She led an active life before surgery, is financially independent, has her own apartment, and lives alone since her husband's death 3 years ago. She belongs to several social clubs and has many friends. Her two daughters are married and live nearby. Before her marriage she was a fashion model and has always liked to design and sew her own clothes. She has taken great pride in her youthful appearance and in being neat and attractively dressed. She used to keep fit by watching her diet and swimming several times a week.

PLAN OF CARE FOR MRS. SUSAN L.

Nursing Diagnosis: *Body Image Disturbance related to structural and functional changes in elimination resulting from colostomy*

Expected Patient Outcomes	Nursing Interventions
Mrs. L. will show awareness of loss as evidenced by: tolerating colostomy care and beginning to inspect the stoma site and appliance over the next 2 days.	• Prepare Mrs. L. for each pouch emptying and stoma care by planning mutually suitable times. • Use proper name, "stoma care," and describe what is seen and done. • Acknowledge the need to look away and that it takes time to gather courage for looking. • Show acceptance for the expression of grief and the need for denial. • Plan with Mrs. L. for a time to inspect the stoma, depending on Mrs. L.'s level of awareness and readiness. • Show Mrs. L. the equipment that is used without expecting participation. • Show personal acceptance through attentive care and brief visits not associated with stoma care.
Mrs. L. will resolve emotions as evidenced by: expression of frustration, anxieties, and fears.	• Encourage expression of feelings about the change in appearance and elimination. • Assist by mentioning possible threats to Mrs. L.'s social life and desire to be attractive so these can be explored. • Offer some initial information on successful management of elimination and available appliances. • Assist the daughters in their understanding of Mrs. L.'s initial response, stoma care, and management of elimination; stress the importance of their visiting, acceptance, and support.
Mrs. L. will acknowledge changes as evidenced by participation in stoma care before discharge from the hospital and by using proper terminology.	• Encourage proper use of terminology; for instance, colostomy, stoma. • Encourage gradual participation in stoma care; plan with Mrs. L. daily inspection of stoma with verbal description of what she sees. • Offer praise for accomplishments. • Discuss possible social contacts; encourage plans for visitors.
Mrs. L. will manifest constructive integration of body image as manifested by: • Discussing appearance of open stoma as part of self.	• Encourage verbalization of stoma appearance.
• Beginning to manage altered elimination.	• Teach ostomy care, management of elimination, and odor control.
• Resuming contacts with friends during visiting hours.	• Praise accomplishments.
• Planning how to adjust clothing for neat appearance.	• Facilitate and assist in discharge planning for attractive clothing, social activities.

Continued.

VII

Expected Patient Outcomes	Nursing Interventions[17]
• Demonstrating understanding of elimination, ostomy care, and control of odor.	• Introduce enterostomal therapist as available resource and support.
• Accepting daughters' involvement in ostomy care.	• Involve daughters in colostomy care if Mrs. L. agrees.
• Talking positively about adjustments in lifestyle after discharge.	• Reinforce positive statements about body appearance and management of elimination. • Discuss participation in recreational and exercise regimen.

REFERENCES

1. Beard SA, Herndon DN, and Desai M: Adaptation of self-image in burn-disfigured children, *J Burn Care Rehabil* 10:550-553, 1989.
2. Bernado LM, Conway A, and Bove M: The ABC method of emotional assessment and intervention: a new approach in pediatric emergency care, *J Emerg Nurs* 16(2):70-76, 1990.
3. Ciliska DJ: *Beyond dieting: psychoeducational intervention for chronically obese women: a non-dieting approach,* Eating Disorders Monograph (5), New York, 1990, Brunner/Mazel.
4. Dewis ME: Spinal cord injured adolescents and young adults: the meaning of body changes, *J Adv Nurs* 14(5):389-396, 1989.
5. Dropkin MJ: Coping with disfigurement and dysfunction after head and neck cancer surgery: a conceptual framework, *Semin Oncol Nurs* 5(3):213-219, 1989.
6. Foster RLR, Hunsberger MM, and Anderson JJT: *Family-centered nursing care of children,* Philadelphia, 1989, WB Saunders.
7. Hopwood P, Maguire GP: Body image problems in cancer patients, *Br J Psychiatry* 153(suppl 2):47-50, 1988.
8. Jourard SM: *Personal adjustment: an approach through the study of healthy personality,* New York, 1963, Macmillan Publishing.
9. Jureidini J: Psychotherapeutic implications of severe physical disability, *Am J Psychotherapy* 42(2):297-307, 1988.
10. Kim MJ, McFarland GK, and McLane AM: *Pocket guide to nursing diagnoses,* ed 4, St Louis, 1991, CV Mosby.
11. Kinley BG, Burge JC: Dieting restriction in young women: issues and concerns, *Ann Behav Med* 11(2):66-72, 1989.
12. Koff E, Rierdan J: Perceptions of weight and attitudes toward eating in early adolescent girls, *J Adolesc Health* 12:307-312, 1991.
13. Leppa CJ: Cosmetic surgery and the motivation for health and beauty, *Nurs Forum* 25(1):25-31, 1990.
14. Matteson MA, McConnell ES: *Gerontological nursing concepts and practice,* Philadelphia, 1988, WB Saunders.
15. Mason KJ: Congenital orthopedic anomalies and their impact on the family, *Nurs Clin North Am* 26(1):1-16, 1991.
16. Moses N, Banilivy MM, and Lifshitz F: Fear of obesity among adolescent girls, *Pediatrics* 83(3):393-398, 1989.
17. Olds SB, London ML, and Ladewig PA: *Maternal newborn nursing: a family-centered approach,* ed 3, Menlo Park, 1988, Addison-Wesley.
18. Olson B, Ustanko L, and Warner S: The patient in a halo brace: striving for normalcy in body image and self concept, *Orthop Nurs* 10(1):44-50, 1991.
19. Price B: *Body image nursing concepts and care,* New York, 1990, Prentice Hall.
20. Rix KJB, Smith RP, editors: The psychopathology of body image, *Br J Psychiatry* 153(suppl 2), 1988.
21. Roberts SL: *Behavioral concepts and the critically ill patient,* ed 2, Norwalk, Conn, 1986, Appleton-Century-Crofts.
22. Samond RJ, Cammermeyer M: Perceptions of body image in subjects with multiple sclerosis: pilot study, *J Neurosci Nurs* 21(3):190-194, 1989.
23. Santopinto MDA: The relentless drive to be ever thinner: a study using the phenomenological method, *Nurs Sci Quart* 2(1):29-36, 1989.
24. Utz SW, Hammer J, Whitmire VM, Grass S: Perceptions of body image and health status in persons with mitral valve prolapse, *Image: J Nurs Scholar* 22(1):18-22, 1990.
25. Whaley LF, Wong DL: *Nursing care of infants and children,* ed 4, St Louis, 1991, CV Mosby.
26. Whitehouse AM, Freeman CPL, Annandale A: Body size estimation in anorexia nervosa, *Br J Psychiatry,* 153(suppl 2):23-26, 1988.
27. Williamson ML: The nursing diagnosis of body image disturbance in adolescents dissatisfied with their physical characteristics, *Hol Nurs Pract* 1(4):52-59, 1987.
28. Winkelstein ML: Fostering positive self-concept in the school-age child, *Pediatr Nurs* 15(3):229-233, 1989.

VII

Personal Identity Disturbance

Personal Identity Disturbance is the inability to distinguish between self and nonself, or to differentiate self as a unique human being living in a social environment.

OVERVIEW

A Personal Identity Disturbance results from confusion about who one *really* is or from adopting a negative identity that clashes with individual or societal expectations. A serious threat to the self-concept, the nature of the Personal Identity Disturbance varies with the cause of the condition and surrounding circumstances. The intensity may range from relatively mild to severe—from someone experiencing a midlife crisis to someone suffering from a prolonged episode of psychosis.

Less extreme, but still painful, disturbances in personal identity may occur with maturational and situational crises.[6] Confusion about "who I really am" is a normal part of growth as one proceeds through various developmental stages.[4] However, in transition between stages people often experience strong feelings of anxiety, conflict, ambivalence, and frustration related to their fears about the loss of familiar roles and responsibilities and the challenges of new ones. Their sense of self is shaken as they respond to their own expectations and those of others about their "new" self.[2] They must struggle to reformulate their identity as they accomplish developmental tasks.

Life circumstances also dictate the adjustment of personal identity. Some examples of events that affect identity are the death of a spouse, loss of a job, status as a minority member of society,[13] relocation or immigration to a different cultural setting, family violence,[6] and onset of chronic illness. Some people experience little disturbance in personal identity, and others have great difficulty as they try to cope with crisis.

More extreme disturbances in identity are characterized by severe confusion about or even denial of one's identity.[5] Mental illnesses such as schizophrenia, mania, depression, borderline personality, and multiple personality disorders may result in severe disturbances in personal identity.[1,12] In these disorders, a combination of physiological, psychological, sociocultural, and spiritual factors interact to disrupt personal identity and functional behavior.[8,11,15] Afflicted individuals lose the ability to perceive self and environment realistically, to differentiate themselves from the environment. They seem to view the interaction between self and environment through a distorted lens. This distortion of reality transforms their sense of knowing who they are into their being a stranger to themselves, a condition of being "not-me." The strangeness becomes reinforced by others who react in a puzzled, anxious, or rejecting way to the "strange identity."[9] As the disturbed individuals become more and more estranged from their original identity, they become highly anxious and confused about the world. Unable to integrate their behavior with the demands of society, their fragmented, diffuse sense of self leads to the total disintegration of their personality.

In addition to interpersonal dynamics, pathophysiology can cause a personal identity disturbance. Any disruption in the brain's normal structure and function may affect the sense of personal identity.[3] Psychoactive drugs such as cocaine, narcotics, hypnotics, hallucinogens and alcohol may cause extreme but usually temporary changes in identity. Memory loss, such as in Alzheimer's disease, has grave and permanent effects on identity. Traumatic injuries to the brain and cerebrovascular accidents may cause identity disturbances. Virtually any insult to the brain that affects perception, cognition, or motor functioning may ultimately result in a personal disturbance.[1]

ASSESSMENT

The nurse begins to assess the patient's sense of personal identity while taking a thorough nursing history and conducting a health assessment. The nurse must obtain information from the patient about functional health patterns, particularly pertaining to Cognitive—Perceptual and Self-Perception—Self-Concept patterns. A comprehensive assessment of the individual, including physical, psychological, sociocultural, and spiritual dimensions, is necessary because the possible causes of a Personal Identity Disturbance are so varied and related factors are crucial in determining treatment and outcomes.[10]

The diagnosis of Personal Identity Disturbance is based on the subjective and objective data the nurse assesses through the interpersonal relationship with the patient. Therefore establishing a therapeutic relationship is key.[9] The nurse continues the in-depth assessment by asking open-ended questions that provide the patient an opportunity to share thoughts and feelings about self and personal identity. Examples of assessment questions are in the box on this page.

As the nurse talks to and observes the patient, the patient will reveal his/her sense of identity through verbal and nonverbal behavior. The nurse then evaluates this information about personal identity in terms of the patient's age, gender and sexual preference, ethnicity, developmental stage, family relations, socioeconomic status, social roles, value system, and residential community. The nurse also considers the appropriateness of the patient's behavioral responses for time and place, the congruence between verbal and nonverbal behavior, and the intensity of accompanying emotions, particularly the level of anxiety. With a disturbance in identity, the patient will empathically communicate some degree of anxiety—

VII

❖ *QUESTIONS TO ASSESS PERSONAL IDENTITY*

How would you describe yourself?

How would you compare your *real* self to your *ideal* self? (How you really are to how you would like to be.)

Is the way you see yourself *now* different from the way you saw yourself in the *past?* If so, what are the differences? What caused the changes?

How do you see yourself changing in the future? What would you like to change about yourself?

Do you feel comfortable with who you are? If not, what makes you feel uncomfortable about yourself?

Are the important people in your life comfortable with who you are? If not, what makes them feel uncomfortable?

Do you sometimes feel uncertain or confused about who you really are? If so, when do you feel this way? Tell me about one time.

Do you ever experience a sense of unreality about who you are or about where you fit in the scheme of things? If so, when do you feel this way? Tell me about one time.

Do you ever have a sense of being "not-me?" If so, when do you feel this way? Tell me about one time.

Do you ever feel as if you are really some other person or that you do not really exist? If so, when do you feel this way? Tell me about one time.

from moderate discomfort to overt panic—depending on the cause and extent of the disturbance. The nurse uses the empathic communication to guide further assessment of the patient's sense of personal vulnerability and perceptions of threat from within the self or in the environment. (See pages 492 to 494 for assessment of anxiety.)

The nurse will examine other sources of data that may influence or have an effect on the patient's sense of personal identity, such as social support, environmental stimulation, and community events.[2] The patient's family and friends may provide important information about the client's recent and past behavior that contribute to and validate the nurse's clinical impressions.

Because a person's identity is unique and a disturbance may be manifested in such a variety of ways, no *single* question or observation of behavior will provide sufficient evidence for the nurse to make this diagnosis. Therefore conducting a comprehensive assessment is essential, including a focus on the patient's usual sense of personal identity, feelings about the self, and coping behavior. An exception to this is the patient who exhibits obvious disorientation or confusion or who has suffered a head trauma that resulted in loss of consciousness. Then a screening question such as "What is your name?" may be sufficient to diagnose a Personal Identity Disturbance when the patient's answer is compared with known facts.

❖ Defining Characteristics

The presence of the following defining characteristics indicates that the patient may be experiencing Personal Identity Disturbance:

- Sense of "not being myself"
- Alienation
- Ambivalence
- Confusion
- Disorientation
- Blurred boundaries
- Depersonalization
- Narcissism
- Fear
- Memory loss
- Defensiveness
- Secretiveness
- Suspiciousness
- Delusions
- Hallucinations
- Social withdrawal
- Incongruent verbal/nonverbal behavior
- Inappropriate behavior
- Change in appearance/routine
- Loss of meaning in life

❖ Related Factors

The following related factors are associated with Personal Identity Disturbance:

- Biochemical imbalances in the brain
- Structural changes in the brain
- Ineffective coping
- Deviant lifestyle
- Disturbances in interpersonal relationships

- Changes in perception and cognition
- Traumatic injury to the brain
- Use of psychoactive drugs
- Ingestion/inhalation of toxic chemicals
- Bodily injury/illness
- Impairment of sensory organs
- Stages of growth and development
- Situational crises
- Dysfunctional family processes
- Role conflict and strain
- Discrimination and prejudice
- Homelessness
- Conflict in values and morals
- Cult indoctrination
- Cultural discontinuity

❖ Related Medical/Psychiatric Diagnoses

The following are examples of related medical/psychiatric diagnoses for Personal Identity Disturbance:

- Anxiety disorders
  Panic disorder
  Posttraumatic stress disorder
- Autistic disorder
- Delusional (paranoid) disorder
- Dissociative disorders
  Multiple personality disorder
  Psychogenic amnesia
  Depersonalization disorder
- Gender identity disorder
- Mood disorders
- Organic mental disorders
  Dementias
  Delirium
  Amnesic disorder

Psychoactive substance-induced organic mental disorders associated with axis III physical disorders
  Organic hallucinosis
- Personality disorders
  Borderline
  Bipolar disorders
  Depressive disorders
- Psychotic disorders not elsewhere classified
  Brief reactive psychosis
  Schizoaffective disorder
- Schizophrenia

NURSING DIAGNOSES

Examples of *specific* nursing diagnoses for Personal Identity Disturbance are:

- Personal Identity Disturbance related to brain dysfunction

- Personal Identity Disturbance related to recent homelessness
- Personal Identity Disturbance related to sensory deprivation in a nursing home
- Personal Identity Disturbance related to episodes of sexual abuse

PLANNING AND IMPLEMENTATION WITH RATIONALE

After a diagnosis of Personal Identity Disturbance is made and the related factors are determined, the nurse helps the patient set goals for treatment.[7] The patient's level of awareness about the health problem must be determined first. Patients with a disturbed sense of identity will vary in self-awareness, but most are sufficiently uncomfortable that they acknowledge a problem exists and willingly accept some assistance from the nurse. Therefore the nurse can expect the patient to aid actively in designing the nursing care plan.

The overall objective is to establish a clear sense of identity. This will provide internal self consistency, foster goal attainment, and allow meaningful interaction with others. To achieve this objective, the nurse and patient must focus on several intermediate outcomes. The first outcome is: the patient will express feelings of distress (anxiety) related to a sense of "not being myself." A sense of depersonalization or self-alienation engenders a high level of anxiety. Initially, reducing the anxiety that accompanies a disturbed sense of self takes priority, *because a highly anxious patient is acutely uncomfortable and unable to engage in problem-solving and other therapeutic tasks.* The patient's anxiety may be manifested in many different behaviors such as passivity and withdrawal, extreme nervousness, hallucinations and delusions, bizarre behavior, or incoherent thoughts. Interventions to decrease anxiety are based on the understanding that when the patient's needs are not met and usual ways of coping do not work, the patient may resort to less functional behavior to obtain relief, or dissociate the self from painful feelings or the stressful environment. The nurse must help the patient to identify unmet needs and examine the relationships among unmet needs, ineffective coping, and the resulting uncomfortable feelings. *This decreases anxiety by providing an understanding of the dynamics of particularly stressful situations and clarifies needs, which the nurse can assist the patient to meet in other ways.* Throughout the process of decreasing distress, the nurse uses his/her own healthy sense of self to convey acceptance, empathy, and respect for the patient's unique way of "being in the world." *This builds trust and strengthens the nurse-patient relationship.*

Next, in planning and implementing care, the patient and nurse must consider the predominant factors—developmental, psychosocial, and physical—related to the Personal Identity Disturbance. An outcome that deals with developmental issues is: the patient will examine sense of self according to developmental stage and tasks, and current life situation. A crisis intervention approach that focuses on the present situation may be most helpful. The nurse designs interventions within a time-limited framework to explore the patient's perception of self, evaluate effectiveness of coping behaviors, and determine the availability of social supports. The nurse emphasizes educating the patient about the thoughts and feelings commonly experienced during maturational and situational crises *to decrease feelings of isolation and unreality and to increase identification and normalization.* The nurse draws on knowledge of growth, development, and normative processes (such as the grief process) *to provide a context for the patient to understand and cope with his/her own crisis as part of the human condition.* Within a supportive environment, the nurse encourages the patient to explore different facets of the self, inner conflicts, boundaries between self and environment, and the meaning of life. *In this way the patient can test alternative identities and practice new behaviors in a safe, accepting, interpersonal environment before risking the reactions of others in the "real world."*

When psychosocial factors are most prominent, the patient's problem with identity may be longstanding. Negative feelings about the self and maladaptive social interactions may be entrenched

❖ NURSING CARE GUIDELINES

Nursing Diagnosis: *Personal Identity Disturbance*

Expected Patient Outcomes	Nursing Interventions
The patient will express feelings of distress related to "not being myself."	• Establish a trusting relationship: convey acceptance and respect, confirm the patient's identity, reduce anxiety by eliciting feelings of distress and examining relationships among needs, coping, and feelings, and meet client's needs as possible.
The patient will describe sense of self in terms of thoughts, feelings and conflicts, confusion about identity, alienation from self, disorientation from the environment, and boundaries between self and environment.	• Use crisis intervention techniques to: elicit perceptions of reality, clarify misconceptions, discuss thoughts and feelings, evaluate coping, determine social support, discuss crisis situation, and provide feedback and validation.
The patient will explore identity resources: ego strengths and weaknesses, stage of development, relationships with others, major roles, significant life events and value system.	• Facilitate elaboration of identity: expand awareness of self, identify strengths and weaknesses, assess family dynamics and life history by doing a genogram, and teach information about growth and development and normal life processes.
The patient will demonstrate a clear sense of identity: verbalize affirmation of personal identity, exhibit congruent verbal and nonverbal behavior, practice presentation of self in simulated social situations, and elicit social support from others.	• Support the patient's personal identity: clarify conception and identity of self; discuss relation of identity to verbal and nonverbal behavior; examine adaptive and maladaptive coping behavior; reinforce strengths and skills; use role play, role modeling, and role rehearsal to strengthen identity; and mobilize support system.

VII

in the person's psyche. In this case the best approach is ongoing one-to-one therapeutic interaction. This therapy concentrates on the patient's self-awareness. The outcome is the patient will explore identity resources. With the nurse's help the patient can explore thoughts, feelings, and events related to self and formative relationships.

The patient and nurse discuss family dynamics and significant childhood experiences *to make connections between past events and present emotions and behaviors and increase insight*. The nurse encourages the patient to test perceptions of reality and to learn new coping behaviors. Specifically, the nurse uses therapeutic communication techniques, such as active listening, clarifying unclear meanings, validating perceptions, modeling self-disclosure, and expressing genuine interest. These interventions facilitate the patient's use of identity and coping resources *by expanding self-awareness, building ego strength, challenging faulty beliefs and negative images, and giving positive affirmations from the environment*. In addition to working with the patient, the nurse must interact with the family and others in the community. *Building a strong identity involves group and family participation as the patient reestablishes boundaries, redefines roles, resolves interpersonal conflicts, and reenters the community in a meaningful way*.

To demonstrate the main outcome, the patient will articulate a clear sense of personal identity. Interventions to support the patient's identity are based on *social learning theory and communication techniques that affirm a strong sense of personal competency*. The hallmarks of a healthy identity are the person's affirmed self differentiation, coherent presentation of self, appropriate role behavior, and well-articulated value system. With the nurse's help the patient learns to verbalize thoughts, wishes, and feelings, using "I" statements to convey a sense of differentiation between self and nonself and the presence of intact ego boundaries. Interventions are designed to clarify the patient's self-conception, including the difference between the real and the ideal self *to build realistic expectations for personal competence*. The nurse engages the patient in role play, role modeling, and role rehearsal *to practice and strengthen new interpersonal skills that reflect a clear sense of identity*. The patient is taught to be congruent in verbal and nonverbal behavior, to practice presentation of self in simulated social situations, and to elicit social support from others. As the patient exhibits a coherent personal identity, the nurse reinforces new learned behavior and encourages the patient to seek validation from others in the environment for the healthy self and to mobilize social support. *In this way the nurse prepares the patient for termination of the nurse-patient relationship and continuing growth in the daily life*.

EVALUATION

The nurse evaluates the nursing interventions by measuring the expected patient outcomes. If the nursing interventions are successful, the patient will exhibit a clear sense of identity, a reduction in anxiety and other distressful feelings, consistency in presentation of self and patterns of behavior, congruent verbal and nonverbal behavior appropriate to the sociocultural situation, and the ability to relate to others in a way that can be validated consensually.

When physical factors cause disturbances in personal identity, the disturbance tends to be progressive and permanent or chronic in nature. The nursing care plan must be revised to reflect a focus on orienting the patient to the environment and maintaining personal safety. The use of memory devices, orienting materials, and environmental constraints may be helpful when the brain is severely damaged or cognitive functioning is impaired. In some situations, the use of behavioral techniques, such as positive reinforcement and modeling of targeted behaviors, may *support the less severely affected patient's sense of self*. However, often no interventions will enable the impaired person to regain a true sense of identity. This situation may be devastating when the individual's self-awareness is still somewhat intact. In this instance, the nurse must be sensitive to the patient's pervasive sense of confusion *to prevent accidents or self-harm*. Interventions include anticipating the patient's needs, repeating concrete information and specific directions as necessary, providing environmental stimulation, eliminating environmental hazards, protecting the patient's dignity in social situations, and respecting the patient at all times. Successful outcomes of this plan may be that the patient receives respect as a unique human being, lives a dependent lifestyle in a protective, caring environment, and has a peaceful death.

❖ CASE STUDY WITH PLAN OF CARE

Ms. Lynn C., a 23-year-old graduate student, was admitted to the acute psychiatric unit. She had been found wandering the streets late at night, wearing a bathing suit over her jeans and sweater. When asked, she did not know her name or where she was. College friends reported that she had been acting strangely for the past 2 months. Lynn had called her mother the day before, alternately crying and laughing as she said, "I'm failing all my courses, but it's better that way." On the unit she withdraws from others, repeating, "This isn't like me. I just don't know what to do. My world is over." She is single and attending school full time while working part time as a research assistant. The only child of elderly parents who are in good health, Ms. C. seldom dates and has few close friends. She devotes all of her time to her studies. She has had no previous serious illness or hospitalizations, and her family has no history of mental illness. Ms. C. also has no allergies. A physical examination reveals a healthy adult woman whose vital signs are stable. She stands 5'2" and weighs 117 pounds. There is no evidence of trauma or abnormal neurological findings. Lynn suffered a memory loss for the 24-hour period before hospitalization and still has some confusion about personal identity. However, she is oriented to time and place. She does not hallucinate, but she has a delusion that she is failing in school. (She has an excellent college record and is scheduled to receive an MBA degree in 2 weeks.) Her thought content involves a preoccupation with failing and feelings of unreality and alienation. She experiences moderate anxiety, bouts of crying, and fear about what is going to happen to her. Her replies to questions are hesitant and quiet, and she avoids social contact with others. She expresses no concern about personal appearance. A chemical urinalysis reveals no trace of marijuana, barbiturates, morphine, cocaine, or alcohol.

PLAN OF CARE FOR MS. LYNN C.

Nursing Diagnosis: Personal Identity Disturbance related to maturational crisis (graduation from college) and role conflict

Expected Patient Outcomes	Nursing Interventions
Ms. C. will express distress and anxiety related to impending graduation and change in lifestyle and relationships.	• Establish a therapeutic relationship with Ms. C., assess anxiety level and try to meet her needs for security, confirm her identity by calling her by name, and elicit acknowledgement of distress.
Ms. C. will describe her sense of self and perception of reality through discussing her inner thoughts and feelings and making comparisons of self between past and present.	• Use assessment questions and communication techniques to help discuss Ms. C.'s thoughts and feelings about who she is, who she would like to be, her present situation, and her past experiences. • Assist Ms. C. to explore feelings of personal alienation and unreality.

Continued.

Expected Patient Outcomes	Nursing Interventions
Ms. C. will explore resources: discuss family history; examine her major roles as an adult in the intimacy stage of development; evaluate what graduation means to her; examine her values about family, independence, work, and intimate relationships; list strengths and weaknesses; and discuss college experience.	• Diagram family genogram to define family relationships and explain family process and significant events, especially the role of the only child. • Review dynamics related to tasks and capacities of adult development in the intimacy stage and identity formation in adolescence. • Assist Mrs. C. in comparing strengths and weaknesses, discussing educational achievements in particular.
Ms. C. will exhibit realistic and consistent sense of self: speak with confidence and conviction about self, respond to others appropriately with reference to herself, value her accomplishments in college and life, rehearse presentation of herself in job interview, and relate to her parents as an adult.	• Validate Ms. C.'s identity as a competent young adult woman: discuss her future plans for work and living arrangements, facilitate a family meeting to discuss issues related to this stage of family development, assist Ms. C in engaging in social activities with peers, role play job interview and other new social situations, and evaluate her progress in terms of planned objectives.

REFERENCES

1. American Psychiatric Association: *Diagnostic and statistical manual of mental disorders,* ed 3 revised, Washington, DC, 1987, The Association.
2. Comerci GD: Society, community and the adolescent: how much the problem, how much the solution, *J Early Adolesc* 9(1-2):8-12, 1989.
3. Cummings LJ: Organic psychosis, *Psychosomatics* 29(1):16-26, 1988.
4. Erikson EH: *Identity: youth and crisis,* New York, 1968, WW Norton.
5. Gara MA, Rosenberg S, and Cohen BD: Personal identity and the schizophrenic process: an integration, *Psychiatry* 50(3):267-279, 1987.
6. Hoff LA: *People in crisis,* ed 3, Redwood City, Calif, 1989, Addison-Wesley Publishing.
7. Kim M, McFarland G, and McLane A: Pocket guide to nursing diagnoses, ed 4, St Louis, 1991, Mosby–Year Book.
8. Malone JA: Schizophrenia research update: implications for nursing, *J Psychosoc Nurs* 28(8):4-8, 1990.
9. O'Toole AW, Welt SR: *Interpersonal theory in nursing practice,* New York, 1989, Springer Publishing.
10. Pasquali EA, Arnold HM, and DeBasio N: *Mental health nursing,* ed 3, St Louis, 1989, CV Mosby.
11. Peterson EA, Nelson K: How to meet your clients' spiritual needs, *J Psychosoc Nurs* 25(5):34-39, 1987.
12. Piccinino S: The nursing care challenge: borderline patients, *J Psychosoc Nurs* 28(4):22-27, 1990.
13. Poston WC: The biracial identity development model: a needed addition, *J Counsel Dev* 69(2):152-155, 1990.
14. Snow DA, Anderson L: Identity work among the homeless: the verbal construction and avowal of personal identities, *Am J Soc* 92(6):1336-1371, 1987.
15. Steele K: Looking for answers: understanding multiple personality disorder, *J Psychosoc Nurs* 27(8):6-10, 1989.

VII

Self-Esteem Disturbance

Situational Low Self-Esteem

Chronic Low Self-Esteem

Self-Esteem Disturbance is a disruption in an individual's perceptions or unrealistic self-evaluation/feelings about self or self capabilities, which may be directly or indirectly expressed.[11]

Situational Low Self-Esteem is negative self-evaluation or feelings about self that develops in response to a loss or change in an individual who previously had a positive self-evaluation.

Chronic Low Self-Esteem is a longstanding negative self-evaluation or feelings about self or self capabilities.

OVERVIEW

Maslow[13] specified that the esteem needs, which include self-esteem, are the fourth level of Maslow's hierarchy of needs and noted that everyone in society needs to have a stable, firmly based, high self-esteem. If the individual develops negative feelings about the self, those feelings can seriously hamper an individual's ability to function. Thus self-esteem can be defined as the favorable or unfavorable attitude that an individual develops toward the self.[20] Inherent within the definition are two factors that have implications for developing interventions for Self-Esteem Disturbance. First, the individual learns either favorable or unfavorable attitudes that are expressed as evaluations or feelings about the self. Second, the individual must use cognitive and attitudinal pro-

cesses to learn these evaluations or feelings. Self-esteem, therefore, is the learned attitudes or feelings, either favorable or unfavorable, that an individual perceives about the self. Consequently, the nurse needs to validate with the patient the meaning of a given behavior. Because an individual's self-esteem influences behavior, a disturbance in it can adversely affect that individual's ability to effectively interact with external and internal environments.

Usually when a diagnosis of Self-Esteem Disturbance is considered, the nurse thinks in terms of low or poor self-esteem. However, some individuals may overvalue the self unrealistically.[7] Both low and unrealistically high self-esteem depend on distorted perceptions that frequently have been learned from past experiences. Such experiences do not themselves cause a Self-Esteem Disturbance but provide the parameters in which the distorted perceptions develop. In other words, the past experiences of an individual become cues indicating the need to explore that individual's perceptions regarding the experiences' effect on the self-esteem. The same type of experience for two individuals may strengthen the self-esteem of one and contribute toward Self-Esteem Disturbance in the other. Sometimes, an individual's cultural/ethnic background, age, sex, familial and community mores, and values provide the criteria used to evaluate and develop that individual's self-es-

529

teem, but only if the individual subscribes to them. The expression of negative self-evaluations or feelings may result from a specific situation (Situational Low Self-Esteem) or may be the result of longstanding negative self-evaluations (Chronic Low Self-Esteem).

Situational Low Self-Esteem occurs when individuals report or describe self-evaluations or feelings as a temporary event.[17] It usually can be traced to a specific situation and frequently involves a significant loss to the person, such as a loss of an interpersonal relationship, loss of perceived status, loss of perceived competency, difficulty in meeting expectations, or inability to reach a goal. In some instances, a biological or biochemical disturbance can precipitate such feelings until that abnormality is corrected; examples are strokes in certain parts of the brain and drugs that precipitate abnormal thinking/feeling patterns or biochemical imbalances.

Chronic Low Self-Esteem occurs when individuals, on a longstanding basis, are unable to report or describe self-evaluations or feelings at any time that are positive about the self.[17] This situation develops as a result of negative reinforcers from childhood or from significant losses later in life to which the individual cannot adjust. The extent to which genetics may influence this disturbance has not been determined.

Any of life's experiences may adversely affect an individual's self-esteem or a component of it, depending on how the given individual evaluates its personal meaning.[6] Because of the complexity of the human personality, these factors interact with each other in a uniquely human way, so to determine a given event's effect on the individual's self-esteem, it must be individually verified.

Physiological parameters can also affect a person's self-esteem and include physical losses, medical illnesses, and some psychiatric illnesses.[11,15] Physical losses include, but are not limited to, areas of sexuality and reproduction, physical disfigurement, incapacity, or dismemberment. For example, a man may lose the ability to perform sexual activities, believe he is no longer a man, and feel worthless. Or a woman may think

she has such a disfiguring birthmark that others will socialize with her only out of pity. A man who was a good heavy-equipment operator and who loses an arm and a leg in an accident may think he is a failure because he can no longer work in construction. Chronic medical problems that create a permanent change in an individual's lifestyle or ability to function, and are perceived as having a negative consequence for that individual, can also disrupt an individual's self-esteem. Such problems include but are not limited to chronic renal problems, including the need for dialysis, traumatic injury to the spinal cord resulting in paralysis, chronic pulmonary or coronary diseases, any of the degenerative neurological or skeletal diseases, and cancers. Although an individual is at risk for developing disturbed self-esteem as a consequence of a chronic medical problem, it is also possible to develop enhanced self-esteem because of accomplishments in spite of the problem.

Individuals with mental disorders frequently exhibit Self-Esteem Disturbance.[7] Although many of these are considered to be primarily psychological in nature, several have physiological parameters as well, such as the dementias or intoxication from drugs/alcohol. Although dementias have physiological parameters, it is the difficulty these individuals experience in communicating their perceptions that present the nurse with difficulties in accurately assessing their self-esteem level. Some of the substance abusers may have a distorted high self-esteem, as they are frequently satisfied with themselves, see no need to change either their behavior or their thinking,[12] and in fact may say that it is the responsibility of others to change. It is only as they become dissatisfied with themselves by incorporating a self-esteem that accurately reflects reality that they will be motivated to change.

Psychologically related factors frequently pertain to disrupted or distorted thinking and feeling parameters. These include, but are not limited to, expressions negating the self after a failure, a loss of role or lifestyle, or even success. If failure is attributed to the intrinsic worth of the individual, then the feeling and attitude this fosters may prevent an individual from trying anything new or at least severely restrict the amount of risk the individual is willing to take.

A loss of role or lifestyle could also lead to Self-Esteem Disturbance. Examples include the loss of a job, illness, changes in the ability to care for the self, and changes within the family.[13] For instance, the individual who is laid off from work and is unable to secure a new position may feel that he/she is no longer a valuable member of the family because of the inability to provide for the family. Or the individual may need to take a position with a lower salary or status, which can lower that individual's self-esteem. Another individual, because of infirmities of age, may perceive that he/she is no longer a valued member of society because of the inability to care for the self. Or a mother may feel that she is no longer providing a useful service when her last child leaves home, so that she experiences a lowered self-esteem until she has resolved the change in her role. If the individual cannot resolve the situationally lowered self-esteem, it may become chronically low.

One of the more insidious situations is the perception that the individual no longer has any control over a situation; i.e., that no matter what is done, the situation cannot be changed. This perception, in its varying degrees, immobilizes the individual and becomes devastating to his/her self-confidence and self-reliance and thus lowers self-esteem. Examples of such situations would be those wherein an individual feels victimized; e.g., rape, abuse, robbery, or a violated confidence. Depending on the circumstance, the individual may generalize the experience(s) to all areas and develop Chronic Low Self-Esteem.

Social parameters can affect one's self-esteem and include all types of interpersonal interactions. Any statement or behavior indicating abnormally high or low self-esteem in relation to interpersonal relationships needs to be explored for a Self-Esteem Disturbance. Only a few examples are given here to help identify areas wherein one might develop a disturbed self-esteem. Some individuals develop low self-esteem, either chronic or situational, because of a lack of approval, respect, or love from others.[13,15] That lack, either real or a distorted perception of reality, decreases the individual's ability to function as effectively as he/she could if provided with adequate positive reinforcements. For example, children who do not receive adequate reinforcement for their positive attributes and whose parent(s) repeatedly inform them that they are bad, no good, or unable to do anything right, will learn to express negative attitudes and feelings about the self that frequently result in Chronic Low Self-Esteem. Other psychological factors could include negative interpretations of life events, such as involvement in environmental disasters, change in living condition/residence, or assumption of guilt. Another example is the individual who was kept so dependent on another that he or she did not learn the skills necessary for successful adjustment to life. This individual lacks self-confidence or self-reliance and experiences Chronic Low Self-Esteem as a result.

At some time or another, everyone will interact with someone who exults the self at the expense of others. Such an individual may be experiencing Situational or Chronic Low Self-Esteem. For example, an upper level manager comes into the hospital with an ulcer. During an interview, he says that he has worked his way up through the ranks and has worked hard to get where he is. He considers his former coworkers "bums" for not demonstrating a little initiative in trying to improve themselves. Depending on the length of time this misperception has been held, that individual might be expressing either Chronic or Situational Low Self-Esteem.

Situational Low Self-Esteem may develop when an individual perceives that a significant other is emotionally distancing himself or herself. As a result, that individual may feel that he or she is not worthy of being loved and experiences lowered self-esteem. Other changes in interpersonal relationships, such as the death of a significant other, can bring about the development of Situational Low Self-Esteem. For example, a family

VII

may lose a young child to an incurable illness, but the father, mother, or both may believe they failed as parents even when they did all that they could. Death, divorce, and separation are changes in interpersonal relationships that may also be categorized as losses. Although they may start as factors in the development of Situational Low Self-Esteem, they can be influential in the development of Chronic Low Self-Esteem when an individual cannot reconstitute the previous positive self-evaluation by experiencing positive events.

Many of an individual's values and beliefs are developed in response to his or her cultural and spiritual expressions. An individual's self-esteem is influenced by his or her perceptions of worth to the community, which may or may not take into account his/her positive characteristics or belief in ability to function. For example, a physician and a trash collector may each believe they are valuable members of the community because they both contribute to the maintenance of health within a community. Or, the trash collector may believe that he or she is not as valuable as the physician because of a lack of education. The individual who places a lower value on his or her actions, thoughts, and feelings than on those of others based on cultural and spiritual factors may experience a Self-Esteem Disturbance.

An individual may think he/she is more important than others. The individual who thinks that an institution cannot survive without his or her support may experience an unrealistically high self-esteem. One factor that is not always assessed pertains to the purpose of an individual's life. The individual who has lost or never developed purpose in life may believe there is no reason for his/her continued existence and that life no longer has much meaning or value.

Discrimination or acculturation pressures can also influence the development of an individual's self-esteem, either positively or negatively, as these processes are culturally defined. Immigrants who have not been able to acculturate can develop serious physical or psychiatric conditions and may have a decreased life expectancy, particularly if they do not have a culturally significant

support group. Within this group, the nurse needs to assess for the posttraumatic stress syndrome and the strength of the individual's self-esteem in relation to the culture of origin.

Basically, Self-Esteem Disturbance could develop when an individual perceives any loss as important, regardless of what that loss was. The severity of the lowered self-esteem will be directly related to the perceived value or its meaning to the individual, whether or not there is a perceived replacement, and the degree to which that individual is willing to let go. Such losses may pertain to the body, to an individual's role or lifestyle, or to changes in interpersonal relationships.*

The complexity of self-esteem presents numerous problems in accurately and specifically assessing the extent and severity of Self-Esteem Disturbance and its role in health. The Tennessee Self-Concept Scale, which has a self-esteem subscale, is probably one of the better-known scales for the measurement of self-esteem.[7] However, it is difficult to complete accurately and time consuming to score, so its routine clinical use is somewhat problematical for the nurse. For a tool to be useful to nursing, it needs to provide useful information and be easy to administer and score. One tool that meets these criteria is Rosenberg's Self-Esteem Scale.[20] Rosenberg's Self-Esteem Scale consists of 10 items with scores ranging from 0 (high self-esteem) to 6 (low self-esteem). The items address the individual's perceptions of worth, of being not good, satisfactions with the self, self-respect, being able to function as well as others, being proud of something pertaining to the self, possession of any good qualities, feeling useful, attitude toward the self, and whether the individual is a failure. Snyder[21] used this tool in evaluating group psychotherapy as treatment for depression in women and found that it measured changes in the women's self-esteem during the course of therapy. The tool can identify the severity of the disturbed low self-esteem and provide

---

*References 2, 4-7, 9, 13, 15-17, 19, 20, 22.

some indications about the directions of change or the effectiveness of treatment. A study on client-therapist similarities by Berry and Sipps[1] used it and found that the level of a patient's self-esteem could influence the relationship between the patient and therapist.

In summary, multiple related factors can contribute toward the development of Self-Esteem Disturbance. In Situational Low Self-Esteem the related factors occurred during the recent past. In Chronic Low Self-Esteem the related factors occur over time and the defining characteristics continue over an extended time with little or no improvement. For a diagnosis of Chronic Low Self-Esteem, the defining characteristics indicating a lower than average self-esteem must be present for an extended time and/or the important related factors must have occurred in the distant past.

ASSESSMENT
Self-Esteem Disturbance

In general, any verbalizations by the patient that indicate that the individual has a negative perception about the self or self-capabilities can be used as evidence to support a diagnosis of Self-Esteem Disturbance.[11,15,17] The nurse also needs to validate the meaning of any given behavior with that patient because a specific behavior can express different meanings.

Self-Esteem Disturbance can be suspected when individuals verbalize feelings of inferiority, such as not being as good as most people, or being worthless, no good, or inadequate. Individuals also may make statements indicating that they feel adrift with no direction to their lives, that nobody appreciates them, or that others treat them as if they are insignificant. Individuals may verbalize negative feelings about the self, such as feeling disappointed or dissatisfied with themselves, unlovable, or unhappy. They may specify that they cannot experience pleasure, live up to expectations, feel useful, amount to anything, contribute anything, or think positively about their self. They may indicate one of the following: they are excessively anxious or fearful of the unknown; they have lost control of their lives;

they have nothing in which they can take pride; nothing ever goes right for them; they have only contempt for themselves; or they are no good. Other statements that may indicate Self-Esteem Disturbance include expressions of feelings of being violated, such as after a rape, abuse, robbery, or betrayal of confidence. Verbalizations indicative of Self-Esteem Disturbance also include constant rumination about past failures, defeatist thinking, minimization of strengths, and critical or negative statements about the self. All of these verbalizations generally express negative feelings and attitudes about the self and indicate low self-esteem.[7,11,16,20]

Statements indicating an unrealistically high self-esteem include grandiose statements that elevate the person above others and statements indicating that the individual can do better than what he or she realistically can be expected to do. Clinicians may interpret statements such as these as an attempt to compensate for a low self-esteem. The nurse needs to complete a very careful assessment of the patient's overall self-perceptions to discriminate between Situational or Chronic Low Self-Esteem and an unrealistically high self-esteem. A patient who appears to be satisfied with the self and indicates there is no need to make *any* changes, even though he/she cannot function in the community, may report a high self-esteem.[7,12] Again, these could reflect a defense against a low self-esteem. However, the clinician needs to start where the patient is, acknowledging the patient's perceptions, and plan interventions to assist the patient to change distorted perceptions in the desired direction.

Several behaviors may be indicative of Self-Esteem Disturbance, particularly if they form a pattern rather than occurring occasionally. Such behaviors include: rigid, narrowly focused, or constricted thinking; lack of or refusal to participate in prescribed therapy or therapeutic activities; inability to follow through on treatment or other activities; or setting unrealistic goals that the individual cannot achieve. In addition, the individual may hesitate to offer opinions and viewpoints or to initiate activities. The individual may demon-

VII

strate a decrease in interpersonal interactions, for example, with the family or significant others; or even a decrease in involvement with life. A few individuals may bully others so as to feel better about the self.

Individuals with Self-Esteem Disturbance may reduce spontaneous behaviors and experience difficulty in defending the self or engaging in independent activity. They may also find it difficult to seek out new situations. Such individuals may be underachievers or chronic procrastinators, or take longer than usual to relax in a situation. Sometimes body language may indicate that an individual is guarded and trying to protect the self; for example, eye contact may be poor or the shoulders may curl inward as if to protect the body. An individual's appearance also might indicate a Self-Esteem Disturbance. The patient who does not, but is able to, perform activities of daily living, such as bathing, grooming, feeding, and toileting, may be expressing feelings of unworthiness, a manifestation of Self-Esteem Disturbance. Or perhaps the individual persists in dressing very inappropriately for the activity in which he/she is engaged; e.g., dressing in formal wear, jewels, and furs while engaged in gardening. Again, behaviors indicative of Self-Esteem Disturbance should be verified by verbal statements that the individual is actually experiencing a disturbance in self-esteem. As noted earlier, any of these behaviors can have more than one meaning. It is only by validating the individual's perception of the behavior that the nurse can make an accurate assessment of Self-Esteem Disturbance.*

In addition to assessing for verbalizations and behaviors indicative of Self-Esteem Disturbance, the nurse needs to assess for the presence of this nursing diagnosis when other disturbances of self-perception/self-concept occur. These include, but are not limited to, Fear, Anxiety, Hopelessness, Powerlessness, Body Image Disturbance, and Personal Identity Disturbance. Some of the same defining characteristics for other nursing diag-

noses, such as Hopelessness also pertain to Disturbed Self-Esteem. Research is beginning to identify the role of self-esteem in other diagnoses.[18]

❖ **Defining Characteristics**

The presence of the following defining characteristics indicates that the patient may be experiencing a Self-Esteem Disturbance:[9,11,15-17]

- Anorexia or obesity
- Decrease in sexual relationships and drive
- Frequent expression of body aches and pains
- Overconcern with somatic woes
- Inability to assume responsibilities for self-care
- Homicidal/suicidal behavior
- Timid, seclusive, pessimistic, unassertive, and/or unable to initiate, follow through, or complete a task in a timely fashion
- Despair, guilt, inferiority, inadequacy, failure, defeatism, frustration
- Denial of past/present successes/accomplishments
- Lack of eye contact, energy, attention to appearance, and/or initiative in problem-solving
- Verbalizations of being unworthy of God's love and forgiveness
- Feelings of hopelessness, helplessness, powerlessness, disappointment, worthlessness, isolation, and depression
- Emotional distancing from significant others
- Withdrawal from activities and interpersonal-social relationships
- Reluctance to engage in social interactions
- Resentment of others
- Perception of minimum strengths/assets with refusal to accept positive feedback
- Inability to accept and/or extremely sensitive to criticism
- Lack confidence in social situations
- Difficulties in job performance or perfectionism
- Fear of handling change, making decisions, taking risks, expressing anger, and relating to others

---

*References 6, 7, 15, 17, 23.

❖ **Related Factors**

The following related factors are associated with Self-Esteem Disturbance:[9,11,15-17]

- Physical losses
- Medical illness
- Inability to adjust to alterations in body function
- Inability to adjust to losses of body structure
- Psychiatric illness
- Cognitive/perceptual problems
- Traumatic experiences
- Unresolved emotionally traumatic experiences
- Loss of control
- Negative interpretations of experiences
- Unrealistic expectations of self
- Inadequate knowledge/problem-solving skills for coping with life's stresses
- Loss of role or lifestyle
- Early loss of parent/significant other
- Lack of adequate positive feedback
- Repeated negative interpersonal experiences
- Ridiculed by others excessively
- Inadequate social support
- Perceived loss of relationship with God

❖ **Related Medical/Psychiatric Diagnoses**

The following are examples of related medical/psychiatric diagnoses for Self-Esteem Disturbance:

- Acne
- Amputation of limb
- Arthritis
- Carcinoma
- Cardiac condition
- Chronic obstructive pulmonary disease
- Denucleation of an eye
- Gender identity disorder of childhood
- Generalized anxiety disorder
- Major depressive episode
- Personality disorders (e.g., borderline, avoidant)
- Posttraumatic stress disorder
- Psoriasis
- Renal failure
- Schizophrenia
- Social phobia
- Substance abuse (e.g., alcohol, cannabis, cocaine, opioid, PCP)

Situational Low Self-Esteem

Self-Esteem Disturbance: Situational Low Self-Esteem includes any of the general characteristics indicative of a disturbed self-esteem that are currently present, but were not present before a given situation, and may include expressions of shame/guilt or evaluation of the self as unable to handle situations and events. For example, a mother may state that since her child was seriously injured, she has believed she is not an adequate mother. Or there may be a distinct change in behavior resulting from feelings of insufficiency. For example, a young man may have enjoyed flirting and talking with young women. He stopped this behavior when a girl he had asked for a date two months ago laughed at him and told him not to be ridiculous.

❖ **Defining Characteristics**

The presence of the following defining characteristics indicates that the patient may be experiencing a Situational Low Self-Esteem:[15,17]

- Episodic negative self-appraisal in response to a sudden loss or change
- Self-negative verbalization in response to a sudden loss or change
- Difficulty in making decisions caused by a sudden loss or change
- Expressions of shame/guilt and evaluating self as unable to handle situations/events in response to a sudden loss or change
- See also Self-Esteem Disturbance

❖ **Related Factors**

The following related factors are associated with Situational Low Self-Esteem:

Major loss(es) of:
- Body part/functions
- Significant other
- Job/work/role
- Pet
- Material goods
- Reputation

Major stress or change in life such as:

- Marriage/divorce
- Prison term
- Addition/loss of a family member
- Failure in school/work/significant life event
- Financial problems
- Promotion/demotion

VII

- Adolescent adjust-
  ment
- Sexual difficulties
- Hospitalization
- Occupational
  changes/other major
  moves
- Change in religious
  affiliation/practice

**Environmental fac-
tors such as:**
- Disasters (natural or
  manmade)
- Poverty
- Change in residence
  or living conditions
- Discrimination
- Acculturation

❖ Related Medical/Psychiatric Diagnoses

The following are examples of related medical/
psychiatric diagnoses for Situational Low Self-Esteem:

- Any recent amputa-
  tion or surgical or-
  gan removal
- Brief reactive psy-
  chosis
- Pregnancy

- Psychoactive sub-
  stance intoxication
  (e.g., alcohol, opi-
  oid, cocaine, PCP,
  or other substance)
- Uncomplicated be-
  reavement

❖ Chronic Low Self-Esteem

Chronic Low Self-Esteem includes any of the
previously cited characteristics of Self-Esteem
Disturbance that are longstanding or cannot be
traced to a specific situation (e.g., frequent lack
of success in life's activities, hesitation in trying
new things/situations, alienation from others, and
ruminations about past problems.*

❖ Defining Characteristics

The presence of the following defining characteristics indicates that the patient may be experiencing a Chronic Low Self-Esteem:[15,17]

- Longstanding low
  self-evaluations/
  feelings about self
  and abilities
- Frequent lack of
  success in life
  events/work
- Pattern of hesitating
  to try new things/
  situations

- Long-term alien-
  ation from network
  of community re-
  sources
- Pattern of being
  passive and with-
  drawing from others
- Frequent rumina-
  tions about past
  problems over time
- See also Self-
  Esteem Disturbance

❖ Related Factors

The following related factors are associated
with Chronic Low Self-Esteem:

- Longstanding nega-
  tivity as a fixated
  life response
- Maladaptive fixated
  life response

- Isolated lifestyle
  pattern
- Long-term adverse
  childhood experi-
  ences

❖ Related Medical/Psychiatric Diagnoses

The following are examples of related medical/
psychiatric diagnoses for Chronic Low Self-Esteem:

- Blindness
- Cerebrovascular
  accident
- Chronic skin dis-
  eases
- Deafness
- Obesity
- Overanxious disor-
  der/panic disorder

- Personality disor-
  ders; paranoid, bor-
  derline, narcissistic
- Posttraumatic stress
  disorder
- Spinal cord injury

NURSING DIAGNOSES

Examples of *specific* nursing diagnoses for
Self-Esteem Disturbance are:
- Self-Esteem Disturbance related to adverse in-
  terpersonal relationship with parents
- Self-Esteem Disturbance related to the social
  condition of discrimination
- Self-Esteem Disturbance related to cognitive/
  perceptual problems
- Self-Esteem Disturbance related to inadequate
  knowledge and skills for coping

Examples of specific nursing diagnoses for Situational Low Self-Esteem are:
- Situational Low Self-Esteem related to loss of
  job
- Situational Low Self-Esteem related to divorce
- Situational Low Self-Esteem related to acculturation stresses

Examples of specific nursing diagnoses for
Chronic Low Self-Esteem are:
- Chronic Low Self-Esteem related to long-term
  adverse childhood experiences
- Chronic Low Self-Esteem related to longstand-
  ing negativity as the response to life

---

*References 6, 7, 15, 17, 23.

- Chronic Low Self-Esteem related to an isolated lifestyle
- Chronic Low Self-Esteem related to a maladaptive fixated life response

PLANNING AND IMPLEMENTATION WITH RATIONALE
Self-Esteem Disturbance

Self-esteem is learned as a result of the interaction between an individual's internal processes and the environment. Patients can either confirm or alter an existing perception of the self based on their perceptions of how the staff interacts with them. Patient-staff interactions provide a part of the external environment that patients can use to develop positive and realistic self-esteem. Nurses can use several techniques or approaches to help provide positive patient-nurse interactions, which include, but are not limited to, those specified in this chapter.

First, the nurse must use a nonjudgmental and empathic attitude at all times. This means that the nurse accepts the patient's expressed negative feelings about the self without belittling, criticizing, or demeaning the patient for expressing such feelings. Another technique is for the nurse to express unconditional regard for the patient, which communicates that the patient is of value or worthwhile and that offers positive reinforcement for actual achievements. This also occurs when the nurse is congruent and genuine, and demonstrates real interest, concern, and understanding, without offering false praise. Improvement can also occur when the nurse recognizes the patient's experiences and knowledge while discouraging repeated conversations about past problems and failures.* *With these approaches, the nurse can provide a climate or external environment conducive to patients learning to perceive the self positively.*

If the patient will acknowledge that there is a problem with self-esteem, that patient can work with the nurse and treatment team to identify and work through the causative factors. To do this, develop realistic goals and plans with the patient

---

*References 1, 3, 8, 14, 15.

to change the thinking, feeling, and behavior patterns so that a realistic, positive self-esteem can be achieved. Changing entrenched habits of feeling, thinking, or behaving can be difficult and fraught with lapses. Be patient, persevere, and continue to reinforce the progress the patient makes. The patient can be involved in several different activities that assist in learning to modify a habitual manner of thinking, feeling, and behaving. *Activities that provide help to others or contribute to the good of the community can assist the patients to perceive themselves as a being of worth.* Byers et al[4] found that alcoholic inpatients increased their self-esteem when paired with nursing home residents in a helping-companion relationship over those who went to the library for the same period of time.

The activities in which the patients participate can also be used to improve distorted perceptions about the self. A review of the literature by Gleser and Mendelberg[10] led them to conclude "that physical exercise and sport. . .contribute to the enhancement of self-esteem/self-concept in diverse populations of subjects."

Nurses, through groups and one-to-one relationships, can provide the patients a nonthreatening, supportive environment in which they learn to respect themselves. Topics to be considered for these interventions include clarifying values and beliefs within a positive framework, practicing positive statement about themselves, developing assertiveness skills, learning how their behavior influences the behavior of others, developing congruence between body language and feelings, and learning to accept and use positive criticism for growth and development.[2,3,14,15] *These activities also provide a mechanism whereby the patient can validate his/her perceptions of the emotions, statements, and behaviors of others.* If the perceptions are distorted, techniques for verifying and correcting them can be learned and interpersonal techniques improved.

Sometimes it is necessary to intervene with the significant others and to teach them appropriate interaction techniques. *Family members may not always be aware of how their negative statements and lack of positive verbal and behavioral rein-*

❖ NURSING CARE GUIDELINES
Nursing Diagnosis: Self-Esteem Disturbance

Expected Patient Outcome	**Nursing Interventions**
Patient will perceive self positively as evidenced by: making positive statements about the self and exhibiting congruent behavior; identifying positive relationships and making an effort to maintain and improve them; and setting realistic goals, initiating the needed activities, and following through to reach them.	• Keep a nonjudgmental and empathic attitude. • Express unconditional regard for the patient. • Be congruent and genuine. • Recognize the patient's past experiences and knowledge. • Actively listen. • Discourage repeated conversations about past problems and failures. • Facilitate patient involvement in activities such as helping others, contributing to the community, participating in the creative arts and physical activities, and attending support or self-help groups. • Facilitate patient education to clarify values/beliefs, perceive negative influences, behave assertively, identify how own behavior influences others, develop congruence between feelings and body language, learn to accept and use positive criticism, validate perceptions, improve interpersonal techniques, and identify situations that damage self-esteem. • Teach significant others appropriate interaction techniques. • Encourage patient to engage in psychotherapy: individual or group. • Help patient identify and participate in experiences that are satisfying and rewarding. • Increase opportunities for social interaction. • Help the patient accept responsibility for personal opinions and behavior and then evaluate their outcome in relation to options available.

---

forcements have helped the patient to develop a disturbed self-esteem. *If they develop appropriate interaction techniques, this will assist the patient to maintain the gains reached during treatment and provide a healthier interaction climate for all.*

As noted previously, any situation or intervention can either maintain and improve or decrease a patient's self-esteem, depending on that patient's perception of the event. Nurses infer those changes based on the patient's self-reports and interpretations of the patient's visible emotions/behaviors.

Situational Low Self-Esteem

Interventions for Situational Low Self-Esteem include any of those used for Self-Esteem Disturbance but with a focus on changing distorted perceptions concerning a specific situation. Such interventions include an analysis of the situation, problem-solving techniques, and values clarification. *Reality-based perceptions of a situation provide the mechanism for developing a self-esteem that is congruent with an individual's capabilities and values.*[2,20]

❖ *NURSING CARE GUIDELINES*

Nursing Diagnosis: *Situational Low Self-Esteem (See also Self-Esteem Disturbance)*

Expected Patient Outcomes	Nursing Interventions
The patient will realistically perceive situation and acknowledge factors that decreased self-esteem.	• Assist patient to analyze situational factors to clarify values and correct distorted perceptions.
The patient will engage in corrective activities to restore/improve self-esteem.	• Assist patient to develop strategies to help cope with loss, stress, or environmental factors that can cause low self-esteem. • Assist patient to engage in problem-solving activities and to identify behaviors that will help to restore self-esteem.

❖ *NURSING CARE GUIDELINES*

Nursing Diagnosis: *Chronic Low Self-Esteem (See also Self-Esteem Disturbance)*

Expected Patient Outcomes	Nursing Interventions
Patient will increase frequency of positive statements pertaining to self.	• Assist patient to engage in problem-solving activities and to identify behaviors that will help to restore self-esteem. • Plan for small increments in change.
Patient will engage in corrective activities to restore/improve self-esteem.	• See Self-Esteem Disturbance • Assist patient to analyze situational factors to clarify values and correct distorted perceptions. • Assist patient to identify family and community resources that will help to improve his/her self-esteem.

VII

Chronic Low Self-Esteem

Interventions for Chronic Low Self-Esteem include any of those used for Self-Esteem Disturbance with a focus on changing deep-seated and long-term distortions about the self. *These activities assist patients in examining their life patterns over time to determine the priority of modifying behaviors.* Progress for these patients will be in small increments, and the nurse may need to refer them to other resources for ongoing treatment.[15]

EVALUATION

To evaluate the effectiveness of the interventions, validate the patient's feelings and thoughts about the self. If these are realistically positive, or at least more so than previously, the interventions brought about change in the desired direction. Observations of the patient's interactions with others can provide cues concerning the desired change and can help the nurse identify what to validate with the patient. If a tool was used to assess the patient's initial level of self-esteem, then changes in the scores also can demonstrate the effectiveness of the interventions. The evaluation process can be a learning experience for the patient by identifying continuing problems and providing information for the development of realistic goals concerning future activities.

It will be crucial at this time to help the patient to understand that progress will not continue smoothly but will involve a number of ups and downs. However, self-knowledge and willingness to engage in positive activities even when "down" can provide an overall gradual increase in self-esteem.

Situational Low Self-Esteem interventions can be evaluated similarly to those for Self-Esteem Disturbance. If the interventions have been effective, the patient's self-esteem will return to the previous level or improve. If this does not occur within a reasonable time, the diagnosis may need to be reevaluated for Chronic Low Self-Esteem. Chronic Low Self-Esteem also can be evaluated similarly to Self-Esteem Disturbance. However, the changes toward more positive and realistic self-esteem may be lower and of a smaller magnitude. There also may be lapses in the progress when anything occurs to trigger the old, low self-esteem thinking, emotional, and behavioral patterns. If this should happen, evaluate with the patient what occurred and help to identify approaches or activities to ameliorate the effects of the current traumatizing event.

❖ CASE STUDY WITH PLAN OF CARE

Mrs. Maria M. was admitted to the hospital for a cholecystectomy. She married at 17 and is now 21 with three preschool children. She and her family immigrated from El Salvador 2 years ago and now live in a small two-bedroom apartment while they try to save money to purchase a house. During the past 3 months, the children have taken turns at being sick and fussy. Their medical costs have significantly reduced the family's savings. Mrs. M. is a nonsmoker, abstains from alcohol, and has no known physical problems other than the one for which she was admitted. Her blood pressure is 130/76, respirations 24, temperature 99° F, pulse 88, height 5′4″, and weight 160 lbs. Her abdominal muscles are flaccid, with a tense body. She states that she has not regained her figure or lost the additional weight after her last pregnancy. Her activities include managing the family's finances and the house as well as caring for their three preschool children. She attends Mass on Sunday, and occasionally the family will go on a special outing. Her husband is too tired to do anything other than work at his job during the week. On weekends, he also works at a part-time job to increase their meager income. They do not believe in using baby-sitters, so do not go anywhere they cannot take the children. Mrs. M. has one fairly close friend within the apartment complex who speaks Spanish and has two preschool children. Although both can speak some English, neither could be considered fluent in the language. She writes to her mother in El Salvador and occasionally receives a letter from her. They have no other relatives in the United States.

During the course of several interactions with the nurse, Mrs. M. stated that she was not really worth the attention the nurse was giving her. As the nurse explored this statement, Mrs. M. stated that her husband was working so hard to support them and to help them get ahead and that she was endangering this, because she had let the children get sick so much, and now she needed surgery. She felt as if she could not do anything right because the children's illnesses and her surgery were using up all of their savings. She had felt so tired after her third delivery and just did not have the energy to care for the children as she should have. Then just before she was admitted to the hospital, her husband had stumbled on the children's toys when coming in from work. He could have seriously hurt himself, and then where would they be? Her husband was doing his part, but she was endangering their dreams because she could not keep the children and herself healthy, and had been unable to monitor the children's activities to ensure that no one would get injured. Situational Low Self-Esteem related to the children's illnesses and her surgery, which was using up the family's savings, was one of the nursing diagnoses the nurse formulated.

PLAN OF CARE FOR MRS. MARIA M.

Nursing Diagnosis: Situational Low Self-Esteem related to the children's illnesses and her surgery depleting the family's savings.

Expected Patient Outcome	Nursing Interventions
Mrs. M. will experience improved self-esteem as evidenced by verbalizing positive statements regarding ability to care for children and self, and of her value and worth to her family and husband; and by identifying and verbalizing to her husband her need for rest, expressions of appreciation; and involving self in a culturally related support peer group and other social/religious activities.	• Be nonjudgmental and empathic of Mrs. M. • Be genuinely interested and concerned about Mrs. M. • Discourage repetitious talking about inability to function as a wife and mother. • Explore with and help Mrs. M. identify her strengths. • Help Mrs. M. to analyze her situation and to identify actions she can take to improve it, such as talking with the priest to find out if there are other church activities that she would enjoy. • Have Mrs. M. realistically evaluate the demands of caring for three preschool children. • Provide Mrs. M. with an opportunity to learn assertive behavior within her cultural context. • Explore assumptions behind Mrs. M.'s self-perceptions and reinterpret them with a positive frame of reference. • Assist in exploring appropriate culturally relevant community supports; e.g., peer groups, religious activities.

REFERENCES

1. Berry GW, Sipps GJ: Interactive effects of counselor-client similarity and client self-esteem on termination type and number of sessions, *J Couns Psych* 38(2):120-125, 1991.
2. Bredehoft DJ: An evaluation study of the self-esteem: a family affair program with high-risk abusive parents, *Trans Anal J* 20(2):111-117, 1990.
3. Bulechek GM, McCloskey JC: *Nursing interventions, treatments for nursing diagnoses,* 1985, WB Saunders.
4. Byers PH, Raven LM, Hill JD, and Robyak JE: Enhancing self-esteem of inpatient alcoholics, *Iss Ment Health Nurs* 11:337-346, 1990.
5. Cheney AM: Critical indicators for the nursing diagnosis of disturbance in self-concept. In Kim MJ, McFarland GK, and McLane AM: *Classification of nursing diagnoses. Proceedings of the Fifth National Conference,* St Louis, 1984, CV Mosby.
6. Combs AW, Snygg D: *Individual behavior: a perceptual approach to behavior,* rev ed, New York, 1959, Harper & Row, Publishers.
7. Fitts W: *The self-concept and psychopathology,* Nashville, Tenn, 1972, Counselor Recordings and Tests.
8. Flaskerud JH, Liu PY: Effects of an Asian client therapist, language, ethnicity and gender match on utilization and outcome of therapy, *Community Ment Health J* 27(1):31-42, 1991.
9. Flett GL, Hewitt PL, Blankstein K, O'Brien S: Perfectionism and learned resourcefulness in depression and self-esteem, *Person Individ Diff* 12(1):61-68, 1991.
10. Gleser J, Mendelber H: Exercise and sport in mental health: a review of the literature, *Isr J Psychiatry Relat Sci* 27(2):99-112, 1990.
11. Kim MJ, McFarland GK, and McLane AM: *Pocket guide to nursing diagnoses,* ed 3, St Louis, 1991, CV Mosby.
12. Larson L: *Trust and self-esteem of psychiatric patients as perceived by the patients and psychiatric nurses,* Ann Arbor, Mich, 1985, University Microfilms International.
13. Maslow AH: *Motivation and personality,* ed 2, New York, 1970, Harper & Row, Publishers.
14. McFarland G, Gerety E: Self-esteem disturbance. In Kim MJ, McFarland GK, and McLane AM: *Pocket guide to nursing diagnoses,* ed 4, St Louis, 1991, Mosby–Year Book.
15. McFarland G and others: Self-esteem disturbance. In Thompson J, McFarland GK, Hirsch J, and others: *Mosby's manual of clinical nursing,* ed 2, St Louis, 1989, Mosby–Year Book.
16. Nelson RB: Social support, self-esteem, and depression in the institutionalized elderly, *Iss Ment Health Nurs* 10:55-68, 1989.
17. Norris J, Kunes-Connell M: Self-esteem disturbance: a clinical validation study. In McLane AM: *Classification of nursing diagnoses, proceedings of the Seventh Conference,* St Louis, 1987, CV Mosby.
18. Pillow DR, West SG, and Reich JW: Attributional style in relation to self-esteem and depression: mediational and interactive models, *J Res Person* 25:57-69, 1991.
19. Ratheram-Borus MJ: Adolescents' reference-group choices, self-esteem, and adjustment, *J Person Soc Psych* 59(5):1075-1081, 1990.
20. Rosenberg M: Society and the adolescent self-image, Princeton, NJ, 1965, Princeton University Press.
21. Snyder S: Comprehensive inpatient for the young adult patient, *Psychiatr Hosp* 15:119, 1984.
22. Westermeyer J: Cross-cultural care for ptsd: research, training, and service needs for the future, *J Traum Stress* 2(4):515-536, 1989.
23. Wilson HS, Kneisl CR: *Psychiatric nursing,* ed 3, Menlo Park, Calif, 1988, Addison-Wesley Publishing.

High Risk for Self-Mutilation

High Risk for Self-Mutilation is a state in which an individual is at risk to perform a deliberate act upon the self with the intent to injure, not kill, which produces immediate tissue damage to the body.

OVERVIEW

Self-mutilation includes an array of behaviors, the essence of which is deliberate destruction of tissue without conscious suicidal intent. Moderate pathologic self-mutilation is manifested by behaviors of self-biting, self-scratching, self-hitting, and hair pulling. Major self-mutilation includes eye enucleation, facial skinning and amputation of limbs, breasts or genitals.[6]

Self-mutilation is a patient behavior that occurs in a number of mental retardation, psychiatric and organic diagnoses. Only a few small-scale studies have reported the incidence of self-mutilation. The incidence of this behavior in mentally retarded hospitalized patients is reported as ranging between 9% and 19%.[5] Among patients with personality disorders, it is estimated that 34% of patients with multiple personalities, 24% with antisocial personality, and 26% to 40% with borderline personality had mutilated themselves.[18,19,22] Forty percent of patients with bulimia self-mutilate.[17] The total rate of self-mutilation is reported to be 750 per 100,000.[8]

Self-mutilation has been correlated with childhood experiences of sexual or physical abuse and stormy or violent family interactions.[2,12] Loss of a parent from death or divorce and mental illness in family members, especially alcoholism, is also correlated with self-mutilation in adults.[7,10,20] In a study of 89 patients referred to an intensive case management program, 29 practiced self-mutila-

tion. Of these patients, 71% reported being the victim of sexual abuse and 79% experienced physical abuse. Seventy-one percent of the self-mutilating were adult children of alcoholics.[20]

The reasons given by patients for performing moderate self-mutilating behaviors are to release tension, vent anger, relieve alienation and regain control over racing thoughts, fluctuating emotions and unstable environments.[7,9] Patients engaging in major self-mutilation often indicate biblical influence, demonic possession, heavenly commands, atonement for sin, and sexual determinants for their behavior.[7]

The Deliberate Self-Harm Syndrome has been described and proposed to be included in the psychiatric nomenclature of diagnosis. This syndrome has six essential features[9]:
1. A sudden impulse to physically harm oneself.
2. A perception of existing in an intolerable, uncontrollable situation without an available escape.
3. Mounting anxiety, agitation, and anger in response to the perceived situation.
4. Perceptual and cognitive constriction resulting in a narrowed perspective of the situation and the alternatives.
5. Self-mutilation done in private.
6. Rapid, temporary feeling of relief.

ASSESSMENT

When assessing a patient's risk for self-mutilation, the nurse should analyze the patient data for the presence or absence of early developmental correlates of adult self-mutilation, as well as current behaviors associated with this diagnosis. Sources of data include a nursing history, the nurse's observations of and interaction with the patient, the patient's perceptions of self and interaction with others and feedback from significant others about the patient. Correlates of, and current behaviors associated with, self-mutilation, must be significant in amount or severity to result in a diagnosis of high risk for self- mutilation.

In taking a history, the nurse must gather data regarding the patient's family history of violence, alcoholism, and physical and sexual abuse. The nurse must use effective interviewing and communication skills to sensitively elicit the patient data needed to plan nursing care. Studies have documented diffidence about abuse by the mental health system.[3,4,13] However, inquiry concerning these events validates the experience of the patient and opens up discussion and expression of feelings.

The nurse must assess the patient's ability to express feelings. Expression of feelings such as anxiety, anger or depression can reduce the risk for self-mutilation. However, the manner in which feelings are expressed must allow for management or resolution of the feeling.[1]

Impulse control is another critical assessment parameter. The patient experiencing stress who is able to utilize problem- solving abilities and evaluate his or her behavior increases their control over impulsive behavior and reduces their risk for self-mutilation.[1]

The patient's success and comfort with interpersonal relationships is another essential assessment parameter. Patients at risk for self-mutilation experience a personal identity disturbance, lack of self-differentiation and impaired communication. These difficulties can affect interpersonal relationships. The patient at risk for self-mutilation has difficulty acquiring the knowledge, attitudes and skills for positive interactions with others, including family.

❖ Risk Factors

The presence of the following behaviors, conditions, or circumstances renders the patient more vulnerable to High Risk for Self-Mutilation:

- Past self-injury
- Borderline personality disorder
- Depersonalization
- Fluctuating emotions
- Psychotic states
- Emotionally disturbed children
- Depression
- Mental retardation
- Autism
- Altered impulse control
- Rejection
- Self-hatred
- Guilt
- Separation anxiety
- Dysfunctional family
- Command hallucinations
- Emotional deprivation
- Inability to cope with increased tension
- Need for sensory stimuli
- Identity disturbance
- Sexual or physical abuse
- Battered children

❖ Related Medical/Psychiatric Diagnoses

The following are examples of related medical/psychiatric diagnoses for high risk for self- mutilation:

- Adrenocortical Insufficiency
- Antisocial personality disorder
- Autism
- Borderline personality disorder
- Bulimia
- Congenital analgesia/agnosia
- Cornelia de-lange syndrome
- Dementia
- Depression
- Encephalitis, chronic
- Factitious disorder with physical symptoms
- Lesch- Nyham syndrome
- Malingering
- Mania
- Multiple personality disorder
- Neurosyphilis
- Obsessive compulsive disorder
- Organic mental disorder
- Rett syndrome
- Schizophrenia
- Sensory isolation
- Sexual masochism
- Temporal lobe epilepsy
- Tourette syndrome
- Trichotillomania

NURSING DIAGNOSES

Examples of specific nursing diagnoses for High Risk for Self-Mutilation are:

- High risk for Self-Mutilation related to borderline personality

- High risk for Self-Mutilation related to altered impulse control
- High risk for Self-Mutilation related to command hallucinations

PLANNING AND IMPLEMENTATION WITH RATIONALE

Nursing interventions for patients at High Risk for Self-Mutilation are focused on appropriate expression of feelings, control of impulses and positive interactions with significant others. When selecting nursing interventions, consideration must be given to the specific risk factors such as the presence of psychotic, character or organic disorders; violence and sexual or physical abuse in the family; and destructive feelings that are present.

Environmental, developmental, and cultural factors may also affect selection of nursing interventions.

Appropriate expression of feelings reduces the patient's risk for self-mutilation. Feelings preceding self-mutilation most commonly reported by patients include tension, depression, self-anger, powerlessness, depersonalization, numbing and overwhelming guilt, loneliness, and boredom.[7,9] These feelings mount according to the patient's perception of the situation. Often, before the patient is aware of the situation and the related feelings, an emotional outburst occurs. *Creating a non- threatening environment and a sense of being safe in the environment, and with people, enhances the patient's ability to express feelings.*

❖ *NURSING CARE GUIDELINES*
Nursing Diagnosis: *High Risk for Self-Mutilation*

VII

Expected Patient Outcomes	Nursing Interventions*
Patient will identify feelings and express feelings in a socially acceptable manner.	• Develop trust through establishment and maintenance of a nurse patient relationship. • Utilize the same staff to work with the patient. • Teach patient to name the feeling state being experienced. • Assist patient to identify situations that precipitate feelings. • Teach and support use of defense mechanisms and constructive expressions of feelings. • Instruct patient on the use of relaxation techniques.
Patient will experience fewer episodes of impulsive behavior.	• Teach patient to identify perceived stressors. • Assist patient to replace faulty interpretations of perceived stressors with reality-based interpretations. • Discuss with patient successes in reducing stress utilized in the past. • Instruct and support use of stress reduction techniques and assertive skills. • Develop, with patient, a plan to reduce stress. • Define appropriate behaviors. • Set limits on inappropriate behavior. • Demonstrate, teach and support use of problem solving skills. • Assist patient to identify advantages and disadvantages of alternatives for behaviors. • Teach patient to analyze behavior.

---

*References 1, 4, 5, 11, 14-16, 20, 21.

Continued.

❖ *NURSING CARE GUIDELINES—cont'd*

Expected Patient Outcomes	Nursing Interventions*
• The patient will interact positively with significant others.	• Relay unconditional positive regard for patient. • Assist patient to identify strengths. • Engage patient in clarification of values, appraisal of self and identification of ideal self. • Explore, with patient, situations in which he or she overidentifies with others. • Assess the degree to which the patient's perception of self is affected by dysfunctional relationships. • Demonstrate through role-play positive interactions. • Explore, with patient, alternative methods to improve interaction, e.g., family and group therapy.

Teaching the patient to analyze situations for precipitants, and identification of feelings, facilitates the patient's ability to express feelings appropriately and reduce acting-out behaviors.[16,21]

An essential feature of self-mutilation is lack of impulse control. The patient believes that he or she is trapped in a stressful situation and experiences a narrowed perspective of the situation and the alternatives.[8] The patient experiences an absence of, or an inability to use, problem-solving skill. *Because an increase in stressors may precipitate self-mutilation,* improving the patient's ability to accurately interpret and reduce stressors decreases the risk for self-mutilation. *Increasing the patient's ability to problem-solve and think through consequences expands the range of behavioral responses.*[1,11,16]

Instability of self-image, identity disturbance and resulting dysfunctional relationships are characteristic of the person who self-mutilates. Instability of self-image is often experienced as chronic feelings of boredom or emptiness. Identity disturbance is pervasive and is demonstrated by uncertainty about sexuality, career choice, selection of friends, and values. Interpersonal relationships are intense, unstable and either overidealized or devalued.[9,10] A focus for nursing inter-

ventions is provision of experiences and feedback that foster self-regard. *Identification of strengths and positive interaction between the environment and others influences the estimate one places on oneself.* Additionally, nursing interventions that focus on self-differentiation *enhance the patient's self-identity and ability to interact positively with others.*[14,15]

EVALUATION

Evaluation of the nursing interventions to reduce the risk for self-mutilation is determined by the patient's attainment of the identified expected outcomes. Achievement of the expected patient outcomes is assessed through the nurse's observation of and interaction with the patient, the patient's evaluation of his or her tendency toward self-mutilation and feedback from others. If the identified limitations are no longer present and the patient demonstrates ability to express feelings appropriately, control impulses and interact positively with others, the expected patient outcomes have been achieved and the risk for self-mutilation has been reduced. If expected patient outcomes are not achieved, the patient is assessed for presence of risk factors. A revised plan for care is developed, implemented, and evaluated.

VII

❖ CASE STUDY WITH PLAN OF CARE

Sandra P. is 20 years old, unemployed and currently living with her mother. She has been brought to the mental health clinic by her younger sister who states, "I have had it. If you don't do something, someone is going to get hurt at home." Ms. P. is described by her sister as moody, with frequent outbursts of anger often directed at her parents. Their father recently entered a residential treatment facility for treatment of chronic al-coholism. There is a history of violence within the family. Ms. P. was taken on several occasions to the emergency room for treatment of injuries inflicted by her father. Ms. P. reports feelings of anxiety, emptiness, and boredom; "I can't seem to hang on to friends or a job. Every time I think I have figured out who I want to be with and what I want to do, something happens and I lose my friends and my job."

PLAN OF CARE FOR MS. SANDRA P.

Nursing Diagnosis: High Risk for Self-Mutilation related to Borderline Personality

Expected Patient Outcomes	Nursing Interventions
• Ms. P. will express her feelings appropriately as evidenced by: self-reports of reduction of anxiety, ability to name feelings, ability to match mode of feeling expression to persons and context.	• Establish a contract to establish a nurse-patient relationship delineating length, location and frequency of sessions and expectations for behavior. • Request that Ms. P. monitor and report on situations precipitating feelings. • Analyze situations reported by Ms. P. for identification of precipitants and labeling of feelings. • Explore with Ms. P. alternatives for expressing feelings, utilizing hypothetical situations and/or actual situations described by Ms. P. • Encourage expression and exploration of feelings Ms. P. experiences during nurse-patient interactions.
• Ms. P. will experience fewer episodes of impulsive behavior as evidenced by: use of stress reduction techniques, identification of consequences of behavior, use of problem-solving skills.	• Teach stress reduction techniques, e.g., meditation, progressive neuromuscular relaxation. • Discuss and encourage Ms. P. to use techniques found useful in the past to reduce stress. • Assist Ms. P. to identify alternatives for obtaining and maintaining employment. • Discuss advantages and disadvantages of each alternative identified for obtaining and maintaining employment. • Assist Ms. P. to make a plan for obtaining a job. • Evaluate implementation of plan with Ms. P., identifying consequences of behaviors.
• Ms. P. will interact positively with others as evidenced by: positive self-statements, describes a clearer sense of self, reports satisfaction from interactions.	• Point out Ms. P.'s strengths. • Engage Ms. P. in clarification of values, self-appraisal, and identification of ideal self. • Analyze Ms. P.'s descriptions of troublesome relationships for impact on Ms. P.'s self-definition. • Role-play with Ms. P., positive strategies for interaction. • Provide feedback to Ms. P. regarding positive interaction strategies utilized in nurse-patient relationship. • Discuss with Ms. P.'s family or group therapy.

VII

REFERENCES

1. Anderson M: Clients with altered impulse control. In McFarland G, Thomas M: *Psychiatric mental health nursing practice: Application of the nursing process,* Philadelphia, 1991, JB Lippincott.

2. Bryer J, Nelson B, Miller J: Childhood sexual and physical abuse as a factor in adult psychiatric in-patient illness, *Am J Psych* 144:1426-1430, 1987.

3. Cole C: Routine comprehensive inquiry for abuse: a justifiable clinical assessment procedure, *Clin Soc Work J* 16:33- 42, 1988.

4. Craine L, Henson C, Colliver J: Prevalence of a history of sexual abuse among female psychiatric patients in a state hospital system, *Hosp Commun Psych* 39:300-304, 1988.

5. Emberson J, Walker E: Self-injurious behavior in people with a mental handicap, *Nsg Times* 86:43-46, 1990.

6. Favazza A: Why patients mutilate themselves, *Hosp Commun Psych* 40:137-145, 1989.

7. Favazza A: Bodies under seige: *Self-mutilation in culture and psychiatry,* Baltimore, 1987, Johns Hopkins Press.

8. Favazza A and Conterio K: The plight of chronic self-mutilators, *Commun Mental Health J* 24:22-24, 1988.

9. Feldman M: The challenge of self-mutilation: A review, *Comrehen Psychiatr* 29:252-269, 1988.

10. Figueroa M: A dynamic taxonomy of self-destructive behavior, *Psychotherapy* 25:280-287, 1988.

11. Godfrey M: Clients with personality disorders. In McFarland G, Thomas M: Psychiatric mental health nursing: Application of the nursing process, Philadelphia, 1991, JB Lippincott.

12. Jacobson A: Physical and sexual assault histories among psychiatric outpatients, *Am J Psychiatr* 146:755-758, 1989.

13. Jacobson A, Herald C: The relevance of childhood sexual abuse to adult psychiatric in-patient care, *Hosp Commun Psych* 41:154, 1990.

14. Kim M, McFarland G, McLane A: *A pocket guide to nursing diagnosis,* ed 5, St Louis, 1993, Mosby.

15. McCloskey J, Bulechek G: *Nursing interventions classification,* St Louis, 1992, Mosby.

16. McFarland G, Wasli E, Gerety E: *Nursing diagnosis and process in psychiatric mental health nursing,* ed 2, Philadelphia, 1992, JB Lippincott.

17. Mitchell J, Boutacoff L, and Hatsukami O: Laxative abuse as a variant of bulimia, *J Nervous Mental Disease* 171:174- 176, 1986.

18. Oldham J: *Personality disorders: New perspectives on diagnostic validity,* Washington, DC, 1991, American Psychiatric Press.

19. Putnam F, Guroff J, Silberman E: The clinical phenomenology of multiple personality disorder: Review of 100 cases, *J Clin Psychiatr* 47:285-293, 1986.

20. Rose S, Peabody C, Stratigeas B: Undetected abuse among intensive case management clients, *Hosp Commun Psych* 42:499, 1991.

21. Schultz J, Dark S: *Manual of psychiatric nursing care plans,* ed 2, Boston, 1986, Little, Brown Co.

22. Virkkunen M: Self-mutilation in anti-social personality disorder, *Acta Psychiatr Scand* 54:347-352, 1976.

VII

VIII

ROLE—RELATIONSHIP PATTERN
Impaired Verbal Communication

Impaired Verbal Communication *is the state in which an individual experiences a decreased or absent ability to use or understand language in human interaction. Difficulties experienced in verbal communication must occur over time and be evidenced by observable signs or reported symptoms for a nursing diagnosis of Impaired Verbal Communication to be valid.*

OVERVIEW

Communication is a dynamic, complex, continuous series of reciprocal events through which messages are exchanged, primarily to produce a response from a person or group. It includes all conscious and unconscious behavior that affects another person. Therefore communication is essential in interpersonal relationships. Communication is a major factor that determines an individual's life situations and types of relationships.[12] The communication process is continuous; that is, it has no beginning or end.

The four major components of the communication process are sender, message, receiver, and feedback.

The sender generates and transmits a message. A message is triggered by internal or external stimuli, such as an idea, event, or situation, that are mediated by the senses. The sender can focus consciously on only a few of the many stimuli available at any one point in time. The selected stimuli are analyzed and evaluated through "covert rehearsal" before a message is developed.[13] Covert rehearsal involves the sender's review of perception of self and others and rehearsal of possible actions and expected reactions. Covert rehearsal is mediated by such psychosocial factors as self-concept, values, mood, and culture, as well as by the parts of the central nervous system that connect input with output (for example, sensory end organs, nerve fibers, and the cerebral cortex). After internally rehearsing alternative messages, the sender transmits the one evaluated as potentially most successful.

The message is derived through translation of ideas, purpose, and intention and is formulated into a code that is carried to the receiver through a channel.

The two basic systems of codification of a message are the *analog* and the *digital* system. The *analog* system is nonverbal and is based on similarities in form, color, or proportion between the actual communication and the event represented.[11] Nonverbal communication is as effective and significant as verbal communication and, in some circumstances, even overrides the verbal message. Nonverbal communication fulfills a variety of purposes, such as to augment or replace verbal communication, to display feelings, to regulate the speed of verbal messages, and to reflect the relationship between the sender and receiver.

Nonverbal communication encompasses[13]: *kinesics* (includes the study of body movement, i.e., such nonverbal behaviors as facial expression, eye contact, and gestures); *paralanguage* (includes vocal phenomena such as pitch and range of voice, vocal differentiators, e.g., crying and laughing; vocal identifiers, e.g., "ah" and "uh-hum," and the conveyance of emotions through the voice quality); *proxemics* (includes the study of the relationship of space and social interaction, e.g., four main distances are intimate, personal, social, and public, each indicating the distance, relationship, appropriate messages, and activities between sender and receiver); *touch* (includes physical contact between sender and receiver, which is a significant form of nonverbal communication); and *cultural artifacts* (includes items or substances that reflect a given culture or subculture, e.g., use of cosmetics, jewelry, clothing).

Cultural considerations are very important in the analog system of codification of a message. For example, culture influences the interpretation of eye contact. Eye contact often reflects a willingness to interact. However, extended eye contact can indicate aggression and the deliberate intent to induce anxiety. An absence of eye contact can communicate disinterest, lack of self-esteem, competitiveness, embarrassment, or hurt. Gestures express or emphasize the communicated ideas. How a person feels about another can be indicated through gestures, including the position of the body, and the placement and movements of eyes, hands, and feet. Because gestures are learned through imitation, culture determines the meaning of the gesture. The personal zone ranges from 12 inches to 36 inches. Confidential or personal information is communicated in this zone. Americans use this zone at parties and in close friendships. The effectiveness of touch is influenced by the meaning of touch to a given person within a given culture. The mores of a culture must also be considered when interpreting cultural artifacts. For example, the use of perfume may be interpreted in one culture as an invitation for interaction. However, in another culture that values the body's natural odors, perfume would be considered offensive.

In the *digital* system of message codification, signs and symbols represent concepts and objects. Language is created through manipulation of these signs and symbols. Verbal communication depends on a digital system. To communicate, persons must have the same meanings for words. This involves more than a common language because each word has both a *denotation* and a *connotation*. A *denotative* meaning is the one that is most generally used and the *connotative* meaning is an additional meaning specific to a person. Connotative meaning includes associations, referrents, and emotions derived from personal experience that add to the denotative meaning. Because effective communication depends on similar meanings, the selected words must convey the intended meaning and be understood by the other person.

The receiver perceives and interprets the message based on stimuli in his/her perceptual field. These stimuli include those in the sender's verbal and nonverbal communication and the immediate environment (context). As with the sender, the stimuli are selectively received, reviewed, and interpreted. The receiver's perception is affected by such psychological factors as concept of self and others, feelings, and social and cultural factors.

To organize the complex and dynamic series of events into a communication sequence for interpretation and response, the receiver "punctuates" the interactional sequence by organizing it into a beginning and an end.[2] Disagreement between the sender and receiver about the punctuation of a communication sequence often results in conflict and impaired communication. For example, a student claims that he cheated on an examination because he believes the teacher does not trust him. "I may as well do what I'm accused of," the student states. The teacher views the situation differently. She is distrustful and suspicious in response to the student's behavior.

The receiver responds according to his/her perceptions and interpretations, thereby providing feedback and becoming a sender. Feedback is the receiver's communicated reaction to the sender's message. Feedback regulates the communication process by stimulating modification or correction. Feedback should be clearly and tactfully stated, relevant to the person, culture, and context, and be appropriately timed to facilitate understanding and agreement between communicators. In providing feedback, the original receiver becomes a sender, thereby perpetuating the communication process.

Characteristics of successful communication include:[7,8]

1. Both the sender and receiver are physically able to receive, analyze, and send messages.
2. Appropriate input is selectively analyzed.
3. Consistent verbal and nonverbal communication are used.
4. The sender and receiver have similar meanings for words.
5. The message is appropriate to the context and complete (not overloaded or insufficient in information).
6. The timing of the message coincides with its meaning and the context.
7. The sender and receiver agree on the punctuation of a communication sequence.
8. If indicated, the feedback is clearly stated, relevant to the person, context, and culture, and appropriately timed.
9. The sender can correct the information or the message.
10. Concordant information is established between the sender and receiver, both of whom attain confirmation and gratification.

Many variables can positively or negatively affect the communication process. When these variables consistently exert a negative influence on a person's communication, a pattern of impaired communication results.

ASSESSMENT

When assessing the patient's communication pattern, the nurse should analyze the patient data for the presence or absence of characteristics of successful communication. Sources of data include the nurse's observation of and interaction with the patient, the patient's perceptions of his/her communication with others, and feedback from significant others about the patient's communication ability.[9] Limitations in verbal communication must be significant in amount and frequency to result in a diagnosis of Impaired Verbal Communication.

A variety of factors affect the communication process and are related to Impaired Verbal Communication. These include *growth and development, physical condition, stress, emotional state, perception, culture,* and *communication skills.*

Communication is a major human function, mastery of which involves learning a series of progressive tasks over time. Each stage of human *growth and development* includes physical, social, psychological, and cultural events that can either enhance or interfere with the development of effective communication. Some examples are the rapid physical and cognitive development of a child, the growing independence of the adolescent, the complexity of an adult's roles, and the effects of the aging process.

Physical conditions or medical treatments may affect a person's ability to communicate. Those directly affecting communication include conditions and treatments that interfere with the physical ability to receive and process sensory input or generate output, such as blindness, cerebrovascular accident, cleft palate, endotracheal intubation, laryngectomy, and wired jaws. Communication may be indirectly influenced by physical conditions, such as social withdrawal resulting from embarrassment about physical symptoms.

Stress also affects communication. Stress, a complex phenomenon, is precipitated by internal or external demands that result in neurocognitive, affective, physiological, and behavioral responses.[6] A moderate level of stress enhances learning and increases motivation and productivity. However, excessive stress can cause mental, social, or physical dysfunction, including impaired communication.

Feelings or *emotional states* are states of mind or being that can enhance or impede communication. Expression of feelings such as anxiety, anger, or depression can facilitate communication and interpersonal relationships by allowing others to know us and our feelings. However, expression of feelings can impair communication, most often through the manner used to express the feeling. For example, a staff nurse is angry that her supervisor frequently reminds her about her tasks. If

VIII

she expresses her anger by throwing the temperature chart on the desk and storming out of the nurses' station when the supervisor reminds her to take temperatures, communication has ceased because of her emotional outburst. If she instead responds by saying, "I appreciate and share your concern about getting the work done, but I feel angry when you continually remind me to do my work. I would prefer to be informed of my assignments only once. I will ask for assistance when I need it." The supervisor, in this example, has more information on which to base her supervision of this staff nurse, and the channels of communication remain open.

A person's behavior depends on his/her perceptual field at the moment. *Perception* is a process that includes reception, selection, organization, and interpretation of sensory data. Each component of the communication process is affected by perception. The receiver will only perceive input considered relevant and will then only respond to *some* of the perceived input. The resulting messages sent and received are mediated by perception of self, the environment, the culture, and the receiver. The nervous system, past experiences, values, needs, and the emotional state of the individual all influence perception. Whenever perception is limited because of distortion, omission, or falsification of sensory input, impaired communication results.[8]

Culture also influences the communication process. The culture of the communicators determines the meanings of verbal and nonverbal communication and governs where, what, how, why, and with whom a person communicates. Impaired communication can result from not understanding or considering cultural influences.

Effective communication also depends on communication skills. A variety of effective communication styles and skills have been described in the literature.* Impaired communication may result when the communicator has not learned or fails to use the style and specific skills that enhance the communication process.

---

*References 1, 6, 8, 9, 13.

❖ **Defining Characteristics**

The presence of the following defining characteristics indicates that the patient may be experiencing Impaired Verbal Communication:

- Speech impediment
- Inability to speak
- Hypervigilance or hypovigilance
- Disorientation
- Distorted perception
- Inappropriate selection of words
- Unable to speak dominant language
- Inappropriate message for context
- Illogical speech
- Dissonant information
- Disparate verbal and nonverbal messages
- Ill-timed messages
- Lack of confirmation
- Disagreement on punctuation of communication
- Unresponsive feedback
- Inappropriate feedback
- Withdrawal from interactions
- Inappropriate expression of feelings

❖ **Related Factors**

The following related factors are associated with Impaired Verbal Communication:

- Sensory end organ impairment
- Afferent or efferent nerve impairment
- Developmental physical problems
- Cerebral cortex impairment
- Age-related physical problems
- Mechanical barrier or impairment
- Faulty perception
- Excessive stress
- Emotional state
- Inadequate self-perception
- Poor communication skills
- Social isolation
- Cultural differences

❖ **Related Medical/Psychiatric Diagnoses**

The following are examples of related medical/psychiatric diagnoses for Impaired Verbal Communication.

- Adult respiratory distress syndrome
- Amyotrophic lateral sclerosis
- Aneurysm
- Anxiety
- Autism
- Bell's palsy
- Bipolar disorders
- Bronchial asthma

VIII

- Cancer of larynx
- Cerebrovascular accident
- Craniocerebral trauma
- Cystic fibrosis
- Delirium
- Depressive disorders
- Diphtheria
- Laryngitis
- Multiple sclerosis
- Myasthenia gravis
- Parkinson's disease
- Poliomyelitis
- Psychoactive substance use disorders
- Schizophrenia
- Thoracic surgery
- Thyroidectomy
- Tracheotomy
- Vocal cord paralysis
- Vocal cord polyps and nodules

NURSING DIAGNOSES

Examples of *specific* nursing diagnoses for Impaired Verbal Communication are:
- Impaired Verbal Communication related to sensory end organ impairment
- Impaired Verbal Communication related to developmental physical problem
- Impaired Verbal Communication related to mechanical impairment
- Impaired Verbal Communication related to social isolation

PLANNING AND IMPLEMENTATION WITH RATIONALE

Nursing interventions for patients with Impaired Verbal Communication can be organized into the four major components of the communication process: sender, message, receiver, and feedback. When selecting nursing interventions, the nurse must consider related factors such as physical condition, emotional state, and perceptions that may negatively influence the communication process.

To generate and transmit a message, the patient (sender or receiver) must notice, perceive, and process stimuli. Physical, developmental, and psychosocial conditions of the patient, as well as environmental and cultural factors, can interfere in this stage of communication, thereby becoming the foci of nursing interventions.

Extremely physically ill patients may be unable to participate in assessment or trial of a communication system and their acceptance of communica-tion disabilities may be unstable. *The nurse can help the patient correct, modify, or prevent physical conditions that interfere with reception and interpretation of stimuli.* The environment can be manipulated by the nurse to reduce or increase available stimuli, such as providing music or pictures for the patient in an intensive care unit. The patient's ability to identify and focus on relevant stimuli can be aided directly through the nurse's teaching these skills. Indirect interventions include reducing both excessive stress and the emotions affecting identification of, and attention to, stimuli. The nurse can also intervene to prevent or correct the patient's distortion, omission, or false perception of stimuli.

Effective communication also depends on the ability to send precise, succinct, and understandable messages. The nurse should refer the patient for assistance in correcting, modifying, or preventing physical conditions that interfere with the transmission of messages. The nurse can assist the patient in this stage of communication through demonstrating, teaching, and supporting the patient's use of effective communication techniques (see Table 12). The nurse must identify the patient's cognitive skills and interpretation of nonverbal communication *so that the nurse can modify his/her own communication techniques to coincide with the patient's ability to understand.* The nurse should also assist the patient in mastering any developmental tasks or cultural differences that interfere with the transmission of clear messages. Attempts at communication (verbal and nonverbal) should be encouraged *so that motivation to communicate is not lost.*

The message component of communication involves translation of ideas, purpose, and intent into congruent verbal and nonverbal communication. A number of communication aids may be used to assist a patient unable to speak,[4] e.g., signing systems, individualized communication charts, electronic aids, and writing/drawing. Any aid used should be introduced early in treatment to avoid the patient's rejection of it as second best if speech is not regained. The patient must be taught how to use a communication aid and be

VIII

Table 12 Useful Communication Techniques

Technique Defined	Purpose	Example
REFLECTION		
Conveying to the receiver his expressed thoughts and implied feelings.	Allow patient to develop and evaluate thoughts. Clarify unspoken or incongruent impressions Explore new information.	Patient (P): "I feel so depressed." Nurse (N): "You feel depressed?" P: "My thoughts are disjointed?" N: "Disjointed?"
FOCUSING		
Concentrating on a specific thought or feeling in reference to a particular point.	Sustain goal-directed communication. Draw attention to significant data.	P: "Every morning I feel so bad." N: "Describe how you feel." P: "My husband always puts me down." N: "Give me an example."
VALIDATION		
Confirming one's observations and interpretations.	Accurately appraise patient and message. Prevent inaccurate assumptions.	P: "I don't want to do what my mother tells me to do." N: "It must be hard to disagree with your mother."
SILENCE		
Communicating without verbalization.	Communicate concern, interest, or acceptance. Allow time for collection of thoughts. Allow patient to assume initiative. Reduce emotionally charged content.	P: "Diabetes is going to upset my whole life." N: (remains silent)
SUMMARIZING		
Highlighting the main ideas.	Review progress. Focus thinking. Facilitate conscious learning. Recall important points.	P: "I must leave soon." N: "Today you and I have discussed . . . ."
CLARIFICATION		
Attempting to find the meaning of a communication.	Establish mutual understanding. Promote further communication. Assist patient to be more specific.	P: "Life's not fair." N: "I'm not sure what you're telling me." P: "They are always telling me what to do." N: "Who are they?"
OPEN-ENDED QUESTIONS		
Questions that allow multiple options for response.	Encourage expression of ideas and feelings. Allow patient freedom to structure conversation.	P: "The nurses don't have much to say to me." N: "What would you like to talk about?"

Table 12 Useful Communication Techniques—cont'd

Technique Defined	Purpose	Example
STATING OBSERVATIONS		
Verbalizing what is observed.	Explain connections between verbal and nonverbal behavior. Correct perception.	N: "While you were talking about your daughter's graduation plans, you began to fidget and sweat."
CONFRONTATION		
Description and examination of discrepant behaviors.	Promote self-understanding. Evaluate consequences of behavior. Encourage exploration.	N: "Your words say 'yes' but your body language says 'no.'"
EXPLORING		
Obtaining all pertinent data on a specific subject or feeling.	Establish mutual understanding. Allow patient to develop and evaluate thoughts.	P: "My husband and I had a fight." N: "Tell me what happened." P: "I want to move to Dallas with my parents, but I just don't know." N: "You seem unsure. You don't know what?"
PROVIDING FEEDBACK		
Description of some aspect of an individual's communication and its effect on the receiver.	Become aware of the effects of behavior. Verify, modify, or correct perception.	P: "When you do everything for me I feel helpless. I can feed and bathe myself."

From Thompson J, McFarland G, Hirsch J, Tucker S, and Bowers A: Mosby's manual of clinical nursing, ed 2 St Louis, 1989, Mosby–Year Book.

VIII

❖ *NURSING CARE GUIDELINES*

Nursing Diagnosis: Impaired Verbal Communication

Expected Patient Outcomes	Nursing Interventions
The patient will notice, perceive, and process relevant stimuli.	• Refer patient for help in correcting, modifying, or preventing physical conditions that inhibit reception and interpretation of stimuli or transmission of messages. • Interpret cultural context of stimuli. • Manipulate environment to increase or reduce stimuli. • Teach patient to discern and focus on relevant stimuli. • Reduce faulty perception. • Teach method to reduce stress. • Increase the patient's self-esteem.

Continued.

❖ NURSING CARE GUIDELINES—cont'd

Nursing Diagnosis: *Impaired Verbal Communication*

Expected Patient Outcomes	Nursing Interventions
The patient will send precise, understandable messages through congruent verbal and nonverbal communication.	• Demonstrate, teach, and support patient's use of effective communication techniques. • Assist patient in mastering developmental tasks and reconciling cultural differences. • Point out discrepancies in the patient's verbal and nonverbal behaviors. • Teach appropriate language skills and nonverbal behavior. • Demonstrate and encourage appropriate expression of feelings.
The patient will transmit and receive feedback.	• Provide opportunity and encourage interaction with others. • Help the patient understand the dynamics of relationships. • Increase the patient's awareness of strengths and limitations in communicating with others. • Assist the patient's efforts to provide feedback. • Request the patient ask for feedback. • Help and support the patient's attempts to accept positive and negative feedback from others. • Role play the use of effective communication techniques and evaluate communication.

VIII

encouraged to do so. An essential starting point is establishment of a reliable yes/no response. Any movement that the patient can use consistently may be used. *It is important that everyone knows what the patient's responses are and encourages their use.* Written instructions posted near the patient's bed are helpful. A patient must be assured that assistance can be gained quickly. Beeper alarms sensitive to minimal pressure may be placed near any body part over which the patient has some reliable control. The nurse can intervene by indicating the patient discrepancies in nonverbal and verbal behaviors. The patient's cultural background must be considered when selecting nursing interventions. A cultural assessment may be obtained through interviewing the patient, a family member, or significant other. Through teaching, *the nurse can assist the patient in modifying or learning language skills and nonverbal behaviors of the dominant culture.* Interventions

to reduce stress or modify the feeling states that interfere with congruent messages should also be used.

Feedback is the regulatory process by which communication is modified or corrected, thereby establishing understanding between communicators. Therefore interventions that enhance the patient's ability to provide clear, relevant, and timely feedback should be used by the nurse. *Evaluating the effects of one's own behavior on others and understanding interpersonal relationships are both necessary to send and receive feedback.* In the context of the nurse-patient relationship, the nurse can assist the patient in evaluating strengths and limitations in communication and understanding the dynamics of relationships. The nurse should demonstrate, teach, and support the use and acceptance of feedback, as well as the use of effective communication techniques, including active listening.

EVALUATION

Evaluation of the nursing interventions to alleviate impaired verbal communication is determined by the patient's attaining the identified expected outcomes. Achievement of the expected patient outcomes is assessed through tools such as the Communication Assessment Profile,[3] the nurse's observation of and interaction with the patient, the patient's evaluation of his/her communication with others, and feedback from significant others about the patient's communication ability.

If the previously identified limitations are no longer present and the patient reports satisfaction and confirmation from communication, the expected patient outcomes have been achieved and the problem of impaired verbal communication has been resolved.

If expected outcomes are not achieved, the patient is assessed for presence of defining characteristics of Impaired Verbal Communication. A revised plan of care is developed, implemented, and evaluated.

❖ CASE STUDY WITH PLAN OF CARE

Mrs. Marilyn A. has been recently transferred to a medical unit from intensive care where she was admitted with the diagnosis of cerebrovascular accident (CVA). Her treatment on the medical unit focuses on supportive care and initial rehabilitation, one aspect of which is correction of an alteration in communication resulting from dysarthria. (Dysarthria is a condition in which the musculature used in speaking is paralyzed, weak, or uncoordinated after a stroke or other neurological problem.[10]) Mrs. A.'s speech is slow, halting, and lacks variation in pitch and inflection. She often expresses nonverbal behaviors indicating anger and frustration when she attempts to communicate. A 65-year-old retired elementary school teacher, Marilyn is married and has two daughters and three grandchildren. She has adequate financial resources and an attentive, supportive family. Her medical history includes hypertension of 20 years duration; she smokes one pack of cigarettes per day, but has had no previous cardiovascular illness or hospitalizations. Her physical and emotional health before the CVA were good. Mrs. A. stands 5′4″ and weighs 145 pounds. Her diet is balanced but somewhat high in calories and cholesterol. Her activities include maintaining the home, reading avidly, volunteering as a tutor for children with reading difficulties, and traveling with her husband.

VIII

PLAN OF CARE FOR MRS. MARILYN A.

Nursing Diagnosis: Impaired Verbal Communication related to dysarthria

Expected Patient Outcomes	Nursing Interventions
Mrs. A. will accurately process perceived stimuli as evidenced by verbal and nonverbal responses pertinent to the environment, self, and other persons.	• Refer Mrs. A. to speech pathologist for differential dysarthria diagnosis to confirm unimpaired selection and processing of stimuli.

Mrs. A. will communicate her needs and wants clearly and understandably as evidenced by:
   Congruent verbal and nonverbal communication.
   Speech that varies in pitch and inflection.
	• Provide adequate time for Mrs. A. to initiate or respond to communication from others.
	 • Ask Mrs. A. to overemphasize words she is trying to say.
	 • Initially ask questions that Mrs. A. can answer with few words.
	 • Provide alternatives for expressing needs and wants such as paper and pencil or a communication board that includes pictures that Mrs. A. can point to.
	 • Teach and encourage use of alternate communication system to husband.

Continued.

Expected Patient Outcomes	Nursing Interventions
Lack of anger and frustration when attempting to communicate.	• Demonstrate and encourage nonverbal behaviors that replace or emphasize verbal expression of needs and wants. • Praise use of effective communication techniques. • Obtain books on tape from library. • Acknowledge and encourage appropriate expression of anger and frustration that Mrs. A. encounters in communication.
Mrs. A. will transmit and receive feedback as evidenced by: Request for response to communication. Acceptance of response. Clarification/elaboration of idea. Use of effective communication techniques. Satisfaction with communication.	• Establish a nurse-patient relationship. • Provide opportunity and encourage interaction with others in the medical unit and family members. • Provide feedback to Mrs. A. concerning strengths and limitations in communication. • Use Mrs. A.'s strengths and offer unconditional positive regard to help her accept positive and negative feedback. • Instruct Mrs. A. to request feedback so that she can judge whether she is accurately understood. • Provide opportunities to practice effective communication techniques.

REFERENCES

1. Burgess A: *Psychiatric nursing in the hospital and the community,* ed 5, East Norwalk, Conn, 1990, Appleton & Lange.
2. Crowther D: Metacommunications: a missed opportunity, *J Psycho-soc Nurs Ment Health Serv* 29(4):13-16, 1991.
3. Dormandy K, Van der Gaag A: What color are the alligators: a critical look at methods used to assess communication skills in adults with learning difficulties, *Br J Disord Commun* 24:265-279, 1989.
4. Easton J: Alternative communication for patients in intensive care, *Intens Care Nurs* 4(2):47-55, 1988.
5. Kim M, McFarland G, and McLane A: *Pocket guide to nursing diagnoses,* ed 4, St Louis, 1991, CV Mosby.
6. McFarland G, Leonard H, and Morris M: *Nursing leadership and management: contemporary strategies,* New York, 1984, Wiley & Sons.
7. McFarland G, Naschinski C: Impaired communication: a descriptive study, *Nurs Clin North Am* 20(4):775-778, 1985.
8. McFarland G, Naschinski C: Communication. In Thompson J, McFarland G, Hirsch J, Tucker S, Bowers A: *Mosby's manual of clinical nursing,* ed 2, St Louis, 1989, CV Mosby.
9. McFarland G, Wasli E, Gerety E: *Nursing diagnoses and process in psychiatric mental health nursing,* ed 2, Philadelphia, 1992, JB Lippincott.
10. Palmer J, Yantis P: *Survey of communication disorders,* Baltimore, 1990, Williams & Wilkins.
11. Ruesch J, Bateson G: *Communication: the social matrix of psychiatry,* New York, 1987, WW Norton.
12. Satir V: *Peoplemaking,* Palo Alto, 1972, Science & Behavior Books.
13. Wilson H: *Psychiatric nursing,* ed 3, Menlo Park, Calif, 1988, Addison-Wesley.

VIII

Social Isolation

Social Isolation is actual or potential aloneness, perceived as imposed by others and as negative or threatening

OVERVIEW

Lack of contact with other people results in social isolation. Although an individual that the nurse diagnoses as socially isolated believes that his/her limited involvement with other people is caused by factors outside of his/her control, many others consciously or unconsciously isolate themselves. A good example is people who socially isolate themselves while participating in religious retreats. Another example of self-imposed avoidance of others is people who consciously or unconsciously encourage isolation because of a physical or psychological condition. People who have deficient hearing may avoid others because communication is difficult and, many times, unrewarding, and people who are psychiatrically impaired, such as some schizophrenic patients, may view contact with others as dangerous or threatening. Environmental factors may also cause Social Isolation. A shipwreck, imprisonment, or hospitalization in a communicable disease isolation unit prevents or severely limits human interactions.

Social Isolation is defined as an individual's inability to make contact with others although he/she may need or desire it. Psychological, physical, or sociocultural factors cause this isolation. Isolation is subjective and exists whenever the person says it does and perceives it as imposed by others. Because Social Isolation is subjective, the diagnosis must be validated by the individual.[3] In other words, the nurse might suspect isolation, but until the individual acknowledges it, the diagnosis cannot be confirmed.

Elsen and Blegen[6] suggest five critical requirements for effective socializing: "(1) physiologic abilities to contact and communicate with others; (2) other people with whom to interact; (3) knowledge of the usual methods of communication; (4) a system of language understood by all involved; and (5) the motivation or desire to interact." Limitations or deficiencies in one or more of these areas may indicate the potential for a socially isolated patient.

Social Isolation inherently includes aloneness, loneliness, deprivation, and unhappiness, and involves the loss of social roles, social support, and environmental contact that the individual considers varied, stimulating, and fulfilling.[14]

Many factors may precipitate social isolation. One of the most common causes of social isolation is loss. The loss may be obvious, such as the death of a family member or a friend, or it may be more subjective, such as a move from familiar surroundings or the loss of functional abilities. Loss may also be perceptual—the person feels or thinks that he/she has a limited chance for social interaction. An example of this might be a depressed patient who says that "old friends don't include me anymore," when in fact the friends are acting the same, but the individual perceives them as withdrawn. Loss, both perceived and real, may trigger social isolation.

Another theory underlying Social Isolation is proposed by Goffman.[7] Goffman suggests that certain people or groups of people are stigmatized by society because of discernible defects that cause anxiety for the majority of the population. He speculates that individuals who are perceived as "different" are rejected, thus becoming socially isolated. Examples of this are a person who is

VIII

crippled and must wear braces or a person with an indwelling tracheal tube that causes him/her to hiss when talking. People often withdraw from these afflicted individuals because they do not know how to respond; therefore the afflicted person becomes socially isolated. Stigmatization also occurs when a person has a dreaded disease that causes discomfort in the community because of the population's perceptions about the communicability of the disease. Thus the diseased person is ostracized. A specific example of this is a patient with tuberculosis or acquired immunodeficiency syndrome (AIDS).

Still other psychosocial causes of isolation are alienation and low self-esteem. Alienation and low self-esteem are so interwoven that it is almost impossible to discern which is the cause and which is the effect. However, both cause Social Isolation through a person's feeling that he/she does not belong because he/she is "unworthy" and "apart." These people feel shunned and see themselves as "outsiders." Therefore because they feel and become alienated, other people treat them that way. For instance, this can occur when immigrants have language problems and no support systems or when an elderly couple who moves to a warmer climate finds the social climate cool and unresponsive. These people feel that they do not fit in and tend to blame themselves. Consequently, they do not reach out to others and either consciously or unconsciously make themselves socially unattractive, thereby suffering isolation. Social Isolation is a major concern for elders and may be a precursor to loneliness. Social Isolation may also result in low self-concept, disruption of one's support network, alterations in family process, or deterioration of social skills.[10]

Patients with personality disorders or chronic mental impairments are at a greater risk for Social Isolation than those without such illnesses.[8] Patterns of social isolation may also be predictive of mental disorder[2] and suicide.[12]

Widespread family mobility can influence the prevalence of Social Isolation. For instance, it is not uncommon for families to move to new locations, which sometimes leads to social isolation that may then cause health problems. Although some family members may not become socially isolated, others will. For instance, the father may have new work associates, and the older children may make new friends at school. But the mother who stays home with preschool children in a neighborhood where all the other women work may experience unhappiness as she perceives her social world as very limited. The mother will need much more support from the family members than they will need from her, and her family may eventually begin to resent her clinging to them. The mother might feel rejected and develop tension headaches. This may be her way of dealing with anxiety about the situation and may serve for her to get the attention that she needs from her family.

Changing community standards of involvement that encourage people to be suspicious of others and "not to get involved" further promote Social Isolation. Community standards influence social interaction just as social interaction may influence community standards.

ASSESSMENT

Assessment and diagnosis of Social Isolation depend on objective and subjective data. Feelings of loneliness and isolation need to be validated with the patient. Careful assessment of the individual's social history is indicated when barriers or limitations are identified that inhibit relationships with others. Physical, psychological, and sociocultural factors may influence the patient's ability to develop and maintain relationships with others.[5]

Carpenito[3] suggests that subjective assessment of social isolation would include examination of factors such as feelings of loneliness, desire for more human contact, loss of significant others, barriers to social contact, changes in living arrangements, and adequacy of support systems. Objective assessment may focus on aesthetic problems, physical limitations and disabilities, and environmental issues. Because individuals vary in their responses to isolation and aloneness, definitive objective indicators to this diagnosis are difficult to obtain; therefore subjective patient responses are critical in making this diagnosis.

The nurse must listen carefully to what the patient is saying for subjective cues. Does the patient feel lonely? Has the patient moved recently? Does the patient lack knowledge about available resources? Does the patient have sensory impairment? When does the patient feel most alone? Do physical barriers prevent the patient from participating in desired activities? Does the patient feel rejected? What kind of relationships would the patient like?

Assessment of objective data includes observations for difficulties in seeking help, initiating conversations, or responding to others. Self-report questionnaires may provide data about the patient's perception of his/her social skills, and a social skills checklist may help to identify behavioral patterns.[6] The Past Month Isolation Index (PMI) and the Adult Isolation Index provide a means to measure social isolation in elders.[2] Assessment also includes physiologic parameters such as changes in eating or sleeping habits.

Social Isolation may occur across the life span with a rapid or insidious onset. A young child who has been severely disfigured as a result of a burn injury may experience isolation almost overnight. An elderly male may experience isolation more gradually as his health weakens and social network of family and friends diminishes. Patients experience Social Isolation in a variety of settings for a variety of reasons. Therefore the nurse must be aware of vulnerable populations at risk for Social Isolation, including the elderly, the physically compromised, the psychologically impaired, and those experiencing relocation stress or cultural shock.

It is well documented that social support provided through social networks influences health and well-being.[4,11,13] Social networks such as families, friends, social groups and organizations, and communities can facilitate or inhibit efforts for health protection and promotion. The nurse is able to assist patients in assessing the strengths and limitations of the existing social support systems and subsequently aid these patients in modi-

fying or developing a social support system. Supportive social networks can help decrease feelings of isolation.

❖ Defining Characteristics

The presence of the following defining characteristics indicates that the patient may be experiencing Social Isolation[3,9]:

- Evidence of physical or mental handicap
- Inappropriate or immature interests and activities for developmental stage and age
- Exhibiting unacceptable behavior
- Sad or dull affect
- Hostility in behavior and voice
- Expressions of inadequacy or lack of purpose in life
- Absence of supportive significant others (e.g., family, friends, or social group)
- Withdrawal and inability or refusal to communicate (patient has no eye contact)
- Seeking to be alone
- Verbalization of feelings of aloneness and rejection imposed by others
- Expressions of being "different" and unable to meet expectations of others
- Insecurity in social situations

❖ Related Factors

The following related factors are associated with Social Isolation:

- Alteration in health
- Sensory deficits
- Impaired mobility
- Delay in accomplishing developmental tasks
- Alteration in physical appearance
- Body image disturbance
- Inadequate or loss of personal resources
- Chemical dependence
- Immature interest
- Alteration in mental status
- Unaccepted social behavior
- Impaired communication
- Inability to engage in satisfying personal relationships
- Divorce
- Homosexuality
- Poverty

VIII

❖ **Related Medical/Psychiatric Diagnoses**

The following are examples of related medical/psychiatric diagnoses for Social Isolation:

- AIDS
- Depression
- Obesity
- Organic brain syndrome
- Schizophrenia
- Terminal disease
- Tuberculosis

NURSING DIAGNOSES

Examples of *specific* nursing diagnoses for Social Isolation are:

- Social Isolation related to low self-esteem
- Social Isolation related to altered state of wellness
- Social Isolation related to inadequate personal resources
- Social Isolation related to severe anxiety

PLANNING AND IMPLEMENTATION WITH RATIONALE

Nursing interventions for the socially isolated patient are generally directed at assisting the patient in identifying the causative factors of the isolation, decreasing or limiting the barriers to social contact, promoting social interaction and self-worth, improving meaningful relationships, distinguishing reality from perceptions, and using community resources to limit isolation.

In planning care for the socially isolated patient, the nurse implements similar interventions and outcomes regardless of the cause of the social isolation. The focus is on helping the patient to identify the reasons for the isolation and ways to alleviate it.[17] Nursing interventions should focus on decreasing the sense of isolation and loneliness. This may include assisting the patient in the identification of available social networks or in developing the needed skills to maintain relationships. For instance, these skills may include those related to improving communication or meeting new people. The goal is to have the patient increase opportunities for and achieve success in interpersonal involvements. It is necessary to ex-

plore the possible causes of Social Isolation directly and openly. The nurse must convey an accepting attitude that will increase the patient's sense of self-worth. The nurse should assist the patient in identifying acceptable social behaviors. *Positive reinforcement of those behaviors can enhance self-esteem and encourage repetition of those behaviors.*[16]

For some individuals, social skills enhancement may be helpful. Some patients may feel embarrassed about their appearance and therefore anxious about social situations. A social skills training program would help improve social skills and decrease anxiety in social situations. *Instruction and modeling are necessary for behavioral change.*[1]

Research indicates that a variety of interventions are effective in decreasing Social Isolation in elders, including behavior modification techniques, mutual aid groups, therapeutic groups, and multipurpose senior centers. *Nursing interventions that promote confidence and sharing will decrease loneliness and isolation.*[10]

In planning care, the nurse and patient must consider factors contributing to the isolation as well as discrepancies between the patient's perception and reality. The socially isolated patient may lack objectivity, self-confidence, and self-worth. Nursing interventions that focus on the provision of a supportive and consistent environment help the patient gain confidence. Consistent care promotes open communication. Exploration of patient perceptions and objective observations may assist the individual in gaining an understanding about his/her feelings and responses in social situations. Strengths and weaknesses should be identified, and positive feedback for patient progress should be provided. *Involving the patient in setting goals and planning care increases sense of control and decreases isolation.*[15]

Encouragement of participation in appropriate diversional activities will enhance the patient's interaction with others. Involvement with others is the first step in developing meaningful relationships. Realistic goals need to be planned with the

❖ NURSING CARE GUIDELINES

Nursing Diagnosis: *Social Isolation*

Expected Patient Outcomes	Nursing Interventions
The patient will acknowledge social isolation and identify its causes.	• Engage in active listening. • Ask appropriate questions about perceived social isolation. • Restate the patient's perceptions about the reason he or she is socially isolated. • Assist the patient in validating the causes of social isolation.
The patient will verbalize a willingness to seek to end social isolation.	• Assess the patient's motivation to alleviate social isolation. • Help the patient make correlations between own behavior and alleviation of social isolation.
The patient will formulate a plan to become more involved with others.	• Discuss with the patient the possible opportunities to reach out to others. • Promote realistic course of action. • Encourage some risk taking. • Determine possible barriers to social contacts and ways to surmount these barriers. • Suggest possible resources and actions. • Encourage the patient to develop a realistic time frame for the achievement of his/her goals. • Allow and support the patient to progress at his/her own rate.
The patient will become involved in activities with others.	• Give positive reinforcement for successful involvement. • Assist the patient to examine the elements that have contributed to success and those that have hindered success. • Encourage the patient to continue interpersonal involvement. • Emphasize the need to avoid relapse into social isolation.

VIII

patient so that success and positive feedback will result. The type of activity and frequency of participation will depend on the patient's health status and interests. *Specific periods of planned diversional activities will increase feelings of self-worth and decrease negative self-absorption.*[15]

Knowledge of community resources is essential for socially isolated individuals who experience physical barriers to social contact. Although the socially isolated patients should be supported to maintain his/her independence, assistance is sometimes warranted. Assessment of the patient's present social network may indicate the need for more support in a particular area. For example, a homebound elder may need assistance with grocery shopping or transportation to medical appointments. A socially isolated mother may need assistance with childcare. Enhancement of one's social network may limit feelings of isolation and helplessness and increase feelings of confidence and independence. *Encouragement of self-care activities and promotion of functional independence fosters independent actions and decreases helplessness and isolation.*[16]

EVALUATION

Evaluation involves measuring the expected client outcomes and the reduction of the defining characteristics of Social Isolation. The evaluation process is a mutual ongoing activity between the patient and nurse. Subjective and objective data are validated with the patient. Effectiveness of the nursing interventions is assessed in light of patient outcomes.

For the nursing diagnosis Social Isolation, expected outcomes are achieved when the patient (1) identifies causes and contributing factors of

❖ *CASE STUDY WITH PLAN OF CARE*

Mr. Justin Y., a 60-year-old man, lives alone in an apartment complex for senior citizens. Although Mr. Y. is functionally independent and capable of performing activities of daily living, he has gradually withdrawn from activities outside of his home. Before the death of his wife a year ago, Mr. Y. was actively involved in many of the daily apartment complex activities, enjoyed a large circle of friends, and frequently volunteered to help other residents in the building when a need arose. During the past year, however, Mr. Y. has discontinued all volunteer activities, no longer eats in the main dining room with other residents, and has very limited contact with friends. A community health nurse who is also the health consultant to the apartment complex made a home visit to Mr. Y. after a request from the apartment house manager. Mr. Y. was receptive to the home visit and eager to talk with the nurse.

During the assessment, Mr. Y. explained that since the death of his wife, he had lost all interest in outside activities. He no longer enjoyed being with other residents because he felt as if he were a burden to them. He stated that his vision was getting poor and that his arthritis slowed him down. He felt that he was no longer able to help his friends and that he was probably a disappointment to them. Assessment data revealed that Mr. Y. had neglected to keep his medical appointments during the past year, had been taking his prescribed daily medications sporadically, and had poor nutritional intake for the past several months. It was also determined that Mr. Y. demonstrated low self-esteem resulting from several factors, including the loss of his wife and limitations resulting from his physical condition.

PLAN OF CARE FOR MR. JUSTIN Y.

Nursing Diagnosis: *Social Isolation related in inability to engage in satisfying personal relationships*

Expected Patient Outcomes	Nursing Interventions
Mr. Y. will talk about his social isolation.	• Encourage Mr. Y. to express his feelings. • Help Mr. Y. make correlations between his feelings and his present lack of contact with others.
Mr. Y. will identify reasons for isolation.	• Review with Mr. Y. when he first experienced social isolation. • Identify with Mr. Y. those things he can change and those things outside of his power to change.
Mr. Y. will make a plan with specific evaluation criteria that will decrease his social isolation.	• Help Mr. Y. identify opportunities for interaction. • Encourage Mr. Y. to set up a weekly plan to eat in residents' dining hall five times, take part in at least two group activities, initiate visits to two friends in the building, and keep a record of his increased social interactions.
Mr. Y. will evaluate his present course of action and either continue the present plan or begin a new one.	• Provide support. • Engage in positive reinforcement. • Assist Mr. Y. with referrals if needed. • Allow Mr. Y. to progress at his own rate.

the isolation, (2) employs strategies for increasing meaningful relationships, (3) reduces barriers to social contact, (4) participates in selected diversional activities, (5) expresses increased confidence in social skills, (6) expresses increased self-worth, and (7) identifies community resources that will assist in decreasing the isolation.

If the outcomes are not achieved, reevaluation and modification of outcomes and interventions are indicated. Alternative strategies should be implemented if defining characteristics continue to be present. Referrals to other health care team members and community agencies may be indicated. Follow-up care is necessary for continued support of the patient and accomplishment of the desired outcomes.

REFERENCES

1. Bandura A: *Social learning theory,* Englewood Cliffs, NJ, 1977, Prentice-Hall.
2. Bennett R, editor: *Aging, isolation, and resocialization,* New York, 1980, Van Nostrand Reinhold.
3. Carpenito LJ: *Nursing diagnosis: application to clinical practice,* ed 4, Philadelphia, 1992, JB Lippincott.
4. Cobb S: Social support as a moderator of life stress, *Psychosom Med* 38:300, 1976.
5. Dychtwald K: *Wellness and health promotion for the elderly,* Rockville, Md, 1986, Aspens Systems.
6. Elsen J, Blegen M: Social isolation. In Maas M, Buckwalter KC, and Hardy M, editors: *Nursing diagnoses and interventions for the elderly,* Redwood City, Calif, 1991, Addison-Wesley Nursing.
7. Goffman E: *Stigma,* Englewood Cliffs, NJ, 1963, Prentice Hall.
8. Golden M, Bessant A: Social withdrawal, *Nurs 85* 2(35):1025-1032, 1985.
9. Kim M, McFarland GK, and McLane AM: *Pocket guide to nursing diagnoses,* ed 4, St Louis, 1991, Mosby–Year Book.
10. McConnell ES: Nursing diagnoses related to psychosocial alterations. In Matteson MA, McConnell ES, editors: *Gerontological nursing: concepts and practice,* Philadelphia, 1988, WB Saunders.
11. Meuller D: Social networks: a promising direction for research on the relationship of the social environment to psychiatric disorder, *Soc Sci Med* 14A:147, 1980.
12. Ofstein DH, Acuff FG: Durkheim and disengagement: a causal model of aging suicide, *Free Inquiry Creative Sociology* 7(2):108-111, 117, 1979.
13. Pender NJ: *Health promotion in nursing practice,* ed 2, Norwalk, Conn, 1987, Appleton & Lange.
14. Ravish T: Prevent social isolation before it starts, *J Gerontol Nurs* 11:10-13, 1985.
15. Sparks SM, Taylor CM, editors: *Nursing diagnoses reference manual,* Springhouse, Penn, 1991, Springhouse.
16. Stanhope M, Lancaster J: *Community health nursing: process and practice for promoting health,* ed 2, St Louis, 1988, CV Mosby.
17. Townsend MC: *Nursing diagnosis: a pocket guide for care plan construction,* Philadelphia, 1988, FA Davis.

VIII

Impaired Social Interaction

Impaired Social Interaction is the state in which an individual participates in an insufficient or excessive quantity or ineffective quality of social exchange.[7]

OVERVIEW

People have an innate need for relationships. From the moment of birth, a person learns to relate with others. This ongoing learning process continues until death. Relating with others requires social skill and social sensitivity. Throughout life, a person learns to handle the needs of dependence and independence by maintaining interpersonal relationships. The ability to relate interdependently with others is one indicator of maturity.

Throughout life, people engage in social interactions, which allow them to know themselves more fully. If a person feels inadequate or unable to handle social interactions, the potential for loneliness, isolation, depression, and withdrawal increases. Nursing focuses on the ability of patients to enter in growth-producing relationships.

Effective social interaction occurs when the involved persons maintain a sense of self during mutual interaction. People relate with each other on a variety of levels for a variety of purposes. To understand how people maintain social interactions, three main areas must be studied. These include (1) positive self-concept, (2) accurate perception of reality, and (3) the need for interdependence.

A positive self-concept is essential to maintaining healthy social interaction. According to Orem's Self-Care Deficit Theory of Nursing, self-care is based on every person achieving normalcy.[12] To promote normalcy, an individual must develop and maintain a realistic self-concept. Self-concept incorporates all of a person's beliefs and convictions that constitute self-knowledge and influence his/her interpersonal relationships.[14] Self-concept includes (1) self-awareness, (2) validity of self-concept, (3) feelings about self, and (4) sense of identity.[6] Self-awareness is defined as a person's consciousness of his/her beliefs, values, ideals, and goals. Validity of self-concept implies the capacity to see the self realistically and, to the degree possible, objectively.[6] Feelings about self relate to one's acceptance of self, including personal strengths, limitations, and the ability to realistically evaluate the potential for personal change and growth. Sense of identity involves a positive regard for self and the capacity to know self and not doubt inner identity.[6] Self-concept develops from relationships with significant others throughout the life span. Self-concept powerfully influences human behavior. One must, therefore, understand a person's situation through his/her frame of reference.

A person's perception of reality will also affect social interaction. Perception of reality is healthy when a person's perceptions correspond to reality. This criterion for positive mental health includes (1) freedom from need distortion and (2) social sensitivity.[6] Freedom from need distortion is defined as a correct perception of the environment that is not clouded by unhealthy distortions of needs. In other words, the lens through which one perceives the world is clear enough to allow one to assess, make assumptions, validate those assumptions, and draw conclusions based on those perceptions. Social sensitivity means that an individual can treat the inner life of another person with concern and attention. Social sensitivity also

VIII

implies that conclusions about other persons are free from need distortion. A person's ability to perceive is influenced by degrees of anxiety or threat. A perceived threat to self results in higher levels of anxiety that narrow a person's perceptual field and heighten need distortion. The person acts to protect self, which in turn inhibits social interaction.

Social interaction is also influenced by the human need for interdependence in relationships. This concept involves the capacity for people to give and receive in relationships. Interdependence can be viewed as the balancing point between dependent and independent behavior. Inherent in the concept of interdependence is the human need for autonomy. Autonomy is the capacity to act for oneself. It is only when a person is clear about his/her own boundaries and separateness from the other that effective interdependent social interactions can occur. As a criterion for positive mental health, autonomy involves regulating behavior from within, that is, making decisions based on one's own internalized standards and values.[6]

In summary, persons with positive self-concepts can better perceive their reality without need distortion, resulting in an increased ability to explain their world, inquire into the nature of their world, and take risks. Their interdependence with others enables them to learn and gain satisfaction through their self-competence. Effective social interactions are influenced by a person's interdependence with others. Both self-concept and perception of reality affect social interactions. Through the nursing process, nurses frequently assist patients in correcting, maintaining, or enhancing social interactions.

ASSESSMENT

Defining characteristics of the nursing diagnosis Impaired Social Interaction include subjective and objective data. Subjective data include the patient's verbalization of discomfort in social situations or verbalization of the inability to receive or communicate a satisfying sense of belonging, caring, interest, or shared history.[7] The nurse also assesses a patient for Impaired Social Interaction

by listening for expressions of anxiety. How does the patient experience anxiety in social interactions? Under what circumstances does this occur? How does the patient perceive self when relating with others? The nurse should ask the patient how time is spent each day and assess the patient's quality of relaxation time, close friendships, and his/her degree of comfort in meeting new people.[5] Is the patient threatened by close interactions? What defenses are used? Is it possible that the patient never learned adequate communication and interpersonal skills to feel competent in social interactions? Perceived incompetency can cause feelings of threat to self, heightened anxiety, and narrowed perception, leading to a preoccupation with self-protection. The nurse should observe whether the patient explores his/her world openly and freely. Anxiety can immobilize a patient in social interaction. A patient's interaction with the nurse reflects how he/she interacts in other social situations. The nurse must assess the nurse-patient interaction to understand the patient's situation more fully.

Subjective data revealing the patient's self-concept, perception of reality, and interdependence are key areas of assessment. To assess self-concept, the nurse must listen for patient expressions about self. What messages are heard? Are these messages ambivalent, negative, or positive? The nurse listens for themes and patterns of response that indicate how the patient views self. Does the patient verbalize disappointment with self? Does the patient describe his/her strengths and limitations? Patients with the diagnosis Impaired Social Interaction share an underlying fear of rejection. For a variety of reasons, repeated rejections in social situations can be generalized to all of the patient's interactions. Therefore the patient struggles with the inability to trust self and others. Other assessment questions include, What are the patient's beliefs about self and how do these influence interactions? Is the patient aware of his/her beliefs, values, ideals, goals, strengths, and limitations? Can the patient begin to view self more objectively? What is the potential for a positive self-regard?

VIII

In assessing the patient's perception of reality, the nurse can consider the following guide questions: Is the perception of reality accurate? Does the patient see options available? Are perceptions free from need distortion? Does the patient use defenses that cause need distortion? When does this happen? Does it occur in interaction with the nurse? Does the patient demonstrate social sensitivity toward others? Are conclusions about others free from need distortion? Does anxiety interfere with the ability to perceive accurately?

The nurse assesses interdependence by observing how a patient assumes responsibility for self in social interactions. A patient's sense of self may be so anxiety laden that it inhibits awareness of his/her beliefs, values, and standards. When this occurs, social interactions can become impaired. The patient is unable to maintain a clear boundary between self and the other. This inhibits the patient from viewing the other person as valued and separate and can promote excessive dependence. Because the sense of self is intertwined with anxiety and poor learning experiences, the patient doubts his/her empathic sensitivity to others. The patient may fear self-exposure and avoid relationships. Assessment questions include, Is the patient able to take responsibility for self in social situations? Can he/she make decisions and live by them? Is the patient able to respect his/her own rights and the rights of others? Can the patient give and receive in relationships? Can the patient make decisions according to his/her own internalized standards? What tolerance does the patient demonstrate in handling togetherness and individuality needs? Does the patient seem to borrow strength or a sense of self from others?

Assessment of objective data includes observing patient behavior such as discomfort in social situations or an inability to communicate or use interpersonal skills effectively. Objective data may be obtained from observations of the patient in a clinical setting, reports of significant others, or the patient's history. Assessment is important to establish patterns of patient limitations and strengths and define deficits that inhibit the patient from healthy functioning. Assessment provides a valid basis for the nurse to establish interventions that will enable the patient to attain specific goals. Assessment also provides an opportunity for the nurse to share with the patient the behavior observed so that both can understand the patient's perceived need. Assisting the patient in working mutually with the nurse toward therapeutic goals is in itself a measure to correct Impaired Social Interaction.

Nurses frequently encounter patients in many settings who are struggling with social interactions. For example, a patient with an unexpected illness may have stress that causes him to relate negatively with others. An adolescent in school may face an adjustment problem that disrupts his/her ability to interact effectively. Because nurses function in many settings, they must recognize the potential for Impaired Social Interaction so they can prevent actual impairment and provide a corrective learning experience to struggling persons. Sensitivity to cultural and familial factors is important in nursing assessment because cultural and family practices affect the beliefs, norms, and values the patient embraces.[8]

❖ **Defining Characteristics**[1,4,7]

The presence of the following defining characteristics indicates that the patient may be experiencing Impaired Social Interaction:

- Verbalized or observed discomfort in social situations
- Verbalized or observed inability to receive or communicate a satisfying sense of belonging, caring, interest, or shared history
- Observed use of unsuccessful social interaction behavior
- Dysfunctional interaction with peers, family, and/or others
- Family report of change in style or pattern of interaction
- Presence of a pattern of mild, moderate, or severe anxiety in social interactions
- Presence of a pattern of dependent behavior in social interactions
- Presence of a pattern of superficiality in relationships

VIII

❖ **Related Factors**[1,4,7]

The following related factors are associated with Impaired Social Interaction:

- Limited physical mobility
- Loss of body function
- Hearing or visual deficits
- Chronic Illness
- Terminal illness
- Self-concept disturbance
- Anxiety
- Altered thought process
- Absence of available significant others or peers
- Knowledge deficit about ways to enhance mutuality
- Communication barriers
- Therapeutic isolation
- Environmental barriers
- Sociocultural dissonance
- Language/cultural barriers

❖ **Related Medical/Psychiatric Diagnoses**[10]

The following are examples of related medical/psychiatric diagnoses for Impaired Social Interaction:

- Anxiety disorders
- Chronic physical illness
- Delusional (paranoid) disorder
- Mental retardation
- Mood disorders
- Neurological impairments
- Organic mental disorders
- Personality disorder
- Physical disabilities
- Psychoactive substance abuse disorder
- Schizophrenia
- Sensory impairments
- Somatoform disorders

NURSING DIAGNOSES

Examples of *specific* nursing diagnoses for Impaired Social Interaction are:

- Impaired Social Interaction related to negative self-feelings
- Impaired Social Interaction related to distorted perception of reality
- Impaired Social Interaction related to anxiety in social situations
- Impaired Social Interaction related to a pattern of dependent behavior in interactions

PLANNING AND IMPLEMENTATION WITH RATIONALE

Nursing interventions for patients with Impaired Social Interaction address three key areas: (1) developing a positive self-concept, (2) building social skills, and (3) establishing mutual relationships.

A five-level approach to facilitate growth toward a positive self-concept includes (1) self-awareness, (2) self-exploration, (3) self-evaluation, (4) realistic planning, and (5) commitment to action.[14] This approach intrinsically requires time for meeting with the patient on a regular basis. However, the effectiveness of short-term intervention involving a nurse-patient relationship is documented in recent literature.[2,3] Assisting a patient to become self-aware and to explore how self-perceptions influence social interaction can cause anxiety and perceptions of threat. *Support and acceptance must be included in nursing interventions to assist the patient to become calm and to enter into a working therapeutic relationship. Initially, the patient may require consistent, supportive feedback from the nurse to reduce anxiety and promote trust.*

The nurse must plan interventions that assist the patient in working through feelings and beliefs about self and in developing a positive self-concept. The nurse can help the patient examine feelings, behaviors, beliefs, and thoughts that relate to impaired interactions[9,14] and encourage the patient to express feelings. The nursing interventions must also focus on assisting the patient to determine the significance of his/her experiences, clarify perceptions of self and others, and explore his/her strengths and limitations. The nurse must support patient strengths while he/she aids in the improvement of limitations. As the patient becomes increasingly objective in viewing his/her situation, he/she may define goals, options, and planned change with the nurse's assistance. The nurse should support the patient's self-evaluation by dispelling erroneous thinking or irrational beliefs in a kind and gentle confrontation.[13] Finally, the nurse should support the patient's decision-making and goal-planning processes and positively reinforce any changes that the patient is

VIII

Text continues on p. 571.

❖ NURSING CARE GUIDELINES
Nursing Diagnosis: Impaired Social Interaction

Expected Patient Outcomes	Nursing Interventions
The patient will state self-strengths and self-limitations.	• Assist the patient to explore his/her strengths and limitations.
The patient will discuss feelings associated with perceived self-limitations.	• Identify nonverbals and expression of feelings of which the patient is not aware; support strengths and ability to act for self.
The patient will define goals for growth and personal change.	• Encourage involvement in goal setting and verbalize the patient's responsibility for working toward goals, focus on here and now, and have reasonable expectations for progress.
The patient will practice new behaviors and skills with nurse.	• Provide opportunity for the patient to practice new behaviors and skills.
The patient will test new behaviors in other situations.	• Promote use of new skills in other relationships. • Assess the patient's patterns of behavior and themes, seek mutual understanding with patient about deficits in social skills, and create a teaching plan for social skill development.
The patient will engage in role playing a situation that he/she perceives as difficult.	• Role play social interactions with the patient to promote and reinforce positive social skills.
The patient will demonstrate self-confidence by using new social skills in other relationships.	• Support the patient's growth and encourage use of skills in expanded social situations.
The patient will describe behavior used in social interactions that interferes with effective relationships.	• View the patient as an adult capable of self-determination and self-responsibility.
The patient will understand how patterns of behavior facilitate or inhibit social interactions.	• Express belief and hope that the patient is capable of change and help the patient to understand the dynamics of dependent, independent, and interdependent behaviors.
The patient will develop the ability to make decisions and to accept responsibility for decision making.	• Support the patient's decision-making process and identify alternatives and options not considered by the patient.

VIII

able to make. *These interventions are based on the rationale that beliefs about self and associated feelings can be explored and altered to promote adaptive change and growth.*

Deficits in social skills are revealed as the nurse assesses patient strengths and limitations; the patterns of behavior inhibiting the patient in social situations are thus discovered. After these deficits are identified, the nurse can assist the patient in recognizing and dealing with them. Effective social skills can be learned, practiced, and appropriately implemented.[9,11] Realistic goals for the patient guide the nurse's actions. Ideally, the patient should be involved to the degree possible in the goal-setting process. The nurse and patient should develop a plan in which social skills can be taught to the patient.[5] Within the nurse-patient relationship, social skills can be practiced. The nurse will observe patient use of social skills and assist him/her in considering other approaches to the interaction. Problem situations can also be role played with the nurse for problem solving, discussion, and practice. Often beneficial is the reversal of nurse and patient roles to assist the patient with learning new ways of interaction. *Role playing provides an experiential learning situation through which the patient gains understanding of his/her situation and develops a sense of competence. The patient's growth potential increases with the development of social skills.*

Supportive feedback and encouragement of effective social and interpersonal skills help the patient gain confidence and a sense of independence through the knowledge that he/she can act for the self. The nurse encourages the patient to participate in expanded areas of his/her interest and interaction.[5]

Establishing a mutual relationship with the nurse is one method for the patient to develop and learn how to maintain a new sense of self. The therapeutic nurse-patient relationship is based on the assumption that the process between nurse and patient is mutual and cooperative.[14] The nurse does not assume power for the patient; rather, the patient is viewed as an adult capable of self-care and self-direction.[5,12] *Understanding a patient's*

strengths, as well as his/her limitations, assists the nurse in supporting the patient's actions that build strength while addressing patterns of limitation.*

The patient is invited and encouraged to enter a mutual relationship with the nurse. The patient is supported to use the strengths that subsequently develop in other relationships. Interventions that promote mutuality in the therapeutic relationship include assisting the patient to observe patterns of behavior (dependent, independent, and interdependent) in relationships, describe and discuss feelings associated with the identified patterns of behavior, understand the dynamics of identified behaviors, choose to positively alter existing behaviors, make decisions, and accept responsibility. *The nurse's response must consistently convey respectful feedback and a belief in the patient's capacity for self-determination.*

Ideally, the nurse seeks supervision to assess the nurse's own position in the therapeutic relationship. *Supervision assists the nurse in maintaining a clear role with the patient so that excessive or insufficient interaction with the patient does not occur.* The nurse's consistent goal is to assist the patient to act for self while maintaining effective social relationships.

EVALUATION

Evaluation is ongoing throughout the therapeutic process. It is a mutual process shared by both the nurse and the patient. Ideally, the patient participates in the goal-setting process and can therefore help evaluate the outcomes. In the evaluation process, the nurse and patient refer back to goals and expected patient outcomes. Each shares his/her own evaluation of the outcome. From these separate evaluations, revisions are discussed and incorporated into the therapeutic plan. Evaluation sessions must be held regularly.

Specific outcomes can be evaluated by observing patterns of patient behavior and by patient self-report. The patient develops a capacity to monitor his/her anxiety and to take appropriate actions to promote effective social interaction. Interpersonal relationships are developed based on

VIII

trust and mutuality. The patient's sense of self strengthens to permit clarity regarding his/her position in relationships with appropriate use of social interaction skills. Self-awareness promotes a realistic appreciation of one's strengths and limitations, the capacity to define goals and to make decisions, and sufficient self-objectivity to evaluate one's actions in social interactions. The patient is better able to enter into mutual relationships with others through an increase in self-confidence and autonomy. This enables the patient to expand his/her participation in social relationships.

If outcomes are not achieved, the nurse must reassess the patient situation to determine what is inhibiting progress. Often supervision of the nurse by a colleague or a clinical nurse specialist is sufficient to reassess and analyze the clinical situation, and to determine appropriate nursing interventions that are congruent with the patient's needs. Staff planning conferences contribute toward the development of a nursing care plan carried out consistently by all nurses.

❖ CASE STUDY WITH PLAN OF CARE

Ms. Wendy T. is a 23-year-old single woman who arrived at a community mental health center because she was distracted and unable to concentrate, and experienced problems making decisions. Ms. T. described herself as "alone and lonely." She stated that she found making friends difficult, and she felt a lack of confidence in her ability to maintain relationships. She stated, "When I meet people, I feel uncomfortable and awkward. I am unable to talk to other people. I feel inadequate, so I try to leave." In her work situation, Ms. T. reported that she was having difficulty making decisions. She recently passed up a job promotion because "I could not decide what to do." Wendy described herself as quiet and shy since childhood. She lived with her family and only recently moved away from home to gain employment in the city. She stated that she did not feel prepared for life away from her family. She believes her loneliness interferes with her ability to make decisions. Ms. T. appeared shy and nonassertive in the initial interview and lacked self-confidence in her interactions with others. She was uncomfortable and communicated negative feelings about self. She requested assistance with her problem. The nurse made the nursing diagnosis Impaired Social Interaction related to negative self-feelings and perceived incompetence in relationships.

PLAN OF CARE FOR MS. WENDY T.

Nursing Diagnosis: Impaired Social Interaction related to negative self-feelings and perceived incompetence in relationships

Expected Patient Outcomes

Ms. T. will meet regularly with the nurse in a therapeutic one-on-one relationship.

Nursing Interventions

- Establish a contract providing guidelines for a one-on-one nurse-patient relationship.
- Mutually agree to times, frequency, and place for one-on-one sessions.
- Build a trusting relationship by communicating that Ms. T. is a person of worth and capable of change.
- Construct a family tree to assess and understand Ms. T.'s position in her family relationships and associated emotional responses to such relationships.
- Assess and appreciate family cultural background, mores, norms, and values.

Expected Patient Outcomes	**Nursing Interventions**
Ms. T. will develop self-understanding by describing perceptions of situations, including feelings, behaviors, and thoughts.	• Use empathic approach to help Ms. T. identify feelings. Observe and comment on verbal and nonverbal expressions of behavior in a supportive and respectful manner. • Encourage Ms. T. to identify feelings as they occur in discussion with nurse, to accept and understand feelings, and to talk feelings through with nurse. • Point out ways expression of feelings is avoided. • State hunches and conclusions about what Ms. T. is experiencing. Ask for feedback about this analysis.
Ms. T. will explore meaning of behavior and assess self-strengths, self-limitations, and deficits in social relationships.	• Assess Ms. T.'s strengths, limitations, and patterns of behavior. Listen for behavioral themes expressed in nurse-patient interaction. • Support strengths. As Ms. T. demonstrates readiness, share perceptions of behavior and respond empathically. • Assist Ms. T. in understanding the meaning of her behavior. Share knowledge and experiences to enhance understanding.
Ms. T. will evaluate how to develop effective social skills and set realistic goals to achieve desired change in behavior.	• Encourage goal-setting in realistic and achievable steps. • Support self-evaluation by affirming realistic goal-setting or by kind confrontation of erroneous thinking.
Ms. T. will develop a realistic plan to achieve goals and demonstrate willingness to take action.	• Support self-care activity and assist in evaluating changes in behavior that will promote effective relationships with others. Stress that Ms. T. has a mutual relationship with nurse. • Devise plan to teach social interaction skills and role play in practice experiences. • Encourage use of effective social skills in other relationships. Refer to young adult groups, and support the patient to build a social network.

VIII

REFERENCES

1. Carpenito LJ: *Handbook of nursing diagnoses,* ed 4, Philadelphia, 1991, JB Lippincott.
2. Carr V, Farran CJ, and Maxson E: Development of a model for short-term psychiatric hospitalization, *Arch Psychiatric Nurs* 2:153-158, 1988.
3. Farran CJ, Carr V, and Maxson E: Goal-related behaviors in short-term psychiatric hospitalization, *Arch Psychiatric Nurs* 2:159-164, 1988.
4. Gordon M: *Manual of nursing diagnosis: 1991-1992,* St Louis, 1991, Mosby–Year Book.
5. Haber J, Hoskins P, Leach A, and Sideleau B: *Comprehensive psychiatric nursing,* ed 3, New York, 1987, McGraw Hill Book Company.
6. Jahoda M: *Current concepts of positive mental health,* New York, 1958, Basic Books.
7. Kim MJ, McFarland GK, and McLane AM: *Pocket guide to nursing diagnoses,* ed 4, St Louis, 1991, Mosby–Year Book.
8. Leininger M: Leininger's theory of nursing: cultural care diversity and universality, *Nurs Sci Quart* 4:152-160, 1988.
9. Manderino MA, Bzdek VM: Mobilizing depressed clients, *J Psychosoc Nurs Ment Health Serv* 24(5):23-28, 1986.
10. McFarland GK, Thomas MD: *Psychiatric mental health nursing: application of the nursing process,* Philadelphia, 1991, JB Lippincott.
11. Morris MM, Myton CL: Ego function: enhancement through social interaction, *J Psychosoc Nurs Ment Health Serv* 24(12):17-22, 1986.
12. Orem D: *Nursing concepts of practice,* ed 4, St Louis, 1990, Mosby–Year Book.
13. Sideleau BF: Irrational beliefs and interventions, *J Psychosoc Nurs Ment Health Serv* 25(3):18-24, 1987.
14. Stuart GW, Sundeen SJ: *Principles and practice of psychiatric nursing,* ed 4, St Louis, 1991, Mosby–Year Book.

Altered Role Performance

***Altered Role Performance** is a disruption in role functioning, e.g., inadequate role transition, role distance, role conflict, or role failure, as perceived by self and others.*

OVERVIEW

The social context of life and living requires that each person function in a variety of roles. Each role is characterized by a set of behaviors that guide interactions and transactions involving the self and others. Roles are influenced by social forces, norms, and values that affect conduct in a given situation, society, or culture. A basic principle is that any role held by an individual will have a relationship to roles held by others. Some roles are more clearly defined and enacted in circumscribed, time-limited situations, such as tennis player. Others, such as father, are more diffuse and change with growth and development, family structure, and general shifts in social norms and values.[10]

Roles and role performance are learned and acquired. The functionalists view roles as persisting over time in any given society, with socialization guiding role development with positive and negative reinforcements. On the other hand, the interactionists see society as a framework within which people interact dynamically. Each person is simultaneously involved in interpreting another's behavior and constructing responses based on perceived cues, such as expectations, feelings, and beliefs, transmitted in the interaction.[2] Together these two perspectives explain major forces that contribute to persistent general expectations for role behavior as well as those influences that individualize role performance and give rise to change.

In nursing, it is important to understand how social roles develop and evolve because they influence a sense of well-being in the person as well as influence life goals and health. Roles give meaning and value to life and foster a sense of belonging and contributing within society. Roles are action and interaction oriented and can be viewed as motivating forces in stimulating biopsychosocial integrity. Roles are associated with shared beliefs and values, and with personal likes or dislikes about social behavior, and they are an integral part of the self-concept.[9] Nurses, in recognizing the significance of role performance and its relevance to health, can promote learning and coping when patients encounter role changes.

The various roles an individual performs can be classified as *primary, secondary,* or *tertiary.*[10] *Primary roles* are based on sex and relate to age and to stages in the developmental process. The individual rarely has a choice in being male or female and is expected to perform according to his/her developmental stage; for example, being in the social position of child. Social norms and expectations shape primary roles, and role behavior must meet generally recognized social standards. Transitional life stages such as preadolescence, characterized by expected changes in age-related role behavior, are stressful and confusing as the individual experiences ambiguities and conflicts.[12] Children and families may require professional guidance during transitional periods of development.

Secondary roles have an element of choice and tend to be task oriented to meet certain functions associated with life stages; for example, the role of husband/wife or father/mother. Other secondary roles are based on achieved positions such as

VIII

574

being a teacher. These roles relate to work or occupations that require specified skills and knowledge for role competence and are instrumental in providing sustenance for self and others. Roles in general have an affective component in that they meet personal ambitions for success and recognition and give meaning and satisfaction to life and living. Life circumstances may require changes. The experience of role loss or role acquisition can be traumatic, with the grieving process resulting from role loss. Or the person may need to learn new sets of behaviors with associated feelings of uncertainty, anxiety, and insecurities about role expectations. Because secondary roles have an element of choice and usually persist over long periods of time, individuals invest personal energies that are achievement oriented to yield material rewards and personal growth and satisfaction. When life changes occur, such as promotion, unemployment, marriage, divorce, or illness, the individual must master significant role changes and may require professional services to promote healthful adjustment.

The third category of roles, *tertiary roles,* is more transitory. These tend to be associated with responsibilities or obligations taken on by choice for a limited period of time; e.g., being president of a club. Tertiary roles are often linked to secondary roles. When such a role is changed or lost, considerable stress can occur, affecting other roles and possibly leading to negative self-perception.

A number of conditions influence each role as it is learned, acquired, or maintained. Goals designated to meet perceived expectations, social rewards, or other personal gains direct role behavior. Role performance requires a set of circumstances such as artifacts, tools, or designated space. Further, any role requires the participation of others to complement and facilitate role performance. Added to external circumstances are feelings of success and accomplishment based on immediate feedback or known recognition by others. There are also feelings of confidence that certain external circumstances can lead to success and

that others are interested and willing to offer support, thus making the performance worthwhile. If circumstances do not facilitate role performance, conflicts, insecurities, and role failure may arise, resulting in disturbance of role performance. Felt obligations and perceived expectations are powerful forces that constantly shape, guide, and give purpose to role behavior. Thus the circumstances of illness or altered health may create stressful changes in roles and role-determined relationships.

In a multicultural society such as that of North America, cultural attitudes, values, and beliefs may prescribe role behavior that can be quite different for similar social positions.[2] To expect role sharing in case of illness or disability may not be acceptable or compatible with the existing belief system and ethnic orientation. The secondary role of husband/wife or parent/child may have cultural sanctions or taboos that regulate behavior during childbirth or at times of death. For example, a Vietnamese family may not be able to provide home care for an aging mother with a terminal cancer, because their duty would be to keep doors and windows open at all times regardless of the severe winter coldness. Similarly a Jewish husband may not be able to coach his wife during labor and delivery, because at that time he must attend to certain religious practices associated with birth. Cultural and religious beliefs and practices have a strong influence on role performance and must be recognized when role functions are threatened by illness and when the health care system is organized and dominated by majority rules and standards for role performance.

Altered Role Performance can be described as four types, each involving stress: *altered role transition, role distance, role conflict,* and *role failure.*[8]

Role transition occurs in developing new roles or when existing roles change because of altered circumstances that affect role behavior. Developmental crises occur when growth and maturation bring about changes in capabilities and expectations for roles and role mastery and the individual is not prepared to cope with or cannot cope with the experienced changes. Developmental periods of role transition usually are anticipated, but the guidance for role mastery may be insufficient or inadequate or expectations may be unrealistic. Altered Role Performance can then occur.

An individual may have adequate role behavior (for example, in mothering an infant), but when this role behavior differs from socially prescribed expectations, this is described as role distance.

One of the more common alterations in role performance arises in role conflict. Conflict can arise when expectations for role performance are incompatible or incongruent within a certain role. This situation would be considered intrarole conflict. Another type of intrarole conflict can arise when role expectations are incongruent with beliefs and values the individual holds. Other sources of role conflict the individual can encounter are incompatibility or incongruity, between different roles that a person occupies.[2] Such role stress is defined as interrole conflict. In these situations the person cannot meet certain role expectations for one role, because another role requires behaviors that are incompatible or incongruous with the other role.

In role failure, there is evidence of absence or ineffectiveness in performing the functions of a role or in experiencing role satisfaction. Failures in secondary roles are usually more serious, because important life goals may be threatened. However, failure in any role may be very stressful to the individual experiencing it. Many reasons may exist for role failure. The person's ability to function in a given role may change when injuries or illness (including mental illness) impose limitations or when age-related factors indicate a lack of maturity in younger years and limitations in senior years. Conditions in the environment may also change, resulting in a lack of resources, support, or even purpose for a given role. Roles may be vaguely defined or ambiguous, leading to uncertainty and confusion about role expectations, which contribute to perceived role failure. Inability to function in a role as a result of illness or disability may require relinquishing a valued role, and role loss may be experienced.

ASSESSMENT

Changes in health status or transitional periods of development are likely to affect role performance. As the ability to perform a given role is altered or if the individual cannot meet expectations for role performance, role stress arises and he/she will experience role strain.[2] This strain can further compromise the individual's ability to cope with physical and mental illness or with developmental expectations. Family members often assume the caregiver role affecting role functions within the family. Caregivers may experience considerable role strain during family illness or when disability occurs in the family.[11] What changes in role functions have occurred and how are caregivers coping with these? The patient's physical condition, the age of the caregiver, the health of the caregiver, family commitments, and loss of work (income) can be important causes of caregiver stress.[1]

Assessment requires knowledge about the significance of role performance in the self-concept as well as knowledge about the person's perceived health and well-being. Knowledge is also needed about what to expect in terms of cultural beliefs, social norms, and the individual's life stage, level of development, and actual role performance. In the assessment process, the nurse must consider ethnic and cultural beliefs, values, and norms. These can play a significant part in the perceptions of role ambiguities and associated stresses.[3] For example, an Italian mother insists on feeding her convalescent child pasta, when the child is on a medical regimen at home requiring a modified diet. Assessment must include the mother's knowledge base, her values and beliefs, and her perception of her care-provider role in this new context. The presence of defining characteristics of inadequate role performance must be determined.

Assessment requires effective interactive skills to elicit the nature of what the patient is experiencing related to personal perceptions of how role performance is affected and what this means for attainment of life goals or personal ambitions. The nurse who offers an opportunity to discuss the patient's primary, secondary, and tertiary

VIII

roles will convey (1) an interest in role performance, (2) a holistic approach to the patient's life situation, and (3) an understanding of expressed views or concerns. In clarifying role perceptions with the patient, the nurse can determine the hierarchy of importance of secondary and tertiary roles as perceived by the patient. Apart from eliciting information about role perception from the patient, the nurse may also have an opportunity to observe role behavior in certain situations.

The nurse must assess role transition, role distance, role conflict, and role failure. In relation to role transition, for example, during the early teen years a transition from childhood to adolescence is expected. The secondary role of becoming a high school student and making decisions about participation in certain sports, such as playing hockey, a tertiary role, require supportive circumstances from peers and guidance from teachers and parents. Assessment must consider whether the individual has completed previous studies at primary school, indicating readiness to cope with a higher level of education. In case of enrollment in sports, the nurse needs to assess the student's previous experience and his/her physical abilities along with access to sports activities, time schedules, needed equipment, and parental supports. Focusing on how the student perceives encountered role changes is important; for example: "Now that you are in high school, do you see that the way you used to learn is different? In what ways? What makes being in high school fun? How do you think the others in your class want you to behave? What about the teachers? What do they expect?" Such questions can determine whether the student has a sense of orientation to the changed role and is coping to make needed adjustments. Or the nurse may find that the student has fears and unrealistic perceptions based on a lack of preparation or knowledge.

How a woman perceives and performs her role as a mother caring for an infant may satisfy the infant's and the mother's needs. However, the expectations for how the infant ought to be "mothered" based on prescribed cultural/social norms are different. The mother may swaddle her infant, yet the cultural norm prescribes freedom of movement as a developmental prerequisite. Thus the mother will experience role strain when her behavior meets with disapproval and she receives instruction to change her way of caring for the infant. The nurse can assess role distance by observing role functions and by questioning role perceptions. When both functions and perceptions differ from prescribed norms, the nurse can make a diagnosis of Altered Role Performance (role distance).

In relation to role conflict, if, for example, a teacher is expected to regularly attend afternoon meetings of the teachers' association and also is expected to supervise students during afternoon sports activities, conflict will result because these two expectations are incompatible. Assessment will need to identify the kinds of expectations exerted on role behavior and how and why conflict arises. The individual teacher may experience conflict, because he/she is unaware of regulations or policies that could resolve the conflict, or the teacher may lack problem-solving skills that can meet both responsibilities—attending meetings and supervising students. A nurse working in a hospital is expected to care for patients admitted for induced abortions. The nurse knows that such patients require supportive nursing care, yet the nurse might find abortions to be unacceptable on moral grounds. This nurse will experience conflict related to a personal belief that is perceived as incongruent with expected role functions. Assessment will need to focus on identifying the nature of the conflict and on exploring how the person is trying to cope with the experienced role strain. Coping may be inadequate if it is characterized by avoiding expected role functions. The nurse may have somatic complaints such as headaches which may be evidence of subconscious avoidance that does not deal with the sources of conflict. The nurse may lack problem-solving skills in seeking alternatives for satisfactory role performance. The nurse in the intrarole conflict situation above could seek to work on a unit where he/she will not encounter abortion cases. During acute or chronic illness, the patient role may be in conflict with many other roles the person holds.

Assessment will need to center on eliciting the

VIII

patient's perceptions of role expectations for secondary and tertiary roles. As different roles are discussed, the nurse needs to listen for evidence of experienced role strain. Expressions such as "I want to be a good mother/father and a good teacher, but it does not seem to work" or "Having to stick to my diabetic diet will never work when I am back in my business" may indicate frustration and possible role conflict. To determine the person's ability to function in a variety of roles, the nurse may need to assess the patient's level of knowledge about available alternatives and problem-solving skills for conflict resolution.

The nurse must assess role failure and its causes. For example, the college student may fail to perform in the student role because of a reading disability, immaturity, lack of support, or lack of a goal for studies.

Characteristic behaviors may be expressed as dissatisfactions with a role, for example: "I do not like being a mother" or "I do not wish to return to my job as secretary." The patient (a mother) may be observed as performing role expectations ineffectively, for example, feeding/diapering the infant improperly. If she neglects the infant this may indicate absence of expected mothering behavior. Patients may express their felt inadequacies as "I am no good at this" or "I can never learn to do this right." The patient may express felt confusion and ambiguity about role performance in statements such as "My mother told me to lie down when breast-feeding, and now you tell me to sit up when breast-feeding. How am I supposed to know what is right?" Questioning the patient about role expectations may reveal a lack of knowledge about role functions. Assessment also should focus on needed equipment, social supports, and environmental factors that promote comfort when role functions are performed. The mother may fail in breast-feeding if her husband does not approve of this function or if she has no role model for learning. To assess adequacy or inadequacy for a given role, a checklist of role ex-

pectations can be developed and can assist the nurse in conducting a comprehensive assessment of role performance.

❖ Defining Characteristics[4]

The presence of the following defining characteristics indicates that the patient may be experiencing Altered Role Performance:

Role transition
- Feelings of anger or depression
- Change in usual pattern of responsibility
- Change in capacity to perform role
- Inability to achieve desired role
- Refusal to participate in role
- Change in others' perception or expectations of role

Role distance
- Uncertainty about role requirement
- Lack of knowledge of role
- Different role perceptions

Role conflict
- Confusion
- Frustration in role (intrarole or interrole conflict)
- Ambivalence about role
- Inadequate problem-solving skills
- Incongruent, incompatible role expectations

Role failure
- Withdrawal
- Loss of role skills
- Inability to achieve desired role
- Refusal to participate in role
- Difficulty in learning new role

❖ Related Factors

The following related factors are associated with Altered Role Performance:
- Physical illness
- Decline in physical strength/ability
- Alcohol or drug abuse
- Mental retardation
- Cognitive difficulties
- Low self-concept
- Developmental crisis
- Severe stress during change in occupation
- Inability to deal with changed expectations in new role
- Role incompatibility
- Lack of adequate role model
- Role ambiguity, incongruity

- Inability to learn new role requirements
- Inadequate social support
- Inadequate resources
- Very frustrating social situations
- Cultural transition

❖ **Related Medical/Psychiatric Diagnoses**

The following are examples of related medical/psychiatric diagnoses for Altered Role Performance:

- AIDS
- Alzheimer's disease
- Bipolar disorders
- Cerebrovascular accident
- Chronic obstructive pulmonary disease
- Congenital heart disease
- Degenerative disorders, e.g., multiple sclerosis
- Depressive disorders
- Mental retardation
- Myocardial infarction
- Organic substance disorder
- Paranoia
- Schizophrenia
- Sensory organ impairment, e.g., blindness, deafness
- Severe osteoporosis
- Trauma, e.g., fractures, burns

NURSING DIAGNOSES

Examples of *specific* nursing diagnoses for Altered Role Performance are:

- Altered Role Performance related to inadequate social support
- Altered Role Performance related to lack of role model
- Altered Role Performance related to low self-concept
- Altered Role Performance related to alcoholism

PLANNING AND IMPLEMENTATION WITH RATIONALE

Nursing interventions for Altered Role Performance are individualized for each patient situation. The type of alteration, the evident characteristics, and related factors will determine nursing actions that can enhance role performance and/or reduce stresses associated with experienced role strain. In setting goals for desired role mastery or required role changes, the patient, significant others, and the nurse are mutually involved in the planning process. It is the patient who has to attain perceived satisfaction in role adjustments to meet personal goals, ambitions, and/or social expectations.

Inadequate Role Transition

The experience of stressful role transition may occur during developmental stages or when life events, such as illness or disability, require role changes. The patient is expected to relinquish previous role behavior and/or to master new role behavior. So that they can develop realistic goals for adjustment, the nurse and patient may need to explore *the patient's perceptions of what has changed and how this change is affecting different roles*. The nurse can assist the patient in identifying losses of previously held and valued role functions, with a focus on why these are no longer feasible related to altered capabilities or changes in life situation. *In determining the type of role that is changed and its importance to the patient, the nurse can anticipate a grieving response. Grieving requires expression and resolution before the person can recognize the need for a new role and direct energies toward learning. Encouraging expression of emotions and verbalization of perceived losses will facilitate grieving.*[5] The patient may require information about changed capacity as well as role options available for consideration. For example, a letter carrier with a hip disorder may need to understand how the decreased walking capacity affects the current role and may need to know that letter sorting is a possible alternative in employment. The nurse can encourage the patient to seek needed information and to explore options.

Anticipating life stages and associated roles, such as becoming a mother or reaching retirement age, will focus nursing interventions on anticipatory guidance and preparatory teaching. Prenatal classes provide a group setting for discussion of expectations regarding infant care and demands of

VIII

time and energy for the mothering role. Nurses as group leaders can facilitate expression of concerns and give direction to focus discussion on known expectations, norms, and values related to the role. The community nurse may suggest group sessions for older people nearing retirement age or offer counseling regarding assessment of capabilities and interests and encourage development of new and meaningful secondary or tertiary roles. *Anticipatory guidance and preparatory teaching will facilitate role transition and can prevent stresses when role changes do take place. Both knowledge and skill serve to enhance confidence in role perception and mastery in role performance.*

Because roles are interdependent and complementary, significant others may need assistance to focus on their functions in clarifying role behaviors and expectations when patients experience role transitions. For example, the roles of husband and wife are complementary. With the experience of a myocardial infarction, both roles require adjustments and clarification.[7] *By assisting expression of altered role perceptions and possible role strain as well as by facilitating clarification of expectations for complementary role functions, the nurse can offer guidance and reduce or prevent role insufficiency.* The nurse can encourage significant others to communicate recognition of desired role behavior. To provide reinforcement. The nurse can support them in their efforts to discuss anticipated behaviors, sentiments, sensations, and goals involved in the patient's role change and their own complementary functions. *Increased role awareness and effective communication will facilitate role transitions.*

Role Distance

When Altered Role Performance is recognized as role distance, nursing interventions will be designed to reduce or alleviate role distance. *Because the patient may not be aware that role functions differ from expected cultural or social norms, the nursing approach will need to focus on clarifying perceptions and fostering awareness of prevailing expectations. Because cultural beliefs and values can play a significant part in the patient's orientation toward a given role such as mothering, the nurse must make an effort to understand the patient's value system. To do this the nurse explores the reasoning and perceptions associated with the observed role function, such as the previously mentioned swaddling of the infant. By showing respect for the practice in its cultural context, the nurse can then guide the patient into discussing and comparing traditions of the past with current methods of infant care and their rationale.*

Another example of role distance occurs when a mother of a premature infant treats the infant as, and expects the infant to behave as, a normal full-term infant. The nurse may need to focus first on the mother's wish to perceive her infant as full term to avoid her felt disappointment. *When the nurse shows acceptance of the mother's feelings and encourages expression of disappointment, the patient will achieve readiness to focus on the infant's actual needs and the mother's ability to meet those.* Teaching strategies may include role clarification with discussion of and information on role expectations, role modeling with demonstrations of handling the premature infant, and referral to reference groups of other parents with premature infants.[6] *Added knowledge and skill can reduce role distance.*

Role Conflict

When role conflicts are encountered, resolution of conflict becomes the expected patient outcome for planned nursing interventions. As a first step, conflict situations require a thorough exploration of the type of conflict the patient experienced. *The patient needs to recognize sources of stress to determine incompatibility or incongruities causing conflict.* As nurse and patient together identify conflicting expectations, perceptions can be clarified, rectified, or reinforced. For example, the teacher experiencing intrarole conflict can be advised to plan with colleagues for sharing of responsibilities in the supervision of sports activities and in attending association meetings. *Mutual efforts and a compromise may allow for time to* meet with role-related activities and thus reduce frustrations arising from a felt conflict.

For interrole conflicts, the nurse can assist the patient in assessing the felt demands on time and efforts in relation to both roles. *Supportive guidance may help the patient to recognize priorities in relation to felt ambitions or desired goals for role performance.* For example, the mothering role requiring playtime with children may be assigned priority over the teaching role requiring "extra time" for pupils. Reflective counseling can help the patient in accepting differences in role perception, thus reducing felt strain about conflicts.

Incompatibilities and incongruities about roles may require joint family or group meetings in which the nurse can facilitate discussion and exploration of conflicts and assist the group in clarifying mutual expectations. *Verbalization of felt strain and experienced stress can foster mutual understanding, acceptance, and goal setting for resolution of experienced conflict. As the nurse facilitates open communication among all participants in role sets, they learn to solve problems and become prepared to prevent or resolve future role conflicts.*[13]

Role Failure

In role failure planned interventions will address the lack of knowledge and skills for a given role and assist the patient to achieve satisfactory role competence. *Reasons for the patient's inability to meet role expectations must be explored and mutually acknowledged so that realistic learning goals can be developed.* Assessing the patient's readiness to learn and setting mutually acceptable goals are prerequisites for all teaching strategies. Role failure implies that the patient has tried to achieve a role and has not succeeded or that the patient's ability or health status has changed, resulting in role failure. The patient is most likely feeling disappointment and distress. *Facilitating expression of these feelings and also recognizing strengths and abilities that the patient possesses for the desired role can mobilize confidence and energies for the learning task.*

A *jointly developed list of tasks for expected role performance (for example, mothering an infant) may provide guidance for focusing on definable tasks and the associated knowledge and skills. By discussing each task (for example, feeding an infant) the nurse can assess and reinforce existing knowledge and provide additional information.* The nurse can demonstrate how to hold the infant for spoon-feeding while he/she discusses position and utensils that facilitate the feeding process. *Because many role functions cannot be fully described because they involve social interactions, role modeling becomes an important teaching strategy. Using opportunities to model interaction with the infant may stimulate the mother to interact likewise. Interpreting the infant's behavior may sensitize the mother in recognizing the cues the infant gives for her behavior.* The nurse also should seek every opportunity for praising the mother's efforts and effectiveness in appropriate role behavior. *Recognition and praise provide reinforcement of learning and build confidence and competence in role performance.*

When role failure is related to a change in ability to meet expectations, the nurse may assist the patient and others within the role set to examine whether modifications in role performance are feasible and acceptable to all concerned. For example, a teacher with early Alzheimer's disease may be able to perform selected teaching responsibilities with small groups or individual students while avoiding large groups and public speaking responsibilities.

The nurse also can use role rehearsal as a teaching strategy. *This approach allows the patient to anticipate role behaviors and sentiments and to try out behaviors that can correct previously identified inadequacies in an imaginary role play without actual pressures or obligations for role performance.*[14] The nurse can act as the designated role partner to provide the patient with responses and cues for experimental learning. This teaching strategy may be particularly useful in working with teenagers who fail to assume an appropriate student role or with parents who fail to

❖ NURSING CARE GUIDELINES
Nursing Diagnosis: Altered Role Performance

Expected Patient Outcomes	Nursing Interventions
The patient will experience less stressful role transition as evidenced by: verbalizing role loss and expressing satisfaction about functioning in a changed or new role and demonstrating appropriate knowledge and skill for role mastery.	• Assist the patient in identifying role loss or change. • Facilitate grieving response to experienced role loss. • Inform the patient about altered functional capacity and how it affects the role performance. • Explore available options for role change or adjustments. • Offer anticipatory guidance for life-stage role transitions.
The patient will demonstrate reduced or alleviated role distance as evidenced by: expression of awareness and ability to meet role expectations.	• Explore and clarify perceptions of role performance. • Show respect for existing belief systems and values that support role expectations. • Demonstrate role behaviors that patient needs to learn. • Make referral to appropriate reference group.
The patient will demonstrate resolution of role conflict as evidenced by: reduced stress and frustration and verbalization of a resolution of role conflicts.	• Assist the patient in exploring encountered role conflict and in identifying sources of stress. • Offer clarification and rectify misunderstandings. • Assist the patient in reaching a compromise if necessary. • Offer supportive guidance for determining priorities. • Suggest family or group meetings to clarify conflicting role expectations. • Foster effective communication and problem-solving skills.
The patient will resolve role failure as evidenced by satisfactory role competence.	• Assist in identifying reasons for role failure. • Teach the patient knowledge and skills by using role modeling and role rehearsal. • Involve others in clarifying expectations and giving feedback. • Offer praise for accomplishments. • Assess the patient's readiness to learn required role functions. • Facilitate expression of disappointment about encountered failure. • Assist the patient in recognizing strengths and abilities.

VIII

work out their respective roles in raising children. In most cases of role failure the nurse can facilitate learning to overcome inadequacies. *The nurse's support and assistance can help the patient to gain satisfaction from competent role behavior.*

EVALUATION

Evaluation of the resolution of Altered Role Performance is ongoing and requires participation by the patient and significant others. Nurse and patient together assess which goals are met and the need for modifications. In case of role transition the patient relinquishes previous role behav-

ior and shows role mastery, with expressed satisfaction in accomplishing role expectations. In case of role distance the patient expresses awareness of role expectations and shows ability to assume expected role functions. In case of role conflict the patient identifies sources of conflict and engages self and others in problem-solving activities that set realistic priorities and/or find acceptable compromises for mutually satisfying role expectations. In case of role failure, the patient learns to perform role behaviors competently and expresses confidence and satisfaction about role attainment.

❖ *CASE STUDY WITH PLAN OF CARE*

Mrs. Mary M. was looking forward to the birth of her second child; however, in her thirty-second week of gestation she went into premature labor and gave birth to a son who weighed 1.9 kg. The infant was transferred to the neonatal intensive care unit (NICU). The medical diagnosis was prematurity, with a good prognosis for normal development. Mary made infrequent visits to the NICU. The nurse observed that she did not want to touch the infant. She was tearful during some visits and did not initiate questions about the infant's

care. She expressed, "He looks so tiny. How can I take care of him? He is so different from the way Susie was. I am afraid of him; he seems so fragile. He needs a lot of extra care and all these feedings!" Mary has a supportive husband and a 3-year-old daughter. Both are looking forward to having the baby at home. She considers herself a "good mother" for her daughter but has had no previous experience in caring for a premature infant. She was hoping to remain active in her career as a teacher by doing substitute teaching.

VIII

PLAN OF CARE FOR MRS. MARY M.

Nursing Diagnosis: Altered Role Performance (inadequate role transition) related to stressful and frustrating role changes encountered in mothering a premature infant

Expected Patient Outcomes	Nursing Interventions
Mrs. M. will experience less stressful role transition as evidenced by:	
Expressing grief and disappointment about loss of the expected mothering role	• Encourage regular visits to NICU and plan to stay with Mrs. M. during visits, making her feel welcome. • Facilitate expression of sadness and show acceptance of Mrs. M.'s disappointment. • Assist Mrs. M. in comparing her previous full-term child with the premature infant to identify similarities and differences in role expectations.
Engaging in learning to care for her premature infant.	• Introduce Mrs. M. to the equipment surrounding her infant; explain its function in assisting her infant to grow. • Allow time to observe and model the care giving, and simultaneously discuss and interpret the infant's behavioral cues.

Continued.

Expected Patient Outcomes	Nursing Interventions
	• Encourage gradual engagement in care tasks—diapering, feeding, comforting.
	• Explain the special needs of the infant.
	• Provide contact with other mothers who care for their infants in the NICU.
	• Offer praise for accomplished care and reflect on the infant's responses that indicate comfort and progressive growth.
Demonstrating confidence and satisfaction in mastery of her mothering role for the infant before he is discharged.	• Encourage visits by both parents and facilitate husband's involvement and positive reinforcement of mothering skills.
	• Provide opportunities to discuss concerns and provide information on the infant's anticipated progress and development.
	• Make referral to community nursing service for needed support or counseling after discharge.
	• Assist Mrs. M. to verbalize satisfaction and confidence in her mother role.

REFERENCES

1. Caradoc-Davies TH, Dixon GS: Stress in caregivers of elderly patients: the effect of an admission to a rehabilitation unit, *NZ Med J* 104:226-228, 1991.
2. Hardy ME, Conway ME: *Role theory: perspectives for health professionals,* New York, 1978, Appleton-Century-Crofts.
3. Hernandez GG: Not so benign neglect: researchers ignore ethnicity in defining family caregiver burden and recommending services, letters, *Gerontologist* 31(2):271-272, 1991.
4. Kim MJ, McFarland GK, and McLane AM: *Pocket guide to nursing diagnosis,* ed 4, St Louis, 1991, Mosby–Year Book.
5. McFarland GK, Wasli EL, Gerety EK: *Nursing diagnosis and process in psychiatric mental health nursing,* ed 2, Philadelphia, 1991, JB Lippincott.
6. Moorhead SA: Role supplementation. In Bulechek GM, McClosky JC: *Nursing interventions: treatment for nursing diagnosis,* Philadelphia, 1985, WB Saunders.
7. Musolf JM: Easing the impact of the family caregiver's role, *Rehab Nurs* 16(2):82-84, 1991.
8. Nuwayhid KA: Role transition, disturbance, and conflict. In Roy SC, Andrews HA: *The roy adaptation model, the definite statement,* Norwalk, Conn, 1991, Appleton & Lange.
9. Robertson SM: Self-concept disturbance. In McFarland GK, Thomas MD: *Psychiatric mental health nursing, application of the nursing process,* Philadelphia, 1991, JB Lippincott.
10. Roy SC, Andrews HA: *The roy adaptation model, the definite statement,* Norwalk Conn, 1991, Appleton & Lange.
11. Titler MG, Cohen MZ, and Craft MJ: Impact of adult critical care hospitalization: perceptions of patients, spouses, children, and nurses, *Heart Lung* 20(2):174-182, 1991.
12. Whiting SMA, Antai-Otong DJ: Development of the person. In Johnson BS: *Adaptation and growth psychiatric-mental health nursing,* ed 2, Philadelphia, 1989, JB Lippincott.
13. Whitlatch MS, Zarit SH, and von Eye A: Efficacy of interventions with caregivers: a reanalysis, *Gerontologist* 31(1):9-14, 1991.
14. Wistrom FE: Role playing, *J Psychosoc Nurs Ment Health Serv* 25:21, 1987.

Anticipatory Grieving

Dysfunctional Grieving

Anticipatory Grieving is the state in which an individual grieves before an actual loss.[14]

Dysfunctional Grieving is a maladaptive process that occurs when grief is intensified to the degree that the person is overwhelmed, becomes stuck in one phase of grieving, and demonstrates excessive or prolonged emotional responses to a significant loss.[6,14,18]

OVERVIEW

To be able to understand the meaning and significance of Anticipatory Grieving, as well as complicated or Dysfunctional Grieving, one must be familiar with the manifestations of normal, uncomplicated grief.[17,24] Normal grieving encompasses a range of feelings, moods, and behaviors that follow loss, the removal or departure of someone or something that was meaningful to the person; e.g., death of significant other, death of pet animal, loss of job, loss of home.

Normal grief includes feelings of sadness, anger, guilt and self-reproach, anxiety, loneliness, fatigue, helplessness, shock, yearning, emancipation, relief, and numbness, and there is nothing necessarily pathological about any of them.[29] The symptoms of normal grief include the syndrome of sensations of somatic distress that can occur in waves that last from 20 minutes to an hour at a time—feelings of tightness in the throat, choking, shortness of breath, sighing, empty feeling in the stomach, decreased muscular power, and subjective distress such as tension or mental pain.[18]

Four aspects of the process of normal grieving

that have been identified are shock and disbelief, developing awareness, restitution, and resolution of the loss.[6] Kubler-Ross[16] describes five aspects of Anticipatory Grieving: denial and isolation, anger, bargaining, depression, and acceptance. She states that these behaviors do not necessarily occur in sequential order and that the grieving process does not always include each of these aspects. Engel[6] describes patterns of loss that occur as a sequence of "psychological processes" in which there is the recognition of the loss, attempts to deal with it, and then the final resolution of the loss. Four tasks of mourning that must be accomplished to reestablish equilibrium and to complete the process of mourning after a significant loss are[29]: (1) to accept the reality of the loss; (2) to experience the pain of grief; (3) to adjust to an environment in which the deceased is missing; and, (4) to withdraw emotional energy and reinvest it in another relationship. Two years of mourning may not be unusual when a close relationship has been lost. The duration of a grief reaction seems to depend on the success with which a person does the grief work.[18] Kubler-Ross[16] cautions against the belief that stages are sequential or that an individual must experience each of them to achieve satisfactory resolution of loss.

Anticipatory Grieving refers to the grieving process that takes place before the actual experience of a loss. It is the response that occurs in preparation for the actual loss.[7] The nursing diagnosis Anticipatory Grieving is based on the timing of the grief.[21] Anticipatory grieving refers to a state in which an individual grieves before an actual loss.[14]

Any kind of change—physical, psychological, or social—may be perceived as a loss.[7] It is important to recognize that potential significant losses include loss of body part(s), function(s), or image or the impending loss of one's own life. Other potential losses include loss of a significant other because of geographical separation, change in marital status, or diagnosis of a terminal illness.[22] Bowlby[2] believes that the loss of a loved one is one of the most painful experiences of human suffering. Anticipatory Grieving also may occur with the perceived potential loss of a pet, prized material possession, or social role.[22]

Lindemann[18] recognized anticipatory grief as a response to separation when a family member left for military service. He described this anticipatory grief as a syndrome in which concern for adjustment after the potential death of a loved one is so great that the individual experiences the same process of grieving as though an actual death had occurred.

The experience of loss is a subjective one. The intensity of response to a potential loss is influenced by the meaning of the loss for the individual. The very same loss can be of great significance to one person and of little importance to another.[7] One's previous experiences with life-threatening illness, cultural and spiritual beliefs, and socioeconomic background are examples of factors that affect an individual's response to an anticipated loss.[7,30] Feelings, behaviors, and patterns of grief and mourning that occur during the experience of Anticipatory Grieving are somewhat similar to feelings, behaviors, and patterns that occur with normal grieving.[7]

Resolution and restitution of the losses associated with Anticipatory Grieving, however, are also somewhat different from the resolution and restitution that occur with normal grieving. Anticipatory Grieving that is related to terminal illness has a definitive end point—death, whereas post-loss grieving can be prolonged.[7] Another difference between the resolution of normal grieving and that of Anticipatory Grieving is that during

Anticipatory Grieving there can always exist some hope that action can be taken to prevent the significant loss. This is in contrast to the experience of normal grieving, in which action does not alter the fact that the loss has occurred. The terminally ill person who is experiencing Anticipatory Grieving does not reach a period of reestablishment, such as in normal grieving. Resolution occurs with the acceptance and recognition of impending death.[7,16]

Anticipatory Grieving may facilitate adjustment to the actual loss by lessening the intensity of grieving that is felt after the loss takes place.[7] Anticipatory Grieving related to the impending death of a significant other can allow for preparation to cope with grief and to begin to let go of a relationship. However, it has also been observed that Anticipatory Grieving intensifies attachment behaviors and that the actual death of a significant other is felt as a shock.[2,27] The repeated cycle of anticipatory grief may compromise the survivor's ability to cope effectively with the grieving process.

Shock and disbelief are characteristic behaviors during the period of recognizing the anticipated loss.[2,6] Denial is the most likely mental mechanism to occur at this time. Denial may be manifested by initial intellectual acceptance and by extremely appropriate behaviors. It also may manifest itself by overt attempts to block out factual information related to the loss. Kubler-Ross[16] sees this form of denial as a temporary defense that precedes partial acceptance.

Engel[6] describes the stage of developing awareness of loss as being characterized by feelings of acute sadness, anxiety, helplessness, and hopelessness. Tearfulness may accompany feelings of anguish and despair. Anger, bargaining, and depression, as described by Kubler-Ross[16] are likely to occur during this time.

Dysfunctional Grieving occurs when an individual has failed to proceed through the stages or phases of normal grieving in response to experiencing an actual or perceived object loss.[14] Avoidance of the intense distress and emotions associated with the grief experience is a major obstacle to the completion of grief work. Lindemann[18] used the term *morbid grief reactions* as representing distortions of normal grief.

The term *pathological grief* has been used to describe grief that has intensified to a degree at which the person is overwhelmed and resorts to maladaptive behavior. Or the person may remain interminably in the state of grieving without further progression of the mourning process toward its completion.[11] Pathological mourning refers to processes or behaviors that do not move progressively toward assimilation or accommodation. Instead they lead to stereotyped repetitions or extensive interruptions of healing.[11] Unresolved grief can be referred to as the clinical condition that can follow a loss of a significant person. This unresolved grief can be characterized by any one of three dimensions[17]: (1) inhibition, suppression, or absence of the grief process; (2) exaggeration or distortion of certain symptoms or behaviors that normally occur with grief; and, (3) prolongation of normal grieving. Other descriptions of dysfunctional grieving include the inability to attain the phase of acceptance, which is a necessary component for successful adaptation to loss. Dysfunctional Grieving may also be characterized by prolonged, excessive denial as well as prolonged depression. Dysfunctional Grieving can lead to mental illness, especially clinical depression.[22]

ASSESSMENT

The perceived potential loss of a significant object that is of value is the central related factor for understanding the response of *Anticipatory Grieving*. An understanding of loss assists in the assessment in cases of individuals who are anticipating the loss of an object or person that is of significance to them.

Assessment of *Anticipatory Grieving* includes the recognition that medical, surgical, and obstetrical diagnoses may represent perceived potential losses for both the identified patient and the patient's significant others. Diagnoses such as cancer, end-stage renal disease, coronary artery disease, myocardial infarction, chronic obstructive pulmonary disease, and diabetes may activate the process of Anticipatory Grieving because of the potential losses involved. Surgical interventions pose a threat to loss of body image, body functions, and life itself. Prenatal complications and fetal abnormalities also may be contributing factors in the experience of Anticipatory Grieving.

Defining characteristics of Anticipatory Grieving include the expression of distress with the recognition of the potential loss of a significant object.[14] The nurse should determine the patient's perception of strengths and weaknesses for coping with the perceived loss. It must be recognized that responses to the current situation are influenced by the individual's past experiences with loss, illness, and death. The nurse must be aware that past problem-solving abilities, socioeconomical and educational background, and cultural and spiritual beliefs also influence one's ability to cope with a potential loss.[7,20,28,30] How much time has elapsed since the individual learned of the potential loss? The behaviors during the interval of learning of the loss and the present time must be noted. Likewise, disruptions in the current lifestyle, such as finances, living arrangements, and transportation, that are related to the anticipated loss must be monitored. These disruptions may be affecting both the patient and significant others.[7,20]

Denial of the potential loss is a defining characteristic that occurs most frequently during the stage of shock and disbelief. This stage, which follows the recognition of the potential loss, is characterized by behaviors that are directed toward insulating and protecting the individual from the intensity of feelings that are generated by the anticipated loss.[6] Denial also may occur during later phases of the Anticipatory Grieving experience, and the patient's use of denial sometimes may be related to the use of denial by health care professionals.[16]

Ambivalence is another defining characteristic of Anticipatory Grieving.[7] During the early stages of Anticipatory Grieving, the element of hope that is held by significant others may be closely related to feelings of ambivalence toward the patient.

Sleep and appetite disturbances as well as changes in activity level and communication patterns may occur in both the patient and significant others. The stage of grieving that the patient and significant others are experiencing must be determined. The patient and significant others may differ in their stages of grieving.[7,20] Possible conflicts that may result from these differences should be noted.

The manifestations of grief are highly individual, and they include progression as well as regression in the attempt to achieve the realization of the anticipated loss as well as resolution of the anticipated loss.[25]

For *Dysfunctional Grieving,* initial assessment includes identification of the stage of grieving that the patient is currently experiencing. Are the defining characteristics of Dysfunctional Grieving present? Does the patient appear to be stuck in a particular phase of grieving?

It is important to obtain information about the causes and circumstances of the loss. The following questions should be addressed: When did the loss occur? What is the patient's perception of the loss? What is the patient's perception of adaptation to the loss? What are the responses of the patient's significant others? What is the patient's social network? Persons over 75 years of age are at greatest risk for a decrease in the social network, so assessment of actual or potential social resources is especially important.[19] What are the patient's past life experiences and past problem-solving skills?

Pollock[24] emphasizes that when adults, children, and adolescents have difficulties coping with the death of a significant other, it is necessary to obtain specific information about the loss and the specific circumstances surrounding the loss.

Inhibition, suppression, or absence of emotional reactions to a loss needs to be recognized. Lindemann[18] observed that difficulty in showing reactions to a loss sometimes occurs when an individual is forced to deal with important tasks re-

lated to the loss or when the individual initially helps to maintain the morale of others. Lazare[17] uses the phrase "the social role of the strong one" to describe people who assume the designated role of ignoring their own grieving needs in order to provide psychological support to others who are mourning. The absence of Anticipatory Grieving may be a related factor in the absence of emotional reactions to a loss.

Bowlby[2] believes that the avoidance of conscious grieving in response to the death of a significant other eventually results in some form of depression. Assessment for possible precipitants of this depression includes: (1) an anniversary of a death that has not been mourned; (2) another loss, of an apparent minor kind; (3) reaching the same age as the significant other who died; and (4) a loss suffered by a compulsively cared-for person with whose experience the failed mourner may be identifying.

Indicators of prolonged normal grieving, which may include the excessive reliving of past experiences, the feeling that the loss occurred yesterday, and general themes of loss, need to be assessed. Social factors that may contribute to Dysfunctional Grieving must likewise be assessed. Social negation of a loss may occur when an individual has an abortion or miscarriage and the experience has not been defined as a loss by members of the person's social network. Be aware of *socially unspeakable* losses, a defining term that is used to refer to losses that are mourned by the bereaved but are not seen as socially appropriate to discuss. Examples[15,17] of these kinds of losses include death by suicide, abortion, miscarriage, children lost to adoption and the death of an illicit lover.

Social isolation[8] is another factor that may contribute to Dysfunctional Grieving. Some precipitants of social isolation are geographical separation from significant others, a breakdown of the extended family, diminished importance of religious institutions, and the loss of an entire support system through death.

Excessive or distorted emotional reactions are an indication of Dysfunctional Grieving. Assess for extreme anger or hostility or prolonged or excessive denial. Severe hopelessness, excessive guilt, and self-blame may lead to suicidal ideation and intent.

Alterations in eating habits, sleep patterns, activity level, and libido are important to observe. Green[8] notes that increased illness in a previously well person may be indicative of Dysfunctional Grieving. Increased smoking and excessive alcohol consumption may also be indicators of bereavement difficulty. Although increased somatization is common among some ethnic groups, persistent somatic complaints may be indicative of the need for help.

Lazare[17] states that patients may complain of physical distress under the upper half of the sternum. The complaints are described as, "There is something stuck inside" or "I feel there is a demon inside of me." The nurse should recognize that a patient's refusal to follow a prescribed treatment regimen can indicate Dysfunctional Grieving.

Parental Dysfunctional Grieving processes and unconscious family maneuvers to alleviate guilt or to control fate can be contributing factors to unresolved grief in children.[18] Be aware that children may express a need for help in coping with loss by displaying aggressive or hostile behavior, problems in school performance, regressed behavior, and somatic complaints.[8]

Assessment of Dysfunctional Grieving includes consideration of the effect of the loss on the entire family system. Worden[29] believes that unresolved grief may be a key factor in family pathology and contribute to pathological relationships across the generations.

Anticipatory Grieving
❖ Defining Characteristics[14]

The presence of the following defining characteristics indicates that the patient may be experiencing Anticipatory Grieving:

- Expression of distress at the potential loss
- Disinterest or difficulty in carrying out activities of daily living
- Denial of potential loss: shock, disbelief, and avoidance of focus on loss
- Physiological symptoms: changes in eating habits, emptiness in stomach, choking sensation, or decreased muscular power
- Alterations in sleep patterns
- Alterations in activity level
- Altered libido
- Altered communication patterns
- Preoccupation with self
- Social withdrawal
- Anger
- Hostility or irritability toward others
- Guilt
- Self-accusation of negligence
- Feelings of loss and loneliness
- Sense of unreality
- Ambivalence
- Hope for preventing loss
- Realization or resolution of impending death or loss

❖ Related Factors

The following related factors are associated with Anticipatory Grieving[14,25]

- Perceived potential loss of significant object that is of value; e.g.,
  Physiophychosocial well-being
  Body part
  Body function(s)
  Impending death of self
  Significant other
  Social role
  Personal possessions
  Pet animal
  Griever's own physical health
- Griever's lifestyle (e.g., energy depletion, sleep, etc.)
- Unique meaning of loss to be experienced
- Nature of relationship and roles to be lost
- Degree of unfinished business
- Griever's coping skills
- Griever's ethnic, religious, cultural background
- Griever's fears about death
- Patient's attitude toward illness
- Patient's knowledge of illness
- Patient's ability to communicate
- Specific family characteristics (e.g., norms)
- Family strain

VIII

❖ **Related Medical/Psychiatric Diagnoses**

The following are examples of related medical/psychiatric diagnoses for Anticipatory Grieving:

- AIDS
- Anxiety disorder
- Carcinoma
- Chronic obstructive pulmonary disease
- Coronary artery disease
- Diabetes
- End-stage renal disease
- Mood disorder
- Myocardial infarction

Dysfunctional Grieving
❖ **Defining Characteristics**[2,8,11,14,15]

The presence of the following defining characteristics indicates that the patient may be experiencing Dysfunctional Grieving:

Inhibition, suppression, or absence of emotional reactions
- Difficulty expressing loss
- Delayed emotional reactions

Prolongation of normal grieving
- Excessive reliving of past experiences
- Interference with life functioning
- Prolonged alterations in concentration and/or pursuit of tasks
- Feeling that loss occurred only yesterday
- Unabated searching behavior for lost person or object
- Diminished participation in religious and ritual activities

Excessive or distorted emotional reactions
- Extreme anger or hostility
- Prolonged or excessive denial
- Developmental regression
- Extreme feelings of low self-esteem
- Severe feelings of identity loss
- Excessive idealization of dead person or lost object
- Excessive guilt and self-blame
- Suicidal ideation
- Severe hopelessness
- Prolonged panic attacks
- Prolonged depression
- Alterations in eating habits, sleep and dream patterns, activity level, or libido

Somatic expression of fear
- Choking sensations
- Difficulties in breathing

Other characteristics
- Somatic symptoms representing identification with the person who died
- Physical distress under upper half of sternum, accompanied by expressions such as "There's something stuck inside" and "I feel there's a demon in me"
- Recurrence of depressive symptoms and searching behavior on specific dates
- Refusal to follow prescribed treatment regimen

❖ **Related Factors**

The following related factors are associated with Dysfunctional Grieving[8,14,15,17,23,29]:

- Absence of anticipatory grieving
- Stressful and prolonged anticipated loss
- History of delayed or prolonged grief
- Loss of significant person, animal, or prized possession
- Negation of the loss by others
- Social isolation
- Assuming role of "the strong one"
- Uncertainty over the loss
- Loss of or change in significant social role
- Chronic mental or physical illness
- Inadequate social supports
- Loss of meaningful body function, part, or physiopsychosocial well-being
- Multiple losses, with unresolved grief
- Unexpected or sudden loss of significant other
- Secondary gains from grieving
- Overidentification or unfinished business with deceased
- Inability to attend to grieving because of other tasks
- Dysfunctional Grieving process exhibited by parents
- Unconscious family maneuvers to alleviate guilt or control fate
- Fear of the mourning process
- Socially unspeakable loss(es)

VIII

❖ Related Medical/Psychiatric Diagnoses

The following are examples of related medical/psychiatric diagnoses for Dysfunctional Grieving:

- AIDS
- Anxiety disorder
- Carcinoma
- Cerebrovascular accident
- Chronic obstructive pulmonary disease
- Congestive heart failure
- Coronary artery disease
- Mood disorder
- Schizophrenic disorder

NURSING DIAGNOSES

Examples of *specific* nursing diagnoses for Anticipatory Grieving are:

- Anticipatory Grieving related to perceived potential loss of body function
- Anticipatory Grieving related to perceived potential loss of significant other

Examples of *specific* nursing diagnoses for Dysfunctional Grieving are:

- Dysfunctional Grieving related to inadequate social supports
- Dysfunctional Grieving related to multiple losses with unresolved grief

PLANNING AND IMPLEMENTATION WITH RATIONALE
Anticipatory Grieving

Nursing interventions for patients and their significant others who are facing a potential loss must take into consideration the unique needs of each individual. The goal of nursing interventions for these people is to facilitate their participating in constructive anticipatory grief work.

Discussion of thoughts and feelings related to the perceived potential loss is one outcome that indicates that the patient and significant others are participating in constructive anticipatory grief work. People who anticipate a significant loss are in a state of crisis that is felt as a state of disequilibrium[1]; that is, they no longer experience a state of harmony, adjustment, or balance. Grieving spouses have emphasized the need to verbalize and ventilate their feelings. *Nursing interventions*

that encourage the patient and significant others to talk to the nurse about the meaning of the loss and to each other serve to decrease some of the anxiety that is associated with the crisis of the anticipated loss. Decreased anxiety enables those who are facing a potential loss to examine their current situation and to compare it with possible similar past experiences with which they coped successfully.[1] When patients and significant others are able to discuss their thoughts and feelings about the impending loss throughout the grieving process, they increase the likelihood of being able to integrate the positive and negative aspects of the perceived loss. It should be noted, however, that intense and prolonged anger can prolong a sense of meaninglessness about the death of a significant other, so monitoring the level of anger is very important.

The ability to make informed decisions is another component of constructive anticipatory grief work. People who are facing a potential loss also are confronted with decisions related to the loss. Avoid forcing the patient or significant others to make decisions. Focus on nursing interventions that facilitate exploration and discussion of available options. In some situations it is possible to provide the opportunity for people facing a potential loss to talk with others who already have experienced the loss or also are facing a future similar loss. *Sharing mutual concerns in a supportive setting can contribute to the process of making informed decisions.*[7]

Verbalization of information needs also contributes to constructive anticipatory grief work. Grieving spouses and families of terminally ill patients place a high priority on the need for ongoing information.[10] Nursing interventions that encourage the ongoing identification of information needs and avoid defensive and judgmental responses to criticisms of health care providers facilitate successful resolution of the grieving process.

Interventions that promote the use of appropriate resources are essential. Patients may initially overlook the resources within their own social

VIII

❖ *NURSING CARE GUIDELINES*
Nursing Diagnosis: Anticipatory Grieving

Expected Patient Outcomes	Nursing Interventions[5,7,25,28]
The patient will discuss thoughts and feelings related to the anticipated loss.	• Encourage the patient to describe perceptions of the potential loss and assist in understanding the reality of the impending loss • During the stage of shock and disbelief, provide a quiet and private environment for expression of emotions. • Assure the patient that it is normal to experience intense feelings and reactions. • Monitor intensity and duration of expressed anger as one means of screening for potential poor adjustment to loss. • During the stage of developing awareness, encourage the patient to discuss feelings with significant others. Be as informative as possible while being supportive. • Encourage the patient to reminisce and to explore the possible positive as well as negative aspects of the anticipated loss.
The patient will verbalize information needs on an ongoing basis.	• Encourage the patient to describe understanding of current health situation and to verbalize fears and concerns. • Avoid defensive and judgmental responses to criticisms directed at health care providers. • Recognize that information needs will continue during the period of mourning, as the patient begins to accept the reality of the impending loss.
The patient will make informed decisions.	• Do not force decisions. • Facilitate exploration and discussion of available options. • Provide opportunity for contact with others who have experienced or are anticipating a similar loss. • Assist in reality testing and in needed planning.
The patient will use appropriate resources.	• Facilitate exploration of available assistance from family, friends, clergy, and other community resources. • Encourage consideration of participation in groups with others who have experienced similar losses (e.g., ostomy groups, Reach for Recovery, I Can Cope). • Inform the patient and significant others of resources for financial assistance or for legal consultation.

network. For example, they may benefit from a suggestion to initiate contact with the clergy. *Referrals to support groups with others who are anticipating or have experienced a similar loss decrease the feelings of aloneness and isolation that*

may occur. The patient and significant others may be unaware of community resources that can assist with financial or legal problems related to the anticipated loss.

Maintaining constructive interpersonal relation-

❖ *NURSING CARE GUIDELINES—cont'd*

Expected Patient Outcomes	Nursing Interventions
The patient will maintain constructive interpersonal relationships.	• Acknowledge to the patient and significant others that the pattern of their past relationships with each other will be similar to their relationship with each other as they experience their anticipated loss. • Acknowledge to the patient and significant others that they may differ in the stage of grieving they are each experiencing. • Offer hope for their ability to cope with potential loss. • Encourage and teach the patient and significant others good health habits. • Foster an environment in which the loss can be experienced within a spiritual context.

ships is a crucial component for participating in constructive anticipatory grief work. It is helpful to acknowledge to the patient and significant others that their past patterns of relating with each other will be very similar to the way in which they continue to interact as they face the potential loss. *Interventions that offer hope that they will be able to cope with the impending loss promote the mobilization of coping strengths.*

The stressfulness of coping with the anticipated loss may cause the patient and significant others to overlook health practices that promote wellness. Nursing interventions that emphasize the importance of good health habits, such as adequate dietary intake, rest, and activity, are of particular value to the patient's significant others. *Health practices that promote a sense of well-being have a direct effect on one's ability to maintain constructive interpersonal relationships.*

The period of mourning may exacerbate feelings of helplessness in both the patient and significant others. *Interventions that encourage reminiscence and review of previous shared life experiences, as well as projections of what the future will be or is hoped to be, can lead to the anticipated loss being experienced within a spiritual context.*[3]

Dysfunctional Grieving

The overall goal for patients who are experiencing Dysfunctional Grieving is to facilitate the normal grieving process. Nursing interventions should be based on the unique needs of each individual patient.

Normal grief work includes working through the phases of normal grieving and acknowledging awareness of the loss that has occurred. *Assess the present stage of grieving to determine appropriate subsequent nursing interventions for assisting the patient to progress through the phase in which he or she is "stuck."* Keep in mind that stages in grieving are not necessarily sequential in their occurrence. There may be overlapping of phases as well as progression and regression. Encourage the patient to describe current objects that are of value as well as factual information that is related to the loss or losses the patient has or is experiencing. If the patient conveys feelings of guilt, convey reassurance that feelings of guilt are part of normal grieving.

Acknowledgment of awareness of the loss that has occurred is a component of normal grief work. *A question such as "What is your understanding of your current health situation?" fre-*

VIII

❖ *NURSING CARE GUIDELINES*

Nursing Diagnosis: Dysfunctional Grieving

Expected Patient Outcomes	Nursing Interventions*
The patient will work through phases of normal grieving.	• Assess the present stage of grieving, what aspect of normal grieving has yet to be completed, and barriers to the grieving process. • Assist the patient to progress through the phase in which there is a lack of progress. • Spend time with the patient, allowing for maximum opportunity to express feelings. • Encourage description of current objects of value or facts that are related to the loss. • Reassure the patient that feelings of guilt are part of normal grieving. • Be aware of times, such as holidays, when pain of grieving person maybe heightened.
The patient will acknowledge awareness of loss.	• Encourage the patient to describe perceptions of current adaptation. • Provide opportunity for description of experiences that preceded current loss. • Assess possible needs met by denial and observe for responses from health care providers that could be reinforcing maladaptive denial. • Point out reality in a nonthreatening manner without arguing with the patient or significant others. • Present the patient with increasing factual information. • Use guided visual imagery; e.g., conversing, or writing letter to deceased. • Use role play to reenact funeral if appropriate, in order to facilitate the normal grieving process.
The patient will demonstrate nonexcessive and nonprolonged emotional reactions.	• Encourage description of current and anticipated problems related to the loss. • Monitor for suicidal ideation/intent. • Permit open expression of feelings without becoming defensive and assist patient to understand possible reasons for these feelings. • Support verbalization of ambivalence and facilitate review of positive and negative aspects of the loss. • Point out universality of the need for normal grieving. • Evaluate the need for referral for brief psychodynamic psychotherapy.

*References 4, 9, 12, 12, 26, 29

❖ NURSING CARE GUIDELINES —*cont'd*

Expected Patient Outcomes	Nursing Interventions
The patient will participate in recommended treatment modalities.	• Evaluate the influence of denial on the patient's adherence to recommended treatments. • Defer teaching related to adaptation to loss until the patient demonstrates decreased denial. • Clarify factual information and correct misinformation about the loss. • Facilitate contact with others who have successfully adapted to a similar loss. • Offer hope for successful adaptation to the loss. • Encourage time for relaxation and rest to restore energy expended in the process of grieving.
The patient will develop goals that are congruent with the loss.	• Encourage description of future expectations. • Promote patient's recognition of past and present strengths that can be used for coping with the current loss. • Promote description of possible strategies for coping with the current loss. • Consider the use of role playing to facilitate the patient's awareness of possible alternatives and consequences of decisions. • Assist the patient in mobilizing his/her support system and identify replacements for void caused by death. • Evaluate the need for referral to resources such as family therapy. • Assist the patient and family to determine the nature of other currently occurring situational, developmental, or transitional stressors and to identify resources to deal with stressor. • Support the family's internal resources and strengths, such as the ability to work together to meet individual and group needs. • Assist the patient and family members to work through perception of the loss and develop positive meaning of loss if possible. • Promote the coordination of resources to help the patient develop new skills, make readjustments in lifestyle, and make new emotional investments. • Work with patient so that he/she can begin to meet own emotional needs. • Provide feedback about therapeutic process to patient and summarize realistic goals for future.

quently elicits useful information for assessing the extent to which a patient is able to acknowledge awareness of loss. Encourage the patient to describe his or her observations of current adaptation and experiences that led up to the current loss. Look for needs that may be met by denial, and be sure that health care providers are not inadvertently contributing to maladaptive denial. Gently point out reality by presenting increasing facts about the situation. Avoid arguments with the patient or significant others when there is a difference in perceptions of what has happened or is happening in relation to the loss.

The demonstration of nonexcessive and non-prolonged emotional reactions is an expected outcome for the patient who is experiencing Dysfunctional Grieving. Encourage the patient to describe current and anticipated problems that are related to the loss. *It is not uncommon for people who are experiencing excessive and prolonged emotional reactions to a loss to have suicidal ideation or intent. Therefore it is important to assess for suicidal thoughts or plans.* Permit an open expression of feelings without becoming defensive when these are actually expressed. Assist the patient to begin to understand possible reasons for these emotional responses. *Feelings of ambivalence may decrease when the patient is provided with an opportunity to discuss the positive and negative aspects of the loss that is being experienced. Recognize that a referral for brief psychodynamic therapy is sometimes indicated to assist in the resolution of excessive and prolonged emotional reactions.*

Participation in recommended treatment modalities is an outcome for patients whose Dysfunctional Grieving has included avoidance or noncompliance with a recommended treatment plan. It is important to evaluate the influence that denial may have on the patient's participation with recommended treatments. Defer teaching related to adaptation until there is evidence of a decrease in denial. *Sometimes the lack of adherence to proposed treatments is a result of the patient's lacking factual information about his/her loss. It may be necessary for the nurse to collaborate with other members of the health team to clarify factual information and to correct misinformation about the loss. Interventions that facilitate contact with others who have successfully adapted to a similar loss increase the likelihood of the patient participating in recommended treatment modalities.* Offering hope for successful adaptation can be a crucial nursing intervention at this time.

It is essential that the patient who has experienced Dysfunctional Grieving be able to develop goals that are congruent with the loss. *Nursing interventions that encourage description of future expectations and promote the patient's recognition of past and present coping strengths contribute to the patient's being able to develop goals that are congruent with the loss.* Encourage the patient to explore possible strategies for coping with the loss. Role playing can be a useful intervention for examining possible alternatives and consequences of tentative decisions. Referrals to resources such as support or self-help groups and referrals for family therapy may assist the patient to restructure his/her life in a constructive fashion. Nursing interventions that coordinate resources to help the patient develop new skills, make readjustments in lifestyle, and make new emotional investments also contribute to the patient being able to develop goals that are congruent with the loss.

EVALUATION

One indicator of the patient's participation in constructive *anticipatory grief* work is the ability to discuss thoughts and feelings related to the potential loss. The patient and significant others should also be verbalizing their information needs on an ongoing basis. Are the patient and significant others making informed decisions in relation to the potential loss? The ability to use appropriate resources and to maintain constructive interpersonal relationships is another indicator of participation in constructive anticipatory grief work and a healthy movement through anticipatory grief.

The patient should be experiencing less or no *Dysfunctional Grieving.* Is there an absence or reduction of the defining characteristics of Dysfunctional Grieving? Be sure that excessive, prolonged, distorted, or delayed emotional reactions are no longer present. The patient should be moving through the phases of normal grieving without spending an excessive time in any one phase.

VIII

❖ CASE STUDY WITH PLAN OF CARE

Mr. Max M. is a 51-year-old widowed man. He maintained an extremely stoic demeanor when he was admitted to the head and neck surgical service for a partial pharyngectomy and laryngectomy approximately 2 weeks after a diagnosis of squamous cell cancer was made. His preoperative evaluation included a speech pathology observation that he was an excellent candidate for using an electrolarynx. His postoperative treatment plan included a series of radiation treatments. Approximately 3 weeks before the conclusion of his radiation therapy, he began to avoid using the electrolarynx, stating that "Everybody I know who uses one of these makes themselves a complete bore." He resorted to using his note pad to communicate. Nurses observed him to be increasingly angry and impatient with various members of his treatment team. For example, one day he threw his electrolarynx at his speech pathologist. He walked slowly with his head held down. There was minimal eye contact, and he appeared to be reluctant to "open up" with staff and other patients. The patient has had non-insulin dependent diabetic disease for 15 years and a 20-year history of alcohol abuse but has been "dry" for 5 years. He has smoked one pack of cigarettes per day for 30 years. Mr. M. has worked in various aspects of radio broadcasting since the age of 21 years. Before admission, he was employed by a local station as a newscaster and part-time disc jockey. He has been a widower for 1 year, since his wife died suddenly of a myocardial infarction. His only daughter was killed in a car accident 5 years ago. The patient describes himself as somewhat of a loner since his wife's death. He is an agnostic with a personal philosophy of "enjoy life while you can." He enjoys model plane building, traveling, and playing golf.

PLAN OF CARE FOR MR. MAX M.

Nursing Diagnosis: *Dysfunctional Grieving related to absence of anticipatory grieving and actual loss of body part (larynx), prized possession (voice), and multiple previous losses*

Expected Patient Outcomes	Nursing Interventions
Mr. M. will work through the phase of acknowledging awareness of the realization of his loss as evidenced by discussing the treatment experience.	• Encourage Mr. M. to describe perceptions of his current postoperative adaptation. • Encourage description of experiences that preceded the loss of Mr. M.'s voice, including the sudden death of his wife. • Promote discussion of other factors that Mr. M. perceives to be related to his current loss.
Mr. M. will demonstrate nonexcessive and nonprolonged emotional reactions to recent losses as evidenced by engaging in normal grieving.	• Assess for possible suicidal ideation/intent. • Permit open expression of feelings of anger and assist Mr. M. to begin to try to understand possible reasons for these feelings. • Point out the need for universal grieving. Evaluate the need for referral for brief psychotherapy to provide further opportunity for Mr. M. to discuss his adaptation to his recent losses.
Mr. M. will agree to resume use of electrolarynx.	• Encourage Mr. M. to describe current and anticipated problems related to the loss of his voice. • Evaluate the influence of denial on Mr. M.'s avoidance of using the electrolarynx. • Collaborate with the health team to clarify factual information of Mr. M.'s health situation in terms of diagnostic findings and prognosis. • Convey recognition that Mr. M.'s knowledge of communication skills as a broadcaster (such as enunciation) will assist in his adaptation to the electrolarynx.
Mr. M. will develop goals that are congruent with his losses.	• Encourage Mr. M. to describe his plans for the future, including employment as well as social and recreational activities. • Support Mr. M.'s plans for contacting the radio station to investigate alternative employment possibilities. • Encourage Mr. M. to explore possibilities for decreasing the social isolation he had experienced before his surgery.

REFERENCES

1. Aguilera D, Messick J: *Crisis intervention: theory and methodology,* ed 6, St Louis, 1989, Mosby–Year Book.
2. Bowlby J: *Attachment and loss,* vol 3, New York, 1980, Basic Books.
3. Collison C, Miller S: Using images of the future in grief work, *Image J Nurs Scholar* 19(1):9, 1987.
4. Cook AS, Oltjenbruns KA: *Dying and grieving: lifespan and family perspectives,* New York, 1989, Holt, Rinehart, & Winston.
5. Dracup K, Breu C: Using nursing research findings to meet the needs of grieving spouses, *Nurs Res* 27:212, 1978.
6. Engel G: *Psychological development in health and disease,* Philadelphia, 1968, WB Saunders.
7. Gerety EK: Grieving, anticipatory grieving, dysfunctional grieving. In McFarland GK, Thomas MD: *Psychiatric mental health nursing,* Philadelphia, 1991, JB Lippincott.
8. Green M: Roles of health professionals and institutions. In Osterweis M, Solomon F, and Green M, editors: *Bereavement reactions, consequences, and care,* Washington, DC, 1984, National Academy Press.
9. Haig RA: *The anatomy of grief: biopsychosocial and therapeutic perspectives,* Springfield, Ill, 1990, Charles C. Thomas Publishers.
10. Hampe S: Needs of the grieving spouse in a hospital setting, *Nurs Res* 24:113, 1975.
11. Horowitz MJ and others: Pathological grief and the activation of latent and self images, *Am J Psychiatry* 137:1157, 1980.
12. Jacob SR: Facing it alone, *J Psychosoc Nurs Ment Health Serv* 29(11):20-24, 1991.
13. Kelly B: Emily: a study of grief and bereavement. *Health Care Women Int* 12:137-147, 1991.
14. Kim MJ, McFarland GK, and McLane AL: *Pocket guide to nursing diagnoses,* ed 4, St Louis, 1991, Mosby–Year Book.
15. Kovarsky SR: Loneliness and disturbed grief: a comparison of parents who lost a child to suicide or accidental death, *Arch Psychiatric Nurs* 3(2):86-96, 1989.
16. Kubler-Ross E: *On death and dying,* New York, 1969, Macmillan.
17. Lazare A: Bereavement and unresolved grief. In Lazare A, editor: *Outpatient psychiatry: diagnosis and treatment,* ed 2, Baltimore, 1989, Williams & Wilkins.
18. Lindemann E: Symptomatology and management of acute grief, *Am J Psychiatry* 101:141, 1944.
19. Lund DA, Caserta MS, and Pelt JV: Stability of social support networks after later-life spousal bereavement, *Death studies* 4(1):53-73, 1990.
20. McFarland GK, Gerety EK: Grieving, anticipatory. In Kim MJ, McFarland GK, and McLane AL: *Pocket guide to nursing diagnoses,* ed 4, St Louis, 1991, Mosby–Year Book.
21. McFarland GK, Gerety EK: Grieving, anticipatory; grieving, dysfunctional. In Thompson J, McFarland G, Hirsch J, Tucker S, and Bowers A: *Mosby's manual of clinical nursing,* ed 2, St Louis, 1989, CV Mosby.
22. McFarland GK, Wasli EL, and Gerety EK: *Nursing diagnoses and process in psychiatric mental health nursing,* Philadelphia, 1992, JB Lippincott.
23. Miller F, Dworkin J, Ward M, and Barone D: A preliminary study of unresolved grief in families of seriously mentally ill patients, *Hosp Commun Psychiatry* 41(12): 1321-1325, 1990.
24. Pollock G: The mourning-liberation process in health and disease, *Psychiatr Clin North Am* 10(3):345, 1987.
25. Rando TA: Understanding and facilitating anticipatory grief in the loved ones of the dying. In Rando TA, editor: *Loss and anticipatory grief,* Lexington, Mass, 1986, Lexington Books.
26. Sanders CM: *Grief: the morning after,* New York, 1989, John Wiley & Sons.
27. Solsberry V, Krupnick J: Adults' reactions to bereavement. In Osterwies M, Solomon F, and Green M, editors: *Bereavement reactions, consequences, and care,* Washington, DC, 1984, National Academy Press.
28. Welch D: Anticipatory grief reactions in family members of adult patients, *Issues Ment Health Nurs* 4(2):149, 158, 1982.
29. Worden J: *Grief counseling and grief therapy, a handbook for the mental health practitioner,* ed 2, New York, 1991, Springer Publishing.
30. York C, Stichler J: Cultural grief expressions following infant death, *Dimens Crit Care Nurs* 4(2):120, 1985.

High Risk for Violence: Self-Directed or Directed at Others

High Risk for Violence: Self-Directed or Directed at Others is a state in which an individual may verbally threaten or physically act against a target that is either a person (self or other) or something in the environment.[13]

OVERVIEW

Violence exists within a complex matrix for which the parameters are not readily identifiable. A part of the complexity results from the affected society's determination of what it considers and does not consider to be an appropriate aggressive or violent response to a perceived threat. This means that the society accepts the use of some aggressive behaviors while instituting sanctions against others who engage in actual violent behavior. Those sanctions may be violent also, but accepted by the society as necessary restraints against forms of violence that threaten the community.

Society recognizes that appropriate levels of aggression (violence can be viewed as extreme aggression) or violence are needed, or humankind would have difficulty surviving: such behavior enables an individual or group to defend against a perceived threat. For instance, a soldier is trained to kill the enemy with the least possible risk to self and may even win medals for doing so. When those same skills are used in a civilian setting, that soldier can be convicted of assault or murder and suffer the civilian consequences for those acts because society considers this maladaptive behavior, or a deleterious use of that individual's skills.

When an inappropriate aggressive or violent response occurs, the individual can become involved in the legal and health care systems. If the individual enters the health care system, other health care problems usually exist and compound the risk for violence. Thus the nurse must be able to assess a patient's risk for violence as well as that patient's health care needs when entering the health care system. Without that assessment, appropriate interventions to mitigate the deleterious outcomes of violent behavior will not be instituted.

Although there is no comprehensive theory capable of explaining violence, research and applicable analyses have identified certain conditions that, if present, indicate a higher probability of violence. First, young males are more prone to violence than any other maturational group. Next the nurse can determine the need to further assess the risk for violence by asking straightforward questions in the following areas: whether there is any recent history of violence; whether the patient is involved with the legal system; whether the patient has experienced a significant physical, emotional, or psychological trauma; and whether there has been a use of recreational drugs.[7,13,15,17] If the patient/significant other reports any of these conditions, the nurse can more specifically assess the risk factors.

ASSESSMENT

Violent behavior exists sporadically and usually for brief periods of time. A patient entering the health care system may be at risk for violence and needs at least a cursory assessment of risk for violence. Therefore the nurse needs to assess patient factors that might trigger a violent reaction. The initial assessment can be quickly accomplished by determining whether any of the following risk factors are present. First, if the patient is a young male, a further assessment is warranted as young males are more prone to violence than any other maturational group. Next the nurse can ask fairly straightforward questions in basic areas to determine the need to further assess the risk for violence; for example, questions related to whether the patient has recently harmed self or others or damaged property. This will aid in determining a prior history of violence, particularly recent violent behavior. "Do you have any current criminal charges pending or have you been convicted of criminal charges?" This will address the patient's involvement with the legal system. "What crises or major problems have you experienced lately?" This will help to identify a significant negative effect on the individual's perception of self/self-esteem, such as a loss of position, development of a serious illness, or any other negative situation. "What recreational drugs do you use?" Drugs and violence are often associated. If any of the preceding risk factors are present, additional assessment activities can further determine the possibility of an individual expressing violent behavior. In assessing the risk for violence, several other common risk factors are listed below and should be assessed.

❖ Risk Factors

The presence of the following behaviors, conditions, or circumstances renders the patient more vulnerable to a High Risk for Violence[1,3-6,9-11,14-17]:

- Gender/age (young male)
- Medical conditions (e.g., brain tumor/damage, Temporal lobe epilepsy, nutritional deficiencies,

- History of violent behavior
- Hostile environment (actual or perceived)
- Low tolerance to stress
- Rage reactions
- Suspiciousness of others

low neuroleptic blood level)
- Body language
  Rigid or taut body
  Clenched teeth or fists
  Very rapid, shallow breathing
  Increased pacing
  Increased excitement or agitation
  Irritability
  Defiance
  Argumentative
  Hostile/threatening verbalizations
- Psychiatric disorders (e.g., dementias, psychoactive substance-induced, paranoid schizophrenia, depressive disorders, anxiety disorders, personality disorders, confusion/panic
- Experiences of violence within the family/community
- Fear of self or others

- Recent aggressive behavior
- Suicidal/homicidal behavior
- Temper tantrums
- Antisocial behavior
- Bullying others
- Intense interpersonal bonding
- Abusive behaviors
- Belief that behavior is not under personal control
- Boasting about previous violent episodes
- Feeling that one's honor has been violated
- Hopelessness
- Increasing anxiety levels
- Lack of self-control/poor impulse control
- Vulnerable self-esteem
- Belief that violence is justified
- Religious frenzy/trances

❖ Related Medical/Psychiatric Diagnoses

The following are examples of related medical/psychiatric diagnoses for High Risk for Violence:
- Brief reactive psychosis
- Delusional disorder, jealous or persecutory types
- Intermittent explosive disorder
- Mood disorders, manic or depressed states

- Obsessive compulsive disorder
- Organic mental syndromes and disorders
  Organic personality syndrome
  Alcohol/drug intoxication or withdrawal,

VIII

such as from amphetamines, cocaine, hallucinogenic substances, nicotine, and phencyclidine.

- Panic disorder
- Personality disorders
  Paranoid
  Antisocial
  Borderline
- Posttraumatic stress disorder
- Schizophrenia, paranoid

NURSING DIAGNOSES

Examples of *specific* nursing diagnoses for High Risk for Violence are:
- High Risk for Violence related to recent aggressive behavior
- High Risk for Violence related to increased agitation
- High Risk for Violence related to poor impulse control
- High Risk for Violence related to recent suicidal behaviors

PLANNING AND IMPLEMENTATION WITH RATIONALE

If the nurse completes an adequate assessment, he/she can implement effective interventions that will mitigate the deleterious effects of violence. When the nurse misses or does not pay attention to a patient's risk factors, violence can erupt with injury or harm occurring to the individual, others, or the environment. Then steps must be taken quickly to mitigate the severity of the violent episode. One, however, cannot always be in a position to perceive or determine an individual's High Risk for Violence. Therefore, if violence does occur, evaluate what happened and determine what might be done in the future to prevent its recurrence. Determine whether the patient comes from another culture, particularly countries wherein violence is known to occur, this could necessitate a modification in treatment modalities and expected outcomes.[17]

Violent episodes consist of three phases: preassault, assault, and postassault.[11] The *preassault phase* occurs before the actual violent behavior and includes the reason for the violence. Individuals with brain damage or who are experiencing psychotic states may react with violence for no apparent reason. Their provocation arises from an internal stimulus such as confusion, delusion, hallucination, or misperception. *Adequate interventions during the preassault phase will abort or significantly reduce the probability, severity, or duration of the assault phase.* Multiple interventions, broadly grouped as environmental manipulations, how the nurse approaches the patient, and medications, are available. Determining which to use will depend on the nurse's assessment of the situation.

Experience has demonstrated that environmental manipulations can diffuse a situation that might generate violent behavior. Such interventions include the reduction of stimuli by lowering lights, decreasing noise levels, requesting that people speak softly, and providing quiet areas where individuals can go to regain control of themselves. Environmental factors that reduce an individual's ability to control violence include poor air quality, such as from tobacco smoke, excessive heat and humidity, and noise.

At times, it is necessary to intervene directly with the patient to redirect the focus of a perceived threat to one less threatening. The nurse can suggest that a patient take a shower, preferably cool. The effect of this intervention can help the patient to regain control of feelings. If the patient is breathing rapidly and shallowly, coach the patient to breathe more slowly and deeply. This helps the patient to relax. Physical activities (sports, using a punching bag, walking, kneading dough or clay, or any similar activity) help the patient to redirect the focus from a perceived threat to an appropriate and socially acceptable way of expressing the feelings. *The approaches and interactions of nursing personnel with patients may actually precipitate violent behavior, particularly if the patient perceives the approach/interaction as threatening or confrontational.* It is therefore important not to get into a power struggle with a patient about who is "the boss" or to alter nonthreatening behavior to achieve social propriety. A nonthreatening, nonconfrontational

VIII

approach allows the patient to feel less threatened, thus decreasing the perceived need for violence. If the nurse can obtain the patient's perception of the situation, the patient will frequently help to abort the violent behavior. This necessitates careful listening on the part of the nurse and recognizing that many patients have learned when they are losing control. A patient's request for medication, to engage in an activity, or to be restrained/secluded in an attempt to control violent behavior should be carefully assessed to assist the patient in controlling his/her behavior.

Additionally, *aspects of cognitive therapy are being used to manage anger.* Some of the strategies of this approach can include teaching patients to question the evidence they are using, helping them to examine options and alternatives and to perceive positive aspects of the situation, "decatastrophizing" the event, assisting them to move away from all-or-nothing thinking, rehearsing the event mentally to practice more effective coping skills, and using specific assignments for patients to do between therapeutic sessions.[12] This treatment approach is a ". . . practical approach that provides a logical concreteness that clients often seem to need to help them establish boundaries."[12]

Medication can also be beneficial for the control of violence.[2] These medications continue to be improved and new ones added. The nurse's responsibilities in drug treatment are to observe for adverse reactions to the drugs, to make certain the patient takes the medication as prescribed, and to assess the need for and administration of prn medications. If a prn medication is needed frequently, the patient needs to be evaluated for a medication change. The nurse should also provide the patient with health teaching about the benefits and risks of taking the prescribed medication. The patient who perceives the need to take medication to help control violent behavior will comply with the medication regimen to a greater extent than one who does not. If the preceding interventions are not effective and if the patient provides external cues to impending violence, the assault phase of violence may occur.

During the assault phase, the first priority is to obtain physical control of the patient to prevent injury to self/others or environmental destruction. To do this, it is best if a trained team works together to physically control and then restrain/seclude the patient.[1,8] Explain to the patient in a calm, soothing voice what is being done and the reason for it. Although the patient may not appear to be responding to what is being said, it does influence the individual's perception of the event.

When a patient is in restraints/seclusion, the nurse needs to provide that patient with the means to maintain adequate hydration, nutrition, and personal hygiene. It may be necessary to directly assist the patient with some of these functions. If medication is being given during this period, it is usually given intramuscularly to facilitate a rapid effect. With the ending of the violent behavior, the postassault phase occurs.

The *postassault phase* involves the evaluation of the assault or violent episode and the responses of those who participated in or witnessed the event. *Because of the intense feelings an assault provokes in those who experience/witness a violent event and the need to clarify perceptions regarding the violent patient and the staff's response to the event, postassault sessions are crucial.* First, determine whether the violent behavior was general and nondirected or goal directed. If the patient incidently injured someone or disrupted the environment, the violent behavior was general and nondirected. Patients with this type of behavior may have an underlying medical problem, acute delirium, or panic behavior. Treatment and control of the underlying problem usually will enable the patient to control the violent behavior. Depending on the problem, the patient can also be taught to recognize and to avoid situations or stimuli that will trigger the problem causing the violent behavior.

In goal-directed violence, the patient chooses a target, for reasons that may or may not make sense to another individual. Patients who use this type of violence often have mental illnesses or feel threatened. Determine the patient's perceptions of the event. It is not unusual for the patient to feel that the staff overreacted or was punishing/persecutory. The patient may also believe that he/she was still in control of personal behavior and should not have been given medication or restrained/secluded. Without clarification of these perceptions, the patient may feel justified regarding the expressed behavior and continue to express hostility. With clarification, the patient may feel remorseful about the event and regain behavioral control.

A variety of educational and psychotherapeutic interventions exists that can assist patients in changing their perception of the need for violence. Educational interventions can decrease patients' stress, vulnerability, and hypersensitivity by teaching them skills to improve their interpersonal and community functioning. These interventions include, but are not limited to, job-seeking skills, skills for independent living, skills for use of time, social and interpersonal skills, and the need to comply with a treatment regimen. Psychotherapeutic interventions assist patients to improve behavioral control by increasing anxiety tolerance, developing the ability to postpone gratification, improving impulse control, developing realistic expectations, accepting responsibility for one's actions, becoming self-reliant, acquiring a sense of autonomy and individuality, and constructively verbalizing feelings. If working with a cross-cultural patient, the nurse must determine the need and conditions for using available translators.[17] If the nurse can identify the cultural significance of the various nursing procedures and potential therapeutic modalities, the nurse can develop appropriate modifications of treatment and expected treatment outcomes. Westermeyer[17] advocates gently confronting cross-cultural patients within a social network that includes the family,

❖ *NURSING CARE GUIDELINES*

Nursing Diagnosis: *High Risk for Violence: Self-Directed or Directed at Others*

Expected Patient Outcomes	Nursing Interventions
	Preassault Phase
The patient will abort or rapidly diffuse impending violent behavior as evidenced by: verbalization of feelings/behavior indicating that the staff and/or the patient are able to control the situation; decreasing the need to use violence in solving problems; using socially appropriate activities that express anger; verbalizing changes in cognitive values indicative of a decreasing need to use violence in solving problems.	• Evaluate patient for presence of risk factors. • Determine cultural/community parameters for violence. • Consult with a clinician with a similar background or proficiency in client's language if different from your own. • Structure the environment to reduce stimuli by any means available. • Determine patient's perception pertaining to the need for violence. • Listen to what the patient says. • Allow the patient to set interaction distance. • Provide those aspects of cognitive therapy (e.g., questioning evidence being used, examining options and alternatives, rehearsing more effective coping skills) that have been helpful for managing assaultive behavior and that reinforce the changing cognitive values. • Interrupt a treatment session or interview to allow the patient to regain control of self. • Verify that the patient takes medication as prescribed. • Use medication as needed before patient becomes violent.

Continued.

❖ *NURSING CARE GUIDELINES—cont'd*

Expected Patient Outcomes	**Nursing Interventions**
	Assault Phase
The patient will incur no personal injuries and inflict no injuries to others during the episode.	• Use adequately trained staff to physically control the patient when necessary. • Restrain/seclude the patient as ordered. • Explain to the patient what is being done and why. • Medicate as ordered. • Monitor closely for adverse reactions to the medication or the situation. • Assist patient to maintain adequate hydration, nutrition, and personal hygiene.
	Postassault Phase
The patient will experience a decreased risk of violence as evidenced by fewer, less intense, and shorter violent episodes, with decreased probability of injury; increased ability to sort out the feelings and thoughts related to violent episodes; increased ability to identify risk for violence and initiate activities, as able, to diffuse or control that potential.	• For general, nondirected violence: treat the underlying condition in collaboration with the physician and avoid situations that trigger violent episodes. • For goal-directed violence: determine patient's perception of need for violence, implement appropriate educational and psychotherapeutic treatments to diffuse or control the risk for violence, hold community and staff postassault sessions, and train the staff to work as a team in the management of the aggressive/assaultive patient.

VIII

as these patients can be very sensitive to feeling rejected/alienated and have a vulnerable self-esteem. These are risk factors for violence.

Staff also need to evaluate their feelings and activities. Without assigning blame or prejudice, a realistic assessment of how they might have handled the situation differently can help staff respond more effectively in the future. These sessions also help to identify staff training needs in managing the aggressive/violent patient.

It is generally recognized that all staff need training if they are to effectively manage the aggressive/violent patient. Identified areas of train-

ing include, but are not limited to, risk factors associated with the High Risk for Violence, nonjudgmental communication skills, techniques for diffusing a violent situation, principles of psychological assessment and intervention, cultural bases for violence, legal and ethical issues, and techniques for increasing staff teamwork.

EVALUATION
Preassault Phase

For evaluating the objective parameters of the preassault phase, the intervention is effective if the violent behaviors were aborted or quickly diffused. For the subjective parameters, patients will believe that the staff can control violent situations and feel that their environment is safe. One area that can be evaluated sometimes is the changing cognitive values expressed by the patient, either verbally or behaviorally, that demonstrate a decreased need to solve problems with violence. When evaluating the *assault phase,* interventions are effective if personal injury or property damage was prevented or limited. A consequence of violence that is not contained is personal injury that could lead to serious injury, death, or the destruction of property. Thus a measure of effective interventions includes a decrease in the intensity/duration or an absence of the violent episodes. In some instances, patients with severe psychoses or toxic drug reactions can remain violent for several days, or may be violent frequently, and may require intensive treatment and ongoing evaluations to bring the behavior under control. The subjective parameters for evaluating intervention effectiveness include the perceptions of both the patient and the staff. If the patient perceives the interventions as beneficial and not punitive and the staff perceive their interventions as therapeutic, then those interventions were effective. The *post-assault* evaluation includes not only determination of the effectiveness of past interventions, but also the identification of appropriate interventions for continued treatment and prevention. The assessment for continued treatment becomes the foundation for successful treatment of violence and will function adequately only if it is done by the treatment team. Positive outcomes include an overall decrease in the frequency and intensity of violent episodes. Interventions are also effective if the frequency of patient or staff injuries decreases. Probably one of the most rewarding outcomes occurs when a patient identifies and then initiates activities to diffuse or control a situation that could lead to violence. If both the patient and the staff perceive the staff as competent to control violent behavior, then the patient perceives the environment as safe; the interventions were effective. Also, interventions will be successful if the underlying risk factors were addressed, treated, and brought under control.

❖ CASE STUDY WITH PLAN OF CARE

VII

Mr. Jonas J., a 21-year-old, black male with a diagnosis of paranoid schizophrenia, was admitted to a psychiatric unit because of an unprovoked assault on a family guest and because of increasing interpersonal problems. On admission, he said that he was just trying to make the guest stop lying about him. He denied any hallucinations or delusions, but when he was alone, he was observed by nursing staff to move his lips as if talking to himself. At other times, he was observed smiling to himself and nodding his head as if he were responding to some sort of internal stimuli. Mr. J. paced the halls continuously with downcast eyes. When he attended unit activities, he maintained a distance of at least 6 to 8 feet between himself and another person and would not participate even when gently encouraged to do so. Appearance, behavior, conversation, cognition, and mood were in keeping with the diagnosis of paranoid schizophrenia. Mr. J. played basketball in high school and liked to talk about how aggressively he had played and how much he now missed playing the sport. Since high school, he has not developed any strong friendships and tends to prefer solitary pursuits, such as physical fitness, except for occasional get-togethers to play basketball. After finishing high school, he worked as an automobile mechanic until being fired 2 weeks ago. His parents stated that he was fired because of insubordination and numerous complaints about hostility from customers. However, Mr. J. stated that he was fired because his supervisor did not like him and had figured out a way to get rid of him. After his firing, Mr. J. stayed in his room listening to music and making no efforts to seek reemployment because he thought his previous employer would make certain he could not get another job. About 2 months ago, he broke up with his girlfriend "because she wanted to be better than I was." He had made no attempt to find another girlfriend and had ceased participating in family activities. His parents thought he was angry, but he denied having any strong feelings about his ex-girlfriend or his family.

Continued.

PLAN OF CARE FOR MR. JONAS J.

Nursing Diagnosis: *High Risk for Violence: Directed at Others as evidenced by paranoid delusions*

Expected Patient Outcomes	Nursing Interventions
Mr. J. will abstain from violent behavior against others as evidenced by his identifying and verbalizing reasons for his violent behavior, recognizing signs/symptoms indicative of impending violence and informing staff of this, taking his medication as prescribed, participating in prescribed activities, and perceiving situations based on reality.	• Monitor for increased pacing, clenched teeth or fists, or other signs of impending violence. • Approach Mr. J. in a nonconfrontational, nonthreatening manner. • Medicate as prescribed and give prn medication if symptoms increase. • Teach the patient the risks/benefits of taking medications. • Explore with Mr. J. his need and reasons for behaving violently. • Teach Mr. J. appropriate ways to express his feelings of aggression and violence. Make provisions for him to use some of these methods on the unit. • Assign one-on-one nurse to work on control of suspiciousness and violent behavior. • Interrupt session if he needs to gain control of himself. • Encourage Mr. J. to participate in prescribed therapies, set limits on aggressive/assaultive behavior during sessions, test Mr. J.'s perceptions of reality while teaching him how others perceive him, and encourage use of socially acceptable means of expressing violence. • Assign Mr. J. to nursing support groups or therapy groups.

REFERENCES

1. Cahill CD, Stuart GW, Laraia MT, and Arana GW: Inpatient management of violent behavior: Nursing prevention and intervention, *Ment Health Nurs* 12:239-252, 1991.
2. Eichelman B: Toward a rational pharmacotherapy for aggressive and violent behavior, *Hosp Community Psychiatry* 39:31, 1988.
3. Garbarino J, Kostelny K, and Dubrow N: What children can tell us about living in danger, *Am Psychol* 376-383, April, 1991.
4. Gorney R: Interpersonal intensity, competition, and synergy: determinants of achievement, aggression, and mental illness. In Pasternack SA, editor: *Violence and Victims*, New York, 1975, Spectrum Publications.
5. Hausman P: *The right dose: how to take vitamins and minerals safely,* Emmaus, Penn, 1987, Rodale Press.
6. Kim MJ, McFarland GK, and McLane AM: *Pocket guide to nursing diagnoses,* ed 4, St Louis, 1991, Mosby–Year Book.
7. Lanza ML: Origins of aggression, *J Psychosoc Nurs Ment Health Serv* 21:11-16, 1983.
8. Morton PG: Staff roles and responsibilities in incidents of patient violence, *Arch Psychiatr Nurs* 1:280, 1987.
9. *The New Jerusalem Bible,* New York, 1985, Doubleday.
10. Pearson M, Wilmont E, and Padi M: A study of violent behavior among in-patients in a psychiatric hospital, *Br J Psychiatry* 149:232, 1986.
11. Rada RT: The violent patient: rapid assessment and management, *Psychosomatics* 22:101, 1981.
12. Reeder DM: Cognitive therapy of anger management: theoretical and practical considerations, *Arch Psychiatr Nurs* 5:147-150, 1991.
13. Roper JM, Anderson NLR: The interactional dynamics of violence, part I, *Arch Psychiatr Nurs* 5:209-215, 1991.
14. Ryden MB, Bossenmaier M, and McLachlan C: Aggressive behavior in cognitively impaired nursing home residents, *Res Nurs Health* 14:87-95, 1991.
15. Swanson JW, Holzer CE III, Ganju VK, and Jono RT: Violence and psychiatric disorder in the community: evidence from the epidemiologic catchment area surveys, *Hosp Community Psychiatry* 41:761-769, 1990.
16. Thomas SP: Toward a new conceptualization of women's anger, *Ment Health Nurs* 12:31-49, 1991.
17. Westermeyer J: Cross-cultural care for ptsd: research, training, and service needs for the future, *J Trauma Stress* 2:515-536, 1989.

VIII

Altered Family Processes

Altered Family Processes is the state in which a family that normally functions effectively experiences a dysfunction.

OVERVIEW

In spite of major societal changes in recent years, the family remains the basic social unit in American society. Families vary significantly in lifestyles, power relationships, values, health status, social and intellectual competence, and structure. The diverse, dynamic nature of families allows us to understand why the family has been defined and conceptualized in many ways by several disciplines. However, for this discussion, family will be defined as two or more individuals who are emotionally involved with each other and live in close geographic proximity.[9]

Although their structures vary widely, families do share common characteristics. They all are social systems with their own cultural attitudes, values, and beliefs. Each family also has its own set of rules, structure, and basic functions. Furthermore, every family moves through certain developmental stages throughout the family life cycle.[8]

Duvall[8] identifies the eight stages within the family life cycle: (1) married couple, (2) childbearing family, (3) families with preschoolers, (4) families with school-children, (5) families with teenagers, (6) launching center families, (7) middle-aged families, and (8) aging families. During each of these stages, family members accomplish certain stage-critical family development tasks. For example, during the eighth stage the parents may need to cope with living alone or adjust to retirement. These adjustments are considered normal or developmental. Family developmental tasks refer to growth responsibilities that families must achieve during each stage to meet biological requirements, cultural imperatives, and aspirations and values.[8]

Families perform certain functions within society, including the provision of affection, security, affiliation, socialization, and control.[8] In addition, Schuster and Ashburn[24] suggest that family functions include reproduction; socialization; protection and security; sexual fulfillment; economic security; conferral of status and roles; social contact; the provision of belongingness, love, and affection; physiological needs; recreation; and religious needs. By performing these effectively, the family meets the needs of its members and society.

Healthy, well-functioning families demonstrate certain characteristics or strengths. Otto[20] provides a framework for assessing the strengths that indicate a well-functioning family. The absence of one or more of these characteristics may indicate an alteration in family processes. Otto's 12 family strengths follow:

1. Fulfillment of the family members' physical, emotional, and spiritual needs
2. Sensitivity to the needs of the family members
3. Effective communication of thoughts and feelings
4. The provision of support, security, and encouragement
5. The initiation and maintenance of growth-producing relationships and experiences both within and without the family
6. The creation and maintenance of constructive and responsible community relationships
7. Growth with and through children
8. Flexibility in the performance of family roles

9. Helping oneself whenever possible and accepting aid when self-help does not suffice
10. Mutual respect for the individuality of family members
11. Growth through crises experiences
12. Family unity, loyalty, and interfamily cooperation

Family therapy models provide theories on both normal and dysfunctional family processes.[29] The family systems and communication-strategic models are all commonly used. Although these models overlap, distinctions can be made between them. In the family systems theory, a healthy family is viewed as not only withstanding stress, but also changing and growing with the experience. A dysfunctional family is unable to meet this challenge. In the structural model, alterations in family processes result when the family structure becomes unbalanced. The communication-strategic model postulates that family dysfunctions occur as a result of inadequate communication and interaction patterns.[29]

ASSESSMENT

Nursing process applied to the family enables the nurse to systematically intervene with a family, decide on mutually acceptable goals and objectives, and plan, implement, and evaluate care. The family can be analyzed through the use of several theories, including systems, developmental, structural-functional, and interactional approaches. These theories provide the basis for a systematically organized family assessment. However, the complexity of the family phenomena may necessitate a combination of these theories to adequately assess the family process.[9]

Several approaches to family assessment are identified in the literature. Helvie[12] advocates analysis of the structural characteristics of the family, such as family type, organization, boundaries, differentiation, specialization, and territoriality. In addition, internal and external family processes would be analyzed from an exchange theory perspective. Clemen-Stone, Eigsti, and McGuire[5] suggest a structural-process approach to family assessment. Structural parameters include

division of labor and power, communication, boundaries, relationships with others, means of giving and obtaining emotional support, rituals and symbols, and personal roles. The process parameters focus on how decisions are made within the family system, how the family structure evolves, and how family functions are performed.

Friedman[9] identifies the five basic functions of the family as the affective function (maintenance of each member's personality), socialization and social placement function, reproductive function, economic function, and health care function (provision and allocation of physical necessities and health care). The six major categories described in the Friedman Family Assessment Model include the family's specific identifying data, present and past family developmental stages, environmental data, the family structure, family functions, and the family's coping abilities.[9]

1. Identifying data
   (a) Family composition
   (b) Type of family form
   (c) Cultural (ethnic) background
   (d) Religious identification
   (e) Social class status
   (f) Recreational or leisure-time activities
2. Developmental stage and history of family
   (a) Present developmental stage
   (b) Tasks needing completion
   (c) Family's history
3. Environmental data
   (a) Characteristics of the home
   (b) Characteristics of the neighborhood and community
   (c) Family's geographic mobility
   (d) Family's associations and transactions with the community
   (e) Family's social support systems or network
4. Family structure
   (a) Communication patterns
   (b) Role structure
   (c) Power structure
   (d) Family values
5. Family functions
   (a) Affective function

(b) Socialization function
(c) Reproductive function
(d) Economic function
(e) Health care function
6. Family coping
   (a) Functional coping strategies
   (b) Short- and long-term family stressors

Two tools that can be used to help assess the family process are the genogram and the ecomap.[5] The genogram is a diagram of the family constellation that shows the intergenerational relationships among family members. Genograms are schematically similar to a family tree and provide a means to obtain information about family relationships, health status of family members, and family reactions to socio-cultural and spiritual variables affecting their lives.[5,9] The ecomap graphically depicts the family's relationships and interactions with the external environment. These tools assist the family in visualizing how either internal or external forces may be affecting the family's health and well-being. In addition, families with long-standing relationship problems may be aided by an assessment through Satir's family-life chronology model.[23]

A number of validated family assessment tools are available to assist the nurse in data collection. These include: (1) Family APGAR,[26] (2) Family Functioning Index,[22] (3) Family Environmental Scale,[19] and (4) Family Dynamics Measure.[15]

Given the pluralistic nature of our society, cultural perspectives on health and illness vary in families. To provide culturally appropriate nursing care, nurses need to understand factors that affect family health and illness behaviors.[2,17] Cultural assessment provides meaning to behaviors that might otherwise be perceived negatively. Cultural assessment models enable the nurse to assess cultural factors in a systematic manner.[3,10,30] Cultural patterns of the family also influence how it copes with crises.[1] Because the family unit is viewed as a primary source in the development of its members' attitudes, beliefs, values, and patterns of behaviors, conducting a cultural assessment would assist the nurse in providing culture-specific care.

Many stressors can affect family functioning and family well-being. Some of these stressors originate within the family itself, whereas others develop externally. For some families, certain events may precipitate a crisis. A crisis is defined as an upset in a previously steady state. Crises may be maturational or situational.[5,21] Maturational (developmental) crises are "normal" crises or transition points during physical, social, psychological, and intellectual growth.[5] Examples of developmental crises would include marriage, parenthood, adolescence, middlescence, and retirement.

Situational crises also occur throughout life but do not occur during specific maturational processes and are generally not anticipated. A situational crisis is external, sudden, and unexpected. Therefore the family's risk for developing distress increases because the members are unprepared to deal with the changes accompanying these situational events.[5] The occurrence of a family crisis is determined by the family's perception of the event, the availability and adequacy of family support, and the family's ability to cope. Situational and developmental crises may occur simultaneously, thereby increasing the chances for stress in the family system even more. An example would be adolescent parenthood.

Health problems contributing to alterations in family processes include traumatic injuries, degenerative diseases, any disease or illness resulting in disability or incapacitation such as chronic renal failure or cerebrovascular accidents, or the birth of an infant with a defect.

❖ **Defining Characteristics**

The presence of the following defining characteristics indicates that the client may be experiencing Altered Family Processes[4,14]
- Family unable to meet physical, emotional, spiritual, or security needs of its members
- Inappropriate level and direction of energy
- Family fails to accomplish current or past developmental task
- Inability to express or accept wide range of feelings

- Inability to express or accept feelings of members
- Family unable to adapt to change or deal with traumatic experiences constructively
- Inability to accept or receive help appropriately
- Inability of family members to relate to each other for mutual growth and maturation
- Parents do not demonstrate respect for each other's child-rearing practices
- Rigidity in function and roles
- Family does not demonstrate respect for individuality and autonomy of its members
- Ineffective family decision-making process
- Failure to send and receive clear messages
- Inappropriate boundaries
- Family uninvolved in community activities
- Inappropriate or poorly communicated family rules, rituals, or symbols
- Unexamined family myths

❖ **Related Factors**

The following related factors are associated with Altered Family Processes[4,14]:

Situational transition and/or crises	Developmental transition and/or crises
• Disaster	• Birth of an infant with a defect
• Economic crisis	
• Change in family roles	• Loss of a family member
• Trauma	• Addition of a family member
	• Retirement

❖ **Related Medical/Psychiatric Diagnoses**

The following are examples of related medical/psychiatric diagnoses for Altered Family Processes:
- AIDS
- Cancer
- Chronic renal failure
- Dementia
- Psychoactive substance use disorders (e.g., alcohol dependence)
- Schizophrenia
- Terminal illness
- Traumatic injury

NURSING DIAGNOSES

Examples of *specific* nursing diagnoses for Altered Family Processes are:
- Altered Family Process related to history of inadequate coping methods
- Altered Family Process related to situational crisis: terminal illness of family member
- Altered Family Process related to economic family crisis (inadequate financial resources)

PLANNING AND IMPLEMENTATION WITH RATIONALE

Nursing interventions for clients with Altered Family Processes are directed at acknowledgement of and adaptive responses to change in family roles, identification of effective coping patterns, participation in decision-making processes, and identification and utilization of community resources. Nursing interventions focus on the reduction of defining characteristics and promotion of effective family processes.

Initial nursing interventions will assist the family in reducing or resolving the crisis. The use of a systematic assessment tool will provide adequate background information and include information about the family as a unit, the ill family member, and the health care environment.[7] An understanding of family theory and family nursing research is crucial to planning effective interventions for the family.[11] The nurse and family develop plans and goals together. In general, healthy families demonstrate the traits of good self-esteem; a sense of nurturance, acceptance, encouragement, and support; good communication; commitment to family; quality time spent together; problem-solving skills; and a shared religious orientation.[6,28] Family strengths should be reinforced and used in times of stress. Because of the family crisis or situation, division of labor and role responsibilities may be altered. To promote smooth role transition, nursing interventions may address competence, knowledge, and skills needed for a particular family role. How the family defines its situation is a major factor in how it responds to crisis or illness.[25] *Families experienc-*

❖ *NURSING CARE GUIDELINES*

Nursing Diagnosis: *Altered Family Processes*

Expected Patient Outcomes	Nursing Interventions
The family will express feelings freely and appropriately.	• Assess situation or crisis for causative factors. • Encourage family to verbalize feelings. • Discuss with family appropriate ways to demonstrate feelings.
The family's energies will be directed toward a purpose.	• Assist family in dealing with situation/crisis. • Promote an open trusting relationship with family.
The family members will become involved in problem-solving processes that are directed at a resolution.	• Acknowledge your own feelings about the family and their situation.
The family will express understanding of the illness or trauma treatment regimen and the prognosis.	• Facilitate family strengths. • Maintain effective communication between staff and family. • Initiate a multidisciplinary team conference to facilitate problem-solving and open communication.
The family members will accept and allow ill member to handle crisis or situation in his/her own way.	• Create a supportive environment for the family. • Encourage family to visit patient. • Encourage family to participate in patient's care.
The family will reduce or resolve crisis or situation.	• Promote wellness through health teaching. • Teach family the skills required for care of the patient.
The family members will develop mutual support.	• Facilitate understanding in other family members of the ill member's feelings. • Provide positive reinforcement for effective use of coping mechanisms.
The family will experience cohesion. The family will be able to adapt to change.	• Initiate referrals as needed, such as social service, financial counselor, home health care, psychiatric nurse, support groups.

VIII

ing a crisis need to preserve and identify the normality of the experience and maintain competency, mastery, and self-esteem.[16]

Family assessment data provide cues about previous family coping strategies. Lewis[18] notes that families have their own schedules for coping and for accepting extrafamilial help. Family coping over time is very complex; healthy functioning and dysfunction are not a simple linear cause-effect outcome.[31] *Because many factors influence family functioning, rigid intervention regimens based on assumptions of family care may not be effective.*[16] *Interventions that work with one family may alienate another.* Families cope in different ways at different times. Factors that influence family coping include characteristics of the event, perceived threat to the family, available resources, and past experiences.[13] *It is important to note that the family's perspective on crisis and illness may be very different from the perspective of the ill family member or of nursing. Thus nursing interventions should focus on the family as the unit of care and address the family's need for information, confidence, assurance of good care for the ill family member, and hope.*[16] *Expediting communication within the family and promoting mutual goals facilitates meeting reciprocal needs in a family crisis and promotes effective family coping.*[27]

Many factors influence family functioning and decision-making: past unresolved issues, repeated hospitalization of an ill family member, and depletion of economic, physical, and emotional resources. The ill family member's need to maintain control may be in opposition to the family's need to care for the ill member. Families need to negotiate role division and clarify how decisions will be made. *Nursing interventions that promote the maintenance of family control and self-esteem, provide information for informed decision-making, and facilitate open lines of communication may ease the distress and dysfunction in the family unit.*[5] Teaching the family practical coping skills, strategies for caring for the ill family member and for themselves, and how to negotiate with the health care delivery system may also be indi-

cated. *Family conferences with health care personnel will enhance communication and decision-making. Family-centered nursing care promotes self-care capabilities and decision-making about health care matters.*[5]

Assessment of the family's support system is essential in mobilizing assistance when needed. Some families that have closed, rigid boundaries may not know how or have the desire to seek extrafamilial support. Other families desire assistance but lack the knowledge and skills needed to obtain support. *Nursing interventions can promote utilization of intrafamilial and extrafamilial support through education, referral, and consultation with other health care providers and community agencies.* For the family experiencing Altered Family Processes, continuity of care and follow-up are essential nursing activities. *Access to additional coping resources will increase family self-confidence and competence and decrease isolation and low-self esteem.*[27]

EVALUATION

Evaluation involves measuring the extent to which expected outcomes are met. The evaluation process is ongoing and shared by the nurse and family. The nurse must examine the family's outcomes to determine the effectiveness of the interventions. For families with an Altered Family Process resulting from illness of a family member, behaviors indicating that predetermined objectives have been realized include (1) family expresses feelings freely and appropriately, (2) family members are involved in problem-solving processes directed at appropriate solutions for the situation or crisis, (3) energies are being directed toward a purpose, (4) family expresses understanding of illness or trauma, treatment regimen, and prognosis, (5) family members are allowing and encouraging ill member to handle situation in his/her own way, (6) family members acknowledge change in family roles and assume responsibility for those changes, (7) family members identify coping patterns, and (8) family members identify and contact available resources as needed.

❖ *CASE STUDY WITH PLAN OF CARE*

Mr. Elmer B., a 75-year-old man, resides with his 74-year-old wife in their own home in the country. Mr. B. recently suffered a cerebrovascular accident that has left him with partial paralysis of the left side. He needs assistance with activities of daily living and is confined to a wheelchair at this time. Family finances are limited. Mrs. B. is a very proud woman who prefers to manage her husband's care by herself and has refused assistance up to this point. She has discontinued all activities and interests outside the home to care for her husband. Although Mr. B.'s health status continues to improve daily, Mrs. B. fears that something may happen if she spends any time away from him. Mr. and Mrs. B. have an adult daughter who is married and living in the same town. She has offered to assist her par-

ents both financially and physically. Mrs. B. refuses to discuss these issues with her daughter. Mrs. B. feels that her husband's care is her responsibility and does not want her daughter to take on this "burden." The family physician is concerned about a deterioration in Mrs. B.'s health. Her blood pressure is elevated, she complains of insomnia, and she reports poor nutritional intake. She appears exhausted and states this to the physician, but she does not want her husband or daughter to know how she feels. She has always taken care of her husband and does not want to change that now. The family physician refers the entire B. family to a community health nurse who diagnoses Altered Family Processes related to the illness of a family member (a situational crisis).

PLAN OF CARE FOR THE B. FAMILY

Nursing Diagnosis: *Altered Family Processes related to the illness of a family member*

Expected Patient Outcomes	**Nursing Interventions**
The B. family will communicate openly and freely.	• Assess the family system. • Identify and support the B. family's strengths.
The B. family members will develop mutual respect.	• Promote trust among family members.
The family will deal constructively with the crisis.	• Encourage the B. family to verbalize feelings.
The B. family will readjust to roles.	• Discuss family members' role adjustments and their ability to adapt.
The B. family will solve problems effectively.	• Teach the B. family problem-solving methods
The B. family will seek assistance when needed.	• Teach coping skills to the B. Family.
The B. family will verbalize need for continued support.	• Provide emotional support to the B. family.
The B. family will identify and mobilize support system.	• Discuss with family members the effect of the crisis on the family. • Positively reinforce adaptive family behaviors.
The B. family will contact community agencies for assistance.	• Refer the B. family to community agencies, support groups, and family therapists as needed.
The B. family will identify the need for help and respite care for Mrs. B.	• Arrange for home health aide services that are within the B. family budget.

If family outcomes are not met, intervention strategies need to be reevaluated. Alternative interventions should be implemented if defining characteristics of Altered Family Processes continue to be present. Referrals to other health care team members may be indicated. Further assessment of the family's ability and readiness to accept assistance is indicated.

REFERENCES

1. Ablon J, Ames GM: Culture and family. In Gillis C, Highley BL, Roberts BM, and Martinson IM, editors: *Toward a science of family nursing,* Menlo Park, Calif, 1989, Addison-Wesley.
2. Anderson JM: Health care across cultures, *Nurs Outlook* 38(3):136-139, 1990.
3. Bloch B: Bloch's assessment guide for ethnic/cultural variations. In Orgue MS, Bloch B, and Monrroy LS, editors: *Ethnic nursing care: a multicultural approach,* St Louis, 1983, CV Mosby.
4. Carpenito LJ: *Handbook of nursing diagnosis,* ed 2, Philadelphia, 1987, JB Lippincott.
5. Clemen-Stone S, Eigsti DG, and McGuire SL: *Comprehensive family and community nursing,* ed 2, New York, 1987, Mcgraw-Hill Book Co.
6. Curran D: *Traits of a healthy family,* New York, 1983, Ballantine.
7. Duespohl TA: *Nursing diagnosis manual for the well and ill client,* Philadelphia, 1986, WB Saunders.
8. Duvall EM: *Marriage and family development,* ed 5, New York, 1977, JB Lippincott.
9. Friedman MM: *Family nursing: theory and assessment,* ed 2, Norwalk, Conn, 1986, Appleton-Century-Crofts.
10. Giger JN, Davidhizar RE: *Transcultural nursing: assessment and intervention,* St Louis, 1991, Mosby–Year Book.
11. Gillis C: Family and research in nursing. In Gillis C, Highley B, Roberts B, and Martinson I, editors: *Toward a science of family nursing,* Menlo Park, Calif, 1989, Addison-Wesley.
12. Helvie C: *Community health nursing: theory and practice,* New York, 1981, Harper & Row.
13. Hill R, Hansen D: The family in disaster. In Baker G, Chapman D, editors: *Man and society in disaster,* New York, 1962, Basic Books.
14. Kim MJ, McFarland GK, and McLane AM: *Pocket guide to nursing diagnoses,* ed 4, St Louis, 1991, Mosby–Year Book.
15. Lasky P. and others: Developing an instrument for the assessment of family dynamics, *West J Nurs Res* 7:40-57, 1985.
16. Leavitt MB: Transition to illness: the family in the hospital. In Gillis C, Highley B, Roberts B, and Martinson I, editors: *Toward a science of family nursing,* Menlo Park, Calif, 1989, Addison-Wesley.
17. Leininger M: *Qualitative research methods in nursing,* Orlando, Fla, 1985, Grune & Stratton.
18. Lewis FM: Family level services for the cancer patient: critical distinctions, fallacies and assessment, *Cancer Nurs* 6:193-200, 1983.
19. Moos R, Insel P, and Humphrey B: *Preliminary manual for family environmental scale,* Palo Alto, Calif, 1974, Consulting Psychologists Press.
20. Otto HA: Criteria for assessing family strength, *Fam Process* 2(2):329-337, 1963.
21. Parad HJ: *Crisis intervention: selected readings,* New York, 1965, Family Services Association of America.
22. Pless IB, Satterwhite B: A measure of family functioning and its application, *Int J Epidemiol* 1:271-277, 1973.
23. Satir V: *Conjoint family therapy,* Palo Alto, Calif, 1967, Science & Behavior Books.
24. Schuster CS, Ashburn SS: *The process of human development: a holistic approach,* Boston, 1980, Little, Brown & Co.
25. Schwenk T, Hughes C: The family as patient in family medicine: rhetoric or reality? *Soc Sci Med* 17:1-16, 1983.
26. Smilkstein G: The family Apgar, *J Fam Pract* 6:1231-1239, 1978.
27. Sparks SM, Taylor CM, editors: *Nursing diagnoses reference manual,* Springhouse, Penn, 1991, Springhouse.
28. Stinnett N, Chessar B, and DeFrain J, editors: *Building family strengths: blueprints for action,* Lincoln, 1979, University of Nebraska Press.
29. Thompson J, McFarland G, Hirsch J, Tucker S, Bowers A: *Mosby's clinical nursing,* ed 2, St Louis, 1989, CV Mosby.
30. Tripp-Reimer T, Brink P, and Saunders J: Cultural assessment: content and process, *Nurs Outlook* 32(2):78-82, 1984.
31. Young R: The family-illness intermesh: theoretical aspects and their application, *Soc Sci Med* 17:395-398, 1983.

Altered Parenting

High Risk for Altered Parenting

Altered Parenting occurs when the ability of the nurturing figure(s) to create an environment that promotes the optimal growth and development of another human being is compromised.[13]

High Risk for Altered Parenting occurs when the ability of the nurturing figure(s) to create an environment that promotes the optimal growth and development of another human being is potentially compromised.

OVERVIEW

Parenting is a learned behavior, primarily based on the observations and perceptions of child rearing in one's own childhood home and those of friends. The mobility of families in today's society has often separated the nuclear family from the resources available in the extended family of earlier generations, which provided opportunities to observe and participate in infant and child care and even the birthing process. In response to the loss of primary experiences of child rearing in developmental years, many communities have developed support groups to provide knowledge regarding the birth process and parenting skills.[4,6] In addition, situations related to ineffective individual or family coping may contribute to potential or actual alterations in parenting behaviors.

The characteristics of an adequate family environment include "basic life supports for the physical survival of the child, stimulation of the child's emotional, social and cognitive achievements, promotion of stability of intra-psychic development of the child to ensure adequate control over impulses, reality testing, affect regulation and moral stability, and the ability to disengage from the family constellation as part of a process of life-long individuation."[15] Adequate parenting is the ability to provide such an environment for all the children of the family.

The roles of parents within the structure of the family system are set by the culture surrounding it. The stereotype of the "typical American family" based on an idealized representation of the nuclear family is a development of the mid-twentieth century owing more to the power of American advertising than to reality based on census statistics. The type of family structure where the parents live together with two or three children and carry out the "traditional" roles of father leaving for work daily in a successful career and mother functioning as homemaker and nurturer of the family is increasingly a thing of the past.[16] Although this structure has been offered as the model for viewing the family in both sociological and political arenas, the nuclear family may function erratically in the long-term process of child rearing. During times of stress, the functioning of the entire family system may be threatened because resources are limited to a very few individuals and their support contacts within the larger community. Several additional family structures, such as blended families, foster families, communal families, and single-parent families, should be considered as acceptable alternatives to the nuclear family in today's society. Within any of these types of family structure there may be deviations from the accepted norms of the community. The most common deviations today are schoolaged parents, in either single- or two-parent families, and homosexual parents.

The primary task of parenting is the socialization of the child.[4] This includes providing an environment that offers sufficient food, shelter, and safety for adequate growth as well as stimulating cognitive and social skills needed for interaction with others. It is the parent's job to reflect reality to the child and teach what is acceptable and unacceptable behavior.[18] The specific needs change as the child matures.[7] Nurturing, as evidenced by frequent holding, touching, smiling, and talking, is needed during infancy. Toddlers and preschoolers need firm, consistent, yet flexible, control strategies as well as expanded play activities and a cognitively rich physical and social environment. Children of all ages need a parent who is a mediator of environmental stimulation, responsive to their behavior, sensitive to and accepting of their emotions, and available.

Although many people assume that parenthood is a natural phenomenon and all adults instinctively react to the presence of a child in a nurturing fashion, becoming a parent creates a period of instability in a family system that requires transitional behaviors. The period of transition to parenthood may be divided into four phases: the anticipatory phase, the honeymoon phase, the plateau phase, and the termination phase.[11] The anticipatory phase begins with the commitment to form a stable family unit and ends with the birth of the first child. During the early part of this phase various activities prepare the adults to assume parenting responsibilities. Among these are the revision of each partner's roles, redefinition of family rules, reassignment of tasks necessary to survival of the family, and development of behaviors expressing both intimacy and individuality.

When pregnancy occurs the couple begins to demonstrate specific preparations for parenting. An increase in passive and dependent behaviors of one or both parents has been noted in the literature. This has been interpreted as a final testing opportunity to take on a dependent role before becoming the one on whom the infant will be dependent.[11] If the dependency needs of the potential parent are not accepted and met by significant others, a sense of insecurity or inability to meet the dependency needs of the child may develop. Another behavior occurring during this time is an increase in fantasies and recall of unresolved childhood conflicts. These are connected with the task of resolving the separation from one's own parents before becoming a parent. The couple is dealing with the fact that although they are still a son or daughter of their respective parents, they are no longer children. At the same time they are developing a relationship with the unborn infant and beginning to identify parenting behaviors they wish to display.[11] Additional tasks during the late anticipatory phase concern concrete preparation for the care of the child: obtaining clothing and furniture and making decisions about how the child will be fed and which partner will care for the infant during which periods of the day. Failure to deal with these issues may reflect inability to understand the specific requirements of parenthood in providing for the basic needs of the child.

The honeymoon phase is the period after the birth of the child when the attachment between parent and child is formed through intimacy and prolonged contact.[11] This is a period of intensity, with each parent exploring the relationship with the new individual now present. Ambivalence is a result of the reality of changes in lifestyle created by the helplessness of the infant, the tremendous energy required to meet its needs, the disparity between the "idealized" child and the actual child, and the feelings of helplessness and vulnerability produced by the need to care for the infant's total needs. One study[12] has shown significant differences between expectations and the actual processes of parenting during the first 3 weeks after birth.

Balancing the individual ambivalence created during this phase with the other individual needs and those of the relationships between parent and child and between the parent's needs as a couple requires either direct or indirect support from external sources.[11] Friends, relatives, community or church support groups, and other resources offer validation of the universality of the new parent's perceptions and reactions, provide occasional release from the responsibilities and intensity of the parent-child relationship, function as emotional sounding boards to help in the acceptance of concerns and self-doubts, give concrete information about child care, care of the self, and resources in the community, and enhance the parents' enjoyment of the child by sharing these experiences. When external support resources are not available to the parents during this honeymoon phase, the likelihood of inability to make a successful transition to parenting increases and professional interventions may be necessary to promote a family system that can nurture the optimum growth and development of all members.

The plateau phase may be described as the protracted middle phase where parental roles are refined and exercised throughout the period of the child's dependency. Although the term plateau gives rise to an image of stability, the act of parenting through the various stages of childhood and adolescence is one of constant change. The parents must learn to juggle the ever-changing balance of dependence and independence within the child and maintain the environment to provide for the physical needs of the family. The ambivalence created during the honeymoon phase may remain, to some extent, throughout the entire parenting experience. Children rarely meet the expectations of their parents, frequently create situations in which the parents feel helpless, and continue to require expenditure of physical and emotional resources that produce scarcity in other aspects of the family systems. The stresses that develop during the extended period of parenting may increase to the point where survival of the family system or of individuals within the system is threatened.

Two principles necessary to survival are altruism and reciprocity.[5] Altruism relates to the cost-benefit ratio. When benefits are given to another, it involves a cost to the giver. The parent-child relationship is assumed to include giving without considering the cost; thus parenting is perceived to be based on altruism. However, even an altruistic relationship is based on reciprocity. Reci-

procity may be of three types: generalized, balanced, or negative.[5] Generalized reciprocity is defined as a one-way flow that requires nothing in return in order to continue and may be viewed as an altruistic expression. This type of reciprocity is expected in parents of infants and young children who depend on the adults in their environment for survival. The cost of helping a child grow and develop is sufficiently balanced by the growth and development of the child. Balanced reciprocity is a direct and real exchange of resources and occurs between parent and child as the child becomes older and develops a degree of independence. Balanced reciprocity may be expressed as directly as requiring the child to perform certain tasks for spending money or as indirectly as the child offering statements of appreciation or gifts that represent an emotional expenditure. Negative reciprocity is an attempt to get something for nothing. Persons who perceive themselves never to have experienced sufficient altruistic reciprocity may approach parenthood with the expectation of having this need met by their children. The child's role then becomes one of provider rather than receiver, and a situation of negative reciprocity has been instituted in which both parent and child expect needs to be met without having to give in return. During this prolonged phase of parenting it is essential that internal and external sources of support to the family system be available as the potential for developmental and situational crises recurs.

The final phase of parenthood is disengagement, in which parent-child roles are revised.[11] As children assume independent roles in the adult world, parents must reassess the emotional and physical resource allocation they have made in the past. More resources are now available to be placed in the parental dyad and in meeting individual needs. Removing these resources from the children initiates feelings of loss and may reawaken former ambivalent feelings. The children may be unable to accept the total loss of dependence and expect to have available the same level of generalized reciprocity that existed in childhood. Negotiating the balance between depen-

VIII

dence and independence with adult children becomes as threatening to the survival of the family system as any earlier crisis, and the need for sufficient internal and external supports still exists.

No single style of parenting has been shown to be an "ideal" to be emulated in all situations. Although in the past parents tended to rear their children as they had been reared, current societal trends have produced an overwhelming number of books, pamphlets, instructional courses, and self-help groups aimed at providing answers to difficult parent-child interactions.

Parenting styles have usually been classified on two types of continuums: permissive-restrictive and democratic-authoritarian.[16] An alternative is a multi-dimensional model that reflects the need to consider the parents' natural behavior as well as the characteristic behavior of the child. Thus permissive parenting behavior may be indicative of either an overindulgent, or an indifferent, parent, as well as one who values creativity and responsible freedom. In such a multi-dimensional model, parenting behaviors expressing love may range from permissive, to democratic, to authoritative, and finally to possessive and overprotective. These behaviors are child-centered and accepting in nature. Behaviors that are essentially hostile to the child may range from indifferent to neglectful, to demanding, to antagonistic, to authoritarian and dictatorial. These behaviors are centered on the needs of the parent and are rejecting of the child.

Although family systems and specific parenting behaviors may have changed as communities have moved toward a mobile, urban society, the basic parenting functions remain. Parents continue to have the responsibility to provide for the physical survival of the child, to protect the child from dangers to his/her safety, to help the child develop a sense of security and self-esteem, and to function as a socializing agent to encourage the child to participate in the community and to seek continuity. Meeting the responsibilities of parenting requires access to physical, social, and emotional resources within both the family structure and the community. When either the re-

sources or access to them is limited, the ability to function as a parent is compromised and intervention from health care professionals may be required.

ASSESSMENT

Although Altered Parenting may occur in any family structure, some individuals or families are perceived to be at higher risk for developing or experiencing difficulties in parenting. Any situation or condition of either parent or child that intensifies the stress within the family unit increases the risk for Altered Parenting.

Because parenting behaviors are the result of the interaction of many factors in the history of individual parents, the parents' relationship to each other, and their relationship to their own parents and to their children, as well as the multiplicity of factors within the current situation, it is difficult to assess the degree to which parenting is successful. All aspects of the functional health patterns need to be assessed. However, some should be focused on the child while others should focus on the parent(s) or on the relationship between parent and child. Information about the nutritional, elimination, activity, and rest patterns of the child may be essential in identifying the presence of maltreatment. Assessment of the health perception, cognitive, and value patterns of the parent(s) will provide information relating to etiology and intervention strategies. The nurse should assess both the child and the parent(s) in the areas of self-perception, role-relationship, and coping-stress tolerance patterns. The nurse should emphasize the assessment of social and economic factors, as these have been demonstrated to be significant in contributing to the maltreatment of children.

The Graduated Resource Assessment Model for assessing parental behaviors has two components: the relationship assessment continuum and the resource assessment continuum[5]. The initial element to be assessed is the attachment capacity of both parent and child within the relationship. Attachment capacity must be present to some extent in both parent and child or this distortion will result in rejection. Assessment of the attachment behaviors is conducted through obtaining historical information and observation of current behaviors relating to pregnancy, bonding at birth, and the progressive expansion of reciprocity in the parent-child relationship.

Assessment of the resources available to the parent-child relationship is the second step in the model. The presence or absence of resources and their appropriate use can predict the degree to which parenting behaviors may be successful. Resource assessment has three elements: physical resources limitations, social support systems, and emotional resources present in both parent and child. Physical resources include not only the physical health and capacity of each member of the family but also aspects of the physical environment, such as economic resources and their use to promote physical means of survival for the child. Assessment of the social support systems available explores extended family, neighborhood, and community resources available and used by the family to survive stressors. The third element to be assessed is the emotional resources present in both parent and child. Emotional resources represent the extent to which a person is able to respond to another in either a generalized or balanced reciprocal relationship. This resource pool may be a result of the parent's childhood, the parent's or child's personality characteristics, or factors present in the current relationship. This element also includes the educational variables of intellectual abilities and fund of parenting alternatives available.

Many other assessment tools have become available within the last 5 years. Hansen and MacMillan[8] reviewed a wide selection of these, grouping them into categories corresponding to the specific behaviors known to be associated with maltreatment of children. The categories identified were: identification of abuse and neglect, child management, anger and arousal, knowledge and expectations, problem-solving and coping skills, and social support. The use of multiple assessment procedures or information sources is emphasized. For example, Anderson[2] developed the Parenting Profile Assessment based on the Ecological Integrative Model of Child Maltreatment as a means of identifying potential abusive mothers. Anderson found 20 items related to the mother, the family, and discipline methods to be discriminating between abusive and nonabusive mothers. These items are included in the listing of related factors.

Altered Parenting
❖ Defining Characteristics

The presence of the following defining characteristics indicates that Altered Parenting may be present:

- Inappropriate caretaking behaviors (e.g., feeding, elimination, rest)
- Physical or psychological abuse
- Inappropriate visual, tactile, or auditory stimulation of the child
- Growth and developmental lag in the child
- Frequent accidents or illnesses of the child
- Lack of parental attachment behaviors
- Inattention to infant/child needs
- Frequent verbalizations of dissatisfaction or disappointment with the child
- Frequent identification of negative characteristics of the child
- Frequent attachment of negative meanings to characteristics or behavior of the child
- Verbalization of resentment toward the child
- Signs of depression, apathy, disturbed, or bizarre behavior in the child
- Rejection of caregiver or over-compliance by the child
- Verbalization of frustration with parenting role or role inadequacy
- Inappropriate or inconsistent discipline
- Abandonment

❖ Related Factors

The following related factors are associated with Altered Parenting:

- Little or no prenatal care
- Parental absence or inability to function because of illness

VIII

- Inability or unwillingness to assume parenting responsibilities
- Ineffective coping with anger
- History of ineffective or abusive relationships with own parents
- Poor problem-solving techniques
- Poor education level (high school or less)
- Chaotic or inappropriate family relationships
- Situational crises (e.g., financial)
- Lack of external resources
- Daily stressors because of poverty, unemployment
- Unrealistic expectations for self, spouse, child
- Lack of knowledge, cognitive functioning, or role identity as a parent
- Not wanting child

❖ Related Medical/Psychiatric Diagnoses

The following are examples of related medical/psychiatric diagnoses for Altered Parenting:
For Parent
- Borderline personality disorder
- Antisocial personality disorder
- Bipolar disorders
- Psychoactive substance dependence/abuse
- Medical illnesses; e.g., cancer, tuberculosis

High Risk for Altering Parenting
❖ Risk Factors

The presence of any of the following behaviors, conditions, and circumstances renders the parents more vulnerable to High Risk for Altered Parenting:
- Little or no prenatal care
- Parental absence or inability to function because of illness
- Inability or unwillingness to assume parenting responsibilities
- Ineffective coping with anger
- History of ineffective or abusive relationships with own parents
- Poor problem-solving techniques
- Poor education level (high school or less)
- Chaotic or inappropriate family relationships
- Situational crises (e.g., financial)
- Lack of external resources

- Daily stressors because of poverty, unemployment
- Unrealistic expectations for self, spouse, child
- Lack of knowledge, cognitive functioning, or role identity as a parent
- Not wanting child

❖ Related Medical/Psychiatric Diagnoses

The following are examples of related medical/psychiatric diagnoses for High Risk for Altered Parenting
- Any major illness leading to parental physical or emotional incapacity, e.g., cerebrovascular disease, schizophrenia

NURSING DIAGNOSES

Examples of *specific* nursing diagnoses for Altered Parenting are:
- Altered Parenting related to unwanted child
- Altered Parenting related to ineffective skills for coping with anger
- Altered Parenting related to lack of external support resources
- Altered Parenting related to unrealistic expectations for child

Examples of *specific* nursing diagnoses of High Risk for Altered Parenting are:
- High Risk for altered parenting related to lack of knowledge
- High Risk for Altered Parenting related to developmental lack of parental skills
- High Risk for Altered Parenting related to daily stressors resulting from poverty

PLANNING AND IMPLEMENTATION WITH RATIONALE

Harris and associates[10] suggest that intervention in family systems can progress through four stages: crisis, stabilization and consolidation, transition, and normalization. The crisis stage develops when health care professionals become involved in the family system as a result of assessed actual or potential breakdown in parenting behaviors that has produced a threat to the safety or security of the child. Treatment issues during this first stage center on potential need to remove the child from the parent, psychological support for the parent, creation of an expectancy of change by the parent, and the initiation of new parenting behaviors. *Specific interventions should be designed to meet selected goals. For instance, when there appears to be a lack of attachment behaviors, helping the parent learn to enjoy play activities and the natural developmental achievements of the child will create the feeling of successful parenting and lead to better bonding.* Age-paced newsletters and other literature can support the development of an adequate knowledge base to enhance effective parenting. Role identity as a parent can be developed by identifying, acknowledging, and praising parental strengths. A nursing history provides opportunity to recognize successful parenting strategies and discussion of alternatives.

During the second stage new parenting behaviors are stabilized and consolidated into the family expectations. This stage requires maintaining the assistance with the cognitive and emotional demands made on the parent as a result of changing expectations and role within the family. *Increased social and physical support from extended family members, friends, or community helpers such as church or school personnel may be essential during this stage* in maintaining assistance with emotional demands on family.

In the transitional stage the parents signal a readiness to undertake independent child care. Supportive interventions are needed during this period *to support the changed role identity and to encourage perceptions of competent performance of parenting behaviors.*

The final stage of treatment interventions focuses on developing the"normal" behaviors of an adequate parent-child system. The parents exhibit nurturing behaviors in addition to usual household and work routines and the child responds with normal gains in growth and developmental tasks. During this stage appropriate plans are developed to maintain contact with health professionals *to obtain routine supervision, health care, and anticipatory guidance during the childhood and adolescent years.*

The overall goals of nursing interventions may remain the same throughout the treatment process, but the specific interventions must be modified as the parents and family progress toward attaining a more stable family system. Goals and interventions discussed in this chapter have addressed only the needs of the parents. The nurse must recognize that the child or children of the family must be included in treatment activities. (See Altered Growth and Development or Ineffective Family Coping.) Nursing goals and the principles of nursing interventions are similar in both actual and High Risk for Altered Parenting behaviors. Specific interventions must be designed to meet the identified needs of the individuals involved.

Planning for the treatment of family systems that exhibit either actual or High Risk for Altered Parenting behaviors should focus on selecting specific interventions to assure that the following goals are met: provision of safe environment for the child; promotion of parent-child attachment behaviors; provision of an adequate knowledge base for effective parenting; development of realistic expectations for self, spouse, and child within the family system; and development of role identity as parent.

The provision of a physically and psychologically safe environment for the child is the basic function of a parent. Child abuse and neglect are the extreme deviations on a continuum of parenting adequacy. Deficiencies in this area may range from routinely ignoring a child's diet or personal hygiene, to homes with multiple safety hazards, to severe physical abuse. Lutzker[14] describes specific interventions designed to focus the awareness of the parent(s) on the child's need for personal hygiene, adequate nutrition, and home safety and cleanliness. In situations where the parent(s) cannot provide for the minimum safety and physiologic needs of the child, mechanisms designed by the community must be engaged to remove the child to a safer environment.

Bonding and attachment are two concepts that have received much attention in recent years and may be seen as the two most significant parenting

VIII

❖ *NURSING CARE GUIDELINES*

Nursing Diagnosis: Altered Parenting

Expected Parent Outcomes	Nursing Interventions
The parent will provide a safe environment for the child.	• Monitor degree of risk to child's safety and contact appropriate authorities if child's safety seems jeopardized.
The parent will develop parent-child attachment behaviors.	• Encourage touching behaviors by parents. • Encourage play activities between the parent and child. • Encourage age-appropriate caretaking activities by parents.
The parent will have an adequate knowledge base for effective parenting.	• Identify knowledge deficits in specific areas, such as growth and development, discipline, caretaking activities, resources, and alternatives. • Identify learning readiness and capability of the parent. • Provide cognitive information to the parent at an appropriate level, and provide an opportunity for the parent to test new information. • Create a positive learning environment for the parent.
The parent will develop realistic expectations for self, spouse, and child within the family.	• Identify present expectations for self, spouse, and child. • Identify areas of failure to meet expectations. • Provide opportunity for expression of feelings about unmet expectations, and encourage speculation about reasons for unmet expectations. • Help parent to develop realistic expectations. • Develop strategies to increase possibilities of having expectations met (e.g., discussing expectation with spouse or child or identifying steps that must occur in order to meet expectations).
The parent will develop role identity as parent.	• Help parent identify major components within role identity (e.g., child of own parents, spouse, career) perceptions of specific parenting behaviors, and source of "ideal" parenting behavior. • Observe parent-child interactions for congruency between verbalized "ideal" and actual behavior. • Provide opportunity for exploring role identity through individual counseling or group interaction. • Provide opportunity for the parent to observe or experience effective parent behaviors. • Provide opportunity for the parent to implement alternative parenting behaviors.
The parent will have emotional, social, and physical support.	• Identify specific areas of needed emotional, social, and physical support. • Identify specific strengths of parent and support systems. • Provide information about additional resources available for parents to meet needs. • Act as liaison or advocate as needed in obtaining help from appropriate resources.

VIII

abilities.[5] Bonding may be defined as a undirectional process, flowing from parent to child, that begins during pregnancy and peaks during the first few days after birth. The process of bonding begins with planning, confirming, and accepting the pregnancy and progresses through the steps of feeling fetal movement, accepting the fetus as an individual person, giving birth, hearing and seeing the baby, touching and holding the baby, and caring for the baby. *The development of bonding is facilitated by bodily contact between parent and child, eye contact, fondling, and caring for the child during the period immediately after birth.*[6]

Attachment is a process that develops during the first year of the child's life and depends on a successful bond being in place.[5] Attachment activities appear to be based on the need to maximize opportunities for survival, and the process reflects the growing trust and security the child finds in the parents. The attachment relationship is reciprocal, containing elements of both generalized and balanced reciprocity. Little consideration is given to the cost of parenting, but small actions undertaken by the child, such as smiling in response to the parent's voice, provide sufficient reward. *Assessment of bonding and attachment behaviors provides information about the parent-child relationship and the abilities of the adults to function in a parenting capacity.*

The majority of interventions found in the literature focus on some aspect of providing an adequate knowledge base for effective parenting.[1,3,17,19] *Lack of information, lack of role models, lack of external resources and ineffective coping skills may all be decreased through appropriate patient education methods.* It is essential to develop the specific teaching strategy based on the parents' needs, cognitive level, previous information, previous life experiences, and emotional/psychological development. Attempting to teach *techniques* to parents without understanding the underlying dynamics may be ineffective. In many cases, the interactions may not appear genuine, and children are quick to sense this. Dependence on a technique to solve the problem may

also lead to further blame of self or the partner if the desired results are not obtained. Hardy[9] has demonstrated the effectiveness of a well-designed family support and parenting education program.

Many parents have unrealistic expectations of their role and abilities as a parent, of their spouse's role and abilities, and the child's role and ability in the relationship. This may lead to increased frustration and anxiety as the expected behaviors are not manifested. Because anxiety is frequently transformed into anger, the potential for disruption of the parenting function is great. *Helping the parent to identify the source of the anger and develop more realistic expectations defuses the anxiety and offers opportunity to develop alternative behaviors.*

The role of the parent is one of the most complex within our society. Understanding and acceptance of the parenting role is not an automatic reaction to becoming a parent. Parenting is a learned behavior. In many communities the opportunity for observing parenting behavior is limited, and persons are forced to rely on their perception of how they were parented. *Interventions that provide information about alternative parenting behaviors and opportunity to discuss the changes in lifestyle required as a parent broaden the perspective of the parent and aid in internalizing the parenting role.*

Many of the defining characteristics of Altered Parenting are the result of insufficient emotional, social, or physical support. Persons whose own basic needs for safety, nutrition, or love have not been met will be unable to meet the needs of another. After specific areas of deficiencies have been identified, the nurse may offer information about services available to provide the support needed.

EVALUATION

Evaluation of the extent to which specific interventions are helping the parent meet the identified goals must be ongoing. Each interaction between nurse and parent contains the opportunity to assess and evaluate the change in attachment behaviors, expectations, and role identity. Descriptions

Text continued on p. 626.

VIII

❖ CASE STUDY WITH PLAN OF CARE: ALTERED PARENTING

Alan, a 6-week-old infant, was brought to the hospital with multiple injuries resulting from repeated stabbings with a meat fork. He sustained a pneumo-hemothorax and liver lacerations but was quickly stabilized. Mrs. Angie A., his mother, explained that she had been unable to quiet him. He had cried all morning, although she had fed him, changed him, and rocked him. He usually enjoyed his bath, and she had thought that might calm him. However, his crying increased until it was intolerable. After she injured him, she called for an ambulance. The nursing history was obtained from Mrs. A. in the pediatric intensive care unit after the baby had been admitted.

RELATIONSHIP ASSESSMENT CONTINUUM

1. Parental childhood attachments: Mrs. A. stated she had had a good relationship with her parents and was particularly close to her father. She saw him as always being available to help her when she had problems. She was the youngest child and did not remember any experience of taking care of infants.

2. Pregnancy: Alan was a wanted child of a planned pregnancy. There were no problems with the pregnancy, and all appropriate preparations were made for his becoming part of the family.

3. Delivery and postpartum experiences, early bonding: Both Mr. and Mrs. A. had participated in natural childbirth classes and had decided to use a birthing room rather than a hospital delivery room. However, Mrs. A.'s labor lasted longer than they had anticipated and she required some medication. It was believed that it would be safer for the baby to use the delivery room. Mr. A. was present at the delivery, and both Mr. and Mrs. A. were able to hold Alan soon after his birth. Mrs. A. reported positive feelings about caring for Alan, although she expressed some nervousness because he seemed so little. During the interview she continued to look at Alan and call him by name. She cried during much of the interview and asked if she could touch him.

RESOURCE ASSESSMENT CONTINUUM

1. Physical limitation of parent: Mrs. A. stated that she had never had any physical problems and enjoyed participation in active sports. She had missed being able to play tennis during her later pregnancy. She indicated that she seemed to be more tired since Alan's birth and couldn't do everything she should.

2. Physical limitation of child: Alan appeared to be a healthy child before the injuries occurred. His weight was within normal limits. The current injuries appeared to be managed with the prompt medical attention received. No long-term physical effects were expected.

3. Physical limitations of environment: None apparent.

4. Social support systems: Both Mr. and Mrs. A.'s parents were still living but in distant cities. They had come for a few days after Alan was born but had not been able to stay. They called frequently, and Mrs. A. stated that she believed she could usually call either her mother or her mother-in-law if she had any "real" problems. Mr. A. had a good job with an income sufficient to support the family in comfort. However, his job included extensive travel at times, and he had been away from home for the last 5 days. Mr. and Mrs. A. had just moved to their present home a few months before Alan was born, and Mrs. A. stated that she didn't know the neighbors very well and hadn't kept in touch with friends in the city from which they moved.

5. Emotional limitations of parents or child: Mrs. A. appeared to be warm and affectionate toward both Alan and her husband when she spoke of them. She expressed primarily satisfaction and pleasure in her marriage and her child. She did verbalize some disappointment with her ability to immediately understand what the baby needed and to perform all the household tasks and other activities she had enjoyed before she become pregnant. She acknowledged that her husband's success in his job depended on his availability to travel, but stated she felt "down" when he wasn't home. She also stated that they had a "modern marriage" and that Mr. A. helped with Alan's care and household tasks when he was home, and that she planned to return to work when "the children" were old enough.

6. Intellectual limitation of parents or child: Both parents were college graduates and had participated in "expectant parent" classes. Mrs. A. stated that even though neither she nor Mr. A had ever been around small children, they had read child-rearing information and thought they knew what to expect from children at different ages. They had discussed how they would discipline their children in principle as well as other activities involving raising them.

PLAN OF CARE FOR MRS. ANGIE A.*

Nursing Diagnosis: *Altered Parenting related to unrealistic expectations for self, inadequate knowledge, lack of positive parental role identity, and lack of adequate social support*

Expected Parent Outcomes	Nursing Interventions
Mrs. A. will provide a safe environment for the child as evidenced by no further attempts to harm him.	• Provide for Alan's care while in hospital. • Observe interaction between Mrs. A. and Alan to ensure safety. • Follow hospital policy regarding the reporting of child injury.
Mrs. A. will develop parent-child attachment behaviors as evidenced by appropriate touching and eye contact.	• Allow Mrs. A. to touch and hold Alan as soon as possible. • Allow and encourage Mrs. A. to be involved in Alan's daily care as soon as possible.
Mrs. A. will have an adequate knowledge base for effective parenting as evidenced by appropriate responses to Alan's crying.	• Identify Mrs. A.'s knowledge about why babies cry and caretaking strategies for crying and provide information on how to cope with her feelings when Alan cries. • Provide opportunity for Mrs. A. to test new information. • Create positive learning environment.
Mrs. A. will develop realistic expectations for self, spouse, and child within the family as evidenced by ability to verbalize needs and expectations.	• Help Mrs. A. to identify expectations for herself, Mr. A., and Alan. • Help Mrs. A. to identify areas of failure to meet her expectations, such as her inability to understand Alan's needs or that her husband would be as available to help her as she believed her father had been. • Provide Mrs. A. with an opportunity to express her feelings about unmet expectations. • Encourage Mrs. A. to speculate about reasons for unmet expectations. • Develop strategies to increase possibilities of having expectations met (e.g., discussing expectations with Mr. A. and identifying steps that must occur to meet expectations).
Mrs. A. will develop role identity as parent as evidenced by nurturing behaviors.	• Help Mrs. A. identify major components within role identity (e.g., child of own, parents, spouse, and career), perceptions of specific parenting behaviors that are successful with crying babies, and source of "ideal" parenting behavior. • Observe interactions between Mrs. A. and Alan for congruency between verbalized "ideal" and actual behavior when Alan is crying. • Provide opportunity for Mrs. A. to observe and experience effective parent behaviors with crying babies. • Provide opportunity for Mrs. A. to implement alternative parenting behaviors.
Mrs. A. will experience emotional, social, and physical support as evidenced by decreased isolation and anxiety.	• Help Mrs. A. identify specific areas in which she needs additional emotional, social, or physical support. • Help Mrs. A. identify her specific strengths and support systems. • Provide information about additional resources for Mrs. A. to meet needs. • Act as liaison or advocate as needed in obtaining help for Mrs. A. from appropriate resources, such as contacting Mr. A. and arranging for his immediate return.

VIII

*This care plan focuses on the parent who has demonstrated Altered Parenting behaviors, Mrs. A. The spouse, Mr. A., is viewed as a part of her support system. If further assessment indicates that Mr. A. also needs help in developing appropriate parenting behaviors, the plan should be altered.

of parent-child interactions, reactions to new disciplinary procedures, and relating experiences with community support agencies or groups provide the data from which evaluations can be made. When evaluation shows that one stage of a goal, such as identification of alternative caretaking activities, has been reached, nursing interventions need to be designed to support the next stage, stabilizing and consolidating the behavior. Including the parent in the evaluation process also reinforces the positive changes and becomes a valuable part of the treatment interventions.

REFERENCES

1. Ammerman RT: Etiological models of child maltreatment: a behavioral perspective, *Behav Modif* 14:230-254, 1990.
2. Anderson CL: Assessing parenting potential for child abuse risk, *Pediatr Nurs* 13:323-327, 1987.
3. Azar ST, Siegel BK: Behavioral treatment of child abuse: a developmental perspective, *Behav Modif* 14:279-300, 1990.
4. Bigner JJ: *Parent-child relations: an introduction to parenting,* New York, 1989, Macmillan Publishing.
5. Bolton FG: *When bonding fails: clinical assessment of high-risk families,* Beverly Hills, Calif, 1983, Sage Publications.
6. Carpenito LJ: *Nursing diagnosis: application to clinical practice,* ed 4, New York, 1992, JB Lippincott.
7. Halpern R: Poverty and early childhood parenting: toward a framework for intervention, *Am J Orthopsychiatry* 60:6-17, 1990.
8. Hansen DJ, MacMillan VM: Behavioral assessment of child-abusive and neglectful families: recent developments and current issues, *Behav Modif* 14:255-278, 1990.
9. Hardy JB, Streett R: Family support and parenting education in the home: an effective extension of clinic-based preventive health care services for poor children, *J Pediatr* 115:927-931, 1989.
10. Harris JA, Haslett NR, and Bolding DD: Nonorganic failure to thrive: a distortion of caregiver-infant interaction. In Stuart IR, Abt LE: *Children of separation and divorce: management and treatment,* New York, 1981, Van Nostand Reinhold.
11. Hrobsky DM: Transition to parenthood: a balancing of needs, *Nurs Clin North Am* 12:457-468, 1977.
12. Humenick SS, Bugen LA: Parenting roles: expectation versus reality, *MCN* 12:36-39, 1987.
13. Kim MJ, McFarland GK, and McLane AM: *Pocket guide to nursing diagnoses,* ed 4, St. Louis, 1991, Mosby–Year Book.
14. Lutzker JR: Behavioral treatment of child neglect, *Behav Modif* 14:310-315, 1990.
15. Pfeffer CR: Development issues among children of separation and divorce. In Stuart IR, Abt LE: *Children of separation and divorce: management and treatment,* New York, 1981, Van Nostand Reinhold.
16. Scipien GM, Chard MA, Howe J, and Barnard MU: *Pediatric nursing care,* St Louis, 1990, CV Mosby.
17. Showers J: Behaviour management cards as a method of anticipatory guidance for parents, *Child: Care Health Dev* 15:401-415, 1989.
18. Simon J: The single parent: power and the integrity of parenting, *Am J Psychoanal* 50:187-198, 1990.
19. Webster-Stratton C: Enhancing the effectiveness of self-administered videotape parent training for families with conduct-problem children, *J Abnorm Child Psychol* 18:479-492, 1990.

VIII

Parental Role Conflict

Parental Role Conflict is the state in which a parent experiences role confusion and conflict in response to crisis.

OVERVIEW

Current nursing philosophy encourages family-centered care for all patients, including children. Open visiting hours, overnight stays, and increasing home responsibilities because of shorter hospital stays have allowed parents much exposure to many aspects of their child's care. Some health professionals ask parents to be involved in their child's care, although others discourage it.

Studies have shown that illness and hospitalization involving children are stressful for parents. A child's illness will have an effect on the entire family.[6,7] Parents may struggle with feelings of guilt, helplessness, depression, and anger as they attempt to cope with stressful events within the family unit. Acute stress may be compounded by the effect of the continual daily chronic strain of coping with the limitations of illness.[10,12] Because parents usually play a critical role in offering the sick child support and stability[13] it is important to focus on the stressors and needs of parents.

Parental stress associated with hospitalization has been identified as complex and multifaceted.[1] Miles and Carter[10] developed a model for understanding parental stress in an intensive care unit setting based on theories of Lazarus and others. This conceptual framework of stressors affecting parents includes situational factors of uncertainty about prognoses, future normality, and duration of hospitalization; personal factors related to parental past experiences; and environmental factors related to the physical and psychosocial aspects of

the treatment context. It has been shown that if the needs of parents are not met they may be unable to adequately support their child.[13] Lazarus and Folkman[8] state that stressors arise from factors within both the individual and the environment. Individuals are not passive recipients of environmental demands but continually perceive and evaluate them in relation to their own needs and resources. Parents must meet the needs of other children as well as those of the sick child and maintain their own health as well. Culturally, parental role expectations may be in conflict with the depersonalized institutional rules and regulations. Stress is therefore a relational concept of a balance between the demands of the individual, such as a parent, and the resources to meet these demands without unreasonable and destructive cost. This balance will determine whether the transaction is appraised as irrelevant, benign, or stressful, the latter involving judgments of harm-loss, threat, or challenge.[8] Harm-loss refers to damage that has already occurred; threat refers to anticipated change; and challenge indicates some hope of changing or mastering the situation.

Psychological stress has been described by Lazarus and Folkman[8] as a "particular relationship between the person and the environment that is appraised by the person as taxing or exceeding his/her resources and endangering his/her well-being". They have described coping as the process of managing both the demands from the person-environment relationship identified as stressful and the emotions they generate. Chronic illness, in particular, can diminish even the strongest psychological and physical stamina, and successful psychological management of the ill child is influenced by the parents' ability to cope. Anxious parents are not as effective in providing emotional support for their child,[1] and events generating uncertainty could hamper parents' appraisal of events and their coping mechanisms.[11] Studies[2,4,9,13-15] have shown that nurses need to communicate more effectively with parents about their role in their child's care, emphasizing the importance of parental support for those parents willing to participate. Parents for example, need help in working with their lack of confidence about their role, such as decreasing the child's pain.[3] Communication is essential for the processes of change, learning to trust, and reevaluating situations, and parents have emphasized the importance of clear, honest, open communication of information, repeated as many times as needed.[6]

Parents have perceived the hospitalization of their child as being stressful and as demanding many adaptations in their parental roles.[6,10] Neither nurses nor parents have been able to agree on the parents' role in giving care to the sick child, and parents' concept of their role in hospital has not always been congruent with that of the health team.[2,10,14] Most mothers were willing to help more than the nurses would allow. The majority of mothers in Algren's[2] sample wanted to be included in care, including staying with the child during procedures, yet had not received any communication from the staff about their role and involvement in care. Goodall[5] found that most nurses expressed confidence in working with children and families but were threatened by the presence of parents during difficult procedures. The most important nursing behavior identified by the largest number of parents in Miles and Carter's[9] sample was to give permission to parents to stay with their child as much as possible. Involvement in care was also the most helpful coping strategy, along with receiving information and communicating with staff. This supports the necessity of early communication and documentation about parents' role in the plan of care. Mishel[11] stressed that events generating uncertainty included ambiguity, lack of clarity, and unpredictability. Visintainer and Wolfer[13] found that children whose mothers were provided with information before admission and periodically throughout the child's stay showed better adaptation and recovery in the hospital. Mothers receiving continual support and information about routines, procedures, and their role in the child's care experienced significantly less emotional distress. They were more satisfied with the information given and the child care received and felt more helpful to their child than the control mothers did. These findings provide strong support for the benefits of systematic preparation and support for hospitalized children and their parents.

In summary, studies have shown that serious childhood illness and hospitalization create considerable stress for parents. Although the studies found do not address the effect of a sick child in the home setting, authors such as Hymovich[7] stress the similar needs of parents in managing the child's illness at home. Parents experience confusion and incongruity with the health care team related to their parenting role with a child who is ill. Parents, mainly mothers, who were given information and ongoing support had better adapted children and were themselves more satisfied with their child's experience.

ASSESSMENT

Whenever a child becomes ill, stress is created within the child's entire family. Whether the illness is acute, chronic, or fatal, treated at home or in the hospital, it will have some effect, not only on the child but on all members of the family. Research indicates that parents are especially susceptible to feelings of stress and concern during this period, ranging from periods of guilt for having been somehow responsible for the child's illness to fear of what he/she will undergo and lack of knowledge about the illness and its treatment. Parents often have financial concerns, fear that the child will die, and worry that the child will reject the parent. Sometimes marital conflicts are intensified by a child's illness. Conflicts of responsibility between being at home and being with the child are often unresolved. A parent may resent the burden of coping with the illness and, by extension, resent the child. All of these factors work singly or together to produce the response in the parents to the situation in which they find themselves when they are met by the nurse. The nurse needs to consider all of these aspects when considering the nursing assessment.

The major characteristic of a person experiencing Parental Role Conflict is expressed concern or feeling of inadequacy about providing for the child's emotional or physical needs during hospitalization or in the home. Parents may talk about disruption in caretaking practices and routines. They may identify concerns about changes in their own role, in how the family is functioning and communicating, and in general family well-being. Parents who are experiencing Parental Role Conflict may express a sense of loss in decisions about their child's well-being. Some parents may withdraw from being involved in the routine care of their child even after considerable encouragement and support is given by others. Some parents may express feelings of guilt, anger, fear, anxiety, or frustration about the effects of the child's illness on the whole family. The extent to which these characteristics are evidenced in any parent may well be a function of several related factors and of the effect the illness has on the entire family.

The degree of Parental Role Conflict will be a function of the interaction of a number of variables, including environmental, situational, and personal factors.[10] Environmental stressors include intimidation by invasive or restrictive treatment methods (including isolation or intubation) and by the nature of the specialized care centers (including sights and sounds of equipment, restrictive policies of institutions). In the home, environmental stressors include intimidation by the equipment and procedures required to meet specialized patient needs (for example, apnea monitoring, postural drainage, hyperalimentation). Parents separated from a child with chronic illness might experience a different kind of stress response than those separated from a child with a more acute illness. The nature of the parental response may be influenced by the experience the parents have with the medical world and by the amount and quality of professional support received. Such factors as the age of the child and the child's developmental level and personality characteristics can influence the parents' response. The nature of the marital relationship and the dynamics of the family (including its structure, the number and age of other children, its values and communication patterns) will influence parental response to stress.[7] Other personal factors that could influence parental response include costs of medical care, concurrent stressors such as debt, unemployment, job change, recent changes in dwelling place, concurrent illness in other family members, and the health of the parents themselves.

Standardized assessment tools to be used globally to measure stress related to Parental Role Conflict have not been developed. Researchers have looked at component parts of this parental experience. Miles and Carter[9] developed a parental stressor scale for use in pediatric intensive care units. However, Mishel[11] claims there is a paucity of measurement tools available to measure parental response, not in the least because more research needs to be done to identify the significant perceptual variables influencing the parental response. Currently, stress theory and role theory provide some baseline framework from which to view the diagnosis of parental role conflict.[8] Consistent with this work, important assessment areas are the nature of the situation in which parents find themselves and the effect of that situation on their ability to maintain the parental role as is consistent with their usual practices.

Subsequent important areas for assessment include

1. *Appearance*. Briefly note apparent age, sex, race, deportment, overt signs of distress or composure.
2. *Parents' perception of the problem*. Ask parents to explain in their own words their perception of the situation as they experience it.
3. *Factors influencing the situation*. Assess parents with respect to the nature of the stressors that are influencing their situation.

VIII

What are the environmental factors (including care environment, child's condition, procedures being completed), the contextual issues (including child's level of development, knowledge of the child's condition, degree of sophistication in using the health care system), and, as appropriate to the situation, the personal factors (including family composition and structure, support systems available, past coping strategies, personal and financial resources, and other social influences)?

After eliciting data related to the nature of the stressors influencing parental functioning, ask the parents to describe in their own words how they feel their ability to carry out their "usual" parental role has been compromised and what their perception of their needs and expectations is. Provide parents with an environment that allows them to express their fears and concerns openly with little fear of recrimination.

❖ Defining Characteristics

The presence of the following defining characteristics indicates that the parent may be experiencing Parental Role Conflict:

- Lack of confidence about physical care
- Anxiety, uncertainty about diagnosis/prognosis
- Decreased involvement in decision-making
- Concerns about cultural practices not considered
- Concurrent stressors concerning multiple role demands
- Concerns about the effect on family process

❖ Related Factors

The following related factors are associated with Parental Role Conflict:

Illness stressors
- Unclear diagnosis
- Inadequate knowledge of procedures
- Uncertain prognosis
- Symptom management ineffective
- Multiple health care professionals

Personal stressors
- Multiple roles
- Own health status
- Decreased parental role

- Concurrent family stressors

Family stressors
- Financial debts
- Marital conflict
- Inadequate social supports
- Family routine disruptions

Environmental stressors
- Invasive procedures
- Cultural practices/beliefs excluded
- Unrealistic staff expectations
- Decreased decision-making

❖ Related Medical/Psychiatric Diagnoses

The following are examples of related medical/psychiatric diagnoses for Parental Role Conflict:
- AIDS
- Back pain
- Comatose
- Confused
- Depression
- Developmentally nonverbal
- Impaired verbally
- Migraine headaches
- Poorly controlled epilepsy
- Progressive multiple sclerosis
- Rheumatoid arthritis
- Schizophrenia
- Terminal cancer

NURSING DIAGNOSES

Examples of *specific* nursing diagnoses for Parental Role Conflict are:
- Parental Role Conflict related to unclear diagnosis of child
- Parental Role Conflict related to marital conflicts
- Parental Role Conflict related to unrealistic staff expectations
- Parental Role Conflict related to multiple roles

PLANNING AND IMPLEMENTATION WITH RATIONALE

The overall outcome anticipated with a diagnosis of Parental Role Conflict will be reduction in the factors that influenced the feelings of compromised role functioning and expressed satisfaction with role functioning. Hymovich[7] maintains that to recover from the crisis presented by a child's illness, parents are called on to accomplish certain tasks. These tasks become the basis for specific patient outcomes:

1. Verbalize understanding and ability to manage their child's illness.
2. Demonstrate ability to assist their child in understanding and coping with the illness.
3. Demonstrate ability to meet the needs of all family members as well as those of the ill child. Consistent with this is the need to maintain their own health and the individual integrity of each family member.

The extent to which parents are able to express satisfaction with their role and to express feelings of reduced stress will be influenced by the degree to which they resolve these challenges. The extent to which these challenges are resolved depends heavily on the unique characteristics of the situation in which the parents find themselves and the internal and external resources available to them to meet these situational demands.

The nature of the nursing response depends on the characteristics of the parents' situation as assessed by the nurse and the specific expected outcomes established by the parents and the nurse for the particular situation. In a global sense, all nursing interventions would be directed at assisting the parents to identify their unique sources of stress and reducing the effect of those stressors on the particular situation. The nature of the child's illness, whether acute or chronic, would also influence the strategies employed in the nursing response.

To understand and manage their child's illness, parents need specific information about the child's illness and its treatment.[7] Even well-educated *parents may have misconceptions about their child's illness.* Clear, concise information provided at timely intervals with validation on the part of the nurse of the parents' understanding of the information provided can greatly *reduce the effect of environmental, situational, and personal stressors acting on parents.* When children are to be cared for in the home, parents need detailed explanations of the care they are expected to give and of resources available to them. Likewise,

when a child is hospitalized, parents not only need detailed information about the care and treatment given but should be allowed to participate in providing direct care for their children. *Providing direct care is one way in which parents can cope with anxiety and guilt about their child's illness and gain a sense of control over the environment.*

Consistent with the need for information is the need for guidance and support as the parents try to cope with their child's illness. *Parental anxiety may decrease understanding and alter perceptions;* therefore the nurse needs to be aware that repetition of all information given may be necessary.[7] The nurse should reassure parents that forgetfulness and confusion are a normal part of the stress response and should encourage them to write down questions and concerns to discuss with the health care team. When the need for repetition is great, parents may be provided with written information.

Parents will need assistance to help their child cope with the illness. Understanding the normal expected behavioral and emotional reactions of children in various age groups to hospitalization is necessary. Children may exhibit anger, rebelliousness, and confusion as they try to cope with their illness.[9] *Parents who are familiar with the range of emotional and behavioral responses they may encounter will be better able to cope with such behaviors if they occur.* Parents can assist the staff in interpreting their child's normal reactions to stressful situations and in using this information to determine how far in advance to prepare the child for specific procedures and how much detailed information to give. Parents should be encouraged to be honest in the information they give children. They should be educated about the value of play in helping the child to deal with feelings he/she cannot put into words. Parents should be taught to facilitate their child's play for the purpose of coping with stress.[7]

The illness of a child affects the whole family, and parents must meet the needs of other family members as well as their own needs. The characteristics of the family and the stability of the family unit will influence the parental response and

VIII

❖ NURSING CARE GUIDELINES
Nursing Diagnosis: *Parental Role Conflict*

Expected Parent Outcomes	Nursing Interventions
The parents will express understanding and ability to manage child's illness.	• Provide education regarding the environment, illness, and procedures. • Include the parents in giving care to the child. • Encourage the parents to express fears and concerns.
The parents will demonstrate ability to assist child to understand and cope with illness.	• Explain normal reactions of children to illness and hospitalization. • Enlist the parents' help in explaining treatment regimen and plan procedures with child. • Educate the parents in value of play therapy and encourage same.
The parents will demonstrate ability to meet needs of self and other family members as well as of ill child.	• Provide support and encouragement for the parents to explore stressors that have an effect on them and their needs. • Identify past successful coping techniques. • Identify hospital and community resources. • Assist the parents to plan and implement strategies to reduce stress and meet personal needs. • Remind the parents of need to maintain own health status. • Explore effect of illness on the family unit and future implications; assist the parents in planning for same.

the amount of personal stress associated with the situation. Hymovich[7] points out that if a child's illness is short it is possible for the family to radically alter its lifestyle for a short time until the crisis has passed. However, such changes are hard to maintain for long periods. Parents need to be made aware of the possible emotional needs of siblings of the hospitalized child. Although the effects of a child's illness on siblings has received little attention, research suggests *that siblings may experience a variety of emotional responses, including fear of becoming ill, anger, jealousy, separation effects, and guilt. Parents need to be knowledgeable about these responses so that they can be sensitive to those possible responses in their other children.*

The nurse needs to assess the nature of the personal stressors specific to the situation and, through sensitive dialogue, assist the parents to identify the nature and magnitude of the stressors they are experiencing. To achieve openness, the nurse must create an environment of trust and demonstrate a nonjudgmental attitude. It is useful during these sessions to have parents identify strategies they have used successfully at other times in their lives to manage and control stress. The nurse can then assist the parents to integrate these strategies in planning to meet the demands of the current situation. In the process, the nurse makes the parents aware of hospital and community resources that may be of assistance in planning. Parents also need to be reminded to be in touch with their own health needs if they are to provide ongoing care to the ill child and other family members. *A long-term illness will create a set of demands on parents different from those of an acute event, and parents must be reminded to pace themselves.* In the case of a long-term or chronic condition, the nurse needs to explore with the parents the effect that such a situation will have on the entire family and examine realistically the kinds of changes that may be required in home and family life to meet this demand.

EVALUATION

The nurse will use both observation and interaction with parents to evaluate the extent to which the nursing interventions have been successful. Expected outcomes are achieved when parents: (1) verbalize understanding and ability to manage their child's illness, and (2) demonstrate the ability to meet the needs of all family members and those of the ill child.

❖ CASE STUDY WITH PLAN OF CARE

Mrs. My L. is a 32-year-old mother of 3 who resides in a small town, a 2-hour drive from the nearest large medical center. Her children range in age from 5 through 14 years, and the family has not had any major health problems. Mrs. L. spends full time in the care of her home and family and takes great pride in her role. She came from Viet Nam 6 years ago and speaks minimal English. Mr. L., fluent in English, is employed by a telecommunications company and spends many hours of the work week on the road for business, which leaves much of the family responsibility and home maintenance to Mrs. L. Over the last year Mrs. L. has noticed that their youngest daughter has been pale and lethargic and has been losing weight. She has taken Hong to the family physician several times over the last year, only to be told that Hong has a virus and that rest will cure it. In total frustration Mrs. L. demanded that Hong be seen by a pediatrician and went to the medical center in a large city nearby. The pediatrician has admitted Hong to the pediatric ward of the teaching hospital; she is in a room with three other children. Results of a battery of tests and procedures indicate that Hong has rheumatic fever with kidney involvement, and intravenous antibiotics have been started. Although Mrs. L. is extremely pleased that her daughter is receiving full medical attention, she does not understand the diagnosis, the tests, how long Hong will be in the hospital, and what this means for the future. She has been finding it very difficult to manage the other children and keep the home as well as spend enough time at the hospital. Hong has been crying nonstop since she was admitted to the hospital because she is in pain, lonely, and separated from her family. Today Mrs. L. took a 5:00 AM bus to the city to spend the day with Hong. She found her whimpering, withdrawn, and refusing to acknowledge her presence. The day nurse approached Mrs. L. and said, "I am so glad you're here. I'm so busy this morning; can you give Hong her bath?" and

left the room. Another nurse found Hong and Mrs. L. crying together. Mrs. L. stated through an interpreter that she is exhausted and doesn't know whether she can carry on. She doesn't know how to help Hong, doesn't understand much of what is happening, and thinks she is not doing a good job of anything.

INTERACTIVE ASSESSMENT

1. Appearance: Thirty-two-year-old mother of three children, exhausted and crying.
2. Parent's perception of problem:
   a. Frustrated with family physician's mismanagement of Hong's condition for 1 year.
   b. Pleased that her daughter is receiving full medical attention.
   c. "I am exhausted and don't know whether I can carry on."
   d. "I don't know how to help Hong."
   e. "I feel I am not doing a good job of anything."
3. Factors influencing the situation:
   a. Environmental:
      (1) Unplanned admission to a large medical center.
      (2) Hospital is a 2-hour drive from home town.
      (3) Three other children in Hong's room.
      (4) Diagnostic work-up and medical treatment that involves intrusive tests and procedures (e.g., intravenous antibiotics).
      (5) Medical diagnosis potentially serious. Acute illness superimposed on a chronic illness of 1 year duration: rheumatic fever with kidney involvement.
      (6) Interpreter not offered until Hong began crying.
   b. Contextual:
      (1) Hong is 5 years of age: preoperational thinking.

Continued.

❖ *NURSING CARE GUIDELINES—cont'd*

(2) In pain and suffering separation anxiety. No preparation for hospitalization.

(3) Mrs. L. lacks knowledge about medical diagnosis, tests, future implications for Hong's health and recovery, duration of hospitalization.

(4) Mrs. L. has no previous experience with ill children in hospital or with major health problems in her family.

c. Personal:

(1) Mother of three children, all dependent (5 to 14 years of age).

(2) Comes to hospital alone and by public transportation (friends, financial resources?).

(3) Personal values: Mrs. L. takes great pride in her role as a full-time homemaker.

(4) Quality support from spouse is poor; husband is frequently away on business.

(5) Structured role expectations for Mr. and Mrs. L., Mrs. L. assumes most of the responsibilities of home and family.

(6) Stress of nursing expectations for Mrs. L. to be involved in child's basic care.

(7) Mrs. L. exhausted; left home at 5:00 AM.

(8) Mrs. L. feels inadequate to help Hong and fulfill her other home and family responsibilities.

(9) Mrs. L. feels guilty about not spending enough time with Hong at the hospital.

(10) Mrs. L.'s English comprehension is partial.

PLAN OF CARE FOR MRS. MY L.

Nursing Diagnosis: Parental Role Conflict related to unfamiliarity with Hong's illness and frustration in meeting needs of self and family

Expected Parent Outcomes	Nursing Interventions
Mrs. L. will express that she understands Hong's illness and the rationale for the tests and treatment.	• Assess Mrs. L's knowledge and understanding of the disease process, diagnostic tests, treatment plan, and prognosis, using interpreter • Provide clear, concise information at timely intervals. • Validate Mrs. L's understanding of information. • Encourage Mrs. L. to write down her questions and concerns. • Repeat explanations, correct misconceptions, and involve physician as necessary. • When the need for repetition is great, provide Mrs. L. with written information. • Reassure Mrs. L. that forgetfulness and confusion are a normal part of the stress response.
Mrs. L. will express satisfaction in her ability to meet the needs of herself, her family, and Hong.	• Recognize Mrs. L.'s past and present stressors and coping skills. • Communicate sensitively with Mrs. L. about her home and family responsibilities. • Plan with Mrs. L. how she can modify her role expectations to successfully manage the stresses of her current situation. • Be available and ready to listen to and guide Mrs. L. without being judgmental or making assumptions about her parental role with Hong in hospital. • Assess Mrs. L.'s readiness to be involved with Hong's activities of daily living. • Respect and reassess her wishes for involvement in Hong's activities of daily living.

VIII

Expected Parent Outcomes	Nursing Interventions
	• Talk with Mrs. L. about the responses of her other children to Hong's hospitalization.
	• Explain to Mrs. L. the possible emotional responses and needs of her other children.
	• Help Mrs. L. to respond sensitively to the needs of other family members.
Mrs. L. will demonstrate the ability to assist Hong in coping with the stress of hospitalization, separation from family, and intrusive procedures.	• Explain to Mrs. L. how children of Hong's age normally respond to the stress of illness and hospitalization.
	• Assist Mrs. L. in comforting Hong (holding, touching, talking).
	• Demonstrate (role model) the use of play as a means of helping Hong cope with hospitalization and separation from family and of preparing Hong for intrusive procedures.
	• Acknowledge increased parental anxiety during stressful procedures.
	• Assess Mrs. L.'s willingness to be present during intrusive procedures.
	• Prepare Mrs. L. for what she will see during procedures; assist her in providing comfort to Hong during and after the procedure.
	• Assist Mrs. L. in being honest with Hong, taking into account that young children are best prepared just before procedures.

REFERENCES

1. Alexander D, White M, and Powell G: Anxiety of non-rooming in parents of hospitalized children, *Child Health Care* 15(1):14, 1986.
2. Algren C: Role perception of mothers who have hospitalized children, *Child Health Care* 14(1):6, 1985.
3. Bennet-Branson S, Craig K: Postoperative pain and coping in children and adolescents, *Pain Sympt Manage 6* (3):145 (Abstract No. 11), 1991.
4. Carter M and others: Parent environmental stress in pediatric intensive care units, *Dimen Crit Care Nurs* 4(3):180, 1985.
5. Goodall A: Perceptions of nurses towards parents' participation on pediatric oncology units, *Cancer Nurs* 2(1):38, 1979.
6. Hayes V, Knox J: The experience of stress in parents of children hospitalized with long term disabilities, *J Adv Nurs* 9:333, 1984.
7. Hymovich D: Parents of sick children, their needs and tasks, *Pediatr Nurs* 2(6):9, 1976.
8. Lazarus RS, Folkman S: *Stress, appraisal, and coping,* New York, 1984, Springer Publishing.
9. Miles M, Carter M: Coping strategies used by parents during their child's hospitalization in an intensive care unit, *Child Health Care* 14(1):14, 1985.
10. Miles M, Carter M: Sources of parental stress in pediatric intensive care units, *Child Health Care* 11(2):65, 1982.
11. Mishel M: Parents' perception of uncertainty concerning their hospitalized child, *Nurs Res* 12(6):324, 1983.
12. Patterson K, Ware L: Coping skills for children undergoing painful medical procedures, *Iss Com Pediatr Nurs* 11:113-143, 1988.
13. Visintainer M, Wolfer J: Psychological preparation for surgical pediatric patients: the effect on children's and parents' stress responses and adjustments, *Pediatrics* 56(2):187, 1975.
14. Watt-Watson J, Everenden C, and Lawson C: Parents' perceptions of their child's acute pain experience, *J Pediatr Nurs* 5(5):344-349, 1990.
15. Wolfer J, Visintainer M: Pediatric surgical patients' and parents' stress responses and adjustment, *Nurs Res* 24(4):245, 1975.

VIII

Caregiver Role Strain

High Risk for Caregiver Role Strain

Caregiver Role Strain is a caregiver's experienced difficulty in performing the caregiver role.

High Risk for Caregiver Role Strain is a caregiver's risk for experiencing difficulty in performing the caregiver role.

OVERVIEW

The provision of health care within the family system is a tradition in this country. The national trend toward increased longevity,[8] increased chronicity of health conditions, effort to contain spiraling health care costs, and a decrease in the length of hospital stay, all place an increased emphasis on the informal caregiving system. *Caregiver burden* is a term frequently refered to in the literature in reference to the physical, psychologic, social, and financial stress associated with the caregiving role. Another term for this is caregiver role strain.

Caregiving spans the generations.[9] The care receiver may be of any age, though the literature currently focuses on the elderly. The caregiver is most often female, usually a spouse, daughter or daughter-in-law. These women frequently experience conflict with other roles such as wife, mother, employee and/or community participant.[2] Generally, this group of female caregivers are involved with direct in-home care. Spousal caregivers tend to provide a greater total number of hours of care, use fewer formal care resources, have greater restrictions of health and physical stamina

and report increased social isolation.

Other family members, neighbors, friends, or individuals from the community may be involved with the care receiver.[15] This group is involved at a level of caregiving that accomplishes goals through contracting for services or by provision of intermittent or supervisory care. The length of time in the caregiver role and attitude toward the role can influence the relationship with the care receiver and the quality of care provided.

Entering into the role of caregiver often follows another person's crisis, such as an unexpected surgery, a fall, or a change in health status. There is little if any time to prepare for this role. Most individuals have had no previous caregiving experience. The uncertainty and guilt that surround the circumstances of care begin to set the stage for caregiver role strain.

The response to the caregiver role varies. Tasks may be simple such as assisting with meals or medication to the more complex ones of using technical equipment or dealing with problematic behaviors. Although the literature reports that the psychologic aspects of stress are perhaps more prevalent and amenable to intervention, the caregivers may not always perceive the stress. The stress of care giving is multidimensional and unique to each individual. Thus each care provider is unique and must be viewed as an individual on a continuum over time.[10,14]

Research to date has examined multiple dimensions of the caregiving response. Studies look at subjective and objective portions of burden of care, for example. However, many studies focus on a limited period of time. Additional longitudinal research studies are needed. Little is known about the long-range effects that caregiving might have on marriage, career, or family dynamics.

ASSESSMENT

Each caregiving situation has unique qualities and needs to be assessed on an individual basis. Currently available clinical evaluation tools do not comprehensively measure the complexity of caregiver role strain.[21,22] A suggested evaluation for this cluster of nursing diagnoses might include: nursing history of the care receiver, nursing history of the caregiver, and a formal in-home evaluation. The assessment must focus upon the strengths or capacity of the caregiver and also examine ever-changing environmental factors, such as circumstances of care and financial demands. By using this approach to assessment, an appropriate match of interventions can be achieved.

Nursing History of Care Receiver[12]

The nursing history of the care receiver must be comprehensive. Assessment of activities of daily living,[6] cognitive status,[18] and any behavioral issues is needed to create a baseline from which to measure changes. Determination of the care receiver's prognosis is useful in facilitating the caregiver's planning process. It is useful to ascertain the care receiver's perception of illness, relationship with the caregiver and support system, and willingness to accept help. Reassessment is useful at intervals because changes in care demands, mental status or behavior problems influence susceptibility to role strain.

Nursing History of Caregiver[6-8,12]

A careful history of the caregiver needs to be obtained. It may take some time to develop a level of trust with the caregiver in order to obtain accurate information. The health status of the caregiver often serves as a barometer for role strain. Information to gather includes a baseline

medical history with particular attention to chronic conditions.[1,3] It is sometimes useful to discuss usual health care practices such as medical and dental check-ups, over-the-counter medications that are used and for what purpose, and how minor illnesses are handled. It is also informative to discuss any major illness or disability within the family or support network and the caregiver's perceptions and reactions about this information.

Caregivers often provide information about their level of subjective burden in response to what their perception of the caregiver role encompasses. Whether or not the caregiver has had any caregiving experience or is able to state where information is available, provides useful data. Other roles that the caregiver is involved in need to be identified and prioritized both by time and importance, because conflict between competing roles is a frequent occurrence.[2]

The relationships within the family and support systems must be identified.[4,5,17] The caregiver's willingness to ask for and accept help is crucial to the intervention process. The quality and history of the relationship between caregiver and care receiver requires note. This is important because a negative relationship may lead to role strain.[1]

Finally, data regarding the caregiver's psychologic history needs to be gathered.[7,8] The caregiver may or may not perceive his or her own level of stress. The level of stress may fluctuate, which may also not be perceived by the caregiver. An appropriate stress scale could be useful.[21]

Depression is noted as a concern for those experiencing role strain.[13] It is appropriate to administer a depression scale to the caregiver at intervals to assess change over time. The nurse must assess other parameters related to the caregiver role. For example, it is important to determine the caregiver's spiritual resources. Baseline information about current and past leisure patterns is also useful when planning interventions.

Home/Environment

The home visit[11] provides an opportunity to see the actual caregiving arena and quite often the in-

VIII

teraction of the key players. Areas to note in addition to the usual safety and access concerns include the presence of adaptive equipment and whether or not it is being used appropriately. Is there space for additional equipment? By what means is emergency help obtained for falls, wandering, or caregiver incapacity?

Caregiver Role Strain
❖ Defining Characteristics

The presence of the following defining characteristics indicates that the individual may be experiencing Caregiver Role Strain:

- Feeling exhausted
- Inability to complete caregiving tasks
- Declining health status
- Feeling depressed
- Feeling loss of usual or expected relationship with care receiver
- Grieving
- Increased stress or nervousness
- Increased emotional lability
- Preoccupation with care routine
- Family conflict
- Withdrawal from social contacts
- Change in leisure activities
- Sleep pattern disturbance
- Low self esteem

❖ Related Factors

The following related factors are associated with Caregiver Role Strain:

- Illness severity of care receiver
- Increasing care needs of care receiver
- Addiction or co-dependency of caregiver or care receiver
- Conflicting role demands
- Caregiver health impairment
- No previous experience with caregiver role
- Caregiver not developmentally ready for caregiving role
- Developmental delay or retardation of the care receiver or caregiver
- Marginal family adaptation or dysfunction prior to caregiving situation.
- Marginal coping patterns of caregiver
- Providing direct, on-going in-home care
- Discharge of family member with significant home care needs
- Unpredictable illness course or instability in the care receiver's health
- Psychologic or cognitive problems in the care receiver.
- Past history of poor relationship between caregiver and care receiver
- Care receiver exhibits deviant, bizarre behavior
- Incontinence in the care receiver

❖ Related Medical/Psychiatric Diagnoses

The following are examples of related medical/psychiatric diagnoses for Caregiver Role Strain:
  Experienced by care receiver:
- Alzheimer's disease
- Cerebral vascular accident
- Cystic fibrosis
- Mental retardation
- Multiple sclerosis
- Muscular dystrophy
- Organic brain syndrome
- Parkinson's disease

High Risk For Caregiver Role Strain
❖ Risk Factors

The presence of the following behaviors, conditions, or circumstances renders the individual more vulnerable to High Risk for Caregiver Role Strain:
- See related factors for Caregiver Role Strain

❖ Related Medical/Psychiatric Diagnoses

The following are examples of related medical/psychiatric diagnoses for High Risk for Caregiver Role Strain:
- See related medical/psychiatric diagnoses for Caregiver Role Strain

NURSING DIAGNOSES

Examples of *specific* nursing diagnoses for Caregiver Role Strain are:
- Caregiver Role Strain related to cognitive impairment of care receiver

VIII

- Caregiver Role Strain related to declining health of caregiver
- Caregiver role strain related to incontinence of care receiver
- Caregiver role strain related to inappropriate social behavior of care receiver.

Examples of *specific* nursing diagnoses for High Risk for Caregiver Role Strain are:

- High risk for caregiver role strain related to anticipated length of caregiving demands.
- High risk for caregiver role strain related to no previous experience with the caregiver role.
- High risk for caregiver role strain related to conflicting role demands.
- High risk for caregiver role strain related to history of strained relationship between caregiver and care receiver.

PLANNING AND IMPLEMENTATION WITH RATIONALE
Caregiver Role Strain

Communities have a myriad of resources to offer the caregiver, but the task of learning where they are, how they are accessed, and which are appropriate for an individual situation is overwhelming to the uninitiated. Caregivers come to the role with little or no previous experience and frequently express guilt and uncertainty about their performance and expectations. *The competency level of the caregiver can be enhanced by increasing his/her knowledge base of resources as well as skill level.*

There is a tendency among caregivers to neglect self-care activities and to experience an increased level of stress. This neglect can translate

---

❖ NURSING CARE GUIDELINES
Nursing Diagnosis: Caregiver Role Strain

VIII

Expected Patient Outcomes	Nursing Interventions
The caregiver will state appropriate informal/formal resources.	• Review caregiver's knowledge of availability of resources. • Establish financial eligibility to obtain community resources. • Determine caregiver/care receiver willingness to accept resource support. • Evaluate current family network. • Assist in referral process as appropriate.
The caregiver will be able to verbalize and execute stress-reduction strategies.	• Establish a pattern of "time-out" from caregiver role. • Provide information/access to relaxation tapes, guided imagry, exercises, meditation and/or biofeedback techniques. • Teach time management strategies. • Encourage involvement in church/social activities. • Access community support groups.[20] • Provide time for active listening to caregiver concerns. • Validate feelings of role strain with caregiver. • Encourage consistent health monitoring for caregiver. • Monitor for caregiver depression (depression scale/observe for vegetative signs) • Administer stress scale at intervals.

Continued.

❖ *NURSING CARE GUIDELINES—cont'd*

Expected Patient Outcomes	**Nursing Interventions**
The caregiver will be able to verbalize change in role expectations.	• Examine usual roles within the family system; compare past, present and future relationships within the unit. • Identify the various roles that caregiver engages in. • Assist caregiver to prioritize roles. • Assist caregiver to negotiate roles with other family members. • Educate the family about the process of caregiving. • Assist family members to deal with the disengaged member and changes of status within the family unit. • Acknowledge and validate the caregiver role.

---

into aggravated health problems, increased somatic complaints and depression. *The connection between psychologic/psychosocial/physical problems and the stress of caregiving is often not recognized by caregivers.* The nurse is instrumental in monitoring the caregiver for changes in stress and depression.

The many roles and competing demands for the caregiver's time, resources and energy are presumed to be associated with high levels of stress and burden. There is a tendency for caregivers to be all things to all people as they attempt to fullfil their roles in the same capacity as before they began caregiving. *Assistance and reassurance in prioritizing roles and establishing realistic time management strategies is critical to alleviate some of the perceived strain.* Once the tasks of caregiving are identified they can be negotiated with other family members or met by incorporating other resources into the plan of care.[19]

High Risk for Caregiver Role Strain

When a new caregiving situation arises or a stable one changes, there is a need to re-examine available resources both within the immediate support system and within the community. The caregiver may initially need a "consultant" for information about how to meet the needs of the care receiver, access community resources, and select appropriate services. The family needs to identify who will be the designated primary caregiver, although the task usually falls to the female spouse or eldest daughter. If the caregiver is unable to acknowledge the need or willingness to accept assistance with the caregiving role, it is difficult to initiate additional resources. *Early identification and intervention of those factors predictive of burden can lessen the perception of caregiver role strain.*

The nurse will assist the caregiver to identify the existing strengths and weaknesses of the existing family system. *The relationship between family members, particularly the caregiver and care receiver, is predictive of increased risk for burden.* Families and individuals may find that psychotherapy is helpful to work through unresolved issues and/or learn more effective conflict management techniques.

EVALUATION
Caregiver Role Strain

Progress for this nursing diagnosis is evaluated by the caregiver selecting appropriate resources for care, following evaluation and discussion with the nurse. Further evaluation includes continued demonstration of effective stress reduction technique by the caregiver, a stress scale score that is maintained or improved and positive self-care activities. The caregiver will be able to relate a feeling that the caregiving role is not menial but has

❖ NURSING CARE GUIDELINES

Nursing Diagnosis: High Risk for Caregiver Role Strain

Expected Patient Outcome	Nursing Interventions
The caregiver is able to state appropriate community resources and how to access them.	• Discuss range/availability of community resources appropriate for both present and future needs. • Discuss financial eligibility requirements for resources. • Evaluate willingness of caregiver to access resources. • Discuss and evaluate circumstances in which resources might be incorporated into the care regimen. • Evaluate family and social support network. • Discuss and provide information about appropriate support groups.
The caregiver is able to identify existing strengths/weakness in family dynamics.	• Identify the family relationship between caregiver and carereceiver. • Identify past methods of dealing with crisis. • Offer family/individual therapy for resolution of conflict and/or unresolved issues.

❖ CASE STUDY WITH PLAN OF CARE

Mr. Lennie P. is a 45-year-old white male. The admitting diagnosis is bipolar functional decline disorder and decubitus ulcer. Mr. P. also experiences failure in previous living situation. He is paraplegic, wheel-chair bound and dependent on caregivers for lower body dressing, transfers, bathing, elimination, bed positioning, and health status monitoring. He has poor judgment. Mr. P. is alienated from his family. Currently he has two close friends who have been designated as conservators for his health care and financial management. Mr. P. has assured them that he will be discharged to his home and he can be cared for there with "somebody to come in." Both conservators are employed full time and live some distance from Mr. P.'s house. They are supportive of Mr. P.'s desire to live at home but are uncertain how they could avoid the "hassle we had when he would manipulate the people taking care of him last time . . . things got out of hand because we couldn't be there all the time." The conservators have no experience in direct care, dressing changes, elimination management, or transfer techniques. They are overwhelmed with the unassembled hoyer lift that Mr. P. had delivered to his home. Mr. P. sold his hospital bed when he was admitted to the hospital so his family "wouldn't get the money." A possible nursing diagnosis is High Risk for Caregiver Role Strain.

PLAN OF CARE FOR CAREGIVERS OF MR. LENNIE P.

Nursing Diagnosis: High Risk for Caregiver Role Strain

Expected Patient Outcomes	Nursing Interventions
Caregivers (conservators) will develop an appropriate care management regimen[14]	• Discuss placement alternatives: e.g., in-home vs nursing home; in-home with or without care assistance. • Discuss financial eligibility for selected placement options.[16] Monitor interaction between conservators and Mr. P. Arrange meeting with interdisciplinary team members and conservators to discuss Mr. P.'s care. • Schedule a meeting among occupational therapist and Mr. P.'s caregivers to discuss equipment needs for home use.

VIII

value. Because the caregiving role is often long term, the nurse will meet regularly with the caregiver to continue reinforcement of the positive self care actions and assist in anticipating changes in the needs of the care receiver. Success of this plan depends on collaboration with other health care professionals and a trusting relationship between caregiver and nurse.

High Risk for Caregiver Role Strain

Appropriate selection and use of community and family resources determine the effectiveness of this nursing diagnosis. The caregiver will be able to express a sense of competency in the role.

REFERENCES

1. Archbold PG, Stewart BJ, Greenlick MR, Harvath T: Mutuality and preparedness as predictors of caregiver role strain, *Res Nurs Health* 13:375-384, 1990.
2. Baldwin BA, Kleeman KM, Stevens GL, Raisin J: Family caregiver stress: Clinical assessment and management, *Int Psychoger* 1(2):185-194, 1989.
3. Ballie V, Norbeck JS, Barnes LE: Stress, social support, and psychological distress of family caregivers of the elderly, *Nurs Res* 37(4):217-222, July/August 1988.
4. Bowers BJ: Intergenerational caregiving: adult caregivers and their aging parents, *Adv Nurs Sci* 9(2):20-31, 1987.
5. Brackley MH, Meadows RF: Nursing support of family caregivers, *Dimens Oncol Nurs* 3(1):14-20, Spring 1989.
6. Bull MJ: Factors influencing family caregiver burden and health, *West J Nurs Res* 12(6):758-776, 1990.
7. Bunting SM: Stress on caregivers of the elderly, *Adv Nurs Sci* 11(2):63-73, 1989.
8. Decker SD, Young E: Self-perceived needs of primary caregivers of home-hospice clients, *J Community Health Nurs* 8(3):147-154, 1991.
9. Dyson LL: Families of young children with handicaps: parental stress and family functioning, *Am J Ment Retard* 95(6):623-629, 1991.
10. McFall S, Miller BH: Caregiver burden and nursing home admission of frail elderly persons, *J Gerontol* 47(2):73-79, 1992.
11. Nolan MR, Grant G, Ellis NC: Stress is in the eye of the beholder: reconceptualizing the measurement of care burden, *J Adv Nurs* 15:544-555, 1990.
12. O'Neill G, Ross MM: Burden of care: an important concept for nurses, *Health Care Women Int* 12:111-121, 1991.
13. Pruchno RA, Resch NL: Husbands and wives as caregivers: antecedents of depression and burden, *Gerontologist* 29(2):159-165, 1989.
14. Robinson KM: Predictors of burden among wife caregivers, *Scholar Inq Nurs Pract* 4(3):189-201, 1990.
15. Seigel K, Raveis VH, Mor V, Houts P: The relationship of spousal caregiver burden to patient disease and treatment-related conditions, *Ann Oncol* 2:511-516, 1991.
16. Seigel K, Raveis VH, Houts P, Mor V: Caregiver burden and unmet patients needs, *Cancer* 68:1131-1140, September 1, 1991.
17. Sheehan NW & Nuttall P: Conflict, emotion and personal strain among family caregivers, *Family Relations:* 92-98, Jan 1988.
18. Stephens MAP, Kinney JM, Ogrocki PK: Stressors and well-being among caregivers to older adults with dementia: the in-home versus nursing home experience, *Gerontologist* 31(2):217-223, 1991.
19. Stone R, Cafferata GL, Sangl J: Caregivers of the frail elderly: a national profile, *Gerontologist* 27(5):616-626, 1987.
20. Toseland RW, Labrecque BA, Goebel ST, Whitney MH: An evaluation of a group program for spouses of frail elderly veterans, *Gerontologist* 32(3):382-390, 1992.
21. Vitaliano PP, Young HM, Russo J: Burden: a review of measures used among caregivers of individuals with dementia, *Gerontologist* 31(1):67-75, 1991.
22. Vitaliano PP, Russo J, Young HM, Becker J, Maiuro RD: The screen for caregiver burden, *Gerontologist* 31(1):76-83, 1991.

Relocation Stress Syndrome

Relocation Stress Syndrome is a problem of transition and adaptation to a new physical and/or cultural environment; it is characterized by physiological and psychosocial disturbances related to changes in physical surroundings and social environment following transfer from one location to another.

OVERVIEW

Changes in one's residential environment are common in our highly mobile culture, and may occur throughout the life span.[7] These changes are multifaceted in nature, and often occur within the context of events such as hospitalization, admission to a nursing home, voluntary or involuntary residential moves, job relocation, geographic moves within national boundaries, and cross-cultural migration and resettlement.

Responses during the adjustment period following moves from one environment to another have been referred to in the literature as culture shock,[17] relocation shock,[29] translocation syndrome,[16,39,42] mobility syndrome,[1] separation anxiety,[40] migration stress,[26] and acculturation stress.[22]

Relocation stress syndrome is characterized by such responses as grieving, anxiety, anger, uncertainty, powerlessness, and physiological symptoms. These are experienced within the context of the individual striving for mastery of a new situation and resolution of multiple losses. The adaptation process is a continuum and includes reactions to the event of relocation, and ongoing efforts by the individual to establish new relationships and achieve equilibrium in a new environment. Relocation adjustment is influenced by personality factors, coping style, stability of family constellation, developmental levels of family members, cultural norms, social support, personal and community resources, as well as the person's perceptions about the changes.

For some individuals, relocation is experienced as a stimulating, morale-boosting, growth-producing, and positive process.[5,13] For some elderly, transfer to a new environment may actually improve daily functioning level and well-being.[6,28] For other individuals, relocation threatens self-integrity, and triggers anxiety during the process of reorganization. For the elderly patient or chronically institutionalized individual, transfer to a new environment may result in acute confusion and cognitive deterioration[3,14,15,24] as well as increased aggression.[44]

Frequently, relocation occurs within the context of other life stressors, such as trauma, chronic illness, hospitalization, financial and social losses, altered role performance, retirement, developmental and family crises, job transfers, political upheaval, persecution, and war.* The cumulative effects of these multiple and often interacting stressors often contribute to emotional upheaval and changes in health status, and may challenge the individual's adaptive capacity.

Coping successfully with relocation stress is influenced by presence of an adequate social support system for the individual, a history of previous successful transfers, some degree of perceived personal control over the move (versus a sudden, unanticipated move), predictability of the stressor, the ability to manipulate some aspect of the environment, and pre-transfer preparation for the move by caretakers.[11,41] The extent of

---

*References 18, 29, 35, 38, 43.

change, quality of the new environment, and conditions associated with the move are other variables affecting adjustment.[4]

Post-relocation adjustment is characterized in part by progression through the grief process. Relocation results in losses; disruption; and change in factors such as familiar surroundings, caretakers, social network, activities of daily living, schedules, living arrangements, roles, status, personal identity, and personal comforts. Psychosocial adaptation may also include establishing new cues for orientation and accommodation to another culture, language, or lifestyle. These dual tasks of grieving and adapting to the multiple demands of an unfamiliar environment constitute the major work of relocation adjustment and mastery.[2]

Symptoms of relocation stress are varied, and have included disorientation, anxiety, and behavioral management difficulties in the elderly[3,15,45]; increased levels of aggression in institutionalized psychiatric patients[19,30,44]; decreased school functioning, withdrawal, negativity, and anger in young children and adolescents[8,25,31,36]; and, emotional problems in refugees.[20,21] Relocation alone does not increase morbidity and mortality in the elderly, but interacts with other variables to produce changes in health status.[32] Some studies have shown insignificant changes in physical functioning of the elderly following transfer,[4,6,12] and insignificant changes in mental status.[37] Other findings have indicated an increase in mortality rates, depending on level of functioning.[34]

Hospitalized patients frequently respond to relocation stress with increased helplessness, powerlessness, and anxiety. For example, a patient transferred out of the intensive care unit to the general nursing floor may experience distress when separated from supportive staff and constant monitoring by life-saving equipment.[33,40,46]

Relocation stress may occur within a number of contexts. These include voluntary or involuntary institutionalization, transfers between facilities, hospital discharge to the community, admission to a nursing home,[47] intrahospital transfers of patients between wards, room changes within a ward, out-of-home placement for young children, changes in foster homes, geographic moves within national boundaries, and transcultural migration and resettlement.

ASSESSMENT

The diagnosis of Relocation Stress Syndrome is most closely associated with acute external stressors of changes in the individual's environment and social network. The nurse is encouraged to explore multiple precipitating factors and to assess the patient and family's responses from a systems point of view. As patient's responses are mediated by multiple influences, consideration must be given to the combined impact of concomitant stressors brought about by the hospitalization experience, changes in health status and roles resulting from illness, alterations in cognitive functioning, and degree of acculturation mastery for the immigrant patient.

The coping capacity and adaptation needs of patients can be determined by interviewing the patient and family at the time of admission to the hospital or nursing home and from medical record information documenting the course of the illness, emotional responses, and need for special support (e.g., language translators). Assessing the patient and family's perceptions about the move and changes in the environment and caretakers is important in determining degree of disruption and vulnerability.

The nurse should also assess the timeframe context for patients experiencing relocation. Rapid, unplanned moves, for example, may compromise an individual's adjustment and increase the likelihood of developing Relocation Stress Syndrome if pre-transfer preparation is overlooked. In caring for the elderly and critical care patient being transferred from the intensive care unit to a general nursing floor, the nurse should assess what the patient understands about the changes that will occur in personnel, acuity level, staffing, equipment, and other aspects of the new environment.

For cognitively impaired patients, the elderly, or chronic psychiatric patients, the nurse should obtain a baseline, pre-transfer assessment of mental status and functional status (e.g., ability to participate in activities of daily living). History provided from family or other caregivers familiar with the patient prior to transfer is a valuable source of collateral information. This is useful in evaluating coping skills, activity level, post-transfer cognitive functioning, and overall adaptation to the new environment. This information will be invaluable if the patient is an unreliable historian.

Nursing assessment should also include attention to the patient's grieving. Grieving may be delayed when energy is focused on the external, logistical details of reorganization within a new setting. Because relocation involves adjustment to various types of loss (for example, personal identity loss, social or cultural loss, loss of familiar routines and structure, loss of cherished belongings and personal space, among others), the nurse should observe the patient for dysfunctional or delayed grieving responses.

For the immigrant patient adjusting to a transcultural move, admission to the hospital may heighten acculturation issues and relocation stress. The nurse should assess the patient's cultural identity, degree of acculturation, and fluency with the English language.[10,23] The nurse should also identify the patient's beliefs about health and health practices, ethnic preferences, and social support that could promote comfort and personalized, culturally sensitive care.[10,23]

For children and adolescents who are affected by major geographic moves with their families, or experiencing transfer between foster home placements or out-of-home placements, it is useful for the nurse to assess history of recent, multiple moves. The type, frequency, and significance of major attachment losses (for example, siblings, biologic parents, extended family, schoolmates, playmates, neighbors, grandparents, or pets) must also be determined. Assessing parental or caretaker coping with relocation issues may also provide information about other stressors within the home context and amount of support available to the child or adolescent.

The nurse should also assess the developmental level of the child or adolescent to facilitate better understanding of age- appropriate coping and emotional expression of relocation stress. History from parents or caretakers, schools, and other health care professionals familiar with the child or adolescent may provide valuable information useful in determining the child or adolescent's support and learning needs.

❖ **Defining Characteristics**

The presence of the following defining characteristics indicates that the patient may be experiencing Relocation Stress Syndrome:

- Increased confusion (elderly)
- Sleep disturbance
- Appetite and weight changes
- Alienation and detachment
- Anger
- Increased aggression
- Anxiety
- Dependency
- Feelings of displacement
- Grieving
- Loneliness
- Loss of identity
- Powerlessness
- Uncertainty about the future
- Unfavorable comparison of post and pretransfer setting or staff
- Verbalization of being upset or concerned about transfer
- Withdrawal
- Lack of acculturation behaviors (e.g., learning new language, customs)
- Performance problems in school (child)
- Regressed behavior
- Reluctance to establish new emotional attachments
- Social status ambiguity

❖ **Related Factors**

The following related factors are associated with Relocation Stress Syndrome:

- Repeated moves
- Hospital admission
- Relocation to a nursing home (e.g., elderly)[27]

VII

- Geographic moves (e.g., children moving with families)
- Foster home placement
- Change in residence
- Job transfer with geographic moves
- Lifestyle of multiple moves (e.g., migrant workers)
- Traumatic departures from homeland (e.g., political refugees)
- Voluntary cross-cultural migration
- Foreign student status
- Transfer between wards (e.g., chronic psychiatric patients)
- Discharge to the community (e.g., chronic, institutionalized psychiatric patients)
- Transfer between intensive care unit and step-down unit or general nursing floor

❖ **Related Medical/Psychiatric Diagnoses**

The following are examples of related medical/psychiatric diagnoses for Relocation Stress Syndrome:
- Adjustment disorder with anxious mood
- Adjustment disorder with depressed mood
- Adjustment disorder with disturbance of conduct
- Adjustment disorder with mixed disturbance of emotions and conduct
- Adjustment disorder with mixed emotional features
- Adjustment disorder with physical complaints
- Adjustment disorder with withdrawal
- AIDS
- Cerebral vascular accident
- Major depression
- Post-traumatic Stress Disorder
- Myocardial Infarction
- Sensory deficits (e.g., blindness, deafness)
- Spinal cord injury

NURSING DIAGNOSES

Examples of *specific* nursing diagnoses for Relocation Stress Syndrome are:
- Relocation Stress Syndrome related to move from the coronary care unit to the general nursing unit.
- Relocation Stress Syndrome related to admission from home to a nursing home.
- Relocation Stress Syndrome related to removal from home and placement into a foster home.
- Relocation Stress Syndrome related to transcultural migration and resettlement.

PLANNING AND IMPLEMENTATION WITH RATIONALE

The nursing interventions for Relocation Stress Syndrome are aimed at reducing anxiety, supporting the patient through grieving, adjusting to the changes, and increasing a sense of control. As adjustment to relocation extends beyond a discrete event, interventions must continue after the patient has been transferred to a new setting, with ongoing assessment of patient responses. In addition, the nurse should assess the impact of other stressors facing the patient during this adjustment period.

Establishing a supportive relationship with a patient who has the diagnosis of Relocation Stress Syndrome, or is at high-risk for developing this diagnosis is essential *to maintain a sense of trust, continuity, and security for the patient. Avoiding multiple caregivers before and after the transfer, and allowing the patient time to establish relationships with staff in the new setting will be helpful in reducing anxiety.* Pre-transfer preparation of the patient and family such as orientation to the new environment, teaching about withdrawal of equipment, and introduction to new caregivers, whenever possible, are other examples of anxiety-reducing interventions to mitigate the potential negative aspects of relocation. *The important principle to keep in mind is that anxiety will decrease the patient's ability to learn new behaviors and coping skills needed in the new environment.*

The nurse should plan and implement strategies to support patients through the normal grieving process associated with Relocation Stress Syndrome.[9] This process may be anticipatory in nature, as well as continuing after the event of transfer. *The multiple personal losses associated with moving, readjustment in life-style, and rebuilding a new identity may overwhelm the pa-*

❖ NURSING CARE GUIDELINES
Nursing Diagnosis: *Relocation Stress Syndrome*

Expected Patient Outcomes	Nursing Interventions
Patient will show reduced anxiety, as evidenced by: self-report of decreased tension and acceptance of new circumstances; ability to concentrate, learn new skills, and problem solve in new environment.	• Establish a supportive, nonthreatening relationship with patient to build trust and a sense of security. • Identify sources of patient's current cumulative stress (e.g., retirement, new job) and encourage verbalization about concerns and uncertainty related to move, in order to assess patient's perception of the move and learning needs regarding transfer. • Maintain structure in schedule and activities, limit amount of changes, arrange for consistent caregivers before and after relocation in order to foster predictability, continuity of care, and to lessen sources of anxiety. • Initiate pre-transfer preparation and early discharge planning, explaining planned changes, describing the new setting, and orienting patient to new environment and caretakers to increase a sense of control. • Inform patient about transfer in advance and accompany to new location whenever possible. • Assist patient in acknowledging feelings of loss and discomfort associated with relocation and adjustment to a new environment.
Patient will progress through normal grieving, as evidenced by: identifying losses associated with relocation; reinvesting emotional energy into relationships and activities in new setting.	• Elicit patient's perceptions of relocation adjustment, difficult aspects of the move, potential problems, and dissimilar aspects of the environment. • Determine patient's support systems, and assist him/her in mobilizing resources and identifying coping strengths within self. • Assess patient for dysfunctional grieving responses in order to determine need for psychiatric referral and treatment. • Assist patient in setting realistic social and personal goals in new setting to increase self-esteem and a sense of mastery.

VIII

tient, so the nurse should continually assess for dysfunctional grieving responses. Frequently, the demands of resettlement delay grieving or interfere with the process. Helping the patient identify these losses and giving permission to verbalize emotional discomfort promotes personal coping and problem-solving.

EVALUATION

Evaluation of interventions for Relocation Stress Syndrome should be validated with the pa-tient and caregivers in the new environment. Successful strategies will decrease anxiety, grieving, and loss of control associated with relocation. The patient will show evidence of establishing social attachments and participating in activities and expected roles in the new environment.

❖ *CASE STUDY WITH PLAN OF CARE*

Mrs. Alice R. is an 89-year-old trauma patient who is married, and living with her 90-year-old husband in their own home. While driving, Mrs. R. apparently suffered a syncopal episode, resulting in a single-vehicle accident, during which time she sustained multiple spinal and rib fractures. Both Mrs. R. and her husband were hospitalized on the same nursing unit, but not in the same room. After one uneventful day of hospitalization in the surgical intensive care unit, Mrs. R. was moved to a step-down unit. Her husband remained in critical condition.

Nurses on the step-down unit reported that Mrs. R. seemed anxious, especially because she had to share a nurse with several other patients, and that she seemed distressed whenever the nurse left the room, used the call light excessively, complained constantly of pain, and seemed withdrawn and resistant to activity. In addition, she stated that she preferred the "other unit" and talked about the better care that she received there. Mrs. R. frequently talked about feeling "disconnected from home" as she and her husband had recently planned to move into a retirement center, and had already partially relocated some of their belongings there. When arrangements were made for discharge to an extended care facility, Mrs. R. became tearful and withdrawn.

PLAN OF CARE FOR MRS. ALICE R.

Nursing Diagnosis: Relocation Stress Syndrome related to transfer from the intensive care unit to a step-down unit and partial move from own home to a retirement center.

Expected Patient Outcomes	Nursing Interventions
Mrs. R. will adapt to the new ward as evidenced by: decreased anxiety and withdrawal; greater participation in own care.	• Support Mrs. R. post-transfer, by acknowledging emotional distress in unfamiliar setting. • Allow Mrs. R. to verbalize about feelings and concerns associated with the transfer and changed environment. • Orient Mrs. R. to the new ward, and explain changes in equipment and staffing patterns. • Accompany Mrs. R. if going off the unit for procedures, and explain any changes planned. • Keep the environment calm, and promote comfort for Mrs. R. • Encourage the family to bring in Mrs. R.'s favorite afghan and bedroom slippers. • Provide predictability and consistency in the post-transfer environment.
Mrs. R. will show increased coping with the anticipated multiple relocation events following discharge from the hospital, as evidenced by: participating in decision-making about placement; verbalizing feelings about temporary move to an extended care facility for rehabilitation; describing future plans for life in a retirement center following discharge from an extended care facility.	Initiate early discharge planning before Mrs. R. is discharged to an extended care facility. Assess Mrs. R's understanding of need for placement and planned, multiple moves versus discharge to home directly. Teach the family strategies to support Mrs. R. during the relocation process, (e.g., bringing favorite belongings from home to personalize the environment. Promote Mrs. R's autonomy by allowing control over some aspects of own care, space, and privacy. Assist Mrs. R. in problem-solving and planning realistic goals for self in new setting.

VIII

REFERENCES

1. Anderson C, Stark C: Psychosocial problems of job relocation: preventive roles in industry, *J Soc Work* 33(1):38-41, 1988.

2. Aroian KJ: A model of psychological adaptation to migration and resettlement, *Nurs Res* 39(1):5-10, 1990.

3. Bellin C: Relocating adult day care-its impact on persons with dementia, *J Geront Nurs* 16(3):11-14, 1990.

4. Bonardi E, Pencer I, Tourigny-Rivard M: Observed changes in the functioning of nursing home residents after relocation, *Int J Aging Hum Dev* 28:295-303, 1989.

5. Borup JH: Relocation: attitudes, information network, and problems encountered, *Gerontol* 21(5):501-511, 1981.

6. Borup JH, Gallego DT, Heffernan PG: Relocation: its effects on health, functioning, and mortality, *Gerontol* 20:468-479, 1980.

7. Bridges W: *Making sense of life's transitions,* New York, 1980, Addison-Wesley.

8. Brockhaus JP, Brockhaus RH: Foster care, adoption, and the grief process, *J Psychosoc Nurs Ment Health Serv* 20(9):9-16, 1982.

9. Brooke V: How elders adjust, *Geriatr Nurs* 10:66-68, 126-128, 1989.

10. Campinha-Bacote J: Culturological assessment: an important factor in psychiatric consultation-liaison nursing, *Arch Psychiatr Nurs* 2(4):244-250, 1988.

11. Cohen F, Lazarus RS: Coping and adaptation in health and illness. In Mechanic D, editor: *Handbook of health, health care, and health professionals,* New York, 1983, Free Press.

12. Davis RE, Thorson JA, Copenhaver JH: Effects of a forced institutional relocation on the mortality and morbidity of nursing home residents, *Psychol Reports* 67:263-266, 1990.

13. Dimond M, McCance K, King K: Forced residential relocation-its impact on the well-being of older adults, *West J Nurs Res* 9(4):445-464, 1987.

14. Evans LK: Sundown syndrome in institutionalized elderly, *J Am Geriatr* 35:101-108, 1987.

15. Foreman MD: Complexities of acute confusion, *Geriatr Nurs* 11:136-139, 1990.

16. Harkulich JT, Brugler C: Relocation of institutionalized residents, *Today's Nursing Home* 10(10):24-25, 1989.

17. Hertz DG: Psychological and psychiatric aspects of remigration, *Isr J Psychiatr Relat Sci* 21(1):57-68, 1984.

18. Hull D: Migration, adaption, and illness: a review, *Soc Sci & Med* 13A:25-36, 1979.

19. Jones EM: Interhospital relocation of long-stay psychiatric patients: a prospective study, *Acta Psychiatr Scand* 83:214-216, 1991.

20. Kinzie JD: The psychiatric effects of massive trauma on cambodian refugees, *J Traum Stress* 2(1):75-91, 1989.

21. Kinzie JD, Boehnlein JJ: Post-traumatic psychosis among cambodian refugees, *J Traum Stress* 2(2):185-198, 1989.

22. Lee E: Cultural factors in working with southeast asian refugee adolescents, *J Adolesc* 11(2):167-179, 1988.

23. Leininger M: Becoming aware of types of health practitioners and cultural imposition, *J Transcult Nurs* 2(2):32-41, 1991.

24. Lindesay J, Macdonald A, Stark I: *Delirium in the elderly,* Oxford, 1990, Oxford University Press.

25. Matter DE, Matter RM: Helping young children cope with the stress of relocation: action steps for the counselor, *Elem Sch Guid Couns* 23:23-29, 1988.

26. McElroy A, Townsend PK: Health repercussions of culture contact. In *Medical anthropology in ecological perspective,* ed 2, Boulder, Colorado, 1989, Westview Press.

27. Mikhail ML: Psychological responses to relocation to a nursing home, *J Gerontol Nurs* 18(3):35-39, 1992.

28. Mirotznik J, Ruskin AP: Interinstitutional relocation and its effects on psychosocial status, *Gerontol Soc Amer* 25(3):265-270, 1985.

29. Netting FE, Wilson CC: Accommodation and relocation decision making in continuing care retirement communities, *Health Soc Work* 16(4):266-273, 1991.

30. Osborne OH, Murphy H, Leichman SS, Griffin M, Hagerott JJ, Ekland ES, Thomas MD: Forced relocation of hospitalized psychiatric patients, *Arch Psych Nurs* 4(4):221-227, 1990.

31. Pearson GS: The latency-aged child in out-of-home placement: treatment considerations, *J Child Adolesc Psychiatr Ment Health Nurs* 1(2):82-88, 1988.

32. Petrou MF, Obenchain JV: Reducing incidents of illness posttransfer, *Geriatr Nurs* 8:264-266, 1987.

33. Poe CM: Minimizing stress-of-transfer responses, *Dimens Crit Care Nurs* 1(6):364-374, 1982.

34. Pruchno RA, Resch NL: Intrainstitutional relocation: mortality effects, *Gerontol Soc Am* 28(3):311-317, 1988.

35. Puskar KR: Relocation support groups for corporate wives, *Am Assoc Occup Health Nurs* 38(1):25-31, 1990.

36. Puskar KR, Dvorsak KG: Relocating stress in adolescents: helping teenagers cope with a moving dilemma, *Ped Nurs* 17(3):295-298, 1991.

37. Rajacich D, Faux S: The relationship between relocation and alterations in mental status among elderly hospitalized patients, *Can J Nurs Res* 20(4):31-42, 1988.

38. Ramey L, Cloud J: Relocation success: a model for mental health counselors, *J Ment Health Couns* 9(3):150-161, 1987.

39. Ranz M, Egan K: Reducing death from translocation syndrome, *Am J Nurs* 87(10):1351-1352, 1987.

40. Schactman M: Transfer stress in patients after myocardial infarction, *Focus Crit Care* 14(2):34-37, 1987.

41. Schulz R, Brenner G: Relocation of the aged: a review and theoretical analysis, *J Gerontol* 32(3):323-333, 1977.

42. Smith BA: When is "confusion" translocation syndrome? *Am J Nurs* 86(11):1280-1281, 1986.

43. Starker JE: Psychosocial aspects of geographic relocation:

VIII

the development of a new social network, *Am J Health Promot* 5(1):52-57, 1990.

44. Thomas MD, Ekland ES, Griffin M, Hagerott RJ, Leichman SS, Murphy H, Osborne OH: Intrahospital relocation of psychiatric patients and effects on aggression, *Arch Psychiatr Nurs* 4(3):154-160, 1990.

45. Thomasma M, Yeaworth RC, McCabe BW: Moving day: relocation and anxiety in the institutionalized elderly, *J Gerontol Nurs* 16(7):18-25, 1990.

46. Toth JC: Effect of structured preparation for transfer on patient anxiety on leaving coronary care unit, *Nurs Res* 29(1):28-34, 1980.

47. Young HM: The transition of relocation to a nursing home, *Holistic Nurs Pract* 4(3):74-83, 1990.

VIII

IX

SEXUALITY— REPRODUCTIVE PATTERN
Sexual Dysfunction

Altered Sexuality Patterns

Sexual Dysfunction *is the state in which problems with sexual function exist.*

Altered Sexuality Patterns *is the state in which an individual or partner expresses concern regarding the individual's sexuality.*

OVERVIEW

The problems of Sexual Dysfunction may be related to physical illness or psychological influences that cause a limitation in sexual desire and activity and subsequent difficulties in sexual performance, which is viewed as unsatisfying, unrewarding, or inadequate. Physical illness may influence one's sexuality in a systemic way or interfere with neural, vascular, or hormonal components of the sexual response. Psychological influences may be traced to lack of knowledge about sexuality or sexual technique, guilt, anxiety, fear, relationship issues, or history of sexual abuse.

The diagnosis of Altered Sexuality Patterns is multidimensional. Concerns regarding sexuality can be present at any point along the continuum from wellness to illness and may occur in conjunction with or independent of sexual dysfunction.[5,13]

The diagnoses Sexual Dysfunction and Altered Sexuality Patterns are separate and distinct. However, the central theme of sexuality provides a similar basis for these diagnoses. Some overlapping of content is inevitable, especially in the areas of definition and assessment and, to an even greater degree, interventions, patient outcomes, and evaluation. This section will address both diagnoses, discussing their shared content as well as pointing out the uniqueness of each individual diagnosis.

The term *sexuality* involves more than the physical act of intercourse. It is intrinsic to our very existence. We are sexual beings from birth to death. Sexuality includes all aspects of people that involve being male or female, and it is a dynamic entity that changes over the life span. People remain sexual regardless of their age or health. Sexuality is a basic human characteristic and cannot be separated from life events. Whereas acute or chronic illness, disabling conditions, or the aging process may require adaptations in the way sexuality is expressed, people continue to be sexual beings.[6,10]

The terms *gender identity* and *sex role* can be defined as one's internal sense of being male or female or the way we disclose ourselves to others as men or women. It is the conviction that one feels a part of the male or female sex groups. Although it involves an internal feeling, it also includes an external display of male or female characteristics. This concept of gender identity is not present at birth but is developed through experience and implicit instruction until the identity is in place around age 2 or 3 years.

The change in sexual performance that occurs in Sexual Dysfunction is viewed as unsatisfying, unrewarding, or inadequate. This loss or impairment may be devastating to the person for whom the ability to express sexuality is highly valued. Whether an actual loss has occurred or only the threat of loss exists, there is the potential for crisis, which may be biophysical or psychosocial. The person who has experienced a biophysical crisis such as surgical disfigurement or sexual assault may also undergo a psychosocial crisis as well because that person may have to deal with a change in relationship, an altered body image, or a change in lifestyle. Sterilization, infertility, or hysterectomy may affect a person's sense of worth as a sexual being. A person's inability to perform sexually can also create a crisis.

Sexual Dysfunction might be compared with sexual difficulties in that the latter results in occasional interference with sexual function, discomfort in the sexual relationship, and disinterest in sexual activity, whereas the former results in disruption of sexual function and severely strains the sexual relationship or sexual self-image. Sexual Dysfunction can usually be divided into three categories: disorders of sexual desire, disorders of arousal, and disorders of orgasm. Sex therapy is the most effective way to treat sexual dysfunction.

Altered Sexuality Patterns cover a wide range of defining characteristics and risk factors. A person's adaptation to these occurrences depends on the type of alteration, the meaning of the change to the patient, the patient's coping ability, and the response of his/her significant other. Each of these factors will influence the extent to which the alteration will affect the patient's sexual satisfaction.

Persons may seek values clarification in hopes of relieving guilt or concerns about their sexuality. Teenagers and often adults exhibit a knowledge deficit regarding information or skills related to sexuality. Other problems perceived by patients might include disinterest in sexual activity, inability to please or be pleased by a partner, and problems in the timing of sexual activities.[10]

ASSESSMENT

Before one can understand Sexual Dysfunction or Altered Sexuality Patterns, one must first understand the concept of sexual health.

> Sexual health is the integration of the somatic, emotional, intellectual and social aspects of sexual being in ways that are positively enriching and that enhance personality, communication, and love.[14]

This WHO definition contains several implicit factors, which include the freedom to control reproductive behavior according to one's personal ethics, freedom from physical disorders that could interfere with sexual or reproductive function, and freedom from factors that might interfere with sexual response, such as guilt, misconceptions, or lack of knowledge.

Sexual Dysfunction

Sexual Dysfunction is a common problem affecting most individuals at some point in their lives. Heterosexual and homosexual couples experience dysfunctions with similar causes and defining characteristics. Both Sexual Dysfunction and Altered Sexuality Patterns have the potential of being integrated into nearly every other physiological, psychological, or emotional problem that a person can experience, as well as being primary dysfunctions themselves.

There are differences between men and women in the defining characteristics of Sexual Dysfunctions. In both sexes, however, one of the most common dysfunctions is inhibited sexual desire. The loss or lack of desire may not seem to be a problem to the person who is experiencing it, but if the individual is in a relationship, then the partner might perceive a dysfunction and seek counseling. The cause of this inhibited desire varies widely. Many medications taken by men and women have a negative effect on sexual desire. Also included in this category of related factors would be drug and alcohol abuse. A wide range of psychological factors can have a profound effect on one's libido; these may include stress (personal or stress in the relationship), depression, anger, performance anxiety, or fear of pain associated with intercourse.[4]

A major defining characteristic in men is impotence, more appropriately referred to as *erectile dysfunction*. The degree to which a man might experience this problem varies widely. Primary erectile dysfunctions arise from either physical or emotional problems of sexual development; these are characterized by a man's not being able to achieve or maintain an erection long enough to have intercourse. Secondary erectile dysfunction occurs in a man who has previously functioned successfully. This inability to achieve a satisfactory erection is frequently a source of depression, frustration, and humiliation for the man. The commonly used term *impotence* implies both physical and emotional failure. Subsequently this depression and low self-esteem can also be causes of erectile dysfunction, and therefore it may become unclear which problem came first. Causes of erectile dysfunction may at times be unclear, but it is usually possible to differentiate between psychological and organic origin. Consideration of several issues helps identify causative factors: whether there is complete inability to obtain an erection or inability to maintain an erection; whether the dysfunction is present at all times or is episodic; whether the onset of the dysfunction is associated with significant life events; and whether the man's sexual desire (libido) is intact. Some of the many organic and psychogenic factors appear in the list of related factors.[3,6]

The third common sexual dysfunction in men is premature ejaculation. Individual experiences vary, and there is no precise definition, but it is generally accepted to be a loss of voluntary control over ejaculation. This may occur before entry or after a few thrusts. (This dysfunction occurs in nearly all men at one time or another, particularly when there has been no sexual activity for a long period of time.) As with erectile problems, increased anxiety about the problem occurring with succeeding performances can be a factor, with premature ejaculation becoming chronic.

The previously described factors of anxiety, alcohol abuse, drug use, and control may also relate to a fourth dysfunction known as *retarded ejaculation*. This condition refers to the inability to ejaculate and may be primary (never able to ejaculate) or secondary (unable to ejaculate after previously having been able to do so). Organic factors may also be responsible for this dysfunction; for example, neurological disorders interfering with the sympathetic innervation of the genitals, diseases that cause central thalamic dysfunction, such as Parkinson's disease, and antiadrenergic drugs such as guanethidine and methyldopa.[1,6]

One of the more common dysfunctions in women, in addition to the previously discussed inhibited sexual desire, is orgasmic dysfunction. This may be a primary dysfunction, a woman who has never had an orgasm, or a wide variation of orgasmic problems. Confusion continues about orgasms that are "normal" and those considered to be dysfunctional. Many women have an orgasm only with clitoral stimulation, some during intercourse, and some with a combination of the two. Women may be anorgasmic because of multiple factors. Inexperience, lack of information, insufficient stimulation, poor communication with the partner, and early established patterns that interfere with sexual enjoyment are common causes. As with men, high expectations causing "performance anxiety" may lead to increased difficulty in becoming orgasmic.[12]

Dyspareunia occurs in women and is characterized by painful penetration that may occur at any time during intercourse. The description of the pain or discomfort varies, as does its location (from external to vaginal or abdominal), but it is sufficient to create a dysfunctional sexual experience. The cause of dyspareunia is most often organic. One common cause is vaginal dryness or lack of lubrication, which may be the result of inadequate stimulation or hormonal factors such as decreased estrogen. Other related factors include irritation related to vaginal infections, discomfort from certain contraceptive methods (such as foams, diaphragms, or condoms), or deep pelvic pain from movement of certain uterine ligaments

IX

or from pelvic diseases such as endometriosis, gonorrhea, or cervicitis. Dyspareunia may infrequently result from complex psychological problems usually associated with fear or anxiety.[2]

A small percentage (2% to 3%) of women experience a rather serious but rare dysfunction known as vaginismus. Women with this condition exhibit an involuntary spasm of the muscles surrounding the vaginal orifice whenever vaginal penetration is attempted. The cause of vaginismus is not always clear. Trauma, such as rape, may lead to a conditioned response pattern, but physical causes should be ruled out first.[11]

❖ Defining Characteristics

The presence of the following defining characteristics indicates that the patient may be experiencing Sexual Dysfunction:
- Erectile dysfunction (male)
- Premature ejaculation (male)
- Retarded ejaculation (male)
- Orgasmic dysfunction (female)
- Dyspareunia (female)
- Vaginismus (female)
- Inhibited sexual desire (male and female)
- Alteration in achieving sexual satisfaction (male and female)
- Inability to achieve desired satisfaction (male and female)

❖ Related Factors

The following related factors are associated with Sexual Dysfunction:
- Medical or surgical conditions: diabetes, neurological problems, urological problems, diseases causing central thalamic dysfunction, trauma to spinal cord, trauma to genital area
- Alcohol or drug abuse
- Use of prescription medications
- Decreased physiological drive (with aging)
- Lack of vaginal lubrication: inadequate stimulation, decreased estrogen
- Vaginal infections
- Vaginal irritation
- Deep pelvic pain associated with movement of uterine ligaments, endometriosis, gonorrhea, or cervicitis

- Stress in general
- Stress in relationship
- Depression
- Anger
- Guilt
- Performance anxiety
- Fear of pain associated with intercourse
- Early established patterns that interfere with sexual enjoyment
- Poor communication with partner
- Lack of information
- Inexperience
- Immaturity (for instance, adolescence)

❖ Related Medical/Psychiatric Diagnoses

The following are examples of related medical/ diagnoses for Sexual Dysfunction:
- Anxiety
- Depression
- Diabetes
- Diseases causing central thalamic dysfunction
- Endometriosis
- Genital trauma
- Neurological disorders
- Sexually transmitted diseases
- Spinal cord trauma
- Urological disorders

Altered Sexuality Patterns

The diagnosis of Altered Sexuality Patterns encompasses all conditions or situations in which an individual expresses concern regarding his/her sexuality or in which there is a change in sexual behavior or activities. This diagnosis always occurs when Sexual Dysfunction is present but may also occur independently. There is wide variation in the degree to which a person can be affected and in the manifestations of the altered pattern(s).

Factors related to the diagnosis of Altered Sexuality Patterns can be grouped into two categories—those of psychosocial or environmental origin and those relating to a lack of knowledge about appropriate responses to health-related transitions, changes in body function or structure, illness, or a prescribed medical treatment. Psychosocial or environmental factors may include lack of privacy, lack or absence of a significant other, poor communication with partner, conflicts with sexual orientation or variant preferences, or ineffective or absent role models. Health-related transitions that necessitate an adaptation may be normal life events such as pregnancy, childbirth, or lactation. Although these may be "normal" life events, a lack of knowledge may make it difficult to achieve a satisfactory adaptation, resulting in concern about sexual issues.

There is no consensus in the literature about sexual activity during pregnancy. Factors that influence sexual patterns during pregnancy are change in body image, cultural and societal expectations, reaction to pregnancy, mother/lover role conflict, fear of potential medical complications relating to sexual behavior, and physiological and anatomical changes.

Infertility is directly linked to sexuality and the sexual and reproductive organs. The period of evaluation leading to a diagnosis of infertility is an extremely stressful time for a couple and a diagnosis of infertility influences one's feelings about self as a sexual being.

Other reproductive issues that might result in altered patterns of sexual expression are contraception and abortion. The management of fertility implies the modification of sexual patterns. Abortion may affect sexual behavior in many ways. Physical sequelae are not known to interfere directly with a resumption of previous sexual behavior, but the risk of physical complications can indirectly affect sexual function and subsequent sexual self-concept. Both negative and positive psychological outcomes are possible after an abortion. The literature suggests that the negative consequences are usually short term. In either case there exists the potential for change in the sexual relationship.[13]

The presence of a developmental, physical, or mental disability can raise concerns regarding sexual behavior. This can be a lifelong issue, as when a disability exists from birth, or it can emerge at any stage of life when an injury or disability occurs. Of course these concerns may be present whether or not the disability or injury directly involves the sexual or reproductive organs. When there is a disability one must deal with sex-

ual concerns caused by physical problems that impose limits on movement and sensation, concerns that arise from lack of information, and concerns that arise from limits imposed by society.[9]

Certain medical conditions can, by virtue of their physiological consequences to all body systems, cause one to experience Altered Sexuality Patterns. Both the disease process and the treatment have the potential of disrupting sexual patterns because of physiological changes or tissue injury. Body image changes are "viewed as incompatible with maintaining a sexual relationship." Various therapies and drug treatments may also interfere with the ability to function sexually. Illness-related anxiety causes a decrease in the sex drive and sexual response as does depression or grief. Illness may also cause physical separation from one's sexual partner.

Cardiovascular disease, like many other chronic illnesses, has the ability to affect patterns of sexuality as well as most other facets of daily living. Patients who experience a myocardial infarction frequently express concern about their sexuality. Resumption of sexual activity after a coronary episode is influenced significantly by the presence of cardiovascular symptoms and fears of sudden death. The effect of a coronary episode on sexual functioning may be felt for up to a year.[7]

In a long-term illness such as chronic renal disease, psychosocial issues, including changes in sexual patterns, become critical concerns. Progressive deterioration occurs that affects all body systems. This deterioration plus anxiety and change in body image cause sexual desire and functioning to diminish. Frequently there is a decrease in sex drive or performance related to uremia, which causes lethargy, listlessness, and peripheral neuropathy. The treatment, renal dialysis, imposes more biological and psychological stressors. Sexual Dysfunction and other sexual concerns are frequently reported in patients undergoing dialysis. The alternative treatment, renal transplantation, may alleviate dysfunctional problems, but the psychosocial factors still have a negative effect on sexual functioning.

Research studies indicate that diabetic men have a higher incidence of sexual dysfunction

IX

than nondiabetic men. However, it should not be assumed that all of the sexual concerns reported in diabetes are organic. Such factors as use of certain medications, alcohol abuse, or poor control of the diabetes may create changes in sexual patterns. Diabetic men may experience erectile dysfunction, which is thought to be neurological in origin. Women report sexual problems and concerns related to first-stage arousal and vaginal lubrication that are sometimes additionally complicated by the presence of vaginitis.[8]

Therapies prescribed in treatment of patients with cancer often cause changes in sexual self-concept, sexual functioning, and sexual relationships. Changes in body image may cause feelings that negatively affect a person's ability to function sexually because of a negative self-perception. Other factors that may cause Altered Sexuality Patterns in patients with cancer are loss of body function, loss of a body part, loss of fertility, and the side effects caused by chemotherapeutic agents.

The consequences of sexual assault or rape are both physical and emotional. Rape causes an intense emotional reaction that interferes with resumption of sexual activity and causes changes in sexual patterns. The physical sequelae of rape (trauma to genital and other body areas, pregnancy, and sexually transmitted disease) also lead to Altered Sexuality Patterns.

The physical consequences of sexually transmitted disease (for example, vaginitis, cervicitis, lower abdominal pain, skin or mucous membrane lesions, or acquired immunodeficiency syndrome) interfere with sexual functioning. Prescribed treatments may also alter patterns of sexuality in that they may necessitate abstinence for a period of time. Emotional factors such as feelings of guilt, shame, or stigma also cause changes in previously established patterns of sexual expression.[13]

The generic tool for assessment of both Sexual Dysfunction and Altered Sexuality Patterns is the sexual history. The subjective information obtained by this method is the most helpful in identifying a diagnosis and formulating a care plan. The approaches to obtaining the sexual history are

varied and may be adapted according to the type of problem, the skills of the interviewer, and expressed needs of the patients. It will help to define expectations and behavior patterns of the patient and to identify misconceptions, areas of difficulty, and need for teaching and counseling.

The nurse must have clarified personal values before he/she can be effective in the sexual health assessment or in subsequent nursing interventions to assist these patients. When discussing sexual issues, an open, nonjudgmental attitude is the key to facilitating communication. It is necessary for the interviewer to be skilled in the techniques of questioning, reflection, clarification, and validation to accurately interpret what the patient is expressing about his/her sexuality.[9]

The process of obtaining the sexual history may be therapeutic in itself. During the interview the nurse gives permission to the patient to talk freely and openly about sexual concerns; answers some questions, which may provide information to the patient; and may be able to confirm that the patient's concerns are acceptable.

It is essential that the setting provide privacy, confidentiality, and freedom from interruptions. Active listening is an important technique used in interviewing to obtain a sexual history. One uses this method to validate the message to be sure the listener understood correctly. Because of implicit messages throughout life, people have a "built-in" system of censorship. Suggesting answers or asking questions in a way that assumes or acknowledges the possibility that the patient has engaged in a particular activity makes it easier for the patient to discuss matters about which he/she might feel guilty or embarrassed. An example of this might be "Many men have had some homosexual experience in their lifetimes. Have you any concerns about this activity, Dave?" It is important to use language in a way to facilitate, not inhibit, communication. The use of appropriate terminology can convey professionalism and knowledge. It is important, though, to clarify euphemisms from colloquial language that the patient uses and to adapt to it, because correcting the patient may inhibit communication. Positive feedback used effectively lets the patient know that the nurse has heard the information and is accepting of the patient as a person. The use of positive feedback need not indicate that all behaviors are condoned.

Several different approaches can be used in eliciting the sexual history. Assist the patient in relating the information in chronological order. For patients with a diagnosis of Altered Sexuality Patterns, a brief sexual history may be sufficient. Inquire as to the patient's current sexual role (for instance, husband) and how the patient feels about himself/herself as a sexual being, and then address concerns directly related to sexual function.

If Sexual Dysfunction is present, a more detailed history of the sexual problem is indicated. This would encompass a description of the problem as perceived by the patient, the patient's ideas about possible causes of the problem, and some discussion of the patient's expectations from treatment. Additionally, data should be collected and reviewed from the patient's physical findings, medical diagnoses, and mental status. It may also be appropriate to include the sexual partner in the assessment process.

❖ Defining Characteristics

The presence of the following defining characteristics indicates that the patient may be experiencing Altered Sexuality Patterns:
- Change in sexual behaviors or activities
- Verbal expression of concern regarding sexual behavior or activities

❖ Related Factors

The following related factors are associated with Altered Sexuality Patterns:
- Medical conditions; e.g., diabetes, cardiac disease, renal disease, cancer, sexually transmitted disease (for example, acquired immunodeficiency syndrome)
- Trauma; e.g., sexual assault
- Disability; e.g., developmental, physical, mental, or emotional
- Childbearing; e.g., infertility, pregnancy, childbirth, postpartum period, lactation, contraception, abortion

- Knowledge deficit or skill deficit related to alternative responses to health-related transitions, altered body functions or structure, illness, or medical treatment
- Ineffective or absent role models
- Conflicts with sexual orientation or variant preferences
- Poor communication with partner
- Impaired relationship with significant other
- Lack or absence of significant other
- Lack of privacy

❖ Related Medical/Psychiatric Diagnoses

The following are examples of related medical/psychiatric diagnoses for Altered Sexuality Patterns:
- Cancer
- Cardiac disease
- Childbearing
- Diabetes
- Disability
- Renal disease
- Sexually transmitted diseases (e.g., AIDS)

NURSING DIAGNOSES

Examples of *specific* nursing diagnoses for Sexual Dysfunction are:
- Sexual Dysfunction related to activity intolerance
- Sexual Dysfunction related to body image disturbance
- Sexual Dysfunction related to posttrauma response
- Sexual Dysfunction related to rape-trauma syndrome

Examples of *specific* nursing diagnoses for Altered Sexuality Patterns are:
- Altered Sexuality Patterns related to anxiety
- Altered Sexuality Patterns related to impaired physical mobility
- Altered Sexuality Patterns related to rape-trauma syndrome
- Altered Sexuality Patterns related to self-esteem disturbance

PLANNING AND IMPLEMENTATION WITH RATIONALE

There are many types of nursing roles within the area of sexual health. Depending on the educational background and the skills of the nurse, there are opportunities to provide for the sexual health care needs of patients in multiple settings and situations. Patients may range from individuals, to groups, to communities, in home, hospital, or community-based settings.

The sexual health *assessment initiates the process of helping the patient with his/her potential or actual expressed need.* Patients with both Sexual Dysfunction and Altered Sexuality Patterns may not directly seek help for their sexual problems. They may, rather, divulge their concerns during the sexuality portion of a more general health assessment.

There are many roles at different levels that enable nurses to assist patients with problems of sexual health. One of the most frequent interventions is education, or providing information. After the assessment process is complete, and based on the patient's needs, the nurse may intervene with appropriate information. *Many patients benefit from basic knowledge of anatomy, physiology, and the sexual response cycle.* The childbearing experience offers many opportunities for teaching women about their bodies and the changes that they experience during pregnancy, labor and delivery, and lactation. This is also an excellent time to get women to talk about how they feel about their bodies and to give information regarding expressions of sexuality during this time. Teenagers need teaching and anticipatory guidance with regard to healthy sexuality, reproduction, contraception choices, and sexually transmitted diseases. Certain prescription drugs are known to cause sexual changes in many people. Teaching should be done to ensure that these patients will be aware of these potential side effects and how they may affect their lives.

Another major role for nurses is counseling patients in regard to their sexuality. Counseling is the process of creating an atmosphere wherein the patient can feel comfortable and express thoughts and feelings openly. With the help of the nurse-counselor *the patient can clarify the sexual problem and, one hopes, change the situation to reach a greater level of satisfaction.* Sexual counseling may be individual or for a couple. Persons with both Sexual Dysfunction and Altered Sexuality Patterns benefit from counseling in many situations. An example might be a patient recovering from a myocardial infarction who becomes fearful of having intercourse. Discussing the situation with the nurse-counselor and acting on suggestions offered over a period of time, the patient would gradually decrease his/her anxieties and relax so that he/she could enjoy sexual intimacy while observing for the warning signs of cardiac stress.

Validating that the patient and the patient's sexual behavior are "normal" is an important role that the nurse can play. This may seem obvious, but many people wonder if their activities (for instance, masturbation, oral-genital sex) or even their fantasies are "perverted" or "dirty," and when a patient is able to open up to a health professional, it may be that the patient is merely seeking validation of what is acceptable. *In allowing this and in ensuring the privacy and confidentiality that was displayed during the assessment process, the nurse becomes a patient advocate.* It is the responsibility of the nurse to encourage patients to participate in decision making regarding their treatment plan and to support these decisions. By exhibiting a nonjudgmental and professional attitude, the nurse maintains the patient's dignity.

Nurses, as members of the health care team, may act as a referral source for patients with sexual problems. Referrals may include support or self-help groups, educational resources, or other professionals.

Occasionally, nurses seek additional educational and clinical preparation and become sex therapists. These professionals offer intensive specialized therapy to patients with Sexual Dysfunction or Altered Sexuality Patterns.

EVALUATION

The effectiveness of the specified nursing interventions will depend on the patient's ability and willingness to accept the guidance and information provided. The time required to achieve the

❖ *NURSING CARE GUIDELINES*
Nursing Diagnosis: Sexual Dysfunction

Expected Patient Outcomes	Nursing Interventions
The patient will seek and obtain appropriate medical/nursing intervention.	• Complete sexual history assessment. • Make appropriate referrals for patients exhibiting any actual or potential condition that requires medical intervention. • Assess and monitor the patient's and partner's level of knowledge and understanding of his/her dysfunction(s).
The patient will have increased knowledge and understanding of factors related to dysfunction(s) experienced.	• Provide the patient (and partner, when appropriate) with accurate information to increase the level of awareness.
The patient will exhibit behavior change that will result in more satisfying sexual function.	• Provide the patient with a safe, nonjudgmental atmosphere. • Offer the patient (couple) the opportunity for clarification of feelings concerning sexuality. • Offer specific suggestions, when appropriate, for alteration in sexual activities that might result in elimination or reduction of dysfunction.
The patient will maintain a sense of personal dignity, and the patient's concerns regarding his/her sexuality will be alleviated.	• Provide the patient (couple) with privacy and maintain confidentiality. • Involve the patient (couple) in decisions about plan of care. • Validate the patient's feelings of normalcy.

IX

❖ *NURSING CARE GUIDELINES*
Nursing Diagnosis: Altered Sexuality Patterns

Expected Patient Outcomes	Nursing Interventions
The patient (or couple) will seek and obtain appropriate counseling/ intervention.	• Complete sexual history assessment. • Make appropriate referrals for patients exhibiting any actual or potential condition that requires medical intervention. • Assess and monitor the patient's and partner's level of knowledge and understanding of his/her alteration in sexuality.

Continued.

❖ NURSING CARE GUIDELINES—cont'd

Expected Patient Outcomes	Nursing Interventions
The patient will have increased knowledge and understanding of factors related to his/her Altered Sexuality Patterns.	• Provide the patient (and partner, when appropriate) with accurate information to increase the level of awareness.
The patient will exhibit behavior change that will result in more satisfying patterns of expressing sexuality.	• Provide the patient with a safe, nonjudgmental atmosphere. • Offer the patient (couple) opportunity for clarification of feelings concerning sexuality. • Offer specific suggestions, when appropriate, for alteration in sexual activities that might result in greater satisfaction for patient or couple.
The patient will maintain a sense of personal dignity, and the patient's concerns regarding his/her sexuality will be alleviated.	• Provide the patient (couple) with privacy and maintain confidentiality. • Involve the patient (couple) in decisions about plan of care. • Validate the patient's feelings of normalcy.

identified outcomes depends on the contributing or related factors and will vary for each patient. An ongoing assessment of the patient's progress will assist in evaluating the patient's response to a particular intervention (for example, the provision of general information on sexual function) and provide data to guide the implementation of other interventions (for example, specific suggestions for altering sexual activities).

❖ CASE STUDY WITH PLAN OF CARE: SEXUAL DYSFUNCTION

Mr. James K. is a 52-year-old man with diabetes type 2. The nurse took a sexual history as part of a health history after the patient expressed concerns about difficulty maintaining an erection. Onset of diabetes was at age 45 years. Mr. K. has been successful in controlling his diabetes with diet and oral hypoglycemics. He has had concerns related to the sexual dysfunction for several years, and he attributes these concerns to the diabetes. He has not discussed this previously with his physician or any other health professional. Mr. and Mrs. K. have been married for 25 years. They have two children, ages 22 and 18 years. Both are in college and live away from home. Mr. K. reports that he and his wife had a satisfactory sexual relationship and that he "hardly ever had a problem" achieving and maintaining an erection until about 5 years ago. At that time Mr. K. began experiencing an increase in the amount of time needed to attain an erection, and the problem gradually worsened until he was frequently unable to have intercourse. Because of this problem he admitted that he approaches his wife less and less frequently for sex and several months often elapse with no attempt at intercourse. Mr. K. stated that he is quite convinced that the erectile dysfunction is related to his diabetes. He states, "I sure don't know what else it could be." When questioned by the nurse Mr. K. admitted that he has episodic erections on awakening in the morning. Mr. K. is employed as an

❖ CASE STUDY WITH PLAN OF CARE: SEXUAL DYSFUNCTION—*cont'd*

insurance agent and has a good income. He states that his wife was a housewife until their son went to college 5 years ago. She then went to work as a receptionist in a busy law office. The sexual assessment also revealed that Mr. K. drinks almost no alcohol and is engaged in a moderate exercise program of walking 2 to 3 miles, 3 days a week. One nursing diagnosis formulated is Sexual Dysfunction related to diabetes.

PLAN OF CARE FOR MR. JAMES K.

Nursing Diagnosis: *Sexual Dysfunction related to diabetes*

Expected Patient Outcomes	Nursing Interventions
Mr. K. will understand factors related to sexual dysfunction.	• Provide information regarding actual and potential physiological effects of diabetes. • Provide Mr. K. with appropriate information regarding erectile dysfunction in diabetic men. • Provide information about sexuality and aging.
Mr. K. will increase awareness of feelings of ambivalence regarding changes in family roles.	• Refer Mr. K. to social worker for counseling regarding his feelings about his family transitions, especially his wife's employment.
Mr. and Mrs. K. will achieve increased intimacy and sexual satisfaction through a successful sex therapy program.	• Counsel Mr. and Mrs. K. about exploring ways of achieving intimacy through means other than sexual intercourse. • Refer Mr. and Mrs. K. to sex therapist for intensive therapy.

❖ CASE STUDY WITH PLAN OF CARE: ALTERED SEXUALITY PATTERNS

Mrs. Susan J. is a 29-year-old primiparous woman. Her child, a healthy girl, is 6 weeks old. Mrs. J. had a normal vaginal delivery with no complications. She chose to breast-feed her baby and was supported by her husband in this choice. Postpartal recovery has been uneventful. The nurse took a sexual history as part of a routine postpartum checkup. Mrs. J. disclosed that she had many concerns and questions about the resumption of sexual activity after delivery. She fears personal injury and pain from breast tenderness and the episiotomy repair. She is unable to state when she thinks it would be safe to resume sexual relations with her husband. Mrs. J. expresses anxiety about confusing sexual feelings that she experiences while nursing her baby. She is concerned that her husband is losing patience with her disinterest in sex. Mrs. J. is uncomfortable with her physical appearance and feels that she will have difficulty losing the weight gained during pregnancy. Mrs. J. reports that she is continuously tired and that except for trips to the grocery store has not been away from her house since coming home from the hospital. One formulated nursing diagnosis is Altered Sexuality Pattern related to childbearing.

Continued.

IX

PLAN OF CARE FOR MRS. SUSAN J.

Nursing Diagnosis: *Altered Sexuality Pattern related to childbearing*

Expected Patient Outcomes	Nursing Interventions
Mrs. J. is reassured that satisfactory physical recovery from childbirth has been achieved.	• Explain physiological process of recovery from childbirth.
Mrs. J. will understand factors related to her Altered Sexuality Patterns.	Provide information concerning safe resumption of sexual activity. • Provide information concerning the physical demands of lactation.
Mrs. J. will exhibit change in behavior that will result in greater sexual satisfaction.	• Offer suggestions for gradual return to previous sexual patterns. • Offer suggestions to reduce depression and fatigue.
Mrs. J. is reassured regarding concerns about sexuality.	• Address issue of changes in body that are causing altered concept of self as a sexual being. • Offer anticipatory guidance about normalcy of increase or decrease in sexual desire or frequency of intercourse. • Support expression of concerns, fears, and feelings relating to sexuality and lactation; reassure as to normalcy of experience.
Mrs. J. will perceive improvement and increased satisfaction in relationship with husband.	• Encourage honest communication with husband, and offer cojoint counseling with husband.

REFERENCES

1. Frank D, Lang A: Disturbances in sexual role performance of chronic alcoholics: an analysis using Roy's adaptation model, *Iss Ment Health Nurs* 11:243, 1990.
2. Glatt A and others: The prevalence of dyspareunia, *Obstet Gynecol* 75:433, 1990.
3. Halvorsen J and others: Male sexual impotence: a case study in evaluation and treatment, *J Fam Pract* 27(6):583, 1988.
4. Jupp J, McCabe M: Sexual desire, general arousability and sexual dysfunction, *Arch Sex Behav* 18(6):509, 1989.
5. Kim M, McFarland G, and McLane A: *Pocket Guide to nursing diagnoses,* ed 4, St Louis, 1991, Mosby–Year Book.
6. Mason D: Erectile dysfunctions: assessment and care, *Nurs Pract* 14(12):23, 1989.
7. McCann M: Sexual healing after heart attack, *Am J Nurs* 89(9):1132, 1989.
8. Morrison H: Diabetic impotence, Nurs Times 84(32), August, 1988.
9. Rowe W, Savage S: *Sexuality and the Developmentally handicapped, vol 7, studies in health and human services,* Lewiston, NY, 1987, Edwin Mellen Press.
10. Sanderson M, Maddock J: Guidelines for assessment and treatment of sexual dysfunction, *Obstet Gynecol* 73:130, 1989.
11. Scholl G: Prognostic variables in treating vaginismus, *Obstet Gynecol* 72:231, 1988.
12. Sheahan S: Identifying sexual dysfunctions, *Nurs Pract* 14(2):25, 1989.
13. Woods N: Human sexuality in health and illness, ed 3, St Louis, 1984, CV Mosby.
14. World Health Organization: *Education and treatment in human sexuality: the training of health professionals,* report of a WHO meeting, Technical Report Series No. 572, Geneva, 1975, World Health Organization.

IX

Rape-Trauma Syndrome

Rape-Trauma Syndrome: Silent Reaction

Rape-Trauma Syndrome: Compound Reaction

Rape-Trauma Syndrome: Rape is the forced violent sexual penetration against the victim's will and consent. The trauma syndrome that develops from this attack or attempted attack includes an acute phase or disorganization of the victim's life-style and a long-term process of reorganization of life-style.[9]

Rape-Trauma Syndrome: Silent Reaction occurs when an individual is raped and is unable to report the rape to anyone because of fears (real or perceived), lack of situational support, lack of knowledge concerning procedures for reporting the rape, inability to articulate the event, and many other factors. The emotional and psychological trauma exists but remains unresolved.[9]

Rape-Trauma Syndrome: Compound Reaction occurs when patients having preexisting psychiatric, physical, social, and financial problems, plus the added stress of rape, experience increased vulnerability and difficulty with everyday living. Consequently, additional problems develop, present problems worsen, or old problems resurface. Depression, suicidal behaviors, increased drug and alcohol abuse, and psychotic behaviors are seen.[9]

OVERVIEW

Rape is "the ultimate violation of the self, short of homicide, and is best understood in the context of a crime against the person and not against the hymen. Rape is an act of violence and humiliation in which the victim experiences overwhelming fear for her very existence as well as a profound sense of powerlessness and helplessness which few other events in one's life can parallel."[16]

Contrary to common belief, rape is not a sexual act but an act of violence, whereby sex becomes the means or weapon for expression.[5,25] Rape is one of the most intrusive, violent crimes that one human being can inflict on another. Survivors of rape report panic, terror, and a sense of domination, powerlessness, and impending death. Yet because of prevailing myths and attitudes of society toward women, rape, and sexuality, survivors are often blamed for their own victimization.[9] After rape, the nurse may be the first to assess the person. If effective interventions are not instituted, survivors may develop serious emotional problems. Therefore it is imperative that nurses examine their attitudes regarding rape and develop a clear understanding of the nursing diagnoses Rape-Trauma Syndrome, Rape-Trauma Syndrome: Silent Reaction, and Rape-Trauma Syndrome: Compound Reaction.

Rape-Trauma Syndrome

Rape-Trauma Syndrome is categorized as a form of posttrauma stress disorder. Because of its relatedness to posttrauma stress disorder, the diagnosis of Rape-Trauma Syndrome has been successfully used in court as evidence of rape having occurred, where physical evidence such as the presence of sperm and vaginal penetration was not present. It is based on the premise that where sex has been forced, survivors show signs of Rape-Trauma Syndrome.[6,7] Even though it is not the nurse's responsibility to determine the legitimacy of the reported rape in assessing survivors, it is important for the nurse to be aware of the circumstances under which rape can occur. Three main types of rape, categorized on the basis of the survivor's lack of consent, are as follows:

- Rape—sex without consent in which the assailant uses blitz or confidence rape. Blitz is rape by a stranger; date and marital rape are examples of confidence rape.
- Accessory to sex—Survivors collaborate in a secondary manner by consenting to sex. Their ability to consent is impaired by cognitive or personality development.
- Stress-sex situation—Sex is agreed on initially but one party decides not to go through with it because of exploitation, but then is not heard.[9]

Myths concerning rape serve to place the responsibility for the rape on the survivor. Promoting optimum nursing care necessitates an understanding of these myths. Some of the most common and damaging myths about rape and the reality of the situation are presented in the box below[24]:

Myth	Fact
Most rapes are spontaneous and unplanned; they occur in dark alleys by strangers.	Most rapes are carefully planned. Often they occur in one's home. The offender is a relative, neighbor, or other acquaintance.
Rape is primarily a sexual crime, one of passion.	Rape is a crime and act of violence that is acted out in part sexually. The rapist often threatens with a weapon, physical and verbal abuse, and even death.
Rape happens only to young women.	Rape survivors have been as young as 4 months and as old as 92 years and more. All women, men, and children, regardless of their age, race, or educational or economic status, are at risk for being raped.
Women secretly want to be raped. They ask for it by the way they dress.	Rape is often a brutal, terrorizing, and humiliating experience. Women fear being raped. The way a woman dresses does not make her a more likely target.
Children and adolescents provoke the attack because of their promiscuous and seductive behavior.	Children do not ask to be sexually abused. The adult, and not the child, is responsible for the abuse.
Children make up stories about sexual abuse as retaliation, or to gain attention.	Children rarely make up stories about sexual abuse. They need to be taught not to keep secrets from their parents or care providers.

Rape-Trauma Syndrome: Silent Reaction

Failure to report the incident of rape stems from various issues and differences among age groups. Small children who have been sexually abused may not have an understanding of what occurred or may be overcome with fear. Others believe threats of harm and retaliation by the rapist or do not want to lose a reward that was promised for keeping the incident a secret. A 5-year-old boy reported performing fellatio with his mother's paramour. When asked if a special treat was offered for keeping it a secret, he quickly retracted his story, saying he had invented the entire incident. Later, he confided to the nurse that he enjoyed trips to McDonald's restaurant and would not be able to do this if the assailant were exposed. In children the silent reaction to rape may be used as a way to cope with the anxiety that may ensue once the rape is disclosed.[10]

Some hearing-impaired individuals who view themselves as being in control of what happens to them in any given situation may fail to report the incident of rape because of problems with communication. Individuals with developmental disorders may not report the incident because of fear of not being believed. Children may also fail to report the incident of rape because of fear of punishment from caregivers for being "bad."

Some adolescents fear that they will not be believed and will be blamed for having provoked the rape. Adolescents have been known to state that they would not report a rape because of guilt associated with being sexually active against their parents' wishes. Preoccupation with not being accepted among peer group members is also reported as a reason for keeping the incident quiet.

Some families react with violence to crisis situations and threaten to harm or even kill the assailant; this may result in the silent reaction by the survivor. Black author Maya Angelou,[4] whose autobiographical best-seller *I Know Why the Caged Bird Sings* gives an account of being raped by her mother's paramour, writes that after the family accidentally found out about the incident, the assailant was tried and found guilty in court. He did not, however, serve a prison term. Shortly after the trial, he was found kicked to death. Guilt-stricken with the thought of possibly causing the death of another human being because of identifying him as the assailant, Maya refused to utter another word. She literally did not speak for years to anyone except her brother.

Being forced to have sex with someone who is young enough to be your own son can be very embarrassing to an elderly woman. There is also tremendous shame in having to discuss the rape with children and grandchildren. Instead, an elderly person may prefer to keep the incident to herself.

Other reported reasons for the silent reaction include knowing the assailant, coupled with fear that the assailant would not be punished and would return to do harm. If survivors feel that they could have used more force or attempted to defend themselves but did not, intense guilt and shame may result in the silent reaction. If the rape is committed while the woman is on a date with a man who is known to her, or who is someone with whom she has been intimate previously, she may not consider it a rape and may not report it. The assailant may not feel that he is committing a crime but in fact may interpret the woman's "no" to the sexual advances as meaning "maybe" or "yes". This is termed *date rape* or *acquaintance rape*.[17] Women also may be subject to rape by their husbands. This is called *marital rape*. The emotional trauma when rape occurs under these circumstances can be the same as in any other type of rape situation.

A sexual assault investigator on staff at a mental institution stated that rape occurs among mentally ill patients, both outpatients and inpatients with ground privileges. The issue of consent to sexual activity may be especially difficult to determine by law enforcement officers if the patient has a history of mental illness such as schizophrenia or affective disorders. With these disorders there is difficulty with interpersonal relationships, decision making, and judgment. Some psychiatric patients use sexual activity to cope with problems, to act out, or as a tradeoff for goods. Therefore, when rape is reported, credibility may be in question from the police and health care providers' perspective. Being aware of this, rape survivors with mental illness may not report the incident, resulting in the silent reaction. Also, the incident of rape may have occurred but may be confused with fantasy and hallucination; consequently, because of the survivor's own confusion and uncertainty about the incident, it is often not reported. When the emotional and psychological trauma of rape is not dealt with, existing emotional problems are intensified.

Rape-Trauma Syndrome: Silent Reaction may occur most often in male survivors because of guilt, shame, and the feeling of powerlessness that may be more intense in male than in female survivors. One of the biggest concerns for male survivors is preoccupation with what others will think of their masculinity. The fear that other people will find out and that they may be labeled as being homosexual is great. Male survivors of rape may also have doubts about their own masculinity.

Denial, wanting to avoid thinking about the rape, and pretending it did not happen may be other reasons for the silent reaction to rape.[9] When drugs and alcohol have been consumed by both the rapist and the survivor, the survivor may experience guilt and self-blame and choose not to report the rape. Individuals with internal locus of control may experience intense guilt and self-blame because of the strong sense of responsibility and personal control experienced in everyday life. The shame, embarrassment, and disappointment toward themselves that these individuals feel may result in the silent reaction.

Rape-Trauma Syndrome: Compound Reaction

Adolescents seem to be at risk for the compound reaction of the syndrome. Adolescence is a period in which the individual is struggling with identity, independence, power, control, sexuality, and other issues. It can be a period of confusion and ambivalence and could lead to what Aguilera and Messick[1] call a developmental crisis. If rape occurs during this period, the increased stressors could cause Rape-Trauma Syndrome: Compound Reaction.

Besides adolescents, other individuals with Rape-Trauma Syndrome: Silent Reaction are also at risk for the compound reaction, especially if raped again. These individuals are unable to openly reveal the source of their stress or share their secret, and they are at risk for mental illness or the resurgence of already existing emotional problems. That is, a person who is raped may not disclose this trauma and may experience Rape-Trauma Syndrome: Silent Reaction. If the person is raped again, it may be revealed and the person may experience Rape-Trauma Syndrome: Compound Reaction. Previous losses in the life of an elderly person who experiences rape may result in Rape-Trauma Syndrome: Compound Reaction.

Cultural and Religious Influences

Cultural and religious beliefs affect how various groups respond to and cope with rape and may cause the silent or compound reaction. Even within cultural groups, individuals do not respond to the trauma of rape in a prescribed manner. Social and economic status within the culture, personality traits, and other factors influence how the individual will respond. Cultural and religious factors are additional areas the nurse needs to explore when assessing survivors. The nurse, however, should exercise caution against stereotyping a member of a particular group.

Because Latinos are the fastest growing minority group in the United States,[21] the cultural and religious beliefs of Latinos as they affect sexuality should be considered. Psychiatrists and sexual-abuse specialists of Latino descent have observed that a significant number of patients who are Latinos are devout Catholics and adhere to the tradition of the church concerning premarital sex. It should be noted that the position of the Catholic Church is to offer emotional support and counseling to survivors and to reinforce the fact that they are not to blame for the rape.

Virginity before marriage is still a high expectation for Latino women. Although the younger generation may have conflicting views, premarital sexual behavior is not practiced without guilt. For female Latinos who are from low socioeconomic background, sexual intercourse may be considered a duty and the sacrifice one has to pay to bear a child. When rape occurs, it is often the female survivor who is blamed for having provoked the man; he is not held accountable because of his "machismo", i.e., he could not control his sexual impulses.

It has been observed that Latino survivors of rape generally do not go through the procedure of reporting the rape to the authorities, nor do they seek counseling. Instead, the trauma of rape is dealt with within the family. This is particularly true because of the language barrier and strong taboo toward sex and its discussion in the home or with outsiders. Latinos who have good command of the English language may still prefer to relate to a counselor who is fluent in their native language.[21] There are few health care providers who are fluent in Spanish. A common question asked by Latino parents from low socioeconomic background is, "Is she still a virgin?" If vaginal penetration is not evident and the hymen is intact, the incident of rape may be minimized. The major concern for the family is that the woman be able to marry while still a virgin. Because of the emphasis on the sexual aspect of the attack rather than the violence, the survivor may experience a deep sense of guilt, shame, and self-blame. This lack of family support can be very disturbing for the survivor.

A number of minority groups, primarily blacks, live in urban areas. Consequently nurses working in emergency rooms of large city hospitals may see a number of blacks and other minority groups who are rape survivors. The nurse will need to guard against stereotypes and myths directed at a particular racial group. For example, there is a myth that for blacks the trauma of rape should be minimal because rape was a common occurrence during slavery. During slavery, rape was a means of subjugation and oppression. Black men were often ordered against their will to copulate with women who were not their partners for the purpose of producing more slaves, and women had no choice in the matter.[15]

ASSESSMENT

Because many of the behaviors exhibited for Rape Trauma Syndrome may be seen in Rape-Trauma Syndrome: Silent and Compound Reactions, it is important to be able to distinguish between these for adequate nursing care. Table 13 presents a symptom rating scale and the box on pp. 669-671 presents an assessment tool which may be useful guides in assisting the nurse to gather important data.

Text continued on p. 671.

IX

Table 13 Rape-Trauma Symptom Rating Scale

5	4	3	2	1
SLEEP DISORDERS				
No sleep; awake all night most nights, sleep-deprived state.	Severe; 1-3 hr sleep per night, early morning waking, stressful nightmares.	Moderate; difficulty falling asleep, nightmares	Mild; episodic nightmares, broken sleep	Sleeping well
APPETITE				
Hardly eating at all; prodded by others to eat	Severe; no appetite, eating out of habit	Moderate change; eating less food less frequently	Very little change; not quite as much food intake as before assault	No noticeable change

Continued.

Table 13 Rape-Trauma Symptom Rating Scale—cont'd

5	4	3	2	1
PHOBIAS				
Succumbed to fear; will not leave home, answer telephone, or talk with nonfamily	Severe; fears dominating life, seeking help, anxiety immobilizing	Moderate suspicion; some fears expressed, change in life-style moderate	Mild suspicion; little change in life-style habits	Calm and relaxed
MOTOR BEHAVIOR				
Uprooting of life (job and home); no activities	Job or home change; reduction in activities, lack of interest or self-control	Restlessness and dissatisfaction with indecisiveness, reduction in activities	Mild restlessness; expressed desire to make changes in work or home life	Calm and relaxed
RELATIONS				
Denial of or from significant other person(s); broken relationship with family, partner, or friend	Severe tension, anxiety; relationship(s) disintegrating	Relationship(s) show stress, nonsupportive, weakened	Relationship(s) intact, strained but supportive	Significant other person(s) supportive, understanding, and patient
SELF-BLAME				
Overcome with shame; feels cannot forgive self	Severe guilt; blames self, feels dirty and cheap	Moderate guilt; feels responsible	Mild guilt; feels it can be overcome	Free of guilt; accepts event
SELF-ESTEEM				
Feels worthless or hates self; completely unsatisfied with self	Disgusted with self	Disappointed with self; feels badly about self	Occasionally doubts self-worth	Feels good about self
SOMATIC REACTIONS				
Compounded symptoms directly related to the assault plus reactivation of symptoms connected to a previous condition (such as heavy drinking or drug use)	Severe symptoms; distressing symptoms described, life-style disrupted	Moderate symptoms; able to function but some disturbance of life-style	Mild symptoms; minor discomfort reported; ability to talk about discomfort and feeling of control over symptoms	No symptoms; none reported and symptoms denied when asked about a specific area

Reprinted with permission from DiVasto P: J Psychosoc Nurs 23(2):34, 1985.[12]

❖ RAPE SURVIVOR NURSING ASSESSMENT TOOL

Today's date _____   Address _____
Time of arrival _____   _____
Mode of arrival _____   Age _____ Sex _____
Accompanied by _____   Date of birth _____
Dr. notified (name) _____   Rape Crisis Center notified:
Consent for treatment obtained?   Yes _____ No _____
Consent for medication obtained?   Yes _____ No _____
Consent for release of information obtained? Yes _____ No _____
Consent for photographs obtained?   Yes _____ No _____

I. Physical status

Temperature _____Pulse _____Respirations _____Blood pressure _____
A. Physical complaints as expressed by survivor (include past significant medical history):

_____
_____
_____
_____

B. Observations of any physical injury (include approximate age of injury):

_____
_____
_____
_____

C. Vaginal examination/rectal examination done:
Yes _____No _____Refused _____
Date of last consenting sexual intercourse _____
Contraceptive used _____ type _____ Date last used _____
Date of last menstrual period _____

II. Emotional status

A. Statement of events of rape as expressed by survivor:

_____
_____
_____
_____

B. Observed behaviors/reaction to rape trauma:

_____
_____
_____
_____

Assessment tool developed by Sonia Hinds, R.N., M.S.N.   *Continued.*

IX

❖ *RAPE SURVIVOR NURSING ASSESSMENT TOOL—cont'd*

III. *Collection of specimens and evidence*

(Use checkmarks to indicate if procedure was done or not done)

Sperm   Yes _____ No _____ (Vulva _____   Vaginal _____   Cervix _____
                                                          Anal _____   Oral _____)

Gonorrhea   Yes _____ No _____ (Vulva _____   Vaginal _____   Cervix _____
                                                          Anal _____   Oral _____   Urethral _____)

Syphilis   Yes _____ No _____
Saliva   Yes _____ No _____
Urine   Yes _____ No _____
Hair collection (pubic)   Yes _____ No _____
Fingernail scrapings   Yes _____ No _____
Testing for:
   HIV (AIDS virus)   Yes _____ No _____
   Acid phosphatase   Yes _____ No _____
   Blood for pregnancy   Yes _____ No _____
   Blood type   Yes _____ No _____

Disposition of and conditions of clothing _____

Specimens given to _____   Time _____

IV. *Treatment*

Vaginal douche   Done _____   Not done _____
Suturing   Required _____   Not required _____
Wound care   Required _____   Not required _____
Hospitalization   Required _____   Not required _____

Other _____

V. *Medication administration*

Allergies _____
Present medications _____   Purpose _____
Last dose taken (date, time) _____
If medications are administered, include amount, purpose, time, dose and
route _____

Survivor's response to medication administered _____
Instructions to the survivor _____

IX

❖ *RAPE SURVIVOR NURSING ASSESSMENT TOOL—cont'd*

VI. *Nursing diagnosis*

(Use checkmarks to indicate the nursing diagnosis that applies; add any other nursing diagnosis present)

_____ Rape-Trauma Syndrome

_____ Rape-Trauma Syndrome: Silent Reaction

_____ Rape-Trauma Syndrome: Compound Reaction

Other _____

VII. *Nursing diagnosis*   ***Nursing interventions***   ***Survivor outcome***

VIII. *Referrals for follow-up care and appointments (include date, time, and with whom):*

IX. *Disposition of survivor* _____
   ***Accompanied by* _____**

   SIGNATURE OF NURSE AND TITLE _____

IX

Rape-Trauma Syndrome

According to Burgess and Holmstrom,[9] Rape-Trauma Syndrome consists of two phases: the acute and the long-term. The acute phase occurs immediately after the attack. It is a period of extreme disorganization or stress reaction with behavioral, somatic, and psychological manifestations. The acute phase is divided into immediate impact reactions, which can be expressed or controlled, and physical and emotional reactions. The second phase, or long-term process of reorganization, often begins 2 to 3 weeks after the attack but varies in length among survivors. It may last 6 to 12 weeks, or a lifetime. The second phase consists of coping behaviors exhibited during the period in which survivors attempt to put their lives back in order. Symptoms in the acute phase often overlap those in the second phase.

The nursing diagnosis of Rape-Trauma Syndrome consists of a host of behaviors, signs, and symptoms. Survivors of rape will have a wide range of responses. The impact of rape on a survivor cannot be determined only by outward reactions and behaviors observed. Every incident of rape occurs under different circumstances; how an individual copes with the trauma of rape is determined by numerous factors.

A number of defining characteristics of Rape-Trauma Syndrome have been identified and are discussed in detail here.[9,11,18]

Initial Reaction

The most common immediate reaction often observed in the emergency room is the survivor's attempt at a composed and controlled demeanor, rather than hysteria, although the survivor is clearly upset. Most survivors sob quietly.

Guilt, Shame, Self-Blame, and Embarrassment. Lack of eye contact and preoccupation with own thoughts are often observed in many survivors. Guilt, self-blame, and embarrassment are not always expressed verbally but are sometimes exhibited by lack of eye contact, withdrawal, and reluctance to talk.

Fear. Feelings of overwhelming fear of being beaten or mutilated and fear for one's own existence are also common observations. Fear of being killed is reported as common among survivors. Another common concern is fear of contracting sexually transmitted diseases, specifically acquired immunodeficiency syndrome (AIDS). Along with fear of sexually transmitted diseases, fear of becoming pregnant from the rape was also frequently voiced. Fear of "going crazy" is another commonly expressed concern.

Anger. Anger is said to be rarely expressed at the aggressor, but it is often directed inward and demonstrated in statements such as, "I'm so angry at myself for being so stupid . . . . How could I have allowed that to happen . . . . I should have fought harder." Although rape is a violent act and the survivor often experiences intense fear, it has

been noted that there are times when *no* direct anger is expressed toward the rapist. Instead, there is identification with the aggressor. By taking responsibility for the rape, the survivor attempts to regain lost control. As a result there is an increased feeling of guilt and shame. Anger is directed inward, and the anger felt for the rapist is repressed. It may surface later in explosive outbursts displaced toward the police, nurse, and others.[25] Often anger is reflected in complaints by the survivor about having to wait to see the doctor or that too many questions are being asked by the police, social worker, nurse, and others. Survivors often express anger at themselves for not fighting the aggressor with more force to defend themselves. Anger is also voiced at the fact that survivors feel violated and that there was nothing they could do at the time.

Safety. Safety is also a major concern. A survivor may say, "I'm no longer a special person . . . . I no longer feel safe in this world . . . . There is no place that I can go and feel safe anymore . . . . I'm marked for life . . . . Everybody will know." Patients are known to express relief that they are in a hospital and being cared for. Patients fear being left alone and often will ask the nurse not to leave them alone.

Physical Injury. The most frequently observed physical injuries are bruises, scratches, and other minor injuries. Occasionally teeth marks, rope burns, cigarette burns, and open wounds are seen. Women are sometimes choked by the assailant and sustain bruises on their necks. More severe injuries such as stab wounds, fractures, and concussions are less commonly seen.

Long-Term Reorganization Phase

Fears and changes in life-style, appearance, and behaviors develop as a result of specific circumstances of the rape.

Changes in Appearance. Survivors who were able to lose a significant amount of weight before the rape may revert to overeating. This may be an unconscious desire to appear unattractive, creating a distance between self and others, and attempting to prevent future rapes, or it can be interpreted as a way of avoiding intimacy with others. Another means of changing appearance is a change of hair-style. A woman with very long hair decided to cut her hair very short and stated that she would never allow it to grow long again because her hair was used by the rapist to control her.

Sleep Disturbance. Nightmares, insomnia, and fear of falling asleep are reported. For example, a woman who was raped with the lights on in her bedroom was unable after the rape to go to sleep with lights on, because the lights reminded her of the rape.

Changes in Life-Style. Some patients relate that there is a constant feeling of vigilance, always being on guard and anticipating that something bad will happen. Flashbacks of the rape have been reported as long as 7 years after the rape. Thoughts of the rape never seem to leave, and anything can trigger their recurrence. The constant state of uneasiness may cause a decrease in concentration and poor job or school performance. Survivors reportedly have lost jobs and dropped out of school. There is fear of meeting the rapist. Some survivors consider other living arrangements if the rape occurred in the home.

Ego Defenses. Survivors are known to use ego defenses such as depersonalization and dissociation to protect the ego from the reality of rape and regain control and lost autonomy. Depersonalization and dissociation occur when the survivor separates self from the attacks and acts as if it had happened to someone else.[2]

Changes in Sexual Relationships. Being raped does not mean that the survivor automatically will develop and maintain sexual dysfunctions or problems in a relationship. However, a number of rape survivors have difficulty in relationships with their spouse or lover after a rape. These difficulties may arise from lack of trust, or the lover or spouse may be unsupportive and view the survivor as "used merchandise." The rape may serve to heighten preexisting problems with the relationship, resulting in divorce or separation. Difficulties may also arise from frequent mood swings experienced by the survivor.

Additional symptoms of Rape-Trauma Syndrome, such as fatigue, depression, suicide attempts, hostility, somatic complaints, poor concentration, intrusive thoughts, poor self-esteem, and obsessive-compulsive symptoms, have been identified.[27] With the exception of fears and anxiety, most of the symptoms of the trauma dissipate within 3 to 4 months for most survivors. Fears and anxiety seem to linger after 3 to 4 months. Survivors interviewed state that these feelings seem never to leave them. Most survivors suffer immediate depressive reactions that last a few months. However, for some individuals depression persists for years.

Special Population Groups

Rape-Trauma Syndrome transcends all cultures and all age groups throughout the life span. This section addresses Rape-Trauma Syndrome as it affects children, adolescents, the elderly, men, homosexuals, and the mentally ill.

Child Survivors. Children experience rape trauma from not only vaginal penetration but also from other forms of sexual abuse. Such abuse may be fondling of breasts or genitals, fellatio, anal sex, vaginal penetration with an object or body part, masturbation of assailant, and exposure to pornography. These acts may be performed by a stranger, members of the immediate or extended family, caretakers such as babysitters, and people in positions of authority such as a teacher. Some children experience minimal effects; others may suffer severe psychological trauma.

Children 6 months of age or younger have been raped; however, most are over 5 years of age. Male children are also victimized. Children are rarely violently raped. The abuse generally occurs after the assailant has gained the trust and respect of the child.[19] Children who experience incest over a prolonged period may be at risk for a more severe and long-lasting psychological trauma than the child who experiences one incident of rape by a stranger. Numerous incidents of sexual abuse in children go unreported. If the child does not report it or if physical trauma is not evident, the

IX

sexual abuse may not be suspected because changes in behaviors may be attributed to circumstances other than sexual abuse. It must be emphasized that changes in behaviors, when seen by themselves, do not necessarily indicate sexual abuse. The entire situation needs to be assessed.

Adolescent Survivors. Response to rape trauma in the adolescent with Rape-Trauma Syndrome is contingent on the same factors listed for the adult survivor. The older the adolescent, the more the reaction to rape resembles that of the adult survivor. Most adolescent survivors of rape are sullen but in control of their emotions when seen in the emergency room. One factor that has a significant effect on how adolescents react is the attitude and responses of the parents. There is great fear that parents might not believe them.

If the survivor is under the influence of drugs or alcohol when the rape occurs, there may be verbalization of guilt, shame, and self-blame. Occasionally adolescents brought into the emergency room resist staff interaction and examination procedures.

Experts working with adolescent rape survivors feel that all adolescents should be assessed for suicidal ideation. Peer relationships are very important to the adolescent. If the incident of rape is known among peer group members and their relationship disintegrates, the adolescent may consider suicide. Suicidal behavior for adolescents may be seen as a means of controlling their lives and regaining control of their bodies, control that was lost during the rape. The long-term reorganization process for the adolescent is also similar to that of the adult survivor of rape.

Elderly Survivors. Compared to the adult survivor, rape does not seem to occur in as large numbers among the elderly. When rape does occur among the elderly, it is seldom reported. The emotional and physical immediate aftermath of rape in the elderly is similar to that in the adult survivor. Shock, horror, and disbelief are intensified for the elderly survivor because rape seems so unexpected for this age-group. A patient stated, "I can't believe anyone would want to rape a little old lady like me." Conservative val-

ues concerning sex cause intense feelings of shame and embarrassment, making it extremely difficult to discuss the incident with anyone.

Because of the aging process, the elderly are physically less resilient and more susceptible to sustaining serious physical injuries if beaten by the assailant during the rape. Because hormonal secretions have decreased, the vaginal walls may be dry and lacking in lubrication, causing vaginal penetration by the rapist to be extremely painful. Tearing of the vaginal walls and severe bleeding have been reported.

Over the years the elderly person may have experienced several losses, resulting in declining abilities or desire to cope with further losses.[14] After the rape there may be unresolved grieving, along with a loss of self-esteem, power, and control over one's body, as well as depression. The elderly survivor of rape may be faced with the loss of independence as a result of the rape. An elderly person who has been traumatized by rape may be forced to live with children, grandchildren, or other relatives or to move to a retirement or nursing home. This may be devastating for the elderly person, because it could increase feelings of powerlessness and helplessness.

Male (Including Homosexual) Survivors. Rape of males is a reality, although it is much more difficult to acknowledge than rape of females. Male rape survivors are much more likely to experience Rape-Trauma Syndrome: Silent Reaction because of the intense guilt, shame, and preoccupation with masculinity. Failure to report rape has resulted in the lack of proper medical and psychological treatment and emotional support from significant others, all of which may be available to the female survivor.

When males are seen in the emergency room, nurses report that the initial reaction is similar to that for the female survivor. Men are reportedly in control of their emotions but are obviously upset. Nurses report that there is lack of eye contact, a flat affect, and expressed indifference about their fate. Inability to speak because of shock has also been reported. One social worker said, "When seen alone, male survivors are choked up and tearful. In the crowded emergency room, there are too many people, so they just act numb and unemotional." Whereas a female survivor may agree to call a friend or have a volunteer from the rape crisis center accompany her, male survivors prefer to be left alone. Guilt may result from an erection or sexual arousal during the rape, which may raise questions such as, "Am I gay?" Guilt and anger may result from the fact that cues to the attack were missed because of alcohol or drug usage before the rape.

Since anal penetration is the most frequent act of male rape, common complaints observed by emergency room nurses are rectal pain, bleeding, anal fissures, tears in the rectal wall, and chronic bowel problems. Bruises, abrasions, hematomas, concussions, fractures, and injuries to internal organs have been reported. Other physical complaints are similar to those found in the female survivor.

The long-term reorganization process may involve low self-esteem, depression, homophobic panic, confusion over sexual identity and sexual orientation, ambivalence over female relationships, preoccupation with manhood, aggressive assertion of masculinity, feelings of persecution, resurfacing of suppressed rage, obsession with vengeance, disturbing sexual fantasies, immersion in new subcultures, and involvement in anti-male violence movements.[3,13,22]

Female Homosexual Survivors. Lesbians also experience rape and display the same immediate reactions and long-term coping behaviors as other survivors. However, for some lesbian survivors specific issues will determine how they react to and cope with the trauma of rape. Some of these issues are the lack of prior sexual experience with a man; possible prior existing feeling of anger toward men; ambivalence about disclosing lesbianism to health care providers, law enforcement officers, or significant others; and lack of emotional support from family members. It should be noted that a lesbian's assailant, like any assailant, can be either male or female.

Survivors With Mental Illness. When there is a history of mental illness, response to Rape-Trauma Syndrome may be different from that in individuals who are mentally healthy. Schizophrenia and affective disorders result in a disturbance in affect.[2] This disturbance in affect may cause inappropriate display of emotions and responses to a crisis. For example, with schizophrenia or the manic phase of bipolar disorder, the survivor may respond to the trauma with hysterical laughter while recounting gruesome details. The individual with severe mental illness is often exposed to various forms of victimization. Rape for this survivor may be considered to be just another form of victimization, and consequently the effects of rape may be minimized. The immediate reaction to rape for patients with mental illness is often the display of a flat affect. This response is similar to that of individuals who are mentally healthy and who are in shock after the rape, but the response is more exaggerated. It is not uncommon for survivors with borderline personality disorders to self-inflict wounds, causing severe physical pain. Over a period of time of repeating this behavior, the borderline patient does not seem to react to the self-inflicted physical pain. The trauma of rape seems to generate the same type of response. For the individual with mental illness, the trauma of rape may be repressed, thereby compounding mental illness. The end result is Rape-Trauma Syndrome: Compound Reaction.

Rape-Trauma Syndrome: Silent Reaction

The same criteria for Rape-Trauma Syndrome apply to the assessment for the survivor with Rape-Trauma Syndrome: Silent Reaction. Some behaviors exhibited by those who experience Rape-Trauma Syndrome: Silent Reaction are abrupt changes in relationships with men for unexplained reasons, increased anxiety during assessment, such as blocking of association, long periods of silence, minor stuttering, physical distress, and sudden onset of phobic reactions.[9,20] A Planned Parenthood sexuality educator related that several survivors were responding with hypersensitivity to routine pelvic examinations. Questioning revealed that a significant number of

IX

these women had experienced rape or sexual abuse earlier in their lives but did not report it. The unresolved issue of the rape was reflected in their response to the pelvic examination.

A sexual history for all survivors as part of the nursing assessment is a valuable tool in uncovering Rape-Trauma Syndrome: Silent Reaction. All survivors, regardless of the reason for seeking medical attention and whether or not sexual abuse is suspected, should be asked questions regarding sexuality and possible sexual abuse.

Rape-Trauma Syndrome: Compound Reaction

Assessment criteria for the person who experiences Rape-Trauma Syndrome: Compound Reaction are the same as those listed for Rape-Trauma Syndrome. Where there is a prior history of mental illness, drug or alcohol abuse, suicide attempts, chronic illness, or social or financial difficulties, more detailed questioning should be done because the patient is at risk for the compound reaction.

Rape-Trauma Syndrome
❖ **Defining Characteristics:**

The presence of the following defining characteristics indicates that the patient may be experiencing Rape-Trauma Syndrome:

Initial reactions

* Expressed emotions
  Shock, disbelief, and terror
  Fear, anger, and anxiety shown by the following: crying, sobbing, smiling nervously, restlessness, trembling, lack of eye contact, hysteria, and hostility

  Fear for physical safety and of retaliation from rapist
  Feelings of powerlessness, helplessness
  Embarrassment, shame, and guilt
  Mood swings

Child survivors may also experience, in addition to the expressed emotions listed above, the following: fear of punishment, abandonment, rejection, and repercussion; loss of promised reward; excessive fear of strangers and adults; overdressing to protect genitals; hallucinations (i.e., imagining seeing male genitals in a banana, pencil, or spine of book).

Adolescent survivors may also experience, in addition to the expressed emotions listed above, the following: denial, isolation, preoccupation with manhood, obsession with revenge, and feelings of persecution. Homosexual survivors may also experience, in addition to expressed emotions listed above, increased anger toward men and preoccupation with revealing sexual orientation to health care provider.

Mentally ill survivors may also experience, in addition to expressed emotions listed above, the following: flat affect, self-destructive or aggressive behavior, and psychotic or bizarre behavior.

* Controlled reaction
  Composed, unable to show true emotions
* Physical reactions
  General soreness/bruising, generalized body pain
  Symptoms specific to rape: rope burns; cigarette burns; teeth bites; open wounds; scarring of vaginal walls; genitourinary and rectal complaints such as itching, burning, vaginal discharge, bleeding, STD; and soreness of mouth, lips, jaws, throat, neck

  Skeletal muscle tension resulting in the following: headaches, fatigue, sleep disturbances (nightmares, crying and screaming out in sleep, waking up at night, insomnia, enuresis), and startle reactions (edgy, jumpy over minor incidents)
  Numbness, indifference to own fate, withdrawn
  Gastrointestinal disturbances: loss of appetite, stomach pain, distorted food taste, nausea, and overeating

Child survivors may experience, in addition to physical reactions listed above, the following:

- Enlarged vaginal opening
- Somatic complaints

Male survivors may experience, in addition to physical reactions listed above, the following:
- More sustained physical injuries

Long-term process reorganization
- Changes in appearance

Change in hairstyle	Significant weight gain
Increased body muscles for body building classes	Significant weight loss

- Psychological response

Depression, especially close to anniversary date, and loss of self-esteem	Avoidance of gynecological examination
Depersonalization	Obsessive-compulsive behavior
Denial	Daydreaming or intrusive thoughts

- Dreams and nightmares
- Fears and phobias

Fear of returning to location of attack, being alone, with crowds; fear and mistrust of all men	Other fears related to specific circumstances of rape

- Change in sexual activity

  Disturbance with sexual relationships
- Change in social or work relationships
- Changes in life-style

Change in residence	Change of phone number and keeping it unlisted
Social isolation	
Renewed contact with family members	

- Change in behavior (children)

Excessive masturbation	Age-inappropriate sexual vocabulary
Sudden drop in academic performance	Sexual precocity
Hints of sexual activity in artwork	

❖ **Related Factors**

The following related factors are associated with Rape-Trauma Syndrome:
- Age
- Maturational level
- Prior life experiences and ability to cope with stressful life events
- Existing and past stressors
- Circumstances under which rape occurred (blitz, acquaintance, date, or marital rape)
- Sexual orientation of survivor (homosexuals, lesbians, or heterosexuals)
- Sex of survivor (male versus female)
- Emotional support from significant others

❖ **Related Medical/Psychiatric Diagnoses**

The following are examples of related medical/psychiatric diagnoses for Rape-Trauma Syndrome:
- Bone fractures
- Dissociative disorders
- GI disturbances (e.g., perforated anus)
- Major depression
- Posttraumatic stress disorder
- Eating disorders (anorexia nervosa, bulimic disorder)
- Sexually transmitted diseases
- Dissociative disorders
- Conduct disorder
- Substance use disorder

Rape-Trauma Syndrome: Silent Reaction

❖ **Defining Characteristics**

The presence of the following defining characteristics indicates that the patient may be experi-

IX

encing Rape-Trauma Syndrome: Silent Reaction:

- Physical distress
- Minor stuttering
- Failure or reluctance to have gynecological exam
- No verbalization of the rape
- Sudden onset of phobic reactions
- Marked changes in sexuality
- Increased number of nightmares
- Increased anxiety during interview (e.g., blocking, long periods of silence)
- Abrupt changes in relationships with men

❖ **Related Factors**

The following related factors are associated with Rape-Trauma Syndrome: Silent Reaction:

- Intense fear of retaliation, ridicule, and not being believed
- In children (in addition to the above), fear of punishment or loss of promised reward
- Inability to verbalize event
- Lack of understanding of what has occurred or procedure to report rape
- Intense shame, embarrassment, guilt, self-blame
- Internal locus of control
- Protection of "male image"
- Denial
- Protection of loved ones
- Knowing the assailant
- Lack of understanding of circumstances under which rape can occur (e.g., marital, acquaintance, and date rape)
- Lack of emotional support
- In elderly, embarrassment because of difference in age

❖ **Related Medical/Psychiatric Diagnoses**

The following are examples of related medical/psychiatric diagnoses for Rape-Trauma Syndrome: Silent Reaction:

- Anxiety disorders
- Major depression
- Pelvic inflammatory disease (unexplained)
- Sexually transmitted diseases (unexplained)
- Unexplained somatic complaints (e.g., headache, nausea, vomiting, back pain)

Rape-Trauma Syndrome: Compound Reaction

❖ **Defining Characteristics**

The presence of the following defining characteristics indicates that the patient may be experiencing Rape-Trauma Syndrome: Compound Reaction:

- Exacerbation of or increase in:
  - Psychiatric illness (e.g., schizophrenia, affective disorders, or depression)
  - Suicidal ideations or self-destructive behavior
- Reliance on alcohol and/or drugs
- Stressful life situations

❖ **Related Factors**

The following related factors are associated with Rape-Trauma Syndrome: Compound Reaction:

- History of mental illness
- Presence of Rape-Trauma Syndrome: Silent Reaction
- History of drug and/or alcohol abuse
- Inability to handle stress
- Presence of physical illness (e.g., asthma, diabetes, heart condition, or seizure disorder)
- Financial difficulties
- In elderly, multiple prior losses sustained

❖ **Related Medical/Psychiatric Diagnosis**

The following are examples of related medical/psychiatric diagnoses for Rape-Trauma Syndrome: Compound Reaction:

- Affective disorders (bipolar, manic)
- Asthmatic attacks
- Major depression
- Personality disorder (borderline personality)
- Psychotic behaviors
- Schizophrenia
- Seizure disorder
- Substance abuse disorder
- Uncontrolled diabetes mellitus

NURSING DIAGNOSES

Examples of *specific* nursing diagnoses for *Rape-Trauma Syndrome* are:

- Rape-Trauma Syndrome related to lack of emotional support from family and friends
- Rape-Trauma Syndrome related to cultural beliefs concerning sexuality

Examples of *specific* nursing diagnoses for Rape-Trauma Syndrome: Silent Reaction are:

- Rape-Trauma Syndrome: Silent Reaction related to intense fear of not being believed
- Rape-Trauma Syndrome: Silent Reaction related to desire to protect loved ones from shame

Examples of *specific* nursing diagnoses for Rape-Trauma Syndrome: Compound Reaction are:

- Rape-Trauma Syndrome: Compound Reaction related to exacerbation of asthma
- Rape-Trauma Syndrome: Compound Reaction related to recurrence of alcohol abuse

PLANNING AND IMPLEMENTATION WITH RATIONALE
Rape-Trauma Syndrome

Care of the rape survivor is based on four models of nursing intervention: the biological, social, psychological, and cognitive-behavioral models.[8] When a rape survivor arrives in the emergency room, the first priority is a physical assessment to determine whether any physical injuries necessitate immediate attention. *The biological model is directed at treating physical injuries and medical complications such as sexually transmitted diseases (STD). Pregnancy prevention and encouraging the survivor to return for follow-up medical care are also addressed.*[5] Health teaching is a very important task for the nurse in dealing with the rape survivor. The nurse must keep in mind that the anxiety level of the rape survivor may be high, and repetition of information may be needed as well as written information.

Establishing trust is a very difficult task for the survivor, especially if the rape was committed by someone who is known to the survivor. *By providing a caring, accepting, and compassionate attitude, the nurse can help the survivor to reestablish trust.*

The social model of intervention[8] *is directed at providing a social network of family and significant others to provide emotional support.* Some families or significant others may not be understanding or supportive or may overreact. A volunteer from the rape crisis center should be made available for emotional support, especially in the absence of family or significant others. The nurse may need to provide guidance in assisting the family to understand what effects these responses could have on the recovery of the survivor. The nurse could model appropriate verbal interventions for them. Parents of adolescents and spouses may need help in conveying concern rather an instilling guilt. Latino parents who are concerned with whether or not the child is still a virgin need to be helped to focus on the emotional aspects of the abuse rather than the sexual act. They need to be told that the child is still indeed a "senorita" (a virgin, a woman who marries in a white dress), and virginity is given by choice and not taken by force. If parents or significant others are able to put the incident in its proper perspective, they can in turn be supportive of the survivor. The entire family may need to be referred for family therapy. Some couples are referred for marital counseling.

The psychological model of intervention is aimed at assisting the survivor in returning to a healthy level of functioning as soon as possible.[8,23] Survivors appreciate practical things during the crisis. The examination and screening process after the assault can range from 3 to 5 hours. Survivors may be physically and emotionally exhausted and appreciate a cup of coffee, shower, vaginal douche, and clean underwear and other clothing. Having these needs met may help to decrease anxiety. Survivors may be experiencing guilt because they feel they may have used bad judgment with the assailant, fear that they are "going crazy," and displace anger onto the treatment team. It is helpful for the survivor to hear, "You're not to blame," "You're in a safe place,"[26] "You're not going crazy." If anger is directed at the nurse, the nurse must be aware that this is not uncommon and must not be taken personally. Survivors need to be helped to redirect their anger at the rapist.

The emotional trauma of rape may be so severe that survivors may have suicidal ideations. This is

Text continues on p. 681.

❖ *NURSING CARE GUIDELINES: RAPE-TRAUMA SYNDROME*
Nursing Diagnosis: Rape-Trauma Syndrome

Expected Patient Outcomes	Nursing Interventions
	Short-term outcomes
The survivor will be free of medical and physical complications of rape trauma.	• Assist with/or conduct physical assessment. • Collect specimens and evidence as appropriate, after consent is obtained from the survivor. • Educate the survivor regarding possible complications such as STDs and pregnancy. • Stress importance of follow-up medical care and adherence to medication regimen.
The survivor will establish a therapeutic alliance with the primary nurse.	• Convey a caring, accepting, compassionate, and nonjudgmental attitude regardless of the circumstances of the rape. • Let the survivor know you are glad he or she is alive and that he or she is not to blame for the rape.
The survivor will have support of family/significant others.	• Explain the importance of seeking emotional support from family/significant others; assist family members in providing support. • Make referrals for family counseling as needed. • Call rape crisis center volunteer, with survivor's permission, for additional support.
The survivor will experience decreased psychological symptoms such as anxiety, fear, guilt, anger, and lack of trust.	• Encourage the survivor to acknowledge the pain of the terrifying experience by facilitating verbalization of feelings. • Assess rape belief pattern and educate as needed. • Inform about the need to report incident to authorities; respect wish not to do so.
The survivor will not harm self.	• Assess for suicidal ideations. • Use crisis intervention measures as needed.
The survivor will have restored feelings of power and control over life situation.	• Explore strengths and resources, and allow survivor to make decisions pertaining to care where feasible. • Refer/teach assertiveness training techniques and rape prevention measures.
Long-term outcome The survivor will return to prior level of functioning.	• Monitor psychological aftermath of rape using Rape Trauma Symptom Rating Scale (Table 1) during follow-up counseling. • Provide/refer for psychotherapy and rape support groups. • Use desensitizing techniques such as systematic desensitization, confrontation with rapist, thought-stopping technique, guided imagery and flooding as necessary. • Use therapeutic stories to provide insight and empowerment.

IX

❖ *NURSING CARE GUIDELINES: RAPE-TRAUMA SYNDROME: SILENT REACTION*

Nursing Diagnosis: Rape-Trauma Syndrome: Silent Reaction

Expected Patient Outcomes	Nursing Interventions
	Short-term outcomes (include those for Rape-Trauma Syndrome)
The survivor will not develop Rape-Trauma Syndrome: Compound Reaction.	• Assess for predisposing factors of Rape-Trauma Syndrome: Compound Reaction (such as history of mental illness, physical illness, financial problems, drug and/or alcohol abuse), and assist in identifying realistic future plans in coping, or refer to primary therapist or physician for treatment. • Provide individual therapy early to help prevent the Compound Reaction.
The survivor's feelings of self-worth will be restored.	• Give positive feedback for disclosing the rape and for sharing feelings; give hope that there can be healing from trauma. • Refer for pastoral counseling, if so desired, to deal with guilt and self-blame and to reassure that the survivor is not a "sinner."
	Long-term outcome
Same as for Rape-Trauma Syndrome	• Same as for Rape-Trauma Syndrome

particularly important to assess for those with a history of mental illness as well as adolescents. If suicidal ideations are present, psychiatric hospitalization may be needed.

Rape is an act of violence where the rapist seeks to overpower the victim. During rape, the survivor is stripped of power and control. Restoring a sense of power and control is vital to the recovery of survivors. Allowing survivors to make decisions about their care, as appropriate, gives the message that they are competent and in control of their lives. Assertiveness training and rape prevention training are additional ways for restoring control.

For some survivors, follow-up counseling or psychotherapy may be needed to assess for the presence and extent of the psychological aftermath of assault and provide therapy. *The cognitive-behavioral model[8] assesses the survivor's be-

lief pattern about rape and provides intervention measures such as systematic desensitization, thought stopping techniques, psychotherapy and other interventions to facilitate return to prior level of functioning.[23]*

Rape-Trauma Syndrome: Silent Reaction

Survivors who are unable to reveal the rape to someone and obtain emotional support suffer in silence. The result may be the trauma of rape compounded by mental illness, resurgence or complications of present illnesses, and perhaps financial difficulties due to lost wages. Providing an opportunity to reveal the trauma of rape is important and should be a part of all physical assessments and psychiatric evaluations. Children should be taught not to keep secrets regardless of the reward. *Once the silence has been broken, survivors must be assessed for the Compound Re-*

IX

❖ *NURSING CARE GUIDELINES: RAPE-TRAUMA SYNDROME: COMPOUND REACTION*

Nursing Diagnosis: Rape-Trauma Syndrome: Compound Reaction

Expected Patient Outcomes	Nursing Interventions
	Short-term outcomes (include those for Rape-Trauma Syndrome)
The survivor will not harm self or others.	• Assess for suicidal or homicidal ideations. • Protect survivor from hostile, aggressive, and self-destructive behavior.
The survivor will regain control of physical problems or disorders such asthma, diabetes, heart condition, or seizure disorder.	• Refer to primary physician or nurse practitioner for evaluation/treatment of medical problems. • Stress importance of compliance with treatment.
The survivor will regain control of financial difficulties as a result of rape.	• Refer to social services for evaluation and assistance with expenses (lost wages, cost of medical care) relating to the rape. Also, the National Organization for Victim Assistance (NOVA).
The survivor will use problem-solving rather than affective ways of coping, such as alcohol/drug abuse and self-destructive behavior.	• Assess coping pattern, explore problem-solving measures rather than affective or self-destructive measures. • Refer survivor for substance abuse or alcohol detoxification/therapy as needed.
	Long-term outcome
Same as for Rape-Trauma Syndrome.	• Same as for Rape-Trauma Syndrome.

IX

action and measures taken to prevent it. Whether or not signs of the Compound Reaction are present, the survivor should be encouraged to have counseling regardless of how long ago the rape occurred.

Survivors are unable to disclose the trauma of rape for various reasons. Once they have disclosed, survivors should be respected and not made to feel guilty for not revealing this sooner. *The nurse must recognize that disclosure is difficult, and positive feedback and acceptance are*

necessary in helping the survivor to restore feelings of self-worth.

Rape-Trauma Syndrome: Compound Reaction

High anxiety level may interfere with the ability to use adaptive coping mechanisms such as seeking support from family and friends, seeking counseling, or using meditation. The survivor who once relied on drugs and alcohol may easily resort to this again. Getting the survivor back in touch with emotional support from Alcoholics Anonymous or Narcotics Anonymous should be considered. Refer to the discussion under Rape-Trauma Syndrome: Silent Reaction for additional information on patient outcomes and nursing interventions.

EVALUATION
Rape-Trauma Syndrome

Emergency room nurses and nurses on crisis teams usually do not provide follow-up medical or psychological services to rape survivors. Telephone follow-up counseling is sometimes provided. Survivors are referred to rape crisis centers, sexual abuse centers, or their own physician or nurse practitioner for counseling and medical care. Therefore it is difficult for emergency room and crisis team nurses to assess the effectiveness of their interventions on a long-term basis.

In the emergency room, nurses are able to evaluate their interventions on the basis of (1) the decrease in symptoms while the survivor is still in the emergency room, (2) verbalization of understanding of instructions for medication or treat-

ment, and (3) willingness to comply with follow-up visits. Feedback from the survivor or family members on how they feel as a result of interventions is also useful. Interventions can be further evaluated when survivors write letters of appreciation.

Nurses and counselors who provide follow-up counseling can evaluate interventions by assessing the survivor's progress by means of the Rape-Trauma Syndrome Rating Scale (Table 1).

If the outcomes are not met, and the patient is noncompliant and experiences medical problems, in-patient hospitalization will be needed. If the emotional crisis continues and the patient is unable to return to prior level of functioning, in-patient psychiatric hospitalization may be needed, particularly if self-destructive behavior is present.

Rape-Trauma Syndrome: Silent Reaction

The nursing plan of care for this diagnosis can be considered successful if, after disclosing the abuse, the patient does not develop the Compound Reaction and is able to utilize therapy for empowerment, can regain control, and is able to

Text continues on p. 684.

❖ CASE STUDY WITH PLAN OF CARE

Ms. Ann F., a 20-year-old sophomore in college, dated a young man for 3 years. A week after terminating their relationship, they met at a sorority dance. The young man offered to take her home, and she accepted. When they arrived at the dormitory, he forced himself into her room and forced her to have sexual intercourse with him. When it was all over, she cried hysterically. After an hour or so, she got up, showered, changed her clothing, and cried herself to sleep. During the night she woke up screaming because of a nightmare. Her roommate woke up to find her crying, holding her side, and complaining of severe abdominal pain. An ambulance was called, and the college sophomore was rushed to the closest emergency room. While in the emergency room she refused to be examined by a male physician. When the female physician arrived, the survivor was very reluctant to remove her clothing for the examination. In addition, there was stuttering, long pe-

riods of silence, and blocking of association when the physician tried to obtain the medical history. Further questioning by the physician revealed that Ms. F. had been sexually abused at 8 years of age by an uncle but had never told her parents or anyone else, which caused much emotional turmoil. The present rape by her former boyfriend caused her to relive the same feelings of terror and helplessness. The college sophomore reported that her failure to report the second assault stemmed from doubts about knowing whether she could consider the present assault a rape, because the assailant was known to her and she was intimate with him before the assault. She related feeling "dirty," guilty about accepting the ride home, and not deserving of being alive. After a complete assessment the nurse formulated the nursing diagnosis of Rape-Trauma Syndrome: Silent Reaction.

Continued.

IX

PLAN OF CARE FOR MS. ANN F.

Nursing Diagnosis: *Rape-Trauma Syndrome: Silent Reaction related to lack of knowledge concerning acquaintance rape.*

Expected Patient Outcomes	Nursing Interventions
Short-term outcomes (include the first, second, fifth, and sixth outcomes from the Nursing Care Guidelines for Rape-Trauma Syndrome)	
Ms. F. will continue existing situational support from roommate and will obtain support from family members.	• Give roommate positive feedback for offering emotional support. • Explain to Ms. F. importance of seeking additional support from family members. • Assist family members in providing support as needed. • Make referrals for family counseling as needed.
Ms. F. will experience decreased mistrust of men.	• Respect Ms. F.'s wish to be treated by female physician if possible. • Allow Ms. F. to verbalize anger and hostile feelings toward the rapist in nondestructive ways. • Refer for intense, long-term counseling, if needed.
Ms. F. will return to previous sleep pattern, free of nightmares.	• Assess previous sleep pattern. • Discuss realistic ways to achieve uninterrupted sleep.
Ms. F. will be free of guilt and self-blame resulting from the rape.	• Assess rape belief pattern. • Educate about acquaintance rape; let Ms. F. know that she indeed was raped. • Reassure her that she was not to blame for either present or previous rape.
Include first and second outcomes from Nursing Care Guidelines for Rape-Trauma Syndrome: Silent Reaction.	• Include as first and second interventions from Nursing Care Guidelines for Rape-Trauma Syndrome: Silent Reaction.
Ms. F. will experience decreased psychological symptoms such as anxiety and fear.	• Encourage Ms. F. to acknowledge the pain of the terrifying experience by facilitating verbalization of feelings, fears, and anxieties. • Inform Ms. F. about the need to report incident to authorities; respect her wish not to do so.
Long-term outcome	
Same as in Nursing Care Guidelines for Rape-Trauma Syndrome	• Same as in Nursing Care Guidelines for Rape-Trauma Syndrome.

reframe the traumatic experience in a meaningful way.

Rape-Trauma Syndrome: Compound Reaction

The nursing plan of care for this diagnosis can be considered successful if the patient does not harm self or others and is able to utilize available resources and to control any physical, emotional, or financial problems. Ongoing assessment for this diagnosis will be necessary since it could occur many years following the abuse.

REFERENCES

1. Aguilera DC and Messick JM: *Crisis intervention: theory and methodology,* ed 5, St. Louis, 1991, Mosby–Year Book.
2. American Psychiatric Association: *Diagnostic and statistical manual of mental disorders,* ed 3 (revised), Washington, DC, 1987, The Association.
3. Anderson C: Males as sexual assault victims: multiple levels of trauma, *J Homosex* 7:145-159, 1981-1982.
4. Angelou, M: *I know why the caged bird sings,* New York, 1969, Bantam Books.
5. Beebe D.: Emergency management of the adult female rape victim, *AFP* 43(6):2041-2046, 1991.
6. Bownes IT, O'Gorman EC: assault characteristics and posttraumatic stress disorder in rape victims, *Acta Psychiatr Scandinavia,* 83:27-30, 1991.
7. Brozan N: Rape trauma: seeking court acceptance, *The New York Times Style,* August 10, 1985.
8. Burgess AW: Rape trauma syndrome: a nursing diagnosis, *Occupation Health Nurs* 33(8):405-406, 1985.
9. Burgess AW, Holmstrom LL: *Rape: victims of crisis,* Bowie, MD, 1974, Robert J. Brody Co.
10. Burgess AW, Holmstrom LL: Sexual trauma of children and adolescents: pressure, sex and secrecy, *Nurs Clin North Am* 10:551-563, 1975.
11. DC *Rape Crisis Training Manual: Rape trauma syndrome,* Washington, DC, 1986, DC Rape Crisis Center.
12. Divasto P: Measuring the aftermath of rape, *J Psychosoc Nurs* 23(2):34, 1985.
13. Donaldson S: Male rape survivors: a checklist of consequences, unpublished manuscript, 1985.
14. Fields S: How does crime affect the elderly? *Geriatr Nurs* 8(2):80-83, 1987.
15. Genovese ED: *Roll, Jordan, roll: the world the slaves made,* New York, 1974, Vantage Books.
16. Hilberman E: Rape: the ultimate violation of self, *Am J Psychiatry* 133(4):436-437, 1976.
17. Hughes JO: Friends raping friends. Could it happen to you? Project on the status and education of women, pp. 1-8. April 1987, Association of American Colleges.
18. Hyde J: Rape guidelines, *Nurs Standards* 3(49):53, Sept. 2, 1989.
19. Kemp RS, Kemp CH: The common secret. Sexual abuse of children and adolescents, New York, 1984, WH Freeman.
20. Kim MJ, McFarland G, McLane A: Pocket guide to nursing diagnoses, ed 4, St. Louis, Mosby Year Book.
21. Medina C: Latino culture and sex education, Sex Information Education Council US Report, 15(3):1-4, 1987.
22. Mezey G, King M: The effects of sexual assault on men: a survey of 22 victims, *Psychol Med* 19:205-209, 1989.
23. Moscarello R: Psychological management of victims of sexual assault, *Canad J Psychiatr* 35:25-30, 1990.
24. National Organization for Victim Assistance: Sexual assault and domestic violence, pp. 41-62, 1992, The Organization.
25. Notman M, Nadelson C: The rape victim: psychodynamic considerations, *Am J Psychiatr* 133:408-413, 1976.
26. Smith, L: Sexual assault—the nurse's role *AD Nurse* 2(2):24-28, 1987.
27. Steketee MS, Foa EB: Rape victims: post-traumatic stress responses and their treatment: a review of the literature, *J Anxiety Disor* 1:69-86, 1987.

IX

COPING—STRESS TOLERANCE PATTERN
Ineffective Individual Coping

Ineffective Individual Coping is impairment of adaptive behaviors and problem-solving abilities of a person in meeting life's demands and roles.[15]

OVERVIEW

Coping is a process by which a person manages the ever-changing environment. From a beginning awareness that a condition exists, to dealing with the emotions generated by it, to a specific, deliberate action on it, to considering the effects of the action on a life goal, the range of the process is great. For the individual at a given time, the behaviors noted are often the best that he/she can do given a particular genetic, developmental, biological, and situational context. Effective coping implies adaptation to the environment, successful accomplishment of the tasks associated with growth and development, and management of problems. Some aspects of the environment and events in the life cycle are more critical or problematic to an individual and are labeled stressful. A person with an acute health crisis, such as a broken leg or a chronic disease, or someone undergoing treatment for a particular condition, is experiencing stress.[22] Changes in lifestyle, in one's role in the family or work situation, or in one's body can be perceived as stressful. If a person is coping effectively with a stressful event, then the adjustment or recovery is enhanced.

Disease and maladaptation, even death, are believed to be long-term consequences of stress and related to Ineffective Individual Coping. A de-crease in psychological well-being and social functioning are experienced. More immediate effects or outcomes are noted in changes in affect, in quality of interpersonal encounters, and in physiological response.

Lazarus and others[8,16,19] describe a model that focuses on the regulation of the emotions and management of the person-environment transaction. "Coping refers to the person's cognitive and behavioral efforts to manage (reduce, minimize, master, or tolerate) the internal and external demands of the person-environment transaction that is appraised as taxing or exceeding the person's resources."[8, p. 993] Two appraisals precede coping: (1) primary appraisal considers effects on self, goals, values, and commitments. The person asks self about the possibilities of being perceived as incompetent, endangering one's life or health or another's, or losing the love of an important person; and (2) secondary appraisal identifies the actions possible; that is, what can be changed; what cannot be changed but must be accepted; what can improve chances for a positive outcome; and what actions need to be delayed or postponed. During these appraisals one arrives at conclusions regarding the threat to self, meaning of event, predictability, and degree of control possible.

Coping strategies or modes can be divided into two major groupings, problem focused and emotion focused. Problem-focused strategies are actions to identify or change the effects of the event/stress/illness or cognitive activities generated by the event/stress/illness. Emotion-focused strategies are actions to change or control feelings/emotional states generated by the event/stress/illness.

The Ways of Coping Checklist (WOC and WOCR)[16] is an inventory of adult coping strategies in eight categories: problem-focused coping, wishful thinking, distancing, emphazing the problem, self-blame, tension reduction, self-isolation, and seeking social supports. Other studies* have identified strategies, such as increasing activity, making self statements, praying/hoping and relying on religious/philosophical beliefs, ignoring pain, diverting attention, denial, and preoccupation with objects of meaning.

Leventhal and Nerenz[17] have also conceptualized coping as part of a self-regulating system. The first stage of their model is the preattentive stage/appraisal process in which perceptual representation and interpretation occur. The stimulus first enters the perceptual system through the sense organs, where it is registered and a perceptual representation is generated. The sense organs then relay the input to the central nervous system. Emotions affect the process by intensifying body sensations. By further processing, aspects of the stimulus event stimulate the recall and perception memories, which again may activate other memories. The relationships among memory structure, the input, the one's attending to the information determine when the information reaches conscious awareness. Emotional memory structures are more powerful and demand greater attention. The schemata of past experiences assists in interpreting the event, in other words, mental images about what was felt, seen, heard, and smelled, what the symptom was called, how long it lasted, its cause, and its prognosis. The interpretation of the stimulus occurs as it is given labels, causal relationships, time structures, and consequences. Leventhal and Nerenz stress the importance of distinguishing between the types of memory for determining the effect on the coping process. Perceptual memory — memory of the visual, audi-

tory, and tactile sensations of an event — is associated with automatic responding. Therefore interpretation of an event using more of the emotional schemata leads to automatic responding. Abstract and conceptual memory is related to more conscious, volitional responding.

The response or coping stage follows the complex appraisal process. The representations of the event/stress/illness and the interrelated factors direct the plan and actions. For example, the meaning of the label *diabetic* to the patient will give the patient ideas of where to go for help, and in what medication and diet regimen the patient may be asked to participate. Fears, anxiety, or other emotions aroused by the thought of AIDS will promote behaviors to regulate or cope with these emotions. The amount of time believed to be necessary to make a plan of action, or to carry it out, will influence coping actions taken. The patient's ability to postpone satisfaction or to endure will also influence timing.

Health problems are particularly demanding of emotional coping resources. The threat to the self is great. The dependence on others for assistance of all types increases. The feelings generated may overwhelm abilities to do what is necessary; problem-solving is delayed. Lifestyle changes may be easy while in a hospital, but not at work or in the home. If treatment is extended months or habits/daily routines altered for years, the time dimension will affect the plan and action.

The patient tends to repeat actions found useful in the past. Medications used the last time are thought to work this time. Fear may cause the patient to postpone a needed visit to a clinic. Beliefs, values, and goals also influence the strategies used or planned. The nurse deals differently with a cocaine habit of an unemployed, homeless man than with a college student studying to become a chemist.

Perceptions of the self as able to identify problems, make plans, and act greatly affect the patient's use of available resources. In other words, self-esteem is important. Being able to visualize one's self as thin, or not smoking, or free from pain is also useful. One's knowledge and skill base affects coping. Observing others who are

---

*References 1-3, 6, 9, 13, 20, 26, 27

X

successfully handling the event/stress/illness further enhances development. Opportunity to practice or try out for one's self is reinforcing.

The last stage of Leventhal and Nerenz's model is the monitoring stage, which involves the appraisal process again. The patient evaluates the change in distress, the coping responses, and the objective effect on the illness or event. The appraisal is related to several factors. First, the setting of reasonable goals is important. When goals are set too high, are unrealistic and very abstract, are extremely concrete and minute, or demand an unreasonable time sequence, the person may conclude that he/she cannot make a difference and thus effect change. Second, the feedback system is important in the appraisal process. The model has two basic types of feedback: emotional and objective. Leventhal and Nerenz proposed that the key sign of disruption of problem-solving behavior is awareness of affect. As the problem-solving behavior becomes less effective in coping with the stresses, the person focuses less on acquiring and processing information and more on emotional responses. Emotional expressions are pleas for assistance or social support. Reevaluation is signaled by the intense emotions.

Finally, the recurring appraisal/interpretation of the event/stress/illness and the coping are dynamic. Change does occur; transitions are made. Perhaps most important, one perceives things differently, feels more sure of self, plans for self, takes pleasure in the actions taken, sees the progress made, and knows his/her desires.

ASSESSMENT*

The nurse assesses information regarding the patient's experience with the event/stress/illness, the actions being taken to deal with the consequences of the event/stress/illness, and the outcomes desired. Important considerations include the effects of age, sex, specific illness, procedure(s) and/or treatment(s), and socioeconomic status. Of extreme importance are the effects of the support system, including the nurse and other

*References 7, 8, 10, 11, 16, 17, 26

members of the health care team, in making an event less threatening or a situation more tolerable or understandable, in meeting basic needs for food, safety, shelter, and caring, and in validating the fears and emotion being experienced. Specifically, the nurse should address the following parameters: complex situation being experienced; coping style; coping style demanded by a particular event/stress/illness or family/community/culture; degree of anxiety; effects of time on event/stress/illness; opportunity for control over important outcomes; timing of coping strategies; information and/or teaching gaps; and effects of stress on the 11 functional health patterns.

❖ Defining Characteristics

The presence of the following defining characteristics indicates that the patient may be experiencing Ineffective Individual Coping:

- Physiological disturbances
- Abuse of alcohol, drugs
- Participation in potentially dangerous activities
- Engaging in lifestyles with risk to health
- Impairment of social role functioning
  Nonproductive lifestyle
  Lack of functioning in usual social roles
  Non-performance of activities of daily living
  Inappropriate behaviors in social situations
  Self-absorption
  Lack of concern for, and detachment from, usual social supports
- Poor morale
  Unhappiness
  Lack of future orientation
  Hopelessness
  Unacceptable quality of life
  Pessimism
- Defensive patterns
  Inflexibility
  Hypervigilance
  Avoidance
  Inertia
  Refusal or rejection of help

❖ Related Factors

The following related factors are associated with Ineffective Individual Coping:
- Physical or psychological impairment
  Memory loss
  Sensory or perceptual impairment
  Nervous system impairment
  Disease process
  Personality disorder
  Previous psychiatric treatment
  Complications
- Impaired self-efficacy or self-concept
  Powerlessness
  Lowered self-competency
  Lack of hardiness
  Lack of perceived control
  Lack of social support
- Stress event or illness
  Loss of loved one
  Threat to life
  Threat to security, lack of employment
  Life cycle/stage of development
  Pain
  Multiple repetitive stressors over time
  Overload, daily hassles
  Conflict arising from incompatible motives or goals
- Situation or context
  Lack of resources
  Social or cultural instability
  Lack of available treatment
  Exhaustion of available treatments
- Inaccurate appraisal of stress, event, or illness
  Inability to recognize source of threat
  Inability to redefine or interpret threat correctly
  Inability to find meaning for the event
  Inability to identify the skills, knowledge, and abilities self has to cope with the threat
  Lack of clear, realistic goals or outcomes
  Unresolved memories of past threats or negative experiences
- Inaccurate response repertoire
  Difficulty in expressing feeling, especially anger, guilt, and fear
  Use of behavior destructive to self or others

Inability to seek out or to learn new skills and knowledge needed
Inability to deal with tangible consequences of stress event or illness
Increasing emotional responsiveness or lack of objective responsiveness
Defensive avoidance of dealing with threatening situations
Lack of palliative skills
- Inappropriate deployment of coping resources
  Inability to develop alternative goals, plans, actions, and rewards
  Lack of ability to transfer knowledge and skills to actual resolution of problem
  Giving up hope and spiritual values
  Social withdrawal
  Difficulty in using problem-solving skills and decision-making skills
  Lack of assertiveness behaviors
  Impaired communication skills
  Concerns and/or fears about initiating action
  Lack of an appropriate coping response because there is not a cognitive cue to action
  Lack of supportive social network
  Overuse or underuse of certain responses

❖ Related Medical/Psychiatric Diagnoses

The following are examples of related medical/psychiatric diagnoses for Ineffective Individual Coping:
- Adjustment disorder
- Cancer of the breast
- Diabetes
- Heart surgery
- Major depression
- Obesity
- Psychiatric diagnoses
- Schizophrenia, undifferentiated

NURSING DIAGNOSES

Examples of *specific* nursing diagnoses for Ineffective Individual Coping are:
- Ineffective Individual Coping related to rejection by boyfriend and limited social support system
- Ineffective Individual Coping related to lack of employment and social withdrawal

- Ineffective Individual Coping related to lack of clear day-to-day or long-term goals
- Ineffective Individual Coping related to pain associated with recent cholescystectomy, demands of 3-month-old infant, and limited support in home environment

PLANNING AND IMPLEMENTATION WITH RATIONALE

Nursing management for patients with a diagnosis of Ineffective Individual Coping includes (1) managing the environment to reduce sources of threat, pain, or misperceptions; (2) availability of resources to meet basic physiological and safety/security needs; (3) exploring opportunities for the patient to continue, or perhaps find, sources of emotional support from family, friends, or other patients; and (4) promoting the value of patient choice, control, and participation in planning, treatment, and monitoring.

Programs have been developed to manage stress experienced in health settings. The Stress Inoculation Training (SIT)[18] reflects the application of self-regulating theory and cognitive appraisal theory. During the initial state, the patient learns about the event/stress/illness, its effect on performance, and how to monitor thoughts, feelings, and behaviors. In a second stage, the skill acquisition and rehearsal phase, the patient identifies and rehearses problem-solving, taking direct action, and coping skills for regulating emotions and maintaining self-control. The third stage is application and follow-up over time. In this stage the patient gains experience using the knowledge and skills in stressful situations.

The Stress Inoculation Program can be effective, for example, for parents of children undergoing painful medical procedures.[12] For example, the program may give the parent information about leukemia and its treatment and about effective parental coping by using an example of modeling on video. The parent receives training in making helpful self-statements and in relaxation techniques.

Another example is a program supporting patients in preparation for cancer chemotherapy.[5]

The program includes (1) giving concrete information about what is going to happen and using video to provide modeling by a patient coping with the treatment; and (2) discussing what the patient has seen and any other concerns. The nurse encourages the patient to express feelings, makes other coping suggestions, and gives the patient a booklet reviewing the presented material for reference and further reinforcement of concepts presented.

An intervention dealing with patient expectations and the treatment experience provides concrete, objective, factual information in four taped messages during the treatment period.[14] The nurse assists the patient in developing a cognitive appraisal of the experience so that he/she can appropriately solve problems and use emotional skills. In these cases, coping was effective.

The combination of procedural and sensory information reported by Suls and Wan[25] was more effective than sensory or procedure information alone. The authors explained the effect as decreasing perceived threat and providing a readily available cognitive map of what will occur.

Many nursing interventions (relaxation, music, cognitive re-appraisal) applicable to stress management are presented in the literature.[4,23,24]

The plan of care for patients with Ineffective Coping reflects the concept of coping as a process and nursing as assisting in the individual's coping processes. The nursing care plan developed for a patient needs to support and complement the treatment plan.

Having an awareness of what happened, or what is happening, is the first step in being able to resolve the issues for oneself and to take action. *If the stimulus and related actions remain out of conscious awareness, the opportunities to take effective actions are decreased.* A person needs to be articulate about the what, who, when, where, and why of an event/stress/illness.

The nurse assists the patient in identifying these factors and other factors through by active listening as described by Peplau,[21] by questions, and by restating what the patient said. The nurse can use numerous strategies to help the patient recall

❖ *NURSING CARE GUIDELINES*

Nursing Diagnosis: *Ineffective Individual Coping*

Expected Outcomes	Interventions
The patient will accurately appraise the event/stress/illness.	• Assist patient to determine the what, who, why, where, when, and how of the event/stress/illness. • Seek time sequences, beliefs about what should or should not be, and roles of important people involved. • Identify areas that cannot be recalled or described. • Give empathetic responses to expressions of feelings.
The patient will use new facts/or knowledge to redefine the threat/stress/illness.	• Provide precatory information to changes, treatments, tests, etc. Describe the sound, smell, taste, feel, and appearance of the treatment. • Explain the causes of the sensation. • Give information about how long the pain, procedure, or treatment will last.
The patient will appropriately express feelings and identify them as related to the event/stress/illness.	• Assist in identifying feelings with names that are acceptable and understandable to the client. • Validate the feelings expressed. • Encourage description of feelings. • Ask questions and make comments that relate the feelings being experienced to the event/stress/illness.
The patient will have decreased emotional responsiveness.	• Give feedback about the behavior and feeling states observed and expressed. • Offer relief of intense emotions by distraction, distancing, relaxation instruction, listening, and directing activity. • Teach relaxation techniques, distraction, removing self from situation via mind or body, taking time, seeking help, etc. • Provide opportunity for practice and use in real situation.
The patient will have increased objectivity and ability to solve problems, make decisions, and communicate needs.	• Teach problem-solving, decision-making, and communication skills. • Provide opportunity for practice and use in real situations.
The patient will evaluate the strategies used to deal with the event/stress/illness.	• Explore past situations in which effective coping behaviors were demonstrated. • Provide feedback and instruct on how to obtain it from others. • Teach conceptual model for understanding coping and stress.

X

and describe events; e.g., bringing the subject up at each outpatient visit, asking the patient to write down what occurred when he/she took the medications, citing an experience of another patient in learning how to self-administer insulin, or suggesting a book on problem resolution.

The occurrence of an event/stress/illness is an opportunity for the patient to understand it. The patient can perceive the event/stress/illness as resulting in death, pain, and other negative consequences, as resulting in death in 5 years with no treatment, as painful but controllable with medication, as stressful for a week but less stressful if Mom and Dad are there, or as a growing experience if "I can only still work."

In addition, the perception that the event/stress/illness is something within a person's span of control is conducive to effective problem solving and action. *Redefining the threat as something over which a person can achieve some control will further diminish the threat.* The possible actions to be taken quickly multiply as the perception of the event/stress/illness is altered.

The nurse uses learning/teaching principles to enhance the presentation of new facts or information about treatments and procedures. Providing preparatory information for patients undergoing a new procedure or treatment by describing the sound, smell, taste, appearance, and feel (affect-ing all the five senses) is effective. However, if the experience is an old, painful, seemingly recurrent, nonchanging event, the patient may need to work through the event. The assistance of an experienced therapist who may use flooding, imagery, or other psychotherapeutic techniques is advised. *The nurse may assist in the recalling of a past experience with similar circumstances as evidence to the client of his/her capacity to deal with the event/stress/illness.* An exploring of the similarities and differences is also useful. The nurse can correct inaccuracies and misguided information during discussions with the patient.

The effective management of feelings aroused by an event/stress/illness is an important aspect of the coping process. The emotional response is automatic and may not be consciously perceived or associated with the event/stress/illness. The fear, anger, helplessness, hopelessness, or feeling of rejection can overwhelm the more objective, rational processes. The emotions need to be managed before problem-solving can proceed. Giving a name to what one is feeling may be the first step.

The nurse assists the patient to identify the feelings being experienced and may give them a name; e.g., "That was an overwhelming feeling"; "You were afraid of being alone"; "I hear a lot of anger." *Further feedback about the behavior*

X

❖ *CASE STUDY WITH PLAN OF CARE*

Mr. John R., a 29-year-old, separated, black male, walked into the HMO stating he had a severe sore throat, could not eat, had not worked for a day and was feeling "awful." He wanted to see the doctor and get a prescription for an antibiotic. The medical record revealed two episodes within the last 9 months of complaints of a sore throat, culture of organism, and antibiotic treatment. The separation from his wife was a year ago. He had not had a physical in 2 years. During the assessment interview, the nurse gathered the following information. Mr. John R. appeared tired, presented his problem in short, terse statements, was irritable about the clinic's slowness, and expressed a need to get back to work. Within the past 3 weeks he had been required to work overtime because of deadline penalties, and his boss said that the patient's promotion, due in 2 months, depended on his performance now. The patient said that in general things were fine. His wife apparently was happy without him, and he was too busy to care or to think about that relationship now. He made one remark about his boss. "What do you do with a nervous boss?" He described his diet as fast food "taken on the run." He obtains about 6 hours of sleep per night and awakes one to two times near morning. He has infrequent contact with his family, who live in the area.

PLAN OF CARE FOR MR. JOHN R.

Nursing Diagnosis: Infective Individual Coping related to increased stress at work and limited coping strategies.

Expected Outcomes	Interventions
Mr. John R. will report increased information on, and consequences to self, of stressors experienced.	• Give and encourage to read stress management pamphlet. • Raise questions, encourage data gathering, promote an attitude of openness to new information.
Mr. John R. will report change in diet, sleep pattern, and ability to set work limits.	• Monitor diet and sleep pattern. • Note sections of above pamphlet on techniques for stress management and and request that Mr. R. try one during the week and report when he calls back after antibiotic treatment.
Mr. John R. will describe one or two ways to handle nervous boss and deal with self.	• Set time to discuss idea of how to handle "nervous boss" when he calls in after antibiotic treatment.

noted and statements or questions regarding the relationships of feeling states to the perceived threat/stress/illness, further clarify the situation and help the patient perceive it as less threatening.

EVALUATION

Using the expected outcomes as goals, the nurse and the patient together can arrive at a consensus of achievement. To what extent have the defining characteristics been reduced or modified? Probably the most important aspect of the evaluation is the new question raised, the challenge to an old idea held by nurse and patient, or the action avoided—in other words, a discovery of a new goal.

REFERENCES

1. Allen KD, Danforth JS, and Drabman RS: Videotaped modeling and film distraction for fear reduction in adults undergoing hyperbaric oxygen therapy, *J Consult Clin Psychol* 57(4):554-558, 1989.
2. Auerbach SM: Stress management and coping research in the health care setting: an overview and methodological commentary, *J Consult Clin Psychol* 57(3):388-395, 1989.
3. Borden W, Berlin S: Gender, coping and psychological well-being in spouses of older adults with chronic dementia, *Am J Ortho-psychiatry* 60(4):603-610, 1990.
4. Buckwalter KC, Hartsock J, and Gaffney J: Music therapy. In Bulechek GM, McCloskey JC, editors: *Nursing interventions: treatments for nursing diagnoses*, Philadelphia, 1985, WB Saunders.
5. Burish TG, Snyder SL, Jenkins RA: Preparing patients for cancer chemotherapy: effect of coping preparation and relaxation interventions, *J Consult Clin Psychol* 59(4):518-525, 1991.
6. Dagg PKB: The psychological sequelae of therapeutic abortion—denied and completed, *Am J Psychiatry* 148(5):578-585, 1991.
7. De Maio-Esteves M: Mediators of daily stress and perceived health status in adolescent girls, *Nurs Res* 39(6):360-364, 1990.
8. Folkman S, and others: Dynamics of a stressful encounter: cognitive appraisal, coping and encounter outcomes, *J Pers Soc Psychol* 50(5):992-1003, 1986.
9. Geden E, Beck N, Hauge G, and Pohlman S: Self-report and psychophysiological effects of five pain-coping strategies, *Nurs Res* 33(5):260-265, 1983.
10. Gordon M: *Nursing diagnosis: process and application*, New York, 1987, McGraw-Hill Book Co.
11. Grey M, Cameron ME, and Thurber FW: Coping and adaptation in children with diabetes, *Nurs Res* 40(3):144-149, 1991.
12. Jay SM, Elliott CH: A stress inoculation program for parents whose children are undergoing painful medical procedures, *J Consult Clin Psychol* 58(6):799-804, 1990.
13. Jensen MP, Karoly P: Control beliefs, coping efforts, an adjustment to chronic pain, *J Consult Clin Psychol* 59(3):431-438, 1991.
14. Johnson JE, Lauver DR, and Nail LM: Process of coping with radiation therapy, *J Consult Clin Psychol* 57(3):358-364, 1989.

X

15. Kim MJ, McFarland GK, and McLane AM: *Pocket guide to nursing diagnosis,* ed 4, St Louis, 1991, Mosby–Year Book.

16. Lazarus RS, Folkman S: *Stress, appraisal and coping,* New York, 1984, Springer Publishing.

17. Leventhal H, Nerenz DR: A model for stress research with some implications for control of stress disorder. In Meichenbaum D, Jaremko ME, editors: *Stress reduction and prevention,* New York, 1983, Plenum Press.

18. Meichenbaum D: *Stress inoculation training,* New York, 1985, Pergamon Press.

19. Monat A, Lazarus RS: Stress and coping—some current issues and controversies. In Monat A, Lazarus RS, editors: *Coping: an anthology,* New York, 1985, Columbia University Press.

20. Myerowitz BE, Heinrich RL, and Schag LC: A competency-based approach to coping with cancer: In Burich TG, Bradley LA, editors, *Coping with chronic disease,* New York, 1983, Academic Press.

21. O'Toole AW, Welt SR, editors: *Interpersonal theory in nursing practice: selected works of Hildegard E. Peplau,* New York, 1989, Springer Publishing.

22. Petersen L: Special series: coping with medical illness and medical procedures, *J Consult Clin Psychol* 57(3):331-332, 1989.

23. Scandrett S: Cognitive reappraisal. In Bulechek GM, McCloskey JC, editors *Nursing interventions: treatments for nursing diagnoses,* Philadelphia 1985, WB Saunders.

24. Scandrett S, Uecker S: Relaxation training: In Bulechek GM, McCloskey JC, editors: *Nursing interventions: treatments for nursing diagnoses,* Philadelphia, 1985, WB Saunders.

25. Suls J, Wan CK: Effects of sensory and procedural information in coping with stressful medical procedures and pain: a meta analysis, *J Consult Clin Psychol* 57(3):372-379, 1989.

26. Sutton TD, Murphy SP: Stressors and patterns of coping in renal transplant patients, *Nurs Res* 38(1):46-49, 1989.

27. Tarrier N, Main CJ: Applied relaxation training for generalized anxiety and panic attacks, *Br J Psychiatry* 149:330-336, 1986.

Defensive Coping

Defensive Coping is the state in which an individual makes a falsely positive self-evaluation based on a self-protective pattern that defends against underlying perceived threats to positive self-regard.[67]

OVERVIEW

The process of coping—how individuals manage stress in their lives—has received attention from a variety of disciplines. Individuals differ in their responses to stress and may exhibit noticeably different behaviors in the same situation.

When an individual experiences a real or imagined event, he/she responds to regain a sense of equilibrium or well-being.[3,44] The event could be writing an examination, planning a visit to the dentist or being diagnosed with cancer. The event creates demands for a person and evokes a set of response strategies. The strategies are feelings (emotions), thoughts (cognitions), and behaviors (actions) elicited to maintain or regain a sense of balance or well-being. If the person's usual responses to an event do not achieve the desired balance, distress and anxiety occur; in other words, if the demands of the event exceed the resources of the individual, he/she becomes uncomfortable. Other response strategies will be needed to cope with the emerging discomfort and anxiety. Coping with life events is an ongoing, dynamic process that occurs similarly in both life-threatening events and "daily hassles." In this chapter, coping is defined as "the ways in which individuals manipulate their environment in service of themselves or the ways in which they manipulate themselves to better fit the environment."[15]

According to Lazarus and Folkman,[45] coping strategies serve two fundamental purposes. These include (1) managing or altering the problem (event) causing the distress and (2) regulating the emotional response to the problem. The first category is problem-focused coping, and the second is emotion-focused coping. Presently little is known about why an individual chooses a particular strategy or combination of strategies in a given situation.[26] However, we do know that individuals may select the same strategies for a variety of situations and yet select different strategies for the same situation at different times.[39,45,59]

An explanation for the individual response variation has emerged from the work in cognitive appraisal. Cognitive appraisal is the process in which an individual categorizes an event and its various aspects and judges its effect on his/her well-being.[44,45] It is largely evaluative, is focused on meaning, and occurs constantly during the waking hours. When confronted with an event, the individual engages in primary appraisal and judges the event as irrelevant, benign, positive, or stressful by asking the question, "Am I in trouble or will I benefit, now or in the future?" Secondary appraisal involves answering the question, "What can be done about this situation?" and assessing the coping options against the demands of the event. These appraisals may be at a conscious or unconscious level and are conducted through the individual's existing knowledge, experiences, self-concept, needs, attitudes, and life goals. The individual will judge the situation using his/her own unique frame of reference (cognitive map) and personal ideas of what is important.

This interaction between determining what is at stake and whether coping resources are sufficient for the event will shape the degree of stress and

X

the emotional reaction that the individual feels. The stress does not arise from the event itself but rather from the interaction between the person and the environment.[44] Individual variation results from the unique nature of cognitive appraisal.

A person's selection of a coping strategy is based on his/her appraisals. In general, emotion-focused coping strategies are selected when the appraisal concludes that nothing can change a harmful or threatening environment. The problem-solving forms of coping are chosen when conditions are considered amenable to change or challenge. As we learn more about the coping process, we realize that individuals use a wide variety of strategies. The key to understanding any particular individual's responses lies in understanding his/her cognitive appraisal and exploring its specific dimensions. To judge the effectiveness of specific coping strategies or responses requires a clear understanding of the purposes they serve for the individual. Those purposes are derived from the meaning that the person assigns to a particular event through his/her cognitive appraisal.

Meaning may be assigned to an event through an assessment of its perceived harm, threat, or challenge to an individual's sense of self and the occurrences that will maintain the individual's personal integrity. The sense of self (self-system) is the image or picture of oneself as distinct and different from other people.[10,66] It includes the notions of self-concept and self-esteem. Self-concept incorporates the perception of what one is like (self-identity), one's worth as a person (self-evaluation), and one's aspirations for growth and accomplishment (self-ideal).[22] This repertoire of beliefs about one's nature is in part an organization of the interpersonal motives and attitudes that an individual considers centrally important.[25,37] Self-esteem refers to the feelings associated with the self-evaluation or judgment of one's own worth and may emerge from comparisons between what one is like and what one aspires to be.

All individuals presumably have a global self-concept with an associated global self-esteem. This basic level of self-esteem is learned during childhood through the appraisals of significant others, may be relatively stable throughout one's lifetime,[18] and is evidenced in behaviors across a wide variety of situations. Basic self-esteem contains physical, social, personal, family, school, peer, and behavioral aspects. Individuals with relatively high self-esteem are better students, are less depressed, display better physical health, and enjoy better social relationships than those with lower self-esteem.[34] The functional level of self-esteem may change daily as one judges one's performance in a variety of situations (for example, school and work performance, family, peer relationships, and physical well-being). It arises from the ongoing evaluation of interactions with other people and events, the person's notions about what is important, and discrepancies between a person's ideal self and perceived self in specific situations. Functional self-esteem may vary throughout an individual's lifetime as he/she undertakes different tasks and roles, such as marrying or parenting.[63,66] It can exceed or fall below basic self-esteem. Severe, acute, or chronic stress, such as that occurring with illness (acute or chronic) or sudden loss (person or object), may alter functional self-esteem.*

A person's perception of events tends to reinforce his/her self-concept and self-esteem.[63] Self-esteem in adults is influenced by perceived levels of success in employment and interpersonal and parenting roles. Adults may perceive a discrepancy between how they are performing and how they should be performing and therefore experience lowered self-esteem. The resulting behavior may reflect passivity, helplessness, powerlessness, decreased decision making, and despondency. Of particular interest is the concept of defensive self-esteem. Coopersmith[19] described individuals with marked differences between their reported self-view and behavior. Specifically, these individuals reported high self-evaluations in reaction to low underlying self-evaluations resulting from poor performance and low status. Reporting high self-esteem based on denial or avoid-

---

*References 5, 20, 21, 28, 55, 61

ance of negative personal information has been described as "role-faking"[57] to meet perceived demands in a situation. It is a self-protective maneuver that defends against a perceived gap between the ideal and real self.

An event appraised as harmful or threatening to the self-concept will evoke coping strategies to protect what is important to the individual (self-esteem) and defend against a painful experience. Psychoanalytic theory has provided descriptions of mechanisms that defend the self-concept against danger or unpleasant feelings. These defense mechanisms incorporate distorted interpretations of reality, including a distorted self-concept, repression, projection, fantasy, displacement, and sublimation. The literature describing the coping strategies that individuals use during life events provides clear evidence that defensive strategies are indeed used. These mechanisms include daydreaming; use of alcoholic beverages or drugs; sleeping; ignoring, joking about, or denying the situation; blaming oneself or others; just focusing on the day; and getting away by oneself.*

Ego psychological models describe a hierarchy of coping and defense mechanisms, implying that some processes are automatically superior to others.[31,52,68] The implication is that a person has coped with the situation and met the demands successfully or a person has defended and coped ineffectively or inadequately.[47] According to Lazarus and Folkman,[45] this hierarchical assumption should be abandoned, and coping process and coping outcome should be considered independently. The effectiveness of coping and defending must be considered for each person individually. Both can work well or poorly in particular persons, contexts, and occasions.

"No one strategy is considered inherently better than another. The goodness (efficacy, appropriateness) of a strategy is determined only by its effect in a given encounter and its effects in the long term."[45] p. 134

Studies of crisis situations have emphasized the primary importance of maintaining self-esteem to manage the situation.[1,6,33,64] An individual's sense of self can be disrupted by a physical injury or a traumatic event. The resulting need to consider different images of self can threaten self-esteem. Defense mechanisms may be used to avoid or defend against emotional pain, resulting in a retreat from full awareness of what is happening. These defenses may conserve energy by reducing the amount of emotional coping and by providing a buffer that allows time to collect oneself and mobilize problem-focused strategies. In some instances, this can mean holding a distorted view of the personal image and abilities for a period of time. Particularly in unexpected events, seeking relief through avoidance and disavowal—redefining a situation or the self-view—can serve to obliterate the threatening reality of the situation, maintain self-esteem, and allow time for other coping responses to emerge. Also the distress an individual feels often influences thinking and perceiving processes.[36,38] In times of crisis, individuals can have trouble defining who they are and the skills they possess; they may have difficulty making decisions or solving problems. The resulting confusion and anxiety additionally threaten the already vulnerable self-esteem and can cause ineffective coping.[2,14,69]

Defense mechanisms may be helpful in protecting the self from overwhelming unpleasant feelings, particularly on a short-term basis.[6,17,33,64] However, defense mechanisms do close the cognitive field to further input, and they do not allow further cognitive appraisal as new information that could reduce the threat becomes available. The use of these mechanisms is inappropriate when the emotional response (1) prevents seeking and cooperating with treatment for illness, (2) interferes with everyday functioning, (3) evokes behavior that causes more pain and distress than the event itself, or (4) evokes responses that appear as conventional psychiatric symptoms. However, it is important to recognize that not all events are amenable to resolution through problem solving. Many irremediable events (such as natural disas-

---

†References 8, 9, 29, 32, 40, 49, 53, 65, 70

ters, disease, aging, and losses) can demand the use of defensive strategies to manage emotions and maintain self-esteem and a positive outlook in the face of overwhelming loss and harm.

Life events such as illness, bereavement, divorce, job loss, or aging can cause people to use defense mechanisms when the sense of self is threatened. When an individual is uncertain about his/her ability to cope with a particular event or to enact a specific role, he/she may develop self-doubt and fear failure and humiliation. As a defense against failure and low self-esteem, the behavior pattern defensive self-esteem may emerge.

ASSESSMENT

The set of observations previously outlined has contributed to the development of the nursing diagnosis Defensive Coping. The main characteristic of an individual who has this behavior is a tendency to present the self more favorably in response to perceived failure. This may be manifested as a denial of obvious problems or weaknesses and as grandiosity. The individual has a high need for social approval, yet is uncomfortable with intimacy and self-disclosure and is unable to openly acknowledge personal failures. Blame is projected onto someone or something else, and expressions of self-competency are unrealistic or exaggerated. There is difficulty in perceiving reality. In some instances, the person may have a superior attitude toward others and ridicule or laugh hostilely at them. Difficulty in establishing and maintaining relationships is evident. In therapeutic environments, lack of participation in therapy, lack of follow-through, and self-neglect have been reported. This concept of defensive self-esteem is validated in a recent study by Norris and Kunes-Connell[57] in which 15 of 27 subjects with low self-esteem displayed characteristics such as those previously described.

Whether an event is appraised as threatening to one's self-esteem depends on both the environment and the person. Regardless of whether the event is real, anticipated, or imagined or whether the appraisal is realistic or unrealistic, the coping behaviors are based on the perceptions of the individual. Events that occur suddenly or are unpredictable, uncontrollable, or ambiguous present a greater sense of threat. If the event impinges on ideas or goals that are important to the individual, the threat will be heightened. The individual's level of knowledge, skills, and coping abilities will influence feelings of threat. An appraisal of harm or threat occurs when an individual believes or feels that his/her coping resources are insufficient to meet the demands of a particular situation. If a similar situation has happened in the past, the previous experience will provide the frame of reference regarding the ability to manage it. Evidence now leads us to believe that an individual's social support (sense of being cared for) has an influence on feelings of distress.[4,8,9,13] The capability to overcome uncertainty, to maintain motivation, to cope, and to maintain an emotional balance are also considered important personal factors.[16] In general, ego strength and increased self-esteem reduce vulnerability to stress.[45]

A loss or change in significant roles or appraisals that create unrealistic self-expectations may lead to self-esteem disturbance. Self-esteem disturbance is defined as "negative feelings or conception of self including social self or self capabilities."[57] According to Coopersmith,[19] self-appraisals are based on (1) the ability to influence personally significant others (power), (2) the sense of being accepted and valued as worthwhile (significance), (3) the ability to meet performance demands successfully in terms of personal goals (competence), and (4) behaving according to one's moral and ethical beliefs and values (virtue). Situations perceived as harmful or threatening to these dimensions may lead to low self-esteem. The resulting behavior to cope with low self-esteem depends on an individual's coping response style and availability of resources. Generally, individuals will resort to coping strategies they have used in the past.

Almost any medical condition has the potential for being perceived as threatening. Not only may the condition be life threatening, but also the illness and treatment may threaten the person's role in the family, ability to work, or potential for achieving desired goals. The psychosocial effect of illness is vividly described in both professional and popular literature.* The loss of a breast may alter a woman's sense of femininity, the loss of a limb may require an occupational change, and the death of a spouse forces a person to view himself/herself as single. Whether the loss or threat is observable or evident, the self-esteem disturbance can be similar. A woman who has had a hysterectomy may feel a threat to her self-esteem as does a woman who has suffered burns to her hands and face.

How a person copes with a particular acute illness or a permanent disability depends on how the aspects of the event affect the individual and the unique meaning he/she assigns to these aspects. The type of illness; location, rate of onset, and progression of symptoms; degree of reversibility; and functional impairment all have personal meaning for an individual.[41,48] Individuals who perceive their illness as a weakness or failing may attempt to escape by denying it. Illness perceived as an enemy may also evoke coping strategies that defend against attack and danger. Low self-esteem with defensive behaviors has been described by battered women in a women's shelter, alcohol and drug abusers in treatment, hospitalized psychiatric patients, and clients with chronic physical illness.[57]

Assessment needs to occur on two dimensions. First, the nurse needs to assess the interaction between the person and the environment (event) and the effectiveness of the coping strategies. Are the strategies accomplishing the individual's desires without undue harm to self or others? Second, the context surrounding self-esteem must be established to understand the behavioral observations and to ensure that appropriate intervention strategies are initiated.

The immense complexity and variation in human response has, to some degree, hampered efforts to measure coping in a standardized manner. Much ambiguity and confusion exists in the field

*References 4, 12, 24, 42, 45, 46, 58, 60, 62, 71-74

because of inconsistencies in the defining terminology and the boundaries for the concept.[41] A controversial issue in the measurement of coping is the use of specific criteria to define success. Coping success is defined differently by various people.

Much of the work in measuring coping has focused on the process of coping. This approach has resulted in a list of individual specific strategies for a particular situation[27,39,59] or a description of how individuals manage current problem situations.[30] Measurement of the outcomes of coping has included describing how a particular event has changed aspects of life functioning[23,50] or using surrogate measures of emotional distress.[7,51] This last approach is based on the assumption that noncoping will cause measurable emotional distress. Inherent in all measures of coping is the question of what constitutes "normal." What is "normal" when one confronts death, accidents, or life-threatening illnesses?

The standardized measurement of ego strength and psychological defense mechanisms has been methodologically problematic; the validation of existing tools has also been doubtful. Perhaps the best known defense scale is the Defense Mechanisms Inventory (DMI).[35] It was designed to identify defenses used in dealing with conflict and was based on the assumption that the major function of defenses is to resolve conflicts between the perceptions of the individual and his/her internalized values. Gutmann[36] developed an ego styles instrument (TAT) that measures three styles of coping with the environment: (1) active, (2) passive, and (3) magical. The approach is characterized by gross interpretations and distortions of stimuli that reflect misperceptions of the environment and ego regression. Worden and Sobel[74] reported that high ego strength on Barron's Es Scale was correlated with psychosocial adaptation in cancer patients both at the initial diagnosis and 5 months later.

The formal measurement of self-esteem has also suffered from methodological difficulties, including ambiguities and inconsistencies in defining the concept and a wide range of theoretical perspectives.[10] A major issue concerns the appropriateness of using the ratings of both the individual and an objective person. The defining characteristics for Self-Esteem Disturbance include both objective observations and subjective statements from the person, thus suggesting that both types of measures are necessary. Other issues focus on the global nature of measurement devices, the stability of self-esteem, the human need to provide socially desirable information about oneself, and the need for approval. Lawson and McGrath[43] developed the Social Self-Esteem Inventory in an attempt to overcome these shortcomings. This instrument was used in the Norris study cited earlier and has a high level of reliability (T = 0.88). Preliminary work with this instrument supports the idea that self-esteem can be differentiated into basic self-esteem, functional self-esteem and defensive self-esteem. Reviews of self-esteem measures are available by Gilberts[34] and Breytspraak.[10]

Data collected for clinical assessment will depend in large measure on the context of the situation and the time constraints. Ultimately, the goal of assessment is to determine whether the individual's resources correlate with the demands of the event and whether the desirable goals are met. Important areas for data collection are as follows:

1. The nature of the situation (event)
   Determine the specific event at issue
   Assess the event for unexpectedness, predictability, controllability, and duration
   Assess the potential for harm or threat (especially to functional self-esteem)
   Determine the demands of the event
2. The individual
   Appearance: briefly note sex, apparent age, ease of deportment, and overt signs of distress or composure
   Perception of the event: ask the individual to explain in his/her own words the perception of and the (assigned) meaning to the event, including harm or threat to self-esteem
   Coping resources and goals: ask the individual to describe the ability to manage this type of situation; what he/she would consider important objectives (goals)

Self-concept: ask the individual to describe sense of self, including self-worth, personal competence, and achievement ideals or aspirations
3. The context of the situation
   Determine the individual's past experiences with similar events
   Determine available social supports (supportive or tangible)
   Assess the individual's ability to deal with uncertainty, motivation to cope, usual coping patterns, and knowledge and abilities
   Identify other concurrent events
   Identify any discrepancy between ideal self and perceived self in the current situation
4. Coping strategies and outcome
   Identify the emotional, behavioral, and cognitive responses to the event and the purpose they serve for the individual (such as problem solving or emotion controlling)
   Assess the extent to which the desired outcomes are achieved
   Identify the individual's skills, communication patterns, and interactions with others

A key aspect of this assessment is understanding the individual's cognitive appraisal of the situation and the purpose served by his/her specific coping strategies. The environment must be supportive and nonjudgmental for the individual to reveal this information.

❖ Defining Characteristics

The presence of the following defining characteristics indicates that the patient may be experiencing Defensive Coping[11]:

- Denial of obvious weaknesses or problems
- Projection of blame and/or responsibility
- Rationalization of failures
- Hypersensitivity to slight criticism (defensiveness)
- Projection of heightened sense of capabilities (grandiosity)
- Superior attitude toward others

Adapted from North American Nursing Diagnosis Association, 1988 Ballot

- Hostile laughter or ridicule of others
- Difficulty in establishing and maintaining relationships
- Difficulty in testing the reality of perceptions
- Lack of follow-through or participation in treatment or therapy

❖ Relating Factors

The nurse must further examine the assessment data to identify conditions or circumstances that contribute to the development of this nursing diagnosis. The following related factors are associated with Defensive Coping[11]:

- Appraisal of the event by family members/significant others: nature, characteristics, and demands of the event; past experiences with similar event
- Concurrent events (demands) in the family/social system
- Family dynamics/functioning: patterns of interaction and support; patterns of problem-solving
- Coping resources in family/social system: informational, tangible, financial

❖ Related Medical/Psychiatric Diagnoses

The following are examples of related medical/psychiatric diagnoses for Defensive Coping:

- Anorexia/bulimia
- Chronic illnesses requiring a change in lifestyle (e.g., myocardial infarction, chronic obstructive pulmonary disease, AIDS, arthritis)
- Impulse control disorder
- Substance abuse
- Unresolved grieving

NURSING DIAGNOSIS

Examples of *specific* nursing diagnoses for Defensive Coping are:

- Defensive Coping related to a recent promotion (significant additional responsibilities) and the threat to functional self-esteem
- Defensive Coping related to her role as a new mother and her perception of her ability to perform it
- Defensive Coping related to the recent loss of a breast and the threat to sense of self as a woman
- Defensive Coping related to the recent loss of his spouse and the threat to his self-image of being "able to handle anything."

PLANNING AND IMPLEMENTATION WITH RATIONALE

The expected outcome of the nursing interventions is that the individual will feel a sense of balance or well-being. In particular, an individual will feel a reduction in distress and a movement toward a desired goal without undue cost. A major issue is the lack of criteria to judge the success of the individual's coping behavior. As previously discussed, coping success is different for various individuals—it is based, in part, on personal opinion and preferences. In each situation, the efficacy (appropriateness) of the coping strategies must be evaluated for the individual concerned. In one situation, it may be very important for an individual to use denial and avoidance, whereas in another the same strategy creates additional difficulties. The coping outcome must be assessed within the context of the interaction between the event and the person.

The nature of the nursing interventions depends on the nurse's assessment of the interaction between the event and the person and the specific expected outcomes identified by the patient and the nurse. Additionally, the nursing response will be directed toward preventing further loss of self-esteem or confronting and working with the patient to change behaviors consistent with patient readiness.

Whether the defensive self-esteem is used to defend against basic low esteem or functional low self-esteem will also make a difference in the approach. Functional self-esteem is expected to be more amenable to alteration. Enhancing an adult's self-esteem involves, as a first step, exploring the discrepancies within his/her self-concept.[21] In particular, these discrepancies often exist between the person's expectations of the self and his/her perception of current abilities. Second, it is necessary to identify and change the thoughts that cause negative feelings and low self-esteem. These thoughts include minimizing accomplishments, over-generalizing, and magnifying nega-

X

❖ NURSING CARE GUIDELINES

Nursing Diagnosis: *Defensive Coping*

Expected Patient Outcomes	Nursing Interventions
The patient will not suffer further insult to self-esteem.	• Support the individual's humanness, uniqueness, and right to be involved in decision-making. • Seek to understand the patient's perspective of the situation and what is stressful or threatening to him/her (or to the sense of self). • Gently clarify misconceptions. • When possible, reduce stressful aspects of the event. • Encourage maintenance of social networks. • If necessary, confront the patient regarding behaviors that are harmful to others, such as ridicule.
The patient will express a realistic appraisal of the event, its demands, and the coping resources available.	• Assist the patient to explore the nature and characteristics of the event, its demands, and the coping resources required, and identify the discrepancies between the ideal and perceived roles in the situation.
The patient will become comfortable with ideal and perceived roles and develop competency to manage the situation.	• Assist the patient to identify desired goals.
The patient will verbalize a sense of personal integrity and movement toward desired goals.	• Set realistic and concrete goals with the patient. • Identify specific strategies for achieving goals. • Set realistic time frames for reaching goals. • Review capabilities and learning from past experiences. • Explore patterns of thinking (especially negative thoughts). • Teach necessary knowledge and skills. • Acknowledge progress toward desired goals. • Encourage the patient to maintain social networks. • Encourage the expression of fears and concerns.

tives. Involvement in decision making and problem solving, particularly in areas that affect their lifestyles, can enhance self-esteem in older adults.[57] Self-esteem can be enhanced for children and adults through (1) promoting security by defining clear expectations and setting well-defined limits, (2) providing a positive identity through acceptance and recognition, (3) communicating a sense of belonging through strong fam-

ily ties and encouraging group and social concern, and (4) providing purpose by encouraging realistic goal setting and conveying faith in the individual's ability to achieve.[21,66]

Fundamentally, nursing interventions must be based on a clear idea of why the patient exhibits behaviors he/she does. Once the patient is understood, interventions can be generally directed toward reducing the sense of harm or stress and in-

X

creasing the patient's confidence in his/her coping resources.[14] The nurse needs to carefully observe and assess, as well as engage in active listening and supporting. Initially, when the individual perceives an overwhelming threat, he/she will strive to protect the self-concept (image and integrity). Nursing behavior needs to focus on preserving the person's integrity and, at the same time, deal with the behavior the patient has selected (for example, denial, bragging, and joking). The nurse must seek to reduce the stressful aspects of a situation and to gently correct any misconceptions.

When a patient's defensive behavioral choices result from different stages of adapting, and in time the patient moves away from the original closed cognitive stance, the nurse must pace himself/herself with the patient's progression, helping in the patient's adaptation to the situation.[2] This process involves exploring realistic interpretations of the event—why it is threatening, what is required to meet the demands of the situation, and what abilities the individual possesses. In turn, the nurse may need to help the individual acquire new knowledge and skills and to provide support and guidance to aid the patient in maintaining a reasonable emotional balance during the transition period. Specific approaches to assist with functional self-esteem disturbances include designing clearly defined, mutually agreeable goals; identifying specific strategies to accomplish the goals; establishing realistic time frames for achieving the goals; and facilitating the individual's recognition of and challenge of distortions in thinking, especially about his/her ideal self and perceived self in the situation. Other health professionals and community agencies may need to be consulted and the individual's relationships with significant others maintained or strengthened.

If an individual continues to need particular defenses for managing distress, the nurse must think very carefully about more appropriate interventions. In certain instances, interventions aimed at helping the patient "face the truth" could leave a previously "defended" person defenseless and perhaps do more harm than good. In addition, it has been suggested that "well-defended" individuals are not susceptible to intervention. The most appropriate approach is one of support and patience that deals with the aspects of the patient that are more receptive to interventions. This can create a dilemma for health professionals when they believe that the defensive stance retards the person's ability to deal with real threats that are amenable to resolution. The nurse must be aware of the necessity to discriminate between his/her needs and those of the patient.

EVALUATION

The nurse uses both observation of and interaction with the patient to evaluate the effectiveness of the nursing interventions. The desired effect must be defined in the context of the particular situation and the desired outcome identified by the patient. The nurse must be able to separate his/her own idea of effective outcomes from the individual's. Each patient will define coping success differently, and different strategies may be selected for achieving desired goals.

The efficacy of any strategy must be determined on the basis of its success in achieving the desired outcome for the individual and any interventions evaluated accordingly.

❖ *CASE STUDY WITH PLAN OF CARE*

Mr. Edward S. is a 35-year-old male who is married and has two children. He teaches physical education at the local high school. He was admitted to the coronary care unit with a diagnosis of acute myocardial infarction 4 days ago and was transferred today to the general nursing unit. Mr. S. had no history of heart disease and up until admission ran 6.2 miles daily. He prides himself on having the "physical conditioning of a 20-year-old." Mr. S. has had little hospital exposure with the exception of the death of his 70-year-old father from heart disease 5 years before and the birth of his children. During the first few days on the general unit, Mr.

Continued.

❖ *CASE STUDY WITH PLAN OF CARE—cont'd*

S. made frequent trips to the stairwell. When the nursing staff questioned him about these trips, Mr. S. retorted, "Surely, as a health professional, you know that muscles have to be used to be maintained. I've been in bed long enough! It's been 4 days already. A man in my shape needs to be exercising. I have been going up and down the stairs to keep my muscles in shape. After all, I'm the coach and we have a big game next week. I need to be able to keep up with the boys or we won't win the game. What business is it of yours anyway?" The next day, Mr. S. discussed his athletic abilities and his intent to return to the playing field. He ridicules those around him who are not in good physical shape, including the hospital staff. One nurse reports that Mr. S. attributes his hospitalization to that "idiot medical student in emergency who can't tell the difference between chest pain and a cardiac arrest!"

PLAN OF CARE FOR MR. EDWARD S.

Nursing Diagnosis: Defensive Coping related to myocardial infarction and threat to self-esteem

Expected Patient Outcomes	Nursing Interventions
Mr. S. will not experience further insult to his sense of self.	• Encourage Mr. S. to describe the events surrounding his hospitalization and his appraisal and perceptions of the situation.
Mr. S. will demonstrate no increase in climbing the stairs.	• Encourage Mr. S. to describe his perception of his roles at work and what he believes is required to perform these roles.
Mr. S. will discuss his perceptions with the nurses.	• Determine whether there are role inconsistencies between Mr. S.'s ideal self and perceived self secondary to his hospitalization.
	• Assess Mr. S.'s knowledge of cardiac status, exercise, and myocardial infarction.
	• Correct any misconceptions Mr. S. may hold about cardiac physiology and disease.
	• Reduce stressful aspects, such as noise, when possible.
	• Acknowledge Mr. S.'s abilities, achievements, and right to make informed decisions regarding his care.
	• Assist Mr. S. to appraise his situation realistically.
	• Provide information regarding disease rehabilitation and the coping process.
	• Assist Mr. S. to define concrete goals for exercise.

REFERENCES

1. Adams JF, Lindemann E: Coping with long-term disability. In Coelho GV, Hamburg DA, and Adams JE, editors: *Coping and adaptation,* New York, 1974, Basic Books.
2. Aguilera D, Messick L: *Crisis intervention,* St Louis, 1974, CV Mosby.
3. Antonovsky A: *Health, stress and coping,* San Francisco, 1981, Jossey-Bass.
4. Balder L, DeNour AK: Couples' reactions and adjustments to mastectomy, *Int J Psychiatry in Med* 14(3):265-270, 1984.
5. Barnard D: Healing the damaged self, *Perspect Biol Med* 33(4):535-546, 1990.
6. Bean G and others: Coping mechanisms of cancer patients: a study of 33 patients receiving chemotherapy, *CA* 30:257-259, 1980.
7. Beck AT and others: Inventory for measuring depression, *Arch Gen Psychiatry* 4:561-569, 1961.
8. Bishop DS and others: Stroke, morale, family functioning, health status and functional capacity, *Arch Phys Med Rehabil* 67:84-87, 1986.
9. Block AR, Bayers SL: The spouse's adjustment to chronic pain behavior: cognitive and emotional factors, *Soc Sci Med* 19(12):1313-1317, 1984.
10. Breytspraak LM, George LK: Self concept and self esteem. In Mangen DJ, Peterson WA, editors: *Research in-*

X

struments in social gerontology: clinical and social psychology, vol 1, Minneapolis, 1981, University of Minnesota Press.

11. Carroll-Johnson RM: *Classification of nursing diagnoses: proceedings of the Eighth Conference,* Philadelphia, 1989, JB Lippincott.

12. Cassileth BR and others: Psychological analysis of cancer patients and their next of kin, *Cancer* 55:72-76, 1985.

13. Cassileth BR and others: Psychological status in chronic illness, *N Engl J Med* 311:506-511, 1985.

14. Clark S: Nursing diagnosis: ineffective coping. I. A theoretical framework. II. Planning Care, *Heart Lung* 16(6):670-674, 1987.

15. Cobb S: Social support as a moderator of life stress, *Psychosom Med* 38:300-314, 1976.

16. Coelho GV, Hamburg DA, and Adams JE: *Coping and adaptation,* New York, 1974, Basic Books.

17. Cohen F, Lazarus RS: Active coping processes, coping dispositions and recovery from surgery, Psychosom Med 35:375-389, 1973.

18. Colenda C, Dougherty L.M.: Positive ego and coping functions in chronic pain and depressed patients, *J Geriatr Psychiatry Neurol* 3(1):48-52, 1990.

19. Coopersmith S: *Antecedents of self esteem,* San Francisco, 1967, Freeman, Cooper.

20. Coute MA and others: Personal stress and personal attitudes in chronic illness, *Arch Phys Med Rehabil* 64:272-275, 1983.

21. Crouch MA, Straub V: Enhancement of self esteem in adults, *Fam Community Health* 6:65-78, 1983.

22. Curbow B and others: Self-concept and cancer in adults, *Soc Sci Med* 31(2):115-128, 1990.

23. Derogatis LR: *Scoring and procedures manual for PAIS,* Baltimore, 1976, Clinical Psychometric Research.

24. Draup K: Psychosocial aspects of coronary heart disease, *West J Nurs Res* 4(3):257-271, 1982.

25. Epstein S: Anxiety, arousal and the self concept. In Sarason GI, Seilberger CD, editors: *Stress and anxiety,* Washington, DC, 1976, Hemisphere Publishing.

26. Feifel H, Strack S, and Nagy VT: Coping strategies and associated features of medically ill patients, *Psychosom Med* 49:616-625, 1987.

27. Folkman S, Lazarus RS: An analysis of coping in a middle-aged community sample, *J Health Soc Behav* 21:219-239, 1980.

28. Foltz AT: The influence of cancer on self-concept and quality of life, *Semin Oncol Nurs* 3(4):303-312, 1987.

29. Freidenbergs I and others: Psychosocial aspects of living with cancer: a review of the literature, *Int J Psychiatry Med* 11:303-329, 1981.

30. Freidenbergs I and others: Assessment and treatment of psychosocial problems of the cancer patient: a case study, *Cancer Nurs* 3:111-119, 1981.

31. Freud A: *The ego and the mechanisms of defense,* New York, 1946, International Universities Press.

32. Friedman BD: Coping with cancer: a guide for health professionals, *Cancer Nurs* 3:105-110, 1980.

33. George JM and others: The effects of psychological factors of physical trauma on recovery from oral surgery, *J Behav Med* 3:291-310, 1980.

34. Gilberts R: The evaluation of self esteem, *Fam Community Health* 6:29-49, 1983.

35. Gleser G, Ihilevich D: An objective instrument for measuring defense mechanisms, *J Consult Clin Psychol* 33(1):51-60, 1969.

36. Gutmann DL: An exploration of ego configuration in middle and later life. In Neugarten and others, editors: *Personality in middle and later life,* New York, 1964, Atherton Press.

37. Hilgard ER: Human motives and the concepts of the self, *Am Psychol* 4:374-382, 1949.

38. Hoff LA: *People in crisis: understanding and helping,* Toronto, 1978, Addison-Wesley.

39. Ilfeld FW: Coping styles in Chicago adults: description, *Human Stress* 6:2-10, 1980.

40. Judd L and others: The prevalence and correlates of poor psychosocial adjustment in patients with chronic airflow limitation, *Proceedings of the Tenth National Nursing Research Conference,* Toronto, 1985.

41. Kahana E, Faischild T, and Hakana B: Adaptation. In Mangen DJ, Peterson WA, editors: *Research instruments and social gerontology, vol I, clinical and social gerontology,* Minneapolis, 1981, University of Minnesota Press.

42. Kiely WF: Coping with severe illness, *Adv Psychosom Med* 8:105-118, 1982.

43. Lawson M, McGrath: The social self esteem inventory, *Educ Psychol Measure* 39:109-125, 1978.

44. Lazarus RS: *Psychological stress and the coping process,* New York, 1966, McGraw-Hill Book Co.

45. Lazarus RS, Folkman S: *Stress, appraisal and coping,* New York, 1984, Springer Publishing.

46. Lewis F: Patient response to illness and hospitalization, *Radiography* 52(602):91-93, 1986.

47. Lindstrom TC: Defence mechanisms and some notes on their relevance for the caring professions, *Scand J Caring Sci* 3(3):99-104, 1989.

48. Lipowski ZJ: Psychosocial aspects of disease, *Ann Intern Med* 71(6):1197-1206, 1969.

49. Mages NL, Mendelsohn GA: Effects of cancer on patients' lives: a peronological approach. In Stone GC, Cohen F, and Adler NE, editors: *Health psychology,* San Francisco, 1979, Jossey-Bass Publishers.

50. Marrow GR and others: Development of brief measures of psychosocial adjustment to medical illness applied to cancer patients, *Gen Hosp Psychiatry* 3:79-88, 1981.

51. McNair PM, Loor M, and Drappelman L: *POMS manual,* San Diego, 1971, Education and Industrial Testing Services.

52. Menniger K: Regulatory devices of the ego under major stress, *Int J Psychoanal* 35:412-420, 1954.

53. Miller MW, Nygren C: Living with cancer: coping behaviors, *Cancer Nurs* 1:297-302, 1978.

X°

54. Moos RH, Tsu VD: The crisis of physical illness: an overview. In Moos R, editor: *Coping with physical illness,* New York, 1977, Plenum Publishing.

55. Morris CA: Self-concept as altered by the diagnosis of cancer, *Nurs Clin North Am* 20(4):611-630, 1985.

56. Neugarten B, Havinghurst R, and Tobin S: The measurement of life satisfaction, *J Gerontol* 16:134:143, 1961.

57. Norris J, Kunes-Connell M: Self esteem, *Nurs Clin North Am* 20(4):745-761, 1985.

58. Northhouse L: The impact of cancer on the family: an overview, *Int J Psychiatry Med* 14(3):215-242, 1984.

59. Pearlin LI, Schoolar C: The structure of coping, *J Health Soc Behav* 19:2-21, 1978.

60. Pearlman RA, Uhlmann RF: Quality of life in chronic disease: perceptions of elderly patients, *J Gerontol* 43(2):25-30, 1988.

61. Platzer H: Body image—helping patients to cope with changes, *Intensive Care Nurs* 3(3):125-132, 1987.

62. Rawlinson E: Quality of life after treatment for laryngeal cancer: the patient's perspective, *Can J Radiog Radiother Nucl Med* 14(4):125-127, 1983.

63. Reasoner RW: Self esteem through the life span, *Fam Community Health* 6:11-18, 1983.

64. Rosenstiel A, Roth S: Relationships between cognitive activity and adjustment in four spinal-cord-injured individuals: longitudinal investigation, *J Human Stress* 35-43, March 1981.

65. Ruberman W and others: Psychosocial influences on mortality after myocardial infarction, *N Engl J Med* 311(9):552-559, 1984.

66. Stanwyck DJ: Enhancement of self esteem in children, *Fam Community Health* 6:51-64, 1983.

67. Turkat D: Defensiveness in self esteem research, *Psychol Rec* 28:129-135, 1978.

68. Valliant GE: *Adaptation to life,* Boston, 1977, Little, Brown.

69. Vincent KG: The validation of a nursing diagnosis, *Nurs Clin North Am* 20(4):631-664, 1985.

70. Viney LL, Westbrook MT: Coping with chronic illness: strategy preferences, changes in preferences and associated emotional reactions, *J Chronic Dis* 37(6):489-502, 1984.

71. Weisman AD: *Coping with cancer,* New York, 1979, McGraw-Hill Book Co.

72. Wellisch D and others: Evaluation of psychosocial problems of the homebound cancer patient, *Psychosom Med* 45:11-21, 1983.

73. Williams GH: Quality of life and its impact on hypertensive patients, *Am J Med* 82(1):48-105, 1987.

74. Worden JW, Sobel J: Ego strength and psychosocial adaptation to cancer, *Psychosom Med* 40(8):585-592, 1978.

X

Ineffective Denial

Ineffective Denial is the conscious or unconscious disavowal of the knowledge or meaning of an event to reduce anxiety or fear, to the detriment of health.

OVERVIEW

Denial is defined as the negation in word or act of some external reality.[9] Denial is distinguished from repression by its focus on external rather than internal conditions.[2,9] To initiate denial the individual must first receive some information that personal well-being is threatened. It is through the mechanism of denial that the person attempts to protect himself or herself from this threatening information.[2]

According to Breznitz[2] some anxiety must initially be evoked by the threat in order to initiate the denial process. The event that is denied cannot be fleeting but must be of sufficient duration for the individual to assess it as a threat, experience some anxiety, and then institute the denial process. Once initiated, denial is the method by which anxiety is kept at a manageable level.

Denial does not always take the same form. Weisman[19] identified three levels of denial as a result of interviewing patients who were facing death. The first level is denial of facts, such as the denial of a life-threatening illness. Such denial usually cannot be sustained indefinitely because it is difficult to deny what is clear and unambiguous.[9] Eventually the patient's worsening physical condition makes it impossible to deny the illness.[19] The second level of denial is denial of implications.[19] This is a common type of denial. It is much easier to deny something that cannot be known for certain, the implications of the illness, than to deny the illness itself.[9] With denial of implications the illness is accepted but what it means

in terms of personal well-being is denied. The third level is denial of extinction.[19] The patient accepts that he/she has an incurable illness but denies that it will result in death.

Weisman's method of classifying denial is only one way of determining what is being denied. Breznitz[2] uses an information processing model to classify denial. He identifies seven kinds of denial, each related to a stage of information processing: (1) denial of personal relevance: the person recognizes there is danger but does not perceive it to be a personal threat; (2) denial of urgency: the person recognizes there is a personal threat but does not perceive it as current; (3) denial of vulnerability or responsibility: the person perceives the threat as current but does not perceive any difficulty in handling the situation; (4) denial of affect: the person recognizes the threat but does not perceive it as anxiety provoking; (5) denial of affect relevance: the person recognizes the anxiety but attributes it to something other than the threat; (6) denial of threatening information: the person minimizes those aspects of the situation that are particularly threatening or reduces or avoids them; and (7) the most extreme type, denial of information: the person does not allow any information to be received. At any time a person may progress to a different level of denial if objective reality makes it impossible to maintain the previous level.[2]

As can be seen, denial can take many forms. It is not a single act but a complex set of processes.[9] Also, denial is not static, but is dynamic and fluctuating.[9] A person can appear to be denying at one time but have some awareness at another time. Weisman[19] describes this as "middle knowledge," that is, knowing and not knowing at the

X

same time.[20] The problem with this phenomenon is that the patient may vacillate between awareness and denial. This is a good reason for making serial assessments of a patient before assigning the diagnosis of Ineffective Denial. The patient may exhibit denial in one context but not in another.

Denial may allow positive thinking and hopefulness and thus be an important psychological resource for a patient.[10] Someone who is able to view harsh experiences in a positive, challenging light may feel better and perform more effectively in the face of adversity than one who views such events as threats.[9]

Denial may be adaptive or maladaptive. In situations where direct action is needed denial may be maladaptive and indicate Ineffective Coping.[10] However, when the situation does not lend itself to direct action, when there is nothing the person can do to overcome the threat, denial may be an effective means of coping in that by reducing the emotional reaction it allows the individual to engage in other activities.[9,10] Even in situations requiring direct action, as long as the denial is only partial, tentative, or minimal and so does not prevent simultaneous use of problem-focused forms of coping, it may be beneficial.[9,10]

To determine whether denial is indicative of Ineffective Coping the nurse must assess the patient in relation to the outcomes of coping. Lazarus and Folkman[10] identify three outcomes of coping: behavioral outcome, emotional outcome, and health outcome. All three outcomes of coping must be considered when assessing whether coping has been effective.[10] By nature, denial means a favorable emotional outcome. With denial the anxiety and fear that otherwise might be experienced are avoided. This probably allows the person to carry out usual daily activities, resulting in a favorable behavioral outcome. However, it may not lead to a favorable health outcome. Therefore most studies that assess the adaptational outcome of denial do so by assessing whether those who deny have a worse health outcome than those who do not deny.

Denial has positive value at an early stage of coping when the person does not have the resources to cope in a problem-focused way. Denial is a common initial response to a life-threatening illness, and under these circumstances it may not only be beneficial but may even be life preserving. It is commonly used by survivors of heart transplantation, for whom it is thought to serve an important protective function.[13] Studies have shown that patients with a myocardial infarction who use denial during the initial stage of illness are more likely to survive hospitalization than are those who do not deny.[7] Those who exhibit a high level of denial are also likely to experience less cardiac pain,[1] spend fewer days in the intensive care unit,[12] and have fewer signs of cardiac dysfunction during hospitalization.[12] For patients undergoing cardiac surgery, denial was found to have a positive effect preoperatively and immediately postoperatively.[5] The beneficial effects of denial have also been observed in patients hospitalized with unstable angina.[11]

Although in the early stages of an illness denial is an effective means of coping, after the acute stages it may not be beneficial if it prevents the individual from instituting appropriate health practices. There is some evidence to support this. Levine and colleagues[12] found that patients with cardiac disease who were high deniers in the acute stage of illness adapted more poorly to the illness during the year after their initial hospitalization than did those who scored low on the denial scale. They were less compliant with the medical regimen and were rehospitalized for a longer time than were low deniers.

Other studies have found denial to be protective beyond the acute stage of illness.[5,14,16] Shaw[16] found that patients who experienced a high level of denial after myocardial infarction did not experience a poorer outcome in the ensuing 6 months than did those who had a low level of denial. Denial has been found to have a protective effect for as long as a year after hospitalization because of ischemic heart disease. Prince and co-workers[14] studied 320 patients with ischemic heart disease and found that those who denied had a relatively good prognosis as measured by rehospitalization or death in the year after the initial hospitalization. They found that both those who denied and those who did not deny but experienced a high level of stress had a much better prognosis than did those in between. Denial appeared to have a protective effect in spite of evidence that the patients did not comply with medical advice. Why denial is protective under these circumstances is unknown, although it has been suggested that both denial and its positive effect may be related to the release of endorphins.[14]

There is some evidence that even over the long term, denial may be beneficial. Dean and Surtees[4] followed 121 women with breast cancer for 6 to 8 years after a mastectomy. They found that those women who 3 months after the surgery coped by using denial had a better chance of being recurrence-free 6 to 8 years later than those who employed any other type of coping strategy.

Denial is a complex phenomenon. Sometimes it is an effective means of coping, sometimes it is not. The nursing diagnosis of Ineffective Denial should only be used when the patient uses denial to the detriment of health. This is not during the acute stage of illness, when denial is an effective means of coping. If denial continues after the acute stage of illness it may be maladaptive and therefore indicative of ineffective coping. However, even then it may indicate effective coping. More research is needed before it is known under what circumstances denial is maladaptive beyond the acute stage of illness. At this point it is hard to draw any conclusions concerning the long-term effect of denial.

ASSESSMENT

The nursing diagnosis of Ineffective Denial describes a patient who is denying and for whom this denial is maladaptive. To make this diagnosis the nurse must first determine whether the patient is denying and if so, determine whether the denial is indicative of Ineffective Coping. These are difficult determinations to make.

Often behavior that is labeled as denial, on closer examination is not denial at all.[3,17] Just because a patient does not do what a health care provider thinks he/she should does not indicate denial.[17] The patient may be aware of what he/she "should" do and the reasons why, but in spite of this knowledge may decide not to comply. This is not denial, and would probably be clear if the nurse took the time to determine the patient's point of view. Some behavior is labeled denial when in reality there is only inadequate communication.[3,17]

Denial is different from avoidance. Thus the fact that a patient does not mention that he/she has cancer does not indicate denial. The patient may know very well that he/she has cancer but prefer not to talk about it.[9] Thus the nurse needs to be careful not to conclude that a patient is denying based solely on the fact that he/she does not talk about his/her illness. This may indicate avoidance, not denial. If the assessment process is superficial the nurse may incorrectly classify avoidance as denial.[8]

Lazarus[9] also points out that people cannot deny something about which they have not been informed. Thus a person who does not acknowledge cancer is not denying the diagnosis if he/she was never told of it or was not cognitively able to understand what was told.

The fact that a patient delays seeking medical treatment for a symptom does not necessarily indicate denial. Safer and colleagues[15] interviewed 93 patients seeking medical treatment and found that those who delayed coming for treatment had not denied their symptoms. They had thought a great deal about their symptoms and the negative consequences of being ill, such as surgery. Although they were aware of their symptoms, they did not take any action. They displayed inappropriate coping, but not because of denial.

Denial is indicated when a person faced with a threatening situation states unequivocally that he/she is not at all fearful. Based on interviews with patients in a coronary care unit, Hackett and others[7] identified three levels of denial. Major deniers consistently denied fear. A total of 40% of the patients were in this group. Partial deniers initially denied fear but later acknowledged some fear. This was the largest group of patients, 52%

X

of the sample. The remaining 8% of the patients were minimal deniers, who readily admitted fear.

After determining that a patient is denying, the nurse must decide whether the denial indicates effective or Ineffective Coping. There is little clear evidence to indicate exactly when denial constitutes Ineffective Coping. Considerable research has shown that denial is adaptive in the acute stages of illness.[1,5,11-13] Whether it constitutes Ineffective Coping if it extends beyond the acute phase of the illness has not been established. Some research indicates that long-term denial constitutes effective coping[4,5,14,15]; other research indicates that it constitutes Ineffective Coping.[12] Until it is established when denial constitutes Ineffective Coping, this diagnosis should be used cautiously. The nurse can assess whether a patient is denying but, inasmuch as the denial may be an effective coping strategy, should not intervene and attempt to change the patient's method of coping.[6]

Although denial is an effective coping strategy, partial deniers may benefit from some nursing intervention. These patients may be much more apprehensive than they appear.[7] Hackett and others[7] found that such patients did not have as good an outcome in the acute stage of illness as did major deniers; however, they had a better outcome than those who did not deny. They may also have more problems over the long term than either major deniers or patients who face reality and do not deny.[14] Therefore, although denial is an effective means of coping, the nurse needs to be concerned about partial deniers. These patients may have the diagnosis Ineffective Denial. Even if these patients do not admit to having any anxiety, they may have concerns, and if so it is important to provide them with the opportunity to share these concerns.[18] With nursing intervention, any distress they are experiencing may be decreased.

The main characteristic of denial is repudiation of fear or anxiety when faced with a threatening situation. This is not Ineffective Coping. However, denial is not a static phenomenon. The person may be coping effectively using denial in some situations but at other times may experience some fears and anxiety. Even patients who are denying may have problems and concerns.

One factor that will determine whether denial is maladaptive and therefore indicative of Ineffective Coping is the nature of the action that is precluded because of the denial. If direct action is necessary but is not being carried out because of denial, the patient may be coping ineffectively. However, the context of the situation also needs to be considered. Denial only indicates Ineffective Coping in patients beyond the acute stage of illness, and even then it does not always indicate Ineffective Coping.

Denial may be seen with any stressful situation, and therefore may be the response to any serious medical condition. The patient must, however, have appraised the illness as a threat for denial to occur.

In clinical practice the best way for the nurse to assess whether denial is present is to interview the patient. Because denial is a dynamic process, a number of assessments need to be made before the diagnosis is made.[2] Patients may vacillate between awareness and denial, and thus it is easy to misdiagnose denial. In one study it was found that the same patient could both frankly admit fears and deny the seriousness of the illness in the course of a 20-minute interview.[18] This is a good reason for serial assessments of the patient before assigning the diagnosis of Ineffective Denial.

To understand how an individual is coping the nurse must observe the person in many types of encounters and at different times. The nurse needs to consider the context of the situation in which the denial is being used and what is being denied. In addition, more than one person should be involved in assessing the patient, because the nurse's attitude might influence whether the patient appears to be denying. Some nurses are not comfortable with expressions of fear and anxiety by patients, especially those concerning death, and do not encourage disclosure by patients.

❖ Defining Characteristics

The presence of the following defining characteristics indicates that the patient may be experi-

encing Ineffective Denial:
- Necessary direct action not being carried out
- Partial or inconsistent expression of fear and anxiety when in a threatening situation
- Delay in seeking or refusal of medical attention to the detriment of health
- Lack of perception of personal relevance of symptoms or danger
- Lack of recognition of symptoms
- Inability to admit effect of disease on life pattern

❖ **Related Factors**

The following related factors are associated with Ineffective Denial:
- Context of the situation in which denial is occurring
- Nature of the action that is precluded

❖ **Related Medical/Psychiatric Diagnoses**

The following are examples of related medical/psychiatric diagnoses for Ineffective Denial:
- Adjustment disorder with anxious mood
- AIDS
- Cancer
- Diabetes
- Generalized anxiety disorder
- Genetic disorders
- Myocardial infarction

NURSING DIAGNOSES

Examples of *specific* nursing diagnoses for Ineffective Denial are:
- Ineffective Denial related to finding lump in breast
- Ineffective Denial related to learning of diagnosis of cancer
- Ineffective Denial related to recommended changes in lifestyle resulting from diagnosis of cardiovascular disease

PLANNING AND IMPLEMENTATION WITH RATIONALE

It is important that the patient's sense of well-being be preserved. *Denial is a means of controlling anxiety and fear*. The nurse must keep in mind the important role denial plays in preserving the patient's well-being. An important outcome therefore is that the patient remain defended, with anxiety under control.

If the patient indicates problems or concerns, another outcome would be the reduction of same. *The nurse needs to be aware that the patient who is denying may also have some concerns that he/she will share if given the opportunity to do so.* Give the patient time to do this. Once the patient's concerns are known, the nurse may be able to plan specific nursing interventions geared to their reduction. Or there may be nothing the nurse

X

❖ *NURSING CARE GUIDELINES*
Nursing Diagnosis: Ineffective denial

Expected Patient Outcomes	Nursing Interventions
The patient will express low or moderate anxiety.	• Assess the patient's degree of denial and its effectiveness as a coping strategy. • Never confront the patient with the fact that denial is being used.
The patient will express some reduction in problems or concerns.	• Support the patient's behavior. • Provide the patient with opportunities to express any fears or anxieties of which he/she is aware. • Provide the patient with specific information or reassurance as requested or as appropriate.

❖ CASE STUDY WITH PLAN OF CARE

Mrs. Wendy W. is a 27-year-old woman who yesterday underwent a diagnostic dilation and curettage because of intercycle bleeding. Mrs. W. and her husband have been trying to have a child for the past 4 years. This morning Mrs. W. was told by her gynecologist that she has cancer in the wall of the uterus and should have a total hysterectomy tomorrow. She replied, "That's fine doctor; whatever you think is best," and seemed to have no questions. The nurse checked with Mrs. W. 5 minutes after the physician left, and Mrs. W. said, "Have you heard? I have cancer and have to have a hysterectomy tomorrow." When the nurse asked Mrs. W. if she worried about having surgery she replied, "No, I know everything will be fine. I'm not worried." The nurse was concerned about Mrs. W.'s response but left her alone. Two hours later the nurse found Mrs. W. in tears. Mrs. W. asked questions such as: After the operation will I still have periods? Will I still be able to have children? Will I still be attractive to my husband? I know this surgery is common, but is it usual in young women? She said, "I still intend to have children." Mrs. W.'s initial response to the information provided by her physician was complete denial of any fears and concerns related to the diagnosis, the surgery, and the effect of the surgery on her life, particularly with regard to having children. During the course of the 2 hours Mrs. W. had moved from complete denial to partial denial, as evidenced by her beginning to express some concerns and ask questions of the nurse. Nursing interventions were based on the nurse's understanding of the importance of denial in an acute situation. The nurse did not challenge the patient's denial. She did, however, allow Mrs. W. to express her questions and concerns. She panned to provide Mrs. W. with specific information that she requested. If Mrs. W.'s anxiety remains under control the nursing interventions will have been successful.

PLAN FOR MRS. WENDY W.

Nursing Diagnosis *Ineffective denial (partial denial) related to medical diagnosis and effects of surgery on childbearing ability*

Expected Patient Outcomes	Nursing Interventions
Mrs. W. will express concerns and raise questions.	• Assess Mrs. W.'s readiness to raise questions and concerns related to her condition.
Mrs. W. will exhibit low to moderate anxiety.	• Provide Mrs. W. with information as she requests it.
	• Be sensitive to Mrs. W.'s status and readiness to be informed of her condition.
	• Provide a supportive environment that allows Mrs. W. to move back and forth between full and partial denial as needed.
	• Do not confront Mrs. W.'s use of denial.

can do specifically related to the concern. However, the very act of sharing the concern may be therapeutic for the patient. Some patients may want reassurance but not know how to ask for it.[7]

If the patient denies having concerns the nurse should accept this and recognize that denial is an effective coping strategy. Do not try to break down the denial. Direct confrontation is untherapeutic and causes increased patient anxiety, which leads to further denial.[6] It may also destroy whatever relationship the nurse had previously established with the patient. Anyone attempting to break through a patient's denial needs to be prepared to deal with the extreme anxiety that may result.[6] The best action on the part of the nurse may be to do nothing about the denial but maintain the relationship with the patient and be available if the patient has any questions or wants to talk about any problems or concerns.

X

EVALUATION

To evaluate the effectiveness of nursing interventions the nurse should assess the patient for signs of anxiety. Note both verbal and nonverbal indications of anxiety. If the nursing interventions have been successful the patient's anxiety should remain under control. If the patient indicates a high level of anxiety the nursing interventions have not been effective.

REFERENCES

1. Billing E, Lindell B, Sederholm M, and Theorell T: Denial, anxiety, and depression following myocardial infarction, *Psychosomatics,* 21:639-645, 1980.
2. Breznitz S: The seven kinds of denial. In Breznitz S, editor: *The denial of stress,* New York, 1983, International Universities Press.
3. Cousins N: Denial: are sharper definitions needed? *JAMA* 248:210-212, 1982.
4. Dean C, Surtees PG: Do psychological factors predict survival in breast cancer? *J Psychosom Res* 33:561-569, 1989.
5. Folks DG, Freeman AM III, Sokol RS, and Thurstin AH: Denial: predictor of outcome following coronary bypass surgery, *Int J Psychiatry Med* 18:57-66, 1988.
6. Forchuk C, Westwell J: Denial, *J Psychosoc Nurs* 25(6):9-13, 1987.
7. Hackett TP, Cassem NH, and Wishnie HA: The coronary-care unit: an appraisal of its psychologic hazards, *N Engl J Med* 279:1365-1370, 1968.
8. Lazarus RS: Stress and coping as factors in health and illness. In Cohen J, Cullen JW, and Martin LR, editors: *Psychosocial aspects of cancer,* New York, 1982, Raven Press.
9. Lazarus RS: The costs and benefits of denial. In Breznitz S, editor: *The denial of stress,* New York, 1983, International Universities Press.
10. Lazarus RS, Folkman S: *Stress, appraisal and coping,* New York, 1984, Springer Publishing.
11. Levenson JL, Kay R, Monteferrante J, and Herman MV: Denial predicts favorable outcome in unstable angina pectoris, *Psychosom Med* 46:25-32, 1984.
12. Levine J and others: The role of denial in recovery from coronary heart disease, *Psychosom Med* 49:109-117, 1987.
13. Mai FM: Graft and donor denial in heart transplant recipients, *Am J Psychiatry* 143:1159-1161, 1986.
14. Prince R, Frasure-Smith N, and Rolicz-Woloszyk E: Life stress, denial and outcome in ischemic heart disease patients, *J Psychosom Res* 26:23-31, 1982.
15. Safer MA, Tharps QJ, Jackson TC, and Leventhal H: Determinants of three stages of delay in seeking care at a medical clinic, *Med Care* 17:11-29, 1979.
16. Shaw RE, Cohen F, Doyle B, and Palesky J: The impact of denial and repressive styles on information gain and rehabilitation outcomes in myocardial infarction patients, *Psychosom Med* 47(3):262-273, 1985.
17. Shelp EE, Perl M: Denial in clinical medicine: a reexamination of the concept and its significance, *Arch Intern Med* 145:697-699, 1985.
18. Thomas SA and others: Denial in coronary care patients: an objective reassessment, *Heart Lung* 12:74-80, 1983.
19. Weisman AD: *On dying and denying,* New York, 1972, Behavioral Publications.
20. Weisman AD: *Coping with cancer,* New York, 1979, McGraw-Hill.

X

Impaired Adjustment

Impaired Adjustment is the state in which an individual is unable to modify his/her lifestyle or behavior in a manner consistent with a change in health status.[3]

OVERVIEW

The nursing diagnosis Impaired Adjustment is seen in all clinical areas of nursing. It is important to note that this diagnosis appears in the category "Choosing" in *Classification of Nursing Diagnoses*.[4] The nurse should recognize that adjustment impairment does not occur because the patient cannot adjust or because the patient does not perceive a change in health status that results in a limitation. Rather, the individual "chooses" not to acknowledge the modifications necessary to deal with the limitations accompanying the health condition. Ignoring the consequences of the disability denotes a refusal to accept a change in health status, limiting, to various degrees, the activities of daily living and lifestyle. Therefore the individual behaves inconsistently with ability.

People with health limitations have always been a segment of the population in all societies. Disability transcends age, sex, race, and socioeconomic status. Folk tales and classical literary works contain many characters who are lame, blind, or frail. Western medical and nursing literature lists an abundance of conditions, illnesses, and diseases that result in impairment. Disability can be defined as an impairment that interferes with a person's ability to engage successfully in activities of daily living, such as walking, dressing, hearing, or seeing. Because people live longer and more infants with low birth weight survive, chances of developing disability increase.

Although the focus of nursing involves healing[14] the patient, another important aspect is assisting the patient in adjustment to limitations. Therefore rehabilitation is a vital component of nursing action. Unfortunately, adjustment to a change in health status sometimes does not occur. After evaluation, if the nurse decides that rehabilitation has not been successful, one possible explanation is that the patient's adjustment is impaired. To understand Impaired Adjustment, the nurse should refer to several theories that relate to this nursing diagnosis. The main concepts to be considered are change, motivation, self-esteem, and locus of control, with acknowledgement of the role of social support.

Change inherently causes some type of adjustment. Change is everywhere, and all human beings are exposed to its many forms during various times in life. People die, and others are born. We get sick, and we get well. But sometimes people do not get well. When individuals fail to regain their previous level of health, adjustments to the new level are necessary. In other words, the person must change. Essential to change is that the person must acknowledge the problem and the need for change in order to overcome the problem.[12] Many factors are involved in change. In her discussion of barriers that inhibit change, Flynn[7] identified the following elements that hinder a person's adjustment: problems in trust, lack of family or group support, perception of change as a threat to self or family, lack of ability to communicate with and use health care resources, satisfaction with the present situation, and goals that are unrealistic or incongruent with those of health care providers.

Flynn[2] identified another barrier to change—

lack of motivation. The relationship between change and motivation is frequently stressed by both theorists and clinicians. Maslow, whose work focused on motivational aspects of human behavior, theorized that an individual's activity or inactivity resulted from a personal hierarchy of needs.[5] If a need is not satisfied, then a person attempts to change that which blocks the fulfillment of the need. An example is the need for self-actualization being impaired because of an illness that prevents independent function. In this situation, the individual will attempt to meet the need in other ways, such as minimizing the illness or overcompensating in other aspects of functioning. Lavin[11] observed in a clinical setting that highly motivated individuals treat disabilities with impatience, frustration, and sometimes depression. Dolger and Seeman[6] noted that illness was frequently perceived as blocking fulfillment in many spheres of life, and many patients were motivated to remain in control of their lives and live normally, disregarding any limitations of the disability. Many times, the actual change does not upset the person, but the perceived limitation does. Weinstein,[17] when describing the behaviors resulting from the patient's distress over limitations, included (1) ignoring symptoms, (2) not taking prescribed medications, and (3) hoping that symptoms would just disappear without treatment. All of these behaviors hinder successful adjustment. Like most dynamics of human behavior, motivation can be both conscious and unconscious.

Conscious and unconscious aspects also influence a person's self-esteem, which is involved in Impaired Adjustment. Esteem is one of Maslow's broad categories of needs. Therefore when either real or perceived assaults occur that lower self-esteem (such as a condition that limits the person), he/she attempts to control that which inhibits the resolution of the need. In other words, self-esteem influences adjustment. Berland and Addison[2] suggested that people who view themselves as "infallible and invulnerable" fight limitations and have difficulty in adjusting to disability. Self-esteem has been defined and explained by many theories. Psychoanalytic, interpersonal, transac-

tional, and existential-humanistic schools of thought all provide concepts and ideas about the development of an individual's view of self. Closely related to self-esteem are other personality traits, which influence attitudes toward recovery. Most important, one must recognize that self-esteem is a highly complex component of human beings.

Locus of control is another complex concept related to an individual's adjustment to limitations. This theory also stresses perception as more important than real or actual consequences. In locus of control theory, the individual attributes his/her own performance and life situation either to factors from within or outside of the self. Therefore if people have an internal locus of control, they believe that they, themselves, are in control. If they have an external locus, they think and feel that outside forces (such as change or other people) are mainly responsible for what happens to them.[15] In a classic work addressing life after a heart attack, Miller[13] maintained that patients who think they can control certain factors (for example, diet, level of stress and activity, and taking medicine) have an excellent chance for adjustment. In locus of control language, one who perceives oneself as in charge views illness as under one's own control. This belief, of course, is not completely realistic because of its use of absolutes. Generally, people have some, but not complete, control in these situations.

Social support, especially from the family, influences success in adjustment. Cohen and Eisdorfer[5] acknowledge that family, including a family's strengths and effectiveness in coping, affects how people adjust to limiting conditions. A family can provide a stable and loving atmosphere where individuals can accept health status changes and move toward independence. On the other hand, it can be setting where illness and limitations are dangerous because the family itself is unstable.

The reasons some people choose to adjust the limitations accompanying a change in health status and others select not to adjust remains a complex, and not especially well-defined, phenome-

X

non. In summary, factors such as motivation, perception of threat to self-esteem, locus of control, and support systems all affect whether or not an individual adjusts. Loss, similar to beauty, is in the eye of the beholder, and perceived loss is more critical than actual loss. A combination of the concepts relevant to Impaired Adjustments assists the nurse in understanding these patients, but caring for a person with a nursing diagnosis of Impaired Adjustment remains a challenge.

ASSESSMENT

Impaired Adjustment can be seen in all clinical nursing areas. It can occur in patients with heart and lung diseases, orthopedic conditions, complications of infectious illnesses, birth defects, diabetes, and chronic mental illnesses. These are just a few of a long list of conditions that may interfere with activities of daily living. Although most patients with a nursing diagnosis of Impaired Adjustment display physical limitations, the defining characteristics and related factors primarily focus on the patient's psychological state. Therefore the nursing assessment is derived basically from psychological factors, but selected social aspects also should be considered.

Before embarking on the particulars of patient assessment, the nurse must assess his/her own feelings because these patients may resist interventions, causing the nurse to feel angry, frustrated, and helpless. These patients may contend that they "know better" than the medical personnel and then exhibit behavior that negates or belies their knowledge. For example, a nurse works for more than an hour with a diabetic patient regarding diet, and the patient then says, "I know that diabetics should limit the amount of fat and refined sugar in their diets, but I'll probably be able to have a lot if I just figure out how to do it." The nurse feels as though the patient has not listened to a word of the provided education. These patients often say, "Yes, but . . .", which indicates that they understand what has been said but choose not to apply it to themselves. For instance, many patients with heart problems still smoke although they are aware of the adverse effect.[8,13]

There are five general defining characteristics that should be considered in assessing a person for a nursing diagnosis of Impaired Adjustments. These characteristics are related to change, motivation, self-esteem, and locus of control. The two major defining characteristics are the patient's verbalizing nonacceptance of health status change and the nonexistent or unsuccessful involvement in solving problems or setting goals. The nurse can identify both of these areas through keen observations, careful questions, and astute listening. For instance, a nurse observes behavioral indications that a patient with arthritis[1] might be having difficulty in accepting a change in health status. In this case, the nurse could begin a conversation with a comment such as, "I noticed that you didn't seem to agree with Dr. Peters when he was talking about you needing to exercise more. I'm wondering why." To assess the patient's ability to solve problems or set goals, the nurse might ask, "What do you see as the problems caused by your arthritis?" followed by, "And how do you see these problems being handled?" Another method of obtaining this information would be to inquire about the patient's long- and short-term plans and goals regarding the specific limitations.

The latter strategy also addresses one of the minor defining characteristics, the lack of future-oriented thinking. To discover whether the person is suffering from an extended period of shock, disbelief, or anger regarding the limitation, the nurse should ask questions such as, "How do you feel about your condition?", "What do you think regarding your illness?", or "How do you think these limitations will affect your future?" A lack of movement toward independence can be determined through questions about perceived limitations and strengths and a careful observation of how well the person performs activities of daily living.

For a thorough assessment, follow-up questions should be asked of the patient and family. Other staff members' evaluations of the patient can validate the nurse's hunches and conclusions. Feedback from the patient, family, and other staff members is important in processing the data the nurse has gathered.

❖ **Defining Characteristics**

The presence of the following defining characteristics indicates that the patient may be experiencing Impaired Adjustment:

- Verbalization of nonacceptance of health status change
- Extended period of shock, disbelief, or anger regarding limitations

- Nonexistent or unsuccessful involvement in problem solving or goal setting
- Lack of progress toward independence
- Lack of future-oriented thinking

❖ **Related Factors**

The following related factors are associated with Impaired Adjustment:

- Disability requiring changes in lifestyle
- Inadequate support systems
- Sensory overload
- Altered focus of control

- Incomplete grieving
- Impaired cognition
- Lack of motivation
- Low self-esteem

❖ **Related Medical/Psychiatric Diagnoses**

The following are examples of related medical/psychiatric diagnoses for Impaired Adjustment:

- Arthritis
- Chronic health problems requiring changes in usual activities
- Anorexia or Bulimia
- Health problems requiring treatment (e.g., amputation, radical surgery, immobilization of a limb) that may alter functional abilities or body image

- Paralysis
- Severe depression
- Substance abuse
- Terminal illnesses
- Trauma resulting in disfigurement

NURSING DIAGNOSES

Examples of *specific* nursing diagnoses for Impaired Adjustment are:

- Impaired Adjustment related to lack of motivation
- Impaired Adjustment related to paralysis requiring changes in activities of daily living
- Impaired Adjustment related to lack of support from significant others when adjusting to cardiovascular accident and changing activities of daily living/daily routine

PLANNING AND IMPLEMENTATION WITH RATIONALE

The general nursing plan for persons with Impaired Adjustment focuses on the specific assessment findings. For instance, if the defining characteristic "difficulty in goal setting" is identified, then the plan should focus on overcoming this difficulty. Theory provides the rationale for all planning and interventions. *The use of information on change, motivation, self-esteem, locus of control, and support systems should direct nursing plans and interventions.*

The care plan must be individualized to each patient through consideration of the effect that specific related factors have on the patient's physiological and psychosocial responses to the situation. *The way in which a disability affects one's lifestyle and ability to cope will differ for each patient.* For example, two patients who have arthritis may both have severe functional limitations in using their hands and fingers. One of these patients may be a sculptor who does fine, intricate work with his hands; the other may be an author who has always used a typewriter to do her work but now must dictate her work and have someone else transcribe it. The first patient's functional disability threatens his livelihood, and he must seek a new career. The same functional disability creates difficulties and some expense for the second patient, but she can continue to pursue her former career. Both of these patients will experience changes in their lifestyles in varying degrees, their usual coping mechanisms may or may not be effective in dealing with the challenges confronting each of them, and the support systems available in the past and the present may or may not be adequate.

X

❖ *NURSING CARE GUIDELINES*

Nursing Diagnosis: *Impaired Adjustment*

Expected Patient Outcomes	Nursing Interventions
The patient will verbalize awareness of changes in health status and its effect on lifestyle.	• Encourage patient to describe perceived change in health and feelings about change, especially regarding limitations.
The patient will take an active role in identifying goals and the means to achieve these goals.	• Support patient in attempts at goal formulation and problem solving. • Focus on possible ways the patient can exhibit more independence and less dependence. • Assist patient in identifying others (e.g., family, significant others, and health care providers) available to offer assistance. • With the patient, evaluate on a regular basis the progress made in achieving set goals. • Praise the patient's achievements and work with him/her to overcome persistent interferences in attaining goal achievement.
The patient will use strategies that will assist him/her in coping with limitation and losses.	• Assist the patient in developing a sense of self-confidence by focusing on strengths, abilities, and past achievements. • Guide the patient in the identification of various strategies that can be employed. • Support the patient in the identification of ways in which he/she can schedule activities that allow for optimal participation. • Assist the patient in initiating activities from which he/she can gain satisfaction. • Encourage the patient to accept the assistance of family, significant others, and health care providers when necessary.

The long-term goal should *focus on modification of the patient's lifestyle to coincide with the change in health status.* To achieve this goal, specific outcomes must be achieved. The patient must be aware of the change in health status and the demands that the change will place on his/her former lifestyle. It will be essential for the patient to take an active role in identifying short-term goals that must be achieved to adapt his/her lifestyle to the change in health status. Achievement of these short-term goals may require the patient to use new strategies for coping with the change and for implementing a new lifestyle.

EVALUATION

Evaluation criteria should be identified during the planning of the nursing process. The criteria should be qualitative, quantitative, and specific enough to express to others (especially the patient) the achievements of the interventions. In caring for persons with a nursing diagnosis of Impaired Adjustment, one would assume that the goal is the person's becoming better adjusted to the limitations arising from the changes in health status. "Better" is a subjective word, but it does connote movement toward a goal, which in this case is to achieve less impairment and more adjustment. Success may be measured by positive

❖ CASE STUDY WITH PLAN OF CARE

Mrs. Beverly R. is a 61-year-old hospitalized woman who has had a stroke that has primarily affected her balance and walking. This evening she fell while getting out of bed to go to the rest room. This is the fifth time she has fallen in the past 2 days. Although the staff, including her primary nurse and physician, have made several requests that she not get out of bed without a staff member present, each time she laughs and says, "Well, you won't be around to help me next week, so I'm just practicing on my own." Thus far, Mrs. R. has not injured herself, but the staff expresses concern that she doesn't seem aware of her limitations, even though dangers and risks of overreaching her ability have been explained to her. Mrs. R. is due to leave the hospital for home in 3 days. Physically, she has made excellent progress and has been active in physical therapy. The staff thinks that her goal of "being as good as new" is unrealistic in the short time that she expects, and yet they do not want to discourage her enthusiasm and optimism about recovering. Mrs. R. is pleasant and cooperative in all her treatments but has not accepted her health limitations. Tomorrow she is scheduled to meet with the staff and her two daughters for a discharge planning meeting. The visiting nurse has also been invited to attend. The nursing diagnosis is Impaired Adjustment related to disability requiring changes in lifestyle and altered locus of control because of physical limitations.

PLAN OF CARE FOR MRS. BEVERLY R.

Nursing Diagnosis: Impaired Adjustment related to disability requiring changes in lifestyle and altered locus of control because of physical limitations

Expected Patient Outcomes	Nursing Interventions
Mrs. R. will verbalize her strengths.	• Identify Mrs. R.'s strengths with her and her family.
Mrs. R. will verbalize a more realistic view of her limitations.	• Identify with Mrs. R. her limitations and explore her difficulty in accepting them.
Mrs. R. will acknowledge that some things are outside of her control.	• Engage Mrs. R. in discussion about things that are now in and out of her control.
Mrs. R. will share her feelings of frustration and distress over her loss of control.	• Encourage, acknowledge, and accept both Mrs. R.'s positive and negative feelings.
Mrs. R. will recognize that being limited does not mean "the end."	• Accept Mrs. R.'s current level of adjustment and work with her from that point.
Mrs. R. will identify appropriate support systems to aid in her rehabilitation.	• Identify with Mrs. R. and her family the support services available.
Mrs. R. will identify long- and short-term goals.	• Explore realistic expectations with Mrs. R. and her family.
Mrs. R. will continue to attempt independent activity, but with appropriate assistance from staff or family.	• Coordinate with the hospital staff, the family, and the visiting nurse to aid in activities.

X

actions or fewer negative behaviors. The nurse must decide ahead of time the measures of success, or he/she will have no criteria with which to justify the feeling that the nursing interventions have been successful.

REFERENCES

1. Arthritis Foundation: *Understanding arthritis: what it is, how it's treated and how to cope with it,* New York, 1984, Charles Scribner's Sons.
2. Berland R, Addison R: *Living with your bad back,* New York, 1983, St Martin's Press.
3. Carroll-Johnson RM: *Classification of nursing diagnoses: proceedings of the Eighth Conference,* Philadelphia, 1989, JB Lippincott.
4. Carroll-Johnson RM: *Classification of nursing diagnoses: proceedings of the Ninth Conference,* Philadelphia, 1991, JB Lippincott.
5. Cohen D, Eisdorfer C: *The loss of self: a family resource for the care of Alzheimer's disease and related disorders,* New York, 1986, WW Norton.
6. Dolger I, Seeman B: *How to live with diabetes,* New York, 1986, WW Norton.
7. Flynn J: Change theory. In Flynn J, Heffron P, editors: *Nursing: from concepts to practice,* ed 2, Bowie, Md, 1988, RJ Brady.
8. Hoffman N: *Change of heart: the bypass experience,* San Diego, 1985, Harcourt Brace Jovanovich.
9. Jarvis L: *Community health nursing: keeping the public healthy,* Philadelphia, 1981, FA Davis.
10. Kim M, McFarland G, and McLane A: *Pocket guide to nursing diagnoses,* St Louis, 1991, Mosby-Year Book.
11. Lavin J: *Stroke: from crisis to victory,* New York, 1985, Franklin Watts.
12. Lowery BL: Psychological stress, denial and myocardial infraction outcomes, *Image* 23(1):51-55, 1991.
13. Miller R: *How to live with a heart attack,* Radnor, Pa, 1973, Chilton Book Co.
14. Quinn JF: On healing, wholeness, and the Haelan effect, *Nursing Health Care* 10(10):552-55, 1989.
15. Scarr S, Weinberg R, and Levin A: *Understanding development,* San Diego, 1986, Harcourt Brace Jovanovich.
16. Schroeder M: Theories of personhood. In Flynn J, Heffron: *Nursing: from concept to practice,* ed 2, Norwalk, Conn, 1988, Appleton & Lange.
17. Weinstein A: *Asthma: the complete guide to self management of asthma and allergies for patients and their families,* New York, 1987, McGraw-Hill.

X

Post-Trauma Response

Post-Trauma Response is the intense, sustained emotional response of an individual to a traumatic experience or natural or man-made disaster.

OVERVIEW

Post-Trauma Response is characterized by a range of emotional responses from fear and anger to flashbacks and psychic numbing. Post-Trauma Response (PTR) affects those who participated in war-related combat, those who are victims of rape, childhood physical and/or sexual abuse, kidnapping, automobile accidents, and natural and man-made disasters, and those whose emotional or physical survival or that of loved ones is threatened.

PTR can have an acute or a long-term phase or both. In the acute phase, the individual may experience shock and disbelief followed by intense fear and anxiety. Some individuals appear calm and controlled during this phase, giving the impression of coping well. However, it may be difficult for some individuals to express feelings or acknowledge the extent of the trauma to self and others. For example, some rape victims refuse to think or talk about the sexual assault because of the severe humiliation they have experienced.[1] Other trauma victims may be discouraged from expressing feelings because of cultural or religious beliefs. In general, a victim of PTR will in the acute phase express feelings of terror, shock, disbelief, embarrassment, and anger.

In the long-term phase, which begins within a few days to several months after the traumatic event, the individual may have flashbacks (revisualizations of the traumatic scene that seem real), intrusive thoughts, and nightmares in which the event is reenacted. Victims may be preoccupied with the traumatic event and have difficulty concentrating on work or other matters of daily living. Some continue to deny and will develop emotional numbing that may lead to total amnesia for the event. Others feel depressed and hopeless.[2,3]

Long-term effects of trauma from childhood physical or sexual abuse can have a significant effect on the personality and interpersonal relationships of the adult survivor.[9] The individual may develop chronic feelings of low self-esteem, suicidal feelings and acts, substance abuse, and physically abusive adult relationships. Dissociation, a psychological defense mechanism by which the individual separates the self emotionally from the traumatized body, may persist into adulthood, resulting in sexual dysfunction or, in its extreme form, multiple personality disorder.[2,5]

Childhood physical and sexual abuse has been linked to the development of borderline personality disorder, which is characterized by unstable mental images of self and others, impulsive behavior, and rocky interpersonal relationships. The question debated here is whether the personality disorder was established before the experience of a traumatic event, making the individual more vulnerable to PTR. More research and clinical finding are needed to answer this question.

Several films about the Vietnam War have portrayed the consequences of PTR. Veterans have been depicted as having flashbacks of being shot or watching their friends die in battle. The sights, sounds, and smells of the battlefield remain vivid in their memories for years. For some the war has never ended because of the daily intrusion of flashbacks and nightmares into their cognitive and emotional lives.

In contrast, some victims of PTR remain in denial about the event. Although it serves an important role in healthy coping, denial can render the individual emotionally numb, disinterested, and withdrawn from life.[3,5] Unfortunately these victims often "slip through the cracks" of the support systems that are designed to help them adjust to the traumatic experience. When family and friends try to reach out, the sufferer who is denying may react with hostility and rejection, further widening the gap and aggravating maladaptive responses.

Those who survived disasters in which others died or were seriously injured may suffer the long-term consequences of PTR. They may feel guilty for being spared when others died, ashamed that they did not do enough to save others, and helpless.

Alcohol and drug abuse may result when the victim of PTR tries to cope with the effect of the trauma. In an attempt to avoid or numb self from anxiety, depression, and shame the person may drink alcohol or use other drugs. However, substance abuse tends to aggravate the symptoms of PTR, and the victim becomes increasingly alienated from pretrauma relationships and commitments.

Impaired interpersonal relationships occur in the long-term phase. The individual may withdraw from friends and family. He/she may feel increasingly limited in interactions with people, self-conscious, and distrustful of others.

ASSESSMENT

PTR is experienced after an individual has been the victim of a life-threatening disaster or threat of any kind to personal well-being or to well-being of loved ones. Most healthy, emotionally stable people experience some degree of shock, anxiety, and ongoing fear after an event such as an automobile accident or criminal assault. A victim failing to express some anxiety or fear after a traumatic episode should be regarded as highly unusual by the nurse. However, depending on the role played by the victim of the disaster, the reaction may be difficult to assess.

For instance, the driver of a car who survives an automobile accident in which others were seriously injured or were killed may be unable to express the conflicting, confusing feelings of the threat to his own life and his sense of responsibility for his passengers. The driver may have assisted the others immediately after the accident, exposing himself to the gruesome sight of physical trauma and to the sounds of pain and suffering. The driver may have suffered personal injury and may not have noticed it until the police and rescue squads arrived to assist him and the other victims. The driver may feel shock and disbelief, fear, guilt, and shame but may not express any concern for self, only for the passengers. This person may develop flashbacks, nightmares, and intrusive thoughts in the aftermath of the accident. The nurse needs to be aware of the potential for a delayed response in this and other cases.

However, victims of childhood sexual and physical abuse may be incorrectly diagnosed with a personality disorder and not receive appropriate therapy in the wake of a later traumatic event. It is essential that the nurse take a thorough history, including questions about child abuse, to accurately diagnose and treat all trauma victims.

The nurse must consider many factors of the individual with PTR. What was the nature of the trauma? Was the individual alone or with others? Was there physical trauma? Did a loved one die? Did the individual experience loss of personal property, livelihood, or social status? These questions can give important information about the likelihood of a mild or severe emotional response by the individual.

As stated earlier, it is unusual for one to fail to express some degree of anxiety and depression in the aftermath of a trauma. However, not all victims of trauma experience the serious and unremitting reactions associated with PTR. What makes one person more likely than another to develop PTR?

Predisposing factors include the existence of psychopathology or emotional problems before the traumatic event. Individuals who are characteristically anxious, have low self-esteem, or suffer from depression or impaired reality testing may be prone to PTR. Those who as children were discouraged from expressing feelings or who view public demonstrations of grief as inappropriate for cultural or religious reasons may deny and restrict themselves from the benefits of discussing the event with others.

The socially isolated person is at higher risk for PTR than people with established social networks and positive family relationships. Earlier experiences of trauma, especially during childhood, may result in impaired coping mechanisms to handle any additional tragedy. However, having survived previous traumas with the outcome of improved self-esteem and healthy coping, the individual may be more prepared for the range of feelings that accompany a dramatic life experience.[6]

When children are the victims of a disaster, the nurse must consider the child's current developmental stage and the effect on the child's continuing emotional development. Twenty-five survivors of the Chowchilla school bus kidnapping in 1976 were the subjects of a 4-year follow-up study.[7] The children who experienced the most severe reactions to this trauma were assessed as having had prior vulnerabilities, such as family dysfunction and social isolation. The study also identified important differences in the ways children respond to trauma. Children are more likely to exhibit pessimism about the future, superstitiousness, distorted or incorrect memories about the trauma, thought suppression, post-traumatic play and reenactment, and fear of dying young.

The nurse is most likely to encounter the victim of trauma in the acute care setting shortly after the event, in the community mental health center several days, weeks, or months after the event, or in the rehabilitation setting years after the traumatic experience. Depending on the setting, the nurse will be assessing for symptoms and phase of PTR.

In the acute care setting, the nurse must first observe the patient's physical status and attend to his/her immediate needs for help. The nurse can assess the emotional response simultaneously. Is the patient crying? Can the patient be comforted? Does the patient react with fear and suspiciousness to the ministrations of the nurse and other caregivers? The nurse will want to assess what the patient says about what happened and how he/she feels. If the patient is unconscious, the nurse should speak with family members or friends who arrive with the patient. Are they able to discuss their feelings? How do they seem to be coping with the initial shock, fear, and anxiety? Are they expressing emotions appropriate to the circumstances, or is there an attempt to minimize, trivialize, or gloss over the event? Perhaps the patient and family exhibit severe emotional strain and will need crisis intervention to assist in maintaining control of their emotions. These observations and data can provide valuable information about the patient's coping in the aftermath of trauma.

In the community mental health setting, the nurse should interview the self-referred patient or the one referred by a doctor, a friend, an employer, or a family member. The source of the referral is important in that it frequently indicates how motivated the individual will be to examine personal emotions. A self-referred patient may be more aware of problems in personal coping after the trauma and more motivated to express feelings and to discover new coping behaviors. The patient who seeks treatment on the recommendation of another may not be as aware of personal feelings and may not see the need for professional assistance. This patient may have agreed to seek treatment under duress or to get people "off his back." Whatever the source of the referral, the nurse will be challenged to explore gently but purposefully with the patient his/her reactions to getting help and to the trauma.

The nurse in the rehabilitation setting is likely to encounter individuals, perhaps war veterans, who display chronic dysfunction associated with post-trauma response.[4,8] The patient may have been coping maladaptively for years through drug or alcohol abuse, social isolation, and, possibly, sociopathic behavior. The sufferer may have been unable to make the transition from the military setting or the combat zone to civilian life. The patient may be depressed and may display the cognitive impairments associated with PTR: flashbacks, intrusive thoughts, poor reality testing, and poor concentration. The nurse in the rehabilitation setting will be focusing the assessment on the patient's functioning in the physiological, psychological, interpersonal, and occupational areas.

Nursing assessment of the patient with PTR is an ongoing, dynamic process. Regardless of the setting in which the nurse encounters the patient, the patient's response in particular areas should be addressed (see box below).

❖ **Defining Characteristics**

The presence of the following defining characteristics indicates that the patient may be experiencing Post-Trauma Response:
- Flashbacks of the traumatic event triggered by visual, auditory, and olfactory stimuli
- Nightmares
- Intrusive thoughts
- Impaired concentration, memory, and cognition
- Emotional numbing including amnesia for and confusion about the event
- Denial of the effect of the trauma

Physiological impairment associated with the trauma

- Nature of the injury; long-term disability
- Patient's response to medical regimen
- Medications used and abused to cope with pain
- Prostheses or devices used to compensate for impairment
- Involvement in rehabilitation program
- Actual or potential effect of injuries on body image and self-esteem

Emotional functioning

- Ability to express feelings associated with the traumatic event
- Evidence of prolonged denial
- Receptivity of patient to caregivers and significant others
- Use of drugs or alcohol to cope with feelings
- Degree of anxiety, despair, depression, and helplessness exhibited
- Suicidal thoughts and actions
- Adaptive and maladaptive coping patterns
- Significant developmental history related to previous experiences of trauma
- Preexisting mental health disorder

Cognitive functioning

- Presence of flashbacks, intrusive thoughts, and nightmares
- Inability to concentrate on work, academic, or recreational tasks
- Inability to discuss issues other than the trauma
- Substance abuse and evidence of chronic neurological damage

Interpersonal relationships

- Quality of interpersonal relationships before the traumatic event
- Significant others with whom patient maintains regular contact
- Receptivity of patient to efforts of significant others
- Evidence of alienation from pretrauma relationships and activities
- Effect of substance abuse on communication skills

Environmental and community supports

- Supportive responses from patient's work/professional colleagues, organizations, church groups, and school
- Community supports available to the patient (for instance, victim's support group, rape crisis center, Veterans' Administration)
- Patient receptivity to use of community supports

X

- Generalized fear and anxiety related to the possibility of the trauma recurring and associated with nonrelated experiences
- Guilt
- Dissociation
- Impaired interpersonal relationships; social withdrawal
- Abusive adult relationships
- Impaired occupational or academic functioning; withdrawal from activities and commitments
- Alcohol and drug abuse
- Helplessness and hopelessness; suicidal thoughts and actions
- Common characteristics in children and adolescents: posttraumatic play and reenactment, impaired time orientation for traumatic event and related events, limited view of the future; fear of dying young, superstitiousness, and pretrauma family dysfunction

❖ Related Factors

The following related factors are associated with Post-Trauma Response:
- Disasters such as floods, fire, and earthquakes
- Participation in war-related combat
- Rape
- Assault
- Childhood physical and/or sexual abuse
- Torture
- Kidnapping
- Catastrophic illness
- Accidents
- Preexisting emotional disorders
- Previous experience of trauma
- Limited community supports

❖ Related Medical/Psychiatric Diagnoses

The following are examples of related medical/psychiatric diagnoses for Post-Trauma Response:
- Borderline personality disorder
- Disfiguring third-degree burns
- Generalized anxiety disorder
- Mood disorder
- Multiple personality disorder
- Multiple physical trauma
- Suicide attempt
- Victim of homicidal attempt

NURSING DIAGNOSES

Examples of *specific* nursing diagnoses for Post-Trauma Response are:
- Post-Trauma Response related to Vietnam combat experience
- Post-Trauma Response related to positive HIV test
- Post-Trauma Response related to physical abuse experienced during childhood
- Post-Trauma Response related to severe automobile accident

PLANNING AND IMPLEMENTATION WITH RATIONALE

The nursing plan of care for the patient experiencing Post-Trauma Response should focus primarily on providing the patient with emotional support and assisting in the integration of the traumatic experience into the patient's life in order to achieve specified outcomes.

Outcome: The patient will express feelings appropriate to the effect of the trauma on his/her life. Initially the patient may not be receptive to expressing his/her feelings and reactions about the trauma. The nurse must respect the patient's need to avoid or deny feelings. *Denial is an expected and healthy coping mechanism in the initial phases of recovery. Denial can assist the patient in doing what is necessary to regain strength and a positive self-image.*[3] The nurse can be available when the patient feels the need to talk about the trauma, anticipating that when recovering from injuries or when the threat of the disaster occurring again is passed, the patient may become more emotional. Healthy denial may give way to outbursts of anger, anxiety, and depression. *A consistent, supportive response from the nurse is necessary to assist the patient in sorting through confusing and overwhelming feelings.*

Outcome: The patient will experience increasingly longer periods free of impaired concentration. The patient will need assistance in performing cognitive functions and concentrating on tasks because of the occurrence of intrusive thoughts and flashbacks. *The nurse's presence and acceptance of the patient's experience will help him/her to be open to learning techniques that will im-*

X

❖ *NURSING CARE GUIDELINES*

Nursing Diagnosis: *Post-Trauma Response*

Expected Patient Outcomes	Nursing Interventions
The patient will express feelings appropriate to the effect of the trauma on his/her life.	• Allow the patient to focus on recovery of physical health while medical status is compromised. • Introduce discussion of the emotional effect of the trauma as the patient seems ready. • Explain to patient and family that as physical recovery progresses, more extreme emotional responses may occur. • Assist the patient to deal with altered physical status. • Help the patient verbalize feelings of loss, inadequacy, low self-esteem, and distorted body image.
The patient will experience increasingly longer periods free of impaired concentration.	• Encourage the patient to talk about the traumatic event and how it interferes with current life goals. • Accept patient's fears associated with thoughts and revisualizations; provide an understanding response that acknowledges how real these thoughts seem to the patient. • Teach relaxation techniques—progressive relaxation, deep breathing, imagery. • Expose the patient to other calming activities—listening to music, drinking warm milk before bedtime, and taking walks. • Encourage structured time during the day and involvement in meaningful activities to reduce occurrence of intrusive thoughts.
The patient will maintain old and develop new interpersonal relationships.	• Arrange family meetings while the patient is hospitalized to discuss how family can support and assist the patient. • Encourage involvement in unit activities, occupational rehabilitation, and hobbies. • Offer support through frequent one-to-one contact. • Encourage the patient to discuss fears related to interpersonal closeness. • Discuss with family and significant others the meaning of the patient's withdrawal. • Empathize with the family's pain while encouraging family members to maintain involvement with the patient.

prove concentration and encourage returning to work or academic responsibilities.

Outcome: The patient will maintain old and develop new interpersonal relationships. The family and friends will benefit from the nurse's explanations of the patient's difficulties. The patient may need to reexamine some relationships that may be self-defeating or abusive with the nurse's assistance. Survivors of childhood physical and sexual abuse often seek out such abusive relationships in an attempt to repeat the trauma, possibly to master and control the outcome. *The patient needs to*

❖ *NURSING CARE GUIDELINES—cont'd*

Expected Patient Outcomes	Nursing Interventions
The patient will abstain from drug and alcohol use.	• Refer for psychiatric evaluation and treatment with psychoactive drugs. • Refer for individual or group psychotherapy. • Refer to Alcoholics Anonymous or Narcotics Anonymous. • Encourage family support and involvement in Al-Anon or other survivor support groups. • Maintain drug-free environment except for prescribed, therapeutic medications. • Discourage involvement with drug abusers or alcoholics not engaged in rehabilitation efforts. • Encourage the patient to discuss uncomfortable feelings the patient may try to avoid through substance abuse. • Discuss and teach alternatives to substance abuse that may provide the patient with a more satisfying state of well-being (for instance, spiritual renewal, physical exercise, yoga, and meditation).
The patient will integrate the traumatic experience into perception of self and own life.	• Encourage the patient to discuss the trauma and to express feelings of fear, anxiety, sadness, confusion, and guilt. • Discourage the patient from using feelings about trauma to avoid responsibility for self and life goals. • Allow the patient time out from activities as needed, but encourage discussion of feelings that trigger the need to withdraw. • Contact community resources (such as Survivors of Trauma, Victims' Assistance, and Veterans' Administration), and encourage the patient to utilize them. • Encourage the patient to share the experience with others and to offer support to those who also are victims of trauma.

evaluate the positive and negative aspects of these relationships, discarding some, and resuming relationships with those who will accept and support him/her through recovery. New and healthy relationships may be fostered by the patient's involvement in support groups.

Outcome: The patient will abstain from drug and alcohol use. Patients who have difficulty expressing emotions about the trauma often turn to drugs or alcohol to induce a sort of psychological numbing to the experience. *Appropriate psychopharmacologic agents are available to assist the patient in coping with the anxiety, depression, and impaired concentration that result from trau-*

matic experience. Verbalization of feelings, relaxation techniques, and support groups often fill the void the patient feels.

Outcome: The patient will integrate the traumatic experience into his/her perception of self and life. A long-term task for the patient is the integration of the traumatic experience into a realistic perspective. Some patients feel their lives are ruined by the trauma and feel hopeless about overcoming the deleterious effects. *The nurse must understand and explore these attitudes, while encouraging the patient to consider prior skills, qualities, and supports that may be employed in the aftermath of the trauma. Renewal of*

X

spiritual connections may assist the patient to feel unity with other victims, from whom emotional strength can be garnered and to whom the patient may be a source of hope. The stage of acceptance of the trauma and its effect on life is the end stage of the grieving process; the nurse must help the patient understand that this is a slow but necessary stage to complete.

Finally, the nurse must be aware of how he/she is affected emotionally by the patient with PTR. The intense nature of the patient's reactions and needs for support may be draining. The nurse may feel revulsion at the patient's injuries or description of the experience. Some nurses identify with the patient and begin to fear being traumatized themselves.

It will benefit the nurse to share feelings with colleagues, to be aware of the need for intermittent breaks from work with patients with PTR, and to be aware of fears based on personal painful life experience. Attending to personal emotional needs will enable the nurse to continue the important supportive and rehabilitative work with the patient.

EVALUATION

Evaluation of the patient with PTR is based on the patient's reports of feelings and the nurse's observations of behavioral responses. Collaboration among nurse, patient, significant others, and caregivers will yield the most information about the patient's progress. In general the nurse will want to evaluate the patient in these areas:

Response to medical regimen; resolution of physiological injuries
Emotional coping; management of anxiety and adaptation to altered body image
Cognitive abilities
Abstinence from drug and alcohol use
Interpersonal relationships
Integration of trauma into life experience and self image

❖ CASE STUDY WITH PLAN OF CARE

Ms. Ruth C. referred herself to the community mental health center 5 months after an automobile accident in which the car she was driving was hit head-on by a car driven by a drunk driver. Ms. C., a 25-year-old law student, sustained a broken leg and clavicle and cuts to her upper body, including her face. She was hospitalized for 2 weeks after the accident, then spent 1 month with her parents in her hometown. When she returned to her law classes she found that she could not concentrate on her studies, was afraid of driving an automobile, and felt depressed and tearful whenever she thought of or talked about the accident. She felt embarrassed by the temporary scars that were visible on her face and hands and felt uncomfortable when anyone asked about them. She had been refusing offers to socialize with her friends and would cut short calls from her family. She stated, "I don't understand why I'm so upset. Why can't I concentrate at school? Why am I so fearful? I should feel lucky to be alive, but I'm so angry." Ms. C. had no significant medical illnesses or injuries before the accident. When Ms. C. was in her freshman year of college, her father lost his job in the local steel mill. Her mother returned to work, and Ms.

C. returned home to help the family care for the two younger children, who were in elementary and junior high school. Ms. C. took courses for the next 2 years at the local community college and eventually returned to the state university 60 miles from home to complete her undergraduate degree. During the 2 years living at home, Ms. C. stated she observed the strain on her parents' relationship and feared that they might divorce. There was no preexisting mental health or emotional disorder. Ms. C. has a close relationship with her family, although she was never encouraged to talk about her feelings. She has two close girlfriends—one from law school, and the other from home—with whom she has shared her fears and reactions about the accident. She had been dating a man in one of her classes for about 1 month before the accident but had not returned his calls since the accident. Ms. C. belongs to a Unitarian Church near the law school and attends services regularly. She had been involved in an ethical discussion group at the church before the accident. A Victims of Trauma support group meets monthly through the community mental health center.

PLAN OF CARE FOR MS. RUTH C.

Nursing Diagnosis: *Post-Trauma Response related to automobile accident*

Expected Patient Outcomes	Nursing Interventions
Ms. C. will express feelings about accident.	• Establish a trusting, supportive relationship with Ms. C. through twice-a-week sessions for a period of 6 to 8 weeks. • Provide an attitude of acceptance for the range of feelings Ms. C. expresses. • Encourage Ms. C. to continue to talk with her two friends about the accident. • Refer Ms. C. to the Victims of Trauma support group.
Ms. C. will accept altered body image related to injuries.	• Encourage Ms. C. to continue with medical treatments and other self-care programs appropriate to her recovery. • Encourage Ms. C. to express feelings about facial scars and explore ways of increasing comfort with her appearance while they heal.
Ms. C. will maintain interpersonal relationships.	• Encourage Ms. C. to meet with friends for a few hours each week in nonthreatening social situations. • Explore concerns about contact with family; encourage Ms. C. to write letters if phone calls are awkward. • Support attendance at church activities.
Ms. C. will regain cognitive abilities.	• Assist Ms. C. to set up a realistic study schedule that will not tax her physically and emotionally. • Discuss options for reducing credit load or requesting extensions on papers, assignments, and examinations. • Teach relaxation exercises; encourage Ms. C. to revive self with calming activities (for instance, listening to music and meditation).
Ms. C. will integrate effect of accident into her total life experience.	• Encourage Ms. C. to review her previous life history and realistically evaluate what are permanent versus temporary changes in life goals, skills, and accomplishments. • Encourage Ms. C. to attend Victims of Trauma meetings and to offer self as a source of hope and positive coping to other victims. • Discuss stages of grieving process with Ms. C., and encourage her to understand the importance of dealing with the tasks of each stage to resolve the acute and long-term effect of the trauma on her life.

X

REFERENCES

1. Burgess A, Holstrom L: Rape trauma syndrome, *Am J Psychiatry* 131:981, 1974.
2. *American Psychological Association: Diagnostic and statistical manual of mental disorders,* DSM III-R, Washington, DC, 1987, The Association.
3. Horowitz M: *Stress-response syndromes,* New York, 1976, Jason Aronson.
4. Kulka R and others: *Trauma and the Vietnam war generation,* New York, 1990, Brunner Mazel.
5. McCann L, Pearlman L: *Psychological trauma and the adult survivor,* New York, 1990, Brunner Mazel.
6. Rutter M: Psychosocial resilience and protective mechanisms, *Am J Orthopsychiatry* 57:316, 1987.
7. Terr L: Chowchilla revisited: the effects of psychic trauma four years after a school bus kidnapping, *Am J Psychiatry* 140:1543, 1983.
8. Wilson J, Harel Z, and Kahana B, editors: *Human adaptation to extreme stress: from holocaust to Vietnam,* New York, 1988, Plenum Press.
9. Wyatt G, Powell G: *Lasting effects of child sexual abuse,* Newbury Park, 1988, Sage Publications.

Family Coping: Potential For Growth

Ineffective Family Coping: Compromised

Ineffective Family Coping: Disabling

Family Coping: Potential For Growth is the effective management of adaptive tasks by family members involved with the client's health challenge, together with readiness for health and growth as a family, individually and collectively.[15]

Ineffective Family Coping: Compromised is insufficient, ineffective, or accommodated family support, comfort, assistance, or encouragement that may alter the family member's (patient's) or family's competence in adaptive tasks related to the presenting health challenge.[15]

Ineffective Family Coping: Disabling is defined as a family member's behavior that incapacitates the patient or family to therapeutically adapt to the presenting health challenge.[15]

OVERVIEW

In our society the family unit is highly valued and family relationships are given high priority. Moreover, important decisions, including health care decisions, are made within a family context.[8]

Diagnoses related to family coping are guided by the Family Systems Theory. This theory offers a conceptual framework that focuses on the family and the complexity of interacting family variables. These interacting variables include family structures, typology, vulnerability, subsystem boundaries, transactional patterns, dynamics, life-cycle stages, cognitive appraisal skills, problem-solving abilities, coping, and socialization, especially with extrafamilial resources.

According to the family systems theory, the matrix of identity is the family; therefore, when one family member experiences a stressful event, the entire family is affected. The family unit's perception of this stressful event, like each individual's perception, is important. The theory, according to Minuchin[25], focuses on family health and competence, rather than on family pathology or problems. Family responses to transitions and hardships are viewed as natural and as a predictable aspect of family life. During stressful events, families learn to cope, and these coping skills become intrafamily strengths, which are then used to protect the family during future transition and change. The works of McCubbin and others[21]

X

suggest that family units, like individual family members, respond to stressful life events and/or crises by adapting or maladapting; in turn, the family can experience either growth or deprivation/disruption.

Family coping is not created in a single moment. It is evolutionary, multifaceted, dynamic, and shaped over time. Family coping responses are learned skills. Such skills can be altered, expanded, created, and tested. Some families are limited in both number and types of family coping responses. Clark[7,8] describes coping responses as action-oriented behaviors and defense mechanisms. Problem solving, attack, as commonly evidenced by anger, and avoidance are examples of action-oriented coping. Sublimation, suppression, and humor are examples of healthy defense mechanisms. Manipulation, intellectualization, displacement, and projection are examples of less healthy defense mechanisms.

Family coping strategies to resolve family hardships created by a stress event are multifaceted because every family is unique.[17-19] Today, this family uniqueness is even more complex because of the gradual increase in types of family structures, which are physiologically, socially, culturally, legally, economically, and spiritually variable.[14,22] These components vary among family units, are interactive within families, and can influence the quality of family coping.

The family's general physiological health status is often guided by family behaviors or coping responses such as eating, sleeping, physical activity, and/or medication patterns. In turn, each of these can be influenced during situational stress by the intensity and duration of other stimuli, such as advanced technology, quality of lighting, and odors.[13,26,31] Authoritative resources relate that families that withdraw or have prolonged depression with sleep disturbances and eating disorders are coping ineffectively. McGoldrick and others[22] further describe physiologic family health patterns associated with ethnicity. For example, the Irish have a high tolerance for alcohol and have used it as a universal disqualifier to cure fever, ease grief, and serve as a social substitute for food. The pub was the focus for life sharing and gatherings, rather than the family table.

Socialization, especially extrafamilial socialization, is enhanced by the family unit's identity as well as family competence in cognitive appraisal. Cognitive appraisal is the family's perceptions that make stressful events meaningful. The greater the variety of extrafamilial experiences as a family, the greater the family resources and competence with cognitive appraisal to draw on during a stressful event.[3,21]

Cultural dimensions that influence family coping responses can include: intragenerational relationships among family members; family values, rules and rituals; family relationships; and family interactions with the external environment.[12,13] Examples are numerous. The Irish view death as an important life transition and give priority to the wake ritual. In contrast, the Italians emphasize weddings, while Jews place priority on the bar mitzvah ritual. Family rules, according to Satir,[29] are cultural, such as rules for withholding anger, affection, and joy. She suggests that there are no bad families, but there are bad rules. For example, a common rule in families with alcohol dependency is that someone or something is responsible for the alcoholism, rather than the alcohol-dependent person. In turn, the family unit ends up living by this rule and by the delusion that the family member is not responsible for excessive drinking.[23,27]

Family coping is challenged by family structures that are becoming increasingly variable and complex.[21,29] Examples include the nuclear family, blended families, extended families, adoptive families, single-parent families, foster families, and step families that can be subcategorized as legitimate, revitalized, reassembled, and combination families. Culture also influences family structures. Americans focus on an intact nuclear family. Black families include kin and community. Italians tend to disregard the nuclear family concept and view their family as a three-or four-generational family. Also, there are family units that gather by self-initiation to provide support but clearly are not the family structures that are recognized legally.

X

Family coping is influenced by various economic and financial factors.[14,16] Examples include families that are homeless, economically impoverished, poor without access, "immediately poor," such as evicted farm families, and chemically dependent. Increasing within today's society are the poor elderly, who are frequent admitters to hospitals and heavy resource users. Cultural values play an important role for selected groups in seeking assistance. For example, African-Americans turn primarily to their own church, Italians rely closely on their family, and Jews value doctors.[22]

Spirituality influences a family's coping response. A family's spiritual dimension is not restricted to religious beliefs and practices, but it does include family faith belief systems, formal or informal.[21,22] Families perceive spirituality as a meaningful resource and helpful in strengthening family coping during a stressful event or a presenting family health challenge.[21]

ASSESSMENT

Family coping is assessed through a family interview. The interview can be formal using a structured process or informal through nonstructured contact with family members. A family genogram is a useful tool in gathering family information. Circular questions, in contrast to linear questions, are becoming a useful clinical tool in assessing differences between individual family members, family relationships, events, and belief systems.[20] Examples of circular questions include: "How does your family show that they are close?"; "Who does your father turn to for support?"; and "When your family was told about your brother's death, what was most helpful?"

In assessing family coping, the nurse is gathering data related to family perceptions associated with the presenting health challenge, family strengths, and family health status. These are influenced by multifaceted and interacting variables: demographic data, including family composition and availability; family roles; type of family decision-making; interactive external family resources, such as economic, social, environmental, and spiritual support; family perceptions or cognitive appraisal of the stress event; previous family coping styles; and family health and health promotion behaviors.

Family Coping: Potential For Growth

This is an example of a wellness-oriented nursing diagnosis. In this situation, a clinical judgment is made about a family in transition from a specific level of wellness to a higher level of wellness.

Defining characteristics of this nursing diagnosis include both objective and subjective data. The nurse assesses for objective data that include but are not limited to healthy family lifestyle behaviors that optimize wellness (such as healthy nutritional patterns, engagement in physical exercise, and absence of chemical abuse), use of appropriate extrafamilial resources, and a movement toward (versus away from or against) the family unit. Subjective data include communication by family members related to growth in family values and relationships associated with the stress event.

Related factors associated with this nursing diagnosis include family typology, vulnerability, life-cycle stage, and ethnicity, as well as previous family experiences with stressful events, expansion of family coping skills, and level of family adjustment. Usually related factors associated with this diagnosis have a history of contributing to family wellness.

Successful coping as perceived by the family does not necessarily mean effective coping.[7,8] For example, when a family uses withdrawal in a stressful event, such as in verbal, physical, sexual, or chemical abuse by family members, family anxiety may be decreased. This may be *perceived* by the family as successful coping; however, the reality of the situation continues, so in reality there is ineffective family coping.

❖ Defining Characteristics

The presence of the following defining characteristics indicates that the family may be experiencing Family Coping: Potential for Growth[1,15]:

Objective	Subjective
• Family choices demonstrate health	• Family shares perceptions of family

or lifestyle that optimize wellness.
- Family explores and/or utilizes appropriate resources from outside of the family circle.

growth in relation to a family member's health challenge.
- Family seeks assistance appropriately.

❖ Related Factors

The following related factors are associated with Family Coping: Potential for Growth[1,15]:

- Family typology
- Family vulnerability and openness for growth
- Family life-cycle stage(s)
- Family history of successful coping with major family stress events and/or crises
- Family's cognitive appraisal of crisis or stress event, especially if perceived as challenging

- Family history of effective problem-solving ability
- Family history of effective coping strategies
- Optimal level of family adjustment to previous family stress event(s)
- Supportive subculture

❖ Related Medical/Psychiatric Diagnoses

The following are examples of related medical/psychiatric diagnoses for Family Coping: Potential for Growth[32]:

- Eating disorders
- Phase-of-life problems
- Posttraumatic stress disorder
- Uncomplicated bereavement

Ineffective Family Coping: Compromised

This can be temporary or long term. Compromised family coping exists when behaviors are insufficient, ineffective, or accommodated. When family coping is consistently marked by a pattern of compromise, family growth is generally minimal or absent. Over time, altered family coping of this type may result in family dysfunction and/or family system(s) breakdown.

Nurses are in a unique position to observe

when a family's healthy coping skills have begun to change. Examples include reported feelings of powerlessness, inability to share feelings and/or utilize support resources, and resignation of personal or family preferences to accommodate a family member during situational crises and/or family life-cycle transitions.[5,6,9] When family behaviors are insufficient, there is usually an inadequate response, which may be verbalized as family inadequacy associated with a knowledge deficit related to family coping skills, family management of the situational stress, and/or family tasks during family life-cycle transitions. When family behaviors are ineffective, there are unsatisfactory outcomes that are generally related to a multiplicity of factors such as mistiming, inappropriate or unhealthy coping skills, inadequate knowledge base, underutilization of extrafamilial resources, and underfunctioning by selected family members.[2,4] When ineffective family coping is associated with accommodation, generally some family members feel that their preferences have been overridden by other family members, which can result in feelings of powerlessness, guilt, and/or distress.[10]

Defining characteristics of this nursing diagnosis include both objective and subjective data. The nurse assesses for objective data, which includes but is not limited to: (1) supportive behaviors by family members that result in unsatisfactory outcomes, such as absence of quality time between a parent and child in response to homecare for a grandmother; (2) decreased personal communication with family members during a time of need as evidenced by nonrelational communication, distressful silence, and avoidance; and (3) functioning by family members that results in neglect, triangulation, and displaced verbal communication.

Subjective data can include family statements such as "My family members are no longer speaking . . .", "I am so tired, I don't think that I can care for my child one more day . . .", or "My mom and dad are busy taking care of grandma since she came to live with us . . . They don't have time to do things with me like we used to . . ." Verbalized preoccupation with the health challenge or the family's situational or developmental crisis is generally evidenced by frequent repetitive thoughts and often includes personal perceptions related to fear, anticipatory grief, guilt, anger, and/or anxiety.[27,28] Knowledge deficits described by the family are usually associated with family coping strategies and supportive behaviors.

Related factors that may affect Ineffective Family Coping: Compromised include but are not limited to the following: chronicity of the health challenge, multiple family stressors that deplete the family's supportive capacity, limited family coping strategies, knowledge deficit associated with misinformation, altered family dynamics resulting in unhealthy behaviors, temporary family preoccupation with the presenting health challenge, family ethnicity (because of such factors as cultural identity, communication, health belief values), lack of mutual family support, temporary family disorganization during role transition, and concurrent situational or developmental crisis within the family circle.

❖ Defining Characteristics

The presence of the following defining characteristics indicates that the family may be experiencing Ineffective Family Coping: Compromised[1,15]:

Objective
- Assistive or supportive family behaviors resulting in unsatisfactory outcomes
- Limited or absent personal family communication during a time of need
- Over protective or underprotective family behaviors
- Triangulation
- Displaced verbal communication

Subjective
- Family verbalizes maladaptive family coping in response to the presenting health challenge.
- Family verbalizes fear, guilt, or anxiety regarding the presenting health or situational challenge.
- Family members describe a knowledge deficit associated with coping skills or effective supportive behaviors.

- Family members communicate that family decision-making is by accommodation or isolation (rather than consensus)

❖ Related Factors

The following related factors are associated with Ineffective Family Coping: Compromised[1,15]:
- Chronicity of health challenge
- Increased multiple stressors that deplete the supportive capacity of family members and family unit
- Physical exhaustion
- Family history of limited and/or ineffective coping strategies
- Guilt
- Anger
- Spiritual distress
- Knowledge deficit by family members related to inadequate information or misinformation
- Altered family dynamics that result in temporarily unhealthy behaviors
- Temporary preoccupation by family members that results in ineffective action
- Unsupportive subculture
- Lack of mutual support among family members
- Temporary family disorganization
- Alterations in family roles
- Concurrent situational or developmental crises within family circle

❖ Related Medical/Psychiatric Diagnoses

The following are examples of related medical/psychiatric diagnoses for Ineffective Family Coping: Compromised[32]:
- Adjustment disorder
- Anxiety disorder
- Avoidance disorder
- Conduct disorder
- Dependent personality disorder
- Malingering
- Occupational problem

X

- Other specified family circumstances
- Parent-child problem

Ineffective Family Coping: Disabling

This occurs when the family perceives itself to be immobilized or incapacitated and is not able to therapeutically adapt to the stressful event. This can be sudden or chronic.

Defining characteristics of this nursing diagnosis include both objective and subjective data. The nurse assesses for objective data, which includes neglect among the family members related to basic human needs or treatment modalities. This is evidenced by lack of dental hygiene, undernutrition, or altered skin integrity related to immobility. Desertion of family members occurs frequently with multiple losses or stress events and when family dynamics are destructive. Sometimes families carry on usual family routines without regard to a family member's needs, such as when an elderly parent is taken into a family but isolated to a bedroom except for meals. In other situations, an authoritarian family member will make decisions that are detrimental to the social well-being or economic well-being of another family member, such as denying participation in religious or community activities or inappropriate institutionalization. Lack of restructuring of a meaningful life for an individual family member can occur when a family member facing the health challenge is overprotected and cultivates learned helplessness. Neglectful relationships with other family members can occur when there is work overload, unrealistic expectations, and/or lack of understanding in developing and maintaining healthy family relationships.

Subjective data can include: (1) reported distortion and/or denial of the family member's health problem; (2) reported feelings of rejection, intolerance, violence, or abandonment among family members; (3) verbalized psychosomatic tendencies within the family system; (4) reported feelings of agitation, depression, aggression, or hostility within the family circle; (5) family members comment about presence of family intolerance, rejection, abandonment, and neglectful relation-

ships; and (6) family members report that the family seems to be immobilized and out of control.[5-9]

When ineffective family coping is disabling, some degree of family dysfunction exists.[2,3] For example, a family can exhibit a closed family system in which family members must be cautious about what they say and to whom they communicate.[11,23] There is generally a family myth that all family members are to think and feel the same way. If additional family stress events occur, family stress increases and the family becomes more disabled in its coping behavior(s). As the family becomes more disabled, isolation from friends, community, church begins to increase. In turn, the family becomes more alone, more neglectful of relationships, less competent in interacting with extrafamilial support systems, and unhealthy in family dynamics.

Related factors that may affect Ineffective Family Coping: Disabling are multiple. These factors include, but are not limited to: family ethnicity (because of such factors as cultural identity, communication, health belief values); family history of limited and/or ineffective coping strategies such as denial, exploitation of one or more of the family members by scapegoating or violence; and highly ambivalent family relationships such as anger, hostility, resentment. Also, chronically unexpressed feelings such as guilt, anxiety, and anger; chronicity of the health challenge, increased multiple stress events that deplete the family's supportive capacity, and family resistance of family and human services place families at risk for Ineffective Family Coping: Disabling. A knowledge deficit related to areas such as stress, coping, healthy family dynamics and functioning, effective communication skills, and available family and human services is also a risk factor. As the number of risk factors increases, the family becomes more prone to disabled family coping, which can result in pathologic family dysfunction.

❖ Defining Characteristics

The presence of the following defining characteristics indicates that the family may be experiencing Ineffective Family Coping: Disabling[1,15]:

Objective	Subjective
• Neglectful care of family members	• Reported distortion and/or denial of a family member's health problem
• Desertion	• Severe anxiety
• Unhealthy coping behavior(s)	• Severe depression
• Lack of a meaning-ful and healthy fam-ily life	• Severe aggression
• Distortion of a fam-ily member's health challenge, including extreme denial re-garding its presence or severity	• Psychosomatic ten-dencies in family members
	• Family intolerance
	• Family rejection
• Family decision(s) or actions that are detrimental to the economic or social well-being of family members	• Family abandon-ment
	• Family powerless-ness
	• Neglectful family relationships

❖ **Related Factors**

The following related factors are associated with Ineffective Family Coping: Disabling[1,15]:

- Lack of support from subculture
- Family history of ineffective coping strategies
- Highly ambivalent family relationships
- Chronically unex-pressed negative feelings among fam-ily members
- Chronicity of the health challenge
- Multiple stress events and/or situa-tional crises
- Depletion of the family's supportive capacity
- Family resistance of or refusal to use supportive services
- Knowledge deficit about healthy family functioning, coping, communication skills, and utiliza-tion of professional services

❖ **Related Medical/Psychiatric Diagnoses**

The following are examples of related medical/psychiatric diagnoses for Ineffective Family Coping: Disabling[32]:

- Alcohol dependence
- Dependent personality
- Explosive disorder
- Factitious disorder
- Major depression
- Malingering
- Multiple personality disorder
- Other specified family circumstance
- Pathologic gambling
- Recurrent social phobia

NURSING DIAGNOSES

Examples of *specific* nursing diagnoses for Family Coping: Potential for Growth include:

- Family Coping: Potential for Growth related to constructive family coping strategies
- Family Coping: Potential for Growth related to various family perceptions and knowledge asso-ciated with organ donation
- Family Coping: Potential for Growth related to successful family life-cycle transition as evi-denced by joining of step families
- Family Coping: Potential for Growth related to family history of problem-solving ability

Examples of *specific* nursing diagnoses for In-effective Family Coping: Compromised include:

- Ineffective Family Coping: Compromised re-lated to chronic nature of health challenge
- Ineffective Family Coping: Compromised re-lated to anger
- Ineffective Family Coping: Compromised re-lated to alteration of family roles
- Ineffective Family Coping: Compromised re-lated to spiritual distress

Examples of *specific* nursing diagnoses for In-effective Family Coping: Disabling include:

- Ineffective Family Coping: Disabling related to family resistance to treatment
- Ineffective Family Coping: Disabling related to chronic nature of illness of family member
- Ineffective Family Coping: Disabling related to family history of ineffective coping
- Ineffective Family Coping: Disabling related to depletion of the family's supportive capacity

PLANNING AND IMPLEMENTATION WITH RATIONALE

The ultimate expected family outcome related to family coping nursing diagnoses is effective family coping. Nursing interventions can be conceptualized into five major areas: (1) ongoing family assessment, (2) promotion of family strengths, (3) facilitation of family education (supportive and informational), (4) enhancement of the continuity of family caring, and (5) facilitation of family resource referrals.

Family Coping: Potential for Growth

Family outcomes for this nursing diagnosis include: enhancement of health promotion behaviors as a family unit; identification by individual

---

❖ *NURSING CARE GUIDELINES*

Family Coping: Potential for Growth

Expected Family Outcome	Nursing Interventions
Family members and the family as a unit will move toward health-promoting behaviors, such as the expression of hope; healthy nutrition, exercise, and sleeping behaviors; control of modifiable risk factors for heart attacks that are consistent with life-cycle transitions and healthy relationships.	• Determine family unit composition, presenting family dynamics, stage of family growth, effect of presenting stressor(s), and range of family coping strategies. • Assist family to identify meaningful health-promotion behaviors. • Establish a healthy relationship with family. • Facilitate new methods for goal attainment to maximize family growth.
Family members will assess their own role in family growth.	• Provide time for family members to interact privately. • Provide information as needed to enhance individual/family growth. • Monitor areas in which knowledge or understanding is inadequate. • Note expressions related to changes in family perceptions, values.
Family unit will utilize additional resources for support, such as community health nursing, family services, health specialists, or support groups.	• Provide appropriate referrals for expanding family resources. • Provide information. • Respect family choices for referrals.
Family members will express positive feelings related to family unit growth.	• Assist family in using effective communication skills (e.g., "I feel . . . ," "I perceive. . . ," "I prefer . . ."); active listening to one another; and honest and direct communication. • Facilitate experiences in which the family can be supportive of one another. • Assist family in expressing and coping with individual and family feelings. • Provide continuity and consistency in family care.

X

family members of their role responsibilities for family growth; utilization of family or human services resources, and positive cognitive appraisal among family members about family growth and the presenting health challenge.

Most families in situational crisis are viewed as healthy but temporarily in need of support; thus the nurse intervenes by promoting family competence or family strengths in order for the family to *problem-solve, strengthen family competence, and cope.*[12,23] Health promotion behaviors are multiple: nutritional, sleep, and exercise patterns; circular questions (versus structural) within the family; respect for family time; and expansion of family coping strategies and/or problem-solving strengths. Family strengths are respected by the nurse; this *fosters the family support system(s) and family health.*

A caring presence among family members *enables trust.*[24] Information related to stress, coping skills, external family resources, etc., *expands the family unit's knowledge base and enhances opportunities for family growth.* When the nurse and family interact and the family feels respected and secure in expressing questions or concerns, *family growth is enhanced.* There is a climate of openness, the exploration of options, and a movement toward each other (rather than against or away from). In turn, families perceive the presenting health challenge as a positive stress (rather than distress).[12]

Ineffective Family Coping: Compromised

Family outcomes for this nursing diagnosis include: identification of unhealthy family patterns; family communication related to perceptions of distress; utilization of family human services resources; and family communication of perceptions related to effective coping, family growth, and caring behaviors.

When family functioning is perceived as compromised, there is distress and limited energy for health promotion within the family circle. Focusing on the presenting health challenge and joining the family[25] *enhances the nurse's effectiveness in therapeutic family interventions.* Assisting family

members to share a family unit perspective, as well as their individual perspectives, *expands the family's cognitive appraisal skills.*

A family with a limited knowledge base about various coping strategies, codependence, family dysfunction, management of situational stress events or life-cycle transitions, attention-focusing skills, and relational communication among family members can be offered informational and supportive education to begin to *examine family behaviors and their effects on others.*[23,27] By avoiding making value judgments and by affirming family strengths or competence in responding to the presenting health challenge, *the nurse fosters security and trust.* Nursing interventions require sensitivity, privacy, prioritization of educational needs (when teaching areas are multiple), and respect for family perspectives and values. In turn, *the family experiences being family within an educational climate, and family growth is promoted.* Selected nursing interventions are offered by Miles,[24] who studied family caring when a child dies; Hickey,[13] OMalley,[26] and Titler,[31] who studied family needs of the critically ill; and Soukup,[30] who studied family stress associated with organ donation.

The nurse plays a significant role in facilitating appropriate referrals based on family assessment, family choice, and respect for unique family needs and values. *The family needs to be supported for competence (not failure), assisted in their understanding that a family specialist's assistance is viewed as normal (not pathologic), and shown that through such an experience most families work to strengthen family competence (not guilt).* Also, *most families are considered healthy, but during multiple stress events or first experiences with a stressful health challenge are in need of temporary supportive assistance by appropriate professionals.*[19,25] Family human service resources/referrals include extended family, friends, community, and professional assistive resources. Examples may include hospice programs, community health nursing, meals on wheels, pastoral ministry, social services, or family therapy/human services. Nurses can be instru-

Ineffective Family Coping: Compromised

Expected Family Outcome	Nursing Interventions
Family members and the family as a unit will move toward health-promoting behaviors such as caring behaviors, relational communication skills, and a decrease in codependent behaviors to maintain family integrity.	• Determine the family unit composition, family dynamics, range of family coping behaviors, and effect of presenting health challenge on family system. • Establish a healthy relationship with family. • Assist the family to appraise the presenting health challenge and the degree of effectiveness of present family coping. • Assist the family to identify roles to maintain family integrity.
Family members will verbalize educational needs and expectations for self and for the family as a unit.	• Assist the family members to verbalize distress from their own perspective and from a family perspective. • Present an overview of potential family educational areas (such as relational communication skills, coping skills, attention-focusing skills, problem-solving skills). • Assist the family to prioritize needs. • Develop a teaching plan related to these needs, including a family assessment of outcomes.
The family will utilize additional resources to preserve the family supportive capacity.	• Provide an overview of appropriate and available extrafamilial resources. • Provide a climate for family decision-making. • Assist the family in accessing resources. • Monitor family perceptions regarding accessing resources and experiences in using extrafamilial resources. • Facilitate changes as needed.
Family members will express positive feelings related to family strengths and growth.	• Assist the family in using effective communication skills, active listening to one another, or honest, clear communication (e.g., "I cope by . . . ," "When this happens, I feel . . . . ," "I prefer . . . ,"). • Facilitate experiences in which family members can practice being supportive and relational to one another (e.g., role playing, script acting, modeling). • Assist the family in expressing present feelings from both an individual and family perspective (for instance "I feel that I am . . ." and "I feel that my family is angry, withdrawing . . ..").
Family members will verbalize satisfaction with the continuity of family care and their competence in developing effective behaviors.	• Provide regular family conferences for supportive and informational sharing. • Facilitate experiences for family to share feelings regarding quality and presence of continuity of family care; refine nursing interventions as appropriate. • Affirm the family's competence in using healthy coping behaviors through honest appraisals and personal affirmations.

X

mental to families in monitoring for system dysfunction/failure after referrals because, *as a family advocate, the nurse continues to assess family perceptions throughout the referral process.* Encouragement to use extrafamilial resources can also be useful *to preserve the supportive capacity of family members over time.* In turn, *the family's capacity to care and to cope is affirmed with a new focus.*

The nurse can assist the family in identifying family strengths and coping strategies that can be assessed as healthy and less healthy. Family coping skills that *contribute to family health* can be learned. Family coping skills can be strengthened by experience (practice), or by altering (refining) or expanding the range of healthy coping strategies. In turn, *when facing future stress events, the family will have more resources on which to rely.* For example, sometimes an extremely disengaged family, with an overfunctioning parent who dominates the family decision-making, can be assisted to teach and share responsibilities, engage in consensus-type family decision-making, and experience relational (versus structural) communication within the family circle. Role playing, script acting, and modeling can be a useful learning strategy because *family members can practice being supportive of one another.*

Multidisciplinary, regularly held family conferences provide enrichment opportunities for the family.[12] Perceptions can be shared related to the presenting health challenge, decision-making, effectiveness of coping behaviors (individual and as a family unit), or utilization of and satisfaction with external familial resources. Other nursing interventions related to continuity of family care include: monitoring family educational growth related to coping, assessing family comfort level in sharing feelings related to positive as well as negative stressors, and follow-up activities related to referrals or use of external family resources. In turn, *continuity of family caring is respected and fostered.*

Ineffective Family Coping: Disabling

Unhealthy Family Coping: Disabling may occur suddenly in response to a stressful event or more subtly when the chronicity of the health challenge has depleted the limited or underdeveloped supportive family capacities. In turn, *safety and care of family members become a high nursing priority,* and immediate protection or support is offered (e.g., protection from further child, spouse, or elder abuse or physical care of the family member who has had physical or mental impairments, such as quadriplegia or Alzheimer's disease). Ongoing nursing assessment requires monitoring for change in the family member's coping behaviors and for positive outcomes within the family.[25,29] Nursing intervention(s) are prescribed (or refined) to meet the family's need *to promote healthy family coping behaviors.* Multidisciplinary collaboration and referrals to family human services are often important nursing interventions. Family assessment provides meaningful data *that will offer significant contributions to family health.* Through the assessment process, *the family members' humanness is respected.*

Referral to family and human services is important to consider early in the intervention process. *Multiple and complex preexisting situational stress events often precipitate the development of disabled family coping* (e.g., abortion, divorce, altered economic status, altered employment, family separation, loss of loved one or personal items, rape trauma, family relocation, and family dismemberment). Ineffective coping can also be caused by medical-related situational stressors, including substance abuse, depression, chronic or terminal illness, altered body image, and emotional disorders. Referring the family to professional services offers *multidisciplinary collaboration and support for changing the family members' unhealthy coping behaviors and fostering their strength.* Through this type of intervention, *the presenting stressor becomes an opportunity for developing family competence, affirming family strengths, and promoting family health.* In this way, Ineffective Family Coping: Disabling has potential to change to Family Coping: Potential for Growth.

Family education, both supportive and informational, is essential in changing unhealthy family coping behaviors. When family coping is disabling, there is frequently family distress and blame, family resistance to educational interventions, and avoidance behaviors. After assessing the family's readiness, the nurse often intervenes by first establishing a supportive relationship within the family, and then assisting family members to describe the current health challenge and the meaning it has had for them and the other family members. The nurse listens attentively to family members' perceptions, such as feelings associated with mandatory attendance at the family dinners. The nurse must be careful not to judge their feelings or expressions, but rather to assist family members in discovering behaviors for healthy family living. For example, a healthy family life requires more than observance of weddings, birthdays, and other social ceremonies. Pearsall[27] encourages families to focus on being together as compared with the "doing obsession." The family is then encouraged to work on one small dimension of the presenting health challenge.

When the presenting health challenge becomes focused on an individual, the nurse assists the family to focus instead on changing their behavior and redirecting tasks so that *the family can actively participate in bringing about healthy behavior changes.* For example, if the mother overfunctions in caring for her ventilatory-dependent quadriplegic teen-aged son, and this has resulted in altered family dynamics and isolation, the teen-aged brother could be encouraged to spend 15 minutes a day with his brother on a specific task, such as communication. This may include the brother blinking his eyes in response to words, phrases, feelings, or needs. In turn, a word, phrase, or needs chart can be used so that both vision and auditory senses are stimulated. Therefore *communication within the family becomes increasingly clear, efficient, and continuous.* By giving other family members responsibility for selected aspects of the patient's care and decision-making, *the burden on primary care-givers can be lessened, while family strengths are increased.*

It is extremely important that an authoritarian family member does not dominate decision-making, as evidenced by remarks such as, "He will do this," "She will do that," or "Joe does not need you for . . ." This authoritarian family member must be consistently helped in reframing negative expressions into positive ones whenever the opportunity presents itself. The overfunctioning family member needs to be affirmed in his/her family role responsibilities and in guiding the family through transition. Other family members' preferences, capabilities, and creative ways of participating or caring must be explored, encouraged, and valued so that *family integrity is revitalized.* Transforming family guilt and faults into family strengths is an important nursing intervention and often *prepares the family for more intense family education* in other areas, such as stress, coping, and healthy family functioning.

A family with a limited knowledge about coping strategies, management of situational stress events or life-cycle transitions, or relational communication skills within the family may or may not be aware of its options. Sometimes education involves *assisting the family to appreciate the need for change.* Pearsall[27] notes the diminishing role of the family attending worship services. The ritual of families dressing up together and sitting, listening, and praying together has been replaced by sleeping through services, either in places of worship or in front of the television. Thus nursing interventions require sensitivity, privacy, prioritization of educational needs (when teaching areas are multiple), and respect for family perspectives and values. In turn, the family experiences being a family in this educational climate, and *family growth is promoted.*

Continuity of family care for a family with disabled coping requires direct nursing interventions. *If the safety of a selected family member or members is a concern,* the nurse immediately intervenes through appropriate referrals that may or may not involve an immediate response. Those requiring immediate response include child or elder abuse, abandonment of an immobilized family member, or family needs related to accessing the

X

❖ NURSING CARE GUIDELINES
Ineffective Family Coping: *Disabling*

Expected Family Outcome	Nursing Interventions
Family members and the family as a unit will develop health-promoting behaviors in response to the presenting health challenge.	• Evaluate the family unit composition, subculture support, presenting family dynamics, range of family coping behaviors, and quality of family communication patterns. • Establish a healthy relationship with the family. • Assist the family to appraise the presenting health challenge and the degree of family effectiveness in meeting this presenting health challenge. • Assess readiness of the family to adopt alternative ways of responding to the presenting health challenge. • Respect each family member's individual responses (e.g., withdrawal, resistance, anger, blame, verbal assault); intervene appropriately and with supportive caring. • Assist the family to identify roles to maintain family integrity while responding to the health challenge.
The family will utilize family and human services to preserve the family's supportive capacity.	• Provide information about appropriate and available external family resources. • Encourage family to focus on small aspects of the health challenge (those requiring the more immediate attention) rather than all dimensions of it. • Provide a climate for family decision-making. • Assist family in locating and using resources. • Monitor family perceptions about resources and their experiences in accessing and using resources; facilitate changes as needed.
The family members will verbalize educational needs and expectations for self and for the family as a unit.	• Assist the family members to verbalize perceptions of coping behaviors from own perspective. • Present an overview of potential family educational areas (e.g., relational communication skills, family stress and coping skills, family dynamics, and healthy family functioning during family transitions). • Assist family in prioritizing needs. • Develop a teaching plan for identified needs, including a family assessment of outcomes.
The family members will verbalize satisfaction with the continuity of family care and their competence in developing effective behaviors.	• Provide regular family conferences for supportive and informational sharing. • Provide opportunities for the family to share feelings about the quality and continuity of family care; refine nursing interventions as appropriate. • Affirm family competence in healthy coping behaviors with honest appraisals and through personal affirmations. • Assist family to select a family day each month dedicated to the renewal of family energy, caring, and connection.

X

medical or professional systems. Regular family conferences in which family members can share their perceptions and freely express feelings about the present health challenge and its effect on each one of them, as well as on the family as a whole, remain an ongoing nursing priority. Other nursing interventions related to continuity of family care include: (1) providing clear and accurate information about the present health challenge and the available community resources and professional assistance; (2) acting as a liaison and family advocate within the multidisciplinary team; (3) assessing and clarifying the family's communication skills for effectiveness and healthy patterns; (4) assessing the family's attempt to cope effectively and affirming healthy coping behavior changes; (5) fostering the expansion of family social skills over time; and (6) monitoring the quality of family satisfaction with selected tasks, referrals, or use of external family resources. Through these measures, *continuity of family caring is provided while the family becomes more competent in developing or expanding healthy coping skills. Over time, the family moves from disabling coping to another form of family coping: Ineffective Family Coping: Compromised or Family Coping: Potential for Growth.*

EVALUATION

Evaluation of nursing diagnoses related to family coping is based on achievement of family outcomes. These may be perceived as satisfactory or unsatisfactory. Refinement of nursing interventions may be required not because the nursing interventions were inappropriate when formulated, but because family dynamics are in constant change, new data are contributed, and new priorities emerge. The evaluation process requires regular and ongoing evaluation with participation by both family and health professionals. Of importance is continuity of care that is provided by the same nurse(s) so that family competence can be strengthened and family growth can be affirmed. Whether family coping related to these nursing di-

agnoses is transitory or long term, opportunities are offered for creative vision and growth for the family as well as for the nurse.

Family Coping: Potential for Growth

Family reporting will provide the nurse and family with the most definitive evaluation of achievement of expected family outcomes related to this nursing diagnosis. Growth areas can include: family stability and security in the present situation, realistic future plans, respect for individual family members' privacy, mutual trust, healthy love without possessiveness, commitment to and shared responsibility for the family unit, support for individual family members, flexibility of family roles, and a sense of play and humor.

Ineffective Family Coping: Compromised

Successful family outcomes related to this nursing diagnosis are achieved when the family (1) demonstrates and communicates a decrease in family distress, (2) demonstrates a deeper commitment to and shared responsibility for family and family members, (3) uses appropriate external familial resources, and (4) perceives and communicates family growth toward effective family coping.

Ineffective Family Coping: Disabling

The measures to evaluate success will be both formative (i.e., family perceptions) and cumulative. Initially, there would be family acknowledgement of the difficulty of the presenting health challenge. Over time healthy family coping skills would be evidenced by open and honest family expressions of feelings (including anger, hopelessness, or frustration) and reported decrease in family distress. Family utilization of professional resources and learning opportunities would be perceived as generally helpful. Finally, the family would demonstrate and verbalize healthy family energy in meeting the presenting health challenge, with a healthy balance between personal and family commitments.

X

❖ *CASE STUDY WITH PLAN OF CARE*

Mrs. Mary F., abandoned by her husband, is a single parent of three children. Jane is 14 years old, a tenth-grade student, and has become increasingly silent and sad within the family circle. Tammy, 6 years old, has frequent temper tantrums, which usually conclude with her voicing her fears to her imaginary friend. Joe, 4 years old, has become very tearful and quiet, with frequent expressions such as, "If I do this, maybe daddy will come back. . ." Mrs. F. is a full-time night nurse, and she often leaves Jane in charge of the children while she sleeps on Saturday and Sunday mornings. Mealtime, a once happy family time, has become a tense ritual in which the family must eat together; it is marked by long periods of distressful silence or emotional outbursts. Family bickering has increased. Television has replaced all forms of family recreation. The presenting health challenge focuses on Mrs. F., a very competent mother and nurse, who was recently diagnosed with the human immunodeficiency virus (HIV) infection related to a professional incident. She is facing a difficult personal and professional challenge, including role transition.

Mrs. F. informs her nursing supervisor that she will be absent from work for a few weeks and that she plans to remove Jane from school to care for the children during this time and perhaps in the future when she is feeling exhausted. The nursing supervisor, through a hospital philosophy of caring for families of patients and employees, assesses the family situation as *Ineffective Family Coping: Disabling* related to multiple losses and stressors contributing to unhealthy coping patterns, nonrelational communication, and ineffective decision-making within the family. Mrs. F., with support from her supervisor, is invited to develop a general family plan of care for her own family in response to this health challenge.

PLAN OF CARE FOR THE F. FAMILY

Nursing Diagnosis: *Ineffective Family Coping: Disabling related to multiple losses and stressors contributing to unhealthy coping patterns, nonrelational communication, and ineffective decision-making within the family.*

Expected Family Outcome	**Nursing Interventions:**
The family members will develop health-promoting behaviors as evidenced by effective decision-making, coping skills, nutritional choices, and relational communications.	• Engage an extra familial professional, chosen by the family, to provide family counseling and therapy. • Establish a healthy relationship with family. • Respect family members' individual responses to the health challenge. • Assist family members in identifying appropriate roles that maintain family integrity while responding to the presenting health challenge. • Assist family to engage in healthy lifestyle decisions such as making healthy food choices. • Teach and support decision-making skills.
The family unit will use family and human services such as professional family therapy, fiscal planning, and child care as needed, to preserve the family supportive capacity and growth.	• Provide a climate for family awareness in locating and using resources. • Facilitate referrals that meet needs (immediate and long term) identified in family needs assessment. • Monitor family perceptions and outcomes related to use of these resources.

X

Expected Family Outcome	**Nursing Interventions:**
The family members will verbalize continuity of caring and growth as evidenced by relational communication, minimization of verbal abuse, and participation in the family plan of care.	• Provide opportunities for the family to share feelings openly and honestly. • Provide regular family conferences for supportive and informational sharing with professionals. • Monitor unrealistic expectations regarding children and encourage use of alternate community resources (e.g., child care, assistance with meals, community nursing). • Facilitate situations that enhance the development of social skills outside of the family circle and that are appropriate for the child and mother. • Affirm family competence in healthy coping behaviors with honest appraisal and personal affirmations. • Encourage family affirmations for times of disability, such as, "We need help to understand why this illness crisis is happening and we must find ways together to find the creativity, strength, and courage to carry on."

REFERENCES

1. American Association of Critical-Care Nurses, Kuhn R, and others, editors: *AACN outcome standards for nursing care of the critically ill,* Laguna Niguel, Calif, 1990, American Association of Critical Care Nurses.
2. Arnold L: Codependency, I: origins, characteristics, *AORN J* 51(5):1341-1348, 1990.
3. Arnold L: Codependency, II: the hospital as a dysfunctional family, *AORN J,* 51(6):1581-1584, 1990.
4. Artinian N: Stress experience of spouses of patients having coronary artery bypass during hospitalization and six weeks after discharge, *Heart Lung* 20(1):52-29, 1991.
5. Baker J: Family adaptation when one member has a head injury, *J Neurosci Nurs* 22(4):232-237, 1990.
6. Boeing M, Mongera C: Powerlessness in critical care patients, *Dimen Crit Care Nurs* 8(5):274-275, 1989.
7. Clark S: Nursing diagnosis: ineffective coping, I. A theoretical framework, *Heart Lung* 16(6):670-674, 1987.
8. Clark S: Nursing diagnosis: ineffective coping, II. Planning care, *Heart Lung* 16(6):677-683, 1987.
9. Copp L: The spectrum of suffering . . . an AJN classic, *Am J Nurs* 90(8):35-39, 1990.
10. Cowles K: Issues in qualitative research on sensitive topics, *West J Nurs Res* 10(2):163-179, 1988.
11. Friel J, Friel L: *Adult children: the secrets of dysfunctional families,* Deerfield Beach, Fla, 1988, Health Communications.
12. Halm M: Effects of support groups on anxiety of family members during critical illness, *Heart Lung* 19(1):62-71, 1990.
13. Hickey M: What are the needs of families of critically ill patients? A review of the literature since 1976, *Heart Lung* 19(4):401-415, 1990.
14. Hogan S: Care for the caregiver: social policies to ease their burden, *J Gerontol Nurs* 16(5):12-17, 1990.
15. Kim M, McFarland G, and McLane A: *Pocket guide to nursing diagnoses,* ed 4, St Louis, 1991, Mosby–Year Book.
16. Krach P: Filial responsibility and financial strain: the impact on farm families, *J Gerontol Nurs* 16(7):38-43, 1990.
17. Lavee L, McCubbin H, and Olson D: The effect of stressful life events and transitions on family functioning and well being, *J Marriage Fam* 49:857-873, 1987.
18. Lazarus R, Folkman S: *Stress, appraisal, and coping,* New York, 1984, Springer.
19. Leahey M, Wright L: *Families and life-threatening illness,* Springhouse, Penn, 1987, Springhouse.
20. Loos F, and others: Circular questions: a family interviewing strategy, *DCCN* 9(1):46-53, 1990.
21. McCubbin H, Thompson A, editors: *Family assessment inventories for research and practice,* Madison, Wisc, 1987, University of Wisconsin, Madison.
22. McGoldrick M, Pearce J, and Giordano J, editors: *Ethnicity and family therapy,* New York, 1982, The Guilford Press.
23. Mellody P: *Facing codependence,* San Francisco Calif, 1989, Harper & Row.
24. Miles P: Caring for families when a child dies, *Pediatr Nurs* 16(4):346-349, 1990.
25. Minuchin S: *Families and family therapy,* Cambridge, Mass, 1974, Harvard University Press.
26. O'Malley P, and others: Critical care nurse perceptions of family needs, *Heart Lung* 20(2):183-188, 1991.
27. Pearsall P: *The power of the family,* New York, 1987, Doubleday.
28. Robinson P, Roe H, and Boys L: The focus of hospitals on family care, *Health Values* 2(2):19-23, 1987.
29. Satir V: *Conjoint family therapy: your many faces,* Palo Alto, Calif, 1967, Science & Behavior.

X

30. Soukup M: Organ donation from the family of a totally brain-dead donor: professional responsiveness, *Crit Care Nurs Q* 13(4):8-18, 1991.

31. Titler M, Cohen M, and Craft M: Impact of adult critical care hospitalization: perceptions of patients, spouses, children, and nurses, *Heart Lung* 20(2):174-182, 1991.

32. Williams J (text editor): *DMS-III-R,* Washington, DC, 1987, American Psychiatric Association.

X

XI

VALUE—BELIEF PATTERN
Spiritual Distress

Spiritual Distress is a disruption in a person's life principle that pervades entire being and integrates and transcends biological and psychosocial nature.[8]

OVERVIEW

Nurses, as dictated by ANA's Social Policy Statement, have a role and a responsibility in the diagnosis and treatment of human responses to actual or potential health problems.[2] Spiritual responses to actual or potential health problems should be of central concern to nurses. A person's spirituality and extent of spiritual needs are personal, intimate, and subjective areas, and no human definition will ever capture the profound and essential meaning of a person's spiritual needs.

Because nurses treat patients holistically, they cannot ignore the spiritual dimension of the person. A person is a composite of body, mind, and spirit, and just as there are physical and psychological needs in every person, there are spiritual needs as well. Nurses are in a key position to assist patients in meeting their spiritual needs. Most often, the nurse has the unique opportunity to spend time with patients and can observe for signs and symptoms of Spiritual Distress.

The spirit is an integral part of the total person and wholly essential if one is to consider the patient a total and integrated being. A person's spiritual dimension is not restricted to religious beliefs and practices, but it does include the religious aspect. It encompasses a person's total existence and is responsible for the actualization of life. The spirit exists and is actualized only in humans. It helps to center and focus a person's life[5]:

It is the spirit of human beings which enables and motivates us to search for meaning and purpose in life, to seek the supernatural or some meaning which transcends us, to wonder about our origins and our identities, to require morality and equity. It is the spirit which synthesizes the total personality and provides some sense of energizing direction and order.

Paloutzian and Ellison[5, 11a] describe spiritual well-being as two-dimensional, involving both vertical and horizontal components. Both dimensions involve transcendence or moving beyond the physical world. The vertical dimension, which measures religious well-being, refers to one's sense of well-being in relation to God. The horizontal dimension, which measures existential well-being, refers to a nonreligious sense of life purpose and life satisfaction.

According to Amenta[1] the spiritual dimension is expressed in many ways. Beliefs, practices, and rituals of formal religion are one form of expression of the spiritual dimension. Other ways of expressing the spiritual dimension are through our relationships with self, with others, and with anything greater or more enduring than the self.

Piles[12] describes the spiritual dimension as that part of the person that seeks to worship someone or something (such as God) outside one's own powers that controls and/or sustains the person, especially in a time of crisis. The spiritual dimension cannot be defined scientifically, but according to Piles[12] it integrates and transcends the biological and psychological nature manifested through observable behaviors.

Fish and Shelly[7] defined spiritual needs as the absence of any factor or factors necessary to establish and maintain a dynamic relationship with God. They perceived three factors as contributing to this relationship with God: meaning and purpose, love and relatedness, and forgiveness.

Spiritual needs arise from one's inner depths and urge one to pursue life-giving questions. They have many definitions, but they are commonly known as a factor that enables or motivates a person to seek, establish, and maintain a relationship with God or a greater meaning that transcends the person. Essentially, all human beings have the same spiritual needs regardless of specific religious beliefs.

Every person's spiritual quest and pilgrimage is a lifelong journey of growth toward wholeness or integration. This process of becoming involves constant growth and change. The journey toward wholeness encompasses a person, his/her individual qualities, and all of his/her strengths, weaknesses, sorrows, and joys. The challenge is to continually move forward with hope and find meaning in life, even in situations that may appear meaningless.

When confronted with an illness, the person may experience a threat to personal wholeness and well-being. It makes no difference whether the illness is physical or psychological, because the body, mind, and inner spirit are united in such a way that what affects one dimension will affect the others. Because of this unity of the human person, an injury or illness has an effect on the whole person. Suffering and illness often force a person to face ultimate issues, questions, and meanings of life. Illness can disrupt a person's life, necessitating adaptation. In the face of illness, a person may be confronted with the reality of one's existence; relationships with self, others, and God; and perhaps even with one's own death. When life brings to us some unforeseen, unwelcome, life-disrupting reality, we fluctuate between confusion and clarity, between courage and cowardice.[13] Confronted with such crises, a person may exhibit signs of Spiritual Distress.

ASSESSMENT

In view of nursing's concern and focus on the total person, nurses should learn to recognize pa-

tients' expressions of Spiritual Distress. The total patient, in all dimensions, is assessed to identify needs and formulate nursing diagnoses, which may include Spiritual Distress. Data the nurse collects will be the basis for a specific patient care plan. The initial assessment can also be the basis for a more in-depth spiritual assessment.

The assessment of a patient's spiritual dimension does not depend on the nurse's religious beliefs or practices. However, it does rely on the nurse's knowledge and use of the nursing process. The nurse-patient relationship provides the context for the assessment of spiritual needs. An ongoing assessment is essential in this relationship, and the nurse must be available for the patient. Through research, Stiles[15] found that nurses described their being available to families and patients as critical to their relationships. The patient's family or significant other can provide important data in assessing Spiritual Distress.

When assessing a patient's spiritual dimension, the nurse should observe any cues or indications that the patient has spiritual concerns. A listening ear and sensitivity to tiny clues are necessary assessment skills in identifying spiritual needs.[12] More explicitly, the nurse should look for clues, behaviors, and attitudes indicating the patient's response to the present situation. Patients' expressions or indications of hope and meaning in their lives and their relationship with self, others, and God as revealed through words or behavior can signify areas of spiritual concern. Physical symptoms such as loss of appetite, sleep disturbances, muscular tension, and inattentiveness to appearance can also be signs of spiritual distress. Rarely do patients exhibit a clear and definite set of signs and symptoms. Defining characteristics for the nursing diagnosis Spiritual Distress predominantly comprise subjective data. Therefore it is imperative that the nurse's skills of listening, exploring, and validating be used throughout this process.

A person's spirituality is frequently expressed through religious beliefs and practices and culture. Illness often disrupts the person's customary expression of these practices. This can lead to isolation, anxiety, doubt, and fear, of which the nurse should be aware.

Any illness poses the potential for Spiritual Distress; however, the more life-threatening the illness, the greater the potential. Persons with a terminal illness or chronic illness also possess a greater potential for experiencing spiritual needs. When the patient is initially confronted with an illness, he/she may express anger toward God or others. Because a High Risk for Spiritual Distress always exists when a patient is confronted with illness, the nurse's assessment skills are paramount.

Several spiritual assessment tools or guides have been developed to elicit data about the spiritual dimension of the person. The assessment tools are not all specific for the nursing diagnosis of Spiritual Distress, but they do elicit data pertaining to spiritual needs or concerns. Stoll[16] proposed a spiritual assessment that focuses on four major areas of the person: concept of God or deity, source of strength and hope, significance of religious practices and rituals, and the perceived relationship between spiritual beliefs and state of health. O'Brien[11] developed a spiritual assessment guide to investigate a patient's spiritual beliefs and practices. The areas in which a patient is assessed are general spiritual beliefs, personal spiritual beliefs, identification with institutionalized religion, spiritual or religious support systems and rituals, and spiritual deficit or distress.

Two tools have been developed to measure spiritual concerns and spiritual well-being. The Spiritual and Religious Concerns Questionnaire (SRQ) was developed by Silber and Reilly[14] to objectively measure hospitalized adolescents' spiritual and religious concerns and needs. It also analyzes beliefs and attitudes. This tool does not directly assess Spiritual Distress, but it can indicate spiritual concerns of adolescents. A high SRQ score might suggest spiritual and religious concerns, leading to further evaluation and intervention. Paloutzian and Ellison developed a Spiritual Well-Being Scale (SWBS) that measures a person's religious and existential well-being.[5, 11a] Although the Spiritual Well-Being Scale does not assess Spiritual Distress, it assesses spiritual well-being, which expresses spiritual health. The scores of the Spiritual Well-Being Scale could indicate areas of spiritual concern.

These assessment guides, along with the nurse's own assessment skills and awareness of spiritual needs, will provide a basis for developing a patient-centered care plan. Although there are no consistent manifestations of Spiritual Distress, the following specific defining characteristics and related factors are frequently observed and identified.

❖ Defining Characteristics

The presence of the following defining characteristics indicates that the patient may be experiencing Spiritual Distress:

- Somatic complaints such as loss of appetite, muscular tension, headaches, and sleep disturbances
- Regarding illness as a punishment
- Alteration in behavior or mood such as anger, crying, withdrawal, anxiety, or hostility
- Expressions of anger toward God (as defined by that person), self, and others
- Expressions of powerlessness
- Inability to accept self
- Engaging in self-blame
- Denial of responsibility for problems
- Expressions of concern over meaning of life, death, or belief systems
- Inability or refusal to participate in usual religious practices
- Questioning significance of existence and suffering
- Questioning relationship with God
- Seeking spiritual assistance

❖ Related Factors

The following related factors are associated with Spiritual Distress:

- Illness or threat to well-being
- Loss of meaningful roles
- Separation from religious, cultural, or family ties
- Belief and value system that is challenged or questioned

❖ Related Medical/Psychiatric Diagnoses

The following are examples of categories of related medical/psychiatric diagnoses for Spiritual Distress:

XI

- Chronic illnesses (physiologic or psychologic in origin)
- Illnesses altering usual activities or roles
- Illnesses requiring treatments threatening to the quality of life or to life itself
- Life-threatening illnesses

NURSING DIAGNOSES

Examples of *specific* nursing diagnoses for Spiritual Distress are:

- Spiritual Distress related to hospitalization interfering with participation in usual religious rites
- Spiritual Distress related to altered lifestyle resulting from chronic illness
- Spiritual Distress related to conflict between value system and recommended treatment for cancer

PLANNING AND IMPLEMENTATION WITH RATIONALE

The next step in caring for patients with Spiritual Distress is the establishment of expected patient outcomes. Expected outcomes direct the identification of an appropriate plan and focus on attaining wholeness and meaning. The outcomes should be measurable, and whenever possible, they should be set mutually with the patient.

Nurses might question the time involved in assisting patients to fulfill their spiritual needs. However, a long period of time is not necessary; nurses should utilize every available opportunity for patient contact. Planning patient care with the patient will help facilitate communication and establish a therapeutic nurse-patient relationship that will enhance the nursing interventions. Patients benefit from a close relationship between nursing and pastoral care staff that allows personnel in these two disciplines to confer on the spiritual care of patients.

Nursing interventions for patients with Spiritual Distress can be classified into nine general areas: presence, active listening, spiritual counseling, values clarification, reminiscence therapy, crisis intervention, truth telling, relaxation training, and music therapy.[3] Each of the interventions requires

that the nurse be available for the patient. The nurse's presence forms the basis for all interventions and underlies the nurse-patient relationship. It is also an intervention itself. Presence involves a willingness to be available to and for the patient. This availability occurs on physical, psychological, and spiritual levels. Throughout this process, the nurse's gift of self is indispensable.

Active listening is a nursing intervention in which the nurse endeavors to hear what the patient is trying to verbally or nonverbally communicate. *Listening means entering the patient's frame of reference and world view and developing an empathic relationship with him/her.*[4] It requires a commitment to the patient and allows the patient to express guilt, doubts, fears, pain, and suffering. *Active listening also gives patients the opportunity to verbally express anger and allows patients to express feelings with another person.*

Because separation from religious, cultural, or family ties is a related factor in Spiritual Distress, nurses must listen to the patient and assess the patient's religious and cultural background. Fehring and McClane[6] suggest that interventions should be directed toward the nurse providing persons, religious and cultural objects, and resources for religious and cultural rituals.

Spiritual counseling presents a challenge to nurses caring for patients with Spiritual Distress. Not all nurses are comfortable with or have the necessary skills to counsel, but these skills can be learned. Nurses should consult other nurses and professionals in other disciplines to learn counseling so that it can be used when necessary. Three examples of basic nondirective counseling skills that can be used along with listening are open questions, reflection or repetition of the client's last few words, and empathy-building.[4] *Spiritual counseling can help a patient establish meaningful relationships with self, God, and others, which are essential components of the spiritual dimension.*

Basic counseling may assist the patient in releasing emotions and feelings to promote healing. The patient is encouraged to reflect on his/her feelings, discover meaning in the present situa-

XI

tion, and express emotions positively. Throughout the counseling process, the nurse must remain open and sensitive to the patient's needs. *Through counseling a patient may come to experience a greater sense of purpose, meaning, and hope in living with an illness. It also helps the patient to come to an acceptance of self.*

Because a challenged value and belief system is a related factor in Spiritual Distress, clarifying the patient's values can be a therapeutic intervention. *Discussion between nurse and patient about values and life issues assists the patient in clarifying his/her own values, beliefs, and decisions. Values clarification can help patients find joy, hope, and meaning in the present situation.*

Reminiscence therapy involves the exploration of past experiences, feelings, and memories that had significance for the patient. Techniques may include the encouragement of verbal expression or writing of past events, especially those that were painful. A prayer for healing these memories may be included here. This prayer entails a person slowly walking back through his/her past. *During this process, people often discover incidents from long before in which anger, guilt, or other emotions were repressed. When these occurrences are discovered, the person stops and prays for healing. The person may also ask for forgiveness, experience a sense of forgiveness, or forgive someone else if necessary.*

Crisis intervention involves problem-solving techniques that assist a person in working through a crisis, regardless of whether it is physical, psychological, or spiritual. It has no specific tools but involves the process of assessment, planning, intervention, and evaluation. *The goal of crisis intervention is to help the patient move through the crisis as quickly as possible and thereby achieve the same level of psychological comfort as before the crisis.*[9]

❖ NURSING CARE GUIDELINES

Nursing Diagnosis: Spiritual Distress

Expected Patient Outcomes	Nursing Interventions
The patient will experience a greater sense of purpose, meaning, and hope in living with an illness.	• Take time to be available to listen to the patient's expressions and feelings. • Provide time to just be with the patient. • Be honest with the patient. • Use counseling techniques. • Pray with the patient when appropriate.
The patient will express decreased feelings of guilt and experience a sense of forgiveness.	• Using reminiscence therapy, encourage the patient to express past hurts and guilt. • Help the patient to "heal memories." • If appropriate, tell the patient that God loves and accepts people as they are.
The patient will verbally express anger and will discuss his/her feelings with another person.	• Reassure the patient that it is normal and acceptable to feel angry toward God.
The patient will accept self.	• Be an available advocate for the patient's needs. • Use touch to comfort the patient.

XI

Continued.

❖ NURSING CARE GUIDELINES—cont'd

Expected Patient Outcomes	Nursing Interventions
The patient will have a sense of belonging even though he/she is separated from religious practices.	• Inform the patient of available religious resources. • Refer the patient to the spiritual advisor of his/her choice.
The patient will have a clearer understanding and perception of personal beliefs and values.	• Use values clarification. • Refer the patient to other disciplines as needed.
The patient will establish meaningful relationships with self, God, and others.	• Encourage the patient to take responsibility for his/her own life. • Encourage the patient to make positive choices. • Encourage contact with other people.
The patient will develop inner peace through a decrease in somatic complaints and emotional distress.	• Instruct the patient in relaxation techniques, music therapy, and centering prayer.

Because communication is invaluable to the nurse-patient relationship, trust, honesty, openness, and feedback are essential in treating Spiritual Distress. *Truth telling can be used as an intervention by nurses in practicing honest communication with patients.*[10] *The intent of truth telling is (1) to promote more effective coping mechanisms for the individual, (2) to provide information for decision making, (3) to enhance trust in the relationship and in the nursing care, and (4) to give patients what rightfully belongs to them.* This intervention uses problem solving to choose options for truthfulness. *Communication is also a technique that the nurse can use to help the patient achieve a sense of belonging even though the patient is separated from religious practices.*

Relaxation training and music therapy as interventions are helpful in promoting a greater level of openness and harmony. This in turn may allow the person to progress in confronting or working through Spiritual Distress. All the above interventions can be used in helping a patient develop inner peace through a decrease in somatic complaints and emotional distress *by enabling the patient to find hope and meaning in his/her life and relationships with self, God, and others.* Finally, the nurse must use his/her active listening and assessment skills in selecting and implementing the most appropriate plan of care for patients with Spiritual Distress.

EVALUATION

Specific nursing actions are planned to assist patients in fulfilling unmet or partially met needs. The effectiveness of the nursing interventions is evaluated by the patient's expected adaptive behavior. The absence of or decrease in the defining characteristics of Spiritual Distress indicates that spiritual needs are being fulfilled to some extent.

Achievement of each of the identified expected outcomes can be determined by the presence of outcome indicators or criteria. For example, a pa-

❖ *CASE STUDY WITH PLAN OF CARE*

Ms. Cindy S. is a single 28-year-old woman admitted to the hospital for surgical repair of the right subclavian artery. She underwent surgery for division of the anomalous artery with reimplantation in the ascending aorta. Cindy studies nursing and shares an apartment with two friends. She has a close relationship with family members, who live in a neighboring town. During the postoperative recuperation period, she developed complications that prolonged her recovery. Cindy became concerned about the effect of the surgery on her ability to finish her studies and on her future career. She grew increasingly nervous and began to ask, "Will I ever be okay?" and "Will I ever be able to finish school and function as a nurse?" Cindy expressed her fear of weakness and feelings of isolation, loneliness, helplessness, and loss of control. These feelings began to find expression in anger related to this major life disruption. She verbalized her anger at God for allowing this to happen to her. Her incapacity deprived her of her normal outlets for expressing and finding support in such concerns. Ms. S. was unable to participate in the practices of her faith, where she usually had found strength in facing life's challenges. Her inability to concentrate and her growing feeling of lethargy added to her frustrations. It was difficult for Cindy to express these fears and concerns to the nursing staff, because very few nurses took the time to relate at that level. The nurses addressed her physical needs but most nurses did not address the deeper needs of the human spirit. One nurse, however, developed a trusting relationship with Cindy, permitting Cindy to express her fears, anxieties, and concerns. Based on the nurse's assessment of Ms. S., the nursing diagnosis Spiritual Distress was formulated and the following plan of care was proposed.

PLAN OF CARE FOR MS. CINDY S.

Nursing Diagnosis: *Spiritual Distress related to a threat to well-being, loss of meaningful role, and separation from religious and family ties.*

Expected Patient Outcomes	**Nursing Interventions**
Ms. S. will have a greater sense of purpose, meaning, and hope in her life and her illness as evidenced by expressing acceptance of the limitations life has presented to her and by verbalizing that illness is not a punishment.	• Take time to be present and available to listen to Ms. S.'s expressions and feelings. • Encourage Ms. S. to verbalize feelings. • Engage Ms. S. in value clarification.
Ms. S. will express feelings of anger verbally and will discuss anger with another person.	• Encourage Ms. S. to acknowledge feelings of anger and to acknowledge and name any feelings she has. • Reassure Ms. S. that it is okay to feel angry toward God and encourage her to express her feelings directly to God. • Encourage honest dialogue with a person Ms. S. trusts. • Reinforce that God loves and accepts people as they are.
Ms. S. will develop a sense of control in spite of separation from religious practices as evidenced by her expressing knowledge of available religious resources.	• Offer consultation with appropriate spiritual advisor (e.g., a chaplain). • Inform Ms. S. of available religious resources. • Pray with Ms. S. as indicated.

XI

tient who develops a greater sense of purpose, meaning, and hope would express positive thoughts and feelings about life and self. Self-acceptance can be revealed through the patient's positive and realistic expressions of accepting his/her humanness and limitations. In the evaluation phase, as in the other phases of the nursing process, an open and caring nurse-patient relationship is essential. For a patient with the nursing diagnosis Spiritual Distress, the nurse's interpersonal skills must be well developed for effective nursing interventions and the achievement of patient outcomes.

REFERENCES

1. Amenta M: Nurses as primary spiritual care workers, *Hospice J 4* (3):47-55, 1988.
2. American Nurses' Association: *Nursing: a social policy statement,* Kansas City, Mo, 1980, The Association.
3. Bulechek GM, McCloskey JC: *Nursing interventions: treatments for nursing diagnoses,* Philadelphia, 1985, WB Saunders.
4. Burnard P: Spiritual distress and the nursing response: theoretical considerations and counselling skills, *Adv Nurs 12* (3):377, 1987.
5. Ellison CW: Spiritual well-being: conceptualization and measurement, *J Psychol Theol 11* (4):330, 1983.
6. Fehring RJ, McLane AM: Value-belief. In Thompson JM and others, editors: *Mosby's manual of clinical nursing,* St Louis, 1989, CV Mosby.
7. Fish S, Shelley JA: *Spiritual care: the nurse's role,* ed 2, Downers Grove, Ill, 1983, Intervarsity Press.
8. Kim MJ, McFarland GK, and McLane AM: *Pocket guide to nursing diagnosis,* ed 4, St Louis, 1991, Mosby–Year Book.
9. Kus RJ: Crisis intervention. In Bulechek GM, McCloskey JC, editors: *Nursing interventions: treatments for nursing diagnoses,* Philadelphia, 1985, WB Saunders.
10. Livingston D, Williamson C: Truth telling. In Bulechek GM, McCloskey JC, editors: *Nursing interventions: treatments for nursing diagnoses,* Philadelphia, 1985, WB Saunders.
11. O'Brien ME: The need for spiritual integrity. In Yura H, Walsh MB, editors: *Human needs 2 and the nursing process,* Norwalk, Conn, 1992, Appleton-Century-Crofts.
11a. Paloutzian RF, Ellison CW: Loneliness, spiritual well-being and quality of life. In Peplau L, Perlman D, editors: *Loneliness: a source book of current theory, research and therapy,* New York, 1982, John Wiley & Sons.
12. Piles CL: Providing spiritual care, *Nurs Educ 15* (1):36-41, 1990.
13. Ripple P: *Growing strong at broken places,* Notre Dame, Indiana, 1986, Ave Maria Press.
14. Silber TJ, Reilly M: Spiritual and religious concerns of the hospitalized adolescent, *Adolescence* 20(77):217.
15. Stiles MK: The shining stranger: nurse-family relationship, *Cancer Nurs 13* (4):235-245.
16. Stoll RI: Guidelines for spiritual assessment, *Am J Nurs* 9:1574, 1974.

XI

A

NANDA-Approved Nursing Diagnostic Categories

PATTERN 1: EXCHANGING

1.1.2.1	Altered Nutrition: More than body requirements
1.1.2.2	Altered Nutrition: Less than body requirements
1.1.2.3	Altered Nutrition: High Risk for more than body requirements
1.2.1.1	High Risk for Infection
1.2.2.1	High Risk for Altered Body Temperature
1.2.2.2	Hypothermia
1.2.2.3	Hyperthermia
1.2.2.4	Ineffective Thermoregulation
1.2.3.1	Dysreflexia
*1.3.1.1	Constipation
1.3.1.1.1	Perceived Constipation
1.3.1.1.2	Colonic Constipation
*1.3.1.2	Diarrhea
*1.3.1.3	Bowel Incontinence
1.3.2	Altered Urinary Elimination
1.3.2.1.1	Stress Incontinence
1.3.2.1.2	Reflex Incontinence
1.3.2.1.3	Urge Incontinence
1.3.2.1.4	Functional Incontinence
1.3.2.1.5	Total Incontinence
1.3.2.2	Urinary Retention
1.4.1.1	Altered (Specify Type) Tissue Perfusion (Renal, cerebral, cardiopulmonary, gastrointestinal, peripheral)
1.4.1.2.1	Fluid Volume Excess
1.4.1.2.2.1	Fluid Volume Deficit
1.4.1.2.2.2	High Risk for Fluid Volume Deficit
*1.4.2.1	Decreased Cardiac Output
1.5.1.1	Impaired Gas Exchange
1.5.1.2	Ineffective Airway Clearance

*Categories with modified label terminology.

†New diagnostic categories approved 1990.

‡New diagnostic categories approved 1992.

1.5.1.3	Ineffective Breathing Pattern
‡1.5.1.3.1	Inability to Sustain Spontaneous Ventilation
‡1.5.1.3.2	Dysfunctional Ventilatory Wearing Response
1.6.1	High Risk for Injury
1.6.1.1	High Risk for Suffocation
1.6.1.2	High Risk for Poisoning
1.6.1.3	High Risk for Trauma
1.6.1.4	High Risk for Aspiration
1.6.1.5	High Risk for Disuse Syndrome
†1.6.2	Altered Protection
1.6.2.1	Impaired Tissue Integrity
*1.6.2.1.1	Altered Oral Mucous Membrane
1.6.2.1.2.1	Impaired Skin Integrity
1.6.2.1.2.2	High Risk for Impaired Skin Integrity

PATTERN 2: COMMUNICATING

| 2.1.1.1 | Impaired Verbal Communication |

PATTERN 3: RELATING

3.1.1	Impaired Social Interaction
3.1.2	Social Isolation
*3.2.1	Altered Role Performance
3.2.1.1.1	Altered Parenting
3.2.1.1.2	High Risk for Altered Parenting
3.2.1.2.1	Sexual Dysfunction
3.2.2	Altered Family Processes
3.2.2.1	Caregiver Role Strain
3.2.2.2	High Risk for Caregiver Role Strain
3.2.3.1	Parental Role Conflict
3.3	Altered Sexuality Patterns

PATTERN 4: VALUING

| 4.1.1 | Spiritual Distress (distress of the human spirit) |

PATTERN 5: CHOOSING

5.1.1.1	Ineffective Individual Coping
5.1.1.1.1	Impaired Adjustment
5.1.1.1.2	Defensive Coping
5.1.1.1.3	Ineffective Denial
5.1.2.1.1	Ineffective Family Coping: Disabling
5.1.2.1.2	Ineffective Family Coping: Compromised
5.1.2.2	Family Coping: Potential for Growth
‡5.2.1	Ineffective Management of Therapeutic Regimen (Individuals)
5.2.1.1	Noncompliance (Specify)
5.3.1.1	Decisional Conflict (Specify)
5.4	Health Seeking Behaviors (Specify)

PATTERN 6: MOVING

6.1.1.1	Impaired Physical Mobility
‡6.1.1.1.1	High Risk for Peripheral Neurovascular Dysfunction
6.1.1.2	Activity Intolerance
6.1.1.2.1	Fatigue
6.1.1.3	High Risk for Activity Intolerance
6.2.1	Sleep Pattern Disturbance
6.3.1.1	Diversional Activity Deficit
6.4.1.1	Impaired Home Maintenance Management
6.4.2	Altered Health Maintenance
*6.5.1	Feeding Self Care Deficit
6.5.1.1	Impaired Swallowing
6.5.1.2	Ineffective Breastfeeding
‡6.5.1.2.1	Interrupted Breastfeeding
†6.5.1.3	Effective Breastfeeding
‡6.5.1.4	Ineffective Infant Feeding Pattern
*6.5.2	Bathing/Hygiene Self Care Deficit
*6.5.3	Dressing/Grooming Self Care Deficit
*6.5.4	Toileting Self Care Deficit
6.6	Altered Growth and Development
‡6.7	Relocation Stress Syndrome

PATTERN 7: PERCEIVING

*7.1.1	Body Image Disturbance
*7.1.2	Self Esteem Disturbance
7.1.2.1	Chronic Low Self Esteem
7.1.2.2	Situational Low Self Esteem
*7.1.3	Personal Identity Disturbance
7.2	Sensory/Perceptual Alterations (Specify) (Visual, auditory, kinesthetic, gustatory, tactile, olfactory)
7.2.1.1	Unilateral Neglect
7.3.1	Hopelessness
7.3.2	Powerlessness

PATTERN 8: KNOWING

8.1.1	Knowledge Deficit (Specify)
8.3	Altered Thought Processes

PATTERN 9: FEELING

*9.1.1	Pain
9.1.1.1	Chronic Pain
9.2.1.1	Dysfunctional Grieving
9.2.1.2	Anticipatory Grieving
9.2.2	High Risk for Violence: Self-directed or directed at others
‡9.2.2.1	High Risk for Self-Mutilation

B

NANDA-Accepted Nursing Diagnoses Categorized by Functional Health Patterns*

I. Health Perception—Health Management Pattern

Altered Health Maintenance

Ineffective Management of Therapeutic Regimen

Noncompliance (Specify)

Altered Protection

High Risk for Infection

High Risk for Injury

High Risk for Trauma

High Risk for Poisoning

High Risk for Suffocation

Health Seeking Behaviors (Specify)

II. Nutritional and Metabolic Pattern

Altered Nutrition: High Risk for More Than Body Requirements

Altered Nutrition: More Than Body Requirements

Altered Nutrition: Less Than Body Requirements

Interrupted Breastfeeding

Ineffective Breastfeeding

Effective Breastfeeding

Ineffective Infant Feeding Pattern

High Risk for Aspiration

Impaired Swallowing

Altered Oral Mucous Membrane

High Risk for Fluid Volume Deficit

Fluid Volume Deficit (1)

Fluid Volume Deficit (2)

Fluid volume Excess

High Risk for Impaired Skin Integrity

Impaired Skin Integrity

Impaired Tissue Integrity

High Risk for Altered Body Temperature

Ineffective Thermoregulation

Hyperthermia

Hypothermia

III. Elimination Pattern

Constipation

Perceived Constipation

Colonic Constipation

Diarrhea

Bowel Incontinence

Altered Patterns of Urinary Elimination

Functional Incontinence

Reflex Incontinence

Stress Incontinence

Urge Incontinence

Total Incontinence

Urinary Retention

IV. Activity-Exercise Pattern

Altered Growth and Development

Fatigue

Bathing/Hygiene Self-Care Deficit

Dressing/Grooming Self-Care Deficit

Feeding Self-Care Deficit

Toileting Self-Care Deficit

Diversional Activity Deficit

Impaired Home Maintenance Management

High Risk for Activity Intolerance

Activity Intolerance

---

*Based on Gordon (1987).

Impaired Physical Mobility
High Risk for Disuse Syndrome
Dysreflexia
Ineffective Airway Clearance
Ineffective Breathing Pattern
Impaired Gas Exchange
Inability to Sustain Spontaneous Ventilation
Dysfunctional Ventilatory Weaning Response
Decreased Cardiac Output
High Risk for Peripheral Neurovascular Dysfunction
Altered (Specify Type) Tissue Perfusion (Renal, Cerebral, Cardiopulmonary, Gastrointestinal, Peripheral)

V. Sleep-Rest Pattern

Sleep Pattern Disturbance

VI. Cognitive-Perceptual Pattern

Pain
Chronic Pain
Sensory/Perceptual Alterations (Specify) (Visual, Auditory, Kinesthetic, Gustatory, Tactile, Olfactory)
Unilateral Neglect
Altered Thought Processes
Decisional Conflict (Specify)
Knowledge Deficit (Specify)

VII. Self-Perception—Self-Concept Pattern

Fear
Anxiety
Hopelessness
Powerlessness
Body Image Disturbance
Personal Identity Disturbance
Self-Esteem Disturbance
Chronic Low Self-Esteem
Situational Low Self-Esteem
High Risk for Self Mutilation

VIII. Role-Relationship Pattern

Impaired Verbal Communication
Social Isolation
Impaired Social Interaction

Relocation Stress Syndrome
Altered Role Performance
Anticipatory Grieving
Dysfunctional Grieving
High Risk for Violence: Self-directed or Directed at Others
Altered Family Processes
High Risk for Altered Parenting
Altered Parenting
Parental Role Conflict
Caregiver Role Strain
High Risk for Caregiver Role Strain

IX. Sexuality-Reproductive Pattern

Sexual Dysfunction
Altered Sexuality Patterns
Rape-Trauma Syndrome
Rape-Trauma Syndrome: Compound Reaction
Rape-Trauma Syndrome: Silent Reaction

X. Coping—Stress Tolerance Pattern

Ineffective Individual Coping
Defensive Coping
Ineffective Denial
Impaired Adjustment
Post-Trauma Response
Family Coping: Potential for Growth
Ineffective Family Coping: Compromised
Ineffective Family Coping: Disabling

XI. Value-Belief Pattern

Spiritual Distress (Distress of the Human Spirit)

C

Nursing Diagnoses for Home Health Care: Classification and Coding Scheme

I. Coding Structure

- HOME HEALTH CARE COMPONENTS: 1st Alpha Code A to T
- NURSING DIAGNOSIS CATEGORY: 2nd/3rd Digit: 01 to 50
- NURSING DIAGNOSIS SUBCATEGORY: 4th Decimal Digit: 1 to 9
- DISCHARGE STATUS/GOAL: 5th Digit: 1 to 3 (Use Only One)
  1 = Improved, 2 = Stabilized, 3 = Deteriorated

II. 50 Nursing Diagnoses - 95 Subcategories

A ACTIVITY COMPONENT
- 01 Activity Alteration
  - 01.1 Activity Intolerance
  - 01.2 Activity Intolerance Risk
  - 01.3 Diversional Activity Deficit
  - 01.4 Fatigue
  - 01.5 Physical Mobility Impairment
  - 01.6 Sleep Pattern Disturbance
- 02 Musculoskeletal Alteration

B BOWEL ELIMINATION COMPONENT
- 03 Bowel Elimination Alteration
  - 03.1 Bowel Incontinence
  - 03.2 Colonic Constipation
  - 03.3 Diarrhea
  - 03.4 Fecal Impaction
  - 03.5 Perceived Constipation
  - 03.6 Unspecified Constipation
- 04 Gastrointestinal Alteration

C CARDIAC COMPONENT
- 05 Cardiac Output Alteration
- 06 Cardiovascular Alteration
  - 01.1 Blood Pressure Alteration

D COGNITIVE COMPONENT
- 07 Cerebral Alteration
- 08 Knowledge Deficit (of:)
  - 08.1 Diagnostic (Laboratory Test)*
  - 08.2 Dietary Regimen
  - 08.3 Disease Process
  - 08.4 Fluid Volume
  - 08.5 Medication Regimen
  - 08.6 Safety Precaution
  - 08.7 Therapeutic Regimen
- 09 Thought Processes Alteration

E COPING COMPONENT
- 10 Dying Process
- 11 Family Coping Impairment
  - 11.1 Compromised Family Coping
  - 11.2 Disabled Family Coping
- 12 Individual Coping Impairment
  - 12.1 Adjustment Impairment
  - 12.2 Decisional Conflict
  - 12.3 Defensive Coping
  - 12.4 Denial
- 13 Post-Trauma Response
  - 13.1 Rape Trauma Syndrome†

---

*Not Used or Unkown

Terminology modifications made in collaboration with Sheila M. Sparks, D.N.Sc., R.N., C.S. Assistant Professor, School of Nursing, Georgetown University.

14   Spiritual State Alteration
    14.1   Spiritual Distress

F   FLUID VOLUME COMPONENT

15   Fluid Volume Alteration
    15.1   Deficit of Fluid Volume
    15.2   Deficit Risk of Fluid Volume
    15.3   Excess of Fluid Volume
    15.4   Excess Risk of Fluid Volume

G   HEALTH BEHAVIOR COMPONENT

16   Growth and Development Alteration
17   Health Maintenance Alteration
18   Health Seeking Behaviors
19   Home Maintenance Management Impairment
20   Noncompliance (of:)
    20.1   Diagnostic (Laboratory Test)*
    20.2   Dietary Regimen
    20.3   Fluid Volume
    20.4   Medication Regimen
    20.5   Safety Precaution
    20.6   Therapeutic Regimen

H   MEDICATION COMPONENT

21   Medication Risk
    21.1   Polypharmacy

I   METABOLIC COMPONENT

22   Endocrine Alteration
23   Immunologic Alteration
    23.1   Protection Alteration*

J   NUTRITIONAL COMPONENT

24   Nutrition Alteration
    24.1   Less than Body Requirement
    24.2   Less than Body Requirement Risk
    24.3   More than Body Requirement
    24.4   More than Body Requirement Risk

K   PHYSICAL REGULATION COMPONENT

25   Physical Regulation Alteration
    25.1   Dysreflexia
    25.2   Hyperthermia
    25.3   Hypothermia
    25.5   Infection Risk
    25.6   Infection Unspecified
    25.4   Thermoregulation Impairment

L   RESPIRATORY COMPONENT

26   Respiration Alteration
    26.1   Airway Clearance Impairment
    26.2   Breathing Pattern Impairment
    26.3   Gas Exchange Impairment

M   ROLE RELATIONSHIP COMPONENT

27   Role Performance Alteration
    27.1   Parental Role Conflict*
    27.2   Parenting Alteration
    27.3   Sexual Dysfunction*
28   Communication Impairment
    28.1   Verbal Impairment
29   Family Processes Alteration
30   Grieving
    30.1   Anticipatory Grieving
    30.2   Dysfunctional Grieving
31   Sexuality Patterns Alteration
32   Socialization Alteration
    32.1   Social Interaction Impairment
    32.2   Social Isolation

N   SAFETY COMPONENT

33   Injury Risk
    33.1   Aspiration
    33.2   Disuse Syndrome*
    33.3   Poisoning
    33.4   Suffocation
    33.5   Trauma
34   Violence Risk

O   SELF-CARE COMPONENT

35   Bathing/Hygiene Deficit
36   Dressing/Grooming Deficit
37   Feeding Deficit
    37.1   Breastfeeding Impairment*
    37.2   Swallowing Impairment
38   Self Care Deficit
    38.1   Activities of Daily Living (ADLs) Alteration
    38.2   Instrumental Activities of Daily Living (IADLs) Alteration
39   Toileting Deficit

P   SELF-CONCEPT COMPONENT

40   Anxiety
41   Fear
42   Meaningfulness Alteration*
    42.1   Hopelessness
    42.2   Powerlessness
43   Self Concept Alteration
    43.1   Body Image Disturbance
    43.2   Personal Identity Disturbance

D

Assessment Guide for Adult Patient

General Information

Name   Address/Phone
Age
Allergies

Pattern Assessment

Assess not only complaints, limitations, and problems but also what is being done to alleviate the problem or problems, as well as positive health practices and current and previous coping skills.

I. Health Perception—Health Management Pattern

- Perception of own health state? Chief complaint?
- Previous illness or surgery?
- Past and current health seeking behaviors?
- Resources for health maintenance?
- Current treatments? On any prescription medications?
- Adherence to therapeutic recommendations?
- Presence of risk factors for injury? Infection?
- Prevention practices?

II. Nutritional and Metabolic Pattern

- Weight loss or gain?
- Nutritional status? Diet?
- Fluid intake?
- Drug and alcohol consumption?
- Ability to swallow?
- Breastfeeding (if applicable)?
- Skin, tissue, or mucous membrane integrity (including oral cavity)?
- Dentures?
- Body temperature?

III. Elimination Pattern

- Bowel elimination?
- Urinary elimination?

IV. Activity-Exercise Pattern

- Physical mobility?
- Fatigue level?
- Self-care ability?
- Growth and development (in relation to age group norms)?
- Recreation and leisure activities?
- Home maintenance?
- Respirations?
- Shortness of breath?
- Coughing?
- Cyanosis?
- Breath sounds?
- Pulse (rate? rhythm? peripheral pulses?)
- Blood pressure?
- Edema?
- Extremities (cold? cyanosis?)
- Changes in mental status?

V. Sleep-rest Pattern

- Sleep habits? Feel rested?
- Rest habits?
- Methods to promote sleep and relaxation?

VI. Cognitive-perceptual Pattern

- Level of consciousness?
- Ability to see, feel, taste, touch, and smell?
- Special aids?
- Pain? Discomfort? How are these managed?
- Hallucinations? Delusions?
- Awareness of both sides of body?
- Health care self-management knowledge?

- Memory?
- Judgment?
- Ability to concentrate?
- Decision-making ability?
- Education?

VII. Self-Perception—Self-Concept Pattern

- Any perceived threat or danger?
- Apprehension? Tension?
- Restlessness?
- Mood change? Depressed? Anxious?
- Ability to mobilize energy on own behalf? Passivity?
- Perceived control over situations?
- Perception and feelings about self? Self-worth?
- Body image? Personal identity?
- Risk factors for self mutilation?

VIII. Role-relationship Pattern

- Significant loss? Grieving?
- Ability to perform roles? Occupation?
- Marital status?
- Interpersonal interactions?
- Significant others? Any interpersonal difficulties? Any caregiver difficulties?
- Family structure and system? Any difficulties?
- Attitude of family and significant others toward illness?
- Parenting practices and problems?
- Communication skills?
- Risk factors for self-harm?
- Risk factors for other directed physical injury (if relevant)?

IX. Sexuality-reproductive pattern

- Sexuality patterns? Satisfaction? Dysfunctions?
- Contraceptives (use or problems)?
- Menstrual history?
- History of sexual abuse?

X. Coping—Stress Tolerance Pattern

- Current stressors? Life challenges?
- Recent major life changes? Recent relocation?
- Response and adjustment to trauma?
- Methods to deal with stressors?
- Resources available to cope with stressors?
- Degree and quality of family support available?
- Potential for family growth during stress?

XI. Value-belief Pattern

- Overall life beliefs and values?
- Religious affiliation and importance of religion?
- Religious practices? Which ones are desired while in hospital?
- Desire for chaplain visit?

REFERENCES

Gordon M: *Nursing diagnoses: process and application,* New York, 1987, McGraw-Hill Book Co.

McFarland G, Wasli E and Gerety: *Nursing diagnoses and process in psychiatric mental health nursing,* Philadelphia, 1992, JB Lippincott.

Weber J: *Nurses' handbook of health assessment,* Philadelphia, 1988, JB Lippincott.

E

NANDA To-Be-Developed Diagnostic Concepts and Definitions

Activity Level, Excessive

Energy which is being displayed to a level that is beyond the usual measure or proportion. An above a "relative normal" state of energy expenditure is a change or a difference that creates stress which in turn results in needs.

Altered Family Processes: Addictive Behavior (Individual & Family)

The state in which the psychosocial, spiritual, and physiological functions of a family unit are chronically disorganized, leading to conflict, denial of problems, resistance to change, ineffective problem-solving, and a series of self-perpetuating crises.

Altered Parent/Infant Attachment

Disruption of the interactive process between parent/significant other and infant that fosters the development of a protective and nurturing reciprocal relationship.

Confusion, Acute

The abrupt onset of a cluster of global, transient changes and disturbances in attention, cognition, psychomotor activity, level of consciousness, and/or sleep-wake cycle.

Confusion, Chronic

An irreversible, long-standing, and/or progressive deterioration of intellect and personality characterized by decreased ability to interpret environmental stimuli, decreased capacity for intellectual thought processes, and manifested by disturbances of memory, orientation, and behavior.

Decisional Conflict, Family: Required

Identifies the disequilibrium which occurs among and within family members when the family unit must reach a consensus within a specific timeframe. Time constraints and associated ethical and/or value-laden consequences may prompt crisis and uncertainty further blocking the decision-making process.

Decreased Adaptive Capacity, Intracranial

A clinical state in which intracranial fluid dynamic mechanisms that normally compensate for increases in intracranial volumes are compromised, resulting in repeated disproportionate increases in intracranial pressure (ICP) over baseline in response to a variety of noxious and nonnoxious stimuli.

High Risk for Disproportionate Increase in Intracranial Pressure

A clinical state in which a person with baseline increased ICP is at risk for developing disproportionately large and sustained increases over baseline ICP (greater than 10 mm Hg over baseline for more than 5 minutes) in response to external stimuli.

From Handout, Tenth Conference for Classification of Nursing Diagnoses, San Diego, California, 1992.

High Risk for Loneliness

A subjective state in which an individual is at risk of experiencing vague dysphoria.

High Risk for Impaired Skin Integrity: Pressure Ulcer

A state in which the individual's skin is at risk of being adversely affected.

Idiopathic Fecal Incontinence

A change in an individual's pattern of elimination characterized by a loss of ability to voluntarily control the passage of feces/gas and occasional/frequent loss of normal stool.

Impaired Feeding Drive

A state in which a nutritionally sound patient has difficulty returning to normal eating patterns during illness or recovery from illness.

Impaired Memory

The state in which an individual experiences an inability to remember or recall bits of information or behavioral skills. Impaired memory may be attributed to patho-physiological or situational causes that are either temporary or permanent.

Ineffective Coping (Communities)

A pattern of community activities for adaptation and problem solving that is unsatisfactory for meeting the demands or needs of the community.

Ineffective Management of Therapeutic Regimen (Families)

A pattern of regulating and integrating into family processes a program for treatment of illness and the sequelae of illness that is unsatisfactory for meeting specific health goals.

Labor Pain

A subjective measure of an unpleasant sensation which lasts the duration of a contraction, and may linger between contractions. The feeling subsides with delivery of a fetus.

Potential for Enhanced Coping (Communities)

A pattern of community activities for adaptation and problem solving that is satisfactory for meeting the demands or needs of the community but can be improved for management of current and future problems/stressors.

Potential for Enhanced Spiritual Well-Being

The process of an individual's developing/unfolding of mystery through harmonious interconnectedness that springs from inner strengths.

Spasticity

The state in which an individual with an upper motor neuron injury experiences increased muscle tone and abnormal reflexes in response to internal or external stimuli which interfere with functional abilities such as mobility, hygiene, eating, dressing, and toileting.

Terminal Illness Response

That time when a terminal illness develops or is diagnosed, and a patient tries to deal with the pending, permanent separation from loved ones, possessions, and his/her own body. If a patient is unconscious, the family, significant other, or caregiver may experience the phenomena alone.

F

North American Nursing Diagnosis Association Guidelines for Submission of Proposed Diagnoses

I. Proposed Diagnoses

The North American Nursing Diagnosis Association (NANDA) solicits proposed nursing diagnoses for review by the Association. Proposed diagnoses undergo a systematic review for inclusion in NANDA's list of approved diagnoses. Approval indicates that NANDA endorses the diagnosis for clinical testing and continuing development by the discipline. Partially developed diagnoses are placed on NANDA's "To Be Developed" (TBD) List.

Classification of Diagnoses. Approved diagnoses are forwarded to the Taxonomy Committee for review and classification. A working definition of the term "nursing diagnosis" was developed by the NANDA Board and the Taxonomy Committee to use in screening accepted diagnoses for fit with Taxonomy I, Revised.

Working Definition. A nursing diagnosis is a clinical judgment about individual, family, or community responses to actual or potential health problems/life processes. Nursing diagnoses provide the basis for selection of nursing interventions to achieve outcomes for which the nurse is accountable (Approved as working definition at 9th Conference).

II. Types of Diagnostic Concepts

Actual Nursing Diagnoses. Actual nursing diagnoses are diagnostic concepts that describe human responses to health conditions/life processes

that exist in an individual, family or community. Actual nursing diagnoses are supported by defining characteristics (manifestations/signs and symptoms) that cluster in patterns of related cues or inferences. Related factors (etiologies) are factors that contribute to the development or maintenance of an actual diagnosis.

High Risk. High risk nursing diagnoses are diagnostic concepts that describe human responses to health conditions/life processes which may develop in a vulnerable individual, family, or community. High risk nursing diagnoses are supported by risk factors that contribute to increased vulnerability.

Wellness. Wellness nursing diagnoses are diagnostic concepts that describe human responses to levels of wellness in an individual, family, or community that have a potential for enhancement to a higher state.

III. Components of Proposed Diagnoses

Label. The label provides a name for a proposed diagnosis. It is a concise term or phrase that represents a pattern of related cues. Diagnostic labels may include qualifiers.

Definition. The definition provides a clear, precise description of the diagnostic concept; delineates its meaning; and helps differentiate it from similar diagnoses.

Defining Characteristics. Defining characteristics are observable cues/inferences that cluster as manifestations of a nursing diagnosis. Defining characteristics are listed for actual diagnoses. A defining characteristic is described as a "critical indicator" if it *must be present* to make the diagnosis. A defining characteristic is described as "major" if it is *usually* present when the diagnosis exists. A defining characteristic is described as "minor" if it provides supporting evidence for the diagnosis but may not be present.

Related Factors. Related factors are conditions/circumstances that contribute to the development/maintenance of a nursing diagnosis.

Risk Factors. Environmental factors and physiological, psychological, genetic, or chemical elements that increase the vulnerability of an individual, family, or community to an unhealthful event.

IV. Literature Support

A narrative review of relevant literature (theoretical and data-based) is required to demonstrate the existence of a substantive body of knowledge underlying the proposed diagnostic concept. Literature citations (or current research) for each defining characteristic, related factor, or risk factor must be included. Differentiation of major from minor defining characteristics must be logically defended and supported by clinical data.

V. Validation

The validity of a nursing diagnosis refers to the degree to which a cluster of defining characteristics describes a condition that can be observed or inferred in client-environment interactions. One or more descriptive studies and/or content validity indices (Fehring, 1986) are required for a diagnosis to be designated as validated. Higher forms of validity are desirable.

VI. Diagnostic Statement

A diagnostic statement with associated outcome criteria and nurse-prescribed interventions must accompany the submission. A three-part statement (label, related factor(s), clinical cues) is required for actual diagnoses; a two-part statement (label and risk factors) is required for high risk diagnoses; and a one-part statement (label) is used for wellness diagnoses.

VII. Qualifiers for Diagnostic Labels (Suggested/not limited to)

Acute—Severe but of short duration.

Altered—A change from baseline.

Chronic—Lasting a long time; recurring; habitual; constant.

Decreased—Lessened, lesser in size, amount or degree.

Deficient—Inadequate in amount, quality, or degree; defective; not sufficient; incomplete.

Depleted—Emptied wholly or partially; exhausted of.

Disturbed—Agitated; interrupted, interfered with.

Dysfunctional—Abnormal; incomplete functioning.

Excessive—Characterized by an amount or quantity that is greater than is necessary, desirable, or useful.

Increased—Greater in size, amount or degree.

Impaired—Made worse, weakened; damaged, reduced; deteriorated.

Ineffective—Not producing the desired effect.

Intermittent—Stopping and starting again at intervals; periodic; cyclic.

Potential for Enhanced (for use with wellness diagnoses)—Enhanced is defined as made greater, to increase in quality or more desired.

Index

A

AACN; *see* American Association of Critical-Care Nurses
AAMD Adaptive Behavior Scale, 277
Abdellah's definition of nursing problem, 2
Abdomen
  bowel elimination and, 222
  cramping in, 377
  surgery of, 377
Abdominal angina, 377, 393
Abdominal muscles, 354
  incontinence and, 256
Abdominis rectus, 354
Abdominis transversus, 354
Abdominoperineal resection, 250
ABG; *see* Arterial blood gases
Abnormal breath sounds, 349-350
Abnormal growth pattern, 275
Abnormal heart sounds, 382
Abortion, 655
Abscess, lung, 120
Abuse
  alcohol, 37, 201, 543
  child, 619, 624-625
  physical, 543
  post-trauma response and, 721, 722, 727
  sexual, 543, 673-674
  substance, 530, 722
Acceptance, grieving and, 585, 586
Accident, 54
  automobile, 347, 728-729
    disuse syndrome and, 339-340
    post-trauma response and, 722
  cerebrovascular; *see* Cerebrovascular accident
  poisoning and, 55
  submersion, 62
Accidental hypothermia, 182
Accommodation, family coping and, 733
Accreditation Manual for Hospitals, 2
Acculturation, self-esteem disturbance and, 531
Acculturation stress, 643
Acid-base disturbances, 153
Acid pH, infection and, 45
Acidosis, 148, 380
  tissue perfusion and, 374
Acquaintance rape, 665
Acquired diseases in growth and development, 273
Acquired immunodeficiency syndrome
  altered protection and, 37
  breastfeeding and, 105
  family coping and, 744-745
  infection and, 47
  oral mucous membrane and, 137
  social isolation and, 560
Action plan, 17
Active listening, 750

Activities of daily living, 293-300; *see also* Activity
  apraxia and, 452
  childhood disability and, 280-281
  impaired adjustment and, 714
  therapeutic regimen and, 80-81
  unilateral neglect and, 453-455
Activity; *see also* Activities of daily living; Activity-exercise
    pattern
  balanced with rest, 425
  body temperature and, 185
  constipation and, 219, 230
  dysfunctional grieving and, 588, 589
  intolerance for; *see* Activity intolerance
  obesity and, 94
  pain and, 434
  physical, violence and, 601
  recreational, 301-307
Activity deficit, diversional, 301-307; *see also* Diversional activity
    deficit
Activity-exercise pattern, 273-418; *see also* specific activity
  activity intolerance in, 318-328
  assessment and, 14
  cardiac output in, 365-374
  disuse syndrome in, 334-340
  diversional activity deficit and, 301-307
  dysreflexia and, 341-348
  fatigue in, 288-292
  growth and development and, 273-287
  home maintenance management and, 308-317
  impaired gas exchange in, 361-365
  impaired physical mobility in, 329-333
  ineffective airway clearance in, 349-353
  ineffective breathing pattern in, 354-360
  peripheral neurovascular dysfunction and, 410-418
  self-care deficits and, 293-300
  tissue perfusion and, 374-398
  ventilation dysfunction and, 399-409
Activity intolerance, 318-328
  assessment in, 319-323
  care guidelines for, 325-326
  defining characteristics of, 322
  evaluation in, 326
  high risk for, 318-328
    assessment in, 320-321
    care guidelines for, 324
    planning and implementation in, 323
    related medical/psychiatric diagnoses in, 321
    risk factors in, 320-321
    specific diagnoses for, 323
  overview in, 318-319
  planning and implementation in, 323-326
  related factors in, 322
  related medical/psychiatric diagnoses in, 322-323
  specific diagnoses for, 323
Acute care setting, 723

771

G